OXFORD MEDICAL PUBLICATION

Oxford Desk Reference
Geriatric Medicine

Oxford Desk Reference
Geriatric Medicine

Edited by

Professor Margot Gosney

Professor of Elderly Care Medicine/Director Clinical Health Sciences
Royal Berkshire NHS Foundation Trust/University of Reading
Reading

Dr Adam Harper

Consultant Geriatrician
Brighton and Sussex University Hospitals NHS Trust
Brighton

Dr Simon Conroy

Head of Service/Senior Lecturer, Geriatric Medicine
University Hospitals of Leicester
Leicester

OXFORD
UNIVERSITY PRESS

OXFORD
UNIVERSITY PRESS

Great Clarendon Street, Oxford OX2 6DP, United Kingdom

Oxford University Press is a department of the University of Oxford.
It furthers the University's objective of excellence in research, scholarship,
and education by publishing worldwide. Oxford is a registered trade mark of
Oxford University Press in the UK and in certain other countries

© Oxford University Press 2012

The moral rights of the authors have been asserted

First Edition published 2012

Impression: 1

British Library Cataloguing in Publication Data
Data available

Library of Congress Cataloging in Publication Data
Library of Congress Control Number: 2012938696

ISBN 978–0–19–959234–0

Printed in Great Britain by
CPI Group (UK) Ltd, Croydon, CR0 4YY

Oxford University Press makes no representation, express or implied, that the
drug dosages in this book are correct. Readers must therefore always check
the product information and clinical procedures with the most up-to-date
published product information and data sheets provided by the manufacturers
and the most recent codes of conduct and safety regulations. The authors and
the publishers do not accept responsibility or legal liability for any errors in the
text or for the misuse or misapplication of material in this work. Except where
otherwise stated, drug dosages and recommendations are for the non-pregnant
adult who is not breast-feeding.

Links to third party websites are provided by Oxford in good faith and for
information only. Oxford disclaims any responsibility for the materials contained
in any third party website referenced in this work.

Dedications

With all large endeavours comes a price and for the three of us, part of this has been borne by our families.
We wish to thank them for their tolerance during the different stages of this book.
We extend our grateful thanks to Mrs Julie Farwell for her patience with us, for her tact and kindness to the authors and her overall determination that this venture would be completed. Without Julie, this project would not have reached fruition.

Foreword

It is a pleasure to be invited to write the foreword to the *Oxford Desk Reference: Geriatric Medicine*, which represents an extremely important addition to the *Oxford Desk Reference* series of specialty texts.

The editors have done an excellent job in commissioning contributions from authors who are acknowledged as leaders in their respective fields.

Nowadays, a prospective reader is faced with a bewildering array of medical information available either in text format or online, but this book provides an up to date series of informative articles on the rapidly changing specialty of Geriatric Medicine. The articles are written in a punchy, succinct style, peppered with useful practical hints and tips from the authors. They are well researched and referenced and where relevant the authors have drawn on the prevalent guidance and evidence base.

The *Oxford Desk Reference: Geriatric Medicine* addresses all the important aspects of Geriatric Medicine, not only the more traditional 'Geriatric Giants' described by Professor Bernard Isaacs but also topical subjects such as comprehensive geriatric assessment, assistive technology and the concept of frailty. All the 'core topics' of the national training curriculum in Geriatric Medicine are covered to some degree including the assessment and management of acute illness, chronic disease and disability, and sub-specialties such as continence, falls, movement disorders, orthogeriatics, palliative care, and psychiatry of old age. The chapters on assessing fitness to drive and the peri-operative assessment of older people provide information of great practical and clinical importance in a straightforward and readily accessible style.

As someone who has an interest in medical education and training, I believe this book will have widespread appeal. The fact that it is crammed with information in a compact format will appeal to medical undergraduates, the broad range of topics will be invaluable to doctors preparing for the MRCP Diploma, the Diploma in Geriatric Medicine and even those preparing for the Specialty Certificate in Geriatric Medicine. General Practitioners, Geriatricians and other physicians will find the book a useful reference source in their everyday clinical practice or in order to prepare a teaching session. Given the demographic change within society and the increasing numbers of older people in the population described by Drs Padiachy and Carroll in their chapter on the global perspective of ageing, it is vital that the medical workforce is conversant with the medical and social problems of older people and this book will be invaluable in this regard.

In the words of Sir William Osler

He who studies medicine without books sails an uncharted sea.

Practitioners in almost all branches of medicine will increasingly be involved in managing older people and I am sure this book will prove to be an indispensable aid to navigate through their many problems and pathologies.

Dr Oliver J Corrado
Consultant Physician, St James's University Hospital, Leeds
and Chair, Geriatric Medicine Specialist Advisory Committee 2009–12

Preface

Geriatric medicine thrives on being a broad subject. The diversity of areas in which a geriatrician needs knowledge and understanding makes writing textbooks challenging. To cover all areas in detail, large tomes have been written. Others have gone for a more succinct approach, where it is only possible to cover key areas briefly. This book aims to find a balance between covering all areas relevant to geriatric medicine in an accessible and readable format. We hope this will make it an ideal first-line reference for those caring for older people, and also for those preparing for examinations, such as the Speciality Clinical Examination. All the sections are written by specialists, with the use of 'Authors' Tips' for passing on snippets of wisdom from years of experience. The topics start with an introduction to geriatric medicine and its evolution into one of the biggest medical specialities in the UK. It then covers the different systems, specifically with regard to older people. It progresses through to cover multidisciplinary working. Finally, it looks into the future, and the expanding role for technology in the care of older people.

Professor Margot Gosney
Dr Adam Harper
Dr Simon Conroy

Acknowledgements

In editing this book, we are indebted to all of our colleagues and friends who have generously given up their time and expertise to write each of the separate sections of the book. We acknowledge that many of them are both national and international experts in their field, and this has helped to enhance both the quality and clarity of the book.

Brief contents

Detailed contents

List of contributors

Dr Aza Abdulla
Consultant Physician & Geriatrician
Princess Royal University Hospital
Orpington

Mr Stephen Abery
Optometrist
Royal Berkshire NHS Foundation Trust
Reading

Dr Asangaedem Akpan
Consultant Physician & Clinical Lead
Warrington & Halton Hospitals NHS Foundation Trust
Warrington

Dr Albert Edward Alahmar
Consultant Interventional Cardiologist
Glenfield Hospital
Leicester

Dr Khalid Ali
Senior Lecturer in Geriatrics
Brighton and Sussex Medical School
Brighton

Professor Stephen Allen
Consultant Physician and Professor of Clinical
Gerontology
The Royal Bournemouth Hospital
Bournemouth

Dr Khaled Amar
Consultant Physician and Geriatrician
Royal Bournemouth and Christchurch Hospitals NHS
Foundation Trust
Bournemouth

Dr David Anderson
Consultant & Honorary Senior Lecturer, Associate
Medical Director
Mossley Hill Hospital
Liverpool

Dr Stuart Anderson
Consultant Neuropsychologist
Hurstwood Park Neurological Centre
Haywards Heath

Professor Vladimir N Anisimov
Head, Department of Carcinogenesis and
Oncogerontology
N.N. Petrov Research Institute of Oncology
St Petersburg

Dr Katherine Athorn
Specialist Registrar in Elderly Medicine
Leeds Teaching Hospitals NHS Trust
Leeds

Professor Riccardo A Audisio
Consultant Surgical Oncologist/Honorary Professor
St Helens Teaching Hospital/University of Liverpool
Liverpool

Dr Claire Ballinger
Deputy Director/Senior Qualitative Methodologist
Research Design Service South Central Primary Care/
University of Southampton
Southampton

Mr Jay Banerjee
Consultant in Emergency Medicine
University Hospitals of Leicester NHS Trust
Leicester

Mr Keith Barton
Consultant Ophthalmic Surgeon
Moorfields Eye Hospital
London

Mr Andrew Bastawrous
Ophthalmology SpR-Mersey Deanery
Royal Liverpool Hospital
Liverpool

Mr Mark Batterbury
Consultant Ophthalmologist/Honorary Senior Lecturer
Royal Liverpool University Hospital/University of
Liverpool
Liverpool

Dr Antony Bayer
Head of Section of Geriatric Medicine
Cardiff University, University Hospital Llandough,
Cardiff/Penarth

Dr Jessica Rhiannon Beavan
Consultant in Stroke Medicine
Royal Derby Hospitals NHS Foundation Trust
Derby

Dr Nigel Beckett
Consultant in Ageing and Health/Honorary Senior Lecturer
Guy's and St Thomas' NHS Foundation Trust
Imperial College London
London

Dr Nick J Beeching
Senior Lecturer in Infectious Diseases
Royal Liverpool University Hospital
Liverpool

Dr Adam de Belder
Consultant Cardiologist
Brighton and Sussex University Hospitals NHS Trust
Brighton

Dr Neeraj Bhala
MRC Health of the Public Research Fellow/Specialist
Registrar in Gastroenterology
Clinical Trial Service Unit (CTSU)/University of Oxford
Oxford

Dr Keith Bodger
Consultant Gastroenterologist
Aintree University Hospitals NHS Foundation Trust
Liverpool

Dr Clive Bowman
Medical Director
Bupa Care Services
Leeds

Dr Anthony Bradlow
Consultant Rheumatologist
Royal Berkshire NHS Foundation Trust
Reading

Dr Stuart Bruce
Consultant Physician
Conquest Hospital
St Leonard's-on-Sea

Professor Alistair Burns
Professor of old age psychiatry
University of Manchester/Manchester Academic Health
Science Centre
Manchester

Dr Eileen Burns
Consultant Physician
St James Hospital
Leeds

Dr Christopher Burton
Senior Research Fellow in Evidence Based Practice
Bangor University
Bangor

Dr Carmen Carroll
Consultant Geriatrician
Salisbury District Hospital
Salisbury

Professor David Challis
Director PSSRU/Professor of Community Care Research
University of Manchester
Manchester

Dr Jasroop Chana
Specialist Trainee in Rheumatology
Royal Berkshire NHS Foundation Trust
Reading

Dr Anthony WC Chow
Consultant Cardiologist and Honorary Senior Lecturer
The Heart Hospital, UCLH
London

Professor Martin Joseph Connolly
Freemasons' Professor of Geriatric Medicine
University of Auckland
Auckland

Dr Simon Conroy
Head of Service/Senior Lecturer, Geriatric Medicine
University Hospitals of Leicester
Leicester

Dr Robert Cooper
Specialist Registrar
Mersey Deanery
Liverpool

Dr Anna Crown
Consultant Endocrinologist
Royal Sussex County Hospital
Brighton

Dr Adam Darowski
Consultant Physician
John Radcliffe Hospital
Oxford

Dr Christopher WH Davies
Consultant Respiratory Physician
Royal Berkshire NHS Foundation Trust
Reading

Dr Kim Delbaere
Senior Research Officer
Neuroscience Research Australia
Sydney

Dr Michael John Denham
Honorary Consultant Physician in Geriatric Medicine
Northwick Park Hospital
Harrow

Dr Ian Donald
Consultant in Old Age Medicine
Gloucestershire Royal Hospital
Gloucester

Dr Kevin Doughty
Deputy Director
University of York
Heslington

Dr Lindsey Dow
Consultant Geriatrician & Stroke Physician
Royal United Hospital
Bath

Mr Michael Eckstein
Consultant Vitreo-retinal surgeon
Sussex Eye Hospital
Brighton

Professor John E Ellershaw
Professor of Palliative Medicine
Marie Curie Palliative Care Institute/
University of Liverpool
Liverpool

Dr Victoria Ewan
Clinical Research Associate
Newcastle University
Newcastle upon Tyne

Mrs Carol Ann Fairfield
Lecturer in Clinical Practice
University of Reading
Reading

Dr Farhat Farrokhi
Physician and Postgraduate Student
University of Toronto
Toronto

Dr Rick Fielding
Locum Consultant Nephrologist
Brighton and Sussex University Hospitals NHS Trust
Brighton

Dr Malcolm Finlay
Senior Clinical Research Fellow
University College London
London

Dr Martin Fisher
Consultant Physician HIV/GU Medicine
Brighton and Sussex University Hospitals NHS Trust
Brighton

Dr Enrico Flossmann
Consultant Neurologist/Honorary Consultant
Neurologist
Royal Berkshire NHS Foundation Trust/The John
Radcliffe Hospital Oxford
Reading/Oxford

Dr Duncan R Forsyth
Consultant Geriatrician
Cambridge University Hospitals NHS Foundation Trust/
Addenbrooke's Hospital
Cambridge

Professor William Duncan Fraser
Professor of Medicine
University of East Anglia
Norwich

Dr Richard JR Frearson
Consultant Physician/Geriatrician and Honorary Senior
Lecturer
Freeman Hospital, Newcastle Hospitals NHS Foundation
Trust/Newcastle University
Newcastle upon Tyne

Dr Paul F Gallagher
Consultant Geriatrician
Cork University Hospital
Cork

Dr James George
Consultant Physician
Cumberland Infirmary
Carlisle

Professor Tony Gershlick
Consultant Cardiologist
University Hospitals of Leicester
Leicester

Ms Elinor Ginzler
AARP Vice President, Health Portfolio
AARP
Washington DC

Dr Adam L Gordon
Consultant and Special Lecturer in Medicine of Older
People
Nottingham University Hospitals NHS Trust
Nottingham

Mr Paddy Goslyn
Social Work Consultant
Reading Social Services
Reading

Professor Margot Gosney
Professor of Elderly Care Medicine/Director Clinical
Health Sciences
Royal Berkshire NHS Foundation Trust/University of
Reading
Reading

Dr Ralph Gregory
Consultant Neurologist
Poole Hospital NHS Foundation Trust
Poole

Mr Richard Gregson
Consultant Ophthalmologist
Nottingham United Hospitals
Nottingham

Dr Joseph E Grey
Consultant Physician/Honorary Consultant in Wound
Healing
Cardiff and Vale University Health Board
Cardiff

Dr Vandana Gupta
Specialist Registrar in Respiratory Medicine
Manchester Royal Infirmary
Manchester

Dr Danielle Harari
Consultant Geriatrician/Senior Lecturer
Guy's and St Thomas' NHS Foundation Trust/Kings
College London
London

Professor Keith Harding
Director Institute for Translation, Innovation,
Methodologies and Engagement (TIME)
Cardiff University
Cardiff

Dr Adam Harper
Consultant Geriatrician
Brighton and Sussex University Hospitals NHS Trust
Brighton

Professor Rowan H Harwood
Consultant Geriatrician
Nottingham University Hospitals NHS Trust
Nottingham

Dr Anna Lucy Hatton
Research Fellow
University of Salford
Manchester

Dr Victoria Haunton
Specialist Registrar Geriatric Medicine
Leicester Royal Infirmary
Leicester

Dr Frances Healey
Joint Head of Clinical Review and Response
National Patient Safety Agency
York

Professor Michael Horan
Professor of Geriatric Medicine
The University of Manchester
Manchester

Dr Trevor A Howlett
Consultant Physician and Endocrinologist
Leicester Royal Infirmary
Leicester

Dr Jane Hughes
Lecturer in Community Care Research, PSSRU
University of Manchester
Manchester

Dr Erisa Ito
Specialist Registrar in Elderly Care Medicine
Southampton University Healthcare NHS Trust
Southampton

Professor Stephen Jackson
Professor of Clinical Gerontology
King's College Hospital
London

Dr Sarbjit Vanita Jassal
Associate Professor and Staff Physician
University Health Network and University of Toronto
Toronto

Dr Andrew PD Jeffries
Specialist Registrar in Rheumatology
Brighton and Sussex NHS Trust
Brighton

Dr Kelsey M Jordan
Consultant in Rheumatology and Honorary Senior
Lecturer
Brighton and Sussex University Hospitals NHS Trust
Brighton

Dr Orla Kennedy
Faculty Director Teaching and Learning (Science)
University of Reading
Reading

Dr Hannah King
Specialist Registrar in Gerontology
Royal Berkshire NHS Foundation Trust
Reading

Dr Margaret EM Kirkup
Consultant Dermatologist
Weston General Hospital
Weston-super-Mare

Dr Joanna Kitley
Clinical Fellow in Neuromyelitis Optica
John Radcliffe Hospital
Oxford

Dr Shiva Koyalakonda
Specialist Registrar in Cardiology
University Hospital Aintree
Liverpool

Dr Ashok Krishnamoorthy
Consultant Psychiatrist
Wrexham Maelor Hospital
Wrexham

Dr Unni Krishnan
Specialist Registrar in Cardiology
Liverpool Heart and Chest Hospital
Liverpool

Dr Siri Rostoft Kristjansson
Research Fellow
University of Oslo/Oslo University Hospital
Oslo

Professor Joseph Kwan
Consultant Stroke Physician
Royal Bournemouth Hospital and Bournemouth
University
Bournemouth

Professor Peter Langhorne
Professor of Stroke Care
Royal Infirmary
Glasgow

Dr Iracema Leroi
Consultant in Old Age Psychiatry/Honorary Senior
Lecturer
Lancashire Care NHS Foundation Trust/
University of Manchester
Preston/Manchester

Dr Miles J Levy
Consultant Endocrinologist
Leicester Royal Infirmary
Leicester

Dr Martin Llewelyn
Senior Lecturer and Consultant in Infectious Diseases
Brighton and Sussex Medical School
Brighton

Dr Gregory YH Lip
Professor of Cardiovascular Medicine
University of Birmingham Centre for Cardiovascular
Sciences City Hospital
Birmingham

Dr Janet Lippett
Consultant Orthogeriatrician
Royal Berkshire NHS Foundation Trust
Reading

Dr Nelson Lo
Consultant Geriatrician
University Hospitals of Leicester
Leicester

Dr Philippa Anne Logan
Associate Professor in Community Rehabilitation
University of Nottingham
Nottingham

Mrs Michelle Long
Therapy Lead and Specialist Physiotherapist in
Neurological Rehabilitation
Princess Royal Hospital
Haywards Heath

Professor Stephen R Lord
Senior Principal Research Fellow
Neuroscience Research Australia
Sydney

Dr Susi Lund
Nurse Consultant End of Life Care
Royal Berkshire NHS Foundation Trust
Reading

Dr Dimitrius Edward Anthony Luxton
Retired Consultant Community Geriatrician
Formerly of Brookfields Hospital
Cambridge

Mr Peter R Malone
Consultant Urological Surgeon
Royal Berkshire NHS Foundation Trust
Reading

Mr Nicholas John Mansell
Consultant Otolaryngologist/Head and Neck Surgeon
Royal Berkshire NHS Foundation Trust
Reading

Professor Finbarr Martin
Professor of Medical Gerontology
King's College London
London

Professor Tahir Masud
Professor of Geriatric Medicine and Consultant Physician
Nottingham University Hospitals NHS Trust
Nottingham

Dr Helen May
Consultant and Clinical Director Medicine for the Elderly
Norfolk and Norwich University NHS Foundation Trust
Norwich

Dr Rachel McCarthy
Head of Audiology
Royal Berkshire NHS Foundation Trust
Reading

Dr Jeremy McNally
Consultant Rheumatologist
Royal Berkshire NHS Foundation Trust
Reading

Dr Amit Kumar Mistri
Clinical Senior Lecturer/Honorary Consultant in Stroke
Medicine
University of Leicester/University Hospitals of Leicester
NHS Trust
Leicester

Dr Alexandra Montagu
Registrar in Geriatric Medicine and General Internal
Medicine
Royal Berkshire NHS Foundation Trust
Reading

Professor Michael DL Morgan
Consultant Physician and Honorary
Professor of Respiratory Medicine
Glenfield Hospital
Leicester

Dr Aung Myat
Specialist Registrar in Cardiology and
NIHR Clinical Research Fellow
The Rayne Institute,
St Thomas' Hospital King's College
London

Professor Julia L Newton
Professor of Ageing and Medicine
Newcastle University
Newcastle

Dr Wan-fai Ng
Clinical Senior Lecturer in Rheumatology
Newcastle University
Newcastle upon Tyne

Dr Samuel Robert Nyman
Lecturer in Psychology
Bournemouth University
Poole

Dr Shaun O'Keeffe
Consultant Geriatrician
Galway University Hospitals
Galway

Dr Denis O'Mahony
Consultant Geriatrician &
Senior Lecturer in Medicine
University College Cork/Cork University Hospital
Cork

Dr Louise Pack
Consultant, Elderly Medicine
Royal Sussex County Hospital
Brighton

Dr Diran Padiachy
Consultant Physician in Medicine for Older People
Poole General Hospital
Poole

Dr Burak Pamukcu
Post doctorate Research Fellow
University of Birmingham Centre for Cardiovascular
Sciences City Hospital
Birmingham

Professor Stuart G Parker
Professor of Health Care for Older People
University of Sheffield
Sheffield

Professor Viviane Pasqui
Maître de Conférences
Université Pierre et Marie Curie-Sorbonne Universités
Paris

Dr Girish K Patel
Senior Clinical Research Fellow
Cardiff University
Cardiff

Dr Michael D Peake
Consultant and Senior Lecturer in Respiratory
Medicine/National Clinical Lead
Glenfield Hospital/NHS Cancer Improvement &
National Cancer Intelligence Network
Leicester.

Dr Ruth D Piers
Researcher
Ghent University Hospital
Gent

Dr Catherine Jane Quarini
Clinical Editor
British Medical Association
London

Dr Terence J Quinn
Lecturer in Geriatric Medicine
University of Glasgow
Glasgow

Professor Muriel Rainfray
Head of Geriatric Medicine Department
Bordeaux 2 University
Bordeaux

Dr Jason M Raw
Consultant Physician and Geriatrician
Fairfield General Hospital
Greater Manchester

Dr Simon Ray
Consultant Cardiologist / Honorary Reader in Cardiology
Manchester Academic Health Sciences Centre/University
Hospitals of South Manchester
Manchester

Dr Helen Roberts
Senior Lecturer in Geriatric Medicine
University of Southampton
Southampton

Professor Louise Robinson
Professor of Primary Care and Ageing
Newcastle University
Newcastle upon Tyne

Professor Thompson Robinson
Professor in Stroke Medicine
University of Leicester/Leicester Royal Infirmary
Leicester

Professor Kenneth Rockwood
Professor of Medicine (Geriatric Medicine & Neurology)
Dalhousie University
Nova Scotia
Canada

Professor Helen Rodgers
Professor of Stroke Care
Newcastle University
Newcastle Upon Tyne

Professor Keith Rome
Professor of Podiatry
AUT University
Auckland

Dr Pierre FM Rumeau
Head of La Grave Gerontechnology Lab
Toulouse University Hospital
Toulouse

Dr Gregor Russell
Consultant in Older People's Mental Health
Lynfield Mount Hospital
Bradford

Dr Jude Ryan
Specialist Registrar in Clinical Gerontology
King's College Hospital
London

Dr Stephen Saltissi
Consultant Cardiologist
Royal Liverpool University Hospital
Liverpool

Dr Andrew Severn
Consultant Anaesthetist
Royal Lancaster Infirmary
Lancaster

Professor Alan Sinclair
Professor of Medicine and Dean
Bedfordshire and Hertfordshire Postgraduate Medical School
Luton

Dr Manav Sohal
Specialist Registrar in Cardiology
Royal Sussex County Hospital
Brighton

Dr Adrian Stanley
Consultant Physician and Honorary Senior Lecturer
University Hospitals of Leicester NHS Trust
Leicester

Dr Andrew Steel
Consultant Physician
Kettering General Hospital NHS Foundation Trust
Kettering

Professor Jimmy Steele
Chair of Oral Health Research and Head of School of
Dental Sciences
Newcastle University
Newcastle upon Tyne

Mr Venki Sundaram
Specialty Registrar in Ophthalmology
London Deanery
London

Dr Jennifer Thain
Specialist Registrar in Geriatrics and General Medicine
Nottingham University Hospitals NHS Trust
Nottingham

Miss Johanna S Thomas
Urology Registrar
Royal Berkshire NHS Foundation Trust
Reading

Mr James Tildsley
Ophthalmology Registrar
Queens Medical Centre
Nottingham

Dr Stacy Todd
Specialist Trainee in Infectious Diseases and Tropical
Medicine
Royal Liverpool University Hospital
Liverpool

Dr William D Toff
Senior Lecturer in Cardiology
University of Leicester
Leicester

Mr Alex Torrie
Trauma and Orthopaedic Registrar
Frenchay hospital
Bristol

Dr Peter Torrie
Consultant Radiologist
Royal Berkshire NHS Foundation Trust
Reading

Dr Jonathan Treml
Consultant Geriatrician
Queen Elizabeth Hospital
Birmingham

Dr Christopher James Turnbull
Consultant Geriatrician
Arrowe Park Hospital
Wirral

Professor Nele J Van Den Noortgate
Head of Department of Geriatrics
Ghent University Hospital
Gent

Dr Michael Vassallo
Consultant Physician
Royal Bournemouth Hospital
Bournemouth

Dr Emma Vaux
Consultant Nephrologist
Royal Berkshire NHS Foundation Trust
Reading

Professor Christina R Victor
Professor of Gerontology and Public Health, Director of
the Doctorate in Public Health (DrPH)
Brunel University
Middlesex

Dr Nadine Vigouroux
PhD in Computer Science
Senior CNRS researcher, IRIT
Toulouse

Dr Harin Vyas
Specialist Registrar in Cardiology
Royal Liverpool University Hospital
Liverpool

Dr Jonathan Waite
Consultant in the Psychiatry of Old Age
Nottinghamshire Healthcare NHS Trust
Nottingham

Professor Angus WG Walls
Professor of Restorative Dentistry
Newcastle University
Newcastle upon Tyne

Professor Christopher D Ward
Professor and Consultant in Rehabilitation Medicine
Royal Derby Hospital and University of Nottingham
Derby

Professor Caroline Watkins
Professor of Stroke and Older People's Care
University of Central Lancashire
Preston

Dr Timothy Webster
Specialist Registrar in Geriatric Medicine
Royal Liverpool University Teaching Hospital
Liverpool

Mr David Whalebelly
Specialist Elderly Care Dietician
Royal Berkshire NHS Foundation Trust
Reading

Dr Graham Whyte
Speciality Registrar in Palliative Medicine
Marie Curie Hospice Liverpool
Liverpool

Dr Kate Wiles
Specialist Registrar in Nephrology
Queen Alexandra Hospital
Portsmouth

Dr Richard Wong
Consultant Geriatrician
University Hospitals of Leicester NHS Trust
Leicester

Dr Mark Woodhead
Consultant in General and Respiratory Medicine/
Honorary Senior Lecturer
Manchester Royal Infirmary/University of Manchester
Manchester

Dr Juliet Wright
Senior Lecturer/Honorary Consultant Elderly Medicine
Brighton and Sussex Medical School
Brighton

List of abbreviations

AAC	alternative/augmentative communication	BAPEN	British Association for Parenteral and Enteral Nutrition
AAFB	acid and alcohol fast bacilli	BBB	blood brain barrier
(AAI(R))	single chamber atrial pacing and sensing pacemaker	BC	bone conduction
AAL	ambient assisted living	BDAE	Boston Diagnostic Aphasia Examination
ABPI	Association of the British Pharmaceutical Industry	BGS	British Geriatrics Society
		BHS	British Hypertension Society
ABPM	ambulatory blood pressure monitoring	BMD	bone mineral density
AC	air conduction	BMI	Body Mass Index
ACCORD	Action to Control Cardiovascular Risk in Diabetes	BNP	brain natriuretic peptide
		BPE	benign prostatic enlargement
ACE	acute care environments	BPSD	behavioural and psychological symptoms of dementia
ACE	angiotensin-converting enzyme		
ACE-I	angiotensin-converting enzyme inhibitors	BSR	British Society of Rheumatology
ACE-R	Addenbrooke's Cognitive Examination	BTS	British Thoracic Society
ACP	advance care planning	CAD	coronary artery disease
ACR	albumin-creatinine ratio	CADASIL	Cerebral Autosomal Dominant Arteriopathy with Subcortical Infarcts and Leukoencephalopathy
ACS	acute coronary syndrome		
AD	Alzheimer's disease		
ADA	American Diabetes Association	CAM	complementary and alternative therapies
ADEs	adverse drug events	CAM	confusion assessment method
ADR	adverse drug reactions	CAP	community acquired pneumonia
ADRT	advance decisions on refusal of treatment	CASE-SF	Clinical Assessment Scales for the Elderly
ADVANCE	Action in Diabetes and Vascular Disease: Preterax and Diamicron MR Controlled Evaluation	CBGD	cortical basal ganglionic degeneration
		CBT	Cognitive Behaviour Therapy
		CBT-I	Cognitive Behavioural Therapy for Insomnia
AED	anti-epileptic drug		
AFO	ankle-foot orthoses	CCB	calcium channel blockers
AGS	American Geriatrics Society	CCP	anti-cyclic citrullinated peptide
AHI	apnoea-hypopnoea index	CDT	Clock Drawing Test
AHP	allied health professions	CEA	carcinoembryonic antigen
AIH	autoimmune hepatitis	CEA	carotid endarterectomy
AKI	acute kidney injury	CGA	Comprehensive Geriatric Assessment
AMD	age-related macular degeneration	CHL	conductive hearing loss
AMTS	Abbreviated Mental Test Score	CI	confidence intervals
ANP	atrial natriuretic peptide	CIMT	constraint-induced movement therapy
ARBs	angiotensin receptor blockers	CJD	Creutzfeldt-Jakob Disease
ARDS	adult respiratory distress syndrome	CMAPs	compound muscle action potentials
AREDS	Age Related Eye Disease Study	CMHT	Community Mental Health Teams
ARR	absolute risk reduction	CNV	choroidal neovascularisation
ARVD/C	arrhythmogenic right ventricular dysplasia/ cardiomyopathy	COM	chronic otitis media
		COMT-I	catechol-O-methyl transferase inhibitors
AS	advance statements	COPD	chronic obstructive pulmonary disease
ASA	American Society of Anaesthesiologists	CPAP	continuous positive airway pressure
ASWs	approved social workers	CPET	cardiopulmonary exercise testing
AT	anaerobic threshold	CPPDD	calcium pyrophosphate deposition disease
ATN	acute tubular necrosis	CQC	Care Quality Commission
AUR	acute urinary retention	CRB	Criminal Records Bureau
AV	atrioventricular	CREST	Clinical Resource and Efficiency Support Team
AVN	atrioventricular node		

CRP	C-reactive protein	EMS	emergency medical services
CRQ	Chronic Respiratory Questionnaire	EPO	erythropoietin
CSCI	continuous subcutaneous infusion	ESRD	end stage renal disease
CSF	cerebrospinal fluid	ET	essential tremor
CT	computerized tomography	EUCROF	European CRO Federation
CTA	CT angiography	EULAR	European League against Rheumatism
CTEPH	chronic thromboembolic pulmonary hypertension	EUS	endoscopic ultrasound
		EXPRESS	Existing PREventive Strategies for Stroke
CTPA	CT pulmonary angiography	FAST	Face Arm Speech Test
CUR	chronic urinary retention	FAST	Frenchay Aphasia Screening Test
CVI	Certificate of Visual Impairment	FASTER	FAST Assessment of Stroke and TIA to prevent Early Recurrence
CVS	cardiovascular system		
DAs	dopamine agonists	FDA	Food and Drugs Administration
DASH	Dietary Approaches to Stop Hypertension	FEES	flexible endoscopic evaluation of swallowing
DAT-SPECT	dopamine transporter		
DBS	deep brain stimulation	FES	functional electrical stimulation
DDD(R)	dual chamber pacemakers	FFA	fundus fluorescein angiography
DDI	dopa-decarboxylase inhibitor	FI	faecal incontinence
DHF	diastolic heart failure	FNA	fine needle aspiration cytology
DKA	diabetic ketoacidosis	FTD	frontotemporal dementia
DLB	dementia with Lewy bodies	GAD	generalized anxiety disorder
DMARD	disease-modifying anti-rheumatic drug	GAT	Goldman applanation tonometry
DOT	directly observed therapy	GBA	glucocerebrosidase
DPP-IV	dipeptidyl peptidase-4	GCS	Glasgow Coma Score
DSE	dobutamine stress echocardiography	GDS	Geriatric Depression Scale
DSM-IV	Diagnostic and Statistical Manual of Mental Disorders	GFR	glomerular filtration rate
		GIP	glucose-dependent insulinotropic polypeptide
DST	Decision Support Tool		
DWC	Disqualification from Working with Children	GLP-1	glucagon-like polypeptide-1
		GON	glaucomatous optic neuropathy
DWI	diffusion weighted imaging	GPCOG	General Practitioner Assessment of Cognition
DWVA	Disqualification from Working with Vulnerable Adults		
		GPP	good practice points
EAC	external auditory canal	HADS	Hospital Anxiety and Depression Scale
EATL	enteropathy associated T cell lymphoma	HAP	hospital acquired pneumonia
EBUS	endobronchial ultrasound	HARP	Hospital Admission Risk programme
ECCE	extra-capsular cataract extraction	HCM	hypercalcaemiamia associated with malignancy
ECF	extracellular fluid		
ECST	major carotid endarterectomy study	HDL	high density lipoprotein
ECT	electroconvulsive therapy	HER2	human epidermal growth factor receptor 2
ED	erectile dysfunction		
EDV	end-diastolic volume	HFNEF	heart failure with normal ejection fraction
EF	ejection fraction	HFREF	heart failure with reduced ejection fraction
EFGCP	European Forum for Good Clinical Practice		
		HLA	human leukocyte antigen
EGFR	epidermal growth factor receptor	HONK	hyperglycaemic hyperosmolar non-ketotic
EHS	European Hypertension Society	HPA	hypothalamic pituitary adrenal
ELSA	English Longitudinal Study of Ageing	HPT	hyperparathyroidis
EmA	antiendomysial antibody	HRCT	high resolution CT
EMA	European Medicines Agency	HRT	Heidelberg retinal tomograph
EMDR	eye movement desensitization and reprocessing	HYVET	Hypertension in the Very Elderly Trial
		IBS	irritable bowel syndrome
EMG	electromyography	IC	intermediate care
EMI	elderly mentally infirm	ICDs	implantable cardiac defibrillators

IDF	International Diabetes Federation	MSA	multisystem atrophy
IFN	interferon	MSU	monosodium urate
IGT	impaired glucose tolerance	MUAC	mid-upper arm circumference
IHD	ischaemic heart disease	MUAP	motor unit action potential
(IL)-6	interleukin	MUR	medication use review
IMCA	Independent Mental Capacity Advocate	MUST	Malnutrition Universal Screening Tool
INR	international normalized ratio	NAB-Scr	Neuropsychological Assessment Battery Screening Module
IOP	intraocular pressure	NAFLD	non-alcoholic fatty liver disease
IPD	idiopathic Parkinson's disease	NCEPOD	National Confidential Enquiry into Patient Outcomes and Deaths
IQCODE	Informant Questionnaire on Cognitive Decline in the Elderly	NCS	Nerve Conduction Studies
ISA	Independent Safeguarding Authority	NEADL	Nottingham Extended Activities of Daily Living
ISH	isolated systolic hypertension	NEFA	non-esterified fatty-acid
KIM-1	kidney injury molecule-1	NES	non-epileptiform seizures
KLORA	key lines of regulatory assessment	NGaL	neutrophil gelatinase-associated lipocalin
LACI	lacunar infarcts	NHANES III	National Health and Nutrition Examination Survey
LADA	late-onset autoimmune diabetes of adults	NHFD	National Hip Fracture Database
LBBB	left bundle branch block	NICE	National Institute for Health and Clinical Excellence
LCP	Liverpool Care Pathway for the Dying Patient	NIHSS	National Institute of Health Stroke Scale
LDCT	low dose CT	NIMGU	non-insulin medicated glucose uptake
LGIB	lower gastrointestinal bleeding	NIV	non-invasive ventilation
LIF	leukaemia inhibitory factor	NLU	nurse-led inpatient units
LMWH	low molecular weight heparin	NMDA	N-methyl D-aspartate
LOS	length of stay	NNT	number of patients needed to treat
LPA	Lasting Power of Attorney	NO	nitric oxide
LRRK-2	leucine-rich repeat kinase 2	NPG	normal pressure glaucoma
LUTS	lower urinary tract symptoms	NPH	normal pressure hydrocephalus
LVAs	low vision aids	NPV	negative predictive value
LVSD	left ventricular systolic dysfunction	NRS	Nutrition Risk Score
MAOB-I	monoamine oxidase-B inhibitors	NSAIDs	non-steroidal anti-inflammatory drugs
MAR	Medication Administration Record	NSCLC	non-small cell lung cancer
mCare	Mobile Telecare	NSF-OP	National Service Framework for Older People
MCCD	Medical Certificate of the Cause of Death	NT proBNP	N-terminal proBNP
MCI	mild cognitive impairment	NTG	normal tension glaucoma
MD	mean difference	nTG-6	neural transglutaminase
MDRD	modification of diet in renal disease	OAE	otoacoustic emissions
MDR TB	multi drug resistant TB	OCD	obsessive compulsive disorder
MDT	multi-disciplinary team	OCT	optical coherence tomography
MELAS	mitochondrial encephalomyopathy, lactic acidosis, and stroke-like episodes	OGD	oesophagogastroduodenoscopy
MHC	major histocompatibility complex	OGTT	oral glucose tolerance test
MHRA	Medicines and Healthcare products Regulatory Agency	OHT	ocular hypertension
MI	motivational interviewing	OME	otitis media with effusion
MI	myocardial infarction	OPCA	olivopontocerebellar atrophy
MMSE	Mini Mental State Examination	OPG	osteoprotegrin
MNA	Mini-Nutrition Assessment	OR	odds ratio
MOCA	Montreal Cognitive Assessment	OSAHS	obstructive sleep apnoea-hypopnoea syndrome
MPS	myocardial perfusion scintigraphy scan	OT	occupational therapy
MRCP	magnetic resonance cholangiopancreatogram	PACE	Police and Criminal Evidence Act 1984
MRSA	Methicillin resistant Staphylococcus aureus		

PACG	primary angle closure glaucoma		PTSD	post traumatic stress disorder
PACI	partial anterior circulation infarct		PVP	percutaneous vertebroplasty
PAP	pulmonary artery pressure		QOF	Quality and Outcomes Framework
PARR	patient at risk of re-hospitalization		RANKL	Receptor activator of nuclear factor kappa-B ligand
PBC	primary biliary cirrhosis		RAPD	relative afferent pupil defect
PBL	peripheral blood leukocytes		RBANS	Repeatable Battery for the Assessment of Neuropsychological Status
PCC	person-centred dementia care			
PCR	protein creatinine ratio		RBBB	right bundle branch blocks
PCT	Primary Care Trust		RCP	Royal College of Physicians
PD	Parkinson's disease		RCT	randomized controlled trial
PD	pharmacodynamics		RDW	red cell distribution width
PDD	Parkinson's disease dementia		REM	rapid eye movement
PDSN	Parkinson's Disease Specialist Nurse		RFID	radio-frequency identification
PDT	photodynamic therapy		RGC	retinal ganglion cells
PE	pulmonary embolus		RIG	radiologically inserted gastrostomy
PEG	percutaneous endoscopic gastrostomy		RLS	restless legs syndrome
PEEP	positive end-expiratory pressure		RNCC	Registered Nursing Care Contribution
PET	positron emission tomography		RNIB	Royal National Institute for the Blind
PFTs	pulmonary function tests		ROS	reactive oxygen species
PHQ-9	Patient Health Questionnaire		ROSIER	Recognition of Stroke in the Emergency Room
PILOT	platelet-orientated inhibition in new TIA			
PIMs	potentially inappropriate medicines		RPE	retinal pigment epithelium
PK	pharmacokinetics		RRT	renal replacement therapy
PLEDS	periodic lateralizing epileptiform discharges		RVI	referral of vision impaired patient
			SADQ-10	Stroke Aphasic Depression Questionnaire
PKP	percutaneous kyphoplasty		SAH	subarachnoid haemorrhage
PMMA	polymethylmethacrylate		SAQOL	Stroke and Aphasia Quality of Life Scale
PMR	polymyalgia rheumatica		SCLC	small cell lung cancers
PND	paroxysmal nocturnal dyspnoea		SDS	Shy-Drager syndrome
POAG	primary open angle glaucoma		SGA	Subjective Global Assessment
PoCA	Protection of Children Act		SGRQ	St George's Respiratory Questionnaire
PoVA	Protection of Vulnerable Adults		SHF	systolic heart failure
POCI	posterior circulation infarct		SHS	sliding hip screw
POMA	Performance-Oriented Mobility Assessment		SIADH	syndrome of inappropriate anti-diuretic hormone
POPS	Proactive Care of Older Persons undergoing Surgery		SIGN	Scottish Intercollegiate Guidelines Network
POSSUM	Physiological and Operative Severity Score		SMR	standardized mortality ratio
			SND	striatonigral degeneration
PPAR	peroxisome proliferator activated receptor		SNHL	sensorineural hearing loss
			SNRI	serotonin noradrenaline reuptake inhibitor
PPI	proton pump inhibitor			
PPV	positive predictive value		SPARCL	Stroke Prevention by Aggressive Reduction in Cholesterol Levels
PRA	plasma renin activity			
Pra	Probability of Repeat Admissions tool		SPA	smartphone application
ProFaNE	Prevention of Falls Network Europe		SPECT	single photon emission computed tomography
PS	performance status			
PSI	pneumonia severity index		SSI	severely sight impaired
PSP	progressive supranuclear palsy		SSRI	selective serotonin re-uptake inhibitor
PTA	pure tone audiometry		SSS	sick sinus syndrome
PTH	parathyroid hormone		START	Screening Tool to Alert to Right Treatments
PTHrP	parathyroid-hormone-related protein			
PTMC	percutaneous transmitral commissurotomy		SUA	serum uric acid

SV	stroke volume		TSF	triceps skin-fold thickness
SWAP	short wavelength automated perimetry		TTE	transthoracic echocardiogram
T1WI	T1 weighted imaging		tTGA-2	tissue transglutaminase-2
T2WI	T2 weighted imaging		UGIB	upper gastrointestinal bleeding
TAB	temporal artery biopsy		UI	urinary incontinence
TACI	total anterior circulation infarct		UP list	Unsuitable Person's list
TAO	thyroid-associated ophthalmopathy		UPDRS	Unified Parkinson's Disease Rating Scale
TARDIS	Triple Antiplatelets for Reducing Dependency after Ischaemic Stroke		VA-HIT	Veterans Affairs High Density Lipoprotein Cholesterol Intervention Trial
TCAs	tricyclic antidepressants		VAP	ventilator associated pneumonia
TGA	transient global amnesia		VCFs	vertebral compression fractures
TIA	transient ischaemic attack		VD	vascular dementia
TIPS	transjugular intrahepatic portosystemic shunt		VEGF	vascular endothelial growth factor
TKI	tyrosine kinase inhibitors		VFS	videofluoroscopy
TMD	temporo-mandibular disorder		VIM	ventrointermedial
TME	total mesorectal excision		V/Q	ventilation-perfusion scintigraphy
TNF	tumour necrosis factor		VTE	venous thromboembolism
TOE	transoesophageal echocardiogram		WASIa	Wechsler Abbreviated Scale of Intelligence
TONE	Trial of Non-Pharmacologic Intervention in the Elderly		WHO	World Health Organization
TRD	treatment resistant depression		XDR-TB	extensively drug resistant TB

What is geriatric medicine

The epidemiology of ageing

The epidemiological approach is an important perspective in developing our understanding of old age, in caring for older people and an ageing population. Epidemiology studies the patterns of health and illness within and between populations and is a key component of public health medicine, which is concerned with the organized efforts of society to improve health at the population level. It is an approach to medicine that emphasizes a population rather than an individual/clinical patient focused perspective. The epidemiological approach contributes to patient care by searching for the identification of 'risk factors' for specific diseases, such as demonstrating the links between smoking and lung cancer. It is also a key contributing discipline to the development of evidence-based healthcare that provides clinicians with guidance on the most effective methods of caring for their patients.

Describing health and disease

Epidemiological studies are concerned with describing and understanding the patterns and determinants of health at a population level. For older people, health is seen as a key component of quality of life and is central to the models of successful ageing advanced by Rowe and Kahn and the World Health Organization's concept of 'active ageing'. Health in later life (and for any specific older person) reflects the interaction of a range of factors, including biological factors such as genetic heritage, individual 'health' behaviours (e.g. diet, alcohol consumption, exercise, or smoking), exposure to environmental/occupational hazards, the availability and quality of health and social care and socio-structural factors such as gender, ethnicity, and social class. The definition of what is meant by health is problematic. We can identify several approaches: health as the absence of disease (a medical model approach); health as the absence of illness (a sociological perspective); health as an ideal or 'optimal state' (the World Health Organization model); and health as a pragmatically defined entity. Each of these perspectives derives from different theoretical conceptualizations of health and generates different types of research questions and different types of 'knowledge' about the epidemiology of ageing. In studying the epidemiology of ageing, disease-orientated measures such as osteoarthritis, dementia, stroke, or generic measures of chronic disease, such as longstanding limiting illness, predominate.

Describing disease: key epidemiological terms

If, for example, we are interested in establishing the 'disease' burden associated with dementia, one requirement would be to determine the number of people with this particular condition. This is defined as the prevalence rate: the number of people with dementia expressed as a rate (usually per 1000 or 100 000) of the total population 'at risk'. We are also interested in the number of new cases arising during a specific reference period (often a year): this is known as the incidence rate. For both measures to be useful, we also need a reliable and valid measure of dementia (see below) and accurate denominators as well as numerators.

Mortality or morbidity? Measuring health in populations

The epidemiologist is concerned with three key attributes when investigating the health of given populations:

- time (over what period are data collected; is time of year/day/week important)
- place (where is the condition more/less common)
- person (are there variations in terms of age, class, gender, ethnicity, etc.).

Thus we require measures of health that facilitate comparisons between individuals, groups, places, and/or different points in time (or some combination of these). Mortality data that provide details of the distribution of death within a given population are the closest to this technical specification. It is the oldest and most widely used index of health status, especially as the outcome is unambiguous, although establishing the cause of death can be problematic. The use of this indicator is not unproblematic as we assume that (a) patterns of deaths within populations mirror the distribution of health and (b) major causes of death are the principal causes of ill-health.

Morbidity measures are concerned with the patterns of non-morbidity health status and general distinguish between 'acute' (self-limiting) and chronic (long-term) conditions. Four key approaches towards the measurement of morbidity may be identified:

- studies of specific conditions such as osteoarthritis or dementia
- studies of 'generic' health status or self-rated health
- studies of disability and chronic disease
- studies using indirect indices based upon the secondary analysis of routine clinical activity data (e.g. use of data for hip fractures to establish the prevalence of osteoporosis).

For the first three approaches we need to have indicators that are reliable and valid measures of the concept we are measuring. It is difficult to measure disease states such as dementia, depression, or arthritis in population surveys. Such chronic conditions represent a spectrum of severity ranging from normal to severe, with prevalence rates influenced by where along the continuum the 'case definition threshold' is set. Measures defined by service access are problematic as not everyone with a condition will be known to services (e.g. only 25% of the expected number with dementia are in contact with services).

There are two elements to the assumption that mortality reflects morbidity: demographic (i.e. the age and gender distribution of health problems) and the relative importance of the health problems identified. By comparing mortality and morbidity data, we can test the veracity of these assumptions. There are approximately 556 000 deaths each year in England and Wales, 80% of which are accounted for by people aged 65+, and 64% by those aged 75+. Mortality is (relatively) high in the first year of life, at 5.8 per 1000 and then remains under this rate until the seventh decade of life. Thereafter mortality rates increase from 20 per 1000 for those aged 65–74 years to 170 per 1000 at age 85+. This age-related increase in mortality is used as evidence to support the notion that ill-health and disease are not simple factors associated with old age but that they are 'caused' by old age. Patterns of mortality and morbidity for age, class, and ethnicity are broadly similar, indicating an age-related increase in health problems; an inverse relationship with social class and the poorer health of minority elders, but mortality is higher for males than females with the reverse trend for morbidity. The most important causes of death for older adults are circulatory disease (accounting for 40% of deaths), respiratory disease

(19% of deaths), and cancers (23% of deaths), whereas heart disease (30%), musculoskeletal disorders (30%), and respiratory problems (10%) are the major causes of physical disability. Dementia, which afflicts c. 5% of those aged over 65, causes few relatively deaths when compared with cancer and heart disease and thus in a mortality-focused prioritization, dementia would not feature significantly as a health problem as it would using a morbidity-focused approach. Mortality and morbidity are therefore not synonymous in later life and we can distinguish three distinct categories:

- high morbidity and high mortality (e.g. heart and circulatory diseases)
- high morbidity but low mortality (musculoskeletal disease and dementia)
- high mortality and low morbidity (cancer).

By combining mortality and morbidity data we can create indicators of 'healthy' or 'disability free' life expectancy (i.e. the number of years that individuals can expect to live free from disability). These types of measures summarize an important concept if we are concerned with examining both quality as well as quantity of life: what percentage of our life will be lived free from disability/ill-health? By examining data collected over long periods of time we can start to investigate if the unambiguous increases in life expectancy are accompanied by spending more (or less time) over the life course with disability or in ill-health. Such data are important for examining the ideas advanced by Fries, who argued that both morbidity AND mortality, will be 'compressed' into the later phases of life so that that there will be more people surviving into 'old age' and that those who do survive will be fitter because the factors that have delayed mortality will also have delayed morbidity. Hence the compression hypothesizes advanced by Fries argues that those people surviving to old age will be fitter for longer, with significant levels of morbidity being limited to a short period at the very end of life. The alternative hypothesis is the opposite idea encapsulated in the concept of 'survival of the unfittest'. By preventing people dying at earlier phases of life, we are increasing (or expanding) morbidity in later life. Evidence in support of either of these hypothesizes are sparse, especially within the UK. However, evidence from the USA does suggest that there is some modest long-term evidence of a reduction in levels of disability over the last two decades, although evidence from Europe is less conclusive.

Explaining age differences in health status: Age, period, and cohort effects

When studying the epidemiology of ageing, age is the independent variable and measures of social, psychological, or physical function, for example, operate as the dependent variable. The prevalence of disability, chronic health problems, and dementia all show an age-related increase. The simple observation of differences between people of different ages in terms of physical or mental health may well reflect the process of ageing (termed an age effect which reflects the maturation of an individual). However, the simple observation that something is more common among older than younger people does not automatically mean that we may attribute the cause of this difference to ageing or the passing of time. What makes understanding ageing especially challenging is that such observations may be alternatively explained as being the result of either period or cohort effects which reflect the influence of historical time. For example, the dietary restrictions for those born during war time may plausibly explain any cohort differences rather than the effects of ageing. Much of our data about the epidemiology of ageing are garnered from cross-sectional research, whereby we make comparisons between people of different ages and infer that the differences observed reflect the effects of ageing. This is problematic because this form of study design cannot differentiate between age and cohort effects. Longitudinal studies, such as the English Longitudinal Study of Ageing (ELSA), are much more powerful designs in studying ageing. Although they are still problematic because of the problems differentiating period and cohort effects, they can demonstrate the magnitude of age-related changes in, for example, cognitive function but can also identify 'risk factors', identify confounding factors such as comorbidity, and demonstrate the populations most afflicted by such changes.

Conclusion: unequal ageing?

Variations in health status within the older age groups demonstrate the well-characterized health variations demonstrated at earlier phases of the life cycle. Melzer et al. demonstrate the existence of socio-economic differentials in both the overall distributions of disability and severe disability, which are evident for all age/gender groups, and claims that achievement of the disability prevalence of the most privileged groups by all older people would result in an absolute increase in the numbers of disabled elders despite projected increases in both population and longevity. Increases in life expectancy, resulting from decreases in mortality, have not been equally shared throughout the population of older people. Women appear to have benefited more than men have, and those from professional occupations have benefited at the expense of those from manual occupations. Although there are no comparable data on ethnicity, it seems highly improbable that increases in life expectancy, improved mortality/morbidity and probability of surviving to reach 'old age' will have been shared equally across the major ethnic groups. Indeed, a key research agenda for those interested in the epidemiology of ageing is to examine increasing importance of ethnicity in the experience of ageing and later life.

Further reading

Breeze E, Fletcher A, Leon D (2001). Socio-economic differentials persist in old age. Am J Public Health 9192: 277–83.

Fries JF (1980). Aging, natural death and the compression of morbidity. N Engl J Med 303: 130–5.

Fries JF (2003). Measuring and monitoring success in compressing morbidity. Ann Intern Med 139: 455–63.

Melzer D, McWilliams B, Brayne C, et al. (2000). Socio-economic status and the expectation of disability in old age: estimates for England. J Epidemiol Community Health 54: 286–92.

Rowe JW, Kahn RL (1997). Successful aging. The Gerontologist 37: 433–40.

Victor CR (2010). Ageing, health and care. Bristol: Policy press.

World Health Organization (2002). Active Ageing: A Policy Framework (http://whqlibdoc.who.int/hq/2002/who_nmh_nph_02.8.pdf).

The global perspective

Population ageing, defined as the percentage of a given population that is 65 years or older, has been developing over many years. However, this demographic change is accelerating at an alarming pace. This will pose significant challenges to the social, health, and economic systems at a national and international level.

Lutz and Sanderson in 2004 stated, 'While the twentieth century was the century of population growth … the twenty-first century … is likely to become the century of population ageing'. The following points support their assertion.

- The global population aged 65 and older was estimated at 506 million in 2008 (7% of the world population). This is projected to increase to 1.3 billion older people by 2040 (14% of the world population).
- The world's older population increased, on average, by 870 000 people per month during 2007–2008. It is projected to expand, in 10 years' time, by an average of 1.9 million per month.
- Currently, Japan has the largest proportion of elderly people, as 27% of its population is 60 years or older. By 2050 this will be true in more than 70 countries.
- Within the next decade, for the first time in history, people aged 65 and over are expected to outnumber children under five.

Trends in population ageing

The shift from high mortality and high fertility rates, typical of rural societies, to the low mortality and low fertility rates of more urban industrial societies has been labelled the 'demographic transition'. Although this transition has occurred later in developing countries, scientists have been surprised by the speed of fertility decline and ageing. It took France more than a century for the population of 65 and older to increase from 7% to 14%, but this is likely to occur within two decades in Brazil and Columbia.

China is a good example of how rapid decline in fertility affects the population ageing. The total fertility rate decreased from six in 1965 to 1.7 by 2002 following strict birth planning policy of one child per family. As a result, the population over 65 is projected to jump from 88 million in 2000 to 199 million in 2025 and to 349 million by 2050.

In 2008, 62% of the worlds people aged 65 and over lived in the developing nations (313 million people). By 2040, this share is expected to exceed 75% (1 billion people).

Europe is still the 'oldest' world region, with the highest population proportion of people aged 65 and over, while sub-Saharan Africa is the 'youngest' region. The HIV/AIDS pandemic has drastically reduced the life expectancy and altered the age structure of the sub-Saharan population. The average life expectancy at birth in South Africa, Zambia, and Zimbabwe is less than 45 years and the proportion of the sub-Saharan population aged 65 and over is only 3% This contrasts sharply with the Western European countries, e.g. UK has a life expectancy of 78.8 years and 16% of the population is aged 65 and over.

The US population is relatively 'young' compared with Europe, with 13% aged 65 and older. However, the baby-boom generation will boost this to 20% by 2030.

In Russia, life expectancy has declined to 65.9 years since the demise of the Soviet Union. This is mainly due to increases in adult male mortality, probably as a result of excess alcohol consumption and suicide.

Globally, life expectancy between males and females differs, owing to the lower mortality of women in every age group and for most causes of death. The average gap between the genders is 7 years and has widened with time. This has important social and economic consequences, as older women are more likely to be widowed and fall into poverty.

Another important theme in global ageing is the rapid proportional increase in the 'oldest old'. The number of those aged over 80 is projected to increase by 233% between 2008 and 2040, compared with 160% for the over 65s and 33% for the total population of all ages. This has economic consequences as the oldest old consume medical resources disproportionate to its overall population size.

Implications of global ageing
Health

The second important global phenomenon is the 'epidemiological transition', where the burden of disease shifts from infectious and nutritional disorders to the chronic, degenerative conditions of coronary heart disease, stroke, cancer, dementia, and visual impairment.

The challenge facing developing countries is allocating limited resources to address chronic diseases and the high prevalence of communicable diseases. Policy-makers need to invest in programmes to address the 'traditional risks' of undernutrition, unsafe sex, unsafe hygiene, and poor sanitation, and also public health education programmes to reduce the modern risks of physical inactivity, obesity, tobacco, and alcohol misuse. The concern is that health services will be overwhelmed by the older population. Currently in the UK National Health Service, 43% of the budget is spent on those aged 65 and over and this group occupies almost two-thirds of general and acute hospital beds.

Studies in the USA show that although the prevalence of chronic diseases is increasing, there has been a decline in disability rates in later life. This is due to improvements in medical care, use of assistive technologies such as wheelchairs and hearing devices and improving education levels. To meet the increased demand for healthcare with limited resources requires innovative policies focused on prevention and early intervention with appropriate use of resources for end-of-life care.

Social

Global ageing coupled with the gender imbalance at old age has implications for marital status and living arrangements. In the 65 and over age group, 60–85% of men are married compared with only 30–40% of women. Research shows that married older people suffer less depression and have lower mortality rates.

Older peoples' living arrangements vary between developing and developed regions. In developed countries, large proportions of old people live alone. In 2007 in Great Britain, 30% of women and 20% of men aged 65 and over lived alone. In developing countries it is traditional for elderly people to live with family, creating multigenerational households. However, this trend is changing in East Asian countries.

The composition of families has changed as a result of prolonged living, increased divorce, remarriage, and single parenthood. The global trend towards fewer children means fewer potential caregivers for older parents. Comparative data have shown that 4–12% of older people live in institutional care in developed countries. Owing to the high costs of institutional care, this is becoming a last resort. The rates of institutional care in Europe have been decreasing as home- and community-based care are increasingly encouraged.

Older people are often valuable contributors to households, providing financial assistance, caring for the young and unwell, and being a crucial source of wisdom and experience. In countries affected by the AIDS/HIV pandemic, older people are often left as the sole caregivers of orphaned grandchildren.

Economic

A major economic challenge of ageing societies is to provide for the needs of frail older people while potentially experiencing a shrinking labour force. The participation in the labour force of the over 65 age group varies from less than 10% in Europe to a third in developing countries. The social security and pension programmes in developed countries allowed the earlier retirement of older workers. Since the 1990s, this downward trend has reversed in developed countries. Data on retirement age trends in developing countries are scarce.

Mandatory pension plans cover more than 90% of the labour force but are limited in developed countries.

The 'pay-as-you-go' pension system funded by payroll taxes has become unsustainable due to the increased ratio of pensioners to contributors. The costs of public pensions is high, with a weighted average of 12.2% of gross domestic product (GDP) in 25 European nations. Therefore, the World Bank has recommended that governments promote defined-contribution pension schemes, personal retirement savings, universal pensions to address extreme poverty, and family support. Families provide the bulk of social support for elderly people, especially in Africa and South Asia. The challenge facing governments of developing countries is to complement this informal support by expanding the formal social security systems given the lack of infrastructure and resources.

Policy-makers need to be proactive and collectively execute changes to socio-economic and health policies in order to meet the challenges of global ageing. Cross-national research into macroeconomics, behaviour, and genetics is vital to explore potential solutions which can help policy-makers.

Further reading

Brainerd E, Cutler D (2005). Autopsy on an empire: understanding mortality in Russia and the former Soviet Union. *J Eco Perspect* **19**: 107–30.

Department of Health (2010). Improving Care and Saving Money. Crown Copyright (www.dh.gov.uk/publication).

Freedman V, Schoeni RF, Martin L, et al. (2007). Chronic conditions and the decline in late life disability. *Demography* **44**:459–77.

Gibson M, Gregory S, Pandya SM (2003). *Long Term Care in Developed Nations*. Washington, AARP Public Policy Institute.

Hungerford T (2001). The economic consequences of widowhood on elderly women in US and Germany. *The Gerontologist* **41**: 103–10.

Kinsella K, He W (2009). *An Aging World: 2008*. International Population Reports. US Census Bureau. Washington, DC, U.S. Government Printing Office.

Kinsella K, Phillips DR (2005). Global aging: the challenge of success. *Population Bulletin* **60**: 1.

Mujahid G, Siddhisena KAP (2009). Demographic prognosis for South Asia: A future of rapid ageing. *Papers in Population Ageing*, no. 6.

Office for National Statistics (2007). General Household Surveyed (www.statistics.gov.uk).

Rochat S, Cumming RG, Blyth F, et al. (2010). Frailty and use of health and community services by community dwelling older men. *Age Ageing* **39**: 228–33.

U.S. Census Bureau, International Data Base (www.census.gov/ipc/www/idbnew.html).

Yang Z, Norton EC, Sterns S (2003). Longevity and health care expenditures. *J Geron* **58**: S2–10.

The history of geriatric medicine

Background

British geriatric medicine arose in the 1940s in parallel with changes in the organization and funding of services for those unable to look after themselves because of sickness, age, or poverty.

The European history of care for the disadvantaged goes back to early Christian teaching on charity with the third-century Greeks establishing separate types of accommodation for the aged, the sick, and helpless poor. Over centuries, Western Europe slowly followed, but tended to accommodate these three categories together in their institutions, which in Britain developed from around 1100 AD.

Poor laws and workhouses

In Britain, monasteries established houses of hospitality for the poor, frail, and sick. The Dissolution of the Monasteries in 1538 disrupted this work until 1601, when the Elizabethan Poor Law was passed making individual parishes responsible for their poor. Further acts were passed over the next 300 years. From 1834 responsibility passed to the new 643 local government bodies or 'unions' that replaced some 15,500 smaller authorities. Even today a Union road or lane serves to remind us of the nearby workhouse of earlier times, perhaps still surviving as a health facility but remembered with fear and suspicion by those who can recall the original function of the building.

The workhouse accommodated those with chronic ill-health, the aged, and the destitute able-bodied. The incapacitated could be bed-bound for the rest of their lives. Two causes of death featured frequently – phthisis (wasting or tuberculosis) and senility (dementia).

The language of the time termed the able-bodied as paupers or fallen women. The able-bodied were granted short stays and worked in the gardens or the laundry. Funding for workhouses came from donations and local charity taxes. Workhouse conditions were harsh, and those with means received care at home from their families and servants.

Author's Tip

Some people may fearfully remember the old workhouse reputation of the local hospital and resist receiving care there.

Geriatric medicine

The term 'geriatrics', meaning healing the old, was coined in 1909 in the USA by Nascher. It was adopted in England by Marjory Warren in 1943 as a result of her work in the 1930s at the West Middlesex County Hospital. She systematically reviewed over 700 people residing in the old workhouse wards. She reached diagnoses, treated the treatable, and launched the attack on the culture of bed rest that had characterized long-term care. Marjory Warren used the term geriatrics to define this new style of practice. The combined approach of active treatment and rehabilitation allowed many to be discharged. Other pioneers made similar achievements. The move away from custodial care and bed rest to active treatment, rehabilitation, and discharge led to the need for acute beds.

In parallel, the start of the Second World War and bombing resulted in the relocation of many thousands. The frail aged were found to manage in seaside hotels and the bed-bound, deemed chronic sick, became the responsibility of the new NHS in 1948.

The Ministry of Health at the time therefore categorized people into the 'infirm,' who were to become the responsibility of the local authority, and the 'sick,' who needed healthcare.

Infirm – and therefore properly the responsibility of the local authority – persons who are normally able to get up and who could attend meals either in the dining room or a nearby day room. This class would include those who need a certain amount of help from the staff with dressing, toilet or moving from room to room and those who from time to time (for example in bad weather) may need to spend a few days in bed.

Sick – and therefore properly the responsibility of the Regional Hospital Board – patients requiring continued medical treatment and also supervision and nursing care. This would include very old people who, though not suffering from any particular disease, are confined to bed on account of extreme weakness.

The Ministry of Health appointed the first consultant geriatricians shortly after 1948 to provide services for this group, a measure also given impetus by the publications of geriatricians of the time.

In 1947 eight of those early pioneers formed The Medical Society for the Care of the Elderly renamed in 1959 the British Geriatrics Society, which by 2010 had over 2500 members.

From workhouse to acute hospital

Initially many geriatricians worked and built their teams in hospitals that had been workhouses. Access to general hospital facilities was limited. Gradually, as new district general hospitals were built, acute geriatric services relocated to the general hospital, leaving rehabilitation and long-stay care in the older buildings.

The transition from workhouse to acute hospital was not free of medical politics. Hostility to geriatricians was shown in publications published by general physicians seeking the abolition of geriatric medicine. Grimley Evans provides an elegant account of the situation.

Service models

Geriatricians, who had established separate services in the workhouse environment, naturally continued their separate teams after moving into the acute hospital. This traditional service model initially involved accepting patients from other acute specialties for long-term care.

The situation mirrored the early experience of Marjory Warren and colleagues because geriatricians who were accepting patients for long stay care realized that different clinical management would have avoided that need. The natural progression was to start accepting patients from the community and controlling their acute care and rehabilitation. Two types of service evolved from about 1970.

Age-related service

This service would run separately and in parallel to the general medical service. The geriatricians would seek to accept patients above a certain age, for example 65, 75, or 80, which varied by location, and when all beds were full the general medical team would admit any further cases. The geriatricians would also accept patients from other acute services and waiting lists for admission.

Integrated service for hospitals

During the late 1970s, doctors increasingly trained and became accredited in geriatric and general medicine to take up appointments as physicians with an interest in older people as part of a general medical team, examples being in Newcastle, Bath, and Oxford. Acute wards and junior medical staff were shared, but the responsibilities for rehabilitation were kept by the geriatrician. Integration of services improved recruitment to the specialty and its perceived status, and this became the dominant model of service in acute hospitals.

Geriatric medicine and community care

The integrated service model has drawn geriatricians more in to sharing the delivery of acute general medicine. The acute medical care of older people with complex needs is thus not always delivered by geriatricians and the reductions in medical bed numbers have reduced the inpatient length of stay. A feature of this model of care and the increasing number of frail older people that it serves has been high readmission rates and 12-month mortality which has caused concern. From the mid-1990s, geriatricians and NHS bodies have responded by devising community geriatrician posts in which the geriatrician is employed by the primary care trust (PCT) and has some acute hospital duties. More recently the concept of interface geriatrics has arisen, in which the PCT and acute trust jointly fund geriatricians who work both at the hospital 'front door' and undertake community duties so that the primary healthcare teams benefit from the specialist skills of the geriatrician.

This latest turn in the evolution of geriatric medicine brings this account to the present day.

Further reading

Conroy S, Ferguson C, Banerjee J (2010). Interface geriatrics: an evidence based solution for frail older people with medical crises. *British Journal of Hospital Med* **71**: 98–101.

Grimley Evans J (1983). Integration of geriatric with general medical services in Newcastle. *Lancet* **i**: 1430–3.

Grimley Evans J (1997). Geriatric Medicine: a brief history. *Br Med J* **315**: 1075–7.

Townsend P (1962). History of the institutional care of the aged. In: (Townsend P, ed.) *The Last Refuge – A Survey of Residential Institutions and Homes for the Aged in England and Wales*. London, Routledge and Keagan Paul, pp. 17–26.

Warren MW (1946). Care of the chronic aged sick. *Lancet* **i**: 841–3.

Acknowledgement

I am grateful to Peter Millard and Michael Denham for their help in this account.

The major influences in geriatric medicine

Introduction

Three different groups, with different but complimentary agendas, challenged the neglect of sick older people in the UK in the mid-twentieth century. The first group, mainly doctors, had two aims: to discover the state of health of older people in hospital and the community, and to reverse the unsatisfactory medical management of the chronic sick. The second group, the Ministry of Health and its successors, had to resolve the problem of 70 000 hospital beds occupied by the chronic sick, which would impede the embryonic NHS. The third group, consisting of philanthropic organizations, wanted to stimulate research into the ageing process. These three components 'kick-started' geriatric medicine.

The medical revolution (a)

Hospital and community surveys

The health of the older people in hospitals was unknown in the early days of the NHS. In the 1940 and 1950s researchers in Birmingham led by Professor Sir Arthur Thomson, Thomas McKeown, and Charles Lowe surveyed regional chronic sick hospitals. They realized the inauguration of the NHS would trigger substantial increases in requests for admission from older patients, which would add to the 14 000 people already on regional medical and surgical waiting lists. They believed older people blocked many local beds but no data existed. Their surveys showed that the vast majority of patients were admitted without adequate preliminary investigation or treatment and the mean duration of stay was nearly 3 years. About half the patients were inappropriately occupying a hospital bed, with many being admitted for purely social reasons. They were often quite mobile and visited local public houses, returning to hospital drunk. Many patients were profoundly apathetic with their only apparent interest being meal times. Thomson was not very optimistic regarding rehabilitation prospects of older infirm inpatients. He concluded that the then current medical dogma that all signs and symptoms must be due to a single disease did not apply to sick older people, because they usually had multiple pathologies each producing its own signs and symptoms. He and his colleagues believed that medical students should be taught about the diseases of old age, that nurse staffing should be increased and ward equipment improved. In spite of these findings, later studies found that fit patients were still being admitted to hospital even though they could have lived in a home without supervision.

A 1960 study of Birmingham chronic sick hospitals by Joseph Sheldon revealed a continued unsatisfactory state of affairs. Old buildings, one of which was nearly 800 years old, were being inappropriately used to nurse older people. Some hospitals had no lifts, nurses had to share toilets with male patients, bedpans were stored for the night in the bath, the same room was used for washing bedpans and domestic crockery, and the mortuary was in the same building as the piggery!

Other researchers in Oxford, Belfast, and Leeds investigated the management of chronic sick patients with mixed physical and psychiatric disease and found significant misplacement of older people in mental and geriatric hospitals, which could be associated with increased mortality. Geriatricians thought they should care for patients with predominantly medical problems, although they might have some mental symptoms, while patients with behavioural disorders should be the prime responsibility of the psychiatrist, although not all psychiatrists agreed. However, there was a general belief that patients with mixed symptoms should have a preliminary assessment in either a special geriatric ward or a joint assessment unit followed by transfer to the appropriate department. Such suggestions worked best where there was trust on each side to take over the care of the patient once the initial mental or physical problem had been sorted out.

The health characteristics of older people in the community were surveyed in England and Wales. A Wolverhampton study by Joseph Sheldon used the ration book register to identify 583 older respondents and found most were still mobile and living at home. The majority of illnesses in the family were managed within its own resources – spouse, children, or neighbours – which could be a heavy burden on younger members of the family. He emphasized the positive contribution made by older people and backed efforts to help them to be independent for as long as possible. Most importantly, he distinguished between 'chronological' age and 'biological' age. Chronological old age officially started when a pension was paid, but biological old age would begin when there was definite limitation of activity, which could be after the age of 70 or even 75 years. Thus a 5- to 10-year age gap could exist between official and natural onset of old age.

An investigation led by William Hobson in Sheffield in 1949–51 examined the state of health and diet of 476 old people. Evidence of previously undiagnosed illness and disability was found but most was of a minor nature. The majority of those surveyed had unrestricted mobility and only a very small proportion were house bound. Many people considered themselves to be fit and this was most marked with married couples. However, one in five of those surveyed were undernourished. The researchers concluded that an adequate well-balanced diet was an important factor in preserving the health of older people. A contemporaneous study commissioned by the Guillebaud Committee also found a beneficial effect of marriage: older people with a living spouse were less likely to be admitted to hospital than those without one.

A seminal study of old people by Peter Townsend in 1958/59 of local authority, private, and voluntary residential homes in England and Wales showed evidence of poor-quality accommodation, some of which was quite unsuitable for residential use, that relationships between residents and care staff were uneven, and the manner with which death was managed within homes and with residents varied widely. The study was repeated in 2005/7 and found many changes. Residents were segregated according to functional ability. They were older, more infirm, and less institutionalized.

The medical revolution (b)

Geriatric medicine

Starting in 1935, a handful of pioneering doctors led by Marjory Warren, Lionel Cosin, Trevor Howell, and Eric Brooke and followed later by Lord Amulree, Norman Exton-Smith, John Agate, Sir Ferguson Anderson, and many others, began the mammoth task of transforming existing medical management of the chronic sick. The problems they faced were medical, social, apathetic attitudes of fellow consultants and management, and non-existent education of medical students regarding the diseases of older people.

- The medical challenges included enormous workloads, many hundreds of inpatients often in widely separated units with few, if any, beds in the main hospital, hundreds of older people on waiting lists for admission, very poor ward accommodation (some still had gas lighting), totally inadequate investigative facilities, and a dearth of medical, paramedical, and secretarial staffs.
- The social obstacles arose from the fact that long-term care of sick older people had become considered a matter for the State. Patients and relatives believed that admission to a chronic sick bed was a 'bed for life', perhaps for as long as 10 or 20 years, and therefore home accommodation was given up. Patients became institutionalized, did not want to go home, and relatives did not want them back. Home support from younger relatives weakened as family size decreased and grown up children went to work. Local social support services were poorly developed and demand far exceeded supply.
- Indifference of local consultants and management committees towards older inpatients could obstruct even minor developments, causing geriatricians to resort to subterfuges to obtain basic improvements such as heating in unheated wards, repairs to leaky roofs, obtaining bed curtains, and even getting basic washing facilities on wards. It took far longer to build new well-designed ward accommodation.

It seems strange in these days to state that the first thing that these pioneers did was to examine their patients and make medical notes, something at odds with then current practice. Investigations and treatments were organized. Very quickly doctors realized that the presentation of illness in older people could be quite different from younger people and in its way more challenging and rewarding. Social factors often complicated discharge. The ethos of admission was changed to medical need and not destitution: a bed was no longer for life.

New approaches to medical services for older people developed according to local conditions:

- Home visits, initially unpaid, were used to assess the urgency for admission of patients on the waiting list. However, as waiting lists disappeared, they were replaced by paid domiciliary visits, made at the request of the general practitioner to provide medical opinion.
- Outpatient departments were increasingly utilized.
- Progressive patient care became widely practised throughout the UK. Patients were admitted first to a treatment ward and then moved to other wards as they improved or required further treatment. The disadvantage was that beds were not always used to maximum efficiency and nursing continuity was lost but, it was argued, it helped patients' morale to be moved as they improved.
- Day hospitals, pioneered by Lionel Cosin, enabled earlier discharge to take place, provided rehabilitation, physical maintenance, follow-up care after discharge from hospital, and allowed minor medical procedures to be undertaken without the need for admission. Their efficiency became much debated with criticism targeting inadequate audit of their function, poor working policies, and insufficient consultant input.

- Self-referral clinics for older people were set up but their value was limited because they were mainly used by those who were well.
- Continuing (long-stay) care, once an integral part of the geriatric service, was largely transferred into the private and voluntary sectors.
- Publications. Increasingly geriatricians published their experiences in major journals. Case studies and statistics of bed usage showed that older patients could be remobilized and discharged, even those who had been confined to bed for many years and 'written off' by general physicians. Only about 10% of patients were ultimately considered long stay. Official data showed that the length of stay steadily decreased, bed turnover increased, and many more patients were admitted, even though the overall bed numbers remained largely unchanged. Geriatric medicine became the fastest growing medical specialty and the UK became the Mecca of geriatric medicine.
- Geriatric subcommittees were set up by the Royal College of Physicians and the British Medical Association, which promoted a fully coordinated geriatric service.
- The Medical Society for the Care of the Elderly (later the British Geriatrics Society) was created to bring together like-minded geriatricians. It published its own journal, Gerontologia Clinica, which was later replaced by Age and Ageing.
- Integration. More recently geriatricians have integrated with general physicians, shared resources with them and taken part in acute medical take.

Geriatricians deemed general practitioners pivotal in the care of older people. They acted as first line of referral when an older person became ill and coordinator of support services. They were encouraged to learn about the management of older people and take the Diploma of Geriatric Medicine of the Royal College of Physicians of London. Unfortunately, older people did not always consult their general practitioner about their symptoms because they felt little could be done for them. Case-finding programmes for untreated disability showed that general practitioners were largely aware of the major disorders affecting older people at home but were less aware of minor problems with sight, hearing, and care of toenails, all of which could impact on quality of life.

An effective social service department was an essential component of a geriatric service, since it provided a range of domiciliary care, such as home helps, meals on wheels, occupational therapy, appliances, residential homes, and day centres, although these services were limited in the early years. Social workers liaised with voluntary organizations such as Age UK, the WRVS, the Red Cross, old people's clubs, and church organizations.

Teaching and academic geriatric medicine

The geriatricians' cri de coeur was the imperative need to improve the teaching of medical students about the ageing process and the diseases of old age. Although attitudes of medical students were initially sympathetic towards sick older people, this changed to indifference on qualification. Factors blamed included the prejudice of universities and medical teachers against geriatric medicine, poor image/role of the geriatrician, and poor working conditions. Geriatricians tackled the problem by using their patients to educate medical students and, hopefully, to instil some enthusiasm for old age in membership candidates.

Multidisciplinary teaching of paramedical and nursing staffs was started. One geriatrician stated bluntly that elderly patients were a mine of interest to an observer with the merest curiosity.

Pioneering geriatricians wrote specialist textbooks: Professor Exton-Smith published *Medical Problems in Old Age* in 1955, while Trevor Howell published *A Student's Guide to Geriatrics* in 1963. Large geriatric medical textbooks began to appear in the 1970s onwards but it was not until the 1980s that chapters on geriatric medicine appeared in general medical textbooks.

Lord Amulree was appointed as geriatrician to University College Hospital in 1949, but this was the first and only London teaching hospital to have such an appointment for many years. The first UK Professor of Geriatric Medicine, Sir Ferguson Anderson, was not appointed until 1965. Further progress was slow but responded to pressure from Sir George Godber, Chief Medical Officer 1961–1973, and Sir Keith Joseph, Secretary of State 1970–1974, who encouraged the foundation of professorial posts (Charing Cross, St George's and University College Hospitals in London, and Birmingham University). Postgraduate research courses were set up leading to the degrees of MSc and PhD. These new professors of geriatric medicine found that in addition to teaching, researching, and fund raising, they had to organize and manage their own units, which made for a very heavy workload. By 1998, almost all the London teaching hospitals had a professorial chair in the speciality, but since then recruitment into academic geriatric medicine has fallen away.

The Ministry of Health

In 1946, the Ministry had 2 years to create the new NHS. It realized that the programme would be seriously impaired by the 70 000 hospital beds occupied by the chronic sick. Previous Ministry annual reports had already shown that basic medical care of older people in hospital, such as the simple matter of classifying patients and creating medical notes, was often woefully deficient. The situation was compounded by the fact that the number and life expectancy of older people was increasing and would continue to do so, which would further increase pressure on health services. More effective use of existing beds, improved medical care of sick older people, and improvements in community services were therefore essential.

- The Ministry set the ball rolling with a presentation by two of their doctors, one of whom was Lord Amulree, to the Parliamentary Medical Committee in 1947. This stated that the vast majority of the chronic sick were older people who were inadequately classified. Priority for admission was generally given to the acutely ill patient at the expense of the older patient, who was feared as a potential 'bed blocker'. Hospital beds were inappropriately occupied by four groups of patients: by those with diseases which had become chronic because they had not been treated soon enough; those with disabilities who could not be sent home; those admitted with preventable diseases; and those who could go home but had no home to return to.
- General physicians were encouraged to treat the chronic sick but failed to do so. Another initiative was for geriatricians to create training centres where physicians could be shown how to treat and remobilize older people. This also was unsuccessful. These failures convinced the Ministry that a speciality of geriatric medicine was required.

- It organized surveys, supported pioneering geriatric medicine physicians, encouraged recruitment, persuaded health authorities to create more geriatric units and consultant posts in the main hospital, promoted modern management of sick older people, organized conferences and seminars on effective geriatric medicine, improved ward design, and stimulated research. By 1988, there were 476 consultant geriatricians, although this was well short of the 750 considered necessary.
- It considered modern geriatric medicine was effective and the number of existing geriatric beds was sufficient provided they were used efficiently.
- The Hospital (later Health) Advisory Service was created by the Secretary of State to act as his 'eyes and ears' regarding care services for older people in hospital and the community.
- Community services were supported. Case finding, screening of older people, and prevention programmes were encouraged. Community accommodation increased but arguments raged about who should pay residential/nursing home costs. Healthcare such nursing was free, but social care, such as help with washing, dressing, and feeding, was means tested. Those with above-threshold savings had to contribute to their support and felt penalized for saving for their old age.
- Although some political heads of the Ministry/Department of Heath were sympathetic towards older people, new political administrations tended to be more concerned about health service costs and introduced almost yearly reorganizations and centralization, which, while giving the appearance of progress, did little to help the development of care services for the older person. Policy makers shied away from specifying targets for the care of older people for fear of being held accountable for failures, and at the same time denied rationing of healthcare. Many policies were considered by commentators to be little more than statements of good intent. An attempt to create a Minister for the Elderly was foiled by lack of government support. Lord Amulree came to believe that bureaucrats should, if possible, be kept away from care of older people.
- London was chosen as the centre for the 1982 World Health Day (7 April) with the theme of 'Adding Life to Years'.

Voluntary and charitable organizations

Philanthropic institutions appreciated that the ageing process and the diseases of old age were ill understood and therefore supported appropriate research.

- In 1943 Viscount Nuffield founded the Nuffield Foundation, one of whose objectives was the care of the aged and poor, and set up the National Corporation for the Care of Old People (later the Centre for the Policy on Ageing), whose chairman was Seebohm Rowntree. The Foundation created a Research Committee, which gave grants to geriatricians and gerontologists.
- The Nuffield supported Vladimir Korenchevsky, a Russian biologist and a student of Pavlov, who became director of the Oxford Gerontological Institute.
- The Ciba Foundation helped to found the International Association of Gerontology, which held its first meeting in 1950 in Liege, Belgium, while its third World Congress was held in London in 1954. Those attending were welcomed by Iain Macleod, Minister for Health, and Joseph Sheldon gave the opening address. The first meeting of

its clinical section was organized by Dr Lyn Woodford-Williams in Sunderland in 1958 and another was organized by Professor John Brocklehurst in Manchester in 1974. The Ciba Foundation established special colloquia on ageing in London, which were attended by many international experts. The King Edward's Hospital Fund supported research into aspects of ageing.

Failures

Despite the major advances in medicine and social care and the influence of powerful personalities and organizations, many core issues remain unresolved to this day.

Age discrimination continues almost unchecked in spite of efforts to reverse this bias. Quality of care has been questioned, older people are not always nursed with due dignity, services are poorly integrated, and those most in need of care are least able to access it.

Clearly defined objectives for a health service for older people have not been established. No NHS staff college has been created which could focus on such issues and the function of a modern hospital service. Whenever financial cuts in health services are required, care for older people is an early target.

Many geriatricians of an earlier generation worry that the loss of continuing care from the NHS will lead to a rediscovering of the conditions found by Marjory Warren in the 1930s.

Further reading

Boucher CA (1957). *Survey of Services Available to the Chronic Sick and Elderly 1954-1955*. Ministry of Health: Reports on Public Health and Medical Subjects No 98.

Denham MJ (2006). The Surveys of Birmingham 'Chronic Sick' Hospitals 1948-1961. *Social History of Medicine* **19**: 279–93.

Department of Health (1991). *On the State for the Public Health for the Year 1990*. London, HMSO, pp. 68–95.

Sheldon JH (1948). *The Social Medicine of Old Age*. London, Oxford University Press.

Townsend P (1962). *The Last Refuge*. London, Routledge and Paul Kegan.

Warren MW (1948). The evolution of a geriatric unit. *Geriatrics* 3: 42–50.

What makes geriatric medicine different?

Background

Old age is characterized by enormous heterogeneity of health and function. It is sometimes suggested that it is suboptimal, even ageist, for the older person with a given condition not to be treated by the same 'organologist' as the younger person. This argument may have some validity for those older people who are physically and mentally vigorous and present with a single acute condition. However, there are a number of reasons why a special set of skills and attitudes is often important when dealing with sick older people, although much of the need for these skills is based on complexity rather than on age *per se*:

• physiological decline and difficulty distinguishing the effects of ageing and disease
• increased frequency of multiple physical illnesses and of polypharmacy
• increased relevance of functional ability and multidisciplinary assessment
• greater difficulty in history taking
• atypical presentations of illnesses
• importance of ethical issues, including capacity, especially at the end of life and in those with dementia.

Importance of attitudes to ageing

Ageing is particularly prone to stereotyping and labelling – by healthcare professionals, by the general public, and by older people themselves. Although age limits on access to treatments are less common, there remains a tendency to presume that problems in older people are an inevitable and chronic consequence of age rather than looking for remediable factors. The pejorative labels used for older people in emergency departments and the particular weariness and apathy many clinicians feel when dealing with an older patient with dementia or from a nursing home (or worse, both) stem from these same attitudes. Older people themselves may fail to mention or downplay ('what can you expect at my age') symptoms they attribute to old age. Positive stereotypes may seem less objectionable but are just as distorting. For some people ageing may lead to serenity, wisdom, and an excellent sex life; many will be less fortunate. Ultimately, nobody ever died of good health and most will have to deal with loss of spouses and siblings as well as with the effects of physical and perhaps cognitive decline.

Decline with age: normal or abnormal?

Ageing inevitably leads to decline in the physiological functions of most systems of the body. Decreased reserve leads to increased vulnerability to disease and often functional decline. There is, however, enormous individual variation in the degree and rate of decline. Some of this is determined by genetic factors, but there is increasing evidence that potentially modifiable environmental factors operating throughout life have a significant impact on the effects of ageing. In particular, the 'disuse syndrome' of increased cardiovascular disease, obesity, fall risk, and muscle weakness produced by a sedentary lifestyle and physical immobility is associated with accelerated ageing. The positive effects of exercise (even in advanced old age, although the earlier the better) support the age-old mantra of geriatricians to 'use it or lose it'.

Presentation of acute illness in older people

The 'giants of geriatrics' – delirium (acute confusion), falls, immobility, and incontinence – are common presentations of conditions such as pneumonia, myocardial infarction, or heart failure. These syndromes share a number of important characteristics.

• They are multifactorial in origin, with an inverse relationship between the baseline vulnerability of the individual and the severity of the acute insult needed to trigger onset of the syndrome.
• They share the risk factors of age, polypharmacy, severity of illness, multiple systems impairments, and functional or cognitive impairment.
• They are associated with poor outcomes, including dependence, admission to long-term care, and death, and patients who present with the geriatric syndromes do worse in general than those with classical presentations of the same underlying illness.
• They require multifaceted rather than simple interventions.

History taking in older people

The interview is the most informative part of the clinical encounter. However, taking an adequate history from an older person may be time-consuming for both clinician and patient. The reasons include

• communication problems (e.g. cognitive problems, deafness, aphasia)
• underreporting of illness
• multiple complaints and pathologies and complex multidrug regimens
• need to clarify terms (e.g. constipation, dizziness)
• possible unreliability of patient story
• presence of family/carers at interview.

A 'poor historian' or someone who seems 'vague' or 'uncooperative' may not hear what the doctor is asking or may not understand what is being asked. But the label of 'poor historian' is perhaps best applied to the doctor relating the history, who has not recognized the barriers to communication and sought an alternative source to elucidate the story. Causes of incomprehension include cognitive impairment, deafness, aphasia, and depression. Those with an extensive history of multiple medical conditions may have difficulty in recalling all details in an organized manner. Maintaining a problem list, mapping the chronology of each complaint and of the response to treatment, and asking the patient to highlight the most significant current problem are often helpful. Clarifying what the patient means is important when they use medical terms or report on previous consultations or diagnoses.

Family members often accompany the older person on a visit to the doctors. This may be helpful, especially when there is a possibility that the patient's story may be unreliable, but there is the potential for the family member's perspective and preferences to dominate the conversation, and there are times where the patient's and the family's interests are divergent. It is important that the patient's privacy is respected and that the degree to which the family are involved in the interview is negotiated with the patient. The clinician should always have even a brief period alone with the patient to ascertain his or her preferences in this regard and to allow discussion on topics such as abuse and incontinence.

Functional status

An essential part of the assessment of older people is to establish how the patient is functioning and how their level of function has changed. Assessing functional status helps to define the impact of illness on the older person's life, and a recent decline in the ability to walk or to self-care is as good a predictor of outcome as age or traditional measures of illness severity. Comprehensive multidisciplinary assessment, with use of standardized assessment tools to facilitate documentation of dependency and communication with other professionals, is the best approach to the complexity of issues facing older people. A helpful practical approach when time is limited is to ask the patient to take you through a typical day – how they get out of bed, dress, what they have for breakfast, and so on. From here, one should then assess how this may have changed as a result of recent illness.

Ethical issues

The need to grapple with ethical problems is a common and demanding feature of caring for older people. Ethical issues are particularly common in those approaching the end of life. In this group, the aphorism that the doctor's role is 'to cure sometimes, to relieve often, to comfort always' is particularly apt in geriatric medicine, and adequate knowledge of the skills and attitudes of palliative medicine is essential for geriatricians.

One common approach to thinking about ethical problems to consider the key ethical principles of: autonomy (what does the patient want?); beneficence (what can be done to help the patient?); maleficence (are there risks associated with a proposed treatment?); and justice (is the proposed treatment fair to the patient and to all other patients?). While this can be a useful starting point, it may give rise to the illusion that a simplistic cook-book approach (a generous helping of autonomy, a sprinkling of beneficence, etc.) will suffice in making ethical decisions. All relevant details of the individual case and circumstances should be sought, considered, and documented before reaching a decision, and adequate time should be allowed for discussions and to give people a chance to consider often complex information.

A transition from a culture of medical paternalism—the view that doctor knows best—to one where respect for patient autonomy is paramount has occurred in Western countries in recent decades. Difficulties may arise when different generations of doctors and patients have assimilated this change to different degrees. Patients' views of what constitutes an important benefit or harm may not be the same as that of their doctors. There is no evidence that older people are less likely than younger people to want their preferences listened to, although they may be less assertive in making this clear. The competent patient has the right to refuse any treatment however beneficial. Hence, consideration of competence and mental capacity is often important in considering the weight to give patients' views. This is particularly important in dealing with older people when there is an increased prevalence of cognitive impairment.

Further reading

Barton A, Mulley G (2003). History of the development of geriatric medicine in the UK. *Postgrad Med J* **79**: 229–34.

Gillon R (1994). Medical ethics: four principles plus attention to scope. *Br Med J* **309**: 184–8.

Grimley Evans J (1997). Geriatric medicine: a brief history. *Br Med J* **315**: 1075–8.

Harris J (2003). In praise of unprincipled ethics. *J Med Ethics* **29**: 303–6.

Powel C (2007). Whither geriatrics? Do we need another Marjory Warren? *Age Ageing* **36**: 607–10.

Rockwood K (2004). Frailty and the geriatrician. *Age Ageing* **33**: 429–30.

Young JB, Philp I (2000). Future directions for geriatric medicine. *Br Med J* **320**: 133–4.

The concept of frailty

Heterogeneity of risk in relation to age

Anyone who has attended a 25-year class reunion will be struck by how people who have lived the same number of years appear to age at very different rates. Genetically identical animals that have been raised in the same environments show evident age-related differences in grooming, greying, and motor performance. Even simple machines that are produced on the same day show variable times to failure.

Variability in human ageing has long been of interest. In the 1950s, a 'longevity factor' was introduced as a random effect term in an equation summarizing mortality in relation to age. It was seen as a consistent characteristic of an individual, such that for those with a low value, the rate of ageing – the chance of dying – will increase only slowly compared with people with a high longevity factor value. Likewise, in 1979 mathematical demographers defined 'frailty' as a random effect which was constant for a particular individual. They saw that the average chance of dying (the population hazard rate) was typically less than the mortality hazard rate for a reference individual. They demonstrated that the relative increase in the hazard rate for a reference individual compared with the population hazard rate reflects variability in the intrinsic ageing rate. People who are long-lived make up a larger proportion of the population over time, as relatively frailer ones died off. Note that these analysts defined frailty as a random effect which is constant for a particular individual, and which remains so even though the risk of dying increases with age.

Heterogeneity of ageing rates is also of interest in gerontology, but geriatricians conceptualize frailty as vulnerability at the individual level, which increases over time. This reflects our motivation to understand individual vulnerability to adverse health outcomes. This motivation extends beyond simple mortality prediction, which is reflected in a bias against risk models that are rooted in age. In geriatric medicine, frailty can usefully be thought of as a method of explaining the differential vulnerability to adverse outcomes of (predominantly older) people of the same chronological age.

The practical application of the concept of frailty

In contrast to the conceptualization of frailty as a multiply-determined, graded vulnerability state that represents loss of physiological reserve, which is largely non-controversial, how best to operationalize frailty still can raise the ire of partisans on the various sides of the issue. Given that any broad classification will sacrifice concision for precision, two broad camps are discernible: the frailty phenotype, which focuses more on the nature of what frail people look like, and the Frailty Index, which focuses more on the nature of the risk. By way of disclosure, my group is squarely in the second camp.

The frailty phenotype

Frail older adults can share many features, which have been summarized in a classical account as a frailty phenotype, which can operationalize the syndrome. Five characteristics are specified – slowness, weight loss, impaired strength, exhaustion, and low physical activity/energy expenditure. Any person with three of these five characteristics is said to be frail, whereas those who have only one or two are 'pre-frail'. People with none of the characteristics are said to be 'robust'. The presence of an identifiable phenotype has spurred research on frailty, which has validated the tripartite distinction. A large number of studies, by several dozen groups, have shown that risk increases between these three grades of robust, pre-frail, and frail.

Despite the widespread research facilitated by the frailty phenotype, it has been criticized for misclassification in relation to clinical judgement – chiefly classifying as not frail people who would clinically be recognized as frail. Most critics argue for considering more than just the five features, specifically calling for adding information about subjective perception of health status, cognitive performance, sensory or physical impairments, current health status needs, or appearance (as consistent, or not, with age). On the other hand, some critics suggest that five items is too many, and propose that single items, such as slow mobility or poor grip strength, might do as well. Interestingly, neither slow mobility nor poor grip strength is included in a three-item frailty measure that consists of weight loss, inability to rise from a chair, and low energy) and that apparently classifies risk as well as the five-item phenotypic definition.

The frailty index

Frail older adults typically also have many things wrong with them. The Frailty Index proposes that the more things people have wrong with them, then the greater their risk of adverse health outcomes, or the frailer they will be. The frailty index was developed from existing biomedical databases, so typically counts a large number of health deficits (40 or more) as are commonly found in health surveys. For this it has been criticized as impractical. Even so, the number of deficits in a Comprehensive Geriatric Assessment (CGA) is typically large. To calculate the Frailty Index score for a given individual, the number of deficits that they have is divided by the total number of deficits considered. For example, in a typical CGA that assayed 50 potential deficits, a person in whom 25 were present would have a Frailty Index of 25/50 = 0.50. This is a very high score, as the maximum observed value of the Frailty Index is about 0.7, no matter how the Frailty Index is constructed (i.e. regardless of which deficits or which number of deficits were considered, or whether the sample was community or institution or hospital based).

Only about a dozen independent groups have cross-validated the Frailty Index, but they have found that the typical increase with age is about 0.03% per year, that it shows a submaximal limit and is highly correlated with mortality. Change in the Frailty Index can be modelled stochastically, and the output conforms to a Poisson distribution. In general, deficits accumulate slowly, but at all levels of deficits – i.e. at virtually all health states – improvement is possible. The clinical usefulness of the limit to deficit accumulation has yet to be tested. There have been few independent head-to-head comparisons of ability of the Frailty Index versus the frailty phenotype to predict vulnerability to adverse outcomes. This particularly needs to be done in clinical samples.

Frailty and complexity: clinical consequences

It is useful to recognize – indeed to celebrate – the complexity of frailty, from which many clinical consequences arise. Thinking of frail elderly patients as complex systems that are close to failure reveals the common sense of geriatric medicine in a new light.

Comprehensive geriatric assessment

Frailty appears to be a multiply determined state, and patients who are frail typically have many things wrong with them. This is recognized in the major intervention of geriatricians, which is the Comprehensive Geriatric Assessment (CGA), a multifactorial evaluation of function, comorbidity, social factors, and medications. The CGA gives rise to an action plan, which allows patient-centred prioritization of how their problems will be addressed. Typically, the focus will be on solving problems that improve cognition, function, mobility, and social interactions, and those that relieve caregiver burden. This is in contrast to more narrowly focused, 'one-thing-wrong-at-once' medical care, which commonly keys on procedures or interventions that can often seem provider-based, and less evidently measure the impact on cognition, function, mobility, social interaction, pain, and mortality risk.

> **Author's Tip**
>
> The rationale for Comprehensive Geriatric Assessment is to get to grips with what a patient has wrong with them, to prognosticate and to set easily communicated goals in an action plan. It is not to develop a long problem list for its own sake.

Atypical disease presentation

Thinking again about frail older adults as complex systems on the verge of failure, it is worth recognizing that any complex system, when it fails, will fail in its highest order functions first. In consequence, the so-called 'geriatric giants' such as instability/impaired balance and impaired function can be seen as a failure of the high order functions of, respectively, upright bipedal ambulation, and apposable thumbs.

> **Author's Tip**
>
> When frail elderly patents are very ill, they move less, even in bed. As they get better, they move more. Systematically tracking mobility and balance can give insight into acute changes in their overall state of health.

Interdisciplinary care

Given the complexity of need of frail older adults, it is easy to see why their care will need to involve a wide range of expertise. There is a considerable challenge in achieving the teamwork needed to make this care integrated and not fragmented. That all teams do not achieve integrated care may help explain why controlled clinical trials can have variable results, but, as yet, the evidence about what makes a team work particularly well or particularly badly is sparse.

> **Author's Tip**
>
> For multidisciplinary teams to achieve more good than harm, they must practice interdisciplinarity: speak a common, accessible language; stay on time; focus on patient outcomes, not team member inputs; leave personality conflicts outside; eschew passive–aggressive behaviour; be risk tolerant.

Medical decision-making

Complex systems have certain rules, of which the most important is that it is not possible for a single intervention to have a single outcome. In consequence, it is important to minimize the anticipated and unanticipated adverse outcomes of any intervention. In prescribing, for example, this is why it makes sense to 'start low and go slow'.

> **Author's Tip**
>
> Evidence produced for patients with single system disorders might not generalize to frail patients: what is good cardiology (e.g. starting five new medications at high doses after a ST segment elevation myocardial infarction) would be bad geriatrics (e.g. introducing more than one medication at once; introducing medications whose adverse effects can be synergistic, not starting low, going slow).

Key issues

Interventions with frail older adults are likely to have both intended and unintended consequences. Unintended consequences can still be anticipated, and mitigated through actions such as:

- only introducing one intervention at a time
- starting low, going slow
- checking with the patient, family and care staff for unintended consequences.

When frail older adults fail, they will fail in their highest order functions first. This accounts for the tendency to fall, become dependent in activities of daily living, become delirious, take to bed, and suffer from social abandonment.

Further reading

Beard RE (1971). Some aspects of theories of mortality cause of death analysis, forecasting and stochastic processes. In (Brass W ed.) *Biological Aspects of Demography.* London, Taylor & Francis, pp. 557–68.

Beswick AD, Rees K, Dieppe P, *et al.* (2008). Complex interventions to improve physical function and maintain independent living in elderly people: a systematic review and meta-analysis. *Lancet* **371**: 725–35.

Fried LP, Tangen CM, Walston J, *et al.* (2001). Frailty in older adults: evidence for a phenotype. *J Gerontol A Biol Sci Med Sci* **56**: M146–56.

Kulminski AM, Ukraintseva SV, Kulminskaya IV, *et al.* (2008). Cumulative deficits better characterize susceptibility to death in elderly people than phenotypic frailty: lessons from the Cardiovascular Health Study. *J Am Geriatr Soc* **56**: 898–903.

Ling CH, Taekema D, de Craen AJ, *et al.* (2010). Handgrip strength and mortality in the oldest old population: the Leiden 85-plus study. *Can Med Assoc J* **182**: 429–35.

Rockwood K, Mitnitski A (2007). Frailty and the mathematics of deficit accumulation. *Rev Clin Gerontol* **17**: 1–12.

Rockwood K, Rockwood MR, Mitnitski A (2010). Physiological redundancy in older adults in relation to the change with age in the slope of a frailty index. *J Am Geriatr Soc* **58**: 318–23.

Evidence-based medicine for older people

What is evidence-based medicine?

In the 1990s evidence-based medicine as a concept began to take hold and grab people's attention. Prior to this period, clinical practice was very individualized indeed, with clinicians left to practise according to their own experience and the teachings they had been exposed to, which may have included up-to-date journal reading and attendance at teaching events. The treatment a patient received would be subject to much variation depending on the individual clinician's learning. 'Gold standard' evidence existed, in the form of randomized controlled trials and systematic reviews, but the results were not widely known, and even less widely adopted into practice. Evidence-based medicine was intended to push clinicians towards practising medicine using the best available evidence to inform their decisions, along with their clinical judgement. If the best available evidence were collated and analysed and subsequently summarized and distributed to the clinical population, less variation in practice would occur and overall patient care would be enhanced. It was never intended to replace clinical expertise and judgement, or turn clinicians into automatons merely following a set of rigid instructions. To begin with, it was received by some as having precisely that intention. Evidence-based medicine has also been accused of being a tool to cut costs for the health service. Time has shown that evidence-based practice is here to stay and is indeed a good thing, helping doctors to make safe and sensible clinical decisions backed up by clinical evidence.

However, it is not without valid criticism, particularly regarding the ways evidence-based medicine is collated and applied to groups of patients for whom it may not be truly applicable to, such as older patients.

Clinical practice guidelines

The Health Act 1999 in the UK brought with it the concept of clinical governance, aimed at attaining excellence and standardization across the NHS. This was an ambitious and creditable goal. Inconsistent and non-standardized practice across the NHS provided patients with less than ideal care and was wasteful and unsafe. Clinical practice guidelines existed in a small way prior to this point, mainly as local guidelines for emergencies or to help learn procedures, but the creation of the National Institute for Health and Clinical Excellence (NICE) changed this. It was set up as a Special Health Authority and was accountable to the Secretary of State for Health in the government. Its intention is to design and distribute best clinical practice guidelines using the best available evidence and the best experts to construct them. There are now other bodies in the UK that perform a similar function, such as The Scottish Intercollegiate Guidelines Network (SIGN) and the Clinical Resource and Efficiency Support Team (CREST), based in Northern Ireland.

Doctors will always be able to access the latest randomized control trials or systematic reviews of the evidence related to their specialty or clinical decisions, and clinical practice guidelines do not replace these. The primary aim of clinical practice guidelines is to review the available evidence, weigh the outcomes, and make a number of recommendations to clinicians to inform their practice.

If standardized excellent care is what we want to see, having these bodies representing Scotland, Northern Ireland, and the UK as a whole should be sufficient.

However, we continue to see various other bodies produce their own clinical practice guidelines covering the same diagnoses as NICE, with differing recommendations. These can include Royal College guidelines, local hospital guidelines, and guidelines from European specialty societies. One single medical condition may have several UK and European guidelines applicable to it. Rather than inform the clinician, it may only serve to confuse.

Guideline generation and variation

All guideline development bodies have access to the same evidence. One might be forgiven for thinking, therefore, that the recommendations would all be the same. This is not the case. Each guideline development body selects a development panel, with people of many differing levels of knowledge, experience, and personal views coming to the table. How do the recommendations come about? There may be many hundreds of papers to read and analyse for each guideline, does each panellist read each paper and come to a conclusion? Once all the papers are read, how are the final recommendations chosen? You could be forgiven for thinking that the strength of individual personalities could play a part in the decision-making process. Personal views regarding the interpretation of the evidence may also come into play.

An example of the variation seen between different clinical practice guidelines occurs with the very common condition of hypertension. Since 2000, four national and international bodies have published guidelines for the management of hypertension. The SIGN 2001 guidelines still stand as their official guidelines. The European Hypertension Society (EHS) published guidelines in 2003, and revised them in 2007, and most recently in 2009. The British Hypertension Society (BHS) published Guidelines in 2004, the same year as NICE published their hypertension guidelines. All four of these guidelines had the same evidence to make their recommendations, yet the recommendations were all different, including the two guidelines published in the same year. In 2006 NICE and BHS came together and produced a combined set of recommendations. This leaves us with the EHS, SIGN, and NICE/BHS guidance to choose from currently. Which do we use? How can SIGN feel no new evidence has emerged to alter their guidance since 2001, yet EHS have altered theirs twice since 2003, and NICE/BHS altered theirs once in that time?

Guideline panels

Clinical practice guidelines tend to follow a standard structure. This will include a statement about the disease to which the guideline applies, followed by stated aims and objectives. The method assessing the levels of evidence will be stated, and then follows the guideline recommendations, in summary form and then in more detail subsequently. The appendices will include the list of panel members and the list of evidence used. There is a great deal of variation between guidelines as to the number and nature of these panel members, even within NICE guidelines alone. Some will have over 20, some fewer than 10. There will be medical and non-medical panellists. Very few have a geriatrician represented on the panels, the NICE Atrial Fibrillation guidelines 2006, being a rare exception. Levels of evidence are assigned to each recommendation using differing methodologies. In the main, systematic reviews and meta-analyses are at the top, and guideline development group opinion at the bottom, often called good practice points (GPPs). It is surprising how many GPPs there are in most NICE guidelines. The NICE Atrial Fibrillation guidelines 2006 have 114 actual recommendations, of which 61 have graded evidence to back them up, and 53 are good practice points decided by the development panel. These are group opinions that are expected to be applied to the older population of patients, as evidence-based medicine practice.

It is also true, however, that much of the reason for all the opinion in clinical practice guidelines, labelled as good practice points, is that there is not enough evidence available to make substantial decisions. The formation of these clinical practice guidelines highlights this repeatedly and uses it as a call to encourage more research to help clarify these areas of difference. It may also be one reason so many guidelines from different bodies have contradictory recommendations.

Guidelines and older people

Clinical practice guidelines are in the main intended to be applicable to all ages, young and old, in order to be non-discriminatory. However, older people are different, carrying with them often multiple comorbidities and frailties. Clinical practice guidelines are often disease specific, yet older people may be living with as many as eight or nine comorbidities. Can we reasonably be expected to apply nine clinical practice guideline recommendations to a single older individual? Would the consequences be beneficial or harmful to that older individual?

If one looks at a typical fully published clinical practice guideline, the references will contain the full list of the studies used to form the guidance. It is not clear, unless each study is analysed in detail, what proportion will have included a reasonable number of older patients in the numbers. It is commonplace still for older patients to be excluded from randomized controlled studies and other research, either directly because of their age, or indirectly because of the high level of comorbidity present in the older patient population. For evidence-based medicine to be useful for geriatricians, we need to know the guidelines we use can be fairly applied to frail older people, and provide the very best standard of healthcare, otherwise adherence to them may result in more harm than benefit.

The external validity of clinical trial evidence is a controversial area of discussion. It is accepted that randomized controlled trials are conducted under very restricted and controlled conditions, and the results obtained may not be observed when any medicine passes into everyday general use. For older patients this can be particularly true. Deciding how to apply the best available evidence to this population can be difficult. An example is the major carotid endarterectomy study (ECST). All the patients enrolled were shown to have the same baseline characteristics, yet some of those randomized to surgery were deemed not fit enough by the surgeon. When these patients were compared with those randomized to no surgery, their outcome was worse. What is not seen on the baseline characteristics that separated these two groups? Randomized control trials find hard to adequately define 'frailty', making their results less externally valid.

Application of guidelines to older people

Frail older patients are some of the most vulnerable members of our society. As we continue to live longer lives, all the while accumulating chronic disease and comorbidity, we will increasingly need the help of the medical profession. Evidence-based medicine can now be applied to older people via judicious use of clinical practice guidelines for all their illnesses. Should we be expected to rigidly stick to these guidelines, or at least have good clinical reason to fail to use them? An older patient with eight or nine comorbid illnesses could find their lives altered significantly by the application of clinical practice guidelines. Medication prescribed would be evidence based, leading to multiple treatments for cardiac, chest, musculoskeletal, neurological, endocrine, and gastroenterological conditions, all from different guidelines. None of these guidelines will take into account the presence of the others. Medication interactions are very possible, even probable, with direct clashes likely, such as dyspepsia guidelines advocating stopping the antiplatelet therapy required for cardiac secondary prevention. Compliance with the many different tablets, liquids, inhalers, injections, and sprays will be an increasing problem as older people try to manage their ever-increasingly complex regimens without mistakes. Older patients will find themselves expected to attend multiple clinic appointments to assess and monitor their comorbidities, and then referred for tests recommended by the guidelines to quantify and measure these illnesses and plan their treatments.

Lifestyle changes are integral parts of all clinical practice guidelines, with older people expected to alter their diets in different ways, depending on whether they have diabetes, renal disease, cardiac disease, or gastroenterological disease, when in fact, they may have all four diseases.

The geriatric medicine specialty is ideally placed to sift through the many clinical practice guidelines, and apply them sensibly, to frail, older people. Our aim must be to maintain optimum health, with adherence to clinical practice guidelines, balanced by awareness of the many limitations of guidelines, and the older patients' individual desire for quality of life as well as quantity of life.

Geriatric guidelines

In recent years recognition for clinical practice guidelines tailored specifically for older patients has emerged. Leading this are the British Geriatrics Society and the American Geriatric Society. Between them they have published eight guidelines so far, including delirium, falls, and pain management in older people. The British Geriatrics Society has also published many good practice guides covering governance issues in older people's care.

Further reading

American Geriatrics Society
http://americangeriatrics.org
British Geriatrics Society
http://www.bgs.org/index.php
National Institute for Health and Clinical Excellence
http://www.nice.org.uk
Scottish Intercollegiate Guidelines Network
http://www.sign.ac.uk

Comprehensive geriatric assessment

Assessment of physical activity

Assessment of physical activity is an essential element of a comprehensive geriatric assessment. The aims of assessment of physical activity include:

- understanding the physical context and impact of the patients illness
- developing an understanding of the nature and importance of specific physical activities in the patient's life
- identifying needs for physical therapy and social support.

Older people often have more than one health problem. Some will need active treatment, others will need observation or palliation. Assessment of physical functioning can help to identify what it is that a patient finds difficult about their illness and can therefore be useful when considering how to maximize the return following medical treatment.

Assessment procedures and standardized clinical assessment tools

Any scheme for the assessment of physical activity for older patients needs to be able to cover the spectrum of functional health states that may be encountered in clinical practice. These can be highly dependent states, such as are commonly found among residents in nursing and residential care home settings, through to states of extreme independence and autonomy, such as the unaided use of public transport systems, including (for example) international travel, and participation in sporting activities.

It is not surprising that there is no standardized procedure or measuring instrument that can cover all of the aims of the assessment of physical activity and all of the physical states that need to be assessed and measured. However, three simple classes of activity which can be easily assessed, which cover most of the spectrum are:

- personal activities of daily living
- instrumental (or extended) activities of daily living
- life space.

Personal activities of daily living

These include all the things we all have to do to ensure we are ready to greet the day, such as getting in and out of bed, on and off a chair (transferring), walking on the flat or up and down stairs, using the bath, shower, and toilet, getting dressed and undressed, and being able to feed oneself.

All of these activities can be performed independently, with the help of an aid or appliance, with the help of another person, or with the help of more than one person. Assessment and measuring tools are available to help structure and quantify the extent of difficulty (or disability) in personal activities of daily living such as the Barthel index.

Alternatively, if a formal clinical instrument or measuring scale is not available, the assessor can structure an assessment by thinking through their own day, from waking up in the morning and getting out of bed to leaving the house or flat by the front door.

Instrumental (or extended) activities of daily living

These include more complex activities that are necessary for daily life, but often include interaction with tools (or instruments), or external services or agencies. Examples include doing the washing, ironing, and cleaning; visiting the shops and buying groceries or other items; preparing food for consumption; using public transport; managing financial affairs; visiting friends or relatives.

The production of simple clinical instruments to provide a measure of these activities is more complex as many of the activities that we do or are unable to do may be culturally defined in some way. A simple example of this is that older men tend to score worse on assessments that include household tasks including food preparation in cultures where these have traditionally been seen as female roles. It is therefore necessary to tailor an assessment of extended daily living activities to take account of the subject's specific personal and cultural characteristics and circumstances.

One assessment instrument that has been designed and used successfully in rehabilitation studies as an outcome measure is the Nottingham Extended Activities of Daily Living (or NEADL) scale, which divides extended daily activities and tasks into Mobility, Kitchen, Domestic, and Leisure activities (see Table 2.1).

Alternatively, if a formal clinical instrument or measuring scale is not available, the assessor can structure and

Table 2.1 The Nottingham Extended Activities of Daily Living Scale

For each individual item, scoring is as follows:

0 = Not at all

1 = With help

2 = Alone with difficulty

3 = Alone easily

MOBILITY Do you...

- walk around outside?
- climb stairs?
- get in and out of the car?
- walk over uneven ground?
- cross roads?
- travel on public transport?

KITCHEN. Do you...

- manage to feed yourself?
- make yourself a hot drink?
- take hot drinks from one room to another?
- do the washing up?
- make yourself a hot snack?

DOMESTIC. Do you...

- manage your own money when out?
- wash small items of clothing?
- do your own shopping?
- do a full clothes wash?

LEISURE. Do you...

- read newspapers and books?
- use the telephone?
- write letters?
- go out socially?
- manage your own garden?
- drive a car?

Nouri F, Lincoln NB (1987). An extended activities of daily living scale for stroke patients. *Clin Rehab* **1**: 233-8. http://www.nottingham.ac.uk/iwho/documents/neadl.pdf

assessment by thinking through their own daily life and leisure activities, to provide prompts to ask about shopping and cooking, washing and ironing, transport, finance, and leisure activities.

In the author's experience, the assessment of the impact of impairments on daily life, and in particular the capacity for independent mobility, can be augmented by considering the patient's life space.

Life space

Life space assessment can be performed formally with the use of a diary as an accurate measure of mobility or mobility limitation. It can be assessed more simply during a consultation simply by asking a series of questions to establish the limits of the subject's independent mobility. For example, someone who does not get out of bed and whose daily living needs are all met with the help of others has probably the most restricted possible life space, being confined not only to one room, but to one item of furniture in that room. Less restricted life space might include living a life which is confined to a single floor of a building (perhaps two rooms), or one in which the subject rarely gets further than the garden gate, the local shops, or the local town centre. At the other end of the scale are the fully independent individuals who regularly leave their house, and perhaps also their city, county, or country using various forms of transport without difficulty or help.

By establishing, using simple questions, the furthest a patient ever roams, and whether there have been recent changes in the dimensions of this 'life space', one can gain a further insight into the impact of any impairment on physical activity to complement more or less formal assessments of personal and instrumental activities of daily living.

Observational assessment of mobility

Sometimes it is useful or necessary to observe a particular physical activity in order to assess the need for assistance or safety performing the activity. An example of this would be observing a patient getting up out of a chair and walking a distance, turning round and returning to the chair. Much clinically useful information can be obtained by simply observing how easy or difficult the task is. Do they need help standing up? Is their balance normal? Do they have difficulty initiating movement, Is the gait asymmetric or festinant? Do the arms swing normally? How many steps do they take to turn through 180 degrees? Do they lean to one side or backwards?

A more formal assessment of gait and balance can be performed using the Tinetti Gait and Balance Assessment instrument, which has value in helping to identify people who are at increased risk of falls, or the Rivermead Mobility Index.

Objective assessment of walking can be performed simply with a stopwatch and a measured walking distance. Traditionally a 10-metre walk or 5-metre walk turn and return can be timed to provide an objective measure of walking speed. Subsequently the test can be repeated to assess changes in movement speed associated with treatment (for example to assess response to treatment for Parkinson's disease). An alternative is the 'timed up and go' test, which is time taken by an individual to stand up from an arm chair, walk 3 metres, turn, walk back, and sit down.

Specific assessment of muscle strength

Much can be inferred about physical functioning through clinical observation, but the specific diagnosis of two emerging new health states, frailty and sarcopenia, can be augmented specifically by the demonstration of impaired muscle strength. This can be simply done using a hand grip dynamometer and if impaired and combined with clinical observation of impaired muscle function (such as poor mobility, or difficulty with transfers) suggests a diagnosis of sarcopenia, contributes to defining a degree of frailty and is associated with a high risk of poor health outcomes.

Further reading

Collen FM, Wade DT, Robb GF, et al. (1991). The Rivermead Mobility Index: a further development of the Rivermead Motor Assessment. *Int Disabil Stud* **13**: 50–4.

Mahoney FI, Barthel DW (1965). Functional evaluation: the Barthel Index. *MD State Med J* **14**: 61–5.

May D. Nayak US. Isaacs B (1985). The life-space diary: a measure of mobility in old people at home. *Int Rehabil Med* **7**: 182–6.

Nouri F, Lincoln NB (1987). An extended activities of daily living scale for stroke patients. *Clin Rehab* **1**: 233–8.

Podsiadlo D, Richardson S (1991). The timed 'Up & Go': a test of basic functional mobility for frail elderly persons. *J Am Geriatr Soc* **39**: 142–8.

Tinetti ME (1986). Performance-oriented assessment of mobility problems in elderly patients. *J Am Geriatr Soc* **34**: 119–26.

Tinetti ME, Ginter SF (1990). The nursing home life-space diameter. A measure of extent and frequency of mobility among nursing home residents. *J Am Geriatr Soc* **38**: 1311–5.

Wade DT, Hewer RL (1987). Functional abilities after stroke: measurement, natural history and prognosis. *J Neurol Neurosurg Psychiatry* **50**: 177–82.

Cognitive function assessment

Introduction

An assessment of cognitive functioning should form part of the assessment of every older adult. Disorders affecting cognitive functioning are common. They may be the primary reason prompting the assessment or may be a complicating factor in the management of other conditions. The extent and detail of the cognitive assessment will vary depending on the clinical presentation being assessed, but the clinician should have a good grounding in the principles of cognitive functioning, and the tools available to assess this, in order to effectively deploy these and then interpret the findings. This section will first outline why assessing cognitive functioning is important. It will then look at what cognitive functioning is, and discuss some of the many tools available to assess it.

Why is it important?

Conditions affecting cognition are common and becoming commoner. It is estimated that in the next 30 years the number of people with dementia in the UK will double to over 1.4 million. Currently, as few as one in three people with dementia receive a diagnosis. The presence of cognitive impairment has been shown to increase the duration of hospital stay. Dementia predisposes people to developing delirium and an episode of delirium increases the subsequent rate of cognitive decline in dementia. Cognitive impairment has been shown to predict poorer outcomes in a range of conditions, from heart failure to hip fractures. Cognitive assessment therefore has two main goals:

1 To identify the presence of a factor that may complicate the treatment and rehabilitation of patients admitted with a range of conditions.
2 To detect dementia and enable access to a range of treatment and support services.

What is cognition?

Cognition is the work of the brain. It can be conceptualized as being divided into a number of different domains. These fall into two main categories: distributed functions, which involve a number of different brain regions or structures working in concert, and localized functions, which are carried out by a specific brain area.

Distributed cognitive functions

Memory

Retrograde memory refers to the ability to recall previously encoded information, whereas anterograde memory is the ability to make new memories. Memory can also be defined by its content: episodic memory is memory for events, related to a specific time, whereas semantic memory is the store of knowledge about the world. Procedural memory is knowledge of 'how to' carry out a task. Memory can also be divided into short and long term. Short-term memory refers to immediate recall, as tested, for example, by digit span. The recall of items after a number of minutes does not test this, but is a function of longer term storage and recall. Memory problems are related to damage in the medial temporal lobe, the diencephalon, and basal forebrain nuclei.

Frontal/executive functioning

This refers to the ability to plan, problem-solve, and exercise judgement, and includes elements of mental flexibility and regulation of social behaviour. Structures involved include the frontal lobes, thalamus, and basal ganglia.

Attention/concentration

This is the ability to direct and sustain attention on the task in hand. It is fundamental to the successful execution of abilities in other cognitive domains. A failure of attention leads to distractibility and disorientation. The reticular activating system and areas of the frontal, parietal, and temporal cortex are involved in attentional systems.

Localized cognitive functions

Language

The language areas are found in the dominant cortex, and include parts of the frontal and temporal lobes. Disorder in the production or comprehension of spoken language is referred to as aphasia, and the specific nature of the aphasia will be determined by the area of the cortex affected. Aphasia can be classified as fluent or non-fluent. The former is associated with damage in Broca's area, the latter with Wernicke's area. While pure forms of aphasia exist, in dementia there is often a more widespread language disorder that does not fit precisely into any specific category. Problems with naming items are common in all forms of aphasia.

Praxis

This is also a dominant hemisphere function, localized in the frontal and parietal lobes. Deficits in this domain are referred to as apraxia. Defined narrowly, this is the inability to carry out motor tasks on request, although they can still be carried out spontaneously. It is also used to refer to an inability to carry out complex motor tasks of everyday living, such as dressing or washing. However, these tasks may call upon other domains such as language comprehension, attention, and frontal-executive skills, and so deficits in these areas are more complex to interpret.

Visuospatial skills

These are a range of skills which are thought to have their origin in the non-dominant parietal lobe. They include constructional abilities, neglect phenomena, and object/face recognition. Deficits in the latter are referred to as agnosia.

Testing cognition

The extent of cognitive testing carried out will be guided by the clinical picture. The history will give an indication of the likelihood of cognitive deficits being present; if the patient finds it difficult to provide a clear account of the events that have led them to the consultation, deficits in attention, episodic memory, or language skills may be suspected. This should prompt a fuller examination of cognitive functioning. An informant history may be invaluable to obtain information about the consequences of cognitive deficits on daily functioning. An understanding of the domains of cognition and which are likely to be affected in any given disorder can help focus the examination on the areas of likely concern. In brief, deficits in attention/concentration are characteristic of delirium, while deficits in anterograde and recent episodic memory would raise the suspicion of Alzheimer's disease. Frontal/executive dysfunction is often seen in vascular dementia and Lewy body/Parkinson's disease dementia.

There is a huge range of instruments used to test cognition and a detailed examination of them is beyond the scope of this section. However, there are now a number of short batteries of cognitive tests that can be used in clinical settings with minimal training. The clinician is advised to familiarize themselves with a few such instruments and to be aware of the purpose they serve and their limitations. Given evidence indicating that clinicians are poor at detecting milder degrees of cognitive impairment during routine assessment, a strong case could be made for incorporating a brief screening battery into every geriatric medicine assessment, even when cognitive impairment is not suspected. This section will now consider some of the cognitive tests available.

Brief cognitive testing batteries

The Mini Mental State Examination (MMSE)

Developed in 1975, this is the most widely used brief cognitive battery. It includes items that test attention, orientation, anterograde memory, language, and constructional skills. It is broadly recognized in clinical settings and can be used to monitor progression of cognitive problems. It can be used to screen for dementia, with a score of less than 24 out of 30 being taken as abnormal. It has a number of drawbacks: it is poor at detecting frontal/executive deficits; can be confounded by age, extent of education, and ethnicity; and takes too long to administer (10 minutes) to use as a routine screening tool in clinic. It underestimates the abilities of black and minority ethnic elders. However, when supplemented with something to test for frontal lobe functioning, it probably provides the most useful compromise between range and brevity among the instruments described here.

The Abbreviated Mental Test Score (AMTS)

This is short, with only 10 items. A score of less than six is taken to be abnormal. However, problems with educational and cultural bias exist, and it is heavily weighted towards items that test memory and orientation. It has no test of executive function. There is also evidence it is administered in an unstandardized way in clinical practice, reducing its value in tracking changes in cognitive functioning. Despite being widely used, it performs poorly on measures of quality both as a screening test and as a more detailed assessment tool, and has little to recommend it.

Clock Drawing Test (CDT)

This is a widely used and very quick cognitive test (1 minute). The patient is asked to draw a clock face, and set the hands to a particular time. It calls upon a range of cognitive skills, including working memory, global attention, visuospatial representation, and executive control. There are many scoring systems, but a binary normal/abnormal division, with a description of the way the patient attempted the task, would be as useful as any in a clinical setting. It may be a useful adjunct to the MMSE.

Mini-Cog

This is a very brief test, consisting of recalling three items, and clock drawing. There is a well-defined scoring system that divides patients into either 'probably demented', or 'probably not demented'. There is a growing body of evidence that it performs well as a screening test, and may be more sensitive at detecting mild dementia than the MMSE. It is also reported to be free from bias due to education, literacy, or culture, and is very quick to administer (3 minutes). As a result, it may be good to consider this as a routine screening test.

The Addenbrooke's Cognitive Examination

This is the longest battery described here, with 100 available points. It contains the MMSE, and will give a score on this, but includes items testing frontal lobe functioning, and more detailed coverage of the other domains. It performs better than the MMSE at detecting early Alzheimer's disease, and is better at detecting the patterns of impairment seen in Lewy body/Parkinson's disease dementia. Its main drawback is its length, as it takes around 20 minutes to administer. However, this is within the scope of what can be achieved in an inpatient setting, and it has the capacity to provide a more detailed and complete examination that the other instruments.

Cognitive Estimates Test

This is a series of questions to which the patient is unlikely to know the correct answer, and to which they are asked to make an 'informed guess', for example, 'how fast do racehorses gallop'. While there are possible confounding factors such as cultural unfamiliarity with items, this is a good bedside test of frontal lobe functioning. Patients with frontal lobe impairment often make bizarre and improbable suggestions as answers.

IQCODE (Short)

This is an informant questionnaire with 16 items which compares reports of current performance on a range of everyday tasks with performance 10 years previously. It takes around 10 minutes, has little educational bias and is well tolerated.

Further reading

Burns A, Craig S, Lawlor B (1999). *Assessment Scales in Old Age Psychiatry*. London, Martin Dunitz Ltd.

Hodges JR (1994). *Cognitive assessment for clinicians*. OUP, Oxford.

Ismail Z, Rajji TK, Shulman KI (2010). Brief cognitive screening instruments: an update. *Int J Geriatr Psych* 25: 111–20.

Parker C, Philp I (2004). Screening for cognitive impairment among older people in black and minority ethnic groups. *Age Aging* 33: 447–52.

Assessment of nutrition

Healthy ageing is essential to maintain a high quality of life and is defined by the World Health Organization (WHO) as the state of complete physical, mental, and social well-being. However, malnutrition among older adults diminishes quality of life by contributing to serious illness, decreased functional capability, and altered self-perception of health and chronic disability. It is widely accepted that malnutrition may arise from a wide range of conditions and thus can be broadly defined as 'A state of nutrition in which a deficiency or excess (imbalance) of energy, protein and other nutrients causes measurable adverse effects on tissue/body form (body shape, size and composition) and function and clinical outcome'.

The prevalence of malnutrition in older adults is widespread across the UK and varies geographically, with higher prevalence in the north (19.4%) than the south (11.2%) of England. Recent statistics from the National Institute for Health and Clinical Excellence suggested that more than 10% of the over 65s in the general population are at medium or high risk of malnutrition, and that this figure rises to 60% in the hospital setting. The 2008 British Association for Parenteral and Enteral Nutrition (BAPEN) nutrition screening survey found that one in three adults admitted to hospitals was malnourished and that those aged 65 plus, had 40% greater risk of malnutrition than those <65 years.

Malnutrition is a complex, multi-organ problem, which, if left untreated, can lead to atrophy and weakness of the skeletal muscles (including the respiratory muscles), reduced heart muscle mass, impaired wound healing, skin thinning with a predisposition to pressure ulcers, immune deficiency, fatigue, apathy, and hypothermia. In response to such unfavourable consequences, older hospitalized patients are further disadvantaged since malnutrition is associated with increased length of stay, higher rates of medical and surgical complications and increased mortality.

Malnutrition is typically taken to mean undernutrition characterized by an impaired nutritional status resulting from either reduced nutrient intakes or altered nutrient metabolism occurring because of the presence of disease; however, it can also result from overnutrition.

The term 'sarcopoenic obesity' has been coined to describe the loss of muscle mass/strength or quality with obesity. As obesity is caused by a mismatch between energy consumed and that expended, and older adults are known to have lower intakes of protein than recommended, this can lead to poor protein turnover and consequently sarcopenia. Low muscle strength is associated with poor functional performance and increased mortality. Therefore, it is not only those experiencing weight loss who are at risk, but also those with poor dietary quality and weight gain.

Despite its widespread prevalence and devastating consequences, malnutrition, whatever its form, cannot be diagnosed by simple physical observations and weight measurements but requires thorough nutritional assessment on admission to hospital.

The goals of assessment of nutritional status are to first identify those who already have, or are at risk of developing, malnutrition, then to quantify the risk of developing malnutrition-related medical complications, and finally to monitor the adequacy of any nutritional therapy. There are, however no gold standard methodologies for determining nutritional status due to both a lack of universally accepted clinical definitions of malnutrition, and of assessment parameters which are not affected by concurrent illness and injury, and finally a difficulty in isolating the effect of malnutrition from the influence of disease on clinical outcome.

It is therefore generally accepted that to overcome the shortcomings of any one marker of malnutrition, a combination should be used, and it has been found that the sensitivity of detecting malnutrition increases when it has been estimated using a combination of at least one anthropometric and one biochemical indice. However, there is currently no guideline or consensus as to exactly which anthropometric and biochemical variable should be routinely used.

Anthropometry

Body mass index (BMI) is routinely used in the clinical setting as part of the nutritional assessment process; however, it has the disadvantage that it does not take into account age, gender, ethnicity, or fat to muscle mass. Its usefulness in the older population is made more complex due to changes in stature, mobility, and oedema, which may mask true weight, especially upon admission to hospital. To overcome this, BAPEN introduced the Malnutrition Universal Screening Tool (MUST), which includes a number of alternative ways of assessing BMI. Apart from BMI, other popular anthropometric indices involve mid-upper arm circumference (MUAC) and triceps skinfold thickness (TSF) measurements. They are considered as reliable measures to assess changes in body composition with high specificity rates. However, they have low sensitivity and predictive validity when compared with BMI measurements and the Subjective Global Assessment (SGA) screening tool, justifying that individual anthropometric measurements should not be used as single predictive measures of nutritional status. The usefulness of anthropometric measurements as a nutrition assessment tool is also dependent upon having reliable and up-to-date anthropometric reference data, which is currently lacking for the older population in the UK.

Increasingly, waist circumference is being used as an indication of nutritional status, with some authors suggesting that weight to height ratio may be a more reliable indicator of disease risk than BMI.

Biochemistry

There are no biochemical markers of protein malnutrition that can be recommended as a routine and reliable assessment of an individual's nutrition status. The ideal nutritional marker has a short half-life and a small total pool with rapid rate of synthesis that responds only to protein intake, is uninfluenced by other disease processes, and can be easily and inexpensively measured.

The most frequently monitored hepatic protein in clinical care involving nutritional screening is albumin, since its assessment is considered by some to be a good predictor of mortality and morbidity. However, apart from being inexpensive and easy to measure, it meets none of the criteria for an ideal nutritional marker mentioned above and many studies have concluded that it is relatively insensitive to acute changes in nutrition and cannot be used to monitor the effectiveness of nutritional intervention.

Prealbumin, or transthyretin, has been considered as the preferred indicator of nutritional status since it correlates with patient outcomes in a wide variety of clinical conditions. Prealbumin is able to give the most accurate interpretation of the patient's catabolic state and nitrogen loss due to its small pool size in the body and its half-life of only 2 days compared with 20 days in the case of albumin. It has a high content of the amino acid tryptophan and a high proportion of essential to non-essential amino acids making it a specific marker for protein synthesis. Furthermore, it is unaffected by hydration status, is less influenced by liver disease than the other serum proteins, and is easily quantified in the hospital setting (Table 2.2).

Dietary assessment

Assessment of patients, current and past intake can be performed using a number of techniques. Retrospective methods, including diet histories, 24-hour recall, and food frequency questionnaires, can be useful in gaining an insight into a patient's usual dietary habits and any changes in these. However they rely heavily on good memory, and require dietetic input and use of nutritional analysis software in order to calculate nutrient intake.

Current and prospective intake can be recorded using weighed diet diaries, considered the gold standard technique, although they place a high clinical burden, and in practice semi-quantitative food charts/diaries/records may be used in their place. Again dietetic input is required and intakes compared with recommendations adjusted for clinical requirements. It is essential that dietary intake is monitored in order to assess the effectiveness of treatment and to review as necessary (see MUST for more guidelines).

Nutritional screening and assessment tools

Several screening tools have been created to enable rapid assessment of patient nutrition status on admission to hospital. These include Subjective Global Assessment (SGA), Mini-Nutritional Assessment (MNA), Malnutrition Universal Screening Tool (MUST) mentioned previously, and Nutrition Risk Score (NRS). Generally, most screening tools incorporate dietary history and record any recent weight loss, or medical condition which may predispose to malnutrition and incorporate some form of anthropometry. A risk score may be calculated, which is used to determine the course of treatment and monitoring progress.

Table 2.2 Albumin versus prealbumin: characteristics of plasma proteins used in nutritional evaluation

Protein	Molar weight	Half-life	Range
Albumin	65,000	20 days	3.30 to 4.80 g per dL (33 to 48 g per L)
Transferin	76,000	10 days	0.16 to 0.36 g per dL (0.16 to 0.36 g per dL)
Prealbumin	54.980	2 days	16.0 to 35.0 mg per dL (160 to 350 mg per L)

Further reading

BAPEN (2003). *Malnutrition Universal Screening Tool.* Malnutrition Advisory Group (www.bapen.org.uk).

Beck FK, Rosenthal TC (2002). Prealbumin: A marker for nutritional evaluation. *Am Fam Physician* **65**: 1575–8.

Bernstein LH, Leukhardt-Fairfield CJ, Pleban W, et al. (1989). Usefulness of data on albumin and prealbumin concentrations in determining effectiveness of nutritional support. *Clin Chem* **35**: 271–4.

Burden ST, Stoppard E, Shaffer J, et al. (2005). Can we use mid upper arm anthropometry to detect malnutrition in medical inpatients? A validation study. *J Hum Nutr Diet* **18**, 287–94.

Corish CA (1999). 'Nutrition and surgical practice'- Pre-operative nutritional assessment. *Proc Nutr Soc* **58**: 821–9.

Corish CA, Kennedy NP (2003). Anthropometric measurements from a cross-sectional survey of Irish free-living elderly subjects with smoothed centile curves. *Br J Nutr* **89**: 137–45.

Elia M (2000). *Guidelines for Detection and Management of Malnutrition.* Maidenhead, Malnutrition Advisory Group (MAG), Standing Committee of BAPEN.

Fergusson RP, O'Connor P, Crabtree B, et al. (1993). Serum albumin and prealbumin as predictors of clinical outcomes of hospitalised elderly nursing home residents. *J Am Geriatr Soc* **41**: 545–9.

Gibbs J, Cull W, Henderson W, et al. (1999). Preoperative serum albumin level as a predictor of operative mortality band morbidity. *Arch Surg* **134**: 36–42.

Gibson RS (2005). *Principles of Nutritional Assessment*, 2nd edn. Oxford: Oxford University Press.

Guigoz Y, Vellas B, Garry PJ (1996). Assessing the nutritional status of the elderly: The Mini Nutritional Assessment as part of the geriatric evaluation. *Nutr Rev* **54**: S59–65.

Klein S, Kinney J, Jeejeebhoy K, et al. (1997). Nutrition support in clinical practice: review of published data and recommendations for future research directions. Summary of a conference sponsored by the National Institute of Health, American Society for Parenteral and Enteral Nutrition, and American Society for Clinical Nutrition. *Am J Clin Nutr* **66**: 683–706.

Koval KJ, Maurer SG, Su ET, et al. (1999). The effects of nutritional status on outcome after hip fracture. *J Orthop Trauma* **13**: 164–9.

Lansey S, Waslien C, Mulhill M, et al. (1993). The role of anthropometry in assessment of malnutrition in the hospitalized frail elderly. *Gerontology* **39**: 346–53.

Mears E (1996). Outcomes of continuous process improvement of a nutritional care program incorporating serum prealbumin measurements. *Nutrition* **12**: 479–84.

Pennington CR (1997). Symposium on 'Assessment of nutritional status in disease and other trauma' – Disease and malnutrition in British hospitals. *Proc Nutr Soc* **56**: 393–407.

Reilly HM, Martineau JK, Moran A, et al. (1995). Nutritional screening – evaluation and implementation of a simple nutrition risk score. *Clin Nutr* **14**: 269–73.

Spiekerman AM (1995). Nutritional assessment (protein nutriture). *Anal Chem* **67**: R429–36.

Zamboni M, Mazzali G, Fantin F, et al. (2008). Sarcopenic obesity: a new category of obesity in the elderly. *Nutr Metab Cardiovasc Dis* **18**: 388–95.

Assessment of urinary incontinence

The key components of assessing an older adult with urinary incontinence (UI) should include a history of the symptoms, a physical examination, urinalysis, blood glucose and calcium, a frequency volume (bladder) diary, and a post-void residual urine volume.

The objective with the assessment is to identify and treat reversible causes, exclude urinary retention, and identify the need for more in-depth investigations.

Using the DIAPPERS acronym, transient and reversible causes can quickly be identified. This is especially useful when the incontinence is of recent onset.

Delirium/confusional states
Infection – urinary (symptomatic)
Atrophic urethritis/vaginitis
Pharmaceuticals
Psychological, especially depression
Excessive excretion (e.g. diuretics, hyperglycaemia)
Restricted mobility
Stool impaction

A careful history (Table 2.3) that includes a medication review will identify delirium, depression, cognitive impairment, polyuria, functional problems, and drugs that can contribute to incontinence. Information about the circumstances surrounding the episodes of incontinence should be sought with the objective of identifying whether environmental factors have a role.

Physical examination (Table 2.4) will identify visual impairment, atrophic vaginitis, faecal loading, urinary retention, abnormal neurological signs, and evidence of moderate to severe arthritis.

The initial assessment can then be completed by obtaining a urine sample for urinalysis, blood glucose and calcium, post-void residual urine volume, and a 3-day bladder diary

Table 2.3 History

Medical conditions	Congestive cardiac failure, diabetes mellitus, neurological conditions
Medications	Refer to Table 14.2 in causes of UI
Fluid intake	Pattern especially prior to bedtime
Past history	Childbirth, recurrent urinary tract infections, surgery, radiation, urinary retention
General symptoms	Onset and duration Type – urge/stress/mixed Frequency of episodes
Lower urinary tract	Dysuria, frequency, urgency and nocturia, hesitancy, poor, incomplete emptying, haematuria, and suprapubic pain
Other symptoms	Constipation, faecal incontinence, depression, neurological features of stroke, Parkinson's disease, spinal cord compression, normal pressure hydrocephalus and multiple sclerosis
Perception	severity, interference with daily life and any concerns
Environmental	Location, structure and ease of use of toilets or substitutes

Table 2.4 Examination

General	Lower limb pitting oedema
Cognition	Mood, motivation, mental test score
Function	Ability to walk with or without assistance, manual dexterity
Neurology	Limb weakness, hyper/hyporeflexia, parkinsonism
Abdomen	Lower abdominal distension, suprapubic tenderness
Rectal	Perianal sensation, anal tone, masses including any faecal loading, prostate size
Pelvis	Perineal sensation, atrophic vaginitis, pelvic prolapse, cystocele,

At this stage, if the cause/causes have not been identified or the incontinence persists after addressing the initial factors identified, then it is necessary to understand whether the incontinence is urge, stress, or mixed. In addition, overflow incontinence may occur in individuals with outflow obstruction. This will now guide targeted treatment and, if necessary, more in-depth investigations and interventions, some of which may be surgical. It is equally important to identify any other factor outside of the urinary tract that contributes to the incontinence, which may be irreversible at this stage, such as dementia, impaired manual dexterity, inability to walk, moderate to significant dependency levels even if mobile, and significant visual impairment.

The final aspect of a complete assessment is identifying from the history, examination, and simple tests who should be referred on for more in depth investigations. See Table 2.5 for indications for referring.

Suggested flow chart for carrying out an assessment:

* initial assessment
* history, physical examination, urinalysis (use the DIAPPERS acronym)
* blood glucose and calcium
* bladder diary over 3 days
* post-void residual urine volume.

If the post-void bladder volume is less than 100 mL, classify incontinence as stress, urge or mixed. If greater than 180 mL, the patient will need investigation for urinary retention and overflow incontinence.

If the above does not lead to resolution of incontinence following treatment or any of the factors in Table 2.4 are present, refer to an appropriate specialist.

Table 2.5 Recommendations for referral

History	Gross haematuria, pelvic pain, recurrent urinary tract infections, acute spinal cord lesions
Examination	Complete urinary retention, marked enlargement of the prostate, marked prolapse, new neurological signs
Tests	Raised postvoid residual urine, microscopic haematuria
Unclear diagnosis	Failure to respond to initial treatment or unclear diagnosis

Further reading

Tan TL (2003). Urinary incontinence in older persons: A simple approach to a complex problem. *Ann Acad Med Singapore* **32**: 731–9.

Assessing fitness to drive

Background

The number of older drivers (those aged over 65 years old) is growing throughout the world. For instance, the total of 65+ drivers will roughly double in the USA by 2030. Although people age at different rates, the product of many variables, including lifestyle choice and genetic predisposition, the principle of entropy dictates that levels of physical and cognitive functioning diminish with age. Nevertheless, 'having a birthday' does not mean one's driving abilities automatically decline.

Physicians play a pivotal role in assessing patients and making decisions about their fitness to drive. While some driving assessments are easy to make, e.g. dramatic vision impairment, most are much more complicated. Driving is critical to help people stay connected to family and friends. If this privilege is taken away, the potential exists for isolation, depression, and even lack of access to basic healthcare. The potential negative effects of non-driving for older adults may be mitigated by the presence of transportation options (e.g. public transportation or specialized transportation services), but many places do not have a robust set of alternatives for non-drivers to use.

This section focuses on the role of physicians in assessing fitness to drive, which, as noted above, often has significant implications for a patient's health, wellbeing, and successful ageing.

The physician's role

The American Medical Association's (AMA) most recent edition of the *Physician's Guide to Assessing and Counselling Older Drivers* provides an overview of the topic and recommends a variety of areas that doctors should evaluate when working with patients. The guidebook also quite properly frames the issue of fitness to drive as a public health issue.

A physician's primary patient focus centres on their physical and cognitive health. However, once a patient's wellbeing has been evaluated and all procedures or medication regimens planned, a secondary screen should always include an assessment of their fitness to drive and any potential impacts of medical intervention on their abilities to navigate the road safely.

The AMA guide identifies key areas of consideration in assessing driving fitness.

Red flags that indicate that further assessment is needed:
- poor personal care
- impaired ambulation
- impaired attention, memory, or cognition.

Tools for assessment of driving-related skills (ADReS) that focus on:
- visual acuity and fields of view;
- cognition
- motor skills and range of motion.

Medical conditions and medicines that may affect driving:
- arthritis
- cataracts
- dementias
- muscle relaxants
- anticholinergics

- neurological conditions, such as stroke and Parkinson's disease.

The role of the driving rehabilitation specialist:
- driver and vehicle evaluation
- adaptive driving instruction
- vehicle modifications.

Counselling the patient:
- identifying any restrictions to ensure safety (e.g. avoiding night driving)
- provide referrals to community transportation providers
- encourage family participation.

The ethical and legal responsibilities of the physician:
- understanding mandatory reporting requirements and licence renewal practices.

Medical professionals need to consider how treatment regimens can affect driving abilities. When doing so, they should explicitly convey this information to patients and make recommendations on their fitness to drive. These recommendations could range from driving limitations (e.g. only driving during the day) to total driving cessation.

Because the consequences of limiting driving can have a direct effect on a patient's quality of life, family member participation must be considered when sharing any driving recommendations with their patients. Family members and friends are the best support system in place to ensure that any doctor suggestions will be adhered to. A family conversation about driving can reassure the patient that all concerns revolve around their wellbeing. Family members and friends can also be instrumental in providing alternative transportation or identifying resources that can assist the patient with their mobility needs.

The regulatory environment

If a patient's medical evaluation identifies a health condition that poses significant risk associated with continued driving, the physician may be subject to a mandatory reporting requirement. Reporting requirements to licensing agencies and law enforcement officials regarding fitness to drive vary significantly around the world, so physicians need to be aware of their local standards and legal obligations. Importantly, all doctors who identify any limitation that requires reporting must notify the patient that a report needs to be submitted. This notification alerts the patient to the seriousness of the finding and should satisfy the legal and ethical obligations of the doctor.

Medical advisory boards

Advisory boards that impartially assess a person's fitness to drive based on medical records can play a valuable regulatory role, but their decisions must be evidence based. There is extensive international research on correlations between age, health status, and crash risk. Although older adults are more frequently killed in accidents, this mortality rate is generally ascribed to their increased fragility and propensity to succumb to injuries that younger adults could survive. Many jurisdictions give advisory boards wide discretion to develop rehabilitation routines that may significantly improve driving abilities. These board members verify fitness to drive through testing; many are given the latitude to fully reinstate licensing or establish restrictions for a person to legally operate a motor vehicle.

Professional support services

There are driving assessment centres where patients may undergo specific tailored assessments. Patients may be referred or self-refer. Referrals of patients to physical and occupational therapists or driving rehabilitation specialists can enhance fitness to drive. Many times, increasing flexibility, strength, and even cognitive processing speed can help revive a person's driving fitness. In addition, there are compensating skills that can be taught and devices that can enhance a person's driving abilities.

Conclusion

An assessment of a patient's physical and cognitive status is critical in determining fitness to drive. This assessment should focus on vision, and cognitive and motor functions. Whenever possible, physicians should consult with family members when a driving assessment suggests that adjustments need to be made. When appropriate, they should refer patients to medical advisory boards that assess fitness to drive based on evidence. And, they should refer patients to physiotherapists/occupational therapists and driving rehabilitation specialists to strengthen their driving skills. In doing so, they can help older adults stay safe on the road, and, when necessary, suggest driving limitations or cessation that is supported by family and friends.

Further reading

American Medical Association (2010). *Physician's Guide to assessing and counseling older drivers.* Washington, DC, NHTSA.

Classen S (ed.) 2010). Older driver safety and community mobility. *Am J Occupational Ther* **64** (March/April).

Cheung, AT, McCartt, Keli AB (2008). *Exploring the declines in older driver fatal crash involvement.* Arlington VA, Insurance Institute for Highway Safety.

Grabowski D, Christine C, Michael M (2004). Elderly licensure laws and motor vehicle fatalities. *JAMA* **29**: 2840–6.

Hennessey D, Janke M (2009). *Clearing a road to being driving fit by better assessing driving wellness.* California DMV: Sacramento.

Insurance Institute for Highway Safety (2001). *Status Report: Older Drivers Up Close: They aren't Dangerous Except Maybe to Themselves.* Arlington VA.

Insurance Institute For Highway Safety (2007). Status Report. Special Issue: Older Drivers. (http://www.iihs.org/research/topics/older_people.html).

Kerschner and Harris (2007). *Federal Highway Administration. Better Options for Older Adults.* United States Department of Transportation.

Loughran DS, Seabury SA, ZakarasL (2007). Rand Institute for Civil Justice. Regulating Older Drivers: Are New Policies Needed? (http://www.rand.org/pubs/occasional_papers/OP189.html).

MacLennan P, Owsley C, Rue L, et al. (2009). *Older adults' knowledge about medications that can impact driving.* Washington, DC: AAA Foundation for Traffic Safety.

Mayo Clinic (2007). Mayo Clinic Foundation for Medical Education and Research. 1998–2008. (http://www.mayoclinic.com).

Rosenbloom S (2003). Older Drivers: Should We Test Them Off the Road? (http://www.uctc.net).

Stutts J, Martell C, Staplin L (2008). *Identifying Behaviors and Situations Associated with Increased Crash Risk for Older Drivers.* Washington, DC, NHTSA.

United States Department of Transportation, National Highway Traffic Safety Administration. (2001). *Family and Friends Concerned About an Older Driver.* (http://www.nhtsa.gov).

United States Government Accountability Office (2007). Older Driver Safety: Knowledge Sharing Should Help States Prepare for Increase in Older Driver Population. (http://www.gao.gov/new.items/d07413.pdf).

Wang C, Carr D (2004). Older driver safety: a report from the older drivers project. *Am Geriatric Soc,* SZ:143–9.

Preoperative assessment of older people

Preoperative assessment serves two, potentially conflicting, purposes.

1 A 'professionally centred' role that allows the clinicians involved to establish risks and benefits of surgery using population-based statistics, to advise accordingly, to plan the resources required, and to eliminate the waste of resources and failure to achieve 'targets' that results from last-minute cancellations of surgery.

2 A 'patient-centred' role that seeks to discover factors in each patient that can be modified by specific interventions in order to reduce the overall risk and improve the chances of a complication-free recovery.

The widespread adoption of preoperative assessment in the NHS has been driven by the first of these considerations. The second purpose has sadly been largely overlooked.

Surgeons usually discuss risks and benefits at the initial consultation. However there are considerations with which the surgeon may not be expert or interested. The preoperative assessment clinic has developed in response to this. This service can take several forms. At its simplest, a nurse undertakes a basic examination to save the need for a doctor on admission. Other models allow for investigation such as chest x-ray or echocardiogram, or for referral to a cardiologist or anaesthetist, according to local protocols. Factors relating to the improvement of the likelihood of full recovery and rehabilitation may need separate evaluation. This is particularly so in the case of older patients with complex medical needs and requires a more sophisticated model.

What is it that harms surgical patients? Inevitably there are surgical and anaesthetic mishaps as well as failures that are 'organizational'. The latter are not considered here.

In general terms, patients who suffer major morbidity perioperatively such as stroke, myocardial damage, or acute kidney injury do so because they do not have functional reserve to sustain them through the metabolic and endocrine assault of surgery or trauma. Surgery leads to an increased oxygen demand, an increased metabolic rate, starvation with catabolism, followed by recovery in which tissues can only be repaired if there is sufficient substrate and oxygen delivery.

Immobility during recovery is associated with risks of thromboembolism and hypostatic pneumonia. Immobility is made worse by musculoskeletal disease, inactivity, or cognitive problems – problems that geriatricians recognize as part of their assessment of 'frailty'.

Thus patients who are vulnerable to frailty are the ones who pose the greatest challenge to the surgical team. The link between the Fried criteria for frailty and perioperative risk is clear.

It is disappointing that geriatric assessment has so far made relatively little impact on the routine practice of preoperative assessment. A recent publication from the Association of Anaesthetists of Great Britain and Ireland, for example, makes no mention of the role. In respect of geriatric involvement in preoperative assessment, the work of Harari et al. deserves detailed consideration. This is because it goes beyond the assessment of risk factors and describes a strategy for reducing individual risk.

Frailty and its associated perioperative risk

Weight loss: Patients who have lost weight have less muscle reserve as a store of protein and less carbohydrate and fat reserves. Malnutrition may be associated with vitamin and trace element deficiency that may impair tissue healing and immune deficiency that may put them at risk of sepsis Their illness may be more advanced, they may be catabolic even before the surgical assault and are at greater risk of pressure sore damage and hypothermia.

Loss of grip strength: This may reflect a more generalised weakness (sarcopenia), arthritis or a cognitive problem. In the recovery period, sustained respiratory muscle activity has to be able to compensate for increased carbon dioxide production, and certain groups of muscles (e.g. accessory muscles) may need to be recruited. The presence of pain in an abdominal or thoracic wound may also put demands on the accessory muscles. Inadequate tidal volumes lead to airway closure, atelectasis, pneumonia and hypoxia. Painful joints may prevent mobilization and cognitive problems may be a barrier to proper use of respiratory muscles.

Self reported exhaustion: Recovery from major surgery requires sustained respiratory activity, an increased cardiac output to deliver oxygen requirements to meet the new demand and a degree of determination, mental and physical, to overcome the challenges of surgery and the risks of immobility.

Reduced walking speed or low physical activity: A slow walking speed may be indicative of all the above factors: fatigue, arthritis, neurological disease, as well as indicating a failure of peripheral circulation and oxygen delivery. It may mask the symptoms of cardiac disease, as well as making assessment of specific cardiovascular risk factors difficult.

Harari et al. claimed that routine 'patient-centred' concerns are not addressed in routine preoperative surgical assessment clinics. The Proactive care of Older Persons undergoing Surgery (POPS) trial showed that older patients attending for major elective orthopaedic surgery had high levels of comorbidity which resulted in complications that delayed discharge from hospital. Using comprehensive geriatric assessment (CGA) in preoperative assessment—usually arranged as a single consultation with a geriatrician and a nurse, but with the option of involving therapists and social workers – the investigators reduced the risk of complications such as delirium, pneumonia, and wound infection compared with a control cohort. The presence of uncontrolled pain at 72 hours was virtually abolished, as was the requirement for assistance with transfer. Furthermore, the median length of stay was reduced by 4.5 days.

Delirium in hospitalized patients can be reduced by attention to a number of factors. Several of them lend themselves to preoperative assessment and treatment, thus:

Risk factors for delirium and their potential for modification by preoperative assessment

Urinary catheter:

Ultrasound measurement of residual urine volume may help in estimating the risk of postoperative retention. In prostatic hypertrophy, drugs such as tamsulosin may prevent postoperative retention. Constipation predisposes to postoperative retention and may be reduced by laxatives. If analgesics such as codeine are implicated, help may be obtained by using alternative analgesics, such as transdermal buprenorphine. It may be appropriate to modify anaesthetic techniques, such as those using spinal opioids, to reduce the risk of postoperative retention – the assessment process can be used to warn the anaesthetist.

Medications:

Elderly patients take drugs that they have taken without apparent problems for years. Nevertheless these drugs may put the vulnerable patient at risk of delirium. Preoperative assessment allows a rationalization of medication. Specifically it allows the gradual preoperative withdrawal of benzodiazepines and drugs which in combination may have anticholinergic properties, as well as alcohol. Where there is felt to be no justification for diuretics, these can also be reduced, and with this change, the risk of dehydration and electrolyte imbalance is reduced.

Ward environment:

The importance of family members in helping a vulnerable patient cope with the distress associated with delirium can be emphasised at the preoperative assessment. Contact with the surgical ward to enable a patient to be familiarised with ward routines may be useful.

Sensory deprivation:

Preoperative assessment allows for hearing aid batteries to be checked and appropriate ward measures being put in place to ensure that the patient with sensory loss is not put at a disadvantage

Dementia:

Where treatment with anticholinesterases is indicated, the preoperative assessment can establish that these drugs are being taken appropriately. Plans to continue with them through the perioperative period can be agreed with the ward. Decisions about suitable sedative drugs for the treatment of delirium or the availability of specialist staff can be made in advance of admission.

'What are my chances, doc?'
'Well, the mortality for this operation is 90%. My last 9 have died, so you should be fine!''

The nonsense of this parody on risk assessment shows the very real difficulty that professionals have when trying to turn studies of multivariate risk analysis into individual risk prediction that enables the older patient to make a valid decision. Decisions on risks have to consider the risk of natural death with age, which can be estimated at a doubling of monthly mortality for every 7 years. The request of a competent older patient for elective surgery— a 'lifestyle' operation – may be reasonable even though the hospital may be criticized in the event of a perioperative

death. Patient-centred considerations may conflict with professional ones.

Considerable effort, and faith, has been placed in studies designed to compare major morbidity risks. They are applicable to older people but they were not primarily designed to provide bookmakers' odds for individual patients. Some are summarized below.

The American Society of Anaesthesiologists (ASA) score is a simple 5-point scale. Its validity suffers from the subjective nature of the assessment, which may in practice not be made until after the anaesthetist has formed an opinion on the likely outcome.

The American Society of Anaesthesiologists (ASA) scoring system

Grade 1: a normal healthy patient with no clinically important co-morbidity or significant medical history

Grade 2: a patient with mild systemic disease

Grade 3: a patient with severe systemic disease

Grade 4: a patient with severe systemic disease that is a constant threat to life

Grade 5: a moribund patient who is not expected to survive

Goldman described nine variables associated with increased perioperative risk of cardiac morbidity, with each factor being given a different weighting.

The Goldman Index

Age over 70

Abdominal or thoracic surgery

Third heart sound or jugular venous distension

Myocardial infarction within 6 months

Rhythm other than sinus

Ventricular extrasystoles >5 /min

Poor general condition

Aortic stenosis

Emergency operation

These have been refined by Lee to provide stratified risk assessed by simple clinical questionnaires: patients scoring for two risk factors are judged to be at high (>7%) risk of a perioperative cardiac event.

Lee's modification of the Goldman index

High risk surgery

Diabetes requiring insulin

History of ischaemic heart disease

History of cerebrovascular disease

Congestive heart failure

Creatinine >2.0 mg/dl (150 μmol/L)

Internet-based algorithms

These have the risk that patients may use them to calculate individual risk, something for which they were not designed. The POSSUM score – the Physiological and Operative Severity Score for the enUmeration of Mortality and Morbidity – has been applied to many surgical specialities.

POSSUM considers physiological and operative variables. The requirement for operative data (e.g. blood loss) safeguards against inappropriate use, but the inquisitive can always enter estimated data.

Screening tools enable specialist staff to recognize potential problems with a view to improving outcome:
- an estimate of the magnitude of the surgical assault—'oxygen demand'
- an estimate of the degree of cardiorespiratory reserve—'oxygen supply'
- strategies to minimize the mismatch of oxygen demand versus supply.

Oxygen requirements - the anaerobic threshold (AT):

Older *et al.* used cardiopulmonary exercise testing with a bicycle ergometer and sampling of inspired and expired gas testing to predict cardiovascular mortality. They measured AT as the point during exercise at which anaerobic metabolism is needed to supplement aerobic metabolism. The increased oxygen delivery that occurs in response to submaximal exercise is believed to mimic the cardiovascular stress of major surgery.

Applied to a surgical population of 548 (mean age 69), 62 of them over the age of 79, a mean anaerobic threshold of 12.6 mL/min/kg was calculated. The reduction of AT with age was not considered to be significant. AT may have value as a predictive tool: cardiopulmonary deaths were virtually confined to patients with an AT of less than 11 mL/kg/min.

The results of AT testing an elderly population can be interpreted as follows:
- there is a threshold for cardiovascular fitness below which the risk of major surgery rises considerably
- extreme age is not an independent predictor of operative cardiovascular risk.

Whatever method of preoperative assessment is used, it is important to use the information wisely in looking at the individual patient and how the information so gathered can be used to ensure a safe outcome.

Further reading

AAGBI (2010). Pre-operative assessment and patient preparation: the role of the anaesthetist AAGBI Safety Guideline. Association of Anaesthetists of Great Britain and Ireland.

Fried LP, Tangen CM, Walston J, et al. (2001). Frailty in older adults: evidence for a phenotype. *J Gerontology* **56A**: M146–M56.

Goldman L, Caldera DL, Nussbaum SR (1977). Multifactorial index of cardiac risk in noncardiac surgical procedures. *N Engl J Med* **297**: 845–50.

Harari D, Hopper A, Dhesi J (2007). Proactive care of older people undergoing surgery (POPS): designing, embedding, evaluating and funding a comprehensive geriatric assessment service for older elective surgical patients. *Age Ageing* **36**: 190–6.

Inouye S (2006). Delirium in older persons. *CN Engl J Med* **354**: 1157–65.

Lee TH, Marcantonio ER, Mangione CM, et al. (1999). Derivation and prospective validation of a simple index for prediction of cardiac risk of major noncardiac surgery. *Circulation* **100**: 1043–9 (www.riskprediction.co.uk).

Older P, Hall A, Hader R (1999). Cardiopulmonary exercise testing as a screening test for perioperative management of major surgery in the elderly. *Chest* **116**: 355–62.

Prescribing in older people

Pharmacokinetics and pharmacodynamics

Introduction

The world's population is ageing and it is predicted that by the year 2031 people over 65 years will represent 30% of the total population. Sixty to 80% of older people are taking medication and between 20% and 30% of these patients are taking at least three drugs. Adverse drug reactions (ADRs) are a leading cause of death in older patients and are often unrecognized and severe. The National Service Framework for older people highlights the need for appropriate prescribing, which includes both the omission of medicines not indicated and the use of those that are indicated.

Pharmacokinetics and the ageing process

Pharmacokinetics describes the liberation, absorption, distribution, metabolism, and excretion of drugs and their metabolites. The physiological changes associated with ageing may affect the pharmacokinetics of drugs and metabolites.

Absorption

Although ageing itself has little effect on gastric emptying, it is affected by drugs (e.g. slowing - anticholinergics; increasing - prokinetics, e.g. domperidone, erythromycin). Most absorption occurs in the small bowel and there is little effect on this with ageing.

Bioavailability and first pass metabolism

Bioavailability describes the availability of a drug to the systemic circulation. Studies of digoxin, paracetamol, lorazepam, bumetanide, and theophylline have not shown any significant difference in bioavailability with age.

Drugs that undergo substantial first-pass metabolism in the liver are extracted from the blood during passage through the pre-systemic circulation, reducing their bioavailability. Ageing is associated with a reduction in first-pass metabolism, probably due to a 20–30% reduction in liver volume and blood flow with age. As a result, the bioavailability of drugs that undergo extensive first-pass metabolism, such as chlormethiazole and propranolol, can be significantly increased. It is therefore recommended that older patients are started on a lower dose of these medications.

Distribution

The volume of distribution (V) is a term used to quantify the distribution of a medication between plasma and the rest of the body after oral or parenteral dosing. A drug with a high V (e.g. morphine) is extensively distributed outside the blood or plasma to other tissues such as fat. With ageing, there is a decrease in the proportion of lean body weight, muscle mass, and water, and an increase in the proportion of fat. As a result, lipid-soluble drugs such as benzodiazepines, morphine, amiodarone, neuroleptics, and amitriptyline have an increased V. This will result in prolonged elimination half-life (t1/2z) and hence a more prolonged drug effect. The V of diazepam, for example, is increased from 1.19 L/kg in young males to 1.65 L/kg in older males, resulting in a more prolonged drug effect, and although no dose reduction regimen has been absolutely defined it is recommended that the dose of diazepam be halved in older people and closely monitored.

For water-soluble drugs, V will fall, and higher concentrations will be reached after initial administration. Loading doses of water-soluble drugs, such as gentamicin and

theophylline, should, therefore, be reduced in older patients if the drug also binds to muscle (e.g. digoxin) when the muscle mass would also be a relevant consideration.

Protein binding

Many drugs are protein bound, with the bound fraction inactive, while unbound drug is free to mediate its effect. Most acidic drugs (e.g. diazepam, phenytoin, warfarin) bind to albumin. With healthy ageing there is no clinically relevant change in plasma proteins. In the presence of chronic disease, serum albumin concentrations fall. This can produce clinically significant increases in the free fraction, and hence concentration, of very heavily protein-bound drugs such as ibuprofen (99.5% bound), benzodiazepines (>90%), and many antipsychotics (>90%) which increases V and hence t1/2z. Phenytoin is a good example of how protein binding is important in old age. It is highly protein bound so that a reduction in serum albumin results in a higher portion of an administered dose existing in free form in the plasma. Measured phenytoin levels do not reflect the increased active fraction, and so a patient with a normal or low laboratory level may show clinical signs of toxicity. Warfarin is also protein bound, and a reduction in the loading dose of warfarin in patients with low serum albumin levels is required.

Basic drugs such as lidocaine and tricyclic antidepressants bind to alpha-1-acid glycoprotein. Acute illness increases alpha-1-acid glycoprotein concentrations, reducing the free fraction, V, and t1/2z regardless of changed in clearance.

Clearance: hepatic

Hepatic metabolism of drugs is dependent on the ability of the liver to extract drug from the blood. Lipophilic drugs are metabolized into hydrophilic compounds, which are eliminated in the urine. Several studies have shown an age-related decline in the clearance of drugs (e.g. propranolol, theophylline) by hepatic metabolism, probably reflecting a reduced hepatic mass, as enzyme activity is preserved.

Induction of enzymes by drugs, such as phenytoin, isoniazid, glucocorticoids, and alcohol, may decrease the bioavailabilty of parent drug compounds. Inhibition of these enzymes results in elevated levels of parent drug, which can lead to increased pharmacological effects and toxicity especially in older patients.

Drugs such as benzodiazepines, paracetamol, and morphine are metabolized by conjugation. There has been little reported on the effect of ageing on conjugation.

Clearance: renal

With ageing, renal mass decreases, as does the glomerular filtration rate (GFR) and there is a reduced ability to concentrate urine and reduced thirst. Comorbidities such as hypertension and diabetes will potentiate the age-associated decline in renal function. GFR decreases at an average rate of 1 mL/min/year, and is often considered the most important age-related pharmacokinetic change. Reduction in GFR with age affects the clearance of many drugs such as digoxin, water-soluble antibiotics, non-steroidal anti-inflammatory drugs, diuretics, and lithium.

Declining renal function in old age cannot be quantified by measuring serum creatinine alone, as this is a reflection of muscle mass as well as GFR, which declines with age. Estimation of GFR is an essential component of good prescribing in older patients. Where drugs have a narrow therapeutic index (e.g. lithium, aminoglycosides, and digoxin), significant toxicity can occur if doses are not adjusted to account for renal disease and reduced excretion. Penicillins, on the other hand, have a wide therapeutic index and so dose modification based on age and renal disease is not necessary.

Elimination half-life (t₁/₂z)

The t1/2z is the time it takes for the plasma concentration to be reduced by 50% during the elimination phase. It is a function of both V and clearance (Cl):

$$t1/2z \; \alpha \; V/Cl.$$

It takes approximately five half-lives to reach steady state during chronic dosing and a similar time to remove the drug when dosing is stopped. For amiodarone with a t1/2z of at least 2 months in older patients, it would take at least 10 months to reach steady state or to remove the drug from the body after the last dose. For lipid-soluble drugs, t1/2z increases with age, due to both reduced clearance and increased V. For water-soluble drugs, such as lithium, the reduced V partially offsets the effect of reduced clearance on t1/2z.

Pharmacodynamics and the ageing process

Pharmacodynamics is the study of the effects of drugs. Drugs exert their effect by binding selectively to target molecules within the body. Drugs can be agonists (e.g. benzodiazepines—GABAa receptor agonists), partial agonists (e.g. buspirone—partial agonist at 5-HT1A receptors) or antagonists (e.g. mirtazapine, alpha-1-adrenergic, 5-HT2, and 5-HT3 receptor antagonist). Receptor activity and expression changes with age, for example there is evidence of reduced β-adrenoreceptor function in advancing age, reducing the cardiac response to β-antagonists and agonists (e.g. propanolol and salbutamol) in older patients.

The ageing cardiovascular system also has reduced aortic and large artery elasticity and compliance, leading to higher systolic, lower diastolic blood pressure, and a tendency towards left ventricular hypertrophy. There is also a reduction in heart rate and in baroreceptor sensitivity. This results in orthostatic intolerance leading to increased postural hypotension and falls. This can be exacerbated by the concomitant use of antihypertensives, and vasodilator drugs (e.g. α-blockers such as doxazosin and tamsulosin).

In the brain, cholinergic function and thermoregulation are impaired with age. Frail older patients are particularly prone to the adverse effects of neuroleptics, such as an increased susceptibility to delirium, extrapyramidal symptoms, and arrhythmias. There is increased sensitivity to the central nervous system effects of benzodiazepines, causing sedation and balance impairment at lower concentrations in older patients.

Conclusions

Ageing is characterized by functional changes in all organ systems that affect the pharmacokinetics and pharmacodynamics of many drugs used in older patients. The high prevalence of comorbidities and number of concomitantly prescribed drugs are also factors in the development of adverse drug reactions. A knowledge and appreciation of ageing processes, and their consequences, is necessary to ensure appropriate and safe prescribing in this age group.

Further reading

Anderson G, Kerluke K (1996). Distribution of prescription drug exposures in the elderly: description and implications. *J Clin Epidemiol* **49**: 929–35.

Brunton LL, Lazo JS, Parker KL (2006). *Goodman Gilman's the Pharmacological Basis of Therapeutics*, 11th edn. London, McGraw Hill.

Department of Health UK (2001). *National service framework for older people*. London, DH (www.dh.gov.uk).

Jackson SHD, Mangoni AA (2003). Age-related changes in pharmacokinetics and pharmacodynamics: basic principles and practical applications. *Br J Clin Pharmacol* **57**: 6–14.

Lazarou J, Pomeranz BH, Corey PN (1998). Incidence of adverse drug reactions in hospitalized patients: a meta-analysis of prospective studies. *JAMA* **279**: 1200–5.

McLean AJ, Couteur DG (2004). Ageing biology and geriatric pharmacology. *Pharmacol Rev* **56**: 163–84.

Rang HP, Dale MM, Ritter JM, et al (2007). *Rang & Dales Pharmacology*. 6th edn. London, Churchill Livingstone.

Medication review and evidence-based prescribing

Background

As the populations of developed countries age, the numbers of frailer, older and sicker people are steadily increasing. In many such patients, this phenomenon brings with it the related phenomena of complex comorbidity and polypharmacy. Research evidence consistently shows that polypharmacy is the single most consistent predictor of adverse drug events (ADEs). One of the ironies of evidence-based practice of medicine is that evidence-based therapeutics may actually promote polypharmacy. Examples of common chronic disorders in patients aged over 70 years and their evidence-derived therapeutics are as follows:

- ischaemic heart disease: aspirin, statin, beta-blocker, angiotensin-converting enzyme (ACE) inhibitor
- diabetes mellitus (type 2): metformin, sulphonylurea, ACE inhibitor, glitazone
- osteoporosis: calcium, vitamin D, bisphosphonate
- chronic obstructive pulmonary disease (COPD) (moderate severity): inhaled corticosteroid, long-acting beta-2-agonist, anticholinergic
- atrial fibrillation (AF): anticoagulant, digoxin (or beta-blocker)
- Parkinson's disease with functional disability: levodopa, monoamine oxidase type B inhibitor.

It is not difficult to appreciate how an older patient with a combination of some or all of these disorders may be prescribed 10 or more regular medicines. The risk of ADEs increases in a virtually linear fashion in tandem with increasing numbers of regular medicines. Therefore, one of the first considerations of the prescriber when dealing with a frail older patient is: what is the therapeutic target of this prescription and is it appropriate for this patient? For example, it is entirely reasonable to prescribe warfarin for a fit, active 72 year old with chronic atrial fibrillation and an independent life expectancy of 12–15 years. Conversely, it is wholly inappropriate to prescribe warfarin for a frail, dependent 87 year old with advanced dementia, who is housebound, with a life expectancy of no more than 18 months.

Medication compliance

Several factors are associated with poor drug compliance in older patients. These include

- lifetime medication need
- complex drug regimen
- drug side-effects
- poor cognitive function
- drugs dispensed from more than one pharmacy
- absence of home services or carers
- particular health and medication beliefs.

These should be considered when addressing drug prescribing and medication review in all older patients. It is generally accepted that poor compliers, i.e. those who take less than 40% of prescribed medication at widely varying intervals, make up approximately one-sixth of patients. Similarly, good compliers (defined as those who seldom miss doses and only occasionally take extra doses inadvertently) also make up about one-sixth of patients. It is generally accepted that regimen complexity rather than the number of tablets *per se* adversely affects patient compliance.

Medication review

Medication review by a physician/prescriber has the following aims:

- optimization of a patient's therapeutics
- ensuring that the therapeutic goals of treatment are clear to the patient, carer (where appropriate), and physician
- assessment of drug compliance
- avoidance of polypharmacy as much as possible
- looking for ADEs.

Medication use review (MUR) by a pharmacist has somewhat different aims from the physician/prescriber:

- patient/carer education about all medicines
- providing the most appropriate drug preparation, e.g. a liquid may be more suitable than a tablet for particular patients
- rationalization of tablets, e.g. a once daily slow-release preparation may be just as effective as a thrice daily preparation of the same drug
- screening for unnecessary or unused medicines
- seeking best value for money.

Both physician/prescriber and pharmacist are concerned about avoidance of inappropriate medication. There are a number of sets of criteria for inappropriate prescribing in older people, principally Beers' criteria and STOPP/START criteria. Although Beers' criteria have dominated the published literature for almost 20 years, there are several shortcomings that do not make them conducive to day-to-day clinical practice, namely their lack of systematic organization, inclusion of several drugs that are no longer prescribed in Europe, lack of mention of many common instances of inappropriate prescribing, and no account taken of errors of prescribing omission. These deficiencies of Beers' criteria led to the validation and publication of STOPP/START criteria in 2008.

Author's Tip

Most large-scale randomized controlled trials that form the basis for evidence-based prescribing are characterized by the lack or (in some cases) the complete absence of people over 80 years with multiple comorbidity. Prescribers must be cautious in extrapolating results of such drug trials to frail, older people.

Evidence-based prescribing and adverse drug events

Evidence-based prescribing is a fundamental part of evidence-based clinical practice, and its inherent value is undeniable. However, prescribing in frail, sicker, older people should not be an exercise in adding every evidence-based medication for every diagnosis, regardless of comorbid illnesses and overall prognosis. There is good evidence that older, sicker, frail people are usually excluded from large-scale randomized controlled trials (RCTs). Yet, in day-to-day practice, the results of RCTs showing clinical benefit from certain drugs continue to strongly influence drug selection for the very patients who are routinely excluded from the same RCTs.

Another issue with interpretation of RCT data is the decision to medicate or not, based on risk reduction.

Absolute risk reduction (ARR) is of much greater clinical importance than relative risk reduction (RRR). Pharmaceutical companies often quote RRR in preference to ARR resulting from their products in target patient populations because RRR is usually a much higher percentage number than ARR. For example, an RCT shows that a drug reduces the 5-year risk of stroke in an at-risk patient group from 20% to 15%. The prescriber may be impressed by a RRR statistic of 25%. However, the ARR statistic is 5% over 5 years, or an average of 1% per annum. The number of patients needed to treat (NNT) for this level of benefit is calculated as follows:

NNT = 100/ARR

In this example, the NNT is 100/(20 – 15), i.e. 20 patients receiving treatment over 5 years to prevent one extra stroke, equivalent to treating 100 patients for 1 year with the drug to prevent one extra stroke per annum. Furthermore, this level of benefit is dependent on the target patient population being closely similar to the intervention population in the reported RCT.

Strict adherence to RCT-based evidence often leads to polypharmacy, the most potent risk factor for ADE's in older people. ADE's in older people are often subtle and non-specific, e.g. worsening of cognitive function, falls, dizziness, new-onset incontinence, anorexia. Prescribers must always have a high index of suspicion of ADEs. Use of WHO-UMC criteria for ADE's (see Table 3.1) often clarifies the presence/absence of an ADE.

Polypharmacy is also associated with geriatric syndromes, such as acute and chronic cognitive impairment, falls, and urinary incontinence. So-called 'prescribing cascades' are another common result of polypharmacy, i.e. the addition of more drugs to alleviate the unrecognized side-effects of other drugs. Instead, the approach should be as follows.

• Ensure there is a clear *prima facie* indication for all drugs.
• Decide whether the overall intention of prescribing for any individual patient is for symptom relief only i.e. palliative, or if it should include a preventive approach on the basis of a probable life expectancy of 3 years or more with good quality of life.
• Consider the probability of drug–drug and drug–disease adverse interactions and endeavour to avoid these.
• Prescribing six or more regular daily medicines should trigger careful medication review and attempts at drug rationalization.
• Assess the patient's compliance on the basis of his/her cognitive status, visual acuity, ability to handle medication containers (bottles, blister packs, Dossette boxes, etc.) understanding of the purpose of each drug and

drug tolerability. Faulty compliance is dangerous for the patient and costly.

• Provide a clearly written or typed medication sheet, explaining the aim of each medication, the time to take each drug, and the duration of each prescription. This provides clarity for the patient and his/her carer.
• Review all medication when there is a major change in clinical status. For example, continuation of statin therapy in a patient just diagnosed with inoperable metastatic malignancy is not appropriate.

Barriers to medication changes

Doctors are often reluctant to change older patients' medication lists, in particular to reduce patients' number of prescription drugs. There are several reasons for reluctance to reduce the number of drugs, including

• fear of destabilizing a patient's condition, particularly if frail
• fear of litigation
• fear of failing to medicate all comorbid conditions
• fear of countermanding a consultant doctor's prescription ('If the consultant prescribed it, it must be right')
• fear of making some older patients confused by introducing a new drug regimen
• fear of inducing withdrawal syndromes with some long-term prescriptions, e.g. benzodiazepine, hypnotics.

Doctors may also be reluctant to introduce new drugs on the basis of:

• Lack of understanding of the magnitude of patient gain from particular drugs, e.g. major stroke risk reduction from anticoagulant therapy in older people with chronic atrial fibrillation.
• Therapeutic focus entirely on symptom relief, with neglect of preventive therapy where it is appropriate, e.g. failure to prescribe low-dose aspirin to an active, independent 81 year old following a recent myocardial infarction.
• A belief that all polypharmacy is intrinsically bad for all older patients at all times. In some instances, polypharmacy may be appropriate, beneficial, and well-tolerated in older people.

Prescribers should not be afraid to change older patients' medication when the circumstances warrant. In particular, suspected adverse drug–drug interactions and drug–disease interactions should be acted upon with cautious observation.

Author's Tip

Adverse drug reactions, drug–drug interactions, and drug–disease interactions may present with non-specific symptoms in older people. Often, the only way to test a theory of drug adversity is to withdraw the suspect drug at the appropriate rate when other causes of presenting symptoms have been excluded. Most older patients are very receptive to trials of medication withdrawal, if the prescriber explains clearly the reasons for proposing to withhold suspect drugs and is committed to careful monitoring of the patient following drug withdrawal.

Balance-of-risk prescribing

Not uncommonly, the prescriber is faced with situations where balance of risk needs to be considered. For example, a patient with a prior history of major haemorrhage

Table 3.1 WHO-UMC criteria* for adverse drug event

Categories of ADE	Time sequence	Other drugs/ disease ruled out	De- challenge	Re- challenge
Certain	Yes	Yes	Yes	Yes
Probable	Yes	Yes	Yes	No
Possible	Yes	No	No	No
Unlikely	No	No	No	No

* Derived from downloaded document at http//www.who-umc.org/graphics/4409.pdf.

from a duodenal ulcer and current atrial fibrillation presents with a minor ischaemic stroke in the absence of other clear-cut stroke risk factors. In this case, does the balance of risk favour avoidance of anticoagulant therapy to prevent recurrence of gastrointestinal bleeding or initiation of an anticoagulant to prevent major embolic stroke? Another example is that of a patient with mild–moderate dementia who is also handicapped by severe tremor due to concurrent Parkinson's disease, leading to very poor hygiene and repeated spillages of hot liquids. In this instance does the prescriber avoid anticholinergic therapy given the likelihood of worsening the cognitive impairment or proceed with therapy given that no other drug therapy is likely to relieve the tremor? There are many other instances where the prescriber must consider the balance of risk of proceeding with or avoiding certain drug therapies. The only guide in these situations is good clinical judgement and discussion with the patient and carer where appropriate. Clearly, patients receiving balance-of-risk medications must be monitored closely for ADE's.

Potentially inappropriate prescribing

Prescribing of potentially inappropriate medicines (PIMs) is a highly prevalent problem in older people. There are two main sets of criteria for potentially inappropriate prescribing, i.e. Beers' criteria and STOPP criteria (Appendix 3.1). The prevalence rates of one or more PIMs in various clinical settings according to Beers' criteria and STOPP criteria are shown in Table 3.2. Prescribing of PIMs is important because:

i   it is avoidable

ii   it is financially costly

iii it significantly increases the likelihood of ADEs (recent research data).

Errors of prescribing omission is the other important component in inappropriate prescribing in older people. Common important errors of prescribing omission are listed in the START criteria (Appendix 3.2). Errors of prescribing omission are also highly prevalent in various clinical settings. In primary care, 23% of independently living older people were not receiving one or more appropriate medicines; among older people presenting to hospital with acute illness, the figure is 44–57%.

Using STOPP/START criteria as a tool for medication review has recently been shown to significantly improve medication appropriateness (measured using the Medication Appropriateness Index) compared with standard pharmaceutical care. Another evidence-based intervention is structured review by a clinical pharmacist with organized feedback to physician prescribers leading to prescription amendments and optimization. This, coupled with individualized counselling of the patient and/or the patient's carer, has recently been shown to significantly enhance medication appropriateness. It remains to be seen whether application of STOPP/START criteria and structured pharmacist review reduces ADE's, drug costs, or healthcare utilization.

Further reading

Gallagher P, O'Mahony D (2008). Inappropriate prescribing in older people. *Rev Clin Gerontol* **18**: 65–76.

Gallagher P, Ryan C, Byrne S et al. (2008). STOPP (Screening Tool of Older Persons Prescriptions) and START (Screening Tool to Alert doctors to Right Treatment). Consensus validation. *Int J Clin Pharmacol Ther* **46**: 72–83.

Goodyer LI (2002). Compliance, concordance and polypharmacy in the elderly. In (Armour D and Cairns C eds) *Medicines in the Elderly*. Pharmaceutical Press, pp. 371–97.

Hanlon JT, Lindblad C, Maher RL, et al. (2003). Geriatric pharmacotherapy. In Tallis RC and Fillit HM (eds) *Brocklehurst's textbook of geriatric medicine and gerontology*, 6th edn. Churchill Livingstone, pp. 1289–96.

Hilmer SN, Gnjidic D (2009). The effects of polypharmacy in older adults. *Clin Pharmacol Ther*, **85**: 86–8.

Laroche ML, Charmes JP, Bouthier F, et al. (2009). Inappropriate medications in the elderly. *Clin Pharmacol Ther* **85**: 94–7.'

Medication review. In *Medicines for Older People: Implementing medicines-related aspects of the National Service Framework for Older People, 2001*, pp. 7–10 (http://www.doh.gov.uk/nsf/olderpeople.htm).

O'Mahony D, Gallagher P, Ryan C et al. (2010). STOPP & START criteria: A new approach to detecting potentially inappropriate prescribing in old age. *Eur Geriatr Med* **1**: 45–51.

Table 3.2 Prevalence rates of potentially inappropriate medications in various settings of clinical care of older people

Criteria	Primary care (%)	Secondary care (%)	Nursing home care (%)
STOPP	21	34–50	60
Beers	13–18	25–32	37

Appendix 3.1 STOPP (Screening Tool of Older People's Prescriptions) criteria for potentially inappropriate medication in older patients.

The following prescriptions are potentially inappropriate in persons aged 65 years of age or older.

A. Cardiovascular System

1. Digoxin at a long-term dose > 125 µg/day with impaired renal function (estimated GFR < 50 ml/min) *(increased risk of toxicity)*.
2. Loop diuretic for dependent ankle oedema only i.e. no clinical signs of heart failure *(no evidence of efficacy, compression hosiery usually more appropriate)*.
3. Loop diuretic as first-line monotherapy for hypertension *(safer, more effective alternatives available)*.
4. Thiazide diuretic with a history of gout *(may exacerbate gout)*.
5. Non-cardioselective beta-blocker with Chronic Obstructive Pulmonary Disease (COPD) *(risk of bronchospasm)*.
6. Beta-blocker in combination with verapamil *(risk of symptomatic heart block)*.
7. Use of diltiazem or verapamil with NYHA Class III or IV heart failure *(may worsen heart failure)*.
8. Calcium channel blockers with chronic constipation *(may exacerbate constipation)*.
9. Use of aspirin and warfarin in combination without histamine H2 receptor antagonist (except cimetidine because of interaction with warfarin) or proton pump inhibitor *(high risk of gastrointestinal bleeding)*.
10. Dipyridamole as monotherapy for cardiovascular secondary prevention *(no evidence for efficacy)*.
11. Aspirin with a past history of peptic ulcer disease without histamine H2 receptor antagonist or proton pump inhibitor *(risk of bleeding)*.
12. Aspirin at a dose of 150 mg per day or greater *(increased bleeding risk, no evidence for increased efficacy)*.
13. Aspirin with no history of coronary, cerebral or peripheral arterial symptoms or occlusive arterial event *(not indicated)*.
14. Aspirin to treat dizziness not clearly attributable to cerebrovascular disease *(not indicated)*.
15. Warfarin for first, uncomplicated deep venous thrombosis for longer than 6 months' duration *(no proven added benefit)*.
16. Warfarin for first uncomplicated pulmonary embolus for longer than 12 months' duration *(no proven benefit)*.
17. Aspirin, clopidogrel, dipyridamole, or warfarin with concurrent bleeding disorder *(high risk of bleeding)*.

*estimated GFR <50 mL/min.

B. Central Nervous System and Psychotropic Drugs

1. Tricyclic antidepressants (TCAs) with dementia *(risk of worsening cognitive impairment)*.
2. TCAs with glaucoma *(likely to exacerbate glaucoma)*.
3. TCAs with cardiac conductive abnormalities *(pro-arrhythmic effects)*.
4. TCAs with constipation *(likely to worsen constipation)*.
5. TCAs with an opiate or calcium channel blocker *(risk of severe constipation)*.
6. TCAs with prostatism or prior history of urinary retention *(risk of urinary retention)*.
7. Long-term (i.e. >1 month), long-acting benzodiazepines, e.g. chlordiazepoxide, fluazepam, nitrazepam, chlorazepate, and benzodiazepines, with long-acting metabolites, e.g. diazepam *(risk of prolonged sedation, confusion, impaired balance, falls)*.
8. Long-term (i.e. >1 month) neuroleptics as long-term hypnotics *(risk of confusion, hypotension, extrapyramidal side effects, falls)*.
9. Long-term neuroleptics (>1 month) in those with parkinsonism *(likely to worsen extrapyramidal symptoms)*.
10. Phenothiazines in patients with epilepsy *(may lower seizure threshold)*.
11. Anticholinergics to treat extrapyramidal side-effects of neuroleptic medications *(risk of anticholinergic toxicity)*.
12. Selective serotonin reuptake inhibitors (SSRIs) with a history of clinically significant hyponatraemia *(non-iatrogenic hyponatraemia <130 mmol/L within the previous 2 months)*.
13. Prolonged use (>1 week) of first-generation antihistamines, i.e. diphenhydramine, chlorpheniramine, cyclizine, promethazine *(risk of sedation and anticholinergic side effects)*.

C. Gastrointestinal System

1. Diphenoxylate, loperamide, or codeine phosphate for treatment of diarrhoea of unknown cause *(risk of delayed diagnosis, may exacerbate constipation with overflow diarrhoea, may precipitate toxic megacolon in inflammatory bowel disease, may delay recovery in unrecognized gastroenteritis)*.
2. Diphenoxylate, loperamide, or codeine phosphate for treatment of severe infective gastroenteritis, i.e. bloody diarrhoea, high fever, or severe systemic toxicity *(risk of exacerbation or protraction of infection)*.
3. Prochlorperazine (Stemetil) or metoclopramide with parkinsonism *(risk of exacerbating parkinsonism)*.
4. PPI for peptic ulcer disease at full therapeutic dosage for >8 weeks *(earlier discontinuation or dose reduction for maintenance/prophylactic treatment of peptic ulcer disease, oesophagitis or GORD indicated)*.
5. Anticholinergic antispasmodic drugs with chronic constipation *(risk of exacerbation of constipation)*.

D. Respiratory System

1. Theophylline as monotherapy for COPD. *(safer, more effective alternatives; risk of adverse effects due to narrow therapeutic index)*
2. Systemic corticosteroids instead of inhaled corticosteroids for maintenance therapy in moderate-severe COPD *(unnecessary exposure to long-term side-effects of systemic steroids)*.
3. Nebulized ipratropium with glaucoma *(may exacerbate glaucoma)*.

E. Musculoskeletal System

1. Non-steroidal anti-inflammatory drug (NSAID) with history of peptic ulcer disease or gastrointestinal bleeding, unless with concurrent histamine H2 receptor antagonist, PPI, or misoprostol *(risk of peptic ulcer relapse)*.

2. NSAID with moderate–severe hypertension (moderate: 160/100–179/109 mmHg; severe: ≥180/110 mmHg) (*risk of exacerbation of hypertension*).

3. NSAID with heart failure (*risk of exacerbation of heart failure*).

4. Long-term use of NSAID (>3 months) for relief of mild joint pain in osteoarthtitis (*simple analgesics preferable and usually as effective for pain relief*)

5. Warfarin and NSAID together (*risk of gastrointestinal bleeding*).

6. NSAID with chronic renal failure* (*risk of deterioration in renal function*). *estimated GFR 20–50 mL/min.

7. Long-term corticosteroids (>3 months) as monotherapy for rheumatoid arthritis or osteoarthritis (*risk of major systemic corticosteroid side-effects*).

8. **Long-term NSAID or colchicine for chronic treatment of gout where there is no contraindication to allopurinol** (*allopurinol first choice prophylactic drug in gout*)

F. Urogenital System

1. Bladder antimuscarinic drugs with dementia (*risk of increased confusion, agitation*).

2. Bladder antimuscarinic drugs with chronic glaucoma (*risk of acute exacerbation of glaucoma*).

3. Bladder antimuscarinic drugs with chronic constipation (*risk of exacerbation of constipation*).

4. Bladder antimuscarinic drugs with chronic prostatism (*risk of urinary retention*).

5. Alpha-blockers in males with frequent incontinence, i.e. one or more episodes of incontinence daily (*risk of urinary frequency and worsening of incontinence*).

6. Alpha-blockers with long-term urinary catheter *in situ*, i.e. more than 2 months (*drug not indicated*).

G. Endocrine System

1. Glibenclamide or chlorpropamide with type 2 diabetes mellitus (*risk of prolonged hypoglycaemia*).

2. Beta-blockers in those with diabetes mellitus and frequent hypoglycaemic episodes, i.e. ≥1 episode per month (*risk of masking hypoglycaemic symptoms*).

3. Oestrogens with a history of breast cancer or venous thromboembolism (*increased risk of recurrence*)

4. Oestrogens without progestogen in patients with intact uterus (*risk of endometrial cancer*).

H. Drugs that adversely affect those prone to falls (≥1 fall in past three months)

1. Benzodiazepines (sedative, may cause reduced sensorium, impair balance).

2. Neuroleptic drugs (may cause gait dyspraxia, Parkinsonism).

3. First-generation antihistamines (sedative, may impair sensorium).

4. Vasodilator drugs known to cause hypotension in those with persistent postural hypotension i.e. recurrent >20 mmHg drop in systolic blood pressure (risk of syncope, falls).

5. Long-term opiates in those with recurrent falls (risk of drowsiness, postural hypotension, vertigo).

I. Analgesic Drugs

1. Use of long-term powerful opiates, e.g. morphine or fentanyl, as first-line therapy for mild–moderate pain (*WHO analgesic ladder not observed*).

2. Regular opiates for more than 2 weeks in those with chronic constipation without concurrent use of laxatives (*risk of severe constipation*).

3. Long-term opiates in those with dementia unless indicted for palliative care or management of moderate/severe chronic pain syndrome (*risk of exacerbation of cognitive impairment*).

J. Duplicate Drug Classes

Any regular duplicate drug class prescription, e.g. two concurrent opiates, NSAIDs, SSRIs, loop diuretics, ACE inhibitors (*optimization of monotherapy within a single drug class should be observed prior to considering a new class of drug*). This excludes duplicate prescribing of drugs that may be need on an as required basis, e.g. inhaled beta-2-agonists (long and short acting) for asthma or COPD, and opiates for management of breakthrough pain.

Appendix 3.2 START (Screening Tool to Alert to Right Treatments) criteria for potentially inappropriate medication omission

These medications should be considered for people ≥65 years of age with the following conditions, where no contraindication to prescription exists.

A. Cardiovascular System

1. Warfarin in the presence of chronic atrial fibrillation.

2. Aspirin in the presence of chronic atrial fibrillation, where warfarin is contraindicated, but not aspirin.

3. Aspirin or clopidogrel with a documented history of atherosclerotic coronary, cerebral, or peripheral vascular disease in patients with sinus rhythm.

4. Antihypertensive therapy where systolic blood pressure consistently >160 mmHg, where life expectancy exceeds 5 years.

5. Statin therapy with a documented history of coronary, cerebral or peripheral vascular disease, where the patient's functional status remains independent for activities of daily living and life expectancy is >5 years.

6. Angiotensin-converting enzyme (ACE) inhibitor with chronic heart failure.

7. ACE inhibitor following acute myocardial infarction.

8. Beta-blocker with chronic stable angina.

B. Respiratory System

1. Regular inhaled beta-2-agonist or anticholinergic agent for mild to moderate asthma or COPD.

2. Regular inhaled corticosteroid for moderate–severe asthma or COPD, where predicted FEV1 <50%.

3. Home continuous oxygen with documented chronic type 1 respiratory failure (pO_2 <8.0 kPa, pCO_2 <6.5 kPa) or type 2 respiratory failure (pO_2 <8.0 kPa, pCO_2 >6.5 kPa).

C. Central Nervous System

1. L-dopa in idiopathic Parkinson's disease with definite functional impairment and resultant disability.

2. Antidepressant drug in the presence of moderate–severe depressive symptoms lasting at least 3 months.

D. Gastrointestinal System

1. Proton pump inhibitor with severe gastro-oesophageal acid reflux disease or peptic stricture requiring dilatation.

2. Fibre supplement for chronic, symptomatic diverticular disease with constipation.

E. Musculoskeletal System

1. Disease-modifying anti-rheumatic drug (DMARD) with active moderate–severe rheumatoid disease lasting >12 weeks.
2. Bisphosphonates in patients taking maintenance oral corticosteroid therapy.
3. Calcium and vitamin D supplement in patients with known osteoporosis (radiological evidence or previous fragility fracture or acquired dorsal kyphosis).

F. Endocrine System

1. Metformin with type 2 diabetes +/– metabolic syndrome (in the absence of renal impairment*).
2. ACE inhibitor or angiotensin receptor blocker in diabetes with nephropathy i.e. overt urinalysis proteinuria or micoralbuminuria (>30 mg/24 h) +/– serum biochemical renal impairment*.

3. Antiplatelet therapy in diabetes mellitus if one or more coexisting major cardiovascular risk factor present (hypertension, hypercholesterolaemia, smoking history).
4. Statin therapy in diabetes mellitus if one or more co-existing major cardiovascular risk factor present.

*estimated GFR <50 mL/min.

Drug development in older people

Introduction

The authors of other topics in this section have highlighted that older patients are an important 'special group' when prescribing drug therapy. This is specifically due to changes to drug pharmacokinetics (PK) and pharmacodynamics (PD) as people age, but in addition older patients are more likely to develop adverse drug reactions (ADRs) through polypharmacy.

Although older patients are more likely to take drugs that have been investigated in large-scale clinical trials, it is incongruous that not only do very few of these clinical trials include older patients but even less are specifically designed to investigate the efficacy and tolerability of these drugs in older people.

This topic will review the current thinking regarding drug development in older people.

Overview of drug development

The development of an individual drug can take at least 10 years and costs approximately £500 million. After 3–4 years of laboratory investigation, a drug will be investigated in a series of clinical trials to support its licence.

- Phase 1: healthy volunteers (50–100) to gauge PK/PD data, dosing and potential ADRs
- Phase 2: patient volunteers (100–200) to further identify best dosing regimen and tolerability
- Phase 3: large-scale clinical trials (>3000) test the drug against placebo or current best therapy to compare efficacy and tolerability.

Once a drug is granted its licence and is marketed, further larger scale clinical trials may be funded to provide additional evidence to support the drug's use in specific situations to extend its licence or alternatively involve pharmacovigilance (Phase 4).

How old is old in clinical trials?

Arbitrarily and perhaps controversially, patients over 65 years have conventionally been considered as older people. The European Medicines Agency (EMA) suggest 65 years as the upper age of adulthood, but a new report resulting from a joint European Forum for Good Clinical Practice (EFGCP) and European CRO Federation (EUCROF) suggests this should be increased to 75 years. The Food and Drug Administration have provided draft guidance to the pharmaceutical industry (September 2009) suggesting that submissions should include clinical data for patients aged 65–74 and for those aged 75 and older to assess the consistency of the treatment effect and safety profile in older people. Less controversial is the clear reality that most countries' populations are becoming older.

Why is there a need for specific clinical trials in older people?

Many clinical trials have excluded older patients. For example, the incidence of cancer in patients aged 60 and older is 61%, but only 25% of this older age group were recruited into trials sponsored by the National Cancer Institute in the USA. Previously, doctors have tended to 'extrapolate' results in younger patients to older individuals. Primarily this is due to the lack of evidence in older patients, but it may also be unwise. As people age, they are more likely to develop cardiac, renal, and liver disease that can significantly influence drug elimination and clearance.

Changes to patients' body composition and plasma proteins also change the way in which drugs are metabolized. Polypharmacy is also an important determinant of the effectiveness and/or risk of drug therapy.

Incidentally this 'extrapolation' of clinical data is often done in a haphazard manner. The STOPP–START criteria have been developed to reduce overutilization (e.g. duplicate treatments) or underutilization (e.g. statin, warfarin) of drug therapy.

What are the barriers to recruiting older patients?

- Arbitrarily defined age limits.
- Patients with comorbidities who are likely to fulfil one or more of the exclusion criteria.
- Anxiety regarding increased risk of ADRs.
- Ethical concerns/family pressure to avoid the uncertainty of a clinical trial.
- Lack of experience among research personnel or unwilling to invest the extra time required.
- Lack of knowledge within the pharmaceutical industry.

How might recruitment be improved?

The pharmaceutical industry is changing as a result of pressure from regulators and others, but also from within.

The FDA, MHRA, and ABPI in addition to the Committee for Propriety Medicinal Products and the International Conference on Harmonisation have provided guidance. For example, the ABPI 2007 guidelines for Phase 1 clinical trials quote 'Trials of *drugs* in elderly subjects are justified if the product is intended for use in the elderly, and especially if its effects and metabolism might differ from those in younger subjects'.

The recent joint EFGCP and EUCROF workshop in April 2010 has further advised changes to the regulation of clinical trials in older people:

- greater expertise within the EMA
- public consultation regarding research into older people
- the inclusion of geriatric expertise in ethics committees
- the inclusion and audit of geriatric issues in research training
- further development of informed consent and assent.

However, it is likely that the use of mandated regulator-imposed studies in older people would meet resistance from the pharmaceutical industry because of the additional cost and subsequent delays in bringing their new product to market.

The EU-funded PREDICT study set out to determine, from principle investigators within the EU, the rationale of including older people in major clinical trials. Eighty-seven per cent of respondents agreed that exclusion based on age alone was now unjustified. As a result of the information provided by this study, the consortium launched the European Charter for Older People in Clinical Trials in February 2010 encompassing six domains:

1 Older people have the right to access evidence-based treatments

2 Promoting the inclusion of older people in clinical trials and preventing discrimination.

3 Clinical trials should be made as practicable as possible for older people.

4 The safety of clinical trials in older people.

5 Outcome measures should be relevant for older people.

6 The values of older people participating in clinical trials should be respected.

Finally, a number of methods have been identified to improve recruitment

- Use methods geared to older patients (e.g. radio advertising rather than email flyers).
- Expand the inclusion criteria to prevent low levels of recruitment reducing the power of the study.
- Actively liaise with family members who may be able to support their older relative.
- Provide more specific informed consent.

What is the future of research into older people?

It is increasingly likely that there will be more dedicated clinical trials to provide a greater evidence base for drug prescribing in older people. In addition, specific conditions, e.g. involuntary weight loss or sarcopenia, will need to be defined more clearly to allow research themes to be developed that will provide evidence to support treating these conditions of old age.

At the time of writing this topic, the author saw a magazine advert by a UK-based pharmaceutical company directed specifically at recruiting older people into Phase 1 clinical trials.

Further reading

Crome P (2003). What's different about older people? *Toxicology* **192**: 49–54.

Evans WJ (2011). Drug discovery and development for ageing: opportunities and challenges. *Phil Trans R Soc B* **366**: 113–19.

Lewis JH, Kilgore ML, Goldman DP, *et al.* (2003). Participation of patients 65 years of age or older in cancer clinical trials. *J Clin Oncol* **21**: 1383–9.

Riddaa I, MacIntyrea CR, Lindley RI, *et al.* (2010). Difficulties in recruiting older people in clinical trials: an examination of barriers and solutions. *Vaccine* **28**: 901–6.

Shah RR (2004). Drug development and use in the older: search for the right dose and dosing regimen. *Br J Clin Pharmacol* **58**: 452–69.

Townsley CA, Selby R, Siu LL (2005). Systematic review of barriers to the recruitment of older patients with cancer onto clinical trials. *J Clin Oncol* **23**: 3112–24.

Ward P (2010). Geriatric Trials Spark Debate: A new report from EFGCP and EUCROF suggests changes to geriatric trials. Applied Clinical Trials (http://appliedclinicaltrialsonline.findpharma.com/appliedclinicaltrials/Regulatory+Articles/Geriatric-Trials-Spark-Debate/ArticleStandard/Article/detail/686207?contextCategoryId=3300&ref=25).

www.predictEU.org

Adverse drug reactions including drug interactions

Adverse drug reactions (ADRs), including drug interactions, are common in older patients and are an important cause of morbidity, mortality, and health resource utilization. It is estimated that up to 35% of community-dwelling older adults and over 50% of nursing home residents experience at least one ADR each year. Between 5% and 20% of hospital admissions of older patients are attributable to ADRs. The incidence of new ADRs in hospitalized older adults is reported to be as high as 6% and is associated with increased length of stay, greater cost and higher mortality. ADRs occur three times more commonly in people aged 65 years and over than in younger individuals, although this may be an underestimation due to considerable discrepancies in the definition, recognition, and reporting of ADRs in older individuals.

An ADR is typically defined as a noxious and unintended event that occurs at doses used in man for prophylaxis, diagnosis, therapy, or modification of physiological functions. Though easy to define, ADRs often manifest as non-specific signs and symptoms in older patients including lethargy (benzodiazepines), fatigue (beta-blockers), and constipation (calcium antagonists), which may not be perceived as being drug induced. At the more severe end of the spectrum, ADRs can result in gastrointestinal bleeding (non-steroidal anti-inflammatory drugs (NSAIDs), renal failure (ACE inhibitors), falls with resultant injury such as fractures, and, psychiatric and behavioural disturbances, e.g. cognitive decline (anticholinergic drugs), hallucinations (levodopa), depression (beta-blockers, indoramine, tetrabenazine, benzodiazepines), and impulse control disorders including pathological gambling, hypersexuality, and obsessive-compulsive behaviours (dopamine agonists). Such behavioural symptoms may not manifest for months after commencing a drug. However, failure to recognize such symptoms as potentially being drug induced often results in the unnecessary prescription of another drug (e.g. an antipsychotic or antidepressant), thereby increasing the risk of further ADRs.

More than 80% of ADRs in older people are 'type A' in nature, i.e. they are attributable to a predictable accentuation of the known pharmacological effect of a drug due to age-related changes in drug pharmacokinetics (absorption, distribution, metabolism, and excretion) and pharmacodynamics (how the body responds to a drug at the receptor or post-receptor level). 'Type A' ADRs are usually avoidable and typically involve commonly prescribed drugs such as anticoagulants, NSAIDs, digoxin, diuretics, hypoglycaemic agents, vasodilators, anticholinergics, sedative hypnotics, and antipsychotics.

'Type B' (idiosyncratic) reactions are less common than 'type A' reactions, although some important 'type B' reactions appear to be more common in older than younger patients, e.g. hepatotoxicity due to co-amoxiclav or flucloxacillin.

Several other factors contribute to the greater propensity for ADRs in older patients.

- Older patients consume an average of five prescription drugs and three non-prescription drugs per day, thereby increasing the risk of drug–drug and drug–disease interactions. Indeed, the number of drugs consumed is exponentially linked to the risk of ADR.
- Age-related changes in homeostatic mechanisms are often accentuated by drugs, e.g. orthostatic hypotension may be more pronounced in older patients taking alpha-adrenergic blocking drugs or diuretics.
- Inappropriate prescribing is common in older patients. Drugs are often prescribed without clear-cut indication, for excessive duration or at too high a dose without consideration for age-related changes in pharmacodynamics (e.g. increased sensitivity to opiates or warfarin), pharmacokinetics (e.g. use of high-dose digoxin or lithium in older patients with renal impairment) and potential for drug–drug and drug–disease interactions.
- Prescribing cascades are common in older patients, i.e. a new drug is prescribed to treat symptoms that are caused by another drug instead of stopping or reducing the dose of the harmful drug.
- Older patients who are attending multiple physicians and multiple dispensing pharmacies are at greater risk of ADRs.

Drug–drug interactions

Drug–drug interactions are often pharmacokinetic in nature, i.e. one drug may affect the absorption, distribution, metabolism, or excretion of another drug with resultant changes in plasma drug concentration and altered clinical response.

The rate of drug absorption can be reduced by anticholinergic drugs (delayed gastric emptying) or increased by metoclopramide (accelerated gastric emptying). The bioavailability of digoxin, warfarin and quinolone antibiotics can be reduced by antacids and cholestyramine.

The most frequent pharmacokinetic drug–drug interactions involve inhibition or induction of hepatic cytochrome P450 isoenzymes, which are responsible for the metabolism of most drugs. Enzyme inhibition can lead to a rapid reduction in drug metabolism with resultant toxic drug accumulation and greater potential for ADRs, e.g. clarithromycin may impede the metabolism of simvastatin through the inhibition of cytochrome P450 3A4 isoenzyme, thereby increasing the risk of myopathy and hepatotoxicity. Similarly, haloperidol may reduce the metabolism of amitriptyline through inhibition of cytochrome P450 2D6, with resultant potential for toxic effects including tachyarrhythmias and orthostatic hypotension.

Hepatic metabolizing enzyme induction may take days to weeks to become clinically apparent. A drug may induce its own metabolism, e.g. carbamazepine induces the cytochrome P450 3A4 isoenzyme (which metabolizes carbamazepine) but may also accelerate the metabolism and clearance of another drug or unrelated substrate. Powerful enzyme inducers include carbamazepine, phenytoin and rifampicin (see Table 3.3). Should these drugs be coprescribed with drugs that are metabolized by cytochrome P450 3A4 (e.g. felodipine, nifedipine, verapamil, atorvastatin, and losartan), the increased P450 3A4 activity (as a result of enzyme induction) can reduce the substrate drug concentrations below their therapeutic levels, thereby increasing the risk of treatment failure. Tobacco can induce the CYP 1A2 isoenzymes, leading to increased metabolism of theophylline, amitriptyline, and warfarin. A complete list of drug–drug interactions involving the cytochrome P450 enzyme system is available in most comprehensive pharmacology texts (see Further reading).

The pharmacodynamic response to one drug may be affected by another drug. Indeed the toxicity of drug

Table 3.3 Inhibitors and inducers of the hepatic cytochrome P450 enzymes

Enzyme inhibitors	Enzyme inducers
Amiodarone	Carbamazepine
Fluconazole, miconazole, ketoconazole	Ethanol
Erythromycin, clarithromycin	Isoniazid
Sulphonamides	Phenytoin
Cimetidine	Phenobarbital
Ciprofloxacin	Rifampicin
Diltiazem, verapamil	Primidone
Fluoxetine, paroxetine	St John's Wort

combinations in older patients may be synergistic, i.e. greater than the sum of the risks of toxicity of each individual drug. The risk of peptic ulcer in older patients using NSAIDs is increased fourfold compared with non-users. The relative increased risk of peptic ulcer in older users of oral corticosteroids is 10%. However, the risk of peptic ulcer in older patients using both NSAIDs and corticosteroids is 15 times that of non-users of either agent. Similar synergistic pharmacodynamic responses can be seen with the combination of anticoagulants and NSAIDs, and in older users of drugs with anticholinergic or sedating properties. Pharmacodynamic interactions may also reduce drug efficacy in older patients, e.g. NSAIDs can reduce the antihypertensive effect of ACE inhibitors, beta-blockers and thiazide diuretics. Some clinically important drug interactions in older patients are detailed in Table 3.4.

Warfarin and drug interactions
Warfarin is clearly beneficial when used for the treatment of venous thromboembolism and for the prevention of cardioembolic disease in older patients with atrial fibrillation, mural thrombus, or heart valve replacements. However, drug interactions with warfarin are numerous. An increase or decrease in the anticoagulant effect of warfarin should be anticipated with coadministration of the drugs listed in Table 3.5.

Drug–disease interactions
Older patients have a higher prevalence of illness than younger patients and are often prescribed multiple drugs to treat multiple concurrent illnesses. However, many drugs may worsen pre-existing conditions due to altered pharmacokinetics and pharmacodynamics in older patients. Some clinically important drug–disease interactions are detailed in Table 3.6.

Prevention of adverse drug reactions in older patients
The following procedures should minimize the risk of ADRs in older patients.
• Establish the correct diagnosis.
• Document all comorbidities and drug history, including previous ADRs and reasons for drug discontinuation.
• Document all prescribed drugs including over-the-counter and herbal preparations. Ensure there is a clear-cut indication for each drug.
• Discontinue unnecessary drugs, but beware of withdrawal.
• Screen for drug–drug and drug–disease interactions, particularly when adding a new drug. The STOPP/START

Table 3.4 Clinically important drug–drug interactions in older patients

Drug	Drug	Interaction	Effect
Antihypertensive agents	Vasodilators, antipsychotics, TCA	Combined hypotensive effect	Orthostatic hypotension, falls
Antihypertensive agents	NSAIDs	NSAID antagonizes hypotensive effect	↓ antihypertensive effect
Calcium channel blockers (CCBs)	Enzyme inducers	↑ clearance of CCB	↓ antihypertensive effect
Potassium sparing diuretics	ACE inhibitors, spironolactone	Combined potassium sparing effects	↓ renal function, hyperkalaemia
Aspirin	NSAIDs, oral corticosteroids	↑ risk of peptic ulceration	Peptic ulceration
Digoxin	Diuretics	Diuretic induced hypokalaemia	↑ effect of digoxin (arrhythmia, toxicity)
Digoxin	Amiodarone, diltiazem, verapamil	↓ clearance of digoxin	↑ effect of digoxin (arrhythmia, toxicity)
Lithium	NSAIDs, thiazide diuretics	↓ clearance of lithium	↑ effect of lithium, lithium toxicity
TCAs	Enzyme inhibitors	↓ clearance of TCA	arrthythmia, confusion, orthostatic hypotension, falls
Phenothiazines	Drugs with anticholinergic properties	Combined anticholinergic effects	Confusion, constipation, urinary retention, dry mouth
Phenytoin	Enzyme inhibitors	↓ clearance of phenytoin	↑ effect of phenytoin
Theophylline	Enzyme inhibitors, quinolones	↓ clearance of theophylline	↑ effect of theophylline (toxicity)
Thyroxine	Enzyme inducers	↑ clearance of thyroxine	↓ effect of thyroxine

TCA, tricyclic antidepressant; NSAID, non-steroidal anti-inflammatory drug.

Table 3.5 Drug interactions with warfarin

Increased anticoagulant effect	Inhibition of warfarin metabolism	Pharmacodynamic augmentation of anticoagulant effect
	Amiodarone	Clofibrate
	Chloramphenicol	Gemfibrozil
	Cimetidine	Phenytoin
	Ciprofloxacin	Salicylates
	Clarithromycin, erythromycin	Tamoxifen
	Fluconazole, itraconazole, Ketoconazole	Thyroxine
	Mefanamic acid	
	Metronidazole, sulphonamides	
Reduced anticoagulant effect	↓ absorption and ↑ elimination of warfarin	Pharmacodynamic antagonism of warfarin
	Cholestyramine, colestipol	Vitamin K

criteria for potentially inappropriate prescribing in older patients list commonly encountered drug–drug and drug–disease interactions.

- Ensure that a new symptom is not an adverse effect of an already prescribed drug.
- Avoid prescription of a drug with a narrow therapeutic index when equally effective alternatives (including non-pharmacological measures) are available, e.g. avoid digoxin for the treatment of atrial arrhythmias in older patients with renal impairment if no contraindication to other rate-controlling drugs such as beta-blockers or calcium antagonists exists, i.e. choose the safest possible agent.
- Establish a therapeutic target for each drug. This is especially important in frail older patients where the potential for clinical benefit and the scientific evidence base for use of the drug may be slim, e.g. it may not be appropriate to prescribe the full battery of recommended secondary prevention in a frail dependent older patient with cardiovascular or cerebrovascular disease and reduced life expectancy because of the high potential for ADRs.
- Start with the lowest effective dose for appropriately prescribed drugs and adjust dose in the presence of

renal or hepatic impairment (refer to *British National Formulary*).
- Review therapeutic targets regularly and discontinue drug if ineffective.
- Arrange periodic follow-up when a drug–drug interaction or drug–disease interaction is anticipated, e.g. monitor serum potassium if prescribed ACE inhibitor and spironolactone, monitor international normalized ratio (INR) if prescribed warfarin and amiodarone.
- Simplify the drug regimen as much as possible and arrange for drugs to be administered under supervision if patient has cognitive impairment.
- Inform patient or caregiver of potential adverse effects of medications.
- Regular review (at least 6 monthly) of long-term therapy is essential in older patients.

Management of drug interactions in older patients

- Discontinue the drug causing the interaction or the drug affected by the interaction. If this is not possible, then decrease the dose or change the time of the administration.
- If necessary, the suspected drug should be substituted with another of similar efficacy but lower potential for interactions.
- Monitor drug concentrations where possible.
- Prescribe drugs on a regular basis with instructions to hold if necessary, rather than 'as required'.
- Document all suspected ADRs and communicate these to other health professionals involved in the care of the patient.

Further reading

Gallagher P, O'Mahony D (2008). Inappropriate prescribing in older people. *Rev Clin Gerontol* **18**: 65–76.

Gallagher P, Ryan C, Byrne S, et al. (2008). STOPP (Screening Tool of Older Persons Prescriptions) and START (Screening Tool to Alert doctors to Right Treatment). Consensus validation. *Int J Clin Pharmacol Ther* **46**: 72–83.

Golan D, Tashjian A, Armstrong E, et al. (2008). Drug metabolism and drug toxicity. In *Principles of Pharmacology, the Pathophysiologic Basis of Drug Therapy*. Lippincott Williams & Wilkins, pp. 49–75.

Mallet L, Spinewine A, Huang A (2007). The challenge of managing drug interactions in elderly people. *Lancet* **370**: 185–91.

Mangoni A, Jackson S (2004). Age-related changes in pharmacokinetics and pharmacodynamics: basic principles and practical applications. *Br J Clin Pharmacol* **57**: 6–14.

Table 3.6 Clinically important drug–disease interactions in older patients

Disease or condition	Drugs	Effect of drug on disease or condition
Cognitive impairment/dementia	Anticholinergics, benzodiazepines, TCAs, antipsychotics, opiates	↑ confusion, delirium
Falls	Benzodiazepines, opiates, anticholinergics, vasodilators, antipsychotics	↑ risk of falls, sedation, gait instability
Orthostatic hypotension	Diuretics, levodopa, anticholinergics, vasodilators, TCAs	Dizziness, syncope, falls, hip fracture
Osteopenia/osteoporosis	Corticosteroids	Fracture
Cardiac failure	Verapamil, disopyramide	Exacerbation of heart failure
Renal failure	NSAIDs, aminoglycosides, radiological contrast	Acute kidney injury
Peptic ulcer disease	NSAIDs, anticoagulants	Haemorrhagic peptic ulcer
Hypertension	NSAIDs, high sodium content drugs	↑ blood pressure
Benign prostatic hyperplasia	Alpha agonists, anticholinergics	Urinary retention

Acute illness overview

The frail older person in the emergency department

Background

In England over the next 20 years, the number of people aged 85 and over is set to increase by two-thirds, compared to a 10% growth in the overall population.

This ongoing demographic shift has already resulted in an increase in the number of older people attending the emergency department (ED) and accessing acute care services. A small proportion of this population is especially vulnerable because of varying combinations of health and social care problems, and can be classified as frail and at increased risk of adverse health outcomes, prolonged hospital stay, or readmission.

Epidemiology

Many frail older people attend EDs every day and constitute an increasing cohort with complex medical needs. Older patients use EDs more than younger patients, use more resources during a visit, present with more urgent clinical problems, and are more likely to reattend.

Hospital statistics for England reveal that nearly 30% of ambulance transfers to EDs are for patients more than 70 years of age, who account for 15% of all attendances. The figures also show that although older patients are seen and assessed as quickly as younger ones, they spend much longer times in EDs and have a higher admission rate.

An ED frailty mapping exercise showed that despite being a very small proportion of the attendees, frail older people accounted for a significant proportion of breaches in the 4-hour emergency access target and constituted a disproportionate fraction of the total acute admissions.

Frail older people have complex needs spanning health and social care, and key markers of frailty such as confusion, immobility, incontinence, and falls need to be identified in this group to improve quality of care.

Presentation

About a third of all presentations are related to injuries associated with a fall, and the majority of the remainder is due to an illness. Important conditions leading to such presentation are discussed below.

Falls

Each year, over 700 000 older people in the UK attend EDs following a fall and account for over 4 million bed days annually in England alone. Injurious falls, including over 60 000 hip fractures annually, are the leading cause of accident-related mortality in older people. Falls may also result in loss of confidence, activity restriction, reduced functional ability, and thus increased dependency on carers and services. A small but important number of unexplained falls are associated with cardiovascular syncope.

National audits show that management of falls and bone health remain suboptimal within EDs and Minor Injury Units (MIUs).

It is important to remember that signs of abuse may be wrongly attributed to falls, and current estimates suggest over 300 000 older people are being abused in the UK at any time.

Delirium and dementia

These are common conditions affecting up to 30% of all older people admitted to hospitals. This may be a manifestation of another underlying serious condition including potentially life-threatening ones such as sepsis, acute coronary syndromes, stroke, and severe metabolic abnormalities. It may be difficult to differentiate delirium from dementia in the ED but for purposes of risk management it is better to rule out causes as in an acute confusional state.

Poor identification and inappropriate management of delirium contributes towards mortality and morbidity, including increased length of hospital stay.

Assessment

Frail older people in EDs should be assessed and managed promptly with special consideration of their physical, emotional, and cognitive states and reference to privacy, dignity, socio-cultural, and religious issues.

Specific assessment needs include pain and need for analgesia, pressure areas, cognitive state, mental health, injuries associated with falls, gait and balance, continence, hypothermia, and social care. It may be difficult to deliver comprehensive geriatric assessment in the ED.

Valid assessment tools, such as Identification of Seniors at Risk, are useful to communicate further management needs in the community to reduce risk of readmission, functional decline, institutionalization, and death in older patients.

In the acute care setting, non-specific presentation and the need for a biopsychosocial model of assessment (as opposed to a biomedical model) pose considerable clinical challenges.

Pitfalls in assessing illness and trauma include the absence of a raised white cell count and pyrexia in sepsis and a normal heart rate in hypovolaemia. Pharmacological agents prescribed for comorbidities also influence such altered responses. Delayed presentation, for example with intracranial bleeds following head trauma and non-visualization of hip fractures on initial radiographic examination, adds to the complexity of assessing the frail older person.

The emotional response to trauma and illness may be just as unpredictable as the physiological. Fears and anxieties over loss of independence may be heightened when frail older people are unwell. Patients with delirium and dementia need special tools for assessment of pain.

The ED represents the interface between primary and secondary care, and the right kind of resources, processes, and information for assessing frail older patients is necessary for maximal efficiency in discharging safely and admitting appropriately.

Management

Pain management using paracetamol and opiates remains the cornerstone because of the renal and gastrointestinal threats from non-steroidal anti-inflammatory drugs. However, regional anaesthesia and inhaled nitrous oxide are good adjuncts for fractures and for a morphine-sparing effect.

Fluid management needs to be judicious with careful balance between speed of replenishment versus inciting iatrogenic pulmonary oedema often aided by pre-existing cardiac and renal impairment. Thus in sepsis, the typical 20 mL/kg body weight initial bolus may need to be halved. At the same time, invasive measurement and monitoring may be inappropriate for the bed- and wheelchair-dependent older patient, including the need for urinary catheterization.

Pharmacological therapy needs to take into consideration changes in pharmacodynamics and pharmacokinetics associated with altered liver metabolism, renal clearance, and accentuated neurological and cardiovascular side-effects.

Frail older patients do not necessarily need admitting to hospital and it is important to try and establish baseline functional state, which off course may be difficult in the absence of adequate accompanying information. Rapid assessment in outpatient clinics and ambulatory care may be good alternatives, allowing the balance between prevention of admission and early specialist assessment.

Geriatric interventions based in the ED have not yet clearly been shown to improve outcomes, including improved discharge rates, lower admission and readmission rates, and decreased visits to the ED.

For those needing admission, specialized geriatric units such as for stroke, delirium, orthogeriatric services, fast track pathways, access to multidisciplinary teams, and integrated health and social care management are paramount in effective care planning, including decreasing length of hospital stay.

Irrespective of specifics, the care of frail older people needs to be integrated across healthcare settings with the ED-based care forming an integral part of that continuum.

Future implications

Newer models of care including an interface approach with peripatetic multidisciplinary geriatric teams supporting the ED may help deliver the care needs of this population by supporting the workforce.

Focused training and development is paramount to improve cognitive and non-cognitive aspects of caring for frail older people and fostering interdisciplinary collaborative working.

Developing geriatric emergency medicine training programmes and establishing clinical champions who will provide leadership in the ED care of frail older people may help in this venture.

Conclusions

Emergency departments need to understand the challenge posed by the changing demographics on the provision and delivery of services that ensure the highest quality care for frail older patients and address the expectations of patients and carers.

Challenging established behaviour and models of care and ensuring the buy in of stakeholder groups will need to be part of this transformational approach that could help sustain and provide for changing demand. Standards on urgent care for older people are described in the *Sliver Book* - http://www2.le.ac.uk/departments/cardiovascular-sciences/people/conroy/silver-book

Further reading

Bridges J, Meyer J, Dethick L, *et al*. (2005). Older people in accident and emergency: implications for UK policy and practice. *Rev Clin Gerontol* **14**: 15–24.

Conroy S, Ferguson C, Woodward, S, Banerjee, J (2010). Interface geriatrics – an evidence based solution for old people with medical crises. *Br J Hosp Med (Lond)* **71**: 98–10.

Davison J, Bond J, Dawson P, *et al*. (2005). Patients with recurrent falls attending Accident & Emergency benefit from multifactorial intervention – a randomised controlled trial. *Age Ageing* **34**: 162–8.

Department of Health (2004). Transforming emergency care in England. (http://www.dh.gov.uk/en/Publicationsandstatistics/Publications/PublicationsPolicyAndGuidance/DH_4091775).

Department of Health (2007). Urgent care pathways for older people with complex needs (http://www.dh.gov.uk/en/Publicationsandstatistics/Publications/PublicationsPolicyAndGuidance/DH_080135).

Downing A, Wilson R (2005). Older people's use of accident and emergency services. *Age Ageing* **34**: 24–30.

Acute care and frail older people

As a result of the demographic shift and NHS policy, there has been a rapid increase in the number of older people attending emergency departments and acute care services. A significant proportion of this population have complex needs and can be classified as frail and at increased risk of adverse health outcomes, prolonged hospital stay, or readmission.

How and why do frail older people present differently?

As with all patients, frail older people access acute care for a variety of reasons, which can be broadly classified as:

- acute intercurrent illness (for example, pneumonia)
- decompensation of a long-term condition (for example, worsening heart failure)
- breakdown in support (for example, loss of carer support).

Any of these can be considered a crisis; there will usually be an underlying medical problem, whether acute, subacute or a long-term condition, and so the preferred terminology is a 'medical crisis'.

Managing medical crises in frail older people is challenging because they usually present non-specifically (falls, immobility, delirium), which can make the immediate diagnosis obscure. Junior doctors are usually the 'first receivers' at the front door (emergency department or acute medical unit), and few will have any substantial training in geriatric medicine and the formulation of the non-specific presentation. The challenge for inexperienced staff or non-specialists is to translate the non-specific presentation into a clinical diagnosis or objective problem, which can then be appropriately managed. For example, a frail older person presenting with a fall could have anything from pneumonia through to proprioceptive loss due to diabetes as the underlying medical problem.

Aside from an understanding of geriatric syndromes, there is a skill involved in assessing frail older people—history taking is challenging, for example because of sensory impairment, dementia, or delirium. Often a collateral history is needed, which may not be readily accessible in the emergency setting, and time pressures may place pressure on staff not to focus on anything other than immediate triage. A positive attitude to managing frail older people is a prerequisite for implementing the appropriate knowledge and skills; healthcare professionals' attitudes towards frail older people could be better, and ageism remains a problem in the health system. Staff who incorrectly attribute a medical crisis to age alone will miss important underlying medical disorders.

Many frail older people have multiple comorbidities. The management of the immediate problem is often complicated by these comorbidities, which also need to be addressed. Take for example an older person presenting with a fall related to postural hypotension, who is taking several antihypertensive agents and has cerebrovascular disease. The challenge for an emergency doctor is to balance treatment of the comorbidities against treatment of the immediate. This will require a global assessment of the patient, a risk–benefit assessment, and often an assessment of capacity. Such an assessment cannot be undertaken quickly, and may require several discussions with the patient, those close to them, and other health or social care professionals.

Multiple comorbidities bring associated polypharmacy. Older people are at higher risk of adverse drug events, drug–drug interactions, and drug–disease interactions. Adverse drug events may account for up to 30% of hospital admissions in older people. Paradoxically, 11–65% of older people also suffer from lack of appropriate prescribing—underprescribing for bone protection, anticoagulation, and other conditions is well described. Managing polypharmacy is also complex and requires access to relevant information, and understanding of any comorbid conditions, their trajectory, and knowledge of the risk–benefit ratio for each drug.

Finally, the frail older person, perhaps more than any other patient group, will present with a complex interaction of biological, psychological, and social factors. They may exhibit 'differential challenge' – the concept that those most in need are least able to access services themselves, either because of illness, poverty, or social isolation.

The non-specific presentation, multiple comorbidities, polypharmacy, homeostatic failure, and differential challenge may all be present when a frail older person presents with a medical crisis. Resolving these complex, interrelated issues is difficult for specialists, let alone relatively inexperienced front-line staff, and is compounded by the time pressures.

So focusing on older people is in effect a 'stress test' of the health system – if the system can manage such complexities well, then managing of younger, fitter patients will be relatively straightforward.

How to manage the acute care of frail older people

It is challenging to organize healthcare services to meet the needs of this vulnerable patient group. To achieve the best outcomes, the management of frail older people should be based on comprehensive geriatric assessment, a multidimensional diagnostic process which outlines an older person's medical, psychological, and functional capability and identifies their risk of functional decline and institutionalization.

There is robust evidence to support in-hospital comprehensive geriatric assessment (CGA) for frail older people with the literature supporting dedicated geriatric units, rather than liaison services. Similarly, there is reasonable evidence to support CGA in the community setting for frail older people. But only one systematic review has attempted to determine the best model of care for patients at the interface between acute hospital and community care; the authors were unable to recommend any one particular model of care over another.

In addition to the lack of a clear evidence based answer as to how best manage care for frail older people at the interface, there has been a major change (at least in the UK) over the last 10–15 years in how acute care for frail older people is delivered. Previously acute care and the ongoing rehabilitation of older people were delivered in acute hospital settings. Now, acute care is delivered predominantly in acute medical units, often over short time periods, with ongoing care and rehabilitation being provided in a variety of community settings (e.g. intermediate care, community hospitals). Some older patients with complex needs who would previously have been managed in hospitals by geriatricians, may not receive a specialist geriatric assessment, even though they may still access other aspects of comprehensive geriatric care (physiotherapy, occupational therapy, etc.). The optimal model of care which brings together acute and community care for frail older people is not well established.

Evidence of the problem

There is a relative paucity of published evidence documenting the outcomes of frail older people who contact emergency care settings. This is partly due to the difficulties in identifying and defining frailty, and partly because hitherto there has been relatively little interest in this group from the acute service perspective. There is some evidence from North America indicating that older people in general are increasing users of emergency services, and that older people from care homes (likely to be frail) make up approximately 2% of all attendees, but there are no such studies from the UK.

Frail older people attending the emergency department are more likely than non-frail older people to be admitted to an acute medical unit or other receiving area within the hospital. Once in an acute medical unit, 90% of frail older people are admitted to base wards, where they have longer lengths of stay and more complications than non-frail older people. When discharged from any setting (emergency departments, acute medical unit, or base wards), frail older people are at increased risk of readmission.

Although such figures might be of interest to health service planners, they do not reflect the experience of the frail older person attending emergency settings. It might be reasonable to infer that multiple, rapid ward changes, a propensity to lengthy admissions, and subsequent readmissions are not a good thing, but there are little published data to give the patient perspective on acute care in the twenty-first century.

Potential solutions

The key is to identify frail older people attending acute care at the earliest possible opportunity, in order to focus attention on their care, for example through specialist care pathways or coordinated case management. Any 'frailty identification tool' to be used in an emergency setting should be simple, quick, and reliable. Most frailty identification tools are designed for use in the research context, and are less useful in the clinical setting.

Once identified, the challenge is next to have a rapid response service that is able to undertake a holistic assessment of the frail older person within a short period of time, with a view to delivering ongoing care in the community setting if appropriate. This requires a multidisciplinary approach, appropriately skilled medical assessment of the patient, ready access to information (such a medication lists), the ability to communicate rapidly with primary care services, and access to community-based teams. Even with this level of assessment and intervention in place, it is unlikely that all of the important issues relevant to the patient's presentation and future care will be addressed, so ongoing care and follow-up is required. Care across primary and secondary care in this fashion requires a different philosophy that belies traditional boundaries. It requires a great deal of cooperation and a system-wide approach which is agreed by all relevant stakeholders—such a system has been termed 'interface geriatrics'. Figure 4.1 outlines a whole systems approach to improving care for frail older people.

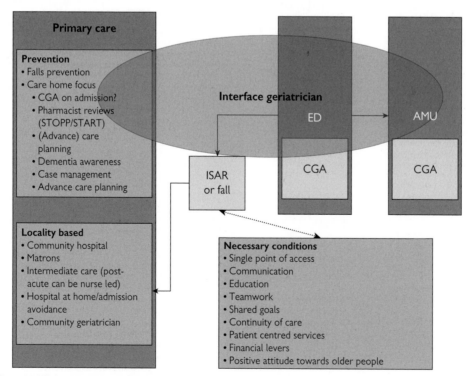

Figure 4.1 Whole system approach: frail older people. AMU: Acute Medical Unit; CGA: Comprehensive Geriatric Assessment; ED: Emergency Department; ISAR: Identification of Seniors At Risk tool.

The interface geriatrics scheme describes some of the activities in primary care that can promote health and potentially reduce crises. However, it acknowledges that crises will occur and that frail older people will still need to access acute care. The Identification of Seniors at Risk tool can be used to identify people at risk of adverse outcome being sent home from the Emergency Department, so that they can access long-term conditions services, such as case managers. For those people requiring admission, there should be rapid access to CGA.

One of the challenges is to deliver specialist geriatric care to patients in acute care settings only (i.e. those in hospital for no more than 72 hours). Most of these patients will be managed on an acute medical unit, with variable geriatric medicine input. Even if there is a geriatrician on duty as the acute physician, it is difficult to deliver a specialist geriatric assessment when also undertaking an acute ward round. This would be the same for any specialist service, although perhaps is more of an issue in geriatric medicine, where adequate time for the assessment is critical.

The role of the interface geriatrician could be extended further. There is reasonable evidence to suggest that a specialist geriatric assessment could lead to different decisions in acute care settings – for example, suggesting that patients could be safely and perhaps more appropriately managed in primary care rather than being admitted. One randomized controlled trial examining the role of CGA for patients being discharged from the emergency department has shown a subsequent reduction in emergency readmissions over 18 months (44% versus 54%; p = 0.007) compared with usual care. In practical terms, a geriatrician who had one foot in the Emergency Department/Acute Medical Unit, and another in the community setting would be able to deliver CGA over time, working with both hospital and community multidisciplinary service/case managers. This helps with continuity of care, a key aspect of effective care for frail older people. For such a scheme to be fully effective, a team of geriatricians would be required to cover different units at different times, and also to cover different community localities.

A weakness of such an approach which seeks to deliver CGA across primary and secondary care, rather than focusing on the delivery of care within discrete units, is that it has a poor evidence base. The few trials which have assessed this method of delivering care to frail older people with medical crises have not provided definitive evidence of clinical or cost-effectiveness.

Although at present there is a relative lack of evidence for such a scheme, the theoretical basis is sound, and is supported indirectly by high-quality systematic reviews. Trials are under way to assess the clinical and cost-effectiveness of such a scheme in the UK.

Summary

There is clear evidence for the benefit of comprehensive geriatric assessment in discrete geriatric units for hospitalized frail older people, but the evidence for liaison and outreach services is less compelling. Effective services aimed at improving outcomes for frail older people in contact with acute hospitals include comprehensive geriatric assessment, continuity of care and an element of case management.

Further reading

Baztán JJ, Suárez-Garc´a FM, López-Arrieta J, et al. (2009). Effectiveness of acute geriatric units on functional decline, living at home, and case fatality among older patients admitted to hospital for acute medical disorders: meta-analysis. Br Med J **338**: b50.

Caplan GA, Williams AJ, Daly B, et al. (2004). A randomized, controlled trial of comprehensive geriatric assessment and multidisciplinary intervention after discharge of elderly from the emergency department – the DEED II study. J Am Geriatr Soc **52**: 1417–23.

Ferguson C, Woodard J, Banerjee J, et al. (2009). Operationalising frailty definitions in the emergency department – a mapping exercise. J Nutr, Health Aging **13**(Supplement 1): S266.

McCusker J BF, Cardin S, Trepanier S, et al. (1999). Detection of older people at increased risk of adverse health outcomes after an emergency visit: the ISAR screening tool. J Am Geriatr Soc **47**: 1229–37.

Mion LC, Palmer RM, Meldon SW, et al. (2003). Case finding and referral model for emergency department elders: a randomized clinical trial. [see comment]. Ann Emerg Med **41**: 57–68.

Parker G, Bhakta P, Katbamna S, et al. (2000). Best place of care for older people after acute and during sub-acute illness: a systematic review. J Health Serv Res Policy **5**: 176–89.

Roberts D, McKay M, Shaffer A (2008). Increasing rates of emergency department visits for elderly patients in the United States, 1993 to 2003. Ann Emerg Med **51**: 769–74.

Stuck AE, Siu AL, Wieland GD, et al. (1993). Comprehensive geriatric assessment: a meta-analysis of controlled trials. Lancet **342**: 1032–6.

Cardiovascular

Cardiac physiology in old age

Introduction

Diseases of the cardiovascular system (CVS) are a common cause of morbidity and mortality in old age. There is no cut-off or age limit when they become more prevalent. However, diseases such as heart failure become more prevalent over 79 years old (Figure 5.1).

Similarly the average systolic blood pressure increases with age (Figure 5.2).

An inherent difficulty in addressing cardiac physiology in older people, given the heterogeneous nature of this population, is the uncertainty with discriminating between 'physiological' and 'pathological' ageing. Older people are different genetically and exposed to different environmental states such as diet and exercise. They also have different coexisting comorbidities and are often subject to polypharmacy.

Changes in the ageing myocardium

There is less reserve capacity in myocardial muscle. Once heart muscle dies, there is no regeneration of new myocardium, and healing occurs by fibrosis. Over time, the number of myocytes decreases, including the conducting tissue. There is also amyloid deposition and atrophy of the sympathetic nerve supply.

Coronary supply of heart muscle

The proximal coronary artery is affected first, with thickening of the subendothelial layer, and later increased stiffness of the coronary vessels.

The vascular endothelium is surrounded by three layers: tunica intima, media, and adventitia. Older people undergo a gradual increase in the thickness of the tunica media in large and medium-sized arteries. There is also an increase in the number of collagen fibres, with disorganized elastin, and deposition of calcium that renders the arteries stiff, rigid, and less elastic.

The cells in the endothelial lining become disorganized, fragmented and invaded by smooth muscle fibres making the lining of the blood vessel roughened and less resilient, as well as thickened, thus narrowing the vessel lumen.

The process of atherosclerosis is similar to the ageing arterial vasculature and the two can be viewed as two ends of a spectrum modified by external factors such as hypertension, hypercholesterolaemia, and smoking.

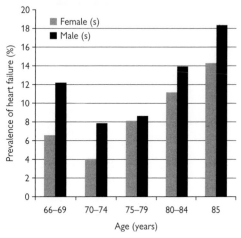

Figure 5.1 The prevalence of heart failure.

Valvular changes with age

Valvular heart disease in old age is usually an acquired pathology rather than congenital. The main age-related valvular changes affect the left side of the heart, with increased thickening and calcification, which can reduce valvular mobility and function.

Rheumatic fever remains a common cause for mitral valve pathology worldwide, although its incidence is decreasing in developing countries. Bicuspid aortic valve is found in about 1% of the population, and along with aortic valve fibrosis that occurs with age, they constitute the major causes of aortic stenosis. Aortic regurgitation is secondary to dilated aortic root that occurs following a variety of causes related to left ventricular dilatation.

Changes in heart rate

With ageing, there is an inevitable decline in pulse rate at rest, and with exercise the maximum heart rate is less than that seen in a younger person. These changes are attributed to the ischaemic damage sustained by specialized conducting nerve tissue the sinoatrial node (SAN) and the

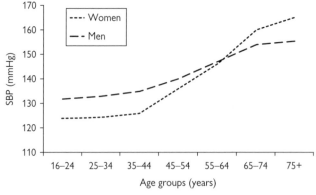

Figure 5.2 Change in systolic blood pressure (SBP) with age. With permission from Professor C. Rajkumar.

atrioventricular node (AVN). These nerve cells are lost and replaced by fibrous tissue. This explains why older people are more at risk of arrhythmias, such as heart blocks or atrial fibrillation.

Changes in ventricles with age
There is a progressive increase in the weight and thickness of the left ventricle with ageing.

Changes in cardiac output with age
Cardiac output is defined as the stroke volume (SV) multiplied by the heart rate. Both SV and peripheral resistance are affected by age. The SV is dependent on the ability of the heart to fill with blood and then contract efficiently. With ageing, the myocardial fibres are stiffer and less contractile, resulting in a suboptimal contractile force.

The stimulating effect of the sympathetic nervous system is blunted in old age, resulting in reduced SV even during exercise. The underlying decline in beta-receptor stimulation of cardiac muscle may be explained by the inability of the receptors to increase the intracellular cAMP (cyclical adenine monophosphate) which is needed for an adequate myocardial contraction. These blunted neuronal responses result in a reduced heart rate response to exercise. In order to maintain cardiac output to meet exercise and metabolic demands, the heart dilates to accommodate an increase in end-systolic and end-diastolic volumes, thus increasing SV.

In exercise states, the increased heart rate results in a reduction of the time when the coronary arteries are perfused (i.e. diastole) and dependence of the heart on increased end-diastolic filling. Clinicians and cardiac physiologists have commonly used the index of ejection fraction (EF) to quantify left ventricle function. EF is defined as the fraction of the end-diastolic volume (EDV) that is ejected per cardiac cycle as the SV:EF = SV/EDV.

Heart failure in old age can be broadly classified into two categories systolic and diastolic, which can coexist.

Changes in blood pressure
There is a rise in systolic blood pressure due the above changes in the loss of elasticity of coronary vasculature along with an increase in peripheral resistance and ventricular hypertrophy. The diastolic blood pressure remains relatively constant with age in the absence of ischaemic heart disease and polypharmacy. The increase in systolic blood pressure (BP) and relative maintenance of diastolic BP results in a wider pulse pressure, which has been associated with an increase in cardiovascular risk.

Older people are also at an increased risk of polypharmacy, which adversely affects their blood pressure and makes them more prone to postural hypotension.

Neural control on heart in old age
Changes in the sympathetic and parasympathetic nervous systems result in a blunted response to drops in blood pressure that occur with standing up and changing posture in older people. These changes are secondary to a downgraded response of the arterial system to the effects of circulating catecholamines. The number of alpha-adrenergic receptors at these arterioles diminishes with age. The downregulation of beta-adrenergic receptor activity has also been suggested as a cause for an impaired sympathetic response in the older population.

The baroreceptor reflexes
There are widely reported well characterized age-related blunted responses to either hypo- or hypertensive episodes in animals and human beings.

Change in arterial distensibility
The previously mentioned changes of the myocardium and vasculature in old age result in blood vessels become stiffer (less elastic, less distensible, and less compliant), and these changes are noted across the whole vasculature to varying degrees. The major arteries affected are the aorta and its main large branches.

Some clinical implications
Arterial changes associated with ageing were considered inevitable and irreversible. Clinical trials such as HYVET (Hypertension in the Very Elderly Trial) suggest that treating conditions such as systolic hypertension in older people has beneficial consequences. At the therapeutic level, there is evidence that certain medications, such as angiotensin-converting enzyme (ACE) inhibitors and calcium channel blockers (CCBs), can improve arterial compliance by increasing the local concentration of nitric oxide.

Conclusions
There are multiple effects of ageing on the cardiovascular system that are partly physiological and partly pathological. There is a generalized loss of arterial compliance due to structural and functional changes with implications for cardiovascular risk. Older people have a reduced heart rate at baseline, and are more prone to left ventricular hypertrophy and increased systolic blood pressure. They respond less to sympathetic stimulation, and their BP-regulating mechanisms, such as baroreceptors, are less responsive to changes in blood volume and postural change.

Older people are at more risk of hypertension, ischaemic heart disease, myocardial infarction, heart failure, cardiac conduction defects strokes, and dementia. These age-related changes have important clinical implications as the presentations of cardiovascular disease can be atypical in older people. Additionally, the management of the cardiovascular system needs to be specifically tailored to the individual as there is a high rate of comorbidity, and polypharmacy.

Further reading
Beckett NS, Peters R, Fletcher AE, et al. (2008). HYVET Study Group. Treatment of hypertension in patients 80 years of age or older. *N Engl J Med* **358**: 1887–98.

Ferrari AU, Radaelli A, Centola M (2003). Ageing and the cardiovascular system. *J Appl Physiol* **95**: 2591–7.

Fleg JL, O'Connor FC, Gerstenblith G, et al. (1995). Impact of age on the cardiovascular response to dynamic upright exercise in healthy men and women. *J Appl Physiol* **78**: 890–900.

Franklin S, Gustin W, Wong ND, et al. (1997). Haemodynamic patterns of age-related changes in blood pressure. The Framingham Heart Study. *Circulation* **96**: 308–15.

Gerstenblith G, Fredriksen J, Yin FCP, et al. (1977). Echocardiographic assessment of a normal adult aging population. *Circulation* **56**: 273–8.

Lakatta EG (1993). Deficient neuroendocrine regulation of the cardiovascular system with advancing age in healthy humans. *Circulation* **87**: 631–6.

Lindroos M, Kupari M, Heikkila J, et al. (1999). Prevalence of aortic valve abnormalities in the elderly: an echocardiographic study of a random population sample. *J Am Coll Cardiol* **21**: 1220–5.

Miller TR, Grossman SJ, Schechtman KB, et al. (1986). Left ventricular diastolic filling and its association with age. *Am J Cardiol* **58**: 531–5.

Pearson AC, Gudipati CV, Labovitz AJ (1991). Effects of ageing on left ventricular structure and function. *Am Heart J* **121**: 871–5.

Rodeheffer RJ, Gerstenblith G, Becker LC, et al. (1984). Exercise cardiac output is maintained with advancing age in healthy human subjects: cardiac dilatation and increased stroke volume compensate for diminished heart rate. *Circulation* **69**: 203–13.

Cardiac investigations

There are a number of investigations available for the diagnosis and assessment of cardiac disease. Cardiovascular disease is common in older people, and investigation and management are similar to those of younger patients. This section groups the principal aims of tests, recognizing that a single test will usually give information relating to more than one aspect of a patient's condition. For example, an echocardiogram demonstrating poor left ventricular function and mitral regurgitation may imply the aetiology of a primary cause, such as the regional wall motion abnormality characteristic of an area of scar from previous myocardial infarction.

The 12-lead electrocardiogram (ECG)

The 12-lead ECG is the simplest cardiac test, yet is central to the investigation of any patient with suspected cardiac disease. It provides a recording of the electrical activity of the heart occurring at the moment that the ECG was recorded. Clues to almost any pathology of the heart can be detected on the 12-lead ECG. However, the ECG is a snapshot in time and only detects pathologies that occur when the recording is made. A normal ECG does not necessarily imply a lack of pathology nor should it replace a good history. However, the ECG does form a basic supplementary tool and further investigations are directed by clinical assessment.

Blood assays

Damage to heart muscle causes the release of enzymes detectable in the blood. Creatine kinase (CK) rises in myocardial infarction (the cardiac-specific isomer CK-MB is normally less than 5% of the total CK fraction). Later on after myocardial injury, other muscle enzymes rise, including lactate dehydrogenase and aspartate transaminase. The development of highly cardiac-specific troponin tests (I or T subunits), produced almost exclusively by myocardium, has almost replaced the older serum markers. A raised serum troponin with a typical history of myocardial ischaemia strongly supports the diagnosis. Nonetheless, pulmonary embolism, renal failure, myocarditis, or severe illness of any cause can lead to increased troponin levels, and caution is needed in the interpretation of a raised troponin with an unusual history.

Measurement of brain natriuretic peptide (BNP), a hormone released in response to rises in left atrial pressure, can help diagnose heart failure. It has not been fully validated in older people and its exact clinical role here remains unclear. It may be useful as a screening test, including in primary care, as a normal assay (<50 units/mL) makes the diagnosis of heart failure unlikely.

Tests for ischaemic heart disease: functional

Coronary disease in older people is common. Non-invasive functional tests are undertaken to detect ischaemia and to assess the functional importance of angiographic disease. Clinical decisions are not based upon pure anatomical appearances from coronary angiograms but correlated with functional tests and symptoms.

Exercise 12-lead ECG

Continuous monitoring of a 12-lead ECG during exercise with intermittent blood pressure monitoring has been the principal screening tool for suspected angina. Cardiac ischaemia is suggested by the development of arrhythmias; a drop in exertional blood pressure; development of ST segment depression of ≥2 mm, particularly in the inferior limb and anterolateral leads; or the development of transient bundle branch block and T-wave changes. Attention is given to any symptoms induced. Despite its widespread use, the exercise ECG has a poor diagnostic yield, with only a 67% sensitivity and 70% specificity at detecting important coronary disease. Mobility issues may limit its usefulness for older people.

Myocardial perfusion scintigraphy (MIBI scan)

The myocardial perfusion scintigraphy scan (MPS) compares cardiac uptake of a radioactive tracer (such as thallium-201 or technetium-99m) in conditions of rest and stress. Stress is induced through exercise or pharmacologically (e.g. with dobutamine). A comparative reduction in regional isotope uptake during stress implies physiologically important coronary disease, with 81% sensitivity and specificity of 67% in a population, the majority of whom were older people. MPS does confer a small but significant radiation dose but is considered relatively non-invasive and safe. It is most useful in patients unable to exercise with a low to moderate likelihood of coronary disease. It is helpful for assessing regional cardiac perfusion in patients with borderline coronary lesions.

Dobutamine stress echocardiography (DSE)

Stress echocardiography relies upon ischaemic cardiac muscle being less contractile than normally perfused myocardium. Echocardiographic images at rest and stress are compared, regional differences in wall motion are then observed in areas of the heart with limited blood supply. In expert hands, stress echocardiography has sensitivity and specificity for the diagnosis of coronary disease similar to MPS. It is non-invasive and safe. Disadvantages of stress echocardiography include the difficulty of obtaining good ultrasound images and the subjective nature of wall motion abnormality detection that may be dependent on the experience of the operator.

Cardiac magnetic resonance imaging: late gadolinium enhancement

Refinements in cardiac magnetic resonance imaging (cMRI) have improved this tool for the detection of myocardial ischaemia. The current state-of-the-art imaging for functional ischaemia uses gadolinium, a tracer which stays in ischaemic tissue for longer than normal tissue, to differentiate normal and ischaemic tissues. The highly detailed scans accurately identify areas of ischemia (Figure 5.3a,b) and can confirm a diagnosis of coronary artery disease. The cMRI also gives detailed structural and functional information of the heart muscle, useful in the diagnosis of myocarditis, cardiomyopathies, complex congenital heart disease, and pericardial disease. It is useful in the assessment and surveillance of valvular and aortic disease (Figure 5.3c,d). However, cMRI scans can take up to 30 minutes and the scanning tunnel is narrow and claustrophobic. Most implanted cardiac devices remain contraindications for cMRI, but there are now MRI-safe pacemakers available. Gadolinium can be dangerous in advanced renal disease, due to the association with the rare but devastating complication of nephrogenic systemic fibrosis.

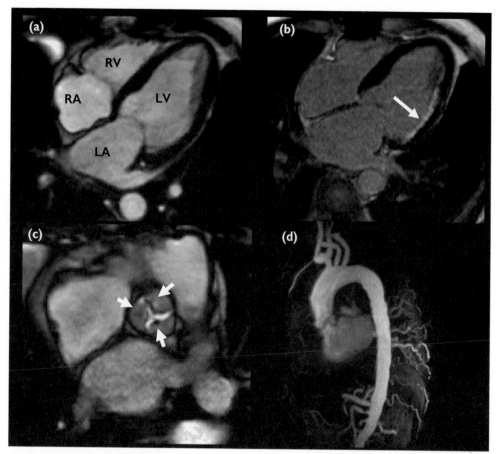

Figure 5.3 Cardiovascular magnetic resonance from an 82-year-old patient with aortic stenosis. (a) SSFP Cine diastolic still image of a four chamber view. (b) Four-chamber view showing area of lateral subendocardial late gadolinium enhancement, indicating the presence of ischaemic scar (white arrow). (c) SSPP Cine systolic still image demonstrating sclerosed aortic valve (AoV). (d) Aortic angiogram, showing diffuse atherosclerosis. Kindly provided by James Moon and Gianni Quateri.

Tests for ischaemic heart disease: anatomical

Coronary angiogram

A coronary angiogram remains the gold standard for diagnosis of coronary artery disease. Small catheters are passed percutaneously from the femoral or radial artery to cannulate the origins of the coronary arteries. Contrast is injected to visualize the extent and severity of any coronary disease using low intensity X-rays, and also to determine left ventricle size and function. High-pressure balloon angioplasty and stenting can be performed at the same sitting. The risk of coronary angiography is small, with around a 0.1% risk of stroke or myocardial infarction, and up to a 0.5% risk of other serious complications, e.g. renal failure, arterial damage requiring repair, etc. However, the risks in older patients may be higher owing to comorbidities, and any risk must be weighed against the importance of establishing a firm diagnosis. The results of a coronary angiogram must be interpreted in light of the patient's symptoms and evidence of inducible ischaemia.

Cardiac CT angiography/CT calcium score

Advances in computed tomography (CT) have allowed imaging of calcium deposits in the wall of coronary arteries, a surrogate for established coronary disease. This technique aims to predict the risk of coronary disease based on quantifying the amount of coronary calcification present and has been well validated. Further advances have enabled detailed reconstructions of the coronary arteries, with the prospect of true non-invasive coronary angiography. A current limitation of this technology in older patients is the relatively poor luminal definition in calcified areas of coronary arteries, which are increasingly common with age. CT angiography is developing into a good screening tool for patients with chest pains, with those who have a normal scan being unlikely to be have serious coronary artery disease.

Tests for structural and functional impairment

Transthoracic echocardiogram

The transthoracic cardiac echocardiogram (TTE) can give accurate and reproducible assessments of cardiac structure and function, including detailed haemodynamic and valvular measurements. It is non-invasive and essentially risk free. Scan interpretation is dependent not only on the images, but also, critically, on the clinical information that accompanies the request. Common indications for a TTE include:

- assessment of ventricular function and regional wall motion abnormalities
- assessment of a murmurs or valvular lesion
- assessment of congenital heart disease
- assessment of pericardial effusion
- evidence of right heart strain for guiding thrombolysis in massive pulmonary embolism
- detection of intracardiac shunts or septal defects using bubble contrast (agitated saline injections) in the investigation of strokes and migraines.

The principal limitation of the TTE is the reliance on good echo 'windows', determined by the patient's body habitus and chest wall. TTE can only detect thrombus or vegetations >5 mm, thus resolution of TTE remains insufficient for firm diagnosis or exclusion of endocarditis.

Transoesophageal echocardiogram

Transoesophageal echocardiogram (TOE) is an invasive procedure, whereby an ultrasound probe is passed down the oesophagus under local anaesthesia and sedation. The probe sits behind the heart in very close proximity to the left atrium, obtaining unobstructed high-resolution images. TOE is usually performed electively. Risks include oesophageal damage (<0.2%) and aspiration (<1%). The high-quality images allow visualization of vegetations in endocarditis of <1 mm accuracy. It also allows detailed assessment of the cardiac valves, the aortic root, and left atrium.

Tests for disturbances of heart rhythm

The 12-lead ECG remains the key to assessing a patient's heart rhythm. A 12-lead ECG of a cardiac arrhythmia will usually suffice for diagnosis without further testing but will often miss paroxysmal arrhythmias.

24-hour Holter recording

The Holter recorder (also known as a loop recorder, 24-hour tape) allows the continuous recording of a patient's ECG over 24 hours, and up to 7 days. The 24-hour monitor is useful in capturing frequently (i.e. ideally occurring on most days) occurring arrhythmias and diagnosis and arrhythmia burden. Correlation of symptoms with arrhythmia is very important, and patients are asked to keep a detailed diary of any symptoms. However, the pick-up rate is low for infrequent rhythm problems, where longer monitoring periods are needed.

Implantable loop recorder

For very infrequent but highly symptomatic arrhythmias, an implantable loop recorder (e.g. Reveal device) can be used. Implantation of these small devices is minimally invasive. They are positioned subcutaneously on the chest wall under local anaesthetic, with a battery life of up to 24 months. Recording is either patient activated or by detection of arrhythmia outside a preset range (either bradycardia or tachycardia). Tracings can be downloaded and analysed in a specialist clinic. Once the information is obtained or battery charge of the device is expired, they can be easily explanted under local anaesthetic.

Electrophysiological study

Patients with heart rhythm disorders may undergo an electrophysiological (EP) study, usually with a view to catheter ablation treatment. Wires are inserted into the heart via the femoral veins under local anaesthesia. Pacing is performed to test for the normal circuitry of the heart. Catheter ablation may be carried out at the same sitting once a firm EP diagnosis has been made. EP studies can be used for risk stratification of ventricular arrhythmia in ischaemic cardiomyopathy, but is relatively poor for other conditions.

Further reading

Ashley EA, Myers J, Froelicher V (2000). Exercise testing in clinical medicine. *Lancet* **356**: 1592–7.

Douglas P, Khandheria B, Stainback R, *et al.* (2008). Appropriateness criteria for stress echocardiography: a report of the American College of Cardiology Foundation Appropriateness Criteria Task Force *et al. Circulation* **117**: 1478–97.

Kaddoura S (2009). *Echo Made Easy.* Churchill Livingstone.

Kim HW, Farzaneh-Far A, Kim RJ (2009). Cardiovascular magnetic resonance in patients with myocardial infarction: current and emerging applications. *J Am Coll Cardiol* **55**: 1–16.

Loong CY, Anagnostopoulos C (2004). Diagnosis of coronary artery disease by radionuclide myocardial perfusion imaging. *Heart* **90**(Suppl 5): v2–9.

Roberts WT, Bax JJ, Davies LC (2008). Cardiac CT and CT coronary angiography: technology and application. *Heart* **94**: 781–92.

Wagner GS. (2007). *Marriott's Practical Electrocardiography.* Lippincott Williams & Wilkins.

Zipes DP, Libby P, Bonow RO, Braunwald E (2007). *Braunwald's Heart Disease: A Textbook of Cardiovascular Medicine.* Saunders.

Hypertension in old age

'A man is as old as his arteries'

Thomas Sydenham
(seventeenth-century London physician).

Introduction

All too often older adults are not recruited to clinical trials, and when one considers the very old, actively excluded. When it comes to hypertension though, there is good evidence of benefit at least in those up to the age of 90 who are relatively robust (i.e. 'free-range', community dwelling older people). This is useful given that hypertension is common in old age and carries with it substantial risk. So does one simply have to make sure of a diagnosis of sustained hypertension, agree on a level of blood pressure as 'hypertensive', and then start treatment? If it was this simple, one has to wonder why such a plethora of articles are published on the subject.

Extrapolating results from clinical trials, however well-designed the trial, to the individual patient in front of the clinician can be challenging. Older adults are a heterogeneous group by whatever criteria we use (e.g. age of retirement, over 70 years). Trial data suggest a fit and healthy 79 year old with a systolic blood pressure of 164 mmHg should be treated but what about an individual of the same age with the same blood pressure in a nursing home who has limited mobility from a previous stroke, troubled with urinary incontinence, and has marked cognitive impairment. This comparison may be extreme but where is the dividing line? What criteria should we use: level of blood pressure, the overall risk to the patient? The eminent epidemiologist Geoffrey Rose once stated that hypertension should be defined as that level at which treatment produces more benefit than harm. Does age have an impact on this?

Pathophysiology

With increasing age the following changes in blood pressure occur:

- systolic blood pressure rises in a linear fashion
- diastolic blood pressure rises until around the age of 55, following which it declines
- consequently the gap between systolic and diastolic pressures (i.e. the pulse pressure) increases.

These changes also account for why isolated systolic hypertension is the commonest type of hypertension seen in older adults.

This age-related change in blood pressure is due to the age associated changes in the vasculature, particularly the aorta and other large arteries. Not that long ago, arteries in older adults were simply thought of as lead pipes and 'hardened arteries' a reflection of the natural process of ageing. The hallmark change of ageing is indeed the increase in central arterial stiffness. This is as a result of

1 increase in the amount of collagen
2 increase in collagen cross-linking
3 increased elastin fragmentation
4 decrease in the amount of elastin.

However, the complexity of the arterial changes that occur with age are becoming better understood and it is interesting to note that these changes (see Table 5.1) are similar to those seen at younger ages with hypertension and in those with atherosclerotic disease. The changes that

Table 5.1 Comparison of the arterial changes seen in ageing, with hypertension and atherosclerosis

	Ageing	Hyper-tension	Athero-sclerosis
Increased arterial stiffness	+	+	+
Endothelial dysfunction	+	+	+
Diffuse intimal thickening	+	+	+
Lipids	−	+/−	+
Increase in VSMC	+	+	+
Macrophages	+	+	+
Increase in matrix deposition	+	+	+
Increase in local Ang II levels	+	+	+
MMP dysregulation	+	+	+
Increase expression of MCP-1/CCR2	+	+	+
Increase in ICAM-1	+	+	+
Increase in calpain-1	unknown	+	+
Increase in TGF-β	+	+	+
Increase in TNF-α	+	+	+
Decrease VEGF	+	+	+
Increase in NADPH oxidase	+	+	+
Decrease in NO bioavailability	+	+	+

VSMC, vascular smooth muscle cells; Ang II, angiotensin II; MMP, matrix metalloproteinase; MCP-1, monocyte chemotactic protein-1; CCR-2, chemokine (C-C motif) receptor 2; ICAM, intercellular adhesion molecule; TGF, transforming growth factor; TNF, tumour necrosis factor; VEGF, vascular endothelial growth factor; NADPH, nicotinamide adenine dinucleotide phosphate; NO, nitric oxide; +, present; −, not present; +/−, possibly present.

occur with age act as a substrate for the development of cardiovascular disease (CVD). Other cardiovascular risk factors such as smoking, hypertension, diabetes, dyslipidaemia, or impaired glucose tolerance accelerate these changes.

As a consequence of the increase in arterial stiffness, there are certain haemodynamic changes that occur. During systole, when a bolus of blood is ejected from the left ventricle, a pulse wave is propagated through the vascular tree. This wave is reflected back towards the heart at branch points or sites of impedance mismatch, e.g. atheromatous plaques. With a stiffer artery, the propagated and reflected waves travel faster, such that the reflected wave returns and augments the systolic pressure and decreases the diastolic pressure augmentation (see Figure 5.4), hence the observed changes of blood pressure with age.

These haemodynamic changes result in an increase in workload for the heart and subsequent changes to left ventricular function with decreased diastolic coronary perfusion. They also result in higher pressures being

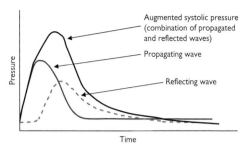

Figure 5.4 Arterial wave form in older adult showing augmentation of the systolic pressure.

transmitted to end organs such as the kidneys and brain and leading to greater structural changes to the artery tree (see Figure 5.5).

Other age-related changes that can have either a direct or indirect effect on blood pressure include:

- reduction in plasma renin activity (PRA)
- increased angiotensin II production in arterial tissue—may explain why drugs blocking the renin–angiotensin system are still effective in older adults
- reduced sensitivity of beta-adrenergic receptors (alpha-adrenergic tend not to change)
- decreased baroreceptor sensitivity—greater risk of orthostatic and post-prandial hypotension
- decreased early left ventricular diastolic filling—increased risk of diastolic dysfunction
- increased left atrial size—increased risk of atrial fibrillation.

More than 90% of older hypertensives have essential, or primary, hypertension. Most cases of secondary hypertension in this age group are drug induced (commonest: corticosteroids, non-steroidals, alcohol, and antihistamines) or have an underlying renal cause, particularly renal artery stenosis. A very small number are due to endocrine or neurological causes.

Epidemiology

> **Author's Tip**
> Hypertension is the most common treatable disorder of older adults.

Given that hypertension is a major risk factor for CVD and the arterial changes that occur with age, it is not surprising that CVD is common in older adults and is the leading cause of death. The rate of doctor-diagnosed CVD in the UK in 2005 for men aged 65 and over was 35%, rising to 45% in those aged 75 and over, in women 21% and 37% respectively. The most important modifiable risk factor for CVD is hypertension. High blood pressure is considered to affect over 16 million people in the UK, the majority of whom are aged 65 or older. It is the direct cause of half of all strokes and heart attacks and accounts for up to 50% of the attributable risk for heart failure. Reducing the average UK systolic pressure by 2 mmHg would save 14 000 lives per year. Failure to actually control blood pressure to target levels in the UK results in around 62 000 unnecessary deaths every year.

Given the changes in blood pressure with age detailed above it is not surprising that hypertension is a common finding in older adults (see Figure 5.6a,b).

With an ageing population, hypertension is becoming more prevalent. In the UK, it has been estimated that the number of people with high blood pressure rose by 2.7% from 2004/2005 to 2007/2008, an increase in absolute terms of just over 330 000. Data from the Framingham Heart study has shown that in men and women aged 55 and not considered to be hypertensive their lifetime risk for developing hypertension by 80 years of age is around 90%.

Prevalence of hypertension is clearly affected by the definition one uses. It is generally accepted that hypertension is defined as a sustained systolic blood pressure of 140 mmHg or more and/or a sustained diastolic blood pressure of 90 mmHg or more. In the UK in 2005, 60% of men aged 65 or more were considered hypertensive rising

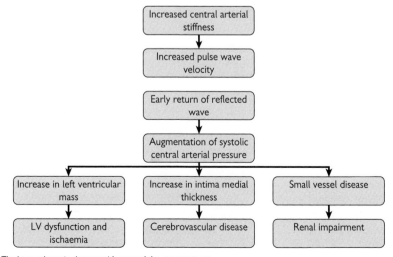

Figure 5.5 The haemodynamic changes with age and the consequences.

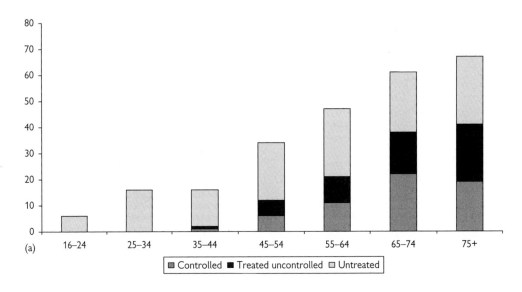

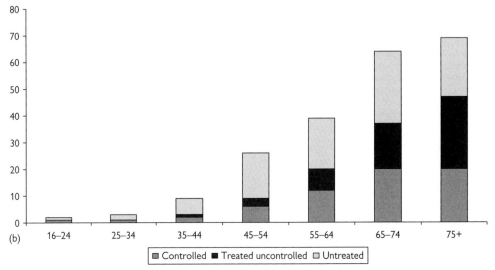

Figure 5.6 Prevalence (%) of hypertension by age for men (a) and women (b) detailing percentage that are controlled, treated but not controlled (systolic blood pressure <140 mmHg and diastolic <90 mmHg), or not treated. Data from the Health Survey for England, 2006.

to 66% for those aged 75 and over. Comparable figures for women were 63% and 69%. Figures of 70–75% have been suggested for those aged 80 or more. It should be stressed that these figures are not based on repeated measurements of blood pressure over a period of time and the true prevalence is likely to be up to a third lower, but this remains a substantial number.

Isolated systolic hypertension (ISH) is defined as systolic blood pressure of 140 mmHg or more and diastolic blood pressure of less than 90 mmHg. This is the commonest form of hypertension in the older adult, occurring in up to 80% of those aged over the age of 70 with similar rates in

men and women. This contrasts with a prevalence of only 20% for those below the age of 50. Although physiologically age-related changes drive this increased prevalence, ISH is not benign. Systolic pressure is a better predictor than diastolic blood pressure for cardiovascular events and total mortality, particularly in older adults. In fact, when diastolic blood pressure is considered in the context of systolic blood pressure, there is the suggestion that a lower diastolic blood pressure for any given level of systolic pressure carries greater cardiovascular risk.

This would suggest that pulse pressure might be a better predictor than systolic pressure. However, there are limitations with this. Pulse pressure has no relation to an absolute level of blood pressure, e.g. a pulse pressure of 60 mmHg can be seen in someone with a blood pressure of 160/100 mmHg and in someone with a blood pressure of 120/60 mmHg. Also, there are no drugs that particularly reduce pulse pressure.

It is agreed that elevated levels of blood pressure are bad. Epidemiological studies suggest that there is a continuous log linear increased risk of cardiovascular events with increasing blood pressure with no clear cut off, at least to the age of 75. One large-scale international study has shown that significantly increased risks of cardiovascular disease begin to appear at a level as low as 115/75 mmHg. This is far lower than the average adult blood pressure in the UK (a mean of 131/74 mmHg for men and 126/73 mmHg for women).

Over the age of 80, it has been shown that high blood pressure is associated with lower mortality. This is likely to represent that those with low blood pressure have other comorbidities that will lead to a loss in weight, e.g. cancer, dementia, heart failure. However, this does not mean that treating individuals aged 80 or more with hypertension is not beneficial (see below for details on this).

Just to make matters more confusing, there is the issue of whether measurements away from the consultation process are better. It has been suggested that ambulatory systolic blood pressure is a better predictor of cardiovascular risk than that measured in the clinic. However, no trials have specifically looked at outcomes based on patients recruited solely according to ambulatory blood pressures, and ambulatory blood pressure monitoring (ABPM) should not form part of routine practice for all patients.

Rather than focus on blood pressure alone, guidelines have suggested that overall cardiovascular risk is considered. The problem with this is that by the age of 75 one can be considered high risk for a cardiovascular event simply by age alone. This raises the question of where the level for intervention should be. The practical answer is that of Geoffrey Rose quoted above. For that, we have to look to the numerous intervention trials performed in this age group, once we have diagnosed hypertension correctly, that is.

Diagnosis

In general, the measurement of blood pressure in the older adult is no different from that in younger individuals: appropriate cuff size, appropriate deflation rate, confirm elevation is sustained, etc. However, certain points should be considered in older adults.

1 Repeated measurements over time are particularly important given the propensity for increased variability.

2 The occurrence of an auscultatory gap is more common, especially in patients with isolated systolic hypertension.

3 Blood pressure should be checked in both arms as there can be as much as a 10 mmHg difference in systolic pressure between arms.

4 Given the prevalence of orthostatic hypotension it is important to take recordings both sitting/supine and standing, especially in those with symptoms.

5 Atrial fibrillation, which is more common in older adults, can lead to inaccuracies in measurement due to beat-to-beat variation in cardiac output.

6 Although rare (less than 2%), pseudohypertension, where the intra-arterial pressure is lower than the measured blood pressure due to failure to occlude a heavily calcified vessel, can lead to inappropriate intervention and needs to be borne in mind.

7 Post-prandial hypotension is frequently forgotten and can be as great as 25 mmHg after a meal in institutional older patients.

It is important to check for other cardiovascular risk factors and comorbidities that would influence drug choice and look for evidence of target organ damage. It is essential to take a full drug history including over-the-counter preparations (especially non-steroidal anti-inflammatory drugs). Studies of non-steroidal usage have been shown to produce a clinically significant increment in mean blood pressure of 5 mmHg in older adults.

Ambulatory blood pressure monitoring

There is evidence to suggest that older adults have a higher prevalence of white coat hypertension, up to double that in younger patients. It is also suggested that it is more frequently seen in females and those with ISH. In the systolic hypertension in Europe (Syst-Eur) trial, the difference between daytime ambulatory blood pressure monitoring (ABPM) readings and clinic blood pressures was as much as 20 mmHg. However, ABPM should not be used routinely but in selected individuals in regard to the following circumstances:

- to confirm elevated BP in those with SBP of 140–160 mmHg
- concern about the presence of white coat hypertension
- detection of postural and post-prandial hypotension
- assessment for drug-induced hypotension
- autonomic failure
- falls.

Treatment

Non-pharmacological treatment

Non-pharmacological methods are a constant feature of recommendations in the management of hypertension. Also, in contrast to drug therapy, there is no contraindication in the majority. The evidence for them has mostly come from trials in middle-aged individuals, but in the few intervention trials in older adults they would appear to be at least as effective. Age-related changes, such as a lack of sensitivity of taste buds, increased rates of depression and anxiety, and a reluctance to make changes to established daily routines, make changes to dietary intake more difficult to initiate. Also, additional comorbidities, such as osteoarthrosis, Parkinson's disease, and cognitive decline make increasing exercise challenging. The main areas to consider are:

1 salt reduction
2 weight reduction
3 increase in physical activity
4 moderation of alcohol consumption.

Stopping smoking must also be encouraged to reduce overall cardiovascular risk.

Older adults are more salt sensitive as a consequence of the changes in the renal handling of sodium with age. Thus, reducing salt intake in older adults can have a greater effect on blood pressure than in younger individuals. The Trial of Non-Pharmacologic Intervention in the Elderly (TONE) in those aged between 60 and 80 showed that reduction in sodium intake resulted in a lower systolic blood pressure of just over 4 mmHg and a 32% reduction in the need for antihypertensive medication. A practical issue with those older adults relying on pre-packaged food for meals is the amount of salt that they contain, making it difficult to achieve a reduction in salt intake. Low salt options are preferable in those with hypertension. In general, one would like to achieve a maximum salt intake of less than 6 g per day (2.4 g of sodium). In the UK, the average intake is currently closer to 9 g per day.

Levels of obesity are increasing both in general and also within older adults. The percentage of those aged 75 and over with a body mass index of 30 or more has more than doubled in the UK in the last 15 years to just over 20% in men and 25% in women. There is a scarcity of data on which to base recommendations in older adults in terms of weight reduction. In TONE, an intended weight loss of 3.5 kg resulted in a decrease in the need for antihypertensive medication by 30%. The trial investigated weight reduction in association with increased exercise. Just under a half of those aged 75 or over are inactive, meaning they engage in no leisure time physical activity. It is estimated that only 6% of this age group engage in vigorous physical activity for 20 minutes on three or more days per week. There is evidence that exercise programmes are beneficial for a range of outcomes, not just cardiovascular ones. Walking (at least 30 minutes per day ideally on most days of the week) is probably the exercise of choice among older adults, although even this can be subject to numerous barriers.

Non-pharmacological measures, particularly in combination, have a place in managing the older adult with hypertension. A multidisciplinary approach setting sensible and achievable goals, involving not just the patient but other family members as well, is most likely to succeed. This is an area that is often neglected but one that has great potential for improvement in blood pressure control. A reasonable set of goals is given in Table 5.2.

Pharmacological Treatment

> **Author's Tip**
>
> If an older cognitively intact adult walks in to see you and has a sustained systolic blood pressure of 160 mmHg or more— TREAT.

Clear evidence exists from many well-conducted randomized controlled trials performed over the last 25 years that antihypertensive medication in patients up to the age of at least 90 is beneficial. The latest was the Hypertension in the Very Elderly Trial (HYVET), which showed benefit in those aged 80 or more. They have all shown similar results,

Table 5.2 Goals of non-pharmacological management in older adults with hypertension

Salt	Reduce to 6 g per day
Diet	Follow the DASH (dietary approaches to stop hypertension) diet
	Consists of diet rich in fruits and vegetables, and low-fat or non-fat dairy.
	Limit caffeine intake to 300 mg per day (3 cups of coffee)
Exercise	30-min walk per day, 6 days a week
Weight loss	If over weight (BMI >25) a 3.5–4.5-kg reduction
Alcohol	Limit to 21 units per week in men, 14 units in women
Smoking	**STOP**

with cardiovascular benefits becoming apparent within 12 months:

- a reduction in stroke events of 25–47%
- a reduction in cardiac events of 13–29%
- a reduction in heart failure of 35–64%
- a reduction in any cardiovascular event of 17–40%.

The latest Cochrane review of January 2010 that included 15 trials and just over 24 000 subjects aged 60 or more showed a reduction in total mortality (at least up to the age of 80) of 10%, a reduction in overall cardiovascular events of 28% with no real difference for those under or over the age of 80. In addition to these clear benefits, there is the suggestion that antihypertensive medication may also reduce the chances of developing dementia. The benefits seen in older adults, in terms of an absolute reduction in events, are greater than those seen in younger individuals. Importantly in the Cochrane review, there was no increase in non-cardiovascular mortality to suggest a major adverse effect from treatment.

Applicability of trial results
The participants in these trials were:
- recruited from older populations from Europe (west and east), USA, Australia, and China
- had diastolic, combined systolic and diastolic, or ISH

BUT
- were less likely to have angina, diabetes, heart failure, dementia, depression, or limitations in their activities of daily living than individuals of a similar age in the general population
- entry level blood pressure was always 160 mmHg systolic or above
- those with orthostatic hypotension were underrepresented.

So the benefit in those that one might consider as 'frail' remains unproven, as it does in those with systolic blood pressures in the range 140–159 mmHg, although guidelines support the introduction of treatment for these levels based on an assessment of cardiovascular risk and the use of ABPM. The problem with those aged 70 or more is that they are at high risk just on their age alone. Also, clinicians remain concerned about those with symptomatic orthostatic hypotension who also have elevated pressures, as it is possible treatment may increase the risk of falls and their associated mortality and morbidity.

One could argue that older adults excluded from these trials were at a greater risk as they had a greater prevalence of risk factors and thus had more to gain. Equally, the greater prevalence of comorbidity might make them more susceptible to side-effects. At some stage the benefit must be lost due to comorbidity resulting in death before any benefit. Where that line is crossed is uncertain and this is where clinical judgement is paramount.

Certainly, those ambulant older adults whom one would not consider to be 'frail' with sustained blood pressures above 160 mmHg systolic or 90 mmHg diastolic should be treated. With regards to those with numerous comorbidities that are impacting markedly on their quality of life, a more individualistic approach will need to be adopted. For those in nursing homes or those with significant cognitive impairment, there is currently no clear evidence of benefit. Having decided upon treatment, the next two issues are which drugs to use and what should be the target blood pressure.

Target blood pressure

> **Author's Tip**
>
> Treatment targets in older adults are based more on wisdom than evidence. Current wisdom suggests below the age of 80 to aim for 140 mmHg systolic but 150 mmHg for those over 80.

There is uncertainty about what is the most appropriate target blood pressure to aim for in older adults. There is also a fear among some that lowering blood pressure too far is harmful.

The recommendations in guidelines to aim for 140 mmHg and below are based on data from younger subjects and usually *post hoc* analyses. In placebo-controlled studies, only one trial out of the many performed in older adults with hypertension have achieved mean blood pressures below 140 mmHg systolic in those on active medication. This study compared treating to below or above 140 mmHg and found no difference in cardiovascular events. The trial was by no means conclusive but does not support aggressive lowering of blood pressure in older adults. For those who are 80 or more, the best data come from the HYVET trial and this had a target of 150 mmHg.

There is often mention of the J-shaped curve in the debate of target blood pressure, particularly with regard to low diastolic pressures and reduced coronary perfusion. Concern has also been raised from observational studies suggesting associations between low blood pressure and white matter lesions in the brain and cognitive impairment.

One has to remember that comorbidities such as cancer, dementia, and heart failure can lead to low blood pressure. The J-shaped curve is probably an epidemiological finding, in that the patients with the lowest systolic and diastolic pressures already have more serious cardiovascular diseases or greater comorbidity than those with higher pressures. Even so, excessive lowering of blood pressure in older adults and in those with established coronary disease is probably best avoided to prevent severe postural hypotension. What should not be the case is that the fear of a J-shaped curve is used as a reason not to treat. Aiming for a target of 140 mmHg in those under the age of 80 and 150 mmHg for those 80 or above would seem to be a fair interpretation of the data and also achievable in the majority, at least in this author's opinion.

Drug choice

> **Author's Tip**
>
> Aim for a drug or combination that works (i.e. gets you close to target blood pressure) and is tolerated.

The majority of trials of antihypertensive treatment in older adults have used thiazide diuretics, beta-blockers, or dihydropyridine (DHP) calcium channel blockers (CCBs), mostly in combination making individual recommendations problematic. HYVET also used an angiotensin converting enzyme inhibitors (ACE-I). The benefits of beta-blockers have been questioned and are no longer supported as first-line treatment (at least in the UK guidelines). It is fair to state that in older adults with uncomplicated

Table 5.3 Indications and contraindications for antihypertensive treatment, adapted from the British Hypertension Guidelines

| Drug Class | Indication | | Contraindication | |
	Compelling	Possible	Possible	Compelling
Alpha-blockers	BPH		CCF	Urinary incontinence Postural/ postprandial Hypotension
ACE-Inhibitors (ACE-I)	CCF, LVSD, Post-MI, Stable CAD, type 1 DM nephropathy, Secondary stroke prevention	Proteinuric CKD, Type 2 DM nephropathy		Bilateral RAS
ARB	ACE-I intolerance, Type 2 DM nephropathy, Post-MI	CCF, CKD		Bilateral RAS
Beta-blockers	MI, CAD, CCF		PVD, COPD, Raynaud's disease	Asthma, Heart block
CCB (dihydropyridine)	ISH		Venous leg ulcers	
CCB (non-dihydropyridine)	CAD		Not with beta-blockers	Heart block CCF
Low dose Thiazide/ Thiazide-like	CCF, Secondary stroke prevention		Hypokalaemia, Hyponatraemia	Gout

BPH, benign prostatic hypertrophy; CAD, coronary artery disease; CCF, congestive cardiac failure; CKD, chronic kidney disease; COPD, chronic obstructive pulmonary disease; DM, diabetes mellitus; ISH, isolated systolic hypertension; LVSD, left ventricular systolic dysfunction; MI, myocardial infarction; PVD, peripheral vascular disease; RAS, renal artery stenosis.

hypertension, the positive evidence for low-dose diuretics exceeds that of beta-blockers. However, the presence of symptomatic coronary artery disease as suggested by angina remains a compelling reason for their use. The majority of data on ACE-Is and angiotensin receptor blockers (ARBs) comes from patients selected on the basis of their cardiovascular risk or presence of diabetes rather than blood pressure *per se*.

There are some general principles that apply when treating older adults due to age-associated changes in pharmacodynamics and pharmacokinetics

- start low and go slow
- keep it simple to improve adherence
- consider comorbidities as this may dictate choice (see Table 5.3)
- if no compelling indications, A/CD approach of the BHS/NICE guidelines is reasonable (see Figure 5.7)
- beware orthostatic hypotension, but it is not a reason to withhold treatment if asymptomatic
- half will require more than one class of drug to reach target, a third will require three
- better to use two at low dose with no adverse effects than one at higher dose and poorly tolerated
- address other cardiovascular risk factors as indicated.

The debate of which antihypertensive treatment to use first is slightly academic as in at least 50% more than one type of class of antihypertensive will be required. In general when no compelling indication/contraindications exist, the A/CD approach supported by the current UK guidelines (Figure 5.7) is sensible. If there are compelling indications (Table 5.3), the approach can be modified.

It is important to remember that older patients can find it difficult to comply with complicated treatment regimens, particularly if they involve multiple drugs and multiple doses. When the patient lives alone, has problems with concentration, understanding and memory, or is mildly demented or depressed, compliance with such regimens becomes even more challenging.

There will be some who fit the definition of resistant hypertension (blood pressure not controlled in spite of three different drug classes). It is more common in older adults although the true prevalence and prognosis is uncertain. It is important to review measurement techniques, adherence and check for potential exacerbating factors (Table 5.4). The use of spironolactone can be considered (Figure 5.7) and is currently being assessed by a clinical trial.

There is still inertia among the medical profession in treating older adults with hypertension to appropriate target blood pressures. The fear of exacerbating falls is one, and although generally supported by the latest systematic review, this should not be a compelling reason to withhold treatment. The benefit of cardiovascular prevention needs to be carefully weighed against the risk of falling. In the UK, one of the biggest drivers to counter this has been the introduction of Quality Framework targets, where primary care physicians receive funding based on reaching set targets such as blood pressure measurement and control. This has had large impact in the UK on control rates for those with hypertension.

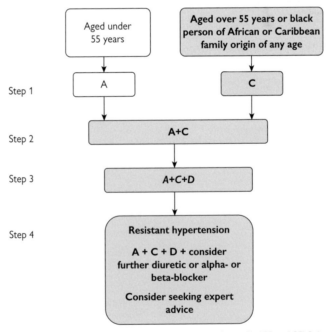

Treatment algorithm—NICE recommendations (A = ARB or ACEI; B = β blocker; C = Calcium channel blocker; D = diuretic.)

| | Aged under 55 years | Aged over 55 years or black person of African or Caribbean family origin of any age |

Step 1	A	C
Step 2	A+C	
Step 3	A+C+D	
Step 4	Resistant hypertension A + C + D + consider further diuretic or alpha- or beta-blocker Consider seeking expert advice	

Figure 5.7 Treatment algorithm based on British Hypertension Society recommendations (A, ARB or ACEI; B, *beta*-blocker; C, calcium channel blocker; D, diuretic). Adapted from the British Hypertension Society Guidelines.

Table 5.4 Issues to consider in resistant hypertension

Measurement errors	Incorrect positioning
	Incorrect cuff size
	Recent ingestion of caffeine
	Pseudohypertension
	Consider 'white-coat effect'
Adherence failure	Non-adherence to lifestyle interventions (especially salt)
	Non-adherence to medication
	Additional OTC medication (e.g. NSAIDs) and other prescribed medication (e.g. steroids, sympathomimetics etc)
Contributing causes	Sleep apnoea
	Secondary causes (especially renovascular disease)
	Paroxsymal hypertension

OTC, over the counter.

Summary

Globally the number of older adults is increasing rapidly and in most societies ageing is associated with a consistent and sustained rise in systolic blood pressure, making hypertension a common finding. It is an important and treatable risk factor for cardiovascular mortality and morbidity even in to late life. Blood pressure lowering needs to take in to consideration the general wellbeing of the individual, but in hypertensive non-frail adults striving for improved blood pressure control will provide benefits. Non-pharmacological methods should be considered. The selection of pharmacological agents should take into consideration an individual's comorbidity and concomitant drug therapy. Age should not be the primary focus. For those starting on treatment most will require two or more drugs to achieve appropriate blood pressure targets.

Further reading

Beckett NS, Peters R, Fletcher AE (2008). Treatment of hypertension in patients 80 years of age or older. *N Engl J Med* **1; 358**: 1887–98.

Blood Pressure Lowering Treatment Trialists' Collaboration (2008). Effects of different regimens to lower blood pressure on major cardiovascular events in older and younger adults: meta-analysis of randomised trials. *Br Med J* **17; 336**: 1121–3.

JATOS Study Group (2008). Principal results of the Japanese trial to assess optimal systolic blood pressure in elderly hypertensive patients (JATOS). *Hypertens Res* **31**: 2115–27.

Lakatta EG, Wang M, Najjar SS (2009). Arterial aging and subclinical arterial disease are fundamentally intertwined at macroscopic and molecular levels. *Med Clin North Am* **93**: 583–604.

Lewington S, Clarke R, Qizilbash N, et al. (2002). Age-specific relevance of usual blood pressure to vascular mortality: a meta-analysis of individual data for one million adults in 61 prospective studies. *Lancet* **360**: 1903–13.

Musini VM, Tejani AM, Bassett K, et al. (2009). Pharmacotherapy for hypertension in the elderly. *Cochrane Database Syst Rev* (4): CD000028.

PATHWAYS Study (2009). Prevention and treatment of resistant hypertension with algorithm based therapy (http://www.bhf.org.uk/default.aspx?page=9984).

Peters R, Beckett N, Forette F, et al. (2008). Incident dementia and blood pressure lowering in the Hypertension in the Very Elderly Trial cognitive function assessment (HYVET-COG): a double-blind, placebo controlled trial. *Lancet Neurol* **7**: 683–9.

Staessen JA, Thijs L, O'Brien ET, et al. (2002). Ambulatory pulse pressure as predictor of outcome in older patients with systolic hypertension. *Am J Hypertens* **15**(10 Pt 1): 835–43.

van Bemmel T, Woittiez K, Blauw GJ, et al. (2006). Prospective study of the effect of blood pressure on renal function in old age: the Leiden 85-Plus Study. *J Am Soc Nephrol* **17**: 2561–6.

Whelton PK, Appel LJ, Espeland MA, et al. (1998). Sodium reduction and weight loss in the treatment of hypertension in older persons: a randomized controlled trial of nonpharmacologic interventions in the elderly (TONE). *JAMA*, **18; 279**: 839–46.

Williams B, Poulter NR, Brown MJ, et al. (2004). British Hypertension Society Guidelines for management of hypertension: report of the fourth working party of the British Hypertension Society, 2004-BHS IV. *J Hum Hypertens* **18**: 139–85.

Williams B, Lindholm LH, Sever P (2008). Systolic pressure is all that matters. *Lancet* **28; 371**: 2219–21 (http://www.ic.nhs.uk/statistics-and-data-collections/health-and-lifestyles-related-surveys/health-survey-for-england).

Woolcott JC, Richardson KJ, Wiens MO, et al. (2009). Meta-analysis of the impact of 9 medication classes on falls in elderly persons. *Arch Intern Med*, 169: 1952–60.

Pulmonary oedema

Introduction

Pulmonary oedema (PO) refers to the accumulation of excess fluid in the lung either within the interstitial spaces or in the alveoli or both. It usually occurs in cardiac diseases with raised left-sided filling pressure as a result of impaired left ventricular (LV) function. However, it is important to understand that the terms PO and LV failure are not synonymous, because PO can occur due to other heart problems in which LV function is entirely normal, e.g. mitral valve disease, or to non-cardiac problems, e.g. adult respiratory distress syndrome (ARDS) (see Table 5.5). However, the most common cause of PO in older patients is LV dysfunction, which is covered in the section on Left ventricular systolic dysfunction in greater detail.

> **Author's Tip**
>
> PO and LV failure are not synonymous

Pathophysiology

When the capillary membrane is intact, intravascular and extravascular fluid equilibrium is principally maintained by the balance between two opposing forces. The hydrostatic pressure head favours fluid efflux and is the difference between the capillary (Pc) and interstitial (Pi) hydrostatic pressure. The plasma colloidal osmotic pressure depends on plasma protein concentration (mainly albumin) and its head of pressure favouring fluid influx is the difference between the osmotic pressure in the capillary (πc) and that in the interstitium (πi).

Normally, the hydrostatic pressure head slightly exceeds osmotic pressure (see Figure 5.8) and there is a net efflux resulting in the formation of some interstitial fluid which is completely drained by interstitial lymphatics. When capillary hydrostatic pressure is raised (usually due to cardiogenic problems increasing LV diastolic, left atrial, or pulmonary vein pressures), the efflux of fluid into the interstitium is increased and overcomes the lymphatic drainage capability. (see Figure 5.9) Excess fluid accumulates as oedema in the interstitium initially and then in the alveoli (PO). This is called cardiogenic or haemodynamic PO. The degree of oedema is increased, and the hydrostatic

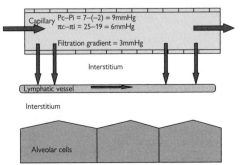

Figure 5.8 Normal haemodynamics. Pc, capillary hydrostatic pressure; π c, capillary osmotic pressure ; Pi , interstitial hydrostatic pressure ; π i , interstitial osmotic pressure.

pressure at which it occurs is reduced when there is hypoalbuminaemia reducing the opposing capillary oncotic pressure.

In contrast, non-cardiac or permeability pulmonary oedema (see Table 5.5) occurs when the capillary endothelium is damaged and leaks protein and fluid into the interstitium +/– alveoli while hydrostatic forces remain fairly normal.

Three stages in the development of pulmonary oedema can be recognized, namely pre-oedema, interstitial oedema, and alveolar oedema, and each has differing tissue changes and radiological appearances (see Table 5.6).

Clinical features of pulmonary oedema
Symptoms

These may arise from the underlying cause as well as from the PO itself. The latter starts with dyspnoea on exertion, then dyspnoea that is worse on lying flat (orthopnoea), often associated with cough and wheeze. As the condition worsens, acute dyspnoea wakes the patient at night (paroxysmal nocturnal dyspnoea, PND) often with frothy sputum, initially clear and later blood tinged (pink) due to extravasation of red cells into the alveolar fluid. Patients become anxious and agitated due to the difficulty in breathing and hypoxia. Central hypoxia may lead to

Table 5.5 Common causes of pulmonary oedema

Cardiac (haemodynamic PO)	Non-cardiac (permeability PO)
LV systolic dysfunction	**Endothelial inflammation**
Ischaemia/infarction	ARDS
Cardiomyopathy	Smoke inhalation
Hypertension	Aspiration
Aortic stenosis	Infection
Aortic regurgitation	**Reactive endothelial damage**
Normal LV systolic function	
Diastolic dysfunction	Pancreatitis
Mitral regurgitation	Head injury
Mitral stenosis	Pulmonary embolism
Tamponade	**Other endothelial injury**
Atrial myxoma	Drugs, e.g. Paraquat, Bleomycin
	High altitude
	Renal artery stenosis

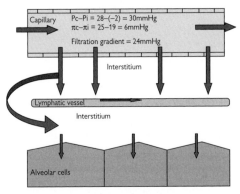

Figure 5.9 Cardiogenic PO. Pc,capillary hydrostatic pressure; πc, capillary osmotic pressure; Pi, interstitial hydrostatic pressure; πi, interstitial osmotic pressure.

Table 5.6 Stages in the development of pulmonary oedema

Stage	Cellular level changes	Radiological appearances
Pre-oedema (congestion) LA pressure 12–15 mmHg	↑ Capillary flow Distended lymphatics	Upper lobe diversion
Interstitial oedema LA pressure 15–24 mmHg	Fluid in peri-alveolar spaces (interstitium)	Fluid in fissure, peribronchial cuffing, Kerley B lines
Alveolar oedema LA pressure >25 mmHg	Alveolar flooding	Fluffy hilar 'bat's wing' shadowing, pleural effusions

confusion and Cheyne–Stokes breathing (periodic hyperventilation and apnoea).

Signs
Common physical signs due to PO itself include sweating, tachycardia, tachypnoea, and central cyanosis. In pulmonary congestion there may be wheeze due to bronchial mucosal thickening and excess bronchial secretion but no crackles. When true oedema occurs fine inspiratory crackles are added, initially at the lung bases but later all over. When the oedema is cardiac in origin (haemodynamic), the classic triad of pulsus alternans, a third heart sound, and pulmonary crackles occurs.

Investigation of pulmonary oedema
Confirmation of the clinical diagnosis and its severity should be sought on a **chest radiograph** (see Table 5.6) and using **arterial blood gases** (usually type I respiratory failure, later Type II). Contributing factors should be identified, e.g. hypoalbuminaemia, anaemia. As soon as possible investigations should be initiated to look for the cause of the PO, although this may be fairly obvious from the **clinical context**, e.g. ARDS in a patient with community-acquired pneumonia or cardiogenic PO following a myocardial infarct in a patient with known LV impairment. The prime initial cardiac investigations are:
- Resting ECG—provides evidence of old infarction or LBBB both favouring LV systolic dysfunction whereas an absolutely normal ECG usually excludes it.
- Echocardiograph—provides vital information about LV size and function, LV hypertrophy, valvular dysfunction, pericardial effusion.

Later investigations may include:
- Cardiac MR/thallium scanning—help identify hibernating (reversibly damaged) myocardium.

> **Author's Tip**
> An absolutely normal ECG essentially rules out LV systolic dysfunction as the cause of PO, but an ECHO is the pivotal test.

Treatment
This section refers to the management of acute PO. For details of longer term treatment and palliative care see the section Left ventricular systolic function. Definitive treatment requires the correction of the underlying cause of the pulmonary oedema.

Initial treatment is aimed at improving the acute symptoms and accompanying haemodynamic/biochemical disturbances and includes:
- Oxygen therapy – by face mask with oxygen concentration/flow determined by repeated blood gases; may require non-invasive ventilation (see below) or ultimately mechanical ventilation on the ITU.
- Intravenous (IV) loop diuretics – usually furosemide. Initial benefit (<1 hour) is due to venodilatation, later benefit is due to renal excretion of salt and water leading to reduced circulatory volume and hence lower pulmonary hydrostatic pressures. Repeated boluses are preferred until the daily dose requirement exceeds 160 mg when continuous infusion is often more convenient and less likely to cause haemodynamic upset or altered hearing especially in the older patient.
- IV (or buccal) nitrate – up titration of dose to optimize reduction in venodilatation/preload (its main effect) and vasodilatation/after load (lesser effect).
- Opiates – IV or IM reduce anxiety and have a venodilatory effect.
- Early non-invasive ventilation (NIV) with positive end-expiratory pressure (PEEP) reduces respiratory distress, short-term mortality and need for intubation in acute cardiogenic PO, especially in older patients who quickly develop respiratory fatigue. NIV with PEEP improves LV function by reducing LV afterload but should be used with caution in cardiogenic shock, RV failure, in COPD and in patients who cannot cooperate. Potential adverse effects include worsening RV failure, hypercapnia, anxiety, pneumothorax, and aspiration.
- Invasive ventilation becomes necessary in patients with increasing respiratory failure despite oxygen via mask or NIV. The ultimate decision on its usage depends upon a consideration of comorbidity and the likelihood of ultimate recovery.
- Medium–large pleural effusions are unusual in acute PO but if present and compromising oxygenation may need tapping. If so this should only be undertaken with imaging control to avoid potentially disastrous pneumothorax or liver damage. Reaccumulation can be made less likely by optimizing hydrostatic pressure and serum albumin.

Prognosis is mainly dependent on the underlying cause and on comorbidity. Very few studies have looked at the factors predicting in-hospital and 1-year mortality. One early study reported 43% overall mortality at 1 year in acute cardiogenic PO in an older population. Subsequent annual mortality is likely to be about 10% despite modern treatment.

Further reading
Armstrong P, Wilson AG, Dee P, et al. (2000). Imaging of diseases of the chest, 3rd edn. London, Mosby (Harcourt), pp. 444–56.

Guyton AC, Hall JE (2000). *Pulmonary Circulation; Pulmonary Oedema; Pleural Fluid. Textbook of Medical Physiology.* Philadelphia, WB Saunders, pp. 444–51.

Libby P, Bonow R, Mann, D, Zipes D (2000). *Braunwald's Heart Disease – A Text of Cardiovascular Medicine,* 7th edn. Philadelphia, WB Saunders, pp. 555–64.

Plotnick GD, Kelemen MH, Garrett RB, et al. (1982). Acute cardiogenic pulmonary oedema in the elderly: factors predicting in-hospital and one year mortality. *South Med J* **75**: 565–9.

Left ventricular systolic dysfunction

Introduction

The left ventricle (LV) is principally a hollow muscular pump, the main function of which is to contract and hence eject blood (the stroke volume) into the aorta. Myocardial contraction occurs due to configurational changes causing shortening of muscle fibres resulting from interaction between the two main contractile proteins, the thin actin and thick myosin filaments. This is triggered by calcium ions which combine with the modulatory protein troponin C to relieve the inhibition of interaction exerted by troponin I.

The term left ventricular systolic dysfunction (LVSD) refers to an impairment of myocardial contraction usually resulting from a reduced number of myocytes, i.e. cellular death due to infarction, infections, infiltration or apoptosis; reduced strength, or force of contraction of viable myocytes (impaired inotropy) due to acute ischaemia, drugs/poisons, e.g. alcohol, infections; or excessive myocardial strain caused by pressure or volume overload. The common causes of LVSD and frequent trigger factors are shown in Table 5.7.

Pathology, pathophysiology and compensatory mechanisms

LVSD may be permanent when it results from myocyte death, e.g. myocardial infarction, or reversible when myocyte integrity is maintained. In the latter case, non-vital cellular functions including contraction are temporarily suspended, e.g. myocardial stunning or hibernation due to acute ischaemia without infarction.

LVSD may affect the whole LV to a similar extent (so-called global LVSD) or pick only certain areas while leaving others intact (regional LVSD). The classical cause of regional LV impairment is ischaemic heart disease (IHD), because each coronary artery has its own fairly well-defined area of supply. This contrasts with the global nature of cardiomyopathy or myocarditis in which all LV myocardial regions are usually equally involved.

> **Author's Tip**
>
> LVSD may be reversible (stunning, hibernation) or permanent (infarction); distribution may be global or regional.

Table 5.7 Common causes of left ventricular systolic dysfunction

Common causes	Triggers
Myocardial damage/death	**Arrhythmias**
IHD (infarction, stunning, hibernation)	Fast AF/flutter
	Acute ischaemia
Cardiomyopathy (Idiopathic, familial, post-partum, drugs)	**Drug discontinuation**
	ACEi
Acute myocarditis	Digoxin
Infiltration (amyloid, sarcoid)	Diuretics
Pressure overload	**Noxious drugs**
Systemic hypertension	NSAIDs
Aortic stenosis	Alcohol
Volume overload	**Respiratory illness**
Aortic/mitral regurgitation	Infection
Intracardiac shunt	Pulmonary embolus
	Anaemia

Whether global or regional, LVSD involves damage to myocytes and extracellular matrix leading to changes in size, shape, and function of the LV and the heart, generally termed remodelling. These changes set in train a number of compensatory mechanisms designed to nullify the adverse effects of the reduced cardiac output resulting from the inevitable reduction in stroke volume. Unfortunately, these compensatory homeostatic mechanisms (see Figure 5.10) are often inappropriate or excessive, tend to aggravate the underlying problem, cause the appearance of a constellation of symptoms and signs termed heart failure, and thus produce a downward spiralling vicious cycle which, unchecked leads to death.

Clinical aspects:

Patients with asymptomatic LVSD progress to overt heart failure over time as a result of the vicious cycle shown in Figure 5.10. LVSD is underdiagnosed in elderly people as reduced exercise tolerance is often attributed to ageing or other comorbidities. LVSD prevalence increases steeply with age rising to 10% or more among persons 70 years of age or older.

When LVSD presents as heart failure it can be usefully classified clinically as forward or backward. Forward left heart failure produces reduced cardiac output with poor systemic circulation resulting in typical symptoms (dizziness, confusion, fatigue, and anuria) and signs (cool extremities, pallor, sweaty, tachycardia, low blood pressure). Backward left heart failure results in pulmonary congestion and oedema causing dyspnoea.

Assessment

- *Subjective functional severity* should be graded according to the New York Heart Association (NYHA) classification, which increments from class I with no limitation of normal physical activity to class IV with symptoms at rest.
- *Objective functional capacity* should be quantified by an exercise test (treadmill or bike) which assesses exercise capacity, exertional symptoms, inducible arrhythmias, and inducible ischaemia. Cardiopulmonary exercise testing (CPET) with gas exchange measurement is being increasingly used to provide additive information on functional capacity, prognosis, and perioperative risk as well as to differentiate cardiac dyspnoea from respiratory causes.
- *Anatomical assessment* by echocardiography is the pivotal investigation. This will confirm the presence of LVSD and its distribution (global, regional). Although an LV ejection fraction (EF) of <45% arbitrarily defines global LVSD, EF may be misleadingly normal in regional LVSD where regional wall motion abnormalities should be assessed. Structural abnormalities especially valvular lesions should be sought to establish the cause of the LVSD.

Other investigations

The ECG may show left bundle branch block or Q waves due to old myocardial infarction but LVSD is very unlikely with an absolutely normal ECG.

Plasma natriuretic peptides including B-type natriuretic peptide (BNP) and N-terminal pro-BNP are secreted by the failing heart, promote diuresis, and may be useful diagnostically, prognostically, and in assessing response

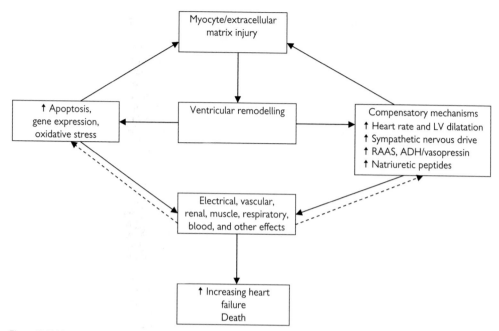

Figure 5.10 Vicious cycle of myocardial damage leading to heart failure.

to treatment. The major source of BNP synthesis and secretion is the ventricular myocardium. Levels increase in response to increased venous return with atrial distension and raised ventricular wall stress. Raised levels are fairly sensitive in the diagnosis of heart failure. Heart failure is unlikely at BNP values of <100 pg/mL and is very likely at BNP values >400 pg/mL. Elevated BNP is not specific for heart failure being also seen in many other conditions, e.g. myocardial ischaemia, left ventricular hypertrophy, cirrhosis, sepsis, and renal failure. BNP rises with age, and elevated levels may occur in advanced age alone. A particular strength of BNP is to rule out heart failure in patients with shortness of breath.

Troponin should be measured when an underlying acute coronary syndrome is suspected. Raised levels indicate myocyte necrosis. Minor rises are frequently seen in severe heart failure without ischaemia especially with renal failure or sepsis but large rises indicate an myocardial infarction or myocarditis.

Cardiac magnetic resonance imaging and radionuclide scanning (MUGA, MIBI, and thallium) may be needed in selected cases to assess LV systolic function as well as viable (hibernating) myocardium and myocardial ischaemia.

Management

An MDT approach to patient care is vital involving both primary and secondary care. Management aims are to reduce mortality due to sudden death or pump failure; improve the quality of life by reducing symptoms, hospital admissions, and drug side-effects; and to provide appropriate advice, support, and education to both patients and their families.

A detailed account of the modern treatment of LVSD and heart failure is beyond the scope of this section but is summarized in the box Treatment options for LVSD and heart failure. Figure 5.11 outlines the management according to the now accepted stages of heart failure.

Notably, treatment of LVSD is becoming increasingly interventional and all patients should be assessed for an implantable cardiac defibrillator (ICD) and/or surgery and the more symptomatic ones for cardiac resynchronization therapy (CRT) as well as receiving non-pharmacological, drug, and palliative therapies (see Treatment options for LVSD and heart failure).

Heart failure drugs: practical tips
Polypharmacy is very common in elderly patients and this may lead to falls and poor compliance. The treatment plan for elderly patients with heart failure must be put in the context of their overall needs. Diuretics often worsen urinary incontinence and cause important biochemical upset (hyponatraemia and hypokalaemia) in older people so maintenance doses should be kept to a minimum by controlling heart rate in AF, optimizing ACE inhibitor dose and treating associated conditions such as anaemia or thyroid abnormalities.

Co-prescription of diuretics with ACE inhibitors or ARBs significantly increases the likelihood of hypotension (especially postural) and hence of falls and collapses.

However, physician reluctance to commence beta-blockers in elderly patients due to concerns about intolerance and comorbidities such as chronic obstructive pulmonary disease and diabetes is often misplaced. Recent evidence (SENIORS and COLA II studies) suggests that they can be used safely in elderly patients with heart failure

---

ADH - antidiuretic hormone; LV -left ventricle; RAAS - renin-angiotensin-aldosterone system
Author's Tip

Try to identify the cause and precipitant of heart failure.

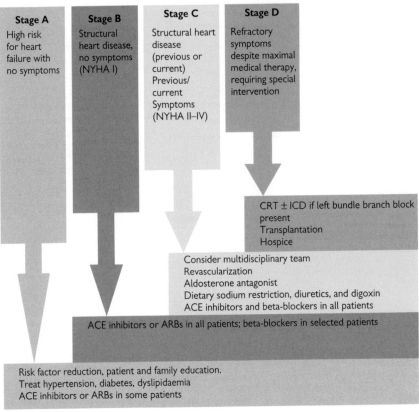

Figure 5.11 Stages of heart failure and treatment. ACE - angiotensin converting enzyme; ARBs - angiotensin receptor blockers; CRT - cardiac resynchronisation therapy; ICD - implantable cardiofibrillator.

Treatment options for LVSD and heart failure

Non-pharmacological:

- Patient education (drugs, weight, alcohol, self-care)
- Fluid restriction (1-1.5L/day); sodium restriction
- Increase exercise (via cardiac rehabilitation team)
- Surgery-correction of cause eg. valve disease, IHD causing hibernation; heart transplantation

Drugs:

- ACEi (ARB if intolerant): improve symptoms/prognosis
- Appropriate beta blockers: carvedilol, bisoprolol, metoprolol and nebivolol improve prognosis and reduce hospital admissions
- Aldosterone antagonists: improve prognosis in symptomatic (NYHAIII-IV) severe LVSD (EF<35%)
- Diuretics: improve symptoms due to fluid retention; no prognostic benefit
- Digoxin: controls exacerbation due to AF; small improvement in symptoms in sinus rhythm due to positive inotropic effect
- Hydralazine/Isosorbide dinitrate combination: to improve prognosis in blacks or when intolerant of ACEi

Devices:

- Cardiac resynchronisation therapy (CRT)
- Implantable cardioverter defibrillator (ICD)
- LV assist devices

Palliative:

- End stage heart failure at home/hospice/hospital

provided care is taken to commence on low doses and titrate up as tolerated.

Further reading

Bristow MR (2000). Beta-adrenergic receptor blockade in chronic heart failure. *Circulation*, **101**: 558–69.

Jessup M, Brozena LS (2003). Heart failure. *N Engl J Med* **348**: 2007–18.

NICE clinical guidance 5 (2003). Chronic heart failure (www.nice.org.uk).

Smith WH, Ball SG (2000). ACE inhibitors in heart failure: an update. *Basic Res Cardiol* **95**: I8–14.

Right ventricular dysfunction

Introduction

Like the left ventricle (LV), the right ventricle (RV) is principally a hollow muscular pump whose main function is to contract and hence eject blood into the pulmonary artery. The RV is connected in series with the LV and should therefore pump the same effective stroke volume. The highly distensible and low-impedance pulmonary circulation allows the RV to do this at low pressures. The RV is the most anterior of the cardiac chambers, situated behind the sternum. The shape of the RV is complex; wrapping itself around the LV it appears crescent shaped in cross-section, and triangular when viewed from the side. The RV has three components: the inlet consisting of the tricuspid valve, the chordae tendineae, and papillary muscles; the apical myocardium; and the infundibulum comprising the outflow tract. In 80% of hearts the RV myocardium is perfused by the right coronary artery. Its low oxygen consumption and more extensive collateral system make the RV less susceptible to irreversible ischaemic injury.

Pathology and pathophysiology

As with the LV, RV dysfunction is predominantly systolic (RVSD) and involves an impairment of RV myocardial contraction due to myocyte loss, impaired inotropy of viable myocytes, or excessive strain (pressure or volume overload). Unlike LVSD, RVSD is usually global because RV ischaemia/infarction is relatively uncommon. Age-related LV impairment (myocyte loss, LV incompliance) and pulmonary changes (with rising PA pressure) mean that presentation with the clinical picture of RV failure is common in the older population.

Causes of RVSD

As for LVSD the causes of RV dysfunction may be split into intrinsic myocardial disease, pressure overload, or volume overload but in addition may result from complex congenital defects. This section will focus on some of the most pertinent pathologies.

Author's Tip

The most common causes of RV dysfunction are LV dysfunction and cor pulmonale

---

Intrinsic myocardial disease

Permanent RV damage due to infarction is rare but transient RV dysfunction in inferior LV infarction is more common (see later). The RV is often involved in generalized cardiomyopathy and there is a specific RV cardiomyopathy (see later). RV infiltration occurs in amyloid, sarcoid, and other similar conditions.

Pressure overload (Figure 5.12, Table 5.8)

Chronic pressure overload in the RV can lead to extensive hypertrophy and fibrosis, with reduced systolic function, dilatation, and hence functional tricuspid regurgitation. The major cause of RV pressure overload is pulmonary hypertension due to left-sided heart failure (see Figure 5.12). Pulmonary hypertension secondary to cor pulmonale is also relatively common and results from reduced pulmonary capillary bed size, particularly in COPD, hypoxic vasoconstriction, pulmonary embolism, or primary pulmonary hypertension.

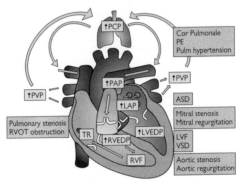

Figure 5.12 (colour plate 1) Backward pressure paradigm; increased pressures from any area of cardiopulmonary circulation can lead to back pressure on the right ventricle, subsequent pressure overload and ultimately RV dysfunction. Stages in backward pressure with pathologies are highlighted. LVEDP, left ventricular end diastolic pressure; LAP, left atrial pressure; PVP, pulmonary venous pressure; PCP, pulmonary capillary pressure; PAP, pulmonary artery pressure; RVEDP, right ventricular end diastolic pressure; RVF, right ventricular failure; TR, tricuspid regurgitation.

RV outflow tract obstruction, infundibular or valvular pulmonary stenosis, leads to pressure overload and can be either congenital or acquired.

Volume Overload (Table 5.8)

The RV adapts better to volume overload than to pressure overload. In valvular defects e.g. tricuspid regurgitation the RV may tolerate the increased volumes longer before RV performance declines. The same is often true when septal defects increase the volume of the right heart. Rarer causes of RV volume overload should also be considered (Table 5.8). Longstanding volume overload leads to RV dilatation and the clinical syndrome of right heart failure, which is associated with an increase in long-term morbidity and mortality.

Clinical signs in RV dysfunction:

As in LVSD, it is clinically useful to divide RVSD into forward and backward failure. Since the RV and LV are in series, forward RV failure produces the same symptoms and signs due to low cardiac output, as does LVSD. Backward RV failure results in systemic, rather than pulmonary, congestion and oedema.

Table 5.8 Causes of pressure and volume overload

Pressure overload	Volume overload
Left-sided heart failure	Tricuspid regurgitation
Pulmonary embolus	Pulmonary regurgitation
Pulmonary hypertension	Atrial septal defect
RV outflow tract obstruction	Ventricular septal defect
Congenital defects	Anomalous pulmonary venous return
	Coronary artery fistula to right heart
	Carcinoid syndrome

The early stages of RV pressure overload lead to RV hypertrophy, clinically apparent by a left parasternal heave, right-sided fourth heart sound, and prominent A wave in the jugular venous pulse. If pulmonary hypertension is present a loud pulmonary component to the second heart sound may be audible. RV dilation due to RVSD and failure causes functional tricuspid regurgitation (TR), leading to a raised JVP, the pansystolic murmur of TR and a pulsatile liver. Right-sided murmurs or gallops become more apparent on inspiration as venous return to the right heart increases (emphysema is an exception). Systemic venous hypertension causes congestive hepatomegaly (pulsatile if TR is prominent) together with peripheral oedema and/or pleural effusion and/or ascites.

Special situations

RV myocardial infarction (RVMI)
The incidence of true RVMI is rare but ischaemic RV dysfunction (usually transient) is not uncommon, complicating 20–50% of inferior LVMIs. Haemodynamically significant RVMI occurs in about 5% of such patients. The clinical triad of elevated jugular veins, hypotension, and clear lung fields should alert the physician to the presence of significant RV impairment without significant LV dysfunction. This leads to a low cardiac output syndrome and heart failure due to an inadequate preload. It is important to treat this with a fluid challenge, rather than diuresis, which will compound matters. Recovery of transient RV dysfunction can be identified on repeat echocardiography.

Author's Tip

Treat low cardiac output syndrome in acute RVMI or inferior LVMI with a fluid challenge, not diuretics

---

Pulmonary embolus
Acute pulmonary embolus (PE) causes an abrupt rise in RV pressure over minutes to hours, which can induce acute RV dilatation and dysfunction. This is seen clinically by raised jugular venous pressure, and often biochemically by the release of cardiac troponins and brain natriuretic peptide. In this context the presence of inverted T waves in leads V1–V3 on the ECG is a strong indicator of RV dysfunction, more so than the transient S1Q3T3 phenomenon. The best investigation for acute RV dysfunction is echocardiography. The optimum treatment for RV dysfunction occurring in this setting of so called submassive PE is still unclear. However when associated with haemodynamic compromise, thrombolysis should be considered since some trials have shown reduced mortality and recurrence rates. For those without haemodynamic compromise, the evidence is less clear, and decisions should be made on an individual basis.

Arrhythmogenic right ventricular dysplasia/cardiomyopathy (ARVD/C)
ARVD is a genetic disorder of desmosomal proteins, causing fibrofatty infiltration of the RV. It rarely presents in the older population, but can cause sudden cardiac death.

Investigation of RV dysfunction
- *ECG.* May show evidence of previous inferior infarction or RV strain (see PE section). A right axis deviation may signify right ventricular hypertrophy.
- *CXR.* Important to identify causes of cor pulmonale or pulmonary oedema due to left-sided failure. Prominent pulmonary arteries with peripheral pruning can sometimes be seen indicating pulmonary hypertension.
- *Echocardiography:* It is more difficult to assess the RV than the LV but in experienced hands an echocardiogram (echo) can usefully assess RV dimensions and systolic function. It can also be used to screen for septal defects, sometimes with bubble contrast, and often allows non-invasive estimation of pulmonary pressures.
- *Nuclear imaging:* Largely superseded by echo and magnetic resonance in the assessment of the RV; ventilation/perfusion scans are still used to screen for PE.
- *Computed tomography:* CT pulmonary angiography (CTPA) is most commonly used to diagnose PE. High-resolution CT may help screen for causes of cor pulmonale. CTPA may also be useful to investigate chronic PEs as a cause of isolated RV dysfunction.
- *Magnetic resonance imaging:* This is the gold standard for assessment of RV volumes and ejection fraction, RV myocardial viability, and infiltrative disease such as amyloid. The main limitations are cost, less widespread availability, and less operator experience.
- *Right heart catheterization:* Less common because of non-invasive imaging but gives direct pressure measurements (especially pulmonary artery pressure), allows estimation of intracardiac shunt size and can be combined with invasive pulmonary angiography/RV biopsy.
- *Invasive pulmonary angiography:* Gold standard for assessment of the pulmonary tree. Largely replaced by safer, non-invasive methods.
- *Myocardial biopsy:* Useful to assess the fatty infiltration of ARVD/C or amyloid when suggested by MR scanning.

Treatment of RV dysfunction
Treatment in RV dysfunction is mainly aimed at the cause. Specific pharmacological therapies used in LV dysfunction, e.g. ACEi, beta-blocker, spironolactone, have no known similar prognostic or symptomatic benefit in isolated RV dysfunction, and are therefore not indicated. Loop diuretics provide symptomatic benefit when fluid overload predominates. Left-sided cardiac lesions, such as valvular defects, may require surgery. Septal defects may now be closed percutaneously. The cause of cor pulmonale should be sought, and if possible treated to reduce pulmonary pressures. Anticoagulation has been proven to help in primary pulmonary hypertension and that secondary to chronic thromboembolism, although the benefit gained should be weighed against the risk of warfarin in those less mobile. Pulmonary valvotomy may be attempted in severe pulmonary stenosis. Surgery to the tricuspid valve is challenging, and reserved for more severe cases. Risk stratification in ARVD/C may lead to implantation of an ICD device.

Marked fluid retention may be treated with intravenous loop diuretics. Short courses of metolazone can be useful in augmenting the diuresis. Daily monitoring of weight and renal function should be performed. It should be borne in mind that the older population are at greater risk of developing renal dysfunction and hypovolaemia as a result of diuretics. It may be necessary to accept mild–moderate renal impairment to keep patients oedema free and mobile. District nurses in the community can be vital to prevent secondary infection in oedematous legs. Occupational therapists may be employed to provide home aids for those that are now less mobile. Community palliative care teams can also provide some support at home.

Prognosis

Defining prognosis in isolated right heart is difficult and depends on many variables. For patients presenting with signs of RV dysfunction due to LV dysfunction and NYHA class 3–4 symptoms, the expected prognosis can be predicted in months to a year.

Further reading

Bleeker G, Steendijk P, Holman E, et al. (2006). Assessing right ventricular function: the role of echocardiography and complementary technologies. Heart **92**: 119–26.

Haddad F, Hunt S, Rosenthal D, et al. (2008). Right ventricular function in cardiovascular disease, part I: Anatomy, physiology, aging, and functional assessment of the right ventricle. Circulation **117**: 1436–48.

Haddad F, Doyle R, Murphy D, et al. (2008). Right ventricular function in cardiovascular disease, part II: pathophysiology, clinical importance, and management of right ventricular failure. Circulation **117**: 1717–31.

Systolic versus diastolic dysfunction

Introduction

Left ventricular systolic dysfunction (LVSD) refers to a decrease in contractile function of the left ventricle (LV) whereas abnormal relaxation of the ventricular myocardium underlies diastolic dysfunction. The former results in 'failure to pump' (systolic heart failure, SHF) and is often associated with progressive dilatation and adverse remodelling, and the latter causes a 'failure to fill' accompanied by concentric hypertrophy and preserved systolic function (diastolic heart failure, DHF).

This section will focus on the pathophysiology, clinical features, diagnosis, and management of diastolic dysfunction which will be contrasted with LVSD (see section Left ventricular systolic dysfunction). Although features distinguishing systolic from diastolic dysfunction are discussed, it is important to recognize that these two entities frequently coexist and that most patients with systolic dysfunction have some degree of diastolic dysfunction. Isolated diastolic dysfunction should be considered in patients with symptoms of heart failure but normal systolic function.

> **Author's Tip**
>
> Systolic and diastolic dysfunction may occur alone but often coexist.

Pathophysiology

Relaxation of the left ventricle in diastole depends on the integrity of cardiomyocytes and the surrounding extracellular matrix. Increased ventricular stiffness results from structural and functional abnormalities of the former and increased fibroblast proliferation and collagen deposition in the latter. Predisposing factors for such ultrastructural changes include advancing age, hypertension, and diabetes mellitus (Figure 5.13).

Diastolic dysfunction results in increased pressures within the left ventricle and the left atrium. The former increases left ventricular filling pressure (see Figure 5.13) and also impedes myocardial perfusion. The latter causes left atrial dilatation and subsequently, atrial fibrillation. With increasing LV filling pressures, the contribution of left atrial contraction to LV end diastolic volume increases, which explains the inability of patients with diastolic dysfunction to tolerate atrial fibrillation. Tachycardia exacerbates

symptoms as shortening of diastole leads to inadequate LV filling.

Epidemiology of diastolic dysfunction

Population-based studies suggest that diastolic dysfunction is more common among women and that the incidence increases with age. Predisposing factors include obesity, hypertension, and diabetes.

Preclinical diastolic dysfunction:

A population-based study of >2000 residents from Olmsted County, MN, indicates a prevalence of 20.6% for mild and 6.8% for moderate to severe preclinical diastolic dysfunction. This increased to 47.6% and 16.5% respectively in a high-risk subgroup (age >65 years and either hypertension or coronary artery disease).

Diastolic heart failure:

The EPICA study analysed a large cross-section of the population (>5400 subjects, age >25 years) and derived the age- and gender-specific prevalence of SHF and DHF (defined according to European Society of Cardiology criteria). In subjects >70 years, the prevalence of SHF was 4% among men and 2% in women, whereas DHF was more prevalent among women (6%) than men (2%). Studies in patients with overt clinical heart failure suggest that 40–70% have evidence of some DHF.

> **Author's Tip**
>
> Frequency of isolated DHF increases with age. Reconsider diagnosis of DHF in the absence of predisposing factors.

Clinical features

The clinical syndrome arising from systolic dysfunction is referred to as heart failure with reduced ejection fraction (HFREF) or SHF, whereas the term heart failure with normal ejection fraction (HFNEF) or diastolic heart failure (DHF) is used to denote the clinical manifestations of diastolic dysfunction. Although SHF and DHF commonly coexist, it is useful to consider clinical parameters which help differentiate between them (Table 5.9).

Table 5.9 Clinical features in systolic heart failure (SHF) versus diastolic heart failure (DHF)

History	SHF	DHF
Coronary artery disease	+++	+
Hypertension	++	+++
Diabetes mellitus	++	++
Examination		
Cardiomegaly	+++	+
S3 gallop	+++	+
S4 gallop	+	+++
Oedema (peripheral)	+++	+
Raised JVP	+++	+

+ infrequent, ++ occasional, +++ frequent.

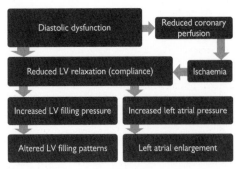

Figure 5.13 Pathophysiology of diastolic heart failure. LV, left ventricle.

Diagnosis

DHF should only be considered in the presence of predisposing factors and relevant clinical features. The importance of this lies in the fact that echocardiographic evidence of asymptomatic diastolic dysfunction is very common in patients over the age of 60 years and alone does not constitute DHF.

A consensus statement issued by the Heart failure and Echocardiography Associations of the European Society of Cardiology in 2007 stipulates three conditions to be satisfied in arriving at a diagnosis of DHF: (i) symptoms and signs of heart failure, (ii) evidence of normal or only mildly reduced LV systolic function, and (iii) evidence of LV diastolic dysfunction. Echocardiographic parameters (Table 5.10) are used in grading the severity of diastolic dysfunction. Transmitral Doppler velocities and tissue Doppler measurements aid more specific classification into mild, moderate, and severe degrees of diastolic dysfunction.

Differential diagnosis

In patients with HFNEF, consideration should be paid to the possibility of constrictive pericarditis. Echocardiography is useful in confirming normal diastolic function in such cases. A review of the history may reveal previous pericarditis, while CT chest is useful to measure pericardial thickness. The gold standard for diagnosis is simultaneous right and left heart catheterization to confirm equalization of diastolic pressures in the ventricles.

Management

Various pharmacological agents have theoretically beneficial effects, including anti-hypertensive treatment with agents affecting the renin–angiotensin–aldosterone axis to prevent disease progression, and negatively chronotropic agents such as beta-blockers to improve ventricular filling by prolongation of diastole. However, the results of randomized trials have been disappointing, partly because the trial quality has been relatively poor. A recent review of the selection criteria of more than 20 trials in diastolic dysfunction concluded that the majority of studies did not adhere to the existing diagnostic criteria for HFNEF (see above). A significant proportion of patients in such studies had SHF with reduced ejection fraction leading to negative results due to underpowered studies.

Table 5.10 Echo findings in diastolic heart failure (DHF)

Echocardiography	DHF		
LVEF greater than 45%	++		
LVH (concentric)	++		
LV dilatation	-		
LA dilatation	++		
Grading of diastolic dysfunction	**Mild**	**Moderate**	**Severe**
Transmitral Doppler (E:A)	<0.75	0.75–1.5	>1.5
TDI (E:E')	<10	>15	>20

LA, left atrium; LV, left ventricular; LVEF, left ventricular ejection fraction; LVH, left ventricular hypertrophy; TDI, tissue Doppler imaging.

Pharmacotherapy in HFNEF

The **PEP-CHF** trial randomly assigned 850 patients ≥70 years of age with diastolic dysfunction to perindopril or placebo. At the end of 1 year, a non-significant 4.4% absolute risk reduction (ARR) in the combined primary end point of all-cause mortality and unexpected hospitalization for HF was noted in the perindopril arm (12% vs 8%), driven entirely by reduced hospitalization. There were also significant improvements in NYHA functional class (secondary end point).

The **CHARM-Preserved** trial recruited 3023 patients with NYHA class II or III heart failure (LVEF >40%) and assigned them to either candesartan or placebo. The patients were also on ACE inhibitors (19%), beta-blockers (56%), and calcium channel blockers (31%). A non-significant 2% ARR (24% vs 22%) in the combined end point of cardiovascular death or hospitalization for heart failure was noted at 37-month median follow-up, again driven entirely by reduced hospitalization.

The **I-PRESERVE** trial studied the effect of irbesartan 300 mg versus placebo in 4128 patients with NYHA class II or III heart failure (LVEF ≥45%). Additional medications included ACE inhibitors (26%), beta-blockers (59%), and calcium channel blocker (40%). After a mean follow-up of 4 years, there was no significant difference in the primary end point of death from any cause or hospitalization for a cardiovascular cause. There were also no significant differences in secondary outcomes, which included death from HF or hospitalization for heart failure.

The **TOPCAT** trial (ongoing), a multicentre, international, randomized, double-blind placebo-controlled trial of the aldosterone antagonist spironolactone aims to recruit 3515 adults with heart failure and left ventricular ejection fraction of at least 45% and to assess a composite end point of cardiovascular mortality, aborted cardiac arrest or hospitalization for the management of heart failure.

Author's Tip

There is a lack of specific prognostically relevant therapy for DHF.

Prognosis

Subclinical diastolic dysfunction

There is evidence that subclinical diastolic dysfunction has adverse prognostic significance. A study of 2042 subjects >45 years followed up for 3.5 years derived hazard ratios for subclinical diastolic dysfunction adjusted for age, gender, and systolic function. The presence of diastolic dysfunction resulted in an 8- to 10-fold increase in mortality in this study.

SHF versus DHF

Data from the Cardiovascular Health Study which recruited 5888 subjects >65 years suggest that for an individual, SHF carries a higher mortality than DHF. However, since in this study the majority of patients (63%) had HFNEF, the overall population attributable risk of DHF was greater than that due to SHF.

A review of 6076 consecutive patients discharged from the Mayo Clinic following decompensated heart failure revealed a numerically lower but statistically insignificant mortality difference at 1 year for DHF versus SHF (29% vs 32%). However, while mortality rates improved with time for patients with SHF, they were static in DHF patients.

Further reading

Ceia F, Fonseca C, Mota T, *et al.* (2002). Prevalence of chronic heart failure in Southwestern Europe: The EPICA study. *Eur J Heart Fail* **4**: 531–39.

Paulus WJ, Tschöpe C, Sanderson JE, *et al.* (2007). How to diagnose diastolic heart failure: a consensus statement on the diagnosis of heart failure with normal left ventricular ejection fraction by the Heart Failure and Echocardiography Associations of the European Society of Cardiology. *Eur Heart J* **28**: 2539–50.

Redfield MM, Jacobsen SJ, Burnett Jr JC, *et al.* (2003). Burden of systolic and diastolic ventricular dysfunction in the community: appreciating the scope of the heart failure epidemic. *JAMA* **289**: 194–202.

Tachyarrhythmias

Tachyarrhythmias in older patients may produce palpitations and symptoms related to impaired haemodynamics (e.g. dizziness, syncope, heart failure). Patients may notice the onset and offset of intermittent tachyarrhythmias. However, permanent rhythm disturbances may be asymptomatic.

Supraventricular tachyarrhythmias

In older patients, supraventricular tachyarrhythmias comprise paroxysmal supraventricular tachycardia, atrioventricular (AV) nodal re-entrant tachycardia, AV reciprocating tachycardia, atrial tachycardia with block, multifocal atrial tachycardia, accelerated junctional rhythm, atrial flutter, and atrial fibrillation.

Paroxysmal supraventricular (atrial) tachycardia (PAT) is a re-entrant tachycardia with regular, narrow QRS complexes at 150–200 bpm. Short asymptomatic episodes of PAT have been reported in 13% of older patients with no evidence of heart disease. If symptomatic, PAT can be treated by vagal manoeuvres, adenosine, verapamil, beta-blockers or, if haemodynamically unstable, DC cardioversion. Antithrombotic therapy is not recommended for PAT, unless atrial fibrillation/flutter is also documented. Radiofrequency ablation of supraventricular tachyarrhythmias is another long-term option that has been commonly used in recent years. Its major advantages include avoidance of pro-arrhythmia caused by therapeutics and low recurrence rates.

Atrial flutter

Typical flutter occurs due to a macro re-entry and has an atrial rate of 250–350 bpm. The degree of AV block determines ventricular response rate. Even where flutter waves are not apparent on the ECG, it should be suspected on any patient with a regular tachycardia of around 150 bpm, with every second flutter wave resulting in ventricular contraction. In the older population, atrial flutter may accompany organic structural heart disease (e.g. ischaemic heart disease). Carotid sinus massage and other vagal stimuli increase the degree of AV block and may expose the flutter waves. Although pure atrial flutter causes a low risk of thromboembolism, patients who have alternating atrial fibrillation and flutter or with valvular heart disease may have higher thromboembolic risk.

Acute treatments for atrial flutter include electrical cardioversion (best option), electrical pacing, chemical cardioversion (e.g. ibutilide, class 1c antiarrhythmic agents) or administration of AV-node-blocking agents (e.g. diltiazem, beta-blockers, or digoxin). Haemodynamically unstable patients need DC cardioversion. For recurrent and drug-resistant atrial flutter, radiofrequency catheter ablation should be considered, as typical atrial flutter has a well-defined anatomic and electrophysiological substrate that can be effectively and safely treated by this.

Atrial fibrillation

Atrial fibrillation (AF) is the most common permanent cardiac tachyarrhythmia in older people. Its prevalence approximately doubles with each advancing decade and reaches to 9% at age 80–89 years from 0.5% at 50–59 years. The Newcastle survey found a prevalence of AF of 4.7%. Risk factors for the development of AF include

- increasing age (OR 2.1 for men, 2.2 for women)
- diabetes (OR 1.4 for men and 1.6 for women)

- hypertension (OR 1.5 for men and 1.4 for women)
- valve disease (OR 1.8 for men and 3.4 for women).

Common causes of AF

Hypertension, ischaemic or rheumatic heart diseases, thyrotoxicosis, infections, pulmonary embolism, electrolyte depletion, excessive alcohol or caffeine consumption, physical or emotional stress, surgery (especially cardiothoracic) are common causes of AF.

> **Authors' Tip**
>
> Medication started for new or paroxysmal AF in the context of acute and reversible pathology, such as sepsis, should be reviewed once the patient is well. Many patients stay on toxic medication such as amiodarone in the long term unnecessarily.

Haemodynamics

AF causes 10–20% reduction in cardiac output and left ventricular systolic performance may decrease critically in older patients with impaired basal myocardial function with the onset of AF with fast ventricular rate. The haemodynamic changes may trigger heart failure and pulmonary oedema. This is especially apparent in patients with diastolic dysfunction, where the atrial contribution to ventricular filling is proportionately more important.

Prothrombotic milieu

AF causes intra-atrial stasis and a prothrombotic state that may lead to thromboembolism. Stroke risk is fivefold increased in patients with AF compared with those without. In the absence of antithrombotic therapy, the annual risk of stroke in patients with non-valvular AF increases from 5% in patients under 65 years of age to 8% in those older than 75 years. The presence of associated risk factors (see below) results in a cumulative stroke risk, with the highest risk (>12%/year if untreated) for those with prior stroke or thromboembolism. The attributable risk of stroke for AF increases with age (1.5% at age 50–59 years; 2.8% at 60–69; 9.9% at 70–79; and 23.5% at 80–89 years).

Management of AF

Antithrombotic therapy is indicated in patients with increased stroke risk which can be predicted by different stratification schemas. The AFFIRM study showed that the rate control in combination with warfarin was not inferior to rhythm control strategy. Criteria for rate control vary with patient age but usually involve achieving ventricular rates between 60 and 80 bpm at rest and between 90 and 115 bpm during moderate exercise. Current guidelines recommend beta-blockers or non-dihydropyridine calcium channel antagonists (verapamil, diltiazem) as first-line agents for rate control of permanent AF.

Beta-blockers may be particularly useful in patients with increased adrenergic tone, such as in postoperative AF. Since digoxin has many disadvantages (e.g. reduced efficacy in increased sympathetic tone, delayed onset of effects in acute settings, no effect on heart rate during exercise), it is now only recommended as a second-line agent in patients with AF and heart failure or reduced EF, or as monotherapy in older sedentary patients in the absence of an accessory pathway. Although amiodarone is usually used for rhythm control, the drug is sometimes used for rate control because of conduction slowing effects.

Paroxysmal AF is defined as AF episodes that generally last for 7 days or less (most <24 h) and characterized with similar stroke risk as permanent AF. Current AF guidelines recommend antithrombotic therapy irrespective of the pattern of AF.

AF patients with both tachycardia and bradycardia attacks are candidates for hybrid therapy, including implantation of a pacemaker and drug therapy.

Stroke risk stratification in AF

A number of tools are available for this in non-valvular AF, including, Framingham, CHADS$_2$ and CHA$_2$DS$_2$Vasc (see Table 5.11). The last of these diminishes the proportion of patients classified in the intermediate risk group compared with CHADS$_2$. Patients with AF associated with valvular heart disease are at higher risk of stroke, and should be on warfarin unless there are contraindications to this (see Table 5.12).

Patients with a CHA$_2$DS$_2$VASc score >1 are at high risk and should be prescribed anticoagulants. For those patients with a CHA$_2$DS$_2$VASc score = 1, either oral anticoagulants or aspirin may be recommended. Antithrombotic therapy may be avoided in low risk patients (CHA2DS2VASc score = 0)

Ventricular tachyarrhythmias

The prevalence of ventricular tachycardias increases with advancing age. A 24-hour ambulatory ECG monitoring study found ventricular tachycardia in 4% of women and 10% of men between 65 and 100 years. Non-sustained ventricular tachycardia was found to be an independent predictor of death (relative risk (RR) 2.8) and MI (RR 3.2). Salvos in themselves are not associated with morbidity and mortality, although can be suggestive of an 'excitable' myocardium and thereby warrant further investigation depending on the clinical circumstances.

VT can be distinguished from SVT with aberrant conduction through the presence of a QRS width over

Table 5.11 CHADS$_2$ and CHA$_2$DS$_2$VASc schemas. MI-myocardial infarction. TIA -transient ischaemic attack

CHADS$_2$		
	Congestive heart failure	1
	Hypertension	1
	Age ≥ 75	1
	Diabetes	1
	Previous stroke/TIA	2
CHA$_2$DS$_2$VASc:		
	Congestive heart failure	1
	Hypertension	1
	Age ≥ 75	2
	Diabetes	1
	Stroke / TIA	2
	Vascular disease (e.g. prior MI)	1
	Aged 65–74 years	1
	Gender (female gender)	1

Table 5.12 The risk of stroke and bleeding under different therapy regimens

Risk of	No medication	Aspirin	Warfarin
Stroke	4.8% p/a*	3.4% p/a[†]	1.6% p/a[†]
Bleeding	0% p/a*	1.9% p/a[†]	1.9% p/a[†]

*AFASAK study, [†]BAFTA study.

0.14 seconds, left axis deviation, capture and fusion beats, and atrioventricular dissociation.

Management of ventricular tachycardia in the older population

Patients with VT and haemodynamic instability (i.e. syncope, hypotension, or angina) require immediate cardioversion. Underlying precipitants should be addressed and potassium levels kept above 4 mmol/L. Parenteral amiodarone or beta-blockers can be used in patients with repetitive monomorphic VT. Amiodarone is probably the most effective antiarrhythmic in the treatment of VT. Transvenous catheter pacing (overdrive pacing) can be useful when sustained monomorphic VT is refractory to cardioversion or is frequently recurrent despite antiarrhythmic medications. Implantable cardioverter defibrillator therapy, radiofrequency catheter ablation, and both together (hybrid therapy) comprise the non-pharmacological therapy of ventricular tachycardias.

Further reading

Frishman WH, Heiman M, Karpenos A, et al. (1996). Twenty-four – hour ambulatory electrocardiography in elderly subjects: Prevalence of various arrhythmias and prognostic implications (report from the Bronx Longitudinal Aging Study). Am Heart J **132**: 297–302.

Fuster V, Rydén LE, Cannom DS, et al. (2006). ACC/AHA/ESC 2006 guidelines for the management of patients with atrial fibrillation: a report of the American College of Cardiology/American Heart Association Task Force on Practice Guidelines and the European Society of Cardiology Committee for Practice Guidelines. J Am Coll Cardiol **48**: 854–906.

Gage BF, Waterman AD, Shannon W, et al. (2001). Validation of clinical classification schemes for predicting stroke: results of the National Registry of Atrial Fibrillation. JAMA **285**: 2864–70.

Lip GYH, Nieuwlaat R, Pisters R, et al. (2010). Refining clinical risk stratification for predicting stroke and thromboembolism in atrial fibrillation using a novel risk factor-based approach: The Euro Heart Survey on Atrial Fibrillation. Chest **137**: 263–72.

Wyse DG, Waldo AL, DiMarco JP, et al. (2002). The Atrial Fibrillation Follow-up Investigation of Rhythm Management (AFFIRM) Investigators. A comparison of rate control and rhythm control in patients with atrial fibrillation. N Engl J Med **347**: 1825–33.

Zipes DP, Camm AJ, Borggrefe M, et al. (2006). ACC/AHA/ESC 2006 guidelines for management of patients with ventricular arrhythmias and the prevention of sudden cardiac death: a report of the American College of Cardiology/American Heart Association Task Force and the European Society of Cardiology Committee for Practice Guidelines. J Am Coll Cardiol **48**: e247–346.

Bradyarrhythmias

Apart from iatrogenic (e.g. drug-induced) or medical causes (e.g. hypothyroidism), bradyarrhythmias are due to sinoatrial (SA) or atrioventricular (AV) node dysfunction or conduction disturbances, which are common in older patients. Ageing causes fibrosis in the cardiac conduction system, and atrophy, amyloid accumulation, and reduced pacemaker cells in the SA node. The number of pacemaker cells in the SA node declines progressively from 60 years, and only 10% of these are still present at 75 years. The prevalence of AV and intraventricular conduction defects is 30% over 65 years. Age-related changes in the His bundle commonly include loss of cells, increase in fibrous and adipose tissue, and amyloid infiltration. Fibrosis of the AV node is the most common cause of chronic AV block in older people.

Sinus bradycardia

Sinus node degeneration is common in older people and is characterized with a sinus rhythm <60 bpm. Sinus bradycardia associated with paroxysmal atrial tachyarrhythmias and sinus arrest is one manifestation of sick sinus syndrome (see below). Hypothermia, hypothyroidism, increased intracranial pressure, or myocardial infarction may also cause sinus bradycardia. Asymptomatic patients with sinus bradycardia do not require treatment, although correction of any reversible predisposing factors may be needed.

Sinoatrial block

SA block is the situation in which the sinus node produces impulses but these impulses cannot depolarize the atrium. Usually SA block is 2:1 conducted. Degenerative conduction system disease, ischaemia, digitalis, or class 1a antiarrhythmic toxicity may cause SA block in older patients. Asymptomatic patients do not require treatment. Pacemaker therapy may be considered in a few symptomatic subjects, especially when symptoms are closely related to SA block.

Sinus node dysfunction: sick sinus syndrome

Sick sinus syndrome (SSS) is a common rhythm disorder in older individuals and closely related to the degeneration of the SA node. The prevalence of SSS is estimated to be 1 in 600 patients over 65 years. In patients with SSS, sinus bradycardia is explained by depressed automaticity in the sinus node itself. Failure of impulse formation or conduction to the atrium causes sinus pauses or arrest, and abnormal automaticity and conduction in the atrium lead to atrial fibrillation and flutter.

The clinical presentations of SSS are insidious and closely related to an inadequate heart rate response to daily physical activities. Symptoms include palpitations, fatigue, syncope, and sudden death.

Patients with SSS usually have inappropriate sinus bradycardia, sinus node pauses or arrests (>3 seconds), SA exit blocks, and atrial fibrillation or flutter episodes. Termination of supraventricular tachycardia is often followed by a long pause. Indeed, alternating brady- and tachycardias are the characteristic of the disease. Management of patients with SSS includes implantation of permanent pacemaker for symptomatic bradycardia, chronotropic incompetence or sinus bradycardia that results from required drug therapy for medical conditions, and pharmacological treatment for tachyarrhythmias (discussed in the Tachyarrhythmias section). A single chamber atrial pacing and sensing pacemaker

(AAI(R)) is the pacemaker of choice in patients with SSS if the conduction system and AV node are normal. If AV node or conduction system disease is present dual chamber pacemakers (DDD(R)) are indicated, as physiological pacing provides less atrial fibrillation and better quality of life. While the incidence of sudden death related to SSS is extremely low and treatment with or without pacemakers does not influence survival, SSS does increase the risk of syncopal collapses and their consequences.

> **Authors' Tip**
>
> SSS accounts for up to 50% of pacemaker implantation indications. Untreated SSS patients experience recurrent syncope. If the conduction system is intact, AAI pacing is the most physiological pacing mode in SSS.

Atrioventricular conduction abnormalities and blocks

AV node and the bundle of His are the main sites where impulse conduction may be delayed or blocked. A delayed conduction below the bifurcation of the His bundle results in bundle branch or fascicular block. However, the expansion of degenerative disease to entire fascicles results in AV block in different degrees.

First-degree AV block is common in the older population (~8%), while second- and third-degree blocks are only seen approximately in 1% of this group. Increased vagal tone, conduction system disturbances, and extrinsic factors (e.g. therapeutic agents such as beta-blockers, calcium channel blockers, digoxin, or antiarrhythmics drugs) may cause first-degree AV block. The presence of a first-degree AV block does not explain bradycardia. However, it is commonly accompanied by other rhythm or conduction disturbances (e.g. second- or third-degree AV block, SSS). Since the first degree AV blocks are well tolerated and the patients are asymptomatic, permanent pacemaker therapy is not normally indicated. However, in a minority of symptomatic patients with a very prolonged PR interval (>300 ms), a permanent pacemaker may be required.

Second-degree AV blocks include three subtypes, Mobitz type I (Wenckebach), Mobitz II, and advanced second-degree or high-degree AV blocks.

In Mobitz type I (Wenckebach) AV block, the PR interval progressively prolongs until a ventricular complex drops. Mobitz type I block usually occurs because of a delay in the AV node, but it may occur in the bundle of His in patients with advanced disease. The ECG shows typically normal QRS complexes. Type I second-degree AV block is often seen during digitalis intoxication and acute inferior myocardial (MI) and it is usually transient and rarely requires pacemaker implantation.

Mobitz type II second-degree AV block is characterized by the presence of fixed stable PP intervals with no measurable prolongation of the PR intervals followed by a dropped QRS complex. Mobitz type II block is usually associated with the degenerative disease of the His–Purkinje system. Since the block's level is at or below the His bundle, Mobitz type II blocks show wide QRS complexes. Mobitz type II blocks are often seen during acute anterior MI, myocarditis, or advanced degenerative conduction system disease. Patients with Mobitz II AV block are often symptomatic and present with syncope due to disturbed cerebral perfusion during blocks (Stokes–Adams attacks).

In patients with advanced second-degree or high-degree AV block an AV conduction ratio exists (e.g. 2:1, 3:1, or 4:1). A prolongation of PR interval before the block is not seen. In 2:1 conducted AV block, a narrow QRS complex and associated periods of Wenckebach block or simultaneous sinus slowing so called 'vagotonic block' indicate the presence of AV nodal block. If QRS complexes are wide, infranodal block should be considered. High-degree AV blocks usually require permanent pacemaker implantation since the block has a potential to progress to complete heart block.

Third-degree AV block (complete heart block) is characterized with blocked AV conduction, AV dissociation, and an escape rhythm with either narrow or wide QRS complexes regarding the anatomical site of the block. For example, an escape with narrow QRS complexes at 60 bpm indicates a block at AV node level, and an escape rhythm with wide QRS complexes <40 bpm suggests a block at His bundle or Purkinje system level. Acute inferior MI, digitalis intoxication, and excessive degenerative disease of the cardiac conduction system may cause third-degree AV block. Recent studies indicate that permanent pacemaker implantation improves survival in patients with complete AV block presenting with syncope.

The randomized UK PACE trial compared VVI(R) and DDD pacing in patients with AV block in patients aged ≥70 years. No significant difference was established in overall mortality or cardiovascular events at 3–5 years of follow-up.

Longer term management of intraventricular conduction defects that appear with acute MI depends upon their type, the infarct location, and the relation between them. Patients needing temporary pacing do not necessarily need a permanent pacemaker. Recent studies established that intraventricular conduction defects appearing with an MI indicate a poor short- and long-term prognosis, except with isolated left anterior fascicular block.

Authors' Tip

Intraventricular conduction defects that can be associated with temporary conditions influence decision-making for permanent pacemaker therapy. Severe symptomatic bradycardia that cannot be explained by temporary conditions almost always requires permanent pacemaker indication.

Current guidelines suggest permanent ventricular pacing in patients with

• persistent second-degree AV block with alternating bundle branch block
• third-degree AV block within or below the His–Purkinje system after ST segment elevation MI
• transient advanced second- or third-degree infranodal AV block and associated bundle branch block
• persistent and symptomatic second- or third-degree AV block.

Pharmacological management

Bradyarrhythmias should be managed carefully and quickly since they may cause haemodynamic instability in older patients. Pharmacological approaches are limited and the first choice is intravenous atropine (0.5–1 mg), which can be repeated within 5-minute intervals up to a total dose of 2–3 mg. If atropine is ineffective, isoproterenol infusion should be considered at 1–4 μg/min. In case of persistent bradyarrhythmia, despite atropine and/or isoproterenol administration, temporary transvenous or permanent pacing becomes necessary.

Bundle branch blocks

Bundle branch blocks are partial or complete interruption of electrical conduction in left or right bundle branches. Left bundle branch block (LBBB) is usually associated with organic heart diseases (e.g. ischaemic or hypertensive heart disease) and its incidence increases in older people. Complete or incomplete right bundle branch blocks (RBBB) are common in healthy older men and may not necessarily indicate serious disease. However, the presence of RBBB in older women is highly correlated with organic heart diseases.

Bifascicular blocks comprise impaired conduction in both left and right bundle branches below the AV node; alternating RBBB and LBBB, RBBB with associated left anterior fascicular block (seen on ECG as left axis deviation), RBBB with left posterior fascicular block (ECG shows right axis deviation).

Pacemakers are not warranted for asymptomatic older people with chronic bifascicular block (either left or right bundle branch block plus left anterior-superior or left posterior-inferior division block), with or without a prolonged PR interval, since complete heart block rarely occurs (<2%) in asymptomatic subjects. Current guidelines indicate that advanced second-degree AV block or intermittent third-degree AV block, type II second-degree AV block and alternating bundle branch block require permanent pacemaker implantation.

Further reading

Epstein AE, DiMarco JP, Ellenbogen KA, et al. (2008). ACC/AHA/HRS 2008 Guidelines for Device-Based Therapy of Cardiac Rhythm Abnormalities A Report of the American College of Cardiology/American Heart Association Task Force on Practice Guidelines (Writing Committee to Revise the ACC/AHA/NASPE 2002 Guideline Update for Implantation of Cardiac Pacemakers and Antiarrhythmia Devices) Developed in Collaboration With the American Association for Thoracic Surgery and Society of Thoracic Surgeons. J Am Coll Cardiol **51**: 1–62.

Lamas GA, Pashos CL, Normand SLT, et al. (1995). Permanent pacemaker selection and subsequent survival in elderly medicare pacemaker recipients. Circulation **91**: 1063–69.

Mangrum JM, DiMarco JP (2000). The evaluation and management of bradycardia. N Engl J Med **342**: 703–9.

Toff WD, Camm AJ, Skehan JD (2005). Single-chamber versus dual chamber pacing for high-grade atrioventricular block. N Engl J Med **353**: 145–55.

Angina

Background

Angina pectoris is caused by a transient mismatch between coronary blood flow and myocardial oxygen demand and is the most common clinical manifestation of cardiac ischaemia. Angina is often the predominant presenting complaint of patients suffering from coronary artery disease (CAD), a pathophysiological process estimated to cause one in every five deaths in the industrialized world. Furthermore, although the overall incidence of acute coronary events is reaching steady state (as a consequence of greater emphasis on public health measures such as smoking cessation, significant advances in revascularization techniques and the pharmacological armamentarium available alongside changes in socioeconomic trends), the prevalence of CAD is expected to rise exponentially during the next decade as a result of:

- an ageing demographic
- an increase in obesity and the incidence of type II diabetes mellitus and the metabolic syndrome
- the emergence of cardiovascular risk factors in younger populations, in particular the 'Westernization' of developing countries.

Pathophysiology

The coronary flow reserve (CFR) refers to the ability of the coronary arteries to augment blood flow in response to increased metabolic demand. In normal subjects this equates to a maximum of four to six times that of the resting coronary blood flow and is determined by:

- the resistance of the epicardial macrovasculature (i.e. the coronary arteries overlying the heart surface)
- the intramural microvasculature
- myocardial and interstitial (i.e. extravascular) resistance
- blood composition.

It follows therefore that myocardial ischaemia can occur as a result of

- a fixed and/or dynamic stenosis within the epicardial coronary arteries (i.e. conductance vessels) leading to a reduction in coronary blood flow
- pathological constriction or abnormal relaxation of the microcirculation (i.e. resistance vessels)
- inadequate oxygen-carrying capacity of the blood (e.g. in severe anaemia or with elevated levels of carboxyhaemoglobin.)

The physical sensation of angina is propagated by the mechanical and chemical stimulation of afferent sensory nerve endings located in the coronary vasculature and myocardium. These nerve fibres extend from the first to the fourth thoracic spinal nerves, which ascend via the spinal cord to the thalamus and on to the cerebral cortex. Angina can take many forms: chronic stable angina, Prinzmetal (variant) angina, microvascular angina, and unstable angina, the last one comprising one end of the spectrum of acute coronary syndromes.

Atherosclerotic plaques are the commonest cause of epicardial coronary artery stenosis (usually 70%) resulting in chronic stable angina. These patients are unable to increase their CFR during exertion and/or emotional stress as a direct result of the mechanical obstruction.

There are several non-atherosclerotic causes of obstructive CAD, although none is as frequent or important as atherosclerosis:

- myocardial/muscular bridging from the systolic compression of those epicardial coronary arteries which have a segmental intramyocardial course
- congenital malformations of the coronary artery (e.g. coronary artery aneurysms or fistulae)
- coronary arteritis secondary to vasculitidies
- coronary artery fibrosis secondary to chest radiotherapy
- coronary intimal fibrosis following cardiac transplantation.

When there is reduced cardiac output, angina may occur in the absence of obstructive CAD, as in

- haemodynamically significant aortic stenosis
- obstructive hypertrophic cardiomyopathy (HCM)
- idiopathic dilated cardiomyopathy
- low output cardiac failure.

Prinzmetal or variant angina is rare. It refers to predominantly non-exertional angina caused by focal coronary vasospasm. This can lead to ST-segment elevation and a mistaken diagnosis of acute myocardial infarction (MI). Although most cases tend to be associated with some degree of fixed coronary stenosis, others have normal coronary arteries on angiography. This condition is typically difficult to treat and several underlying pathophysiological mechanisms have been postulated including:

- inadequate localized production of endothelium-derived nitric oxide (a potent vasodilator)
- low intracellular magnesium levels
- hyperinsulinaemia
- cigarette smoking
- cocaine abuse.

A subset of patients presenting with typical anginal symptoms and a positive non-invasive stress test can have normal or non-flow-limiting disease on coronary arteriography. These individuals may well have microvascular angina caused by dysfunctional small coronary arteries and arterioles (i.e. resistance vessels) which cannot expand the CFR in times of increased metabolic demand. Conditions such as diabetes mellitus, hypertension, and collagen vascular disorders have been implicated.

Syndrome X is another rare condition with typical exertional angina symptoms, ST-segment changes and/or myocardial perfusion defects on stress testing indicative of reversible ischaemia, although anatomically normal coronary arteries on angiography are usually found. There is reduced vasodilatory capacity of the microvasculature associated with endothelial dysfunction; local overproduction of vasoconstrictors; fibrosis and medial hypertrophy of the resistance vessels; impaired adrenergic nerve function; and/or oestrogen deficiency. It typically occurs in postmenopausal women and has an excellent long-term prognosis but can be very difficult to treat. Positive reinforcement and smooth muscle relaxants such as calcium channel blockers are the mainstay of therapy.

Clinical assessment

As well as with cardiac-sounding chest pain, angina should be suspected with exertional dyspnoea. Symptoms are usually provoked by exertion, emotional stress, cold or windy weather, or a heavy meal. Stable angina lasts a few minutes (not seconds), typically settles when the provoking stimulus has stopped and is relieved by glyceryl trinitrate.

While pain or discomfort that is altered by respiration, cough, or postural changes is unlikely to represent angina, decubitus angina occurs while the patient is supine at night. It is thought to relate to increased venous return, which leads to increased myocardial oxygen demand.

> **Authors' Tip**
>
> Especially in the older population, be wary of 'angina equivalent' symptoms such as epigastric discomfort, breathlessness, fatigue, and presyncope.

The severity of angina pectoris can be graded using the system proposed by the Canadian Cardiovascular Society:
- Grade I: No limitation of ordinary activity. Angina with strenuous or prolonged exertion only.
- Grade II: Slight limitation of ordinary activity. Walking more than two blocks on the level and climbing more than one flight of ordinary stairs at a normal pace and in normal conditions.
- Grade III: Marked limitation of ordinary physical activity. Walking one or two blocks on the level and climbing one flight of stairs in normal conditions and at normal pace.
- Grade IV: Inability to carry on any physical activity without discomfort; angina may be present at rest.

Examination is typically normal for patients with angina, though may show evidence of contributory features (e.g. aortic stenosis, anaemia) or flag up findings for alternative causes of the patients' symptoms (e.g. evidence of aortic dissection or pericarditis; superficial tenderness with musculoskeletal pain.)

Investigations
The baseline ECG can be normal in up to >75% of chronic stable angina patients, including some with severe underlying CAD. Non-specific changes are not uncommon, relating to conditions such as left ventricular hypertrophy (itself a risk factor for CAD) or medication (e.g. digoxin). Non-cardiac causes of EGG changes include pulmonary emboli or cerebral haemorrhage. Abnormalities such as Q waves, ST-T wave changes, varying degrees of atrioventricular block, bundle branch block, atrial, and ventricular tachyarrhythmias tend to indicate a poorer prognosis.

Troponins are very specific blood tests indicative of cardiac damage. A 12-hour troponin I or T level tends to be normal in chronic stable angina. Troponins can rise in a number of cardiac and non-cardiac conditions, although they can be a marker for disease severity in these situations. Other causes for a troponin rise include pulmonary emboli; severe sepsis; renal dysfunction; tachyarrhythmia, particularly atrial fibrillation/flutter; and myocarditis. Misinterpretation of the result followed by treatment of patients according to ACS protocols unnecessarily exposes patients to side-effects, notably gastrointestinal bleeding from aggressive dual antiplatelet therapy.

Non-invasive stress testing
Stress testing helps establish the diagnosis of chronic CAD and risk-stratify patients for the likelihood of future adverse events. The National Institute of Health and Clinical Excellence (NICE) 2010 guidance has placed significant emphasis on clinical assessment, and veered away from standard non-invasive stress testing where the likelihood of CAD is high. It remains to be seen whether these recommendations will be adopted nationwide. The guidance advises that for men over 70 years old with atypical or typical symptoms, over 90% will have underlying CAD. For women over 70 years, this is estimated at 61–90% except for women at high risk with typical symptoms, where a risk of over 90% should be assumed.

Exercise stress testing
NICE guidelines discourage the use of this to diagnose or exclude stable angina in patients without known CAD. In established chronic stable angina, it can provide useful prognostic information about the extent of disease and how easily inducible reversible cardiac ischaemia is. Meanwhile, it remains an accessible and readily available tool to screen for and assess those patients with at least a moderate probability of CAD. Limits to its usefulness in older people include the patient's needing a baseline ECG within normal limits and be able to achieve sufficient workload for definitive inferences to be made. The overall sensitivity (68%) and specificity (77%) of exercise stress testing make it relatively inferior to other non-invasive techniques.

> **Authors' Tip**
>
> Interpretation of an exercise stress test result must include examination of exercise capacity (stage achieved and metabolic equivalents), symptoms experienced, exercise-induced arrhythmias, and haemodynamic response alongside ST- and T-wave abnormalities. If uncertain, seek specialist Cardiology review of the result. For a test result to be conclusive patients need to attain 85% of their maximal age-predicted heart rate.

Functional imaging studies are particularly useful following an inconclusive exercise test, or in those poorly ambulant individuals unable to walk on a treadmill and/or with baseline ECG abnormalities (e.g. left bundle branch block). Choice will largely depend on local availability.

Stress echocardiography
Stress can be induced through exercise or by intravenous dobutamine (which increases both heart rate and myocardial contractility and allows for the detection of ischaemia-provoked changes in regional wall motion and systolic wall thickening). Normal myocardium appears hyperdynamic following stress, while ischaemic segments become hypokinetic or akinetic. Sensitivity (0.86–0.82) and specificity (0.84–0.81) of both exercise and dobutamine stress echocardiography is similar to myocardial perfusion scanning and significantly better than exercise electrocardiography. NICE recommends it as a non-invasive functional test to diagnose stable angina in those with an estimated likelihood of CAD in the 61–90% category considered inappropriate for coronary angiography and/or potential revascularization. Advantages include
- simultaneous evaluation of LV function
- determination of LV wall thickness and cavity dimensions
- assessment of valvular heart disease

- accurate localization and quantification of myocardial ischaemia
- no exposure to radiation
- no risk of claustrophobia (compared with magnetic resonance imaging).

It requires good images (adequate images can be obtained in over 85% of patients), which is dependent on operator skill and reporting can be subjective, although in experienced hands the test is usually highly reproducible.

Myocardial perfusion scanning/scintigraphy

The choice between myocardial perfusion scanning/scintigraphy (MPS) and stress echocardiography tends to depend on local preference and availability. Sensitivity (89%) and specificity (75%) are similar to stress echocardiography and superior to exercise electrocardiography. It will be the preferred test in those individuals with LBBB or a ventricular paced rhythm, which can lead to a dyskinetic appearance of the LV on echocardiography and give rise to false-positive findings during stress. MPS can utilize either single-photon emission computed tomography (SPECT) or positron emission topography (PET) to produce images, the latter being most useful in obese patients or those with large breasts, since attenuation correction can be done. Results for the radioactive tracer agents used (thallium, sestamibi, or tetrofosmin) are similar and so can be used interchangeably. Adenosine or dipyridamole (or dobutamine in those with chronic chest problems) are used if patients are unable to exercise adequately. It is a fairly expensive test and labour intensive, as patients may well require separate rest and stress scans to compare images. It is recommended by NICE to diagnose chronic CAD in patients with moderate probability. Advantages include

- determination of how much myocardium is at risk (ischaemic burden) and areas of previous infarction
- estimation of LV ejection fraction
- reliable localization of regional myocardial ischaemia; particularly useful in patients who have had previous revascularization in that territory and in those with underlying LV dysfunction where viable myocardium could potentially be salvaged.

Computed tomography calcium scoring

NICE guidelines advise the use of CT calcium scoring as the first-line diagnostic investigation in those individuals with a 10–29% chance of having CAD and so its role in older patients will be limited. Calcific deposits within the coronary tree are diagnostic of atherosclerosis and the calcium score represents a quantitative index of the total amount of calcium detected by fast CT. The specificity of calcium scoring for obstructive coronary lesions is low (50%), though its sensitivity for atherosclerosis is 90%. Availability and experience with the technique are limited, and as the bulk of data has been derived from predominantly male Caucasian populations, caution must be exercised when making inferences on women and ethnic minority groups. Further drawbacks include:

- a high risk of false-positive results, especially with pre-existing coronary stents and severe calcification
- ideally patients must have a regular heart rhythm at a rate less than 70 bpm
- patients must hold their breath for 15 seconds
- high-dose radiation exposure.

Magnetic resonance imaging

First-pass contrast-enhanced magnetic resonance imaging (MRI) perfusion using adenosine or dypiridamole as a stress agent and MRI to assess stress-induced (either dobutamine or exercise) wall motion abnormalities are increasingly available. Both modalities are recommended as a means of non-invasive functional testing by NICE and both have a high sensitivity (0.84–0.89) and specificity (0.84–0.85) depending on which stress agent is used. Pacemakers and implantable cardioverter-defibrillators (ICDs) are not compatible with the magnet but most vascular stents and heart valve prostheses are safe.

Coronary angiography

Left heart catheterization remains the gold standard test to delineate coronary anatomy, and the extent and severity of coronary atherosclerosis. Patients can be risk stratified simply by the number of large epicardial vessels affected by stenoses: single-, double-, or triple-vessel disease or left main CAD. Significant CAD is defined as ≥70% diameter stenosis of a major epicardial vessel or ≥50% stenosis of the left main coronary artery. Further risk stratification is based on the location (i.e. proximal or distal) of the lesion and the significance of the myocardial territory it serves.

Angina can occur despite the lesion looking less severe with:

- long lesions
- proximal lesions serving large areas of myocardium
- anaemia or added coronary vasospasm giving rise to reduced oxygen delivery
- tachyarrhythmias or left ventricular hypertrophy stimulating greater oxygen demand.

Conversely, there are conditions that allow more severe lesions to remain asymptomatic:

- a well-developed collateral supply
- distal lesions
- previously infarcted myocardium in the territory of the affected vessel.

Coronary angiography (see Figures 5.14–5.16) should be performed when the estimated likelihood of CAD is between 61% and 90%, where the risks of the procedure are acceptable and subsequent revascularization would be viable. It can also be used in those patients with an estimated likelihood of 30–60% when the presence of

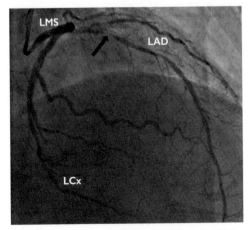

Figure 5.14 Coronary angiogram revealing a tight proximal left anterior descending (LAD) artery lesion (black arrow). LMS, left main stem; LCx, left main circumflex.

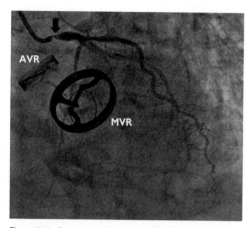

Figure 5.15 Coronary angiogram revealing a tight proximal left main coronary (LAD) artery lesion (black arrow). AVR, aortic valve replacement; MVR mitral valve replacement.

reversible myocardial ischaemia remains equivocal despite non-invasive functional imaging.

Management of chronic stable angina

The fundamental aims of chronic CAD management are twofold: to ameliorate symptoms and ischaemia burden (by tackling the imbalance between myocardial oxygen supply and demand) and to alter prognosis by preventing MI and death (by maintaining atherosclerotic plaque stability). These aims apply to all patients suffering from chronic CAD, whether young or old.

There are five key aspects to achieving these aims:

- identify and treat associated disease states that could potentially exacerbate or precipitate angina
- reduce cardiovascular risk factors
- encourage the uptake of lifestyle changes and promote healthy living
- optimal medical therapy (OMT)

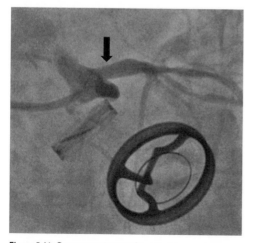

Figure 5.16 Coronary angiogram after percutaneous coronary intervention and coronary stenting of the proximal left main stem lesion (black arrow).

- consider at the point of any OMT treatment failure, coronary revascularization (i.e. percutaneous coronary intervention or coronary artery bypass graft surgery).

These areas of management are interwoven and should be considered simultaneously while tailored to the individual. Moreover, functional status, comorbidity, cognition and insight, tolerance of drug therapy, and the interface between clinician and patient must all be factored in when formulating the overall treatment package, especially in older people. Age should be seen in both a chronological and physiological light, and should not be used in isolation to dictate which patients should receive certain pharmacological or mechanical interventions. Indeed, several recent trials have borne out the morbidity and mortality advantages of effective lipid lowering (e.g. PROSPER), blood pressure control (e.g. HYVET), and beta-blockade (e.g. SENIORS) in specific older cohorts.

Around 10% of all PCI trials involve patients above the age of 70. While risks for the octogenarian will be relatively high compared with a younger individual, PCI remains a highly beneficial treatment modality.

There has been much debate recently over the management of chronic stable angina and whether patients have an initial conservative approach using OMT or a direct invasive strategy utilising revascularization procedures. Results from the RITA-2, COURAGE, BARI-2D, TIME (specifically medical vs invasive therapy in older patients), MASS II, and SWISSI II trials along with two extensive meta-analyses have all helped to fuel the controversy. Ultimately, the decision to refer patients directly for coronary revascularization should be made by specialists. It is fundamentally important to note, however, that an initial pharmacological approach with the option of future revascularization, if required, was not associated with an increase in mortality or MI. In older people, a balance must be struck between the need for a 'quick fix' through revascularization and the potential risks of an invasive procedure. Conversely, patients must accept that 30–50% of those on medication may eventually require an invasive procedure for refractory symptoms.

Regardless of the timing for invasive intervention, OMT remains the cornerstone of CAD management. If tolerated, all patients should be on an aspirin, beta-blocker, ACE inhibitor, and statin, which have all been shown to reduce morbidity and mortality. In terms of symptomatic benefit nitrates, calcium antagonists, and potassium-channel blockers (e.g. nicorandil) should be considered.

Review of all patients treated with medical therapy is mandatory since it is inappropriate to leave patients with symptoms whilst on maximally tolerated therapy and there should be a low threshold for referral for consideration of intervention. PCI and coronary artery bypass graft surgery are low risk in general and provide outstanding symptom relief. Those who continue to suffer refractory symptoms may benefit from newer agents such as ivabradine and ranolazine. Ivabradine is the first specific and selective I_f channel inhibitor. It reduces heart rate by acting on the I_f channel which is highly expressed in the sinoatrial node. Unlike beta-blockers or calcium antagonists, it has no effect on blood pressure. Ranolazine is a piperazine derivative that works on the late sodium current. Its precise mechanism of action remains elusive but it has no haemodynamic consequences and may actually reduce arrhythmias. It can be used as additive symptom relief alongside beta-blockers and/or calcium antagonists.

Those patients with significant angina but who are not candidates for revascularization may benefit from spinal cord stimulation. Here an electrode is inserted in to the epidural space at the level of C7–T1. It then stimulates axons that do not transmit painful stimuli to the brain, thereby overriding those axons that do. An alternative method is to use enhanced external counterpulsation (EECP), which increases the flow of blood back to the heart by serially inflating several cuffs around the legs in a distal to proximal fashion. Again, these treatment options will need specialist supervision.

Conclusions

The management of chronic stable angina in the older population is an important area that is often inadequately focused on. Older patients are often denied revascularization because of preconceptions about risk. Specific issues include frequently less than classical angina symptoms that represent ischaemia; the need to ensure appropriate use of non-invasive stress testing (mobility in older patents may be an issue); comorbidities and polypharmacy that may limit appropriate pharmacotherapy and the increased incidence of potential side-effects from such therapy; and, perhaps most importantly of all, a reluctance to undertake invasive tests and revascularization.

If a patient, regardless of age, has been on maximally tolerated OMT and continues to suffer anything other than minor ongoing ischaemic symptoms, then invasive testing is indicated, providing ischaemia has been confirmed by non-invasive imaging. While older patients may have a higher incidence of adverse sequelae (i.e. as a result of access site complications secondary to an increased incidence of peripheral arterial disease; an increased propensity to bleed following dual antiplatelet therapy especially in conjunction with a significantly low body mass index; reduced renal reserve to an intravenous contrast load or occult comorbid renal dysfunction; and an increased risk of drug interactions) and require a longer convalescence from revascularization (although they are frequently more tolerant than is believed), age itself is not a barrier to successful revascularization and indeed, despite any increase in risk, patients intervened on often do better than those treated medically. For some, symptom relief, and with it an improved quality of life, rather than prognosis is the cornerstone and revascularization may be the best means of achieving this.

We would stress the fundamental importance of fully utilizing the investigative and therapeutic strategies available for chronic CAD to the older population since the prevalence of cardiovascular disease and death associated with it increases steeply with increasing age. Whether this is best achieved in the hands of a cardiologist or a geriatrician (with or without a specialist interest in cardiology) remains a matter open for discussion.

Further reading

Alaeddini J, Shirani J. Angina pectoris. (http://emedicine.medscape.com/article/150215-overview).

Beckett NS, Peters R, Fletcher AE, et al. (2008). Treatment of hypertension in patients 80 years of age or older. N Engl J Med **358**: 1887–98.

Boden WE, O'Rourke RA, Teo KK, et al., for the COURAGE Trial Research Group (2007). Optimal medical therapy with or without PCI for stable coronary disease. N Engl J Med **356**: 1503–16.

Cassar A, Holmes Jr DR, Rihal CS, et al. (2009). Chronic coronary artery disease: diagnosis and management. Mayo Clin Proc **84**: 1130–46.

Flather MD, Shibata MC, Coats AJ, et al. (2005). Randomised trial to determine the effect of nebivolol on mortality and cardiovascular hospital admission in elderly patients with heart failure (SENIORS). Eur Heart J **26**: 215–25.

Morrow DA, Gersh BJ, Braunwald E (2005). Chronic coronary artery disease. Braunwald's Heart Disease. A Textbook of Cardiovascular Medicine, 7th edn. Philadelphia: Elsevier Saunders.

NICE (2010). Chest pain of Recent Onset. Assessment and Diagnosis of Recent Onset Chest Pain or Discomfort of Suspected Cardiac Origin. NICE clinical guideline 95 March 2010. London, NICE.

Pfisterer ME, Zellweger MJ, Gersh BJ (2010). Management of stable coronary artery disease. Lancet **375**: 763–72.

Shepherd J, Blauw G, Murphy MB, et al. (2002). PROSPER study group. Pravastatin in elderly individuals at risk of vascular disease: a randomized controlled trial. Lancet **360**: 1623–30.

The TIME Investigators (2001). Trial of invasive versus medical therapy in elderly patients with chronic symptomatic coronary-artery disease (TIME): a randomised trial. Lancet **358**: 951–7.

Acute myocardial infarction

Cardiovascular disease is the leading cause of premature death in the developed countries and will increasingly become so in developing countries over the next 20 years. Coronary artery disease (CAD) is the most prevalent manifestation of cardiovascular disease. It can present in a wide range of clinical scenarios including classical stable angina, acute coronary syndrome (ACS) with ST segment elevation (STEMI) or without (NSTEMI), silent ischemia, heart failure, and sudden death. Atypical presentations are a particular feature in older patients.

With an increasing ageing population worldwide and particularly in the Western world, where there is increased use of therapeutic modalities to prolong life in older people, this group are likely to represent a higher proportion of CAD and suffer themselves a high incidence of CVD.

This section focuses on the STEMI component of ACS CAD. We will highlight contemporary evidence-based management strategies with emphasis on how the evidence base is applicable to the older population.

It has become clear that for many therapies complications of the treatments are more common in older than in younger age groups, but it has also been repeatedly shown that those older patients who receive evidence-based therapies do better than those of same age cohorts who do not.

Definition

The term myocardial infarction, according to the universal myocardial infarction task force, should be used when there is evidence of myocardial necrosis in a clinical setting consistent with myocardial ischaemia. Although there are a variety of clinical, biochemical, ECG, and imaging criteria to diagnose acute myocardial infarction, it is widely accepted that typical acute chest pain and persistent (>20 minutes) ST-segment elevation or new left bundle branch block (LBBB) reflects an acute total coronary artery occlusion, which is the final step of the process leading to acute myocardial infarction. ACS is now separated by ECG definition into ST and non-ST elevation myocardial infarction driven by the difference in management.

Pathogenesis of STEMI

Occlusion of major coronary artery leads to acute myocardial infarction. Coronary occlusion in the majority of cases is caused by atherosclerotic plaque cap disruption leading to thrombus formation blocking coronary blood flow. Coronary plaque rupture or erosion primarily depends on plaque structure and degree of stenosis. Almost three-quarters of all infarct-related plaques appear to have been mild to moderate stenosis, suggesting the thrombotic component is the most important pathology. Plaques with thin fibrous cap and rich lipid core are deemed vulnerable plaques and prone to cap disruption. Furthermore, inflammation plays an important role in plaque instability, as plasma levels of multiple inflammatory markers including C-reactive protein (CRP) and interleukin-6 have shown strong correlation with outcomes of acute myocardial infarction.

After plaque rupture, exposure to collagen, lipids, and smooth muscle cells leads to activation of platelets and the coagulation cascade system, leading eventually to thrombus formation and coronary occlusion. STEMI has a higher incidence in the early hours, which has been correlated with the increased vascular tone due to beta-adrenergic stimulation and hypercoagulability of the blood during this period.

The natural history of STEMI

Community studies have consistently showed that death due to acute myocardial infarction primarily takes place in the pre-hospital phase, with up to 40% dying before help arrives. This high initial mortality rate seems to have altered little over the years in contrast to hospital mortality. Calling for help is a major public health issue, with many patients delaying this call. Older people may be particularly prone to resisting the need to call for help. In-hospital mortality of STEMI with contemporary therapy is approximately 3%, with 1-year rates up to 9%, a remarkable fall over the last 20 years.

Initial diagnosis and pre-hospital care

Rapid identification of STEMI can reduce the early mortality rate significantly. Chest pain may not be severe and, particularly in older patients, other symptoms such as dyspnoea, faintness, syncope, or fatigue are common.

ST elevation may also be less common in older patients with LBBB as the principle ECG change in a third of patients over 85 years with an acute myocardial infarct. Among STEMI patients in the NRM registry, ST-segment elevation was present on the ECG of 96.3% of patients under 65 years but only 69.9% of those over 85 years. Two-dimensional echocardiography can show regional wall motion abnormalities and help with other causes of chest pain, such as aortic dissection, pulmonary embolism, and pericardial effusion. Suspecting the diagnosis is core to outcome but clearly can be more challenging in older people.

Clinical trials and large registries have shown that for patients over 75 years, elevated heart rate, lower systolic blood pressure, diabetes, and anterior STEMI are independent predictors of early mortality. Other independent predictors are previous infarction, time to treatment, diabetes, weight, and smoking status.

Restoring coronary flow and myocardial tissue perfusion

For patients with STEMI presenting *within 12 hours* after symptom onset and with persistent ST-segment elevation or new (or presumed new) LBBB, early mechanical or pharmacological reperfusion is critical (see Tables 5.13 and 5.14). By general agreement, reperfusion therapy (preferably primary percutaneous intervention, P-PCI) should be considered. If there is clinical and/or electrocardiographic evidence of ongoing ischaemia, even if symptoms started more than 12 hours before PCI may also be considered, especially if the exact timing of symptom onset is unclear. However, there is general agreement that PCI is probably not beneficial in patients presenting over 12 hours from symptom onset in the absence of clinical and/or electrocardiographic evidence of ongoing ischaemia. In a randomized controlled trial in STEMI patients presenting without persisting symptoms between 12 and 48 hours after symptom onset, PCI was associated with significant myocardial salvage, lending some support to an invasive strategy in these patients, but clinical outcomes were not better. In the OAT study, which included 2166 stabilized patients with an occluded infarct-related vessel 3–28 days after symptom onset, PCI did not improve clinical outcome.

Table 5.13 Reperfusion therapy (primary PCI)

Recommendations	Class[a]	Level[b]
Reperfusion therapy is indicated in all patients with history of chest pain/ discomfort of < 12h and with persistent ST-segment elevation or (presumed) new left bundle-branch block	I	A
Reperfusion therapy should be considered if there is clinical and/or ECG evidence of ongoing ischaemia if, according to patient, symptoms started > 12 before	IIa	C
Reperfusion using PCI may be considered in stable patients presenting >12 to 24h after symptom onset	IIb	B
PCI of a totally occluded infarct artery >24h after symptom onset in stable patients without signs of ischaemia	III	B
Primary PCI		
Preferred treatment if performed by an experienced team as soon as possible after FMC	I	A
Time from FMC to balloon inflation should be <2h in any case and <90 min in patients presenting early (e.g, <2h) with large infarct and low bleeding risk	I	B
Indicated for patients in shock and those with contraindications to fibrinalytic therapy irrespective of time delay	I	B
Antiplatelet co-therapy[a]		
Aspirin	I	B
NSAID and COX-2 selective inhibitors	III	B
Clopidogrel loading dose	I	C
GPIbIIa antagonist		
Abciximab	IIa	A
Tirofiban	IIb	B
Eptifibatide	IIb	C
Antithrombin therapy[c]		
Heparin	I	C
Bivalirudin	IIa	B
Fondaparinux	III	B
Adjunctive devixes		
Thrombus aspiration	IIb	B

Treatment-related benefits should rise in an older population, yet data to confirm these benefits are limited, and the multiple comorbidities often seen in older populations (in terms of variable degrees of associated comorbidities) increases treatment-associated risks, albeit these patients do better than those receiving no treatment. Older patients with ST-segment elevation myocardial infarction more often have relative and absolute contraindications to reperfusion therapies, so eligibility for reperfusion declines with age. Even where appropriate therapies have been shown to be valuable in older patients, they are less likely to receive reperfusion even if eligible, something that relates to inappropriate physician bias. Data supporting a benefit from reperfusion in older subgroups have been shown up to age 85 years. The selection of reperfusion strategy is mostly determined more by availability, time from presentation, shock, and comorbidity than by age, although there are higher stroke and bleeding risk w with lysis than with PCI. Additional data are needed on selection and dosing of adjunctive therapies and on complications in

Table 5.14 ESC Recommendation for fibrinolytic therapy

Fibrinolytic therapy[c]		
In the absence of contraindications (see Table 7) and if primary PCI cannot be performed within the recommended time (see above and Figure 2)	I	A
A fibrin-specific agent should be given	I	B
Pre-hospital initiation of fibrinolytic therapy	IIa	A
Antiplatelet co-therapy[c]		
if not already on aspirin oral (soluble or chewable/ non-enteric-coated) or i.v. dose of aspirin plus	I	B
clopidogrel oral loading dose if age ≤75 years	I	B
if age >75 years start with maintenance dose	IIa	B
Antithrombin co-therapy[c]		
with alteplase, reteplase, and tenecteplase:		
enoxaparin i.v. bolus followed 15 min later by first s.c. dose; if age.75 years no i.v. bolus and start with reduced first s.c. dose	I	A
if enoxaparin is not available: a weight-adjusted bolus of i.v. heparin followed by a weight-adjusted i.v. infusion with first aPTT control after 3 h	I	A
with streptokinase:		
an i.v. bolus of fondaparinux followed by an s.c. dose 24 h later or	IIa	B
enoxaparin i.v. bolus followed 15 min later by first s.c. dose; if age.75 years no i.v. bolus and start with reduced first s.c. dose	IIa	B
or a weight-adjusted dose of i.v. heparin followed by a weight-adjusted infusion	IIa	C

older people. A 'one-size-fits-all' approach to care in the oldest old is not feasible, and ethical issues will remain even in the presence of adequate evidence. There is unpublished but intuitively sound evidence that in all older patients PCI may be better than lysis (see below).

In terms of natural history and outcomes, morbidity and mortality rates with STEMI increase with age. In the GUSTO-I trial, the 30-day mortality rate increased 10-fold, from 3.0% among patients over 65 years to 30.3% among those 85 years or older.

The high mortality rate from STEMI in older people is thought to relate to the more frequent occurrence of electric and mechanical acute complications, such as acute mitral regurgitation and acute ventricular septal defect, albeit with early reperfusion therapy these complications are seen much less often nowadays. Indeed, it may be the delay in reperfusion that is patient or physician driven that leads to the excess incidence of acute electrical and mechanical complications in older people. These age-related mechanical catastrophes may also be contributed to by changes in cardiac physiology or decreased vascular compliance, ventricular hypertrophy and remodelling, and diminished response to beta-adrenergic stimulation in older people. Heart failure and pulmonary oedema, complications along this spectrum of adverse occurrences, occur in more than half of patients over 75 years and 65% of patients 85 years or older. Shock (hypotension with hypoperfusion) occurs in more than 10% of patients 75 years or older and is known to be due to ventricular or papillary muscle rupture or to advanced ventricular dysfunction. Myocardial oedema, contraction band necrosis, and intramyocardial haemorrhage are commonly noted at autopsy in older hearts after fibrinolysis. In 706 STEMI patients over 75 years of age, free wall rupture occurred in 17.1% treated with fibrinolytic therapy versus 4.9%

who received PCI and 7.9% who received no reperfusion. Fibrinolytic therapy may have unique adverse myocardial effects in those of advanced age as well as the generic effects of increased stroke risk.

The ability of STEMI treatments to improve outcomes in the very old, given their known physiological differences, is a question for future research. It is important, however, that all patients irrespective of age be considered for early reperfusion to reduce the incidence and severity of STEMI complications.

Primary PCI versus fibrinolytic therapy

Primary PCI (i.e. angioplasty as first therapeutic option in STEMI) is now the preferred reperfusion option provided guideline mandated timings can be met (<150 minutes symptom to balloon and 60–90 minutes door to balloon) Achieving such timings in older people who tend to present later may be a particular challenge, and public education programmes, and even particularly targeted at this group, are needed. Overall for all age ranges and provided the guideline mandated timings can be achieved, outcomes appear better with P-PCI. The overall excess risk of stroke in older people would suggest that a mechanical reperfusion strategy (albeit potent antiplatelet drugs are needed) would be preferable to using an agent such as a lytic with its potent bleeding risk.

One unpublished trial ('SENIOR-PAMI' Grines) randomized 530 patients over 70 years to P-PCI or lysis. Recruitment difficulties resulted in trial discontinuation at 483 patients. The mean age was 78 years. The call to balloon or lytic time was 237 and 210 minutes respectively. There were no significant differences in in-patient CVA (lytic 1.2% P-PCI 2.2%) nor in major bleed (6.2% and 5.6%) ICB (1.3% 0%), but ongoing ischaemia was significantly greater in the lytic arm (31% vs 4.8%). At 30 days there was a difference favouring P-PCI in re-AMI (1.6% vs 5.4% p = 0.039). When the patients were analysed according to age, 70–80 years and over 80 years, there was no difference in any parameter in the over 80 year olds but the numbers were small.

Further studies on the management of STEMI in the oldest old are required. However, in the UK National Infarct Angioplasty Project published by the Department of Health in 2008, two patients treated successfully for their STEMI with P-PCI were over 100 years old. In real-world practice, 'appropriate' older patients with STEMI should be transferred for P-PCI. 'Appropriateness' refers to the consideration of excess comorbidity associated with older people. Many older patients are now treated with P-PCI despite some data suggesting worse outcomes in this group. For example, in over 3000 patients with STEMI treated with primary PCI, in HIJAMI, the Heart Institute of Japan Acute Myocardial Infarction registry, age above 70 was a strong predictor of poor in-hospital and long-term mortality (hazard ratio of 6.8). It needs to be emphasized that those not receiving treatment do worse irrespective of age.

Rescue PCI is defined as PCI performed on a coronary artery which remains occluded despite fibrinolytic therapy. Identification of failed fibrinolysis remains difficult, but 50% segment elevations 60–90 minutes after the start of fibrinolytic therapy has been accepted as a surrogate. In a randomized controlled trial of 427 patients (REACT), the event-free survival after failed fibrinolysis was significantly higher with rescue PCI than with repeated fibrinolytic treatment or conservative treatment. This also applied to a subset analysis of older people.

Antithrombotic treatment

Aspirin should be given to all patients with a STEMI as soon as possible after the diagnosis. Aspirin should be started at a dose of 150–325 mg in a chewable form (enteric-coated aspirin should not be given because of slow onset of action). An alternative way of aspirin administration is the intravenous route (dose of 250–500 mg) but this is rarely done. A dose of 75–160 mg is given orally daily thereafter for life.

Clopidogrel is less studied in patients with STEMI treated with primary PCI. However, there is strong evidence behind clopidogrel usage as an adjunctive antiplatelet therapy on top of aspirin in patients undergoing non-acute PCI with stenting, which is used in >95% of all PCI nowadays.

Clopidogrel should be given as soon as possible to all patients with STEMI who are about to undergo P-PCI. It is started with a loading dose of 600 mg, followed by a daily dose of 75 mg. Prasugrel is a more potent thienopyridine that is increasingly used in P-PCI for STEMI, mostly because of its rapid onset of action, but because of bleeding excess it is contraindicated in patients over 75 years.

GPIIb/IIIa antagonists, which block the final pathway of platelet aggregation, have been studied in several randomized controlled trials in ACS. Most of the studies on the role of GPIIb/IIIa antagonists in STEMI have focused on abciximab rather than on the other two members of the family, tirofiban, and eptifibatide. A review of these trials showed that abciximab reduced 30-day mortality by 32% without affecting the risk of haemorrhagic stroke and major bleeding. However, Abciximab did not have a significant impact on the patency of infarct-related vessels, and its administration upstream of a planned PCI procedure did not offer advantages compared with the administration in the catheter laboratory. The potency of abciximab and its associated bleeding risk (HORIZONS trial) makes the use of bivalirudin a better option, especially in older people.

STEMI complications

These are generally much less common today. Cardiac rupture is characterized by cardiovascular collapse and electromechanical dissociation and it is usually fatal.

Ventricular septal rupture is another mechanical complication which should be suspected when there is sudden severe clinical deterioration confirmed on echocardiography. The definite treatment is emergency surgical repair and intra aorta balloon counter pulsation as a bridge to surgery.

Acute mitral regurgitation is now rare and usually occurs 2–7 days after STEMI. In most patients, acute mitral regurgitation is secondary to papillary muscle dysfunction rather than rupture. The most common cause of partial or total papillary muscle rupture is a small infarct of the posteromedial papillary muscle in the right or circumflex coronary artery distribution. Valve replacement is the procedure of choice for rupture of the papillary muscle, although repair can be attempted in selected cases.

A life-threatening arrhythmia, such as ventricular tachycardia (VT), VF, and total atrioventricular (AV) block, may be the first manifestation of ischaemia and requires immediate action. These arrhythmias may cause many of the reported sudden cardiac deaths in patients with acute ischaemic syndromes. VF or sustained VT has been reported in up to 20% of patients who present with STEMI.

Table 5.15 Class of recommendation and level of evidence tables

Level of Evidence A	Data derived from multiple randomized clinical trials or meta-analyses.
Level of Evidence B	Data derived from a single randomized clinical trial or large non-randomized studies.
Level of Evidence C	Consensus of opinion of the experts and/ or small studies, registries.

Classes of Recommendations	Definition
Class I	Evidence and/or general agreement that a given treatment or procedure is beneficial, useful, effective.
Class II	Conflicting evidence and/or a divergence of opinion about the usefulness/efficacy of the given treatment or procedure.
Class IIa	Weight of evidence/opinion is in favour of usefulness/efficacy.
Class IIb	Usefulness/efficacy is less well established by evidence/opinion.
Class III	Evidence or general agreement that the given treatment or procedure is not useful/effective, and in some cases may be harmful.

Table 5.16 Long-term medical treatment after STEMI

Recommendations	Class[a]	Level[b]
Antiplatelets/anticoagulants		
Aspirin for ever (75–100 mg daily) in all patients without allergy	I	A
Clopidogrel (75 mg daily) for 12 months in all patients irrespective of the acute treatment	IIa	C
Clopidogrel (75 mg daily) in all patients with contraindication to aspirin	I	B
Oral anticoagulant at INR 2–3 in patients who do not tolerate aspirin and clopidogrel	IIa	B
Oral anticoagulant at recommended INR when clinically indicated (e.g. atrial fibrillation, LV thrombus, mechanical valve)	I	A
Oral anticoagulant (at INR 2–3) in addition to low-dose aspirin (75–100 mg) in patients at high risk of thromboembolic events	IIa	B
Oral anticoagulant in addition to aspirin and clopidogrel (recent stent placement plus indication for oral anticoagulation)[c]	IIb	C
Oral anticoagulant in addition to clopidogrel or aspirin (recent stent placement plus indication for oral anticoagulation and increased risk of bleeding)	IIb	C
β-Blockers		
Oral b-blockers in all patients who tolerate these medications and without contraindications, regardless of blood pressure or LV function	I	A
ACE-inhibitor and ARB		
ACE-inhibitor should be considered in all patients without contraindications, regardless of blood pressure or LV function	IIa	A
ARB in all patients without contraindications who do not tolerate ACE-inhibitors, regardless of blood pressure or LV function	IIa	C

Table 5.16 (Continued)

Recommendations	Class[a]	Level[b]
Statins		
Statins in all patients, in the absence of contraindications, irrespective of cholesterol levels, initiated as soon as possible to achieve LDL cholesterol,100 mg/dL (2.5 mmol/L) (see also Table 22)	I	A
Influenza immunization		
In all patients	I	B

Management after STEMI and secondary prevention

Patients who have recovered from a STEMI are at high risk for further events and death, with 10% of post-infarction patients having recurrent infarction within a year, and mortality after discharge remains much higher than in the general population and especially in older people who tend not to be given full contemporary post-MI treatment (e.g. beta-blockade).

Several interventions can improve prognosis in patients who had STEMI (see Tables 5.15 and 5.16). Smoking cessation in this group has been shown to reduce mortality by at least one-third.

Aspirin, beta-blockers, ACE inhibitors, and statins have the strongest evidence of improving prognosis after STEMI. ACEi treatment in older people as most of the trials which demonstrated this benefit (ICIS-1, ICIS 4, SMILE and AIRE) have enrolled small numbers of patients over 75 years. However, optimal medical therapy in older people (albeit there is a chance of excess medication side effects in this group) must be a target.

Conclusion

The contemporary management of STEMI ACS has resulted in a significant fall in subsequent adverse outcomes including mortality. While comorbidities and the increased risk of side-effects and complications of treatments must always be considered in older people, the difference between those who do and those who do not receive treatment, in ALL age groups, is such that age itself should never be a contraindication to reperfusion and contemporary secondary care. The assumption should be that all elderly patients are considered for rapid contemporary treatment for ACS unless there is a valid reason for not doing so.

Further reading

Alp NJ, Gershlick AH, Carver A, et al. (2008). Rescue angioplasty for failed thrombolysis in older patients: insights from the REACT trial. Int J Cardiol 125: 254–7.

Goldberg RJ, Glatfelter K, Burbank-Schmidt E, et al. (2006). Trends in community mortality due to coronary heart disease. Am Heart J 151: 501–7.

Gottwalles Y, Dangelser G, De Poli F, et al. (2004). Acute STEMI in old and very old patients. The real life. Ann Cardiol Angeiol, 53: 305–13.

Gundersen T, Abrahmsen AM, Kjekshus J, et al. (1982). Timolol-related reduction in mortality and reinfarction in patients ages 65–75 years surviving acute myocardial infarction: prepared for the Norwegian Multicentre Study Group. Circulation 66: 1179–84.

Lee KL, Woodlief LH, Topol EJ, et al. (1995). Predictors of 30-day mortality in the era of reperfusion for acute myocardial infarction. Results from an international trial of 41,021 patients. GUSTO-I Investigators. Circulation 91: 1659–68.

Morrow DA, Antman EM, Charlesworth A, et al. (2000). TIMI risk score for ST-elevation myocardial infarction: a convenient, bedside, clinical score for risk assessment at presentation: an intravenous nPA for treatment of infarcting myocardium early II trial substudy. *Circulation* **102**: 2031–7.

Spencer FA, Goldberg RJ, Frederick PD, et al. (2001). Age and the utilization of cardiac catheterization following uncomplicated first acute myocardial infarction treated with thrombolytic therapy (The Second National Registry of Myocardial Infarction [NRMI-2]). *Am J Cardiol* **88**: 107–11.

Stone GW, Witzenbichler B, Guagliumi G, et al. (2008). Bivalirudin during primary PCI in acute myocardial infarction. *N Engl J Med* **358**: 2218–30.

Tunstall-Pedoe H, Kuulasmaa K, Mähönen M, et al. (1999). Contribution of trends in survival and coronary-event rates to changes in coronary heart disease mortality: 10-year results from 37 WHOMONICA project populations. Monitoring trends and determinants in cardiovascular disease. *Lancet* **353**: 1547–57.

Van de Werf F, Bax J, Betriu A, et al. (2008). Management of acute myocardial infarction in patients presenting with persistent ST-segment elevation. The Task Force on the management of ST-segment elevation acute myocardial infarction of the European Society of Cardiology. *Eur Heart J* **29**: 2909–45.

White HD, Barbash GI, Califf RM, et al. (1996). Age and outcome with contemporary thrombolytic therapy: results from the GUSTO-I trial: Global Utilization of Streptokinase and TPA for Occluded Coronary Arteries Trial. *Circulation* **94**: 1826–33.

Indications for cardiac pacing

Background

Cardiac pacing, particularly for bradyarrhythmias, is most often performed in older people, and as the population demographic shifts to a more aged population the number of necessary implants is likely to increase. Cardiac pacing has been used in the treatment of bradyarrhythmias for over 50 years. During that time advances in technology have led to smaller devices and leads, with concomitant improvement in longevity. This combination has made device implantation safer, a fact that is particularly relevant to the older patient population in whom comorbidities are often multiple.

The indications for bradyarrhythmia pacing have altered little over the years, but there has been a proliferation in the use of biventricular pacing as adjunctive treatment in the management of heart failure, and of implantable cardioverter-defibrillators (ICDs) in the treatment of ventricular tachyarrhythmias and prevention of sudden cardiac death. Broadly speaking, bradyarrhythmia pacing is indicated in both sinus nodal and atrioventricular nodal disease but also in some cases of neurocardiogenic syncope and bradycardia-induced ventricular tachyarrhythmia.

Sinus node disease

The so-called sick-sinus syndrome describes a spectrum of disease that encompasses benign sinus bradycardia through sinus arrest and bradycardia–tachycardia syndrome. The latter is characterized by paroxysmal atrial tachyarrhythmias developing in patients with underlying sinoatrial disease. The process of overdrive suppression in these patients often manifests as sinus arrest following the reversion of the tachyarrhythmia to sinus rhythm. It is this sinus arrest that is often responsible for presyncope or syncope erroneously attributed to atrial fibrillation. Chronotropic incompetence is the final manifestation of sinus node disease. Once diagnosed, the decision to pace for sinus node disease is thought to reduce symptoms and perhaps reduce the burden of atrial fibrillation, but is not thought to affect mortality to any great degree. Table 5.17 outlines the indications for pacing in sinus node disease.

With regards to pacing for minimally symptomatic patients with a resting sinus rate of less than 40 bpm who are chronotropically competent, the optimal management is not well defined. It is reasonable to either defer and observe for future symptoms or to offer pacemaker implantation.

The mode of pacing utilized in sinus node disease is subject to debate, but contemporary practice is to implant a dual-chamber pacemaker with the ability to minimize right ventricular pacing. The use of single-chamber ventricular pacing is best avoided because of the increased burden of atrial fibrillation seen in most contemporary studies comparing ventricular with atrial/dual-chamber pacing in sinus node disease. Single-chamber ventricular pacing is also associated with the development of pacemaker syndrome (atrial contraction against closed A-V valves as a result of retrograde VA conduction). This is not a rare phenomenon and can sometimes result in quite debilitating symptoms, including shortness of breath and presyncope. In view of the risk of developing concomitant AV nodal disease single-chamber atrial pacing is not often utilized in the older patient with sinus node disease (the risk is of the order of ~1% per annum). Additionally, it is now accepted

Table 5.17 Indications for cardiac pacing in sinus node disease

Degree of sinus node disease	Management
Sinus node disease manifest as symptomatic bradycardia with documented symptom-rhythm correlation	Pace
Syncope with sinus node disease	Pace
Symptomatic chronotropic incompetence	Pace
Sinus node disease with symptomatic bradycardia with no documented symptom-rhythm correlation	Pace
Minimally symptomatic patients with resting heart rate <40 bpm while awake and with no chronotropic incompetence	Observe or pace*
Sinus node disease without symptoms	Observe
Sinus node disease with symptoms secondary to non-essential medication	Stop medication and observe

*See text.

that persistent right ventricular pacing is detrimental to cardiac performance and most modern dual-chamber devices have facilities to minimize the amount of right ventricular pacing by allowing transient lengthening of the PR interval to encourage as much intrinsic conduction as possible.

AV nodal disease

AV block was the first indication for pacing and remains the most common indication for pacing today. Pacing for complete heart block has been shown to prolong survival particularly where there has been a history of syncope (see Table 5.18).

The indications for pacing in second degree AV block are not as clear cut. It is accepted that Mobitz type II block, particularly with a broad QRS, is a reasonable indication as there is a high rate of progression to higher degrees of block.

Pacing in Mobitz type I block is more controversial but the consensus is that if it is associated with symptoms

Table 5.18 Management of patients with AV block

Degree of AV nodal disease	Management
Chronic, symptomatic third- or second-degree AV block (Mobitz I or II)	Pace
Any iatrogenically induced third- or second-degree AV block (catheter ablation or post valvular surgery)	Pace
Asymptomatic third- or second-degree AV block	Pace
Bifascicular or trifascicular block with a history of syncope	Pace
Symptomatic, prolonged first-degree AV block (see text)	Pace
Asymptomatic first-degree AV block	No action

pacing should be offered. Asymptomatic Mobitz type 1 AV block may not necessarily be benign in older subjects and there is some evidence that pacing this group is associated with better outcome in terms of survival, particularly if there is diurnal block. In patients aged over 45 years, up to 75% of patients will develop higher grades of AV block at 5 years thereby necessitating pacemaker therapy.

First-degree block is not an indication for pacing unless the PR interval is long enough (>300 ms) to cause symptoms related to impaired left ventricular filling or an increase in atrial filling pressure as a result of atrial systole occurring so close to the end of left ventricular systole.

AV block occurring after catheter ablation for arrhythmia or valvular heart surgery is also thought to benefit from pacing as the natural history of AV block in these circumstances is unpredictable.

Bifascicular block and bifascicular block with PR prolongation (so-called trifascicular block)

The key determinant as to whether pacing is indicated in these circumstances is the presence of syncope. The annual incidence of progression to high-grade AV block in patients presenting with syncope is 5–11%, whereas the corresponding figure for those without syncope is as low as 0.6–0.8%. Before pacing it is important to evaluate for other causes, particularly ventricular tachycardia. Pragmatically, if there is good left ventricular function and if there is no history of ST elevation myocardial infarction, then it is reasonable to assume that ventricular tachycardia is not an active problem. In these circumstances 24-hour Holter monitors are not particularly helpful. If there is a history of syncope and either bifascicular or trifascicular block is present, then pacing is indicated with the above caveat.

Pacing in atrial fibrillation

Tachy-brady syndrome is a manifestation of sinus node disease that often requires pacing as described above. In persistent or permanent atrial fibrillation the indications for pacing depend on coupling symptoms to documented pauses. Pauses of greater than 3 seconds during ambulant periods or 4 seconds during nocturnal periods are deemed significant. Patients with presyncope or syncope should be paced if ambulatory monitoring demonstrates that these criteria have been met. It is also reasonable to offer pacemaker implantation if periods of bradycardia coexist with periods of tachycardia such that the use of negative chronotropes is likely to exacerbate bradycardia.

Pacing after myocardial infarction

AV conduction disturbances in the peri- and immediate post-infarction period result from autonomic imbalances and disruption of the blood supply to the conducting tissue. Some of these may be well tolerated and transient but others less well so. Inferior wall infarction is often associated with transient AV conduction disturbance at the level of the AV node and as a result the escape rhythm is usually narrow complex and well tolerated. Conduction disturbance associated with anterior wall infarction can result in block at the level of the bundle of His (or below). The escape rhythm under these circumstances is broad and less reliable. These patients require temporary pacing. On the whole, if the conduction disturbance is transient it does not usually require pacing; if it persists, it does. Persistence is arbitrarily taken as lasting longer than 14 days after infarction. The exception is when AV conduction is transiently disturbed in the presence of new interventricular delay, which carries a poor prognosis if left unpaced, and therefore permanent pacing is required immediately.

Exclusion of reversible causes

Before pacing is offered for either sinus nodal or AV nodal disease reversible causes such as acute myocardial infarction, electrolyte disturbance, drugs (non-essential), and hypothermia must all be excluded and/or corrected. Of particular relevance is the use of drugs such as galantamine and donepezil. It is recognized that they can exacerbate any underlying tendency towards bradyarrhythmia, such that an indication for pacing becomes apparent. These drugs have no disease-modifying potential but can significantly improve symptoms and quality of life in some patients. In such circumstances, if cessation of the drug is likely to cause a significant deterioration, then pacemaker implantation should be advocated. Such decisions are best made on a case by case basis.

Reflex syncope: carotid sinus syndrome and vasovagal syncope

Carotid sinus hypersensitivity is defined as a ventricular pause lasting more than 3 seconds or a fall in systolic blood pressure of greater than 50 mmHg when pressure is applied to the carotid artery at the level of bifurcation. The presence of syncope resulting from the above defines carotid sinus syndrome. Pacing is only indicated if there is a cardioinhibitory response (i.e. ventricular pause) and a history of syncope. When testing for carotid sinus hypersensitivity, it is important that syncope is elicited along with the chronotropic disturbance. In such cases single right ventricular pacing devices usually suffice as the need to pace is rare and often not prolonged, making pacemaker syndrome less of an issue.

Vasovagal syncope is the underlying cause in approximately half of all patients presenting with syncope. There are no class I indications for pacing in this context. In those patients who exhibit a cardioinhibitory response on tilt testing, the data are conflicting. This is primarily because pacing has little (if any) role to play in addressing the vasodepressor component of this syndrome. Many modern dual-chamber devices have rate-drop algorithms which are designed to increase heart rate in response to a sudden fall in heart rate with the aim of increasing cardiac output. Studies of this technology are not robust enough to advocate their routine use. Pacing for the cardioinhibitory component of vasovagal syncope should only be offered if other treatment modalities (education, avoidance of triggering situations, hydration) fail to improve matters, and patients being offered these devices should be made aware that their symptoms are unlikely to abate completely.

Biventricular pacing in heart failure

It has long been recognized that many patients with cardiomyopathies have associated interventricular and AV conduction delays. Bundle branch block alters the sequence of cardiac activation and associated alterations in regional blood flow and myocardial metabolism. These changes lead to inefficient and dyssynchronous left ventricular contraction. Biventricular pacing involves implanting pacing leads in the right atrium (except in permanent atrial fibrillation) and right ventricle as for a standard dual-chamber device. Pacing of the left ventricle is achieved from the epicardial surface with a pacing lead passed via the coronary sinus into an epicardial posterolateral vein. The burden of evidence is such that this treatment modality has been shown to improve symptoms and both morbidity and mortality. Devices can be implanted with or without defibrillatory capacity. The current guidance is that biventricular pacing should be offered to patients who are in NYHA class III–IV heart failure despite optimal medical therapy, and who have an ejection fraction of ≤35% with QRS duration of 120 ms or more. It is also reasonable to implant a biventricular device in a patient with a conventional indication for bradycardia pacing and an ejection fraction of ≤35% if it is thought that they will require a large amount of right ventricular pacing (thereby inducing left bundle branch block).

Pacing for tachyarrhythmias

Overdrive pacing
Broadly speaking, there are three circumstances where rapid overdrive pacing via a temporary pacing wire may be of clinical benefit. First, profound bradycardia can result in critical prolongation of ventricular repolarization which is manifest on the ECG as prolongation of the QT interval. Premature ventricular beats occurring during the period of prolonged repolarization can trigger the R on T phenomenon and then either polymorphic or monomorphic VT. The treatment of the tachyarrhythmia is to cardiovert electrically. Temporarily pacing the right ventricle at an increased heart rate decreases the QT interval, thereby reducing the risk of further episodes. If there is no reversible cause for the underlying bradycardia, permanent pacing is required when matters have stabilized. Second, the same principle applies to managing polymorphic VT (torsades de pointes) associated with iatrogenic or congenital QT prolongation. Finally, the most common form of VT seen clinically is monomorphic VT associated with ventricular scar. The mechanism of this tachycardia is re-entry, and so the re-entrant circuit can be broken by overdrive pacing. Pacing the right ventricle at a rate of 10–20 beats above the rate of tachycardia can be successful in cases where the arrhythmia has proved resistant to pharmacological treatment. Overdrive pacing for monomorphic VT seen in the context of acute myocardial infarction is not a useful treatment, as the mechanism of tachycardia in such cases is usually enhanced automaticity. Such arrhythmias are not amenable to overdrive pacing.

Implantable cardioverter-defibrillators
The evidence for the use of ICDs in both primary and secondary prevention is robust but none of the landmark trials included a significant proportion of older patients.

Ventricular tachyarrhythmias which result in syncope or cardiac arrest will mostly be managed medically in the very elderly population. It must, however, be recognized that chronological age is not necessarily a preclusion to ICD implantation. A significant number of patients aged over 75 years lead active, independent lifestyles and ICDs for secondary prevention should be considered where appropriate. The caveat is that poor left ventricular function or end-stage structural heart disease and not channelopathies are likely to be the aetiological factors. The poor prognosis of these conditions coupled to advanced age and attendant comorbidities will therefore potentially limit the number of ICDs implanted in the older population for secondary prevention.

ICD implantation for primary prevention in older patients is a more difficult area. Based on class I evidence ICDs are of benefit in patients with previous history of myocardial infarction who have a left ventricular ejection fraction of 30% or less. As previously mentioned, most trials excluded the older population. Whether ICDs prevent enough deaths in older patients with sufficient quality of life to justify the risk and cost of implantation when compared with medical management is not known. Contemporary practice is to manage these primary prevention patients medically.

Conclusions
The increased longevity of modern devices and expanding indications for complex pacing outside of the realms of bradyarrhythmias will increase the number of device implants across all age groups but particularly in older people. Complication rates for bradyarrhythmia pacing are generally low (2%) and implantation can improve morbidity and mortality greatly. The threshold for implanting such devices is consequently getting lower. The indications for complex pacing in older people are not based on any great wealth of evidence, and decisions regarding biventricular pacing and implantable defibrillator therapy are best made on a case by case basis.

Further reading
Chan PS, Nallamothu BK, Spertus JA, et al. (2009). Impact of age and medical comorbidity on the effectiveness of implantable cardioverter-defibrillators for primary prevention. Circ Cardiovasc Qual Outcomes, 2: 16–24.

Swindle JP, Rich MW, McCann P, et al. (2010). Implantable cardiac device procedures in older patients: use and in-hospital outcomes. Arch Intern Med, 170: 631–7.

Vardas PE, Auricchio A, Blanc JJ, et al. (2008). Guidelines for cardiac pacing and cardiac resynchronization therapy. Rev Port Cardiol 27: 639–87.

Valvular heart disease

Background
Valvular heart disease is common in older people. Although often asymptomatic, it may be associated with symptoms that markedly impair quality of life and with increased mortality. With advancing age, there are changes in the pattern of valve disease, in the dominant aetiologies and in the presenting signs. Management may also be influenced by comorbidities, which are more prevalent in older people and associated with increased operative risk and limited life expectancy.

Aortic stenosis
Epidemiology
Aortic stenosis (AS) is the most common form of valvular heart disease requiring surgical intervention in the Western world. It is predominantly a disease of older people, in whom the most frequent cause is senile calcific degeneration of a normal tricuspid valve. Less commonly it may be due to calcification of a congenitally bicuspid valve or rheumatic valve disease. The population prevalence of AS is 2–7% in those aged 65 years or older but rises with age and AS may be present in some degree in 30% of those aged over 90 years. Aortic sclerosis, which may be a precursor, is present in around 25% of those over 65 years. AS may have a long asymptomatic phase but after the onset of symptoms, the outlook is poor, with average survival of less than two or three years in the absence of treatment. Sudden death is a well-recognized complication but it is rare in asymptomatic patients.

Clinical features
Typical symptoms include
- exertional breathlessness
- paroxysmal nocturnal dyspnoea and orthopnoea
- angina (may be caused by subendocardial ischaemia)
- exertional dizziness
- falls
- exertional syncope.

  Key signs on physical examination:
- slow-rising pulse may be present but is often masked due to stiff non-compliant vessels
- ejection systolic murmur: amplitude does not differentiate degrees of severity and the murmur may be soft in very severe AS
- loss of second heart sound (specific but not sensitive)
- signs of heart failure (may denote a worse prognosis).

Investigations
Echocardiography, including Doppler studies, is the principal diagnostic tool for diagnosis and assessment of severity. A peak Doppler transvalvular gradient greater than 64 mmHg or a mean gradient greater than 40 mmHg indicates severe stenosis. However, transvalvular gradients may be low despite severe stenosis in the presence of impaired left ventricular (LV) systolic function or with a normal ejection fraction in a small, hypertrophied LV generating a low stroke volume. Severity is therefore best judged by assessment of valve area. A valve area less than 1 cm^2 indicates severe stenosis, 1–1.5 cm^2 moderate stenosis, and 1.5–2 cm^2 mild stenosis. For particularly small or large individuals, indexing to body surface area may be important. An indexed valve area of less than 0.6 cm^2/m^2 indicates severe stenosis.

Low-flow, low-gradient aortic stenosis is defined as a valve area less than 1 cm^2 with a mean gradient of less than 30 mmHg and an LV ejection fraction of less than 40%. This can be due to genuinely severe aortic stenosis with low transvalvular flow, or to moderate stenosis with an impaired LV and inadequate stroke volume, to fully open the aortic valve – pseudo-severe stenosis. Low-dose dobutamine stress echo can be used to distinguish between the two situations. In truly severe aortic stenosis with contractile reserve, dobutamine should result in a 20% rise in stroke volume, with a mean gradient greater than 30 mmHg and a valve area remaining below 1.2 cm^2. In pseudo-severe stenosis with contractile reserve, stroke volume increases but mean gradient remains less than 30 mmHg, while the valve area increases to over 1.2 cm^2. In some patients with no contractile reserve, no parameters change with dobutamine.

Cardiac catheterization and coronary angiography are required in patients considered for surgery, but it is rarely if ever necessary to cross the aortic valve to obtain an invasively measured transvalvular gradient.

> **Authors' Tip**
>
> In aortic stenosis, reduced ejection fraction in the presence of a persistently high valvular gradient (>40 mmHg mean) may be due to afterload mismatch and the LV function should improve with valve replacement

Management
Medical
There is no medical treatment that will reverse or retard the rate of progression of AS. A randomized trial of statins showed no benefit. Antihypertensive therapy with ACE inhibitors or beta-blockers should be used if required to control hypertension but should be introduced with caution in older people.

Surgical
The only effective conventional treatment is surgical replacement of the aortic valve (AVR), which should be considered promptly at the onset of symptoms in patients with severe stenosis. This involves open-chest surgery with cardiopulmonary bypass, but results are excellent with in-hospital mortality of 2.5% overall for isolated AVR and 5.8% in patients over 80 years of age. In patients requiring concomitant coronary artery surgery (about 40%), the corresponding figures are 4.5% and 9% respectively (see Figure 5.17). Consequently, age alone should not be a deterrent to surgery, as survival in those over 65 years of age is only marginally lower than that in an age- and gender-matched general population. However, the comorbidities prevalent in the older population may increase operative risk and impact on survival even after successful surgery. One-year post-operative mortality in patients over 80 years of age is 13% for isolated AVR and 18% for AVR with coronary revascularization. Although the total number patients having AVR and the proportion who are older and at high risk is increasing, one-third of older patients with severe symptomatic AS are not offered surgery. In older patients, bioprosthetic valves are generally preferred, as they have ample longevity and avoid the need for anticoagulation.

Transcatheter aortic valve implantation
For patients in whom surgery is contraindicated or associated with high operative risk, transcatheter aortic valve implantation (TAVI) now offers a viable alternative.

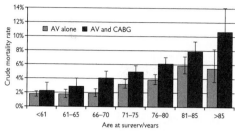

Figure 5.17 Crude mortality for aortic valve surgery, with and without coronary artery bypass grafting (CABG), by age. Reproduced from Bridgewater B, et al. Demonstrating quality: The Sixth National Adult Cardiac Surgery database report (2009), Bridgewater B, Kinsman R, Walton P and Keogh B. Published by Dendrite Clinical Systems Ltd. Henley-on-Thames. ISBN 1-903968-23-2, with permission.

Two CE-marked devices are currently available, a balloon-expandable prosthesis that may be delivered transarterially or transapically, and a self-expanding nitinol prosthesis delivered transarterially (see Figure 5.18). Preliminary data from the UK TAVI registry show good procedural success, with survival of 93.1% at 30 days and 80.3% at 1 year. A randomized trial of TAVI in inoperable patients (PARTNER B) reported a dramatic reduction in 1-year mortality to 30.7%, compared with 50.7% in patients treated conservatively. A trial in patients at high operative risk (PARTNER A) showed TAVI to be non-inferior to surgery in for one-year mortality (24.2% vs 26.8%) but was associated with an increased stroke risk (5.1% vs 2.4%). Extended follow-up and further trials are ongoing.

Balloon aortic valvuloplasty
In patients with severe calcific AS, balloon aortic valvuloplasty (BAV) provides excellent short-term symptom relief but restenosis is common within a few months and there is no survival advantage. The procedure may nonetheless have a role in some circumstances:

- as a bridge to definitive treatment with TAVI or AVR
- to enable complex coronary angioplasty before TAVI
- as a therapeutic trial if attribution of symptoms to AS is uncertain
- for short-term palliative therapy in selected patients.

Aortic regurgitation
Epidemiology
Aortic regurgitation (AR) is caused by inadequate coaptation of the aortic valve cusps during diastole and may result either from a primary abnormality of the valve or from an abnormality of the aortic root resulting in disruption of normal valve closure. A proportion (>50% in severe AR) of the forward stroke volume of the left ventricle leaks back through the aortic valve in diastole. This leads to progressive LV dilatation. Half of patients undergoing valve replacement for chronic pure regurgitation have an abnormality of the aortic valve itself, while the reminder have an abnormality of the aortic root, most commonly of a non-specific cause. Of the valvular causes, endocarditis accounts for about 20%, with the remainder being due to calcific degeneration, commonly in older patients of a morphologically tricuspid aortic valve, as opposed to younger patients in whom bicuspid valves predominate. Rheumatic heart disease accounts for only 6%.

Acute severe aortic regurgitation may be caused by endocarditis and aortic dissection.

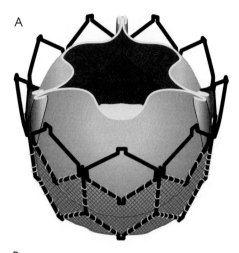

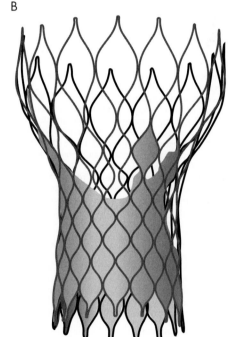

Figure 5.18 Devices used for transcatheter aortic valve implantation. (a) Balloon expandable prosthesis (SAPIEN, Edwards Lifesciences LLC, Irvine, CA, USA). B) Self-expanding nitinol prosthesis (the CoreValve ReValving system, Medtronic Inc., Minneapolis, MN, USA). © John Webb and Alain Cribier, Percutaneous transarterial aortic valve implantation: what do we know?, *European Heart Journal* (2011) **32**(2): 140–7, Fig. 1. By permission of Oxford University Press on behalf of the European Society of Cardiology.

Clinical features
Acute severe aortic regurgitation causes tachycardia, which is often accompanied by pulmonary oedema and cardiogenic shock.

Chronic aortic regurgitation usually has a long asymptomatic phase. Reduced effort tolerance and breathlessness typically occur with the onset of ventricular dysfunction, but some patients remain asymptomatic despite poor LV function.

Examination
- Widened pulse pressure
- High-pitched decrescendo murmur at left sternal edge in expiration—severity of AR correlates with duration rather than intensity of the murmur
- Inferolateral displacement of apex beat
- Bounding pulses—abrupt rise and collapse.

Investigations
Echocardiography is essential to determine the anatomy of the valve and aortic root, the severity of the leak, and LV size and function. Additional imaging of the aortic root with CT or CMR may sometimes be necessary. Cardiac catheterization is required only to assess coronary disease. Although rare, syphilitic aortitis should be excluded by appropriate serological testing. The unexpected finding of AR should always prompt a thorough search for other evidence of infective endocarditis.

Management
Acute severe aortic regurgitation causing circulatory compromise is a surgical emergency. Nitroprusside can be used pending surgery. Beta-blockade and intra-aortic balloon pumping should be avoided.

Asymptomatic patients with severe AR should be followed up annually with echocardiography. Exercise testing may be useful in apparently asymptomatic patients. Surgery should be considered with even mild symptoms or an LV end-systolic diameter of more than 50 mm, end-diastolic diameter of more than 70 mm or an ejection fraction of less than 50%.

Systemic hypertension increases regurgitant flow and should be treated. In asymptomatic patients with severe AR and normal LV function, there is conflicting evidence that vasodilator therapy with ACE inhibitors or nifedipine may slow progression of AR, but it is not routinely used in the absence of hypertension. Vasodilators should, however, be considered as chronic therapy in patients with severe AR and symptomatic LV dysfunction when AVR is contraindicated due to important comorbidities and as short-term therapy to improve haemodynamic status preoperatively in patients with severe symptomatic LV dysfunction undergoing AVR. Patients with AR due to syphilitic aortitis should receive a course of penicillin therapy.

Mitral regurgitation
Epidemiology
In older people, mitral regurgitation (MR) is more common than aortic valve disease. Aetiologically, MR can be divided into organic and functional. In functional MR, the abnormality is of the ventricular myocardium rather than the valve itself.
Primary or organic MR
- Valvular degeneration: Chordal elongation leads to systolic prolapse of one or both valve leaflets. Chordal rupture may lead to a flail leaflet with severe regurgitation.
- Mitral annular calcification: This degenerative process increases with age, particularly in women, resulting in calcific deposits that may distort the annulus and leaflets causing impaired coaptation during systole. Calcific deposits in the mitral annulus, aortic valve and

epicardial coronary arteries are often associated in older people and have common predisposing factors (e.g. hypertension, diabetes, and hypercholesterolaemia).
- Rheumatic heart disease: Regurgitation may be caused by distortion of leaflets and chordal shortening. Endocarditis may damage the leaflets or rupture chords, resulting in acute or chronic MR.

Functional MR
- Ischaemic MR: Acute MR may result from papillary muscle rupture, an uncommon early complication of myocardial infarction. Chronic ischaemic MR is much more common and is caused by altered LV geometry displacing the papillary muscles, in turn pulling on the chords, displacing the leaflets and preventing normal valve closure.
- Cardiomyopathy causing functional MR due to LV dilatation.

Clinical features
Acute MR causes an immediate rise in left atrial pressure and may result in pulmonary oedema. In chronic MR, the rise in left atrial pressure is more modest, as the atrium has time to dilate and accommodate the increased volume load. The compensated phase of chronic MR may last many years but ultimately leads to LV dilatation and failure. Severe symptoms or ventricular dysfunction denote a poor prognosis.

Symptoms of chronic MR include
- gradual onset of breathlessness.
- reduced effort capacity.
- onset of atrial fibrillation (AF) may precipitate cardiac failure.

Key signs on physical examination
Acute severe MR
- Tachycardia, hypotension and shock.
- Systolic murmur, which may be quiet, relatively short and only audible at left sternal edge.

Chronic MR
- Apex beat displaced laterally.
- Pansystolic murmur, maximal at the apex, radiating to the axilla; may be quiet, particularly in ischaemic MR.
- In mitral leaflet prolapse, the murmur may commence in mid-systole and be preceded by a click, as the chords come under maximal tension.
- Secondary pulmonary hypertension may result in a parasternal heave, loud P2 and signs of tricuspid regurgitation.

Investigations
Echocardiography, with Doppler studies, is used to determine the mechanism, severity, and consequences of MR. Transoesophageal echocardiography may be required to determine the precise anatomical and functional mechanism if valve repair is contemplated.

ECG may show a broad, notched P wave if there is left atrial enlargement.

Chest radiograph may show pulmonary oedema in acute MR. In chronic MR, there may be evidence of left atrial and ventricular enlargement. Calcification of the mitral annulus may be seen.

Cardiac catheterization is usually only required preoperatively to assess the presence and extent of any coronary artery disease.

Management

Medical

- Diuretics and nitrates can be used to treat pulmonary oedema in acute MR.
- No medical therapy slows the progression of organic MR. Conventional treatment of heart failure can temporarily improve symptoms but should not delay consideration of surgery.
- Functional MR may be improved by beta-blockers and ACE inhibitors.
- AF should be controlled to alleviate symptoms. DC cardioversion of recent onset AF may be successful. Otherwise, the focus should be on control of the heart rate using beta-blockers, rate-limiting calcium channel blockers, or digoxin.
- Anticoagulation is not required in sinus rhythm but should always be considered in the presence of AF. It may also be required if there is a history of systemic embolism or evidence of left atrial thrombus, and during the first 3 months after mitral valve repair.

Surgical

Non-ischaemic (primary) MR

Intervention is only indicated in the presence of severe MR. The aim is to intervene before the development of limiting symptoms or irreversible LV dysfunction. Surgery is indicated in patients with symptoms due to chronic MR, ejection fraction greater than 30%, and LV end-systolic diameter less than 55 mm. When the ejection fraction is less than 30%, surgery may be considered if symptoms are refractory to medical therapy and there is a high likelihood that repair is feasible with low comorbidity. Valve repair is associated with lower operative mortality and better long-term outcome than valve replacement. Overall in-hospital mortality is 1.9% for isolated MV repair and 3.9% for MV repair with coronary artery bypass graft but increases with age (see Figure 5.19). Most degenerate valves are suitable for repair. Rheumatic valves may be more difficult to repair and often require replacement. If possible, the subvalvular apparatus should be preserved. Valves damaged by endocarditis can often be repaired in expert hands.

Asymptomatic patients with moderate or severe MR should have 6–12 monthly clinical and annual echocardiographic follow-up. Surgery should be considered in patients with evidence of LV dysfunction, and in those with AF or pulmonary hypertension and preserved LV function. In the absence of these features, the role of surgery is less clear

but it may be considered if operative risk is low and repair by an experienced surgeon is likely to be feasible.

Patients with MR due to dilated cardiomyopathy should receive medical therapy for heart failure, with cardiac resynchronization therapy, if indicated. Expert valve repair may occasionally be required for very severe MR.

Ischaemic MR

Acute MR from papillary muscle rupture is life-threatening and requires emergency valve surgery.

Chronic ischaemic MR should be treated with medical therapy for coronary artery disease and LV dysfunction. Surgical intervention may be required in patients

- undergoing coronary artery surgery, with moderate or severe ischaemic MR, irrespective of symptoms
- with symptomatic, severe ischaemic MR, unless LV function is severely impaired.

Mitral valve surgery in these situations improves symptoms but not survival. Valve repair is less durable than in organic MR and chordal-sparing valve replacement may be a better option, particularly in ischaemic MR with localized ventricular remodelling.

In selected patients undergoing mitral valve surgery, concomitant repair of the tricuspid valve and surgical ablation of AF may also be performed, when appropriate.

Percutaneous intervention

Transcatheter techniques have recently been developed, which may be suitable for patients in whom surgery is contraindicated or associated with excessively high operative risk due to severe LV dysfunction, advanced age or serious comorbidity. These include an edge-to-edge clip to oppose the mid-portions of the mitral valve leaflets, creating a double orifice, and a constraining device that may be deployed in the coronary sinus to reduce functional MR. These devices are currently undergoing clinical evaluation but may offer an attractive alternative to surgery for very old or comorbid patients in the future.

Mitral stenosis

Epidemiology

Mitral stenosis (MS) is almost always due to chronic rheumatic heart disease, although 30% of patients have no clear history of rheumatic fever. Rheumatic fever is triggered by oropharyngeal infection with Group A beta-haemolytic streptococci, which induces an immune reaction predominantly affecting the left-sided valves. This is progressive and in time produces a thickened, fibrotic valve with fusion of the commissures, reduced leaflet mobility and a small orifice. The chords may also be matted together and the valve may become heavily calcified. Rheumatic MS is twice as common in women as in men. The incidence of rheumatic mitral valve disease has fallen dramatically in developed countries.

Clinical features

As the valve narrows, a diastolic pressure gradient develops between the left atrium and the left ventricle. Left atrial pressure rises, leading to a passive rise in pulmonary venous pressure. Any situation, such as exercise or infection, that increases heart rate or cardiac output will further increase the transmitral gradient and pulmonary venous pressures, producing breathlessness or even pulmonary oedema. Chronic pulmonary venous hypertension leads to secondary pulmonary arterial hypertension, right heart dilatation, tricuspid regurgitation, and right heart failure.

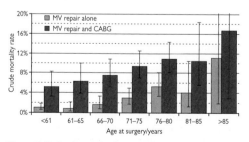

Figure 5.19 Crude mortality for mitral valve repair, with and without CABG, by age. Reproduced from Bridgewater B, et al. Demonstrating quality: The Sixth National Adult Cardiac Surgery database report (2009), Bridgewater B, Kinsman R, Walton P and Keogh B. Published by Dendrite Clinical Systems Ltd. Henley-on-Thames. ISBN 1-903968-23-2, with permission.

Symptoms

The gradual onset of breathlessness and fatigue is often the only symptom and may be far advanced before the cause is recognized. The onset of AF may precipitate acute pulmonary oedema. Some patients present with symptoms of right heart failure or with systemic thromboembolism. Haemoptysis due to severe pulmonary venous hypertension is less common.

Key physical signs

- Malar flush.
- Loud S1 (may be palpable) with opening snap—both may be absent if valve is fibrotic, calcified and immobile.
- Low-pitched delayed diastolic murmur, best heard at apex lying on left side – duration reflects severity but the murmur may be soft or inaudible in older patients.
- Signs of pulmonary hypertension, right ventricular hypertrophy and right heart failure may be present.
- Characteristic signs may be attenuated or even absent in older people and the clinical picture may be of heart failure.

Investigations

- Echocardiography is essential in patients with suspected mitral stenosis and is used to estimate valve area. A valve area of 1.5–2.2 cm^2 indicates a mildly stenotic valve, 1.0–1.5 cm^2 moderate stenosis, and less than 1 cm^2 severe stenosis. Echocardiography also gives important information about the morphology of the other valves, atrial and ventricular sizes, and pulmonary arterial pressures.
- ECG: AF is very common in mitral stenosis. In sinus rhythm a broad, notched P wave may be present.
- Chest radiograph: Appearances change with the progression of MS but in advanced disease may show left atrial enlargement and evidence of pulmonary hypertension or right heart enlargement.
- Cardiac catheterization: Rarely needed except to evaluate the presence and extent of coronary artery disease in candidates for valve surgery.

Management

Medical

Most asymptomatic patients with mild or moderate MS can be reviewed yearly with repeat echocardiograms. They should be advised to seek medical attention if symptoms develop.

Anticoagulation: All patients in AF should be anticoagulated unless there is a clear contraindication. Anticoagulation is recommended in sinus rhythm if the left atrium is enlarged (>5 cm) or there is a history of thromboembolism. The international normalized ratio (INR) should be maintained at 2.5–3.5.

Control of AF: Inappropriate tachycardia shortens diastolic filling time and may aggravate symptoms. Recent onset AF in patients with mild-to-moderate stenosis may respond to DC cardioversion. Otherwise, optimal control of the heart rate during activity is important. Beta-blockers or rate-limiting calcium channel blockers are usually more effective than digoxin.

Symptomatic treatment: Symptoms of breathlessness or congestion may be relieved with diuretics.

The primary indication for intervention in mitral stenosis is the relief of limiting symptoms in patients with a valve area of less than 1.5 cm^2.

Balloon mitral valvuloplasty

In experienced centres, balloon mitral valvuloplasty (percutaneous transmitral commissurotomy—PTMC) is the treatment of choice in patients with favourable anatomy. Contraindications include bilateral commissural calcification, significant mitral regurgitation and atrial thrombus. The results of PTMC are good, with an expected doubling of area for a severely stenosed valve. Restenosis does occur but is usually slow in onset. Successful PTMC can delay valve replacement by around 10 years in suitable patients.

Surgical

In developed countries, surgical mitral valvotomy is now rarely performed, as suitable patients are treated by balloon valvuloplasty. Valves that are unsuitable for balloon dilatation are usually replaced. The mortality of valve replacement is less than 5% in younger patients but more than doubles in older patients with significant comorbidities.

Infective endocarditis prophylaxis

For many years, antimicrobial prophylaxis against infective endocarditis (IE) has been recommended for patients with predisposing cardiac conditions, such as valvular heart disease or prosthetic valves, undergoing dental procedures, or non-dental diagnostic or therapeutic procedures involving the upper and lower gastrointestinal tract, the genitourinary tract or the upper and lower respiratory tract. However, recent guidance from the National Institute for Health and Clinical Excellence (NICE), following re-examination of the evidence, does not recommend antibiotic prophylaxis for any of these procedures.

Patients susceptible to IE should be fully informed of the risk and advised to seek expert advice if they develop symptoms that might indicate IE. They should maintain good oral health and any episodes of infection should be investigated and treated promptly. If a person at risk is receiving antimicrobial therapy because they are undergoing a gastrointestinal or genitourinary procedure at a site where there is suspected infection, an antibiotic should be used that covers organisms that cause IE.

These guidelines are a significant departure from previous practice and have caused some controversy, but they are endorsed by the national specialist societies and Department of Health. The American College of Cardiology and the American Heart Association have also updated their guidelines, but they still judge antibiotic prophylaxis to be reasonable for some dental procedures in patients at the highest risk, including those with prosthetic valves or a past history of IE.

Key points

- Classical physical signs of valve disease may be attenuated by age-related changes in vascular compliance and thoracic anatomy.
- In aortic valve disease, the onset of symptoms denotes a poor prognosis and intervention should be considered promptly.
- Percutaneous therapies for aortic stenosis and mitral regurgitation are evolving rapidly and may offer an alternative for selected patients who are unsuitable or at high risk from conventional surgery.
- In moderate or severe mitral stenosis, balloon valvuloplasty, when feasible, is the treatment of choice for the relief of limiting symptoms.

- Patients with moderate or severe MR should have regular clinical and echocardiographic follow-up to ensure that surgery is offered before the development of limiting symptoms or irreversible LV dysfunction.
- Expert repair of the regurgitant mitral valve, with preservation of the native valve apparatus, is preferable to valve replacement whenever feasible.
- Bioprosthetic valves are preferable to mechanical valves in older patients, as they have ample longevity and avoid the need for long-term anticoagulation.
- Routine antibiotic prophylaxis is no longer recommended for patients with valvular heart disease or prosthetic valves undergoing dental or non-dental diagnostic or therapeutic interventions.

Further reading

Aronow WS, Weiss MB (2008). Aortic disease in the elderly. In (Aronow WS, Fleg JL, Rich MW, eds) *Cardiovascular Disease in the Elderly*, 4th edn. New York, NY: Informa Healthcare, Inc, pp. 419–44.

Bonow RO, Carabello BA, Chatterjee K, et al. ACC/AHA 2006 guidelines for the management of patients with valvular heart disease: a report of the American College of Cardiology/American Heart Association Task Force on Practice Guidelines (Writing Committee to Develop Guidelines for the Management of Patients With Valvular Heart Disease). American College of Cardiology (http://www.acc.org/clinical/guidelines/valvular/index.pdf).

Bridgewater B, Kinsman R, Walton P, et al. (2009). Demonstrating quality: The sixth National Adult Cardiac Surgery database report. Henley-on-Thames, UK: Dendrite Clinical Systems Ltd. (http://www.scts.org/sections/audit/Cardiac/index.html).

Brooks N (2009). Prophylactic antibiotic treatment to prevent infective endocarditis: new guidance from the National Institute for Health and Clinical Excellence. *Heart* **95**: 774–80.

Cheitlin MD, Aronow WS (2008). Mitral regurgitation, mitral stenosis, and mitral annular calcification in the elderly. In (Aronow WS, Fleg JL, Rich MW, eds) *Cardiovascular Disease in the Elderly*, 4th edn. New York, NY: Informa Healthcare, Inc, pp. 445–80.

Leon MB, Smith CR, Mack M, et al. (2010). Transcatheter aortic-valve implantation for aortic stenosis in patients who cannot undergo surgery. *N Engl J Med* **363**: 1597–607.

NICE (2008). Prophylaxis against infective endocarditis: Antimicrobial prophylaxis against infective endocarditis in adults and children undergoing interventional procedures. NICE clinical guideline 64. London, NICE (www.nice.org.uk/nicemedia/pdf/CG64NICEguidance.pdf).

Nishimura RA, Carabello BA, Faxon DP, et al. (2008). ACC/AHA 2008 guideline update on valvular heart disease: focused update on infective endocarditis: a report of the American College of Cardiology/American Heart Association Task Force on Practice Guidelines. *Circulation*, **118**: 887–96.

Smith CR, Leon MB, Mack MJ, et al. (2011). Transcatheter versus surgical aortic-valve replacement in high-risk patients. *N Engl J Med* **364**: 2187–98.

Vahanian A, Baumgartner H, Bax J, et al. (2007). Guidelines on the management of valvular heart disease. *Eur Heart J* **28**: 230–68.

Vahanian A, Alfieri O, Al-Attar N, et al. (2008). Transcatheter valve implantation for patients with aortic stenosis: a position statement from the European Association of Cardio-Thoracic Surgery (EACTS) and the European Society of Cardiology (ESC), in collaboration with the European Association of Percutaneous Cardiovascular Interventions (EAPCI). *Eur Heart J* **29**: 1463–70.

Cardiac rehabilitation

Cardiac rehabilitation (CR) plays a central role in comprehensive management after myocardial infarction, coronary revascularization, cardiac surgery, recent onset angina, chronic heart failure, and symptomatic peripheral vascular disease. It aims to facilitate physical and psychological recovery, reducing avoidable disability and handicap and achieving and maintaining better health and quality of life. An essential goal is functional independence. This is accomplished through a multidisciplinary and multifactorial programme of secondary prevention, structured exercise and education.

Older people are at greatest risk of complications and of prolonged hospital stays (with consequent physical deconditioning and functional decline) after an acute cardiac event or surgery. A growing body of clinical experience and evidence from trials with people up to age 89 years shows that older people with coronary artery disease, congestive cardiac failure, or following cardiac surgery can safely reap very significant benefit from tailored programmes of CR. People whose potential to exercise is limited still have much to gain from the non-exercise components.

Traditionally, CR is provided to groups of patients within a hospital or community setting. There is growing interest in home-based programmes, using self-help material such as the Heart Manual, supported by visits from a nurse facilitator or regular telephone contacts. This approach may better meet the needs of many older people.

Benefits and safety

The pathophysiological benefits of CR probably result from increased fibrinolysis and decreased coagulability, reduced inflammation, improved endothelial function, enhanced insulin sensitivity, and improved autonomic function associated with exercise training and stress reduction, and from the systematic and sustained approach to addressing cardiovascular risk factors.

Five-year mortality rates are 21–34% lower in CR users than non-users aged 65 and over, implying that one 5-year death is averted for every 12 patients receiving CR. Mortality reductions increase progressively in older age groups and with number of CR sessions attended. Women tend to have worse functional capacity at entry and so may derive more benefit than men.

Other outcomes also indicate that CR is at least equally effective in old and young, with fewer readmissions and shorter hospitalizations, increased exercise tolerance and muscle strength (and so likely fewer falls), improved modifiable risk factors (smoking, obesity, blood pressure, lipids), and enhanced psychological wellbeing, functional independence (including return to driving), and health-related quality of life. In chronic heart failure patients, exercise-based CR can improve exercise tolerance, disease-related symptoms and wellbeing, without adversely impacting on left ventricular function.

Cost-effectiveness of CR compares very favourably with other established pharmacological and surgical interventions for secondary prevention, with a mean cost per patient of about £700 (2009 prices), or much less for home-based programmes.

Safety of CR at all ages is well established and complications during supervised exercise are rare, even in the very old. During initial exercise training, ECG monitoring and close supervision is appropriate. Patients with significant cardiac arrhythmias need especially closer surveillance by telemetry or Holter monitoring, and those with severe ventricular arrhythmias or uncontrolled supraventricular arrhythmias should be excluded until effective therapy has been instituted. All patients should be taught self-monitoring of pulse rate and recognition of warning signs. CR is contraindicated in patients with severe ventricular dysfunction or unstable angina, who should only take part after effective treatment is established. It is also contraindicated in patients with severe aortic stenosis.

Phases of cardiac rehabilitation

CR should be initiated once the cardiac condition is stable and before hospital discharge (Phase 1) and continue in the early convalescence period at home (Phase 2). After a few weeks, the patient can enter the formal rehabilitation programme (Phase 3) and then the principles should be practiced indefinitely to achieve long-term maintenance of best possible health (Phase 4).

Phases 1–2

This should include risk factor assessment, emotional support, resumption of self-care activities (facilitated by nurses and occupational therapist), and gentle mobilization. Discharge planning should include education about new medication (benefits and harms) and, where relevant, the importance of continued smoking cessation after leaving hospital. Family members should be actively involved.

In preparation for Phase 3, there needs to be baseline medical assessment (including submaximal or symptom-limited exercise testing, or 6-minute walk), risk stratification and agreement on individualized goals of intervention and an action plan. These are likely to include limiting adverse physiological, psychological, and social effects of cardiac disease, control of symptoms and resumption of customary activities.

Phase 3

This incorporates a planned programme of outpatient intervention, usually running over about 6–12 weeks and typically involving a specialist nurse, physiotherapist and/or psychologist, with other professionals providing their specialist input. A 'menu' of options should be available that can be tailored to the needs of each patient. Centre-based (usually once or twice weekly, within a hospital, gymnasium, or community sport centre setting) and home-based programmes appear equally effective. The Day Hospital might be an appropriate venue for frailer patients.

Exercise prescription should be individualized, and the typical centre-based programme of 30–40 minutes of aerobic exercise, two or three times a week, may need modification because of common comorbidities such as osteoarthritis, stroke, and chronic obstructive pulmonary disease and the increased fatigability in old age. Extended warm-up and cool-down periods are likely to be appropriate. Centre-based programmes usually provide cycle or treadmill exercise and resistance training, while home programmes are usually based on walking, but might incorporate other activities such as swimming or gardening. Supervised exercise helps to boost confidence and graded increase in the intensity of exercise regimens will boost gains in aerobic function and strength.

This phase also incorporates advice about diet, alcohol intake, weight control, stress management, resumption of sexual activity, smoking cessation, and promotion of self-efficacy to boost self-confidence. Further explanations about the purpose and possible side-effects of medication taken for secondary prevention are also appropriate, and drug regimens can be fine-tuned to meet the needs of each patient. This may mean simplifying the regimen to promote compliance and minimize side-effects.

A mixture of individual counselling and group discussions can be used to deliver the educational content and psychosocial support. Health beliefs and cardiac misconceptions need to be identified and addressed. Depression is common in people referred for CR (and associated with higher mortality) and needs to be identified and managed actively. Frailer participants and those with cognitive impairment will need special consideration to ensure they gain benefit and one-to-one sessions may best suit their needs. The involvement of close relatives and carers should be encouraged to increase engagement and improve compliance. Written material should be available to reinforce and amplify the information provided.

Phase 4
A long-term maintenance programme of 'heart-healthy behaviour' should follow. This aims to continue lifestyle changes and to maintain physical fitness (e.g. through membership of local support groups and free access to leisure centres and swimming pools).

Improving uptake
The high prevalence of cardiovascular disease in old age means that the majority of those eligible for CR will be aged over 65 years (and 25% aged >75). Yet older people are less likely to be referred and even when they are they are less likely to attend. Non-referral and non-participation are associated with:

- Patient factors: older age, female gender, less formal education, ethnic minorities, greater functional impairment, more severe cardiac disease, comorbidities (e.g. limited mobility, dementia), conflicting demands on time, denial of severity of illness, not believing it is appropriate for them, psychological distress, overprotective attitudes of relatives and carers.
- Physician factors: ageism, low expectation, and lack of enthusiasm, concerns about risk of exercise.
- Organizational factors:– insufficient places on programme, delayed invitation, inconvenient timing, distance to centre, poor public transport, difficult car parking, financial constraints.

Recognition of these factors allows under-represented groups to be targeted (often those who have most to gain), attitudes to be challenged and organization to be improved. Older cardiac patients have suggested that CR programmes could be improved by including more socialization opportunities, offering varied forms of exercise, enhanced teaching about stress management and adapting teaching strategies to meet their needs. Older men feared physical pain with exercise, whereas older women wanted more emotional support.

Assigning a lead clinician to coordinate activities is of key importance in improving uptake. Ideally the option of hospital or home-based CR should be available, to give patients a choice in line with their preferences. Effective wording of invitation letters is important and regular contact by phone should be encouraged and increases participation. The strongest determinant of entry and compliance with CR programmes is physician recommendation.

Further reading
Clark M, Kelly T, Deighan C (2011). A systematic review of the Heart Manual literature. *Eur J Cardiovasc Nurs* **10**: 3–13.

Dolansky MA, Moore SM, Visovsky C (2006). Older adults' views of cardiac rehabilitation programs: Is it time to reinvent? *J Gerontol Nurs* **32**: 37–44.

Ferrara N, Corbi G, Bosimini E, *et al*. (2006). Cardiac rehabilitation in the elderly: patient selection and outcomes. *Am J Geriatr Cardiol* **15**: 22–7.

Oerkild B, Frederiksen M, Hansen JF, *et al*. (2011). Home-based cardiac rehabilitation is as effective as centre-based cardiac rehabilitation among elderly with coronary heart disease: results from a randomised clinical trial. *Age Ageing* **40**: 78–85.

Royal College of Physicians (2002). *Cardiac rehabilitation. A national clinical guideline. Scottish Intercollegiate Guidelines Network*. Edinburgh: Royal College of Physicians.

Sinclair AJ, Conroy SP, Davies M, *et al*. (2005). Post-discharge home-based support for older cardiac patients: a randomised controlled trial. *Age Ageing* **34**: 338–43.

Suaya JA, Stason WB, Ades PA, *et al*. (2009). Cardiac rehabilitation and survival in older coronary patients. *J Am Coll Cardiol* **54**: 25–33.

Wenger NK (2008). Current status of cardiac rehabilitation. *J Am Coll Cardiol* **51**: 1619–31.

Respiratory

Respiratory physiology in old age

Respiratory physiology cannot be divorced from cardiovascular physiology or from general physiology, either in the young or the ageing individual. This section therefore will 'concentrate' on respiratory physiology but with reference to cardiac and general physiological changes associated with age where needed. Most information on differences between respiratory physiology in young people and respiratory physiology in older people comes from cross-sectional data (i.e. there is almost an absence of longitudinal studies). It is difficult therefore, even in the absence of overt disease, to clearly differentiate between physiological changes of ageing and changes as a result of decades of exposure to environmental insults and challenges to which much of the respiratory system is exposed with every one of approximately 6.5 million breaths per year (or in other ways). Chief among these insults and challenges are the effects of cigarette smoking including passive smoking. Others comprise environmental pollution, nutritional status, previous respiratory infection (probably most importantly childhood infection), and reactive oxidants (the latter possibly also mediated via cigarette smoking).

Structural changes in the older lung
Within the large airways the number of glandular epithelial cells reduces with age. This results in reduced production of protective mucus and hence impaired defence against respiratory infections. The alveoli and alveolar ducts enlarge and the surface area of the alveoli falls by up to 20%. This produces a reduction in respiratory reserve, but this is of little significance in the healthy elderly person. Functional residual capacity, residual volume, and compliance all increase. Perhaps the most important structural change is a quantitative reduction and qualitative impairment of function of the elastin and collagen support of the small airways – 'senile emphysema'. This leads to an enhanced tendency for small airway collapse towards the end of expiration, and hence lack of sensitivity and specificity of isolated bilateral basal crepitations (crackles) as a physical sign in older people.

The respiratory muscles are not immune from general aged-related muscular changes (sarcopenia)—largely comprising a reduction in the percentage of type IIa fibres with consequent reduction in muscle endurance (and perhaps less importantly muscle strength, although impaired muscle strength itself has been suggested as an independent mortality predictor). Finally, increased anteroposterior chest diameter, calcification of rib articulatory surfaces and of costal cartilages, together with the muscle changes above produce impaired thoracic cage mobility.

Functional changes in the older lung
Both longitudinal and cross-sectional data indicate that static expiratory flow volumes fall gradually with age. The FEV_1/FVC ratio of 70% in younger people falls approximately 0.2% per year after the age of 40 years, although the falls are slightly less rapid in men. Apparently paradoxically, FEV_1 declines slightly faster in men.

Cross-sectional studies indicate a difference in arterial oxygen pressure in older people (about 15% lower in older healthy volunteers than in young adults). Although it is unlikely that the small falls in static expiratory flow volumes are relevant to this decline, there is an increase in dead space to tidal volume ratio, and an increase in ventilation/perfusion mismatch, which may both be implicated. The decline in respiratory muscle strength and endurance and reduced compliance of the chest wall already discussed may also be relevant. However, probably the most significant contributors to the fall in arterial oxygen pressure with age are (a) increased closing volume—small airways collapsing sooner during expiration; and (b) changes in the control of breathing. The structural changes leading to increased closing volume are discussed above. Perhaps the most clinically important aspect of this is that with acute illness and consequent reduction in mobility, reduction in deep breaths and hypoventilation of the dependent lobes of the lung may result in failure to clear dependent sputum and thus increased risk of concurrent respiratory infection. This is exacerbated by the observed reduction in mucociliary clearance in old age as well as a possible reduction in the sensitivity of the cough reflex (though the latter has been little studied).

It is well recognized that older people have less ability to perceive acute bronchoconstriction. Indeed, perception of bronchoconstriction appears to fall gradually throughout adult life. This may have clinical consequences in terms of late awareness of respiratory symptoms, late self-referral, and mortality associated with acute bronchoconstriction. The mechanisms leading to this reduced perception are complex but include reduced proprioception of joint movement; reduced tactile sensation; reduction in perception of lung elastic loads; and alterations of central (brain) processing.

Older people are probably not less sensitive (in terms of respiratory response) to hypoxia under most conditions, although there is evidence of reduced respiratory response to hypoxia during sustained hypercapnia.

In common with many other areas of physiology, some of the age-associated changes previously described as consequent upon 'normal' ageing are now thought to reflect, at least in part, deconditioning. The most obvious example is that much of the fall in maximal oxygen uptake (VO_2max) seen in ageing (itself consequent upon a fall in maximal heart rate, cardiac output, and diffusing capacity, plus higher ventilation–perfusion mismatch) can be prevented by regular aerobic exercise. This is important as the decline in VO_2max is associated with a decline in 'reserve', which may not be important on a day-to-day basis (at least until extreme old age) but can become vital during periods of illness as well as being important in post-acute illness rehabilitation.

Although not strictly within the realm of respiratory physiology, the consequences of mouth colonization and aspiration in older people merit consideration here. Frail, functionally dependent elderly people often with multiple comorbidity in community settings, long-term care, and hospital settings have a high prevalence of mouth colonization by Gram-negative (and other potentially pathogenic) bacteria. In addition, the prevalence of spontaneous aspiration may be as high as 33% in community-dwelling older people, up to 50% in residents in long-term care facilities, and in over 50% of older patients presenting with pneumonia. Not surprisingly, therefore, mouth colonization is associated with increased rates of lower respiratory tract infection as well as with medium-term higher mortality in older people.

Further reading

Bellmont M, Portero M, Pampolna R, et al. (1995). Evidence for the Maillaird reaction in rat long collagen and relationship with solubility and age. *Biochim Biophys Acta* **1272**: 53–60.

Bortz WM (1982). Disuse and aging. *JAMA* **248**: 1203–8.

Brook MH, Kaiser KK (1970). Muscle fiber-types how many and what kind? *Arch Neurol* **23**: 369–79.

Cabre M, Serra-Prat M, Palomera E, et al. (2010). Prevalence and prognostic implications of dysphagia in elderly patients with Pneumonia. *Age Ageing* **39**: 39–45.

Cardus JFB, Orlando D, et al. (1997). Increase in pulmonary ventilation–perfusion inequality with age in healthy individuals. *Am J Resp Crit Care Med* **156**: 648–53.

Chilbeck PD, Paterson DH, Tetrella RJ, et al. (1996). The influence of age and cardiorespiratory fitness on kinetics of oxygen uptake. *Can J Appl Physiol* **21**: 185–96.

Connolly MJ (2010). Of proverbs and prevention: Aspiration and its consequences in older patients. *Age Ageing* **39**: 2–4.

Connolly MJ, Charan NB, Neilson CP, et al. (1992). Reduce subjective awareness of bronchoconstriction provoked by methacholine in elderly asthmatic and normal subjects of measured on a simple awareness scale. *Thorax* **47**: 410–13.

Connolly MJ, Crowley JJ, Vestal RE (1992). Clinical significance of crepitations in elderly patients following acute hospital admission: a prospective study. *Age Ageing* **21**: 43–8.

Enright PL, Kraonma RA, Higgins M, et al. (1993). Spirometry reference values for men and women aged 65 to 85 years of age: cardiovascular health study. *Am Rev Respir Dis* **147**: 125–33.

Ewan V, Perry JD, Mawson T, et al. (2010). Detecting potential pathogens in the mouths of older people in hospital. *Age Ageing* **39**: 122–5.

Goodman RM, Yergin BM, Landa JF, et al. (1978). Relationship of smoking history and pulmonary function tests tracheal mucous velocity in non-smokers, young smokers, ex-smokers and patients with chronic bronchitis. *Am Rev Respir Dis* **117**: 205–14.

Janssens JP, Pache JC, Nicod LP (1999). Physiological changes in respiratory functions associated with aging. *Eur Respir J* **13**: 197–205.

Joki S, Saano V (1997). Influence of ageing on ciliary beat frequency and on ciliary response to leukotriene D4 in guinea-pig tracheal epithelium. *Clin Exp Pharmocol Physiol* **24**: 166–9.

Law MR, Hackshaw AK (1996). Environmental tobacco smoke. *Br Med Bull* **52**: 22–34.

Milne JS (1978). Longitudinal respiratory studies in older people. *Thorax* **33**: 547–54.

Milne JS, Williamson J (1972). Respiratory function tests in older people. *Clin Sci* **42**: 371–81.

Newnham DM, Hamilton S (1997). Sensitivity of the cough reflex in young and elderly subjects. *Age Ageing* **26**: 185–8.

Poulin MJ, Cunningham BA, Baterson DH, et al. (1993). Ventilatory sensitivity to CO_2 in hyperoxia and hypoxia in older aged humans. *J Apl Physiol* **75**: 2209–16.

Rahman I, MacNee W (1996). Role of oxidants/anti-oxidants in smoking–induced lung diseases. *Free Radic Biol Med* **21**: 669–81.

Richards JA, Theron AJ, Van der Merwe CA et al. (1989). Spirometric abnormalities in young smokers correlate with increased chemiluminscence responses of activated blood phagocytes. *Am Rev Respir Dis* **139**: 181–7.

Schroll M, Avlund K, Davidsen M (1997). Predictors of the five-year functional ability in a longitudinal survey of men and women aged 75–80. The 1914-population of Glostrup, Denmark. *Aging (Milano)* **9**: 143–52.

Tager IB, Segal MR, Speizer FE, et al. (1988). The natural short history of forced expiratory volumes: effect of cigarette smoking and respiratory symptoms. *Am Rev Respir Dis* **138**: 837–49.

Teale C, Romaniuc C, Mulley G (1989). Calcification on chest radiographs: the association with age. *Age Ageing*, **18**: 333–6.

Turley R, Cohen S (2009). Impact of voice and swallowing problems in the elderly. *Otolaryngol Head Neck Surg* **140**: 33–6.

Verbeken EK, Cauberghs M, Mertens I, et al. (1992). The senile lung; comparison with normal and emphysematous lungs. No 1: Structural aspects. *Chest* **101**: 793–9.

Young RC, Borden DL, Rachel RE (1987). Aging of the lung: pulmonary disease in the elderly. *Age* **10**: 138–45.

Respiratory investigations

Chest radiograph
- Chest radiograph remains routine in evaluating respiratory symptoms as well as a role in screening, e.g. preoperatively.

Computerized tomography (CT)
- Wide use in diagnosis and staging of respiratory diseases
- Concern about high ionizing radiation exposure as it accounts for two-thirds of the radiation dose for diagnostic radiology.

CT pulmonary angiography (CTPA)
- Primary imaging modality for pulmonary emboli (PE) diagnosis
- Multiple thoracic imaging slices are taken
- Radiation exposure is much higher than ventilation–perfusion scintagraphy (V/Q)
- Central PEs better detected
- CTPA confirm PE in about 10% of scans
  - underuse of Well's score and overestimation of PE probability pre-scan important
  - Well's score 'low probability' (<4) with normal D-dimer can rule out PE and need for CTPA
- CTPA in PE diagnosis has a
  - sensitivity of 83% and specificity of 96%
  - positive predictive value is 96% when clinical suspicion is high or low.

High-resolution CT (HRCT)
- HRCT details lung parenchyma anatomy and is the imaging modality for interstitial lung disease, bronchiectasis and pneumocystis pneumonia.
- In intensive treatment unit patients with atypical respiratory presentations, HRCT can help diagnose vasculitis, fungal disease, or other unusual pathologies.
- Typical findings of idiopathic pulmonary fibrosis are peripheral reticular opacities, honeycombing, and lung base volume loss.

Lung cancer screening
Low-dose CT (LDCT)
Lung cancer screening using CT imaging may detect early cancers that the chest radiograph will miss. Screening is frequent in high-risk individuals so a CT low-dose radiation protocol is used. At present, it is unclear whether LDCT affects mortality as research indicates a higher pick up rate of more advanced less treatable disease in screening versus control groups.

Risk prediction models based on epidemiological and genetic biomarkers are being researched currently in their ability to predict 5-year mortality from lung cancer. Genetic markers comprise poor DNA repair capacity or heightened sensitivity to mutagens, e.g. bleomycin.

Lung perfusion scanning (V/Q scans)
If patients have a normal chest radiograph and no known cardiopulmonary disease, V/Q scanning has high sensitivity for PE diagnosis. When clinical factors are taken into account including the Well's score and found to mirror the V/Q results as high or low probability of PE, the diagnosis is likely to be correct. 'Indeterminate' V/Q reports results in patients having more radiological tests than if a CTPA was requested first line.

Pulmonary function tests (PFTs)
Following clinical assessment, PFTs identify airflow limitation (AL), restrictive defects, or whether gas uptake is abnormal (Table 6.1).
- Require patient cooperation and effort
- Older people can provide diagnostically useful spirometry with the exception being significant cognitive impairment
- Test quality is paramount assessing the spirogram forms one part
- A common error is inability to sustain forced expiration (extrapolation or slow vital capacity is required)
- Reference ranges must reflect the patient population.
- Sensitive but relatively non-specific marker of transfer capacity of the lung which is influenced by the surface area/potential for gaseous exchange.
- Reduced, e.g. emphysema, interstitial lung disease, pulmonary vascular disease, pulmonary embolism, and increased, e.g. pulmonary haemorrhage.
- Anaemia reduces Tlco and correction must be made for this.

Arterial gases
Pulse oximetry indirectly assesses arterial oxygen saturation. Oximetry is affected by low blood pressure, pulse rate and abnormal haemoglobin. Arterial blood gas analysis assesses gas exchange, acid–base, and ventilation. Where arterial sampling is unsafe or an option to prevent repeated arterial sampling is sought, venous sampling can be used to estimate pH, pCO_2, pO_2 and bicarbonate providing conversion for venous–arterial differences is undertaken.

Flexible bronchoscopy
Main indications are
- haemopytsis
- radiological lung masses
- mediastinal or hilar lymphadenopathy
- undiagnosed pulmonary infiltrates.

Samples are taken using end bronchial wash or brush, and endobronchial ultrasound. Endobronchial ultrasound is a minimally invasive technique allowing visualization of central airways, identification of airway invasion and safer biopsies of peripheral lesions, mediastinal, and

Table 6.1 Characteristic physiological changes in airflow limitation or restrictive disorders

	Airflow limitation	Restrictive
FEV$_1$, % of predicted FEV$_1$	↓	→/↑
FEV$_1$/FVC (Normal 0.7)	↓	↓/→/↑
FVC	↓/→	↓
Total lung capacity	→/↑	↓
Residual volume	→/↑	↓
Carbon monoxide transfer factor (Tlco)	→/↓	→/↓

hilar nodes. People aged 70 years and above are the most common age group undergoing bronchoscopy and include patients on mechanical ventilation. Older people are more likely to suffer complications like hypoxaemia (saturations below 90%), bleeding, pneumothorax, arrhythmias, and hypotension. Comparing those 80 years and over with a largely middle-aged population, the rate of complications was 10% versus 3% and mortality of 1.2% versus 0.0035%.

Cytological examination of pleural aspirate and pleural biopsy

In suspected malignant pleural effusions
• pleural fluid examination yields diagnosis in about 60%
• pleural biopsy increases diagnostic yield
• CT-guided approaches further increase diagnostic yield.

Thoracoscopy/mediastinoscopy

This involves an incision in an intercostal space or the neck; a camera probe is then inserted to view the pleura or mediastinal tissue and biopsies taken. The main diagnostic indications are
• pleural thickening
• undiagnosed pleural effusions
• mediastinal lymph nodes.

Mediastinoscopy is less commonly performed now with the advent of endobronchial ultrasound guided biopsies.

Further reading

O'Neill J, Murchison JT, Wright L, et al. (2005). Effect of the introduction of helical CT on radiation dose in the investigation of pulmonary embolism. Br J Radiol 78: 46–50.

Rokach A, Fridlender ZG, Arish N, et al. (2008). Bronchoscopy in octogenarians. Age Ageing 37: 710–3.

Stein PD, Fowler SE, Goodman LR, et al. (2006). Multidetector computed tomography for acute pulmonary embolism. N Engl J Med 354: 2317–27.

Toftegaard M, Rees, SE, Andreassen S (2009). Evaluation of a method for converting venous values of acid-base and oxygenation status to arterial values. Emerg Med J 26: 268–72.

Asthma

The prevalence of asthma in old age in the UK is uncertain. Symptomatic asthma requiring treatment has been found to affect between 3% and 7% of the population over the age of 65 years depending on disease definition, survey methodology, and the exact age group studied. Asthma is therefore an important cause of morbidity in older people. Though fatal attacks are relatively uncommon, the recorded mortality rate for asthma in old age has not declined as it has for children and younger adults over the last two decades, probably due to difficulties with diagnosis, consequent undertreatment, late and atypical presentations during exacerbations, and the effects of comorbidities.

Diagnosis

There are no universally agreed diagnostic criteria for asthma at any age so the approach is the same in old age as in younger adults and is well described in national guidelines. In essence, this includes finding a history of intermittent wheezy dyspnoea and the demonstration by physical examination and/or lung function testing, usually spirometry, of reversible airflow obstruction occurring either spontaneously or as a result of treatment.

In patients with clinical features suggestive of asthma, the diagnosis is supported if

• a peak expiratory flow rate diary shows variation more than 20%
• the FEV_1 increases by >15% and at least 150 mL in response to bronchodilator drugs, (with the addition of a trial of 30 mg of prednisolone daily for 10 days if necessary).

For the majority of relatively fit older patients, particularly those in the 65–75 age group with good cognitive function, the standard diagnostic approach works well. However, there are a number of particular problems in frail patients that can lead to a delayed or missed diagnosis of asthma, including:

• some older, usually frail, patients with asthma are more likely to present with the functional consequences of hypoxia during exacerbations. The clinical picture can be dominated by delirium, incontinence, falls or inability to perform activities of daily living
• breathlessness might not be mentioned spontaneously, particularly when there is delirium, dementia, or distraction by other symptoms. Further, older people are often less able to detect a rise in airflow resistance and are therefore less likely to report breathlessness from that source
• the physical signs of asthma (tachypnoea, tachycardia, rhonchi, prolonged expiration, hyperinflation, etc.) are often altered or obscured by comorbidities, such as heart failure, and are more difficult to interpret
• many frail older patients, particularly those with cognitive impairment (Mini-mental State Examination (MMSE) <24/30), dyspraxia or frontal executive dysfunction are unable to perform spirometry or even peak expiratory flow measurements, so objective evidence of changes in airflow obstruction are often lacking.
• there remains a tendency to assume that cough, wheeze and breathlessness in old age must be due to chronic obstructive pulmonary disease (COPD), more so when asthma is chronic and without a clear intermittent history. Indeed, there is an overlap between the two

conditions. Nevertheless, careful information gathering can help to clarify the diagnosis (see Table 6.2)

Treatment

Acute attacks of asthma

An acute attack requires urgent management. Bedside indicators of severity used in younger patients (inability to speak in sentences, clouded consciousness, heart rate above 110 bpm, quiet breath sounds, respiratory rate above 25 per minute, systolic blood pressure below 100 mmHg, central cyanosis, oxygen saturation below 93% on air, signs of exhaustion) remain useful in old age, although older patients with none or few of these features often deteriorate rapidly. Therefore, prompt treatment must be given, as indicated below.

The national asthma treatment guideline should be the basis for management, adjusted to take account of the particular problems in frail older patients.

All patients

• High flow oxygen to maintain oxygen saturation above 94%.
• Nebulized combined beta-agonist and antimuscarinic bronchodilators, such as salbutamol and ipratropium (there is evidence of a proportionally better response to antimuscarinic agents in old age, probably due to an age-related decline in beta-receptor activity). The nebulizer should be driven by oxygen.

Table 6.2 Some clinical features that can help to distinguish asthma from chronic obstructive pulmonary disease (COPD) in older patients

	Asthma	COPD
Smoker	Sometimes	Almost always
Breathlessness	Usually intermittent (can be persistent in chronic untreated asthma)	Usually persistent
Cough and sputum	Intermittent dry cough common, small volume sputum	Common, more persistent cough, often high volume sputum
Nocturnal symptoms	Common	Less common
Age of onset	Often early in life, but can occur for the first time in old age	Always later in life and rarely before the age of 50
Winter exacerbations	Sometimes	Often
Chest radiograph	Often normal (sometimes hyperinflated during exacerbations)	Often abnormal (persisting hyperinflation, bullae, reduced bronchovascular markings)
Spirometry	Variable airflow obstruction. Often normal during remissions	Little or no variability. Usually abnormal except in mild cases

- Systemic high-dose corticosteroid (prednisolone 40–50 mg daily orally, with initial intravenous infusion of 200 mg hydrocortisone 4 hourly if necessary, particularly if the patient is unable to swallow).
- Chest radiograph, mainly to exclude pneumothorax, concomitant pneumonia, and heart failure (many older patients with severe asthma develop heart failure as a complication).
- Arterial blood gases (essential if the oxygen saturation is below 93%) are recommended in all older people with acute asthma as they are more likely to become fatigued, underventilate, retain carbon dioxide and become acidotic.
- Frequent monitoring of vital signs and the overall clinical state to decide whether an escalated level of treatment is required.
- Antibiotics should only be given if there is evidence of a significant bacterial infection.

Some patients

- If the response to the above regimen is slow some patients will respond to the addition of intravenous aminophylline or salbutamol by slow infusion, with the usual precautions.
- In severe cases not responding to standard measures, an intravenous infusion of magnesium sulphate is sometimes beneficial.
- Patients not responding to maximal pharmacological treatment should be considered for ventilatory support, which should normally be conducted in a high-dependency setting, such as an acute lung unit or intensive therapy unit. The indications for ventilatory support include persisting or worsening hypoxia, hypercapnoea, acidosis, exhaustion with reduced respiratory effort, falling peak expiratory flow rate, drowsiness, delirium, respiratory arrest. In that context, some important factors in old age are:
- Age is not in itself a bar to mechanical ventilatory support for severe asthma; a decision to proceed must be based on potential for benefit.
- Any older patients being considered for ventilatory support should be referred to the appropriate team for urgent review earlier and at a lower threshold than young patients.
- If severe comorbidities, such as advanced dementia or malignancy, are present it might not be appropriate to escalate treatment, though such a decision should be made by a senior doctor and needs to be explained carefully to the patient's family.

Maintenance treatment

In general, the long-term management of asthma in old age should be conducted in accordance with national asthma guidelines. Most cognitively intact older patients can obtain satisfactory control by using inhaled corticosteroids with intermittent or regular inhaled bronchodilators. There is evidence that compliance with treatment is very good in that group. Proper inhaler instruction should always be given and technique should be checked and reinforced at follow-up. However, with increasing age and frailty a number of problems arise that create barriers to treatment.

- Patients with significant cognitive impairment are usually unable to learn to use an inhaler device of any pattern. Most people with an MMSE <24/30, or (AMT <7/10, or an abnormal score on tests of global dyspraxia or frontal executive function (such as EXIT25) are unable to learn inhaler technique. Some patients who learned to use an inhaler while their cognition was intact retain the ability in early dementia.
- Impaired vision and loss of manual dexterity also hinder inhaler use for some individuals.
- The inhaler technique of older asthma patients should always be checked during consultation. Many have a poor, or inadequate, technique. These are often patients with mild cognitive problems. Careful instruction can retrieve some of those with reasonably good cognition, though most will continue to have an unsatisfactory technique.
- Patients unable to use an inhaler need assisted dosing by a carer, after appropriate instruction. Metered dose inhalers with spacers, and dry powder inhalers, are suitable for this approach.
- A few patients, usually those with more advanced dementia, are unable to take part in assisted dosing with an inhaler, in which case inhaled medications can be given as nebulized solutions by a carer.
- A small minority of very frail patients, usually with advanced dementia and challenging behaviour, are unable to be given any form of inhaled treatment yet they have asthma of sufficient severity to worsen their clinical state. Such patients can justifiably be given systemic corticosteroids orally, and some appear to benefit from oral bronchodilator drugs, such as salbutamol and aminophylline.

Other aspects of long-term asthma care

The evidence for the use of a range of intervention in asthma is relatively weak in old age, mainly through lack of inclusion of frail older people in trials. A few points can be made with reasonable confidence.

- Clear-cut allergic asthma is rarely seen in old age and there is little evidence of benefit from desensitization or dietary exclusion treatments.
- Some of the oldest old appear less likely to benefit from inhaled cromoglycate or oral leukotriene receptor antagonists, although evidence is sparse. A trial of such treatment can be justified for aged patients with poor control despite standard inhaled therapy.
- Patients who smoke should be encouraged and helped to stop, even in old age.

> **Author's Tip**
>
> Always consider the possibility of asthma in an older person with wheeze and hypoxia, particularly if there is a history of little or no smoking and no other explanation for the findings. A trial of treatment for asthma, including corticosteroids, is usually justified.

Further reading

Allen SC (2009). Practical aspects of inhaler therapy in frail elderly patients. *Eur Resp Mon* **43**: 256–66.

Allen SC, Baxter M (2009). A comparison of four tests of cognition as predictors of inability to perform spirometry in old age. *Age Ageing* **38**: 537–41.

Allen SC, Jain M, Malik N, et al. (2003). Acquisition and short-term retention of inhaler techniques require intact executive function in elderly subjects. *Age Ageing* **32**: 299–302.

British guideline on the management of asthma. (www.britthoracic.org.uk/Portals/0/Clinical%20Information/Asthma/Guidelines/sign101%20revised%20June%2009.pdf).

Dow L, Fowler L, Phelps L, et al. (2001). Prevalence of untreated asthma in a population sample of 6000 older adults in Bristol, UK. *Thorax* **56**: 472–6.

Chronic obstructive pulmonary disease

The prevalence of chronic obstructive pulmonary disease (COPD) in older patients in the UK is not agreed, and depends on the population sampled and the definition used. In some regions it is as high as 10% of men and 7% of women above the age of 75. It is a common condition that results in a considerable burden of morbidity, an excess mortality, and is almost always due to cigarette smoking. The number of people with COPD over the age of 75 years appears to be rising, probably due to the combined effect of better recognition of mild–moderate cases and longer survival resulting from improved management of acute exacerbations, immunization against influenza and pneumococcal infection, better long-term management, control of comorbidities, and smoking cessation.

Diagnosis

There is no single diagnostic test. Patients will usually be smokers or ex-smokers presenting with one or more of breathlessness, wheezing, reduced exercise tolerance, a persistent cough that is often productive of sputum, and a tendency to episodes of winter bronchitis. The symptoms tend to be progressive, with relatively little day-to-day variability.

Physical examination can reveal signs of hyperinflation, expiratory rhonchi, a prolonged expiratory phase, asymmetrical breath sounds, pursed lip expiration, coarse basal lung crackles, central cyanosis, signs of carbon dioxide retention, use of accessory muscles of respiration, and signs of right heart failure. However, in most patients the majority of these signs are absent, and in early cases there may be no abnormal signs.

Differentiating COPD from asthma is summarized in Table 6.2.

Spirometry

The diagnosis is supported by spirometry showing an FEV_1 less than 80% of predicted (for that population) and an FEV_1 to FVC ratio of 70% or less. There is usually much less day-to-day variation in spirometric indices than in patients with asthma.

There are often problems with the performance and interpretation of spirometry in old age.

- Because of the age-related lung compliance changes in old age a significant proportion of healthy non-smokers have an FEV_1 to FVC ratio below 70%. This can lead to overdiagnosis of COPD if the full clinical context is not taken into account.
- However, in more severe cases spirometry provides useful predictive information; older patients with an FEV_1 to FVC ratio below 70 % and an FEV_1 below the 10th percentile for the appropriate population have significantly higher rates of morbidity and those below the 5th percentile have considerably higher mortality.
- Robust normal ranges for spirometry in old age have been established in very few populations, so interpretation must be guarded, particularly when results are close to the purported boundary for normality.
- Most older people with good cognitive function can perform adequate spirometry
- Older patients with evidence of cognitive and/or executive dysfunction (MMSE <24/30, AMTS <7/10, abnormal 'frontal lobe' tests) are much less likely to be able to perform spirometry, and those with an MMSE <20/30 are almost always unable.

Other investigations

A diagnosis of COPD cannot be made from a chest radiograph, but all patients should have a chest radiograph to exclude other pathologies. Many COPD patients will have hyperinflated lung fields (>7 posterior ribs visible overlying the lung fields), flattening of the diaphragm, a horizontal appearance of the posterior ribs, and a 'stretched' appearance to the mediastinum. Bullae are sometimes seen.

A CT scan of the thorax is sometimes needed, mainly to identify large bullae (which can sometimes be resected to improve respirable lung volumes) or to clarify concomitant diagnoses such a malignancy or pulmonary fibrosis.

Heart failure is commonly seen in older people with COPD, either as a coincidental comorbidity or as a consequence of severe chronic hypoxia leading to pulmonary hypertension. An echocardiogram may be a useful means of characterizing and evaluating heart failure in such patients.

Formal reversibility testing with bronchodilators, and sometimes corticosteroids, can be necessary to distinguish COPD from asthma.

Particular diagnostic problems in old age

In addition to the problems with spirometry, frail older people with COPD are more likely than middle-aged patients to present with poorly defined clinical syndromes, particularly during acute exacerbations. The underlying cause is then less clear and can be missed. In particular:

- Worsening hypoxia, with or without hypercapnia, can lead to delirium, incontinence, falls, and immobility. Some simply come to the attention of doctors or nurses because they have reached a critical level of dependence on others.
- The clinical information can be obscured by the signs and symptoms of comorbidities. This is particularly likely when there is heart failure, other pulmonary disease, concomitant sepsis, dementia and cerebrovascular disease.
- Older patients with advanced COPD are often sarcopenic, probably as a consequence of low-grade chronic inflammation, hypoxia and relative inactivity. The weakness, particularly loss of antigravity strength, then tends to dominate the clinical picture.

Treatment

The UK national guideline for the management of COPD should be used to decide treatment at all stages of the disease. It is generally very suited to managing older patients. However, there are a number of issues and questions that are encountered with higher frequency in old age that require mention here.

Long term management

- Most older COPD patients with mild to moderate obstruction (FEV_1 >50% predicted) do not require inhaled drug therapy unless they have frequent exacerbations and/or significant reversibility. They should stop smoking and remain physically active.
- There is evidence that long-term inhaled corticosteroid treatment increases the risk of pneumonia in older people with COPD. Use of such treatment therefore requires the risks and benefits to be weighed up carefully.
- Smoking cessation is beneficial in old age. It reduces the rate of spirometric decline, improves functional

performance, and reduces the frequency of exacerbations requiring admission to hospital. Supported quitting programmes are effective. However, it has been shown that smokers with cognitive impairment are much less likely to be successful.

- Most older people can master the use of inhalers. However, patients with cognitive impairment (MMSE <24) are often unable to learn to use an inhaler consistently (though some with an established technique can manage despite cognitive decline). Such patients often require assistance to use an inhaler with a spacer, or a dry powder inhaler. Those with severe cognitive impairment are usually unable to use any type of inhaler, even with assistance.

- Inhaler technique should always be rechecked when older COPD patients come in contact with doctors and nurses.

- Long-term domiciliary use of assisted nebulized therapy is required for a few patients who are unable to use an inhaler, but should only be continued if there is clear benefit. Nebulizers must be driven by an air pump, not compressed oxygen, in these circumstances.

- Oral maintenance treatments are sometimes required when symptomatic patients with frequent exacerbations are unable to use inhalers. Long-term oral steroid treatment should be with the lowest effective dose, and the usual bone protection precautions.

- Pulmonary rehabilitation has been shown to be effective in patients above the age of 80 years.

- Age is not in itself a bar to long-term or short burst oxygen therapy, so older patients should be properly assessed for eligibility and suitability.

Acute exacerbations

- As described above the acute deterioration is often less clear in old age, particularly in patients with markers of frailty.

- The management of acute exacerbations in old age does not differ fundamentally from that in younger patients. The national guideline should be used. The key elements are nebulized bronchodilator drugs (salbutamol and iprotropium), high-dose corticosteroids, careful use of oxygen supplementation (the aim being to try to keep oxygen saturation above 93% with little or no hypercapnoea when possible, and ventilatory support as appropriate.

- When there is a risk that high-dose systemic corticosteroids will cause excessive fluid retention or decompensation of congestive heart failure, it is acceptable to give high-dose nebulized budesonide as an alternative.

- Good control of comorbidities must not be overlooked during an exacerbation of COPD, and there is narrative evidence that outcomes are better when older COPD patients with complex comorbidities are managed holistically.

- Antibiotics should be given if bacterial infection is suspected (at least one of: dark yellow or green sputum; neutrophil leucocytosis; new inflammatory shadowing on the CXR). Remember that older patients can have bacterial infection without pyrexial or leucocyte responses.

- Age is not a bar to assisted ventilation. However, older people with severe exacerbations tend to deteriorate more rapidly than younger patients, so close monitoring for worsening hypoxia, hypercapnia, acidosis, and haemodynamic deterioration is essential. For those suitable for ventilatory support, discussion with an appropriate high-dependency service should take place as early as is practical.

- Older patients with severe comorbidities, such as end-stage heart failure, advanced dementia, or a fatal malignancy do not usually benefit from ventilatory support. The same is usually true of those with severe end-stage COPD.

- Patients who are considered unsuitable for ventilatory support should be properly identified and their status made clear in case notes.

- It is a vital part of good practice to provide high-quality end-of-life care for those dying from COPD and/or its complications. Advance care planning and structured instruments such as the Liverpool Care Pathway are helpful in that context. Drugs to relieve terminal breathlessness, such as morphine, should not be withheld on the grounds that they can reduce ventilatory drive.

Further reading

Allen SC (2009). Practical aspects of inhaler therapy in frail elderly patients. *Eur Respir Mon* **43**: 256–66.

Ernst P, Wilchesky M, Suissa S (2009). Are current treatment recommendations suited to elderly patients with asthma or COPD? *Eur Resp Mon* **43**: 267–85.

Jarvis S, Ind PW, Shiner RJ (2007). Inhaled therapy in elderly COPD patients; time for re-evaluation. *Age Ageing* **36**: 213–18.

NICE (2004). *NICE Guideline on Chronic Obstructive Pulmonary Disease.* London, NICE (http://guidance.nice.org.uk/CG12).

Vaz Fragoso CA, Concato J, McAvay PH, et al. (2009). Defining chronic obstructive pulmonary disease in older persons. *Respir Med* **103**: 1468–76.

Pneumonia

Community-acquired pneumonia

Definition

Definite community-acquired pneumonia (CAP) is defined as adults admitted to hospital with symptoms and signs of a lower respiratory tract infection associated with new chest radiographic changes for which there are no other explanations.

Suspected CAP is an acute illness with cough and at least one of new focal chest signs, fever >4 days, dyspnoea/tachypnoea. There is no other obvious cause.

Epidemiology

- Incidence is 5–11 per 1000 adult population.
- Incidence varies with age, rising to 34 per 1000 population for those aged ≥75 years.
- 22–44% patients with CAP are admitted to hospital.
- Incidence for patients requiring admission to hospital varies with age, from 1.29 per 1000 persons aged 18–39 up to 13.21 per 1000 persons aged ≥55 years.
- 1.2–10% patients with CAP in hospital are admitted to intensive care.
- Mortality in adults in hospital with CAP is between 5.4% and 14%.
- Mortality in patients admitted to intensive care is >30%.
- Long-term mortality at 5 years is 35.8–39.1%. Higher with increasing age, male gender and nursing home residence.

Risk factors

- Age: increased incidence, hospital admission, and mortality.
- Diabetes: higher incidence, severity, and mortality.
- Smoking: increased risk of bacterial pneumonia and influenza. Caused by alterations in mucociliary transport, humoral and cellular defences, and epithelial cell function.
- Nursing home residents: increased incidence and mortality.
- Alcohol excess: alters respiratory tract defence mechanisms, impairs cough reflexes, and swallowing.
- Drugs: oral steroids may cause higher rates of pneumonia, especially caused by Legionella. Inhaled corticosteroids may also increase pneumonia rates.

Common pathogens

See Table 6.3.

- Organisms found in approximately 30% of hospitalized patients with CAP.
- Older patients: most pathogens have similar frequencies as in young apart from Mycoplasma and Legionella, which are less common.
- The only UK-based study suggests that nursing home residents have the same spectrum of CAP pathogens as others in the community. However, clinicians should be alert to the possibility of aspiration pneumonia in frail older people, such as those coming from nursing homes.

Clinical Features

- Symptoms: cough, sputum, fever, breathlessness, pleuritic chest pain.
- Signs: tachypnoea, tachycardia, localizing signs on chest examination (bronchial breathing, reduced percussion note, increased vocal resonance, and crepitations).

- Older patients: often present with non-specific symptoms such as confusion. Often have significant comorbidities, and pneumonia may be associated with aspiration.

Author's Tip

CAP causes significant morbidity and mortality in the older population. Presentation may be insidious and non-specific.

General investigations

- Radiology: all patients admitted to hospital with suspected CAP should have a chest radiograph as soon as possible to confirm the diagnosis. Ideally this should be performed in time for antibiotics to be administered within 4 hours of admission.
- Chest radiographic evidence of consolidation is necessary for diagnosis of CAP (see Figure 6.1).

The only English-language guideline for diagnosing pneumonia in care home residents comes from the USA and is based upon consensus by a multispecialty consensus panel. It suggests that a diagnosis of probable pneumonia can be made based on two of the following factors being present: new or worsening cough, new purulent sputum, fever >38°C, or over 2°C above normal, or <36°C, dyspnoea, respiratory rate >25, tachycardia, new or worsening hypoxia, pleuritic chest pain, decline in cognition or functional status, or new crepitations or wheezes heard on auscultation. Unlike other pneumonia guidelines, a chest radiograph is not required for diagnosis. The rationale for this is not made clear but, possibly, is a pragmatic decision based on the limited access to radiography in the care home setting and the possible deleterious effects of moving to an acute care setting to obtain a radiograph.

- Oxygen saturation in all and arterial blood gas analysis in all critically unwell patients or hypoxic patients (SpO$_2$ <94%) in keeping with British Thoracic Society (BTS) guidelines.
- Urea and electrolytes to help severity assessment.
- Full blood count, liver function tests.
- C-reactive protein (CRP) to aid diagnosis.

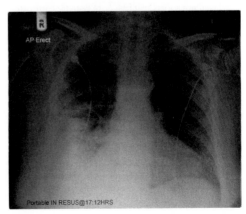

Figure 6.1 Community-acquired pneumonia erect chest radiograph.

Table 6.3 Common pathogens associated with community-acquired pneumonia

Bacteria	Streptococcus pneumoniae	Commonest pathogen involved in CAP (39% hospitalised patients) especially in winter. Associated with herpes simplex peri-oral lesions.
	Haemophilus influenzae	5% hospitalized patients
	Mycoplasma pneumoniae	Occurs in 4-yearly epidemics. Rare in the older person.
	Legionella pneumophila	Consider if recent foreign travel or community outbreak.
	Gram negative bacilli	E.g. *Klebsiella pneumoniae*, *Escherichia coli* and *Pseudomonas aeruginosa*. 1% hospital admissions with CAP. *Klebsiella* more commonly affects men and alcoholics.
	Moraxella catarrhalis	Causes COPD exacerbations but rarely pneumonia.
	Staphylococcus aureus	8% ICU admissions. Associated with influenza infection. More common in winter.
	Chlamydophila pneumoniae	Epidemics may occur in the community. Unclear whether it has direct pathogenic role or is an associated infectious agent.
	Clamydophila psittaci	Acquired from birds and animals. 20% have history of bird contact.
	Coxiella burnetii	Q fever. Epidemics occur in relation to animal sources. Occupational exposure in 8%. Uncommon.
Viruses	Influenza A and B	Epidemics every winter, complicated by pneumonia in 3%. Pandemics occur approximately every 30 years when antigenic shift produces a 'new' virus. Older patients had immunity to the most recent pandemic H1N1 strain in 2009 making it a disease of the young at that time.
	Adenovirus	Airborne/faeco-oral contamination. More common in children

- Procalcitonin (PCT) is a newer biomarker which may be more accurate than CRP in diagnosing bacterial infection and guiding antibiotic therapy.

Differential diagnosis
Important differentials of CAP include:
- Exacerbation of chronic obstructive pulmonary disease (COPD); however chest radiograph is clear.
- Left ventricular failure although CRP not grossly raised.
- Pulmonary embolus although usually no fever or purulent sputum. May need computed tomography pulmonary angiogram to help distinguish. NB D-dimers are often raised in pneumonia.

Microbiological investigations
In low-severity patients, microbiological investigations should be guided by clinical features, e.g. foreign travel, epidemiological factors, and previous antibiotics. In all patients with moderate to severe severity:
- blood cultures, preferably prior to antibiotics
- sputum microscopy, culture, and sensitivity in all patients expectorating.
- urine for pneumococcal antigen
- urine for legionella antigen. *Legionella* culture should be performed on respiratory samples (sputum or broncho-alveolar lavage)
- mycoplasma: ideally polymerase chain reaction (PCR) on respiratory tract secretions or throat swab. Serology widely available although varying sensitivity and specificity
- chlamydophila: PCR and/or antigen detection tests. Complement fixation test is most used serological investigation although varying sensitivity and specificity.
- other: PCR is preferred for detection of respiratory viruses. Paired serological tests can be considered in severely ill patients who fail to improve and no other microbiological cause found
- pleural fluid may be sampled if present.

Severity assessment
Clinical judgement used in conjunction with predictive models. Pneumonia Severity Index (PSI) used in the USA to assess severity, although a major limitation is the complexity of the calculation involved. SMART-COP is another tool used for this purpose developed in Australia. CURB65 is the model recommended by the BTS to score severity in the UK:

Confusion: new mental confusion, AMTS ≤8
Urea: Raised >7 mmol
Respiratory rate: raised ≥30 per min
Blood pressure: low, systolic <90 mmHg, diastolic ≤60 mmHg
65: Age≥65
1 point given for each severity marker.

See Figure 6.2 for guidance on management and treatment.

Author's Tip

CURB65 score together with clinical judgement and assessment of patients wishes/social circumstances should be used to assess severity and guide management in all patients with CAP.

General management
- Oxygen therapy to aim pO_2 94–98%. May vary if coexistent COPD.
- Intravenous fluids if volume depleted.
- Venous thromboembolism prophylaxis.
- Nutritional support.
- Chest physiotherapy if expectorating sputum or has pre-existing lung condition.
- Follow local and national guidelines on CAP.

Antibiotic therapy
Antibiotic therapy is essential and based on severity. Local guidance may differ from that given below. They should be

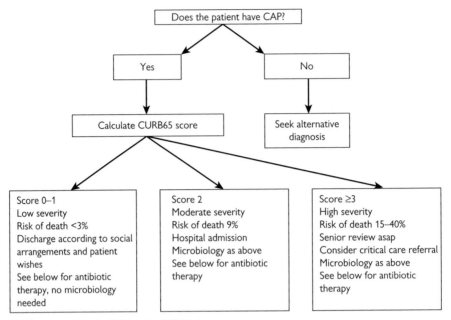

Figure 6.2 Treatment pathway for CAP based on CURB65 score.

administered as soon as diagnosis is made and ideally within 4 hours of admission.

- Low severity (CURB65 0–1):
  - PO amoxicillin 500 mg tds OR
  - PO clarithromycin 500 mg bd OR
  - PO doxycycline 200 mg loading dose followed by 100 mg od.
- Moderate severity (CURB65 2):
  - PO amoxicillin 500 mg to 1 g tds PLUS clarithromycin 500 mg bd. Can be given intravenously if oral route contra-indicated. OR
  - PO doxycycline 200 mg loading dose followed by 100 mg od OR
  - Levofloxacin 500 mg od OR
  - Moxifloxacin 400 mg od
- High severity (CURB65 3–5):
  - Co-amoxiclav 1.2 g iv tds PLUS clarithromycin 500 mg iv tds OR
  - Benzylpenicillin 1.2 g iv qds PLUS levofloxacin 500 mg iv bd or ciprofloxacin 400 mg iv bd OR
  - Cefuroxime 1.5 g iv tds PLUS clarithromycin 500 mg iv bd.

Intravenous antibiotics should be changed to oral when clinical improvement occurs and when temperature normal for 24 hours. Five to 7 days of treatment is sufficient for low–moderate severity. Up to 10 days of antibiotics should be given for high severity or even longer if complications.

Avoid using cephalosporins and fluoroquinolones if possible because of the risk of *Clostridium difficile* diarrhoea, especially in the older person.

Switch to narrow spectrum antibiotics when microbiology results available.

Complications of CAP
- Parapneumonic effusion/empyema: early thoracocentesis indicated. If empyema or pleural fluid pH <7.2, insert chest drain: see BTS guidelines for management of pleural infection.
- Lung abscess: rare complication. May need prolonged e.g. 6-week course of antibiotics.
- Metastatic infection: e.g. septic arthritis, endocarditis, and meningitis.
- Acute respiratory distress syndrome (ARDS): may complicate CAP and usually requires high-flow oxygen, critical care admission, and ventilatory support.
- *Clostridium difficile* diarrhoea.

Follow up
All patients should have follow-up at 6 weeks either with their GP or at a hospital appointment to ensure clinical improvement. A repeat chest radiograph should be performed in patients with underlying risk factors for malignancy, e.g. smoking history or if there are persistent symptoms. Chest radiograph changes may take longer to clear in older people.

Prevention
All patients over 65 years or at risk of invasive pneumococcal disease admitted with CAP should be offered 23-PPV pneumococcal vaccine in convalescence. Patients over 65 and at-risk groups should also be offered the influenza vaccine. Follow Department of Health guidelines for immunization. Smoking cessation advice should be offered to all smokers with CAP.

Hospital-acquired pneumonia
Definition
Pneumonia developing 48 hours after hospital admission. It affects 0.5–1% hospital admissions, increasing length of stay

by 7–9 days. When associated with mechanical ventilation, it is termed ventilator-associated pneumonia (VAP) carrying a mortality of ~50%.

Risk factors
- Age and chronic lung disease/other comorbidities
- Reduced conscious level
- Chest/abdominal surgery
- Mechanical ventilation
- Nasogastric feeding
- Previous antibiotic therapy
- Steroids and immunosuppression

Prevention
- Infection control strategies and hand hygiene.
- Meticulous cleaning and sterilization of respiratory equipment as per guidelines.
- Early postoperative coughing and mobilization.
- Protocols for weaning and reducing sedation in ICU to avoid VAP.
- Non-invasive ventilation (NIV), not intubation, for COPD exacerbations where appropriate.

Causative organisms
- Pseudomonas aeruginosa
- Staphylococcus aureus
- Enterobacteriae, e.g. Enterobacter, E. coli, Klebsiella
- Haemophilus influenzae
- Acinetobacter species
- Meticillin-resistant Staphylococcus aureus (MRSA)
- Streptococcus pneumoniae
- Mixed infections are common especially in VAP

Treatment
- Supportive measures, e.g. oxygen, intravenous fluids, nutrition, and ventilation if appropriate/required.
- Empirical antibiotics based on local guidelines. These depend on susceptibility of local pathogens, length of hospital stay, recent antibiotic therapy and comorbidities.

Aspiration Pneumonia

Definition
Pneumonia following aspiration of gastric or oral contents into the lower respiratory tract. Common in older people and nursing home residents in particular, but difficult to diagnose or exclude with certainty.

Risk factors
- Reduced conscious level, e.g. large stroke, seizures, sedatives, alcohol.
- Impaired swallowing reflex, e.g. motor neurone disease, stroke disease, Parkinson's disease.
- Increased gastrointestinal reflux, e.g. percutaneous endoscopic gastrostomy feeding, recumbent position, nasogastric feeding, vomiting.
- Poor dental hygiene.

Clinical features
- Cough, sputum (may be foul), fever, breathlessness.
- May be chronic and non-specific symptoms in the older person.
- Chest radiographic evidence of consolidation in dependent lobes, usually right lower lobe.
- Usually caused by anaerobic bacteria which are difficult to culture: Bacteroides, Peptostreptococcus, Fusobacterium nucleatum, and Prevotella. Mixed infection common.
- May present with complications, e.g. empyema.

Treatment
- Supportive e.g. oxygen, intravenous fluids.
- Assess swallow.
- Manage underlying cause of aspiration.
- Antibiotics to include anaerobic cover, e.g. co- amoxiclav or metronidazole.

Further reading

Calverley PM, Anderson J, Bartolome C et al. (2007). Salmeterol and fluticasone propionate and survival in chronic obstructive pulmonary disease. N Engl J Med 356: 775–89.

Christ-Crain M, Stolz D, Bingisser R et al. (2006). Procalcitonin Guidance of Antibiotic Therapy in Community Acquired Pneumonia. Am J Respir Crit Care Med 174: 84–93.

Davies CWH, Gleeson FV, Davies RJO (2003). BTS Guidelines for the management of pleural infection. Thorax 58(SII): 8–28.

Hutt E, Kramer AM, Hutt E, et al. (2002). Evidence-based guidelines for management of nursing home-acquired pneumonia. J Family Pract 51: 709–16.

Lim WS, Macfarlane JT (2001). A prospective comparison of nursing home acquired pneumonia with community acquired pneumonia. Eur Respir J 18: 362–8.

Lim WS, Baudouin SV, George RC, et al. (2009). BTS Guideline for the management of community acquired pneumonia in adults. Thorax 64(S): 1–55.

Masterton R, Galloway A, French G et al. (2008). Guidelines for the management of hospital-acquired pneumonia in the UK: Report of the Working Party on Hospital-Acquired Pneumonia of the British Society for Antimicrobial Chemotherapy. J Antimicrob Chemother 62: 5–34.

O'Driscoll BR, Howard LS, Davison AG (2008). BTS Guideline for emergency oxygen use in adult patients. Thorax 63(SIV): 1–73.

Woodhead M, Blasi F, Ewig S, et al. (2011). Guidelines for the management of adult lower respiratory tract infections–full version.; Joint Taskforce of the European Respiratory Society and European Society for Clinical Microbiology and Infectious Diseases. Clin Microbiol Infect Nov; 17 Suppl 6: E1–59.

Tuberculosis

Aetiology

Tuberculosis (TB) is caused by bacteria of the *Mycobacterium tuberculosis* complex, which includes *M. tuberculosis* (most common), *M. bovis*, and *M. africanum*. Mycobacteria are slow-growing aerobic bacilli with high concentrations of lipids in their cell walls. They are referred to as acid and alcohol Fast Bacilli (AAFB) due to their ability to retain carbol fuchsin dye despite attempts to decolorize by acid and alcohol (Ziehl–Neelsen, ZN stain).

TB is spread from person to person by air droplets. Inhaled bacteria reach the lung and grow slowly. The bacilli may spread through the lymphatics or bloodstream, leading to potential sites for extrapulmonary disease. Cell-mediated immunity is activated leading to T cells and macrophages forming granulomas which wall off the mycobacteria. In most people this is asymptomatic and may lead to latent TB (see later). If the immune defences cannot contain the infection, active disease ensues. This may be immediate (mostly young adults and children) or due to reactivation of latent disease many years later in middle aged and older adults.

Epidemiology

- Over 9 million new cases of TB and 2 million deaths are reported globally each year.
- The highest incidence is in sub-Saharan Africa and South East Asia. Rates of disease are increasing in eastern European countries.
- 9000 cases per year in the UK, mostly in London.
- In 2008 in the UK there was an overall 2.2% increase in the rate of disease compared with 2007.
- Most disease was in the non-UK born and age 15–44.
- 639 males and 559 females over 65 were diagnosed with TB in the UK in 2008.
- The incidence rate of smear positive cases in the >65 age group is similar to other age groups.

Risk factors

- Close contacts of infectious (smear positive) cases.
- Travel to or living in areas with high TB prevalence.
- Ethnic minorities from areas with high TB prevalence.
- Immunocompromised/HIV.
- Very young and the older population.
- Chronic poor health and nutrition, e.g. alcoholism.
- Poor or overcrowded housing.
- Silicosis.
- Anti-tumour necrosis factor (TNF) treatment

Clinical features

TB typically presents as pulmonary disease. Symptoms and signs include:

- productive cough
- haemoptysis, especially if cavitating disease
- systemic symptoms, e.g. weight loss, night sweats
- examination may be normal or there may be evidence of cachexia, lymphadenopathy, crepitations, or a pleural effusion.
- TB in the older person may present more indolently with non-specific symptoms and signs.

Investigations

- Chest radiograph (Figure 6.3) classically shows upper lobe infiltrates with cavitation. There may also be

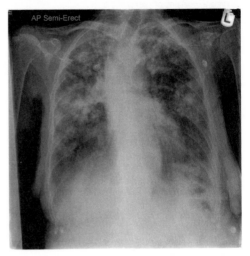

Figure 6.3 Extensive pulmonary TB on chest radiograph.

evidence of lymphadenopathy or fibrotic change and calcification consistent with previous TB infection. The chest radiograph may be atypical in immunocompromised, e.g. HIV patients.

- Sputum ZN stain and culture. Three early-morning samples on consecutive days should be collected. Smear positive cases indicate high infectious risk. Cultures take up to 6 weeks. Samples may also be used for rapid molecular tests for drug resistance.
- Bronchoscopy may be needed to obtain respiratory samples if high clinical suspicion and no sputum available or sputum unhelpful. Endobronchial lesions may be visible.
- Biopsy, e.g. cervical lymph node, mediastinal lymph node, and pleura. Samples should be transported to the laboratory in a dry pot for culture in addition to histology.
- Sample serous fluid, e.g. pleural fluid or ascites for microbiology and cytology; lymphocytosis in an at-risk patient suggests TB.
- Blood tests: Baseline full blood count, urea and electrolytes, and liver function tests should be documented prior to antituberculous treatment. Consider HIV testing. Older patients with TB are more likely to have comorbid illness causing abnormalities in liver and renal function.
- Tuberculin skin test (Mantoux) and new blood gamma-interferon tests unhelpful as fail to separate latent from active disease.

Extrapulmonary TB

Extrapulmonary TB may be more common in the older person and HIV-positive individuals. Imaging helpful, e.g. computed tomography. Common sites include:

- Central nervous system (CNS), the most serious manifestation. Cerebrospinal fluid shows lymphocytes, high protein and low glucose.
- Pericardial.
- Spinal disease or any bone/joint can be affected.
- Abdominal: ileocaecal disease, retroperitoneal lymphadenopathy, and ascites.

- Genitourinary disease indicated by sterile pyuria. Early-morning urine should be sent for TB culture.
- Disseminated disease which is more common in immunosuppressed individuals. Chest radiograph may show a miliary pattern of disease.
- Cryptic disease. Unexplained systemic disease, e.g. failure to thrive, fever, weight loss, sometimes with high erythrocyte sedimentation rate; resolves on trial of antituberculous therapy.

General treatment

Treatment is aimed at curing disease, preventing transmission and preventing resistance.

- All new cases must be notified, even if identified after death.
- Smear-positive patients should become non-infectious after 2 weeks of treatment.
- Material should be sent for culture if at all possible prior to starting treatment.
- Drug treatment is usually in two phases, with an initial phase lasting 2 months and a continuation phase lasting 4 months.
- All patients should have their compliance assessed. If concerns about adherence to treatment, directly observed therapy (DOT) can be considered.
- Inpatients with suspected pulmonary TB should initially be in a side room. Smear-positive cases should be asked to wear a facemask.

Drug treatment

Should be supervised by local TB service with input from TB specialist nurse for compliance monitoring. Four drugs are used for the first 4 months: rifampicin, isoniazid, pyrazinamide, and ethambutol. This is followed by two drugs for 4 months: rifampicin and isoniazid. This regimen is for TB at all sites except CNS disease which requires treatment for 12 months. Drug doses are dependent on weight. Corticosteroids are recommended in CNS disease, pericardial disease, and ureteric disease. Common side-effects of the drugs are listed below. In older patients, drug interactions are especially important.

- Rifampicin: increases clearance of drugs metabolized by the liver, e.g. steroids, sulphonylureas, phenytoin. Maintenance steroids therefore should be doubled. Also causes red discolouration of bodily fluids.
- Isoniazid: major side-effect is deranged liver function. May cause peripheral neuropathy so pyridoxine 10 mg should also be given in patients with diabetes, renal failure, and HIV. Phenytoin clearance reduced in slow acetylators.
- Pyrazinamide: major side-effect is deranged liver function. Hyperuricaemia may also occur.
- Ethambutol: may cause optic neuritis so should be stopped if visual symptoms occur.

Drug resistance

Drug resistance is more common in those previously treated for TB, ethnic minorities, and HIV-positive cases. Isoniazid resistance is seen in 7% patients.

Multidrug-resistant TB (MDR TB) is defined as resistance to rifampicin and isoniazid. Extensively drug-resistant TB (XDR-TB) is MDR TB also resistant to three classes of second-line drugs. Treatment regimes and duration of treatment may need to be altered depending on sensitivities. Specialist advice should be sought for treatment of MDR and XDR-TB.

Screening and contact tracing

- New entrants to the UK are identified for screening at the port of arrival, usually by chest radiograph.
- Contact tracing identifies those with active disease, latent infection and those suitable for BCG vaccination by a combination of Mantoux testing, gamma-interferon blood testing, and chest radiograph according to NICE guidance.
- Mantoux testing involves intradermal injection of tuberculin. It is read at 48 hours and should take into account the patient's BCG history. False-negative results may occur in immunocompromised patients.
- Interferon gamma is released by T cells in response to *M. tuberculosis* antigens. It is more specific than Mantoux testing. Two blood tests: T-SPOT.TB and QuantiFERON-TB are available commercially.

Latent TB

Latent TB occurs when a person has been infected with TB in the past but has not had active disease. The chest radiograph is normal, the patient has no symptoms but the Mantoux and/or gamma interferon is positive. This group may be treated with chemoprophylaxis but in view of side-effects, treatment is usually only given to younger patients (under 35 years) identified by contact tracing.

BCG vaccination

Vaccination is targeted to at-risk groups including infants who live in or whose parents are from a high-incidence area, healthcare workers, new entrants (<35) from high-incidence areas, and TB contacts (<35).

Author's Tip

TB may present indolently in the older population. Treatment may be more difficult due to drug side effects/interactions.

Further reading

The Health Protection Agency (2009). Tuberculosis in the UK: Annual report on tuberculosis surveillance in the UK (www.hpa.org.uk).

Schluger N (2007). Tuberculosis and non-tuberculous mycobacterial infections in older adults. *Clin Chest Med* **28**: 773–vi.

NICE guideline: Clinical diagnosis and management of tuberculosis, and measures for its prevention and control 2006. (www.nice.org.uk)

Pulmonary embolism

Epidemiology

Pulmonary embolism (PE) is a common problem in the older population as the incidence rises with age and risk factors for PE also rise with increasing age.

- Mean age for all patients with PE is 65 years.
- Incidence is 300–500/100 000 aged 70–79 years and 450–600/100 000 aged 80+ years, compared with 60–150/100 000 under 60 years. It is more common in men than women over 75 years.
- PE is commonly found at post-mortem in 13–15% cases and either cause or contributory to death.
- 40% of PE found at post-mortem in older people were not clinically suspected.

Overall mortality from PE is 7–15%, but age over 70 years is an independent risk factor for death from PE.

Aetiology

- Pulmonary emboli form part of the spectrum of venous thromboembolism (VTE) and are due to formation of thrombus often within the deep veins of the lower limbs (DVT). They result from an interaction between genetic factors and external factors.
- Risk factors include patient factors and setting related risk factors (see Table 6.4).

Presentation

- Assessment should include careful history, examination, chest radiograph and ECG. In many patients measurement of D-dimer and arterial blood gas (ABG) will assist decisions about further investigation, treatment and risk stratification.
- In older patients with PE, the most common presentation is with dyspnoea (59–91%), pleuritic chest pain (26–59%), tachypnoea (46–74%), tachycardia (29–76%), haemoptysis, and syncope.
- Syncope is more common in the older population due to hypotension and may also present as an arrhythmia.
- Symptoms may be non-specific in the older person including acute confusion, low grade fever and with symptoms and signs mimicking infection. The diagnosis of PE can be missed in such cases.
- Examination may reveal signs of pleural effusion and right heart strain/failure. Hypotension or shock may be a sign of high mortality risk (massive PE).

Table 6.4 Risk factors for pulmonary embolism

Patient factors	Setting related factors
Age	Immobility/prolonged bed rest
Active malignancy	Fracture hip/leg
Chronic cardiac or respiratory disease	Hip or knee replacement
Stroke	Major general surgery
Obesity	Chemotherapy
Previous venous thromboembolism	
Smoking	

- Arterial PaO_2 >10 kPa is normal in older patients (>12 kPa in younger patients). ABG is normal in 20% PE cases.
- ECG may show sinus tachycardia, atrial fibrillation, and T-wave inversion and rarely signs of right strain.

Clinical probability

An estimation of the pre-test probability is an essential step in helping the clinician decide the likelihood of a PE in a group of patients presenting with similar clinical features. Experienced clinicians may use implicit pre-test probability to assess the likelihood of a patient but this is unreliable for inexperienced doctors and difficult to teach.

Revised Geneva score	
	Points
Age >60 years	1
Previous VTE	3
Surgery/fracture lower limb in last month	2
Active malignancy	2
Unilateral lower limb pain	3
Haemoptysis	2
Heart rate 75–94	3
Heart rate >95	5
Pain on lower limb deep venous palpation and unilateral oedema	4
Clinical probability	Points
• Low	0–3
• Intermediate	4–10
• High	>10

Well's score	
	Points
Signs and symptoms of DVT	3
Alternative diagnosis less likely	3
Heart rate >100	1.5
Immobilisation/surgery in previous 4 weeks	1.5
Previous DVT/PE	1.5
Haemoptysis	1
Malignancy	1
Clinical probability	Points
• Low	≤2
• Intermediate	2–6
• High	>6

Explicit scoring systems have been validated and should be incorporated into management algorithms. The Geneva score uses more objective parameters than the Wells scores.

D-dimer

- Is a degradation product of cross-linked fibrin and may be elevated in plasma if clot is present and should be used in conjunction with pre-test probability.
- A negative D-dimer is useful at ruling out PE in patients with low or intermediate clinical probability but D-dimer levels are higher in older people reducing the specificity in patients over 80 years.

- A positive D-dimer is not specific to VTE and may be elevated in many conditions, e.g. cancer, infection.
- Sensitivity is low in high-probability patients who should undergo a formal diagnostic test such as CT scan or Ventilation/perfusion (V/Q) scan.
- The most sensitive D-dimer tests are the ELISA assays: sensitivity >95%; specificity 40%.
- It is still cost-effective to request D-dimer in older patients. Some studies have used a higher cut-off for D-dimer in older people without losing sensitivity.

Imaging
- Chest radiograph may be normal or show atelectasis, elevated hemidiaphragm, or a pleural effusion.
- Compression ultrasound may identify deep vein thrombosis (DVT) in up to 20% of patients presenting with PE, which may reduce the need for further complex imaging.
- V/Q scanning is influenced by the presence of existing cardiorespiratory disease, prevalent in older people increasing the rate of non-diagnostic intermediate results. Intermediate scans require further imaging, usually CT pulmonary angiography (CTPA).
- Normal/low probability V/Q scan excludes PE in low/moderate-probability patients. High-probability scan is diagnostic of PE if pre-test probability is high.
- Multidetector CTPA scan (see Figure 6.4) is adequate as a stand-alone test, although the PIOPED II study only observed a sensitivity of 83% and specificity of 96%.
- Sensitivity and specificity of CTPA is not affected by increasing age. CT scanning also allows identification of additional pathology and cause of symptoms.
- Patients with renal impairment are at increased risk of contrast-induced nephropathy after CTPA.

Risk Stratification of patients with PE
Current guidelines advocate the stratification into risk of early death usually in-hospital or 30-day mortality based on the presence of markers to identify those at risk of early failing right ventricle (RV) using clinical features, biomarkers of myocardial injury and evidence of RV dysfunction.

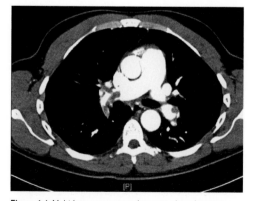

Figure 6.4 Multidetector computed tomography pulmonary angiography showing bilateral pulmonary embolism as filling defects within the pulmonary arteries.

Clinical risk markers include presence of shock or hypotension and their presence alone indicates a higher mortality.
- Biomarkers include troponin (I or T), brain natriuretic peptide (BNP) and N-terminal proBNP (NT proBNP). Elevated markers show good correlation with risk of death and/or complications of PE, especially when combined with echocardiogram evidence of right ventricular (RV) dysfunction (approximately 40% 30-day mortality).
- RV dysfunction is usually detected by echocardiography, which may show paradoxical septal motion, RV dilatation, and tricuspid regurgitation with increased pulmonary artery pressure (PAP) >30 mmHg. CTPA may also show evidence of RV dysfunction and dilated pulmonary outflow.

Risk stratification should help clinicians consider appropriate treatments including thrombolysis for high-mortality risk patients and potentially home treatment in low risk.

Treatment
Anticoagulation
- Low molecular weight heparin (LMWH) should be given as soon as PE is considered based on patients weight and renal function (unfractionated heparin if significant renal impairment).
- Warfarin is usually commenced once diagnosis is confirmed using local prescribing policy. LMWH can be stopped when the international normalized ratio is in target range 2–3 but requires treatment for 5–7 days minimum.
- Patients with malignancy should receive long-term LMWH rather than warfarin, which is associated with lower risk of bleeding and risk of recurrence.
- Anticoagulation should be given for:
  - 3 months if reversible risk factor
  - at least 3–6 months if unprovoked
  - lifelong if recurrent VTE (≥2 episodes).
- In older patients it is especially important to consider the interactions of warfarin with other drugs and to make a careful assessment of bleeding risk.

Thrombolysis
- Patients presenting with high risk of mortality (see Table 6.5) may be considered for thrombolysis.
- All trials show thrombolysis unequivocally improves RV size and dysfunction in 24 hours but does not reduce mortality compared with heparin alone.
- Major bleeding with thrombolysis is high in these patients (9–22%) and increased in patients with cancer, diabetes and abnormal coagulation.

Table 6.5 Risk stratification in pulmonary embolism

PE-related mortality (early and 30-day) risk	Clinical shock and/or hypotension	Right ventricular dysfunction	Biomarkers indicating myocardial injury
High >15%	+	+	+
Intermediate 3–15%	–	+/–	+/–
Low <3%	–	–	–

- First-line treatment is 100 mg of alteplase, 10 mg given as a bolus over 1–2 minutes, and remaining 90 mg over 2 hours followed by iv heparin.

Follow-up

- Patients with PE should undergo follow up at 3–6 months to ensure resolution of symptoms and investigate ongoing symptoms suggestive of underlying cause such as malignancy and to confirm duration of treatment. Routine investigation for malignancy is not cost-effective.
- Repeat echocardiography should be performed if there is RV dysfunction at presentation. Persistent symptoms and evidence of RV dysfunction should prompt consideration of investigation for chronic thrombotic and/or embolic pulmonary hypertension (CTEPH).

Further reading

Torbicki A, Perrier A, Konstantinides S, et al. (2008). Guidelines on diagnosis and management of acute pulmonary embolism. *Eur Heart J* **29**: 2276–315.

Pulmonary rehabilitation

Respiratory diseases, such as chronic obstructive pulmonary disease (COPD), result in progressive breathlessness, activity limitation, and impairment of daily activities. Chronic breathlessness leads to avoidance of activity and the development of disability is associated with superimposed skeletal muscle deconditioning. It is also common for older people with chronic respiratory disease to have other comorbid conditions such as heart failure, arthritis, or obesity which will magnify the impact. Unfortunately, there are no effective disease-modifying treatments for diseases like COPD, so once pharmacological treatment has been optimized, pulmonary rehabilitation becomes an essential component of their management.

Definitions and scope

Various formal definitions of pulmonary rehabilitation exist in the published guidelines. Essentially, pulmonary rehabilitation is a programme of activities for patients and their families aimed at reducing dyspnoea and improving physical performance through a combination of physical training and self-management education. This is usually delivered by a multiprofessional team in the form of a time-limited, hospital-based, outpatient programme. Other models include inpatient or community settings and in some cases even in the patient's own home. In most cases rehabilitation is limited to the formal (reset) model but maintenance classes are also popular with patients. The bulk of experience of pulmonary rehabilitation is with COPD but increasingly there is recognition that rehabilitation can have similar benefits for people with other chronic respiratory diseases, such as chronic stable asthma, bronchiectasis, pulmonary fibrosis, other restrictive disorders, and even lung cancer. The programmes may have to be modified slightly to cope with the diversity.

Content

To be effective, pulmonary rehabilitation must contain individually prescribed physical exercise training. Training sessions should be supervised at least twice weekly and combined with unsupervised home sessions. The training load is increased steadily over the length of the programme. Lower limb training by brisk walking or cycling is the usual method of endurance training with the target intensity of 70–85% of peak performance. This can be supervised in a group setting despite the need for individualized prescription. Resistance exercise training using multigym or free weight training has also been shown to be effective and enhances the benefits of endurance training. In this case, individualized training prescription is also recommended in the form of repetitions at 70% of maximum effort for the respective muscle groups. Other forms of physical training include upper limb exercise and respiratory muscle training but although both of these modalities might be included in a programme, their benefits may be overshadowed by the effects of the more general training.

Many people who attend rehabilitation will have severe breathlessness that restricts their ability to exercise. Consequently, there are several adjunctive strategies that can help get them started or allow them to train beyond their normal ventilatory limit to exercise. Oxygen therapy is the most obvious adjunct to training, as while the practical benefits of providing oxygen to patients who are not hypoxaemic is questionable, there does seem to be a rationale for training on oxygen for those who already use long-term oxygen or who desaturate on exercise. Other devices to increase the training load include helium/oxygen mixtures, non-invasive ventilation, interval training, and one-leg training. These manipulations are only required for patients who are unable to make progress with the traditional training methods.

Apart from the exercise training, the other main component of pulmonary rehabilitation is self-management education. Over the duration of the programme, an education curriculum is delivered by the relevant health professional. The topics may include dyspnoea management, disease education, dietary advice, medicines management, exacerbation avoidance, and relationships and sexuality advice. The rehabilitation setting is also a good opportunity to provide smoking cessation advice and oxygen assessment. These topics are usually presented by the health professional but patient organizations or previous rehabilitation graduates can also make valuable contributions.

Assessment and outcome measures

Pulmonary rehabilitation does not improve lung function. The main benefits to be found in improvements in exercise performance, dyspnoea and quality of life. Wider effects include increased spontaneous physical activity and reduction in healthcare resources. The latter is usually manifest as a reduction in hospital bed days consequent upon better exacerbation management. The routine assessment for pulmonary rehabilitation should involve the baseline assessment of exercise performance and health status in every case. For convenience, most centres used field walking tests such as the 6-minute walk or shuttle walking tests. The latter has the advantage that it can be used for prescription setting. There are a number of health status questionnaires that can be used for rehabilitation assessment. These are usually disease specific questionnaires, such as the St Georges Respiratory Questionnaire (SGRQ) or the Chronic Respiratory Questionnaire (CRQ). Other dyspnoea-specific or activities of daily living questionnaires have also been used successfully. These outcomes have been applied rigorously and have been very important to the development of the field by demonstrating benefit and by providing important tools for programme audit and quality control.

Results

Pulmonary rehabilitation does not improve lung function and probably does not influence survival. However, it has been shown to reliably improve exercise and health status beyond the clinically significant thresholds. It has also been shown to improve spontaneous physical activity and reduce healthcare burden. The benefits of rehabilitation may last for 12–18 months and can be reinforced by repeated courses. The effect size of these benefits is much greater than any pharmacological intervention and hence greatly valued by the patients.

Future directions

Physical capacity to provide rehabilitation for common respiratory conditions is increasing but still inadequate for the potential demand. Inevitably this will mean that local provision in community settings will be required to expand to meet demand. Quality assurance processes will be vital to continued success as this evolves. The economic impact of COPD lies in the repeated admissions to hospital.

Better management of unscheduled care could reduce this burden.

Formal rehabilitation during or immediately following hospital admission can successfully reduce the risk of repeated admissions. Finally, rehabilitation should be part of the integrated care structure for people with COPD. It is one of the cornerstones of the National Strategy for COPD in England and also a component of the Chronic Care Model worldwide.

Further reading

British Thoracic Society (2001). Pulmonary rehabilitation. *Thorax* **56**: 827–34.

Casaburi R, Zuwallack R (2009). Pulmonary rehabilitation for management of chronic obstructive pulmonary disease. *N Engl J Med* **360**: 1329–35.

Department of Health (2010). Consultation on a Strategy for Services for Chronic Obstructive Pulmonary Disease (COPD) in England. Department of Health (http://www.dh.gov.uk/prod_consum_dh/groups/dh_digitalassets/@dh/@en/documents/digitalasset/dh_113279.pdf).

Nici L, Donner C, Wouters E, *et al.* (2006). American Thoracic Society/European Respiratory Society statement on pulmonary rehabilitation. *Am J Respir Crit Care Med* **173**: 1390–413.

Nici L, Raskin J, Rochester CL, *et al.* (2009). Pulmonary rehabilitation: what we know and what we need to know. *J Cardiopulm Rehabil Prev* **29**: 141–51.

O'Reilly J, Jones MM, Parnham J, *et al.* (2010). Management of stable chronic obstructive pulmonary disease in primary and secondary care: summary of updated NICE guidance. *Br Med J* **340**: c3134.

Ries AL, Bauldoff GS, Carlin BW, *et al.* (2007). Pulmonary Rehabilitation: Joint ACCP/AACVPR Evidence-Based Clinical Practice Guidelines. *Chest* **131**(5 Suppl): 4S–42S.

Seymour JM, Moore L, Jolley CJ, *et al.* (2010). Outpatient pulmonary rehabilitation following acute exacerbations of COPD. *Thorax* **65**: 423–8.

Lung cancer

Lung cancer (LC) is the commonest cause of cancer-related death in the Western world. In 2008, 35 000 new cases were diagnosed in the UK. The incidence is falling steadily in men but continues to rise slowly in women, with the male–female ratio now being around 1.4:1. The median age at diagnosis has also been rising slowly over recent years and now stands at 71.5 years with 40% of cases being 75 years of age or more.

Nearly 90% of cases have a non-small cell histology (NSCLC) with the remainder being small cell lung cancer (SCLC). NSCLC is very largely made up of squamous cell, adenocarcinoma, and large cell tumour subtypes.

Presentation and diagnosis

Although the large majority of new cases of lung cancer occur in smokers or ex-smokers, up to 15% arise in people who have never smoked. Patients with COPD are at higher risk over and above that related to their smoking. Thus there should be a low threshold for considering a diagnosis of lung cancer in older smokers and ex-smokers. The commonest symptoms at the time of diagnosis include

- persistent cough (>3 weeks)
- dyspnoea
- chest and/or shoulder pain
- weight loss
- haemoptysis
- fatigue
- persistent hoarseness.

Though in no way age-specific, these symptoms are potentially masked by, or confused for, the symptoms of comorbid conditions that are much more common in older people. The first diagnostic intervention should be a chest radiograph which is abnormal in the vast majority of symptomatic patients, though a normal chest radiograph does not exclude the diagnosis. The optimal management of LC is highly dependent on obtaining both a proper tissue diagnosis and an accurate assessment of the stage of the disease, so with the exception of moribund patients, the large majority will require further investigation. This is best carried out by an expert lung cancer multidisciplinary team, since there is a wide range of procedures now available to individual patients (see Table 6.6). A contrast-enhanced CT scan of the thorax and upper abdomen is a prerequisite for all other investigations. Positron Emission Tomography-CT scanning is now routinely carried out as part of the staging process in fit patients with tumours potentially amenable for radical therapy (see Figure 6.5).

Metastatic disease is detected in well over 50% of patients at the time of diagnosis; the most common sites of distant spread are shown in Table 6.7.

It will be clear that these may cause symptoms and signs that could trigger referral to a wide variety of clinical specialities, indicating the need for a high level of suspicion in the speciality of geriatric medicine.

Survival

The overall survival figures for the entire lung cancer population in the UK are poor with only around 30% of patients being alive at 1 year and 7% at 5 years. These rates are lower than those reported from much of the rest of the Western world, and within the UK itself there is wide variation. A large part of the problem is late diagnosis,

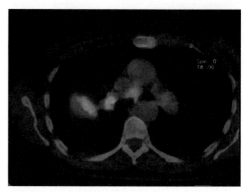

Figure 6.5 (colour plate 2) Fluorodeoxyglucose (FDG) positron emission tomography–computed tomography scan showing high FDG uptake in right mid zone tumour, right hilar and subcarinal lymph glands.

which may be a greater problem in the UK than in some other countries. Despite this, there is a subgroup of patients in whom radical treatment is effective and a much larger group in whom a combination of a modest prolongation of life combined with meaningful improvement in symptoms and quality of life can be achieved.

Treatment

Although the three main therapeutic tools of surgery, radiotherapy and chemotherapy have remained the cornerstone of treatment of lung cancer for many years, all three have developed significantly in recent years and the new 'targeted' therapies are beginning to have a major impact on outcomes for a minority of patients. There have also been significant developments in specialist palliative interventions.

Surgery

Surgical resection is the treatment of choice in patients with stages I and II NSCLC and in some patients with stage IIIA disease. Surgery is rarely indicated in SCLC. Fitness for surgery is of key importance, especially in older people, but age *per se* is not an independent risk factor in terms of outcome and most thoracic surgeons will consider patients for surgery well into their 80s if they are fit and can give

Table 6.6 Tissue sampling options

Fibre-optic bronchoscopy
CT guided needle biopsy
US guided biopsy of supraclavicular lymph nodes
Pleural tap ± CT guided pleural biopsy
Endobronchial ultrasound (EBUS)
Endoscopic ultrasound (EUS)
Thoracoscopy
Biopsy of a metastasis
Open surgical biopsy

Table 6.7 Commonest metastatic sites for lung cancer

Contralateral lung
Liver
Brain
Bone
Adrenal glands
Skin

informed consent. The main comorbidities that impact on fitness for surgery are cardiovascular disease, COPD and cerebrovascular disease.

Chemotherapy
Combination chemotherapy (largely platinum-based) has been demonstrated to have a survival benefit in a number of patient groups and can also result in good improvements in symptoms and quality of life. Most studies have been carried out on patients of good Performance Status (PS; see Table 6.8), a factor of major prognostic significance. The following categories of patients should be considered for chemotherapy.
- SCLC of reasonable performance status (PS 0–2)
- Advanced NSCLC (stage IIIB and IV) of good PS (PS 0–1); benefit in PS 2 patients is less clear
- After surgical resection with stage IIB–IIIA NSCLC and of good PS, plus those with stages IB and IIA disease with tumours >4 cm or positive resection margins.
- Locally advanced NSCLC (stage IIIA and some IIIB) in combination with radiotherapy.

There is little evidence of a systematic increase in toxicity of chemotherapy as a result of increasing age alone, taking into account PS and comorbidities. There is, however, less evidence for the value of adjuvant chemotherapy in patients of 80 years or over.

Radiotherapy
Radiotherapy (RT) can usefully be divided into treatment with either palliative or curative (radical) intent. Palliative RT usually involves between two and five treatment fractions and has a low incidence of side effects. It is particularly effective in controlling symptoms in the following situations:
- pain from bony metastases
- dyspnoea relating to large airway narrowing
- troublesome cough and haemoptysis
- cerebral metastases.

Table 6.8 WHO performance status

0	Able to carry out all normal activity without restriction
1	Restricted in physically strenuous activity but able to walk and do light work
2	Able to walk and capable of all self care but unable to carry out any work. Up and about more than 50% of waking hours
3	Capable of only limited self care, confined to bed or chair more than 50% of waking hours
4	Completely disabled. Cannot carry on any self care. Totally confined to bed or chair

RT with curative intent is used either alone as 'radical RT' in patients with relatively small, localized tumours who are not fit for, or who decline, surgical resection, or in combination with chemotherapy in those with more locally advanced, inoperable tumours who are of good PS. Combination chemo-RT is relatively toxic and the pros and cons of such an approach in patients over the age of 75 needs careful discussion with the patient. RT is not given routinely after surgery, but is used, usually with chemotherapy, in patients where the resection margins are positive or where unexpected involvement of mediastinal nodes is discovered.

'Targeted' therapies
The discovery of a variety of pathways that control tumour growth, spread, and cell death (apoptosis) has led to the development of a host of 'targeted' agents. The only ones that are currently licensed for use in lung cancer are those which target the epidermal growth factor receptor (EGFR) as tyrosine kinase inhibitors (TKI) such as Erlotinib and Gefitinib and the monoclonal antibody VEGF (vascular endothelial growth factor) receptor blocker Bevacizumab. The TKIs have now been approved by NICE for use in certain groups of patients with NSCLC and are particularly effective in patients who have mutations in the EGFR receptor. These are oral agents with very much less serious toxicity profiles than chemotherapy. They can dramatically improve both survival and symptoms in a minority of patients.

Palliative and supportive care
General 'supportive care' is an essential element of the management of all lung cancer patients from very early in their care pathway and Lung Cancer Nurse Specialists can provide a huge amount of support and continuity throughout the care pathway. The involvement of a specialist palliative care team will depend on the needs of the patient at a specific stage of their illness, but the general rule is to involve the palliative care team earlier rather than later and as a matter of urgency for the control of pain. It is important to be aware that there is a wide range of specialist palliative interventions now available for some specific problems in lung cancer. These include
- large airway obstruction: stenting and debulking procedures e.g. laser and rigid bronchoscopic debridement
- SVC obstruction: stenting
- chronic pleural effusions (where pleurodesis has been ineffective): tunnelled indwelling pleural drains
- intractable chest wall pain: nerve block and/or cordotomy.

Multidisciplinary team assessment
As the diagnosis, staging and treatment becomes more complex, the need for proper specialist MDT assessment of every patient where there is a working diagnosis of lung cancer becomes ever more important. It is no longer acceptable for an individual clinician to make major management decisions of the sort involved in the management of lung cancer.

Further reading
Hunt I, Muers M, Treasure T (eds) (2009). *ABC of Lung Cancer.* Wiley-Blackwell, West Sussex.
Information Centre for Health and Social Care. *National Lung Cancer Audit.* Annual report 2009 (www.ic.nhs.uk).
NICE (2005). *Guidelines on the Diagnosis and Treatment of Lung Cancer.* London, NICE (www.nice.org.uk).

Gastrointestinal

Oral hygiene in older people

Key concepts

The importance of teeth

Teeth are important for chewing a wide range of food, and also for social and cosmetic reasons. Tooth retention is associated with better quality of life. A minimum of 21 teeth, arranged in opposable pairs, are needed in order to eat a varied diet. People with fewer teeth will require dentures to eat efficiently. Recent studies have shown that over 20% of nursing home residents have significant unmet oral health needs, and those with dementia often have even poorer oral health. Poor oral health has adverse consequences such as bad breath, toothache, bleeding gums, tooth loss, and poor nutrition. It is therefore important to promote good oral healthcare in the future older population.

Normal ageing of the teeth and mouth

Teeth naturally alter colour with age, both as a consequence of increased levels of mineralization in dentine making it more opaque, and from extrinsic staining related to tea, coffee, and other products. Gum recession may occur, exposing more of the root of the tooth (hence the phrase 'long in the tooth'), making teeth technically more challenging to clean. Teeth will become more worn as a result of chewing and sometimes bruxism. The numbers of taste buds decline from middle age and result in a less sensitive sense of taste, which when combined with reductions in the sense of smell reduces people's enjoyment of food. There are significant reductions in the orofacial musculature, making chewing a more laborious process. Thinning of the oral mucosa may result in increased sensitivity to stimuli and a sense of burning in the mouth. The bone of the jaws may be affected by osteoporosis, although when teeth are present the jaw remains a functional matrix.

Provision of dentistry for older people

The proportion of older people retaining teeth into old age is increasing steadily, and by 2025 75–80% of over 65 year olds are expected to retain some teeth compared with about 55% today. However, higher rates of tooth retention are also likely to put increased pressure on the dental service because these extra teeth will need to be maintained. Older people pay for NHS dental care and much of the work appropriate to this group (e.g. provision of dentures) falls in band C, which currently costs the patient £204 per treatment episode. In some areas NHS dentists are scarce; private dentistry is more expensive (dentures cost from around £500) and may be less accessible on a pension (state pension currently just over £100 per week). Barriers to older people accessing dental care are likely to be complex, and include mobility, cost, perceptions about the necessity or availability of dental care, scarcity of NHS dentists, and illness.

Threats to teeth

Plaque

This is a sticky removable white substance comprising bacteria and extracellular matrix (see Figure 7.1). It mineralizes to form calculus if not removed after about 72 hours. Both tooth decay (caries) and gum disease (periodontitis) require mature plaque to be present to occur.

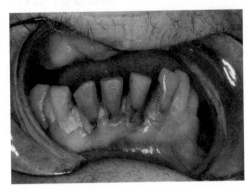

Figure 7.1 (colour plate 3) Plaque on teeth. Victoria Ewan and Konrad Staines, Diagnosis and management of oral mucosal lesions in older people: a review, *Reviews in Clinical Gerontology*, **18**, 2, pp. 115–28, reproduced with permission. Copyright Cambridge University Press.

Periodontitis

A set of conditions characterized by inflammation of the periodontium (the tissue in which the tooth sits comprising gum, tooth surface, supporting ligaments, and alveolar bone) and ulceration of the lining of the pocket around each tooth. It caused by bacteria within plaque which has not been removed, plus vigorous host inflammatory response and can cause loss of attachment and of alveolar bone in which the tooth sits. It is treated by plaque removal (e.g. by flossing, brushing teeth) and chemical disinfectants such as chlorhexidine. Disinfectants alone cannot manage this problem. Periodontitis of 10 teeth could be equivalent to a ~10 × 5 cm cutaneous ulcer and produces a raised C-reactive protein (CRP).

Caries

Cavities develop as a result of demineralization of the tooth. Bacteria within plaques metabolize dietary sugars to produce acids which cause demineralization. Early demineralization is reversible with high fluoride pastes and oral hygiene, but the later stages of disease are associated with pain and abscess formation. Two main bacteria are implicated in the initiation of caries: *Streptococcus mutans* and *Lactobacillus*.

Xerostomia (dry mouth)

Dry mouth is extremely common in hospital patients. It may make chewing and swallowing food difficult (and should be asked about specifically if patients are not eating), and also contributes to caries because saliva acts as a buffer to protect teeth from low pH and wash sugars and acids out of the mouth. It has many causes, including drugs (opiates, antimuscarinic drugs, diuretics, and others), dehydration, anxiety, hyperventilation, oxygen therapy, radiotherapy to head and neck, and Sjögren's syndrome. In practice this condition is difficult to treat satisfactorily. Saliva substitutes or stimulants can be prescribed, certain drugs may be stopped (but equally often are necessary) and constant sipping of liquids or ice chips can help, as can chewing sugar-free gum. However, patients should avoid sugary drinks or sweets because of the higher risk of caries associated with dry mouth. Xerostomia also predisposes to candidal infections and bacterial sialadenitis.

> **Authors' Tip**
>
> Ask patients how many times during the day their mouth feels dry: reporting xerostomia needs to be put into a temporal context.

Other common conditions

- *Black hairy tongue* – benign, due to bacteria and/or fungi producing a black pigment, treated with tongue cleaning and oral hygiene
- *Geographic tongue* – benign, causes stinging often after eating certain foods, cause unknown (see Figure 7.2)
- *Angular stomatitis*: fissuring at the angles of the mouth, often associated with intraoral *Candida* or *Staphylococci* or a combination of both. Look for candidiasis and treat, but also check for anaemia (iron and vitamin B12), diabetes. May need topical antimicrobial therapy as well as topical antifungals. Chloramphenicol eye creams can be useful.
- *Erythroplakia*: red patch, associated with precancerous change; greater risk than leukoplakia.
- *Leukoplakia*: white patch associated with precancerous change
- *Sore tongue*: causes include candida infection, folate/vitamin B12/iron deficiency.

Clinical scenarios

Candidal infections

Candidosis may manifest itself as acute pseudomembranous candidosis (classic removable white plaques), chronic hyperplastic candidosis (white lesions at commissures of mouth, not removable, needs biopsy to exclude dysplastic change, see Figure 7.3), or acute erythematous candidosis (sore, erythematous area commonly affecting palate and dorsum of tongue). Treatment is similar in all cases, and involves topical antifungals, chlorhexidine, improved oral hygiene, and systemic treatment when the above are ineffective. Oesophageal candidiasis may be present in some patients but does not appear to be associated with classic oesophageal symptoms, rather with anaemia and loss of appetite, and the benefits of treatment are unknown. It is associated with malignancy, chronic obstructive pulmonary disease, and recent antibiotic use.

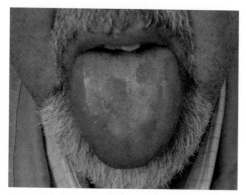

Figure 7.2 (colour plate 4) Geographic tongue. Victoria Ewan and Konrad Staines, Diagnosis and management of oral mucosal lesions in older people: a review, *Reviews in Clinical Gerontology*, **18**, 2, pp. 115–28, reproduced with permission. Copyright Cambridge University Press.

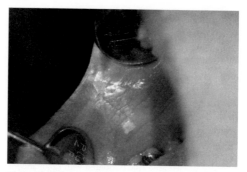

Figure 7.3 (colour plate 5) Chronic hyperplastic candidosis. Victoria Ewan and Konrad Staines, Diagnosis and management of oral mucosal lesions in older people: a review, *Reviews in Clinical Gerontology*, **18**, 2, pp. 115–28, reproduced with permission. Copyright Cambridge University Press.

Oral care in the older person with dentures

Proper care of dentures is needed to maintain a healthy oral environment. Dentures predispose to candidal infections and denture stomatitis (erythema of the mucosal surfaces in contact with dentures, mucosa may become granular in more severe cases. Often related to smoking, nocturnal denture wear, and poorly fitting dentures). Dentures should be removed at night and soaked in a cleaning solution to help to avoid denture stomatitis. They should also be manually brushed to remove food debris and denture plaque before soaking. If a candidal infection is present, dentures need to be soaked overnight in a solution such as sodium hypochlorite at 125 ppm (Milton), as well as simultaneous treatment of the mouth with standard anti-candidal therapy. Good hygiene needs to be maintained as problems may recur. Candidal infections are more common in people with dry mouths and where the dentures are old and/or ill-fitting. Professional dental care to remake dentures may be of help.

Oral care in hospital

Oral care is becoming increasingly recognized as an important strand of hospital care, partly due to the factors mentioned above, but also because certain oral risk factors predispose to hospital-acquired pneumonia (HAP). HAP occurs due to microaspiration of oral secretions which contain potential respiratory pathogens and has a high mortality (20–60%). This tendency to aspirate, combined with a pathological oral bacterial flora and host factors such as advanced age, frailty, and nasogastric feeding tubes, make ideal conditions for HAP. For example, acute stroke patients (who often have some or all of these risk factors) have a ~25% risk of pneumonia. It is not yet known whether improved oral hygiene can reduce the incidence of HAP; limited evidence suggests that this may be the case but larger randomized trials are needed.

Oral care in the palliative setting

Good oral care is extremely important in those who are dying. Common problems include dry mouth, furred tongue, cracked lips, and candidal infections. Drugs which cause dry mouth are often necessary in this group so frequent sips of water and use of ice chips may be the best treatment. Frozen chunks of pineapple can be used to clean the mouth due to enzymatic action. Petroleum jelly can be applied to the lips to prevent cracking. A spray or gel containing chlorhexidine can also be used to prevent candidal infections if the patient is unable to manage using a mouthwash. If chlorhexidine causes discomfort, it can be diluted with water. Cold sores are also common but may present atypically in the dying patient - suspect any painful ulcer and treat with aciclovir.

Bisphosphonate-related osteonecrosis of the jaw (BRONJ)

People who are taking bisphosphonates are susceptible to osteonecrosis of the jaw. Exposed jaw bone for more than eight weeks in those without cancer or radiotherapy treatment but in receipt of bisphosphonate therapy is diagnostic of BRONJ, and 90–95% of cases occur in those with cancer on intravenous bisphosphonates. The risk of developing such lesions is between 1:100 and 1:20, with some evidence of increased risk associated with simultaneous use of tyrosine kynase inhibitors. However, it can also occur in those on longer term oral bisphosphonates (about 1:10 000 patients); the risk in patients who have dental extractions is about 1:300. The pathogenesis of this condition is currently unknown. Nitrogen-containing compounds are more likely to produce BRONJ, including pamidronate, zoledronate, risedronate, and alendronate. All patients who are given these drugs should be warned of this complication and should be told to tell their dentist about their medication (especially those on quarterly intravenous infusions of the more potent agents to manage osteoporosis rather than metabolic bone disease, who may forget), and any outstanding dental work should be completed prior to starting these drugs. There are few data on how best to treat or prevent this condition. One study suggested that conservative management with chlorhexidine 0.12%, intermittent antibiotics, and careful sequestrectomy lead to healing in 53%. Aggressive surgery may exacerbate the problem.

When to refer to a dentist

Hospital doctors can refer in-patients to dentists if necessary. Reasons for referral might include dental pain, tooth loss, suspected oral cancer (erythroplakia, leukoplakia, lump, non-healing ulcer), unresolving periodontitis, or ill-fitting dentures. However, ill-fitting dentures may occur after a period of illness because the dentures were a poor fit initially and the patient has simply forgotten how to manipulate them. Denture wear is a juggling act on the part of the patient, with the muscles of the mouth controlling the position of the denture. Reduced denture stability will impair a patient's ability to chew foods effectively. Residents in care homes can be referred to the Salaried Primary Care Dental Service, who are trained specifically to look after the dental needs of such patients. Some general dentists also provide such care.

Further reading

Scully C, Felix DH (2005). Oral medicine--update for the dental practitioner: red and pigmented lesions. [see comment] *Br Dent J* **199**: 639–45.

Sreebny LM, Schwartz SS (1997). A reference guide to drugs and dry mouth, 2nd edn. *Gerodontology* **14**: 33–47.

Van den Wyngaert T, Claeys T, Huizing MT, *et al.* (2009). Initial experience with conservative treatment in cancer patients with osteonecrosis of the jaw (ONJ) and predictors of outcome. *Ann Oncol* **20**: 331–6.

Gastrointestinal physiology in older age

Although there are no gastrointestinal (GI) diseases specific to older people, many symptoms and diseases become more common in older age groups. The GI tract carries out a complex range of functions, which can all be physiologically affected with increasing age, as well as increased pathology due to different disease entities.

The major role of the GI tract is in the mechanical and chemical breakdown of food, which can be rapidly absorbed and utilized by the body. Another important role is the elimination of waste products, including indigestible food and toxins (e.g. bile pigments).

Changes occur in gastrointestinal physiology with age. Inflammation in the upper gastrointestinal tract increases with age, and the prevalence of gastric atrophy is commoner in older people, partly, but not entirely, related to the increased prevalence of *Helicobacter pylori*. GI transit time is slower owing to age-related changes in the innervation and composition of neuronal tissue in the gut wall. This reduced transit can lead to oesophageal dysmotility, decreased gastric emptying, diverticular disease, and constipation.

Physiological disorders affecting the GI tract in older age include:

- alterations in GI mucosal protection
- effects on nutrition and sensory deficits
- effects on motility
- organ-specific effects.

Gastrointestinal mucosal protection

Throughout the human GI tract there is a balance between aggressive factors and mucosal protective mechanisms. When this equilibrium is disrupted, pathology results.

Mucosal protection in the stomach

There are no overt age-related increases in the endogenous aggressors in the stomach: acid and pepsin. Therefore, the imbalance that leads to diseases seen more commonly in older people, such as cancer or ulceration, is due to an age-associated impairment of mucosal protective mechanisms. Prostaglandins are molecules involved in mucosal protection, via mucus, bicarbonate secretion, and blood flow. Their concentration may be reduced with advancing age. Medications, such as non-steroidal anti-inflammatory drugs (NSAIDs) and aspirin, which inhibit the production of prostaglandins, are used widely by older people, making them particularly vulnerable. Mucus covers the GI tract with an adherent gel, with some barrier properties and a 'sloppy' luminal layer, which acts as a lubricant. The amount of mucus, its quality, and the number of mucus-producing cells in the stomach are reduced with age and *H. pylori* infection, and may contribute to the risk of ulcers in older people. Bicarbonate neutralizes gastric acid and inactivates pepsin by increasing pH. Bicarbonate secretion may be lower in older people, and the ability of the gastric mucosa to produce bicarbonate in response to prostaglandins impaired.

Repair mechanisms

In animal models, ageing is associated with decreased reparative ability in the gastric mucosa, and with delays in both resolution of mucosal injury and regeneration of injured gastric mucosa. It is unclear whether this also occurs in the human stomach. Blood flow to an injured area is important during repair to bring nutrients and remove waste. Reduction in blood flow alone is sufficient to cause ulceration in the mucosa and likely to contribute to human disease. In aged animal models, basal gastric blood flow and flow in response to injury is reduced.

Age-related effects on nutrition

- Food intake diminishes with increasing age, reflecting a lowered metabolic rate and loss of lean muscle mass.
- After the age of 50 years, the calorific requirement drops by approximately 10% each decade.
- The fundamental nutritional requirements (e.g. balanced diet) do not change with age.
- Pathological disease processes affecting any part of the GI tract can present with nutritional sequelae.

Effects of age on smell and taste

- The number of fibres in the olfactory bulb and its receptors decrease with age, reducing the sense of smell.
- This decrease and age-related bone growth in the skull compressing sensory nerve fibres, affects the ability to discriminate between smells.
- Taste (gustatory) defects are largely due to olfactory dysfunction, although ageing can also produce taste loss due to changes in gustatory cell membranes.
- Shrinkage of the maxillary and mandibular bones, and erosion of tooth sockets can exacerbate loss of teeth.
- All of these can result in appetite suppression, and lead to subsequent weight loss and malnutrition.

Anatomical areas

Mouth and pharynx

- Chewing is a complex process involving the lips, tongue, salivary glands, and teeth in order to form a food bolus.
- Loss of acinar cells in the tongue and less fluid from the submandibular salivary glands with age can lead to decreased saliva and consequent dry mouth (xerostomia)
- Swallowing is a coordinated neurological and mechanical process where the food bolus is pushed past the posterior pharyngeal wall through the upper oesophageal sphincter into the oesophagus.

Oesophagus

- The muscular contractions that initiate swallowing slow with age; this increased pharyngeal transit time may lead to dysphagia (difficulty swallowing). As well as increased symptomatic presentation of this in older people, frank food bolus obstruction is more common.
- The strength of oesophageal peristalsis also decreases, with both upper and lower oesophageal sphincters losing tension. Relaxation of the latter can lead to reflux.
- Achalasia is an oesophageal motility disorder involving the smooth muscle of the lower oesophageal sphincter, more common in this age group.
- Barrett's oesophagus, achalasia, and environmental exposures (e.g. smoking and alcohol) are all associated with oesophageal malignancies.

Stomach

- The stomach acts as a reservoir for food, especially for larger meals. With increasing age, it cannot store as much due to reduced elasticity in the stomach wall.

- Gastric emptying of liquids or a mixed meal is delayed in older patients: this is predominantly in the gastric fundus.
- Secretion of gastric juices (hydrochloric acid and pepsin) in the healthy stomach remains constant with ageing.
- However, the incidence of hyposecretory conditions, e.g. atrophic gastritis, are more common in older adults, and can be due to a range of causes (e.g. *H. pylori* infection; autoimmune, e.g. pernicious anaemia).
- Decreased gastric mucosal protection is the major reason for the inability to resist luminal damage. There is decreased secretion of bicarbonate and mucus for an alkaline gel layer, increasing the risk of peptic ulceration and lesions.

Small intestine

- The main function of the small intestine is in absorption of food, by producing a range of enzymes and using secretions from the pancreas and liver.
- Most absorption takes place in the terminal ileum and jejunum via microscopic folds (villi). There is shrinkage and broadening of the villi with age, significantly reducing their surface area and absorptive capabilities.
- Lipid absorption is reduced with older age probably due to less pancreatic enzymes and ability to emulsify. Lactose intolerance is also more common, as lactase levels decrease, resulting in intolerance to dairy products.
- Small bowel motility decreases with age, though this does not affect the smooth muscle or have clinical effects.
- However, small bowel bacterial overgrowth in older age can occur with overpopulation of commensal microbes. This can result in decreased absorption of nutrients (e.g. calcium, folic acid, and iron) and malnutrition.

Large intestine

- Peristalsis slows down, increasing the transit time of waste in the large intestine and can result in constipation. The mucosa and muscle layers of the colon also atrophy with age, leading to weaker peristalsis.
- Sagging of the colonic wall prompts the formation of pouches (diverticulae), exacerbated by lack of dietary fibre.
- Haemorrhoids may develop due to straining and pressure on weakened blood vessel walls in the large bowel.
- The sigmoid functioning and colonic transit are largely unimpaired, but there is decreased rectal compliance and an increased sensory threshold for the urge to defecate.
- Older people are also likely to use laxatives despite no difference in stool frequency compared with younger people.
- Anorectal functioning can be impaired, especially due to pelvic floor dysfunction in women. This can present with faecal incontinence, especially in the institutionalized and those with sensory deficits. Faecal impaction can also occur, due to reduced rectal sensation, limited mobility, weakness, and dementia.
- There is a decline in rates of cell division and repair in the large intestinal mucosa (increasing the risk of pre-malignant polyps and colorectal cancer in particular).

Pancreaticobiliary organs

- Pancreatic exocrine function decreases with age due to lowered cell volume and tissue fibrosis.
- There is decreased secretion of pancreatic proteases and lipases, affecting small bowel absorption.
- The production and flow of bile in the gallbladder decreases with age, affecting absorption of fat.
- Bile also becomes thicker due to increased cholesterol content, resulting in gallstone formation.

Liver

The liver, which plays a key role in metabolism and protein synthesis, has reduced functional capacity with older age. This is due to reduced blood flow and shrinkage, leading to a loss of hepatocyte number and function. This reduces the ability to detoxify harmful substances or inactivate drugs. As well as being more likely to be taking medications, older patients are more likely to have drug-related side effects due to altered pharmacokinetics.

Conclusions

Owing to the large functional reserve of the GI tract, ageing has little direct clinical effect on most organ-specific functions *per se*. However, there are alterations in the equilibrium of normal physiological functions, such as GI mucosal protection. This can be compounded by altered nutritional demands and other sensory changes in the older people patient. Clinicians should be mindful of the effects of altered GI physiology, such as dysmotility, as well as organic disorders, when assessing older people with GI symptoms.

Further reading

Allen A, Newton J, Oliver L, *et al.* (1997). Mucus and H. pylori. *J Physiol Pharmacol* **48**: 297–305.

Barry PP (2000). An overview of special considerations in the evaluation and management of the geriatric patient. *Am J Gastroenterol* **95**: 8–10.

Boyce JM, Shone GR (2006). Effects of ageing on smell and taste. *Postgraduate Medical Journal* **82**: 239–41.

Firth M, Prather M (2002). Gastrointestinal motility problems in the elderly patient. *Gastroenterology* **122**: 1688–700.

Lee A, Veldhuyzen van Zanten S, Lee A, *et al.* (1997). The aging stomach or the stomachs of the ages. *Gut* **41**: 575–6.

Lewis SJ, Potts LF, Malhotra R, *et al.* (1999). Small bowel bacterial overgrowth in subjects living in residential care homes. *Age Ageing* **28**: 181–5.

Newton JL (2004). Changes in upper gastrointestinal physiology with age. Mechanisms of ageing and development, **125**: 867–70.

Newton JL, Johns CE, May FEB (2004). The ageing bowel and intolerance to aspirin. *Aliment Pharmacol Therap* **19**: 39–45.

Orr WC, Chen CL (2002). Ageing and control of the GI tract. Clinical and physiological aspects of gastrointestinal motility and ageing. *Am J Physiol Gastrointest Liver Physiol* **283**: 1226–31.

Vellas B, Ballas D, Moreau J, *et al.* (1998). Exocrine pancreatic secretion in the elderly. *Int J Pancreatol* **3**: 497–502.

Support group: CORE (www.corecharity.org.uk).

Gastrointestinal investigations

Broadly speaking, the aim of investigations is to diagnose the cause of patients' symptoms. However, the patients' fitness to have the investigation and to undergo any consequent procedure must be borne in mind. This is very relevant in gastrointestinal tract (GIT) investigations in the older patient, though most are usually able to undergo most procedures. GI investigations can be broadly categorized into three areas:

- endoscopic
- radiological
- laboratory based.

Endoscopic investigations

The endoscopic request form is an important and valuable document. Apart from demographic information, the request should contain relevant clinical information. This should ensure that the correct procedure is performed.

Upper GIT endoscopy

This common GI investigation may be diagnostic or therapeutic. It may be either an inpatient or an outpatient procedure. Although usually carried out by a doctor, there are increasing numbers of non-medical endoscopists providing an excellent service. It is essential to obtain written consent before the procedure with information regarding rare complications such as perforation (<0.1%) and bleeding. Gastroscopy may be performed under local anaesthetic alone or with the addition of a benzodiazepine, such as midazolam. In an endoscopy suite there must be appropriate resuscitation facilities and reversal agents for medication administered. Patients lacking capacity should be considered for endoscopy if it is in their best interest, as defined by the Mental Capacity Act.

Diagnostic indications

- Suspected upper GIT cancer. (weight loss, abdominal pain, etc.).
- Acute upper GIT bleeding.
- Iron deficiency anaemia (including adult coeliac disease).
- Surveillance of Barrett's oesophagus.

Therapeutic indications

- Banding of known oesophageal varices.
- Control of bleeding by injection, laser, etc.
- Dilatation of oesophagus or pylorus,
- Palliation of oesophageal neoplasia, e.g. stent insertion, alcohol injection, etc.
- Percutaneous endoscopic gastrostomy (PEG) insertion.

Colonoscopy

This investigation is most commonly carried out as an outpatient as preparation of the colon in inpatients is usually ineffective. Clinicians must consider inpatient preparation for very frail individuals. There are many regimens for colonic cleansing but most use either Picolax or Klean-Prep together with a low residue diet. There is little to choose between these two regimens, and the choice may be local. Because of the large volume of fluid consumed, patients often suffer with nausea and satiety. One in four will have an episode of incontinence during preparation. Fluid and electrolyte shifts may be hazardous, particularly in those with cardiovascular and renal comorbidities. Confirmation is required that the patient is fit enough to take the preparation. The risk of perforation is small, at 0.1% for diagnostic procedures and twice this rate in therapeutic colonoscopy. Bleeding is a rare complication; usually following snare polypectomy or hot biopsies the rate of bleeding has been reported as between 0.001% and 0.24%. It is usually obvious at the time of colonoscopy, but can occur up to 14 days after polypectomy. The procedure is most commonly carried out with sedation, often a combination of midazolam and pethidine. The aim is to examine the total colon through to the caecum and terminal ileum.

Diagnostic indications

- Investigation of bloody diarrhoea and rectal bleeding
- Assessment of inflammatory bowel disease
- Biopsy of lesion identified on imaging
- Iron-deficiency anaemia
- Colorectal cancer surveillance in very high-risk patients
- Persistent diarrhoea

Therapeutic indications

- Polypectomy
- Treatment of angiodysplasia and other vascular lesions
- Dilatation of strictures
- Stent insertion to palliate cancer

Flexible sigmoidoscopy

This investigation is frequently employed when a full colonoscopy is not required. The lower bowel is visualized to the splenic flexure. The preparation is simpler, with a phosphate enema given immediately prior to the procedure, and sedation is not usually needed.

Indications

- Bright red rectal bleeding
- Persistent diarrhoea
- In acute colitis when colonoscopy may be dangerous.
- Therapeutic indications: as for colonoscopy

Endoscopic retrograde cholangiopancreatogram (ERCP)

This investigation has a mainly therapeutic role in pancreatic and biliary disease, as the diagnostic role has been largely replaced by MRCP (magnetic resonance cholangiopancreatogram) except where this is contraindicated. Therapeutic options include the palliative stenting of malignant disease or the removal of common bile duct stones. The procedure is carried out under sedation within an X-ray department. Complications include pancreatitis (2%), bleeding and death (<0.5%).

Wireless capsule endoscopy

The patient swallows a disposable capsule, which captures images twice a second as the 'pill' travels through the GIT. Images are downloaded and read. This test is particularly useful in imaging the small intestine and in the work-up of obscure iron-deficient anaemia when both colonoscopy and gastroscopy have been normal. Rarely the capsule may cause obstruction due to a stricture and so preliminary imaging may be needed in high-risk cases.

Enteroscopy

This specialist procedure is an endoscopic examination of the small bowel. The commonest indications are to treat vascular lesions and remove or biopsy other lesions identified at wireless endoscopy.

Endoscopic ultrasound

This investigation is useful in the staging of early oesophageal cancers, rectal cancers, and the evaluation of pancreatic masses. It also has a place in the assessment of faecal incontinence.

Radiological investigations

The request form is vital, the information given on it may colour the report and may guide the reporter if further investigations are required. It is most valuable to discuss the options with the radiologist.

Plain Films

In patients with acute abdominal pain a supine abdominal radiograph and an erect chest radiograph are indicated. This is to look for evidence of perforation or obstruction. Plain films are also useful in the initial assessment and subsequent monitoring of acute colitis.

Contrast studies

Although endoscopic investigations are replacing some radiographic techniques there is still a place for contrast studies, particularly in defining the extent of inflammatory bowel disease or when colonoscopy is incomplete due to technical reasons. By combining a barium solution and some gas the mucosal surface is coated and defined. The investigations for various areas are listed below:

Barium swallow	Oesophagus
Barium meal	Stomach
Barium follow through	Small bowel
Small bowel enema	Small bowel
Barium enema	Large bowel

Ultrasound scanning

Abdominal ultrasound (US) is a non-invasive examination technique that is usually carried out after a 4-hour fast. It is useful in the assessment of jaundice, abdominal pain, abnormal liver function tests, ascites, and an abdominal mass. During the examination, Doppler studies may be employed to delineate blood flow. Liver biopsy is commonly carried out under US scanning. US scanning may help ascitic drainage in locating a safe area to insert the drain. Images may be difficult to interpret in obese patients or due to the presence of excessive bowel gas.

CT scanning

This may be used when US scanning fails to give the required information due to technical problems and in the staging of malignancy. It is also used in the biopsying of abnormal masses. Intravenous contrast is nephrotoxic and so the renal function should be included on the request form. CT colonography may be used as an alternative to a barium enema in frail elderly patients although some patients will still find the technique a challenge.

Magnetic resonance imaging

The presence of pacemakers, metallic clips, etc., is a contraindication to magnetic resonance imaging (MRI). The scanner is noisy and may be claustrophobic. MRI is particularly useful in the evaluation of rectal Crohn's disease and in the staging of rectal cancer. MRCP has largely replaced diagnostic endoscopic retrograde cholangiopancreatography.

Magnetic resonance enteroclysis involves the insertion of a tube through the stomach into the small intestine through which contrast can be given. It is not widely available but may offer an alternative to contrast studies in small bowel evaluation.

Nuclear medicine

There are a wide variety of isotope studies available but most are in specialist centres and may not be easily accessed. The two most common tests are the technetium scan, to look for a Meckel's diverticulum and the indium scan to assess Crohn's disease. A labelled red cell scan is occasionally helpful in obscure GIT bleeding.

Angiography

If colonoscopy and gastroscopy fail to indicate the cause of GIT blood loss angiography may be helpful. When the cause is chronic capsule endoscopy may be more helpful. If Doppler studies suggest mesenteric ischaemia further evaluation with mesenteric angiography and possible intervention may be indicated.

Laboratory and other tests

Some of the following investigations are widely available; however, some others are confined to specialist centres.

Stool testing

Stool is cultured in acute diarrhoea and repeated specimens may be needed to exclude infection. If _C. difficile_ infection is suspected it should be specified on the request form.

Stool may be tested for _H. pylori_ in patients with dyspepsia in the absence of 'red flag' symptoms.

Faecal elastase measurement may be useful in confirming a pancreatic cause for malabsorption.

Faecal occult blood testing has little role outside a bowel cancer-screening programme. It has no value in the investigation of an iron deficiency anaemia.

Blood testing

Apart from the routine haematological and biochemical blood tests some other tests are specific to investigate GIT function. IgA tissue transglutaminase and IgA endomysial antibodies are useful in the investigation of suspected coeliac disease.

A 'Hammersmith screen' is available to investigate chronic secretory diarrhoea associated with gut hormone excess.

Carcinoembryonic antigen testing (CEA) is insufficiently reliable for the screening of colonic tumours due to inadequate positive- and negative-predictive values (with the former leading to excessive investigations, and the latter potentially missing treatable early cancers). It may have a role in monitoring known colon cancer.

Breath testing

C^{13} and C^{14}-urea breath tests can help detect _H. pylori_ infection and more usefully in confirming eradication.

A lactulose breath test is employed when bacterial overgrowth is suspected as a cause for symptoms.

Oesophageal physiology studies

These tests are indicated in the investigation of suspected motility disorders including achalasia. They also maybe used to investigate atypical chest pain and reflux symptoms that are resistant to standard therapies. In the rare instance where an older patient may benefit from antireflux surgery, preoperative studies are vital.

Further reading

Clarke GA, Jacobson BC, Hammett RJ, et al. (2001). The indications, utilization and safety of gastrointestinal endoscopy in an extremely elderly patient cohort. _Endoscopy_ **33**: 580–4.

Goddard AF, McIntyre AS, Scott BB (2000). Guidelines for the management of iron deficiency anaemia. _Gut_ **46**(Suppl IV): 1–5.

Teeth and dentures

Natural teeth

The natural permanent dentition consists of 32 teeth which erupt over a period of 15 years or so, mostly appearing in childhood and adolescence. Human teeth have evolved for a life that is considerably shorter than the one we now expect of them, perhaps for only 30 years or so post eruption. Furthermore, the balance of threats to the dentition has changed over the last couple of hundred years, from those based around wear from an abrasive diet and periodontal (gum) disease, to rapidly destructive dental caries (decay), and its sequelae, as well as a continued threat from periodontal diseases.

By the time people reach old age, few still retain a full dentition of 28 teeth (discounting the third molars which are frequently missing or unerupted). The damage from dental diseases and their sequelae is cumulative. Teeth have very little capacity for repair and none for natural replacement; they are a one-off disposable item. Inevitably, many teeth fail, they break down, wear, or become loose through gum disease or develop an infection that cannot be resolved so are lost and extracted throughout life. Even by the time of retirement most people will have lost some teeth and some will even have lost all of them.

Consequently the dental state of older people is far from uniform. It is also rapidly changing in many countries. In England in 2009, about 6% of the whole population had no teeth at all, mostly in the older age groups, but even among those aged 85 and over, a small majority had at least some teeth. This marks a radical change in the population over the last half century from a position where being old usually meant being toothless to one where retention of some teeth is the norm. However, 6% of a population still accounts for a lot of people, and for those with teeth the number of teeth in old age is often few. As each decade passes the make-up of the older population looks a little different from the decade before, but for the next 30 years older people in much of Europe and North America will be characterized by more people retaining more teeth, but where the teeth remaining often have very complex maintenance needs.

Teeth and function in old age

The consequences of tooth loss are variable and the general appearance of the teeth is not a reliable indicator of good or bad function. From the physician's perspective, function is important as tooth loss can have an impact on diet and nutrition. Studies have observed a close relationship between intakes of key dietary components including dietary fibre and nutrients, such as antioxidant vitamins and dental state. People with few or no teeth tend to have lower intakes of 'healthy' foods such as fruits and vegetables and this has translated to measurably lower blood levels of certain nutrients. The relationship is complex and dietary habits often develop over a long period so the differences may not all be attributed to tooth loss, but there is the capacity for significant dietary limitation, of which the physician should be aware.

Generally people who retain 21 or more teeth (give or take a few) tend to have good functional capacity and relative dietary freedom and are unlikely to require a denture to function. The ability of individuals to tolerate further tooth loss is quite variable. Even where all teeth have been lost before the age of 50 years of age, older people are often well adapted to complete dentures. However, where sudden tooth loss and the need for dentures occurs for the first time at a stage in life when cognitive function and adaptive capacity have reduced, functional problems with an impact on diet, health, and quality of life are a real concern.

Reasons for dental problems and poor function

The section on oral hygiene in older people covers the basic risks to teeth from dental disease, systemic conditions, and poor hygiene, and some of the more common basic mucosal conditions. In this section we will consider the more acute conditions that cause pain or that impact on the ability to function.

Recognising dental pain (toothache)

Classical toothache can arise from the dental pulp (pulpitis) or from infection of the periodontal tissues, usually after the pulp has died and infection spreads out from inside the tooth to create an abscess around the tip of the root. Acute pulpitic, periodontal, and periapical infections all occur in older people and can be very severe. For patients who are already confused, significant dental pain can be very disorientating and make general management difficult.

Pain around the face is not always dental, so for the physician being able to recognize and localize true dental pain can be an important first step. There are five simple diagnostic signs that will rapidly identify a problem that has a dental origin.

- Thermal sensitivity: if, in the absence of obvious physical signs, there is pain brought on and exacerbated by hot or cold stimuli (such as a hot or cold drink) the pain is usually from the pulp. Transient pain lasting just a few seconds following a stimuli is not too much of a concern (see below), but where it lasts for longer than this or is constant but made worse by temperature changes, the pulp may be irrevocably damaged. Early intervention by a dentist is wise to remove the tooth or the pulp as the next stage may be a more serious infection.

- Localization: pain from the pulp may be easy to diagnose on the basis of a thermal response but is difficult to locate. In contrast, a tooth with a periapical or periodontal abscess will usually be tender to touch, sometimes exquisitely so. Gently percussing the candidate tooth with an instrument (a dental mirror is ideal but anything will suffice) will often locate a problem tooth precisely.

- Swelling: an inflammatory swelling on the jaw, whether intra-oral or extra-oral, is usually a sign of a dental infection. In such cases a surgical intervention (extraction or drainage) is likely to be required. This can also be associated with a raised temperature and should provoke a rapid intervention.

- Draining infection: where a tooth has been dead and infected for a while, a small draining sinus adjacent to the tooth is an indication of a chronic infection and usually a dead pulp.

- A broken down tooth: on a quick inspection of the mouth a very decayed or broken down tooth may be obvious. However, many dental problems in older people are related to teeth which are filled or crowned but outwardly look sound, so the absence of an obviously 'bad' tooth is not particularly relevant.

Author's Tip

Each of these is easy and quick to check. Any positive finding would identify a specifically dental problem requiring dental input and usually a straightforward surgical solution. A negative response to each of these does not completely rule out a dental problem.

Other sources of pain and poor function in older people

Other common causes of dental and oral discomfort are described below. Where these are suspected, appropriate dental input should be sought, but none are acute.

- Loose teeth: generally a sign of advanced periodontal disease, loose teeth do not usually cause acute pain but can cause functional problems and eating difficulties.
- Sensitive teeth: teeth showing transient sensitivity to temperature are often relatively healthy and this can often be treated quite easily.
- Temporomandibular disorder (TMD): this can masquerade as toothache but without any of the five toothache signs described above. Pain is rarely acute and often associated with tenderness specifically over the temporomandibular joint or of the muscles of mastication when palpated directly. It can occur in older patients.
- Other pain conditions: a range of chronic pain conditions, from trigeminal neuralgia to atypical odontalgia can present in the absence of any of the specific dental or oral signs described above. None is particularly common but undiagnosed facial pain can be a real concern, with understandable concerns from patients about serious illness or malignancy. Seeking appropriate specialist help and providing a definitive diagnosis and management pathway is an important step in the management process.

Author's Tip

Diagnosing non-dental pain from around the face can be very difficult. If obvious dental causes can be excluded, try and seek expert advice to obtain a definitive diagnosis rather than try to treat undiagnosed pain or make assumptions.

Dentures

Although the proportion of people now wearing complete dentures is now much reduced, it is still significant. Complete dentures rely only on the fit to the mucosa, the shape of the dental ridges and the considerable neuromuscular skills of the wearer to keep them stable. Very poor function with complete dentures is not at all uncommon, particularly where the ridges are poor or the patient's ability to control the denture is impaired, for example after a stroke or with a neuromuscular condition such as Parkinson's disease. In debilitated older people, weight loss

can result in a loss of denture support, and poorly supported dentures can then result in a downward spiral of nutrition due to functional difficulties, or even just reduced levels of pleasure from eating. Age is also associated with a gradual reduction in the height of bony ridges anyway, perhaps exacerbated by conditions such as osteoporosis, where bone density is reduced, with resultant difficulty controlling dentures.

Difficulty with dentures is not something that just has to be accepted. Strategies are possible in an inpatient and outpatient setting to improve function, from the simplest approaches such as a temporary relining in a hospital ward through to the construction of new dentures. The possibility of osseointegrated implants to stabilize complete dentures has revolutionized dental care for older people. Even two lower implants can make a profound difference and this has been recommended as a basic standard of care for edentate people.

Many people who have teeth also wear dentures of various types, so dentures are still a significant issue for many people, even those with natural teeth. In a hospital setting, oral self-care often becomes difficult for the patient, and disease can rapidly become established.

For patients with dentures, the dentures themselves can become a reservoir for infection, most commonly for oral *Candida* species. Even in a healthy patient this is a concern, and dentists always recommend removal of dentures overnight. For ill or debilitated patients, good denture and dental hygiene is even more important. Thorough brushing of all denture surfaces with a toothbrush and toothpaste, or even soap, is simple and can make a huge difference, both in terms of comfort and minimizing the risk of more serious complications. If there are signs of candidal infection, overnight immersion in a dilute solution of Milton can be helpful. More resistant infections can be managed by topical or systemic antifungals but specialist input is recommended to assist with diagnosis and treatment of chronic soft tissue infections.

The mouth is a dirty place carrying a huge bacterial load in the form of dental plaque on teeth and dentures. The risks to older and debilitated people extend beyond the mouth, with emerging evidence of aspiration pneumonia of oral organisms from mouths exhibiting poor hygiene. An emphasis on good dental and denture hygiene is critical to maintaining a healthy, comfortable and functional mouth and minimizing the risks of dental diseases, candidal infections and potentially systemic disease.

Further reading

Patel S, Chong BS (2010). Diagnosis. In (Chong BS, ed.) *Harty's Endodontics in Clinical Practice*, 6th edn. Edinburgh, Elsevier, pp. 17–33.

Polzer I, Schimmel M, Müller F, *et al.* (2010). Edentulism as part of the general health problems of elderly adults. *Int Dent J* **60**: 143–55.

Walls AW, Steele JG, Sheiham A, *et al.* (2000). Oral health and nutrition in older people. *J Public Health Dent* **60**: 304–7.

Dysphagia

Dysphagia, or abnormal swallowing, is a common problem of old age with increased prevalence secondary to specific disorders (e.g. stroke, Parkinson's disease (PD)) and as the ageing process leads to a reduction in physiological reserve (presbyphagia).

Background

The control of swallowing is complex, having cortical, brainstem, and cerebellar controls via crossed and uncrossed pathways through cranial nerves V, VII, IX, X, and XII to skeletal and smooth muscles. The deglutition tract is anatomically close to a number of structures which can obstruct its function (thoracic aorta, mediastinal structures) (see Figure 7.4).

Swallowing function can be divided into three phases: oral, pharyngeal, and oesophageal. Pathology can affect any combination of these stages.

The oral phase requires the coordination of facial muscles, muscles of mastication, the formation of a food bolus by the tongue, and movement to the back of the pharynx to trigger the swallowing reflex. With elevation of the larynx, closure of the vocal cords allows the airway to be protected during the pharyngeal phase. Once the bolus has bypassed the laryngeal inlet safely, oesophageal peristalsis is triggered taking the food/fluid down to the stomach through the gastro-oesophageal sphincter.

With increasing age, swallowing ability is reduced due to diminished oral sensation, increased breathing latency, and general reduction in speed of the swallow process secondary to changes within muscles. Deterioration of swallowing function can occur both in acute systemic illness, (respiratory disease, sepsis, heart failure), as well as in specific localized pathology. In addition, poor dentition and multiple drugs affect saliva production and oral hygiene. The ability to initiate eating and swallowing can also be affected by psychological factors (globus pharyngeus) and cognitive abilities (dementia).

It is useful to divide causes of dysphagia into neurogenic or physical/oesophageal.

Complications

Dysphagia leads to undernutrition, vulnerability to infection particularly pneumonia, increased mortality, and reduced quality of life.

Epidemiology

The frequency of dysphagia (depending on definitions used) in older people may be as high as 20% in the primary care population, 50% of those with acute stroke and

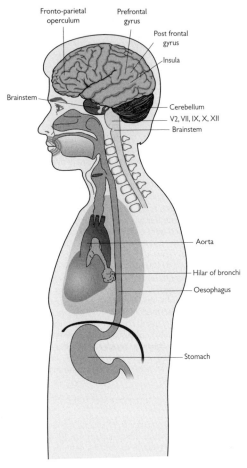

Figure 7.4 Anatomy of swallowing.

Brain	Nerve	Muscle
Cortex	V (Trigeminal)	Facial group
Brainstem	VII (Facial)	Muscles of mastication
Cerebellum	IX (Glossopharyngeal)	Tongue
	X (Vagus)	Pharyngeus complex
	XII (Hypoglossal)	Hyoid
		Oesophagus

Parkinson's disease, 100% with MND, and 60% in the general nursing home population (see Table 7.1).

Environmental exposures

Drugs may interfere with saliva production (e.g. anticholinergics, non-steroidal anti-inflammatory drugs (NSAIDs)), or swallowing function itself (e.g. neuroleptics).

Investigations

The key to diagnosis is the history of onset, duration, description of dysphagia and associated symptoms of regurgitation, dyspepsia, neurological, and other physical abnormalities (e.g. scleroderma), and development of complications (weight loss, anaemia, pneumonia).

Author's Tips

- Dysphagia worsens in acute illness, and additional temporary nutritional support or modification may be required.
- Attention to dental health and oral care is important in reducing pneumonia risk.
- Presence of dysarthria, 'wet' voice or recurrent chest infections should raise the suspicion of dysphagia
- Decisions on long-term enteral support require involvement of the whole MDT and second opinions to ensure best interests are maintained in those people who lack mental capacity

Table 7.1 Causes of dysphagia

Cause	Features
Neurogenic	
Stroke	50% acute, 17% at 1 month, 8% dependent on PEG at 6 months. Recovery depends on other deficits from stroke and complications. Many do recover, but are at risk of decompensation during acute illness
Dementia	32–84%. Progressive; difficult to assess due to combination with food refusal
Multiple Sclerosis	34%. Common in late stages
Parkinson's disease	30–81%. Progressive and at high risk of decompensation if medications omitted
Brain tumour	15–20% depending on type/site
Traumatic brain injury	25%
Huntingdon's chorea	85%. Progressive
Cerebral palsy	Adult prevalence unclear because of wide variance in disability-most studies in children. Mild cases may present with decompensation in older age
Learning difficulties	40–65%
Guillain–Barre syndrome	36–70%. Tends to recover, although some left with long-term problems
Myasthenia gravis	Common; fatigable, reversible.
Sarcoidosis	Rare. Usually secondary to bilateral hilar lymphadenopathy
Motor neurone disease	100% Progressive. Early PEG or RIG, non-invasive ventilation required during procedures if evidence of rapid bulbar deterioration
Post polio syndrome	40%. Mild but maybe progressive
Myotonic dystrophy	Common and usually mild
Physical/oesophageal causes	
Oropharyngeal cancer	75%. May present with other symptoms first
Poor dentition/ ulceration	Painful dysphagia; Ill-fitting dentures, abscesses more likely
Zenker's diverticulum, pharyngeal pouch	Dysphagia with regurgitation
Oesophageal cancer	Presents with dysphagia weight loss, anaemia common
Benign strictures/ oesophageal webs	Presents with dysphagia, anaemia
Achalasia	Present with dysphagia. Classic appearance of 'corkscrew' on barium swallow

Table 7.1 (Continued)

Cause	Features
Physical/oesophageal causes	
Diffuse oesophageal spasm	Painful dysphagia; prognosis good. Treat with PPI's and smooth muscle relaxants (e.g. nitrate)
Scleroderma	May present with other features first. Signs of connective tissue disease
Thoracic aortic aneurysm	Uncommon
Atrial enlargement	Uncommon
Severe kyphosis	Uncommon. Posture may help, regurgitation common
Post neck surgery (Cervical myelopathy)	5–50%. Rates dependent on type of surgery

Neurogenic dysphagia

Bedside assessment using a standardised water swallow test can be used as a screening tool, although validation is limited outside acute stroke. Detailed assessment by speech and language therapists is undertaken incorporating modified textures, auscultation, and pulse oximetry. Further investigations are required for selected patients when silent aspiration is suspected or unclear:

• videofluoroscopy (VFS)
• flexible endoscopic evaluation of swallowing (FEES).

Oesophageal disorders

• Endoscopy
• Barium swallow
• CT/MR

For motility disorders

• Manometry

Pharmacological therapy

There are currently no pharmacological agents used in standard practice for neurogenic dysphagia, although L-dopa, black pepper oil and capsaicin have been trialled.

Calcium channel blockers and nitrates may benefit some oesophageal spasm disorders.

Oral and dental care: antibacterial gel may reduce the risk of pneumonia in stroke patients, but is not widely available. Regular oral care is important.

Non-pharmacological therapy

Speech and language therapy (SLT) interventions

SLT interventions improve recovery in stroke related dysphagia. They may combine a number of modalities of food and fluid consistency trials along with pharyngeal stimulation techniques (e.g. Thermal).

Neurostimulation (pharyngeal electrical and transcranial magnetic stimulation) is currently under investigation.

Compensatory techniques can be taught to patients (chin tuck, head turning).

Nutritional interventions

Oral supplementation is of benefit only in those with undernutrition; however, patients with dysphagia are at high risk and dietetic input should occur at an early stage. Nutritional scores may help to identify those at high risk.

Depending on the cause of the dysphagia and the prognosis, there are a number of options for supplementing nutrition in the short and long term.

- Nasogastric tube feeding (NGT): for short-term nutrition
- Percutaneous endoscopic gastrostomy (PEG): for long-term nutrition
- Radiologically inserted gastrostomy (RIG): for patients at risk of respiratory compromise (motor neurone disease/PD) or where standard PEG insertion is anatomically difficult.
- Nasal or percutaneous jejunal tubes; for those with prior gastrectomy or poor gastric emptying.
- Surgical gastrostomies are rarely used and are associated with higher mortality rates.

The insertion of gastrostomies is associated with significant mortality (1–2%) and morbidity (5–20%) and risks and benefits need to be weighed in the best interests of the person. This is particularly important in those people with dementia where the insertion of PEG tubes does not appear to change and may hasten time to death.

Surgical interventions

Myotomy may be considered in achalasia.

Prognosis

People with dysphagia have poor prognosis because of the underlying cause and the associated complications. The only exceptions to this are some of the benign motility disorders.

Further reading

Bath PM, Bath FJ, Smithard DG (2000). Interventions for dysphagia in acute stroke. *Cochrane Database Syst Rev*, (2): CD000323.

Brady M, Furlanetto D, Hunter RV, *et al* (2006). Staff-led interventions for improving oral hygiene in patients following stroke. *Cochrane Database Syst Rev*, (4): CD003864.

Carnaby G, Hankey GJ, Pizzi J (2006). Behavioural interventions for acute stroke. *Lancet Neurol* **5**: 31–7.

Gosney M, Martin MV, Wright AE (2006). The role of the selective decontamination of the digestive tract in acute stroke. *Age Ageing* **35**: 42–7.

McCullough GH, Wertz RT, Rosenbek JC (2001). Sensitivity and specificity of clinical/bedside examination signs for detecting aspiration in adults subsequent for stroke. *J Commun Disord* **34**: 55–72.

Rohkamm R (2004). *Color atlas of Neurology*, 2nd edn. Thieme Clinical Series. New York, Thieme.

Royal College of Physicians and British Society of Gastroenterologists (2010). Oral feeding difficulties and dilemmas. A guide to practical care, particularly towards end of life. Report of a working party.

Liver disease

Increasing numbers of older people are being diagnosed with chronic liver disease (CLD) and increasing numbers of younger people with CLD are surviving into older age. Geriatricians are therefore seeing escalating numbers of patients with abnormal liver function. Although the aged liver maintains function remarkably well, there are some minor changes which make it more susceptible to injury and less able to regenerate.

Acute liver failure

Acute liver failure is exceptionally rare in older people, and as such evidence-based treatment is lacking and should follow that of younger people where appropriate. The most likely causes are viral and drug-induced hepatitis. Acute failure secondary to hepatitis A virus is more severe in the older patient, with more complications and an increased mortality.

Ischaemic hepatitis is increasing in the older population. It is seen in approximately 1% of critical care patients with a mean age of 70 years. Aminotransaminases and lactate dehydrogenase (LDH) levels rise dramatically as a result of hypoxia, hypotension, decreased perfusion, or venous congestion. Although it is potentially reversible, it carries a high mortality rate of 45%. It is an exceedingly rare cause of acute liver failure in older people.

Chronic liver disease

Clinical presentation

Older people are more likely to have non-specific symptoms which are easily attributed to other comorbidities or medication side effects, and a high index of suspicion is required. Abnormal liver function tests (LFTs) of unknown cause is the commonest reason for referral to a hepatologist and are often identified unexpectedly. Older people are more likely to have clinical signs of chronic liver disease (CLD) than younger people, possibly due to unrecognized longstanding disease.

Investigations

LFTs are often classed as hepatic (elevated alanine transaminase (ALT)) or obstructive (elevated bilirubin and alkaline phosphatase (ALP)) but in practice this is unreliable as most CLDs cause a mixed picture. Table 7.2 describes the causes to consider when investigating abnormal liver function. Table 7.3 describes the investigations to consider when the cause is not apparent.

Author's Tip

Advancing age has no independent effect on serum alkaline phosphatase, bilirubin, transaminases, gamma-glutamyl transpeptidase, or coagulation. Therefore abnormalities should be investigated with diligence.

The liver screen includes investigations to establish liver disease severity, such as the full blood count, coagulation, and ultrasound. Liver biopsy should not be discouraged because of advancing age as there is no age-associated increase in mortality with this procedure. Alpha-1 antitrypsin, ferritin, HFE genotyping, serum caeruloplasmin, and urinary copper are rarely diagnostic in the older person but are considered if other screening tests are negative.

Table 7.2 Causes of abnormal liver function tests

Common	Uncommon	Rare
Non-alcoholic fatty liver disease	Viral hepatitis	Cholangiocarcinoma
Alcoholic liver disease	Primary biliary cirrhosis	Haemochromatosis
Drugs (commonly statins, antibiotics, NSAIDs)	Autoimmune hepatitis	Alpha-1-antitrypsin deficiency
Gall stones	Hepatocellular carcinoma	Primary sclerosing cholangitis
Right ventricular failure		Wilson's disease
Malignancy		Ischaemic hepatitis

Investigations to consider for CLD

Full blood count and coagulation; Glucose and lipids

Alkaline phosphatase sub type

Immunoglobulins and auto antibodies

HBsAg, HBeAg, HBV DNA, HCV Ab, HCV DNA

Alpha fetoprotein

Abdominal ultrasound / CT; ERCP / MRCP

Liver biopsy

General management

General principles apply to all individuals with CLD, irrespective of advancing age. There are however several issues which may need to be considered.

Orthostatic hypotension may result from treatment with diuretics, laxatives and fluid restriction. Treatment is challenging, particularly if fluid restriction is necessary.

Incontinence: both urinary and faecal, from diuretic and laxative use and treatments such as ursodeoxycholic acid.

Polypharmacy: when patients develop cirrhosis and start medications such as beta-blockers, diuretics and laxatives as well as treatments for the cause of the CLD. In general, caution is required when prescribing to people who show decreased synthetic function of the liver (low serum albumin or abnormal clotting), when dosages may need reducing and liver function should be monitored.

Osteoporosis is common in individuals with cirrhosis; screening should be considered in all older people with CLD, especially in those with previous fracture, on steroid treatment, undergoing transplantation or with primary biliary cirrhosis (PBC).

Encephalopathy may be more subtle in older people because of coexisting cognitive impairment or delirium. Evidence specific to older age is lacking. Lactulose, used to improve cognition and quality of life, may cause incontinence, malabsorption, dehydration, and electrolyte disturbance.

Ascites resistant to diuretics may be treated with paracentesis. For refractory ascites, a transjugular intrahepatic portosystemic shunt (TIPS) may be required. Recent evidence refutes previous claims that encephalopathy was more common in those over 60 years following TIPS.

Oesophageal varices have similar short- and long-term survival rates in young and older adults. Injection sclerotherapy may result in higher rebleeding rates, more complications, and increased mortality rates in older than in younger people. There is a poor evidence base for terlipressin and octreotide in older patients, with decisions made on an individual basis; terlipressin is contraindicated in those with vascular disease.

Transplantation in adults aged over 60 years is increasing but there is little data for those over 70 years. While older age *per se* is not a contraindication, more rigorous screening in this group (coronary disease, malignancy, diabetes) results in higher risk patients being excluded. Consequently, for those over 60 years compared with younger patients, there are similar rates for survival, post-transplantation hospital stay, repeat admissions, infections, rejections, and repeat transplantation. Factors associated with poor survival in the older patients are low serum albumin, high bilirubin, abnormal clotting, being an inpatient prior to transplantation and a raised Child–Pugh score. Malignancy is the commonest cause of death in older patients compared with infections in younger people.

Chronic liver diseases

Non-alcoholic fatty liver disease
The incidence of non-alcoholic fatty liver disease (NAFLD) is rising dramatically. Risk factors include diabetes, hypertension, and dyslipidaemia. Over one-quarter of people with NAFLD are over 60 years and it is more severe in older people. Symptoms and signs are typically non-specific. Diagnosis is based on the presence of risk factors, the absence of other causes, and a bright or cirrhotic liver on ultrasound. Biopsy may be required to confirm the diagnosis but raised serum insulin and C-peptide levels can support the diagnosis. Treatment consists of lifestyle modification and addressing risk factors. There is emerging evidence for the use of insulin-sensitizing medication and other pharmacological agents, but at present further evidence is required.

Alcoholic liver disease
Almost one-third of people with alcoholic liver disease (ALD) present over the age of 60 years. Patients are typically asymptomatic but dizziness is the most common symptom when symptoms are present. Histology shows more advanced disease in older people than younger on presentation. Acute withdrawal can be subtle and easily missed. Treatment does not differ between age groups although the effects of benzodiazepines in the older patient can be prolonged.

Autoimmune liver disease
Both autoimmune hepatitis (AIH) and primary biliary cirrhosis (PBC) are more common in females and typically present after the menopause. Patients present with non-specific symptoms such as fatigue or pruritus, asymptomatically or rarely with advanced disease. AIH can be diagnosed with a raised immunoglobulin (Ig)G and positive autoantibodies (antinuclear, smooth muscle, type 1 liver kidney microsomal) Treatment of AIH is usually with prednisolone, azathioprine, or a combination of both, with excellent response rates in older people. PBC is associated with raised IgM and anti mitochondrial antibodies. The management of PBC is generally symptomatic; ursodeoxycholic acid may benefit some patients but evidence that it prolongs survival is inconsistent.

Viral hepatitis
Hepatitis B (HBV) is uncommon in older adults but outbreaks have been reported in care homes related to shared razors, sexual contact, and non-disposable syringes. Older people are less likely to have been vaccinated against HBV and are less likely to have an effective immune response. Hepatitis C (HCV) is more common in older people who have had previous transfusions. Presentation is usually asymptomatic but possible symptoms include malaise, nausea, vomiting, and abdominal pain. Diagnosis is through serology tests. Treatment with interferon is effective in older patients but is more likely to cause side-effects (fatigue, anorexia, and depression). Antiviral agents are effective in older people for both HBV and HCV. Older people with HCV progress to cirrhosis faster than younger patients and have an increased risk of hepatocellular carcinoma (HCC).

Hepatocellular carcinoma
Up to one-third of patients with HCC are over 70 years. It typically presents as an acute deterioration in liver function in someone with existing CLD, and 90% of older people with HCC have a raised alpha-fetoprotein level. Treatment outcomes are similar in younger and older patients and age *per se* should not preclude resection, transplantation, embolization, or radiofrequency.

Other chronic liver diseases
- Primary sclerosing cholangitis typically affects younger males and is rare in older people.
- Alpha-1-antitrypsin deficiency rarely presents in older age but is more likely in lifelong non-smokers.
- Haemochromatosis typically presents in middle age but there is evidence that males who are homozygous for the C282Y gene are surviving into old age, and the therapeutic effect of menstruation may result in females presenting post-menopausally.
- Wilson's disease is extremely rare in older people.

Further reading

Al-Chalabi T, Boccato S, Portmann B, et al. (2006). Autoimmune hepatitis (AIH) in the elderly: A systematic retrospective analysis of a large group of consecutive patients with definite AIH followed at a tertiary referral centre. *J Hepatol* **45**: 575–83.

Brind A, Watson J, James O, et al. (1996). Hepatitis C virus infection in the elderly. *Q J Med* **89**: 291–6.

Bullimore DW, Miloszewski KJ, Losowsky MS (1989). The prognosis of elderly subjects with oesophageal varices. *Age Ageing* **18**: 35–8.

Collier J, Curless R, Bassendine M, et al. (1994). Clinical Features and prognosis of hepatocellular carcinoma in Britain in relation to age. *Age Ageing* **23**: 22–7.

Frith J, Day C, Henderson E, et al. (2009). Non-alcoholic fatty liver disease in older people. *Gerontology* **55**: 607–13.

Garcia C, Garcia R, Mayer A, et al. (2001). Liver transplantation in patients over sixty years of age. *Transplantation* **72**: 679–84.

Newton J, Jones D, Metcalf J, et al. (2000). Presentation and mortality of primary biliary cirrhosis in older patients. *Age Ageing* **29**: 305–9.

Potter J, James O (1987). Clinical features and prognosis of alcoholic liver disease in respect of advancing age. *Gerontology* **33**: 380–7.

Nutrition and nutritional intervention

Nutrition is essential to health and wellbeing. The physio-logical requirements for nutrients changes throughout our lives. Periods of growth during pregnancy, childhood, and adolescence make different nutritional demands. On reaching maturity our primary requirement is for main-tenance and repair, while the physiological changes associ-ated with the ageing process create changed priorities to maintain health and combat disease.

Malnutrition and particularly undernutrition are often overlooked as factors in the development and progression of disease. Timely assessment and treatment of malnutri-tion should be an integral part of clinical management. The challenge therefore is to optimize nutritional interventions for the changing needs of an older population (see Table 7.3).

Factors affecting ability to meet nutritional requirements

However good the available diet is for a person, if they are unable to eat it or extract the nutrients from the food it is of no nutritional value. The goal as clinicians is to remove the barriers to good nutritional status and to optimize the nutritional status of the patient (see Table 7.4).

Table 7.3 Older people's nutritional requirements

Age (years)	Estimated average energy requirements megajoules (kcal)/day	
	Male	Female
60–64	9.93 (2380)	7.99 (1900)
65–74	9.71 (2330)	7.99 (1900)
75+	8.77 (2100)	7.61 (1810)

Nutrient (reference nutrient intake)	Male (50+ years)	Female (50+ years)
Protein (g/d)	53.3	46.5
Thiamin mg/d	0.9	0.8
Riboflavin mg/d	1.3	1.1
Niacin mg/d	16	12
Vitamin B6 mg/d	1.4	1.2
Vitamin B12 µg/d	1.5	1.5
Folate mcg/d	200	200
Vitamin C mg/d	40	40
Vitamin D µg/d	10 (after age 65)	10 (after age 65)
Calcium mg/d	700	700
Magnesium mg/d	300	270
Iron mg/d	8.7	8.7
Zinc mg/d	9.5	7.0
Selenium µg/d	75	60

Department of Health: Nutrition of older people COMA 1992.

Table 7.4 Factors influencing ability to meet nutritional needs

Sensory	Sight
	Hearing
	Taste
	Smell
	Touch
Musculoskeletal	Mobility
	Dexterity
	Dentition
	Swallowing
Gastrointestinal (GI)	GI secretions: saliva/stomach acid/bile/pancreatic secretions
	Gut motility
	Intestinal absorption and elimination
Psychological	Isolation
	Depression
	Cognitive impairment
Socio-cultural	Access to food
	Economic factors
	Religious and cultural beliefs and preferences
	Decreased social contacts

Given this range of factors influencing nutritional status in older people, it is evident that in a population where there are complex clinical conditions nutritional manage-ment requires highly skilled practitioners with extensive knowledge of their specific needs.

Healthy eating and disease prevention
The Eat Well Plate (Food Standards Agency) provides a food group-focused approach to nutrition. Each of the five food groups is proportionally represented. Additional information to support this is also provided in the Food Standards agency '8 steps to a healthy diet'. The recently updated leaflet 'The Good Life' (FSA) provides healthy eating and lifestyle advice for those over 50 years old with a focus on heart health and bone health. This information provides a simple model that is easily adapted to help manage type 2 diabetes, hyperlipidaemia and obesity.

Factors to consider with food based change
• Patient knowledge about nutrition, their condition and how the two interact.
• Patient skills and abilities to implement dietary change.
• Patient motivation—the extent to which the patient is able psychologically to pursue the changes in both the immediate and longer term if necessary.

Non-clinical factors increasing risk of nutritional deficiency
Three key factors emerged from the National Diet and Nutrition Survey of Older Adults (1998):
• low income
• poor dentition
• living in institutions.

The findings showed that these populations were more likely to have diets deficient in a range of nutrients. Of particular concern were vitamin C, folate, thiamine, riboflavin, vitamin D, and iron. It is likely that subclinical deficiencies are more common in the at risk populations. Poor wound healing, fatigue, anaemia, cognitive impairment, and increased risk of fracture are known consequences of vitamin deficiency.

Supplementation of vitamin D in patients over 65 years is recommended at a level of 10 µg/day with further recommendation to consume foods rich in vitamin D and calcium to promote bone health. Supplementation of other nutrients (e.g. folic acid for megaloblastic anaemia) may be effective short-term measures but fail to address poor dietary intake as a possible cause.

Protein and energy malnutrition

Screening for malnutrition using tools such as the Malnutrition Universal Screening Tool (MUST) highlights those at risk of becoming malnourished (see Table 7.5).

Sarcopenia, frailty and anorexia of ageing

Muscle declines in an ageing population. Sarcopenia (loss of muscle mass and quality) can be seen as a consequence of disease (e.g. cancer, chronic obstructive pulmonary disease, heart failure) but is also seen as a result of inactivity. The speed with which muscle deteriorates increases in older people and is even more rapid in hospitalized patients.

Features for doctors and nurses to look for suggestive of malnutrition run from the most basic observations, such as whether the patient looks thin, to other features, such as whether their clothes are too baggy, any watches or rings look loose, and the same for dentures. Assessment in a clinical setting can also use a combination of grip strength, gait speed, and bioimpedance analysis apparatus (other measures are available). Those patients in the lower fifth of the standard are at high risk of decline.

The impact of loss of muscle is a reduction in strength and power leading to an increased risk of falls and reduced weight-bearing activity. As inactivity becomes the norm, appetite stimulation is decreased with lower intake of foods a likely consequence. With increasing frailty, the likelihood of disability as a result of clinical, psychological, and social factors increases.

Anorexia of ageing is the extreme decline in intake where the individual has become almost completely dependent. Physiological changes in gut function leading to early satiation have been identified as contributory factors. Cholecystokinin produced in response to lipid levels in the gut increases the perceived level of satiety and may decrease intake as the patient feels full.

Treatment to prevent the downward spiral should start at the earliest opportunity. Assessment of usual intake through a combination of diet recall, assessing frequency of eating, usual foods eaten, and portion sizes through interview and written records (if available). A combination of nutritional improvements to quality and quantity of foods and drinks and a programme of exercise routines designed to increase and strengthen muscle should be adopted. The consumption of protein foods at mealtimes together with low volumes of protein- and energy-rich liquids between meals and the encouragement of protein intake after exercise help the development of muscle mass. These measures may help to improve mood and confidence as well as nutritional status. Appetite stimulants and other therapies to enhance muscle development can complement the nutrition and exercise programme.

Refeeding syndrome

Patients who have had significant recent weight loss, are underweight, and have had poor or no oral intake for ≥5 days may be at risk of developing refeeding syndrome. This is characterized by abnormal biochemistry, particularly electrolytes, phosphate, and magnesium, on consumption of food. Feeding to the patient's energy requirements produces an insulin response, drawing potassium into the cells and reducing circulating levels. Electrolyte levels become abnormal and may be associated with rapid drops in magnesium and phosphate. This can precipitate cardiac arrhythmias associated with hypokalaemia and other complications associated with hypophosphataemia and low magnesium.

Prior to feeding it is advisable to supplement with thiamine and to correct any existing biochemical deficiency. Feeding should be introduced slowly, aiming to provide no more than 10 calories/kg over 24 hours, and in the case of high-risk patients this may need to be reduced. Daily review of biochemistry is advisable and correction through additional supplementation of potassium, phosphate and magnesium as indicated. As intake increases and body stores are replenished the monitoring should continue but less frequently.

Nutrition and acute illness

The hospital diet traditionally provides around 1800–2000 calories on average per day if the patient is eating all meals and snacks. The estimated average requirement for an older adult ranges between 1800 and 2400 kcal/day. However, activity levels for hospital patients are estimated to be at least 15% lower than people living freely. If a patient is only managing half of their food, we can see their intake will be somewhere around 900–1000 calories per day. The cumulative effect of poor intake and increased demand can quickly escalate weight loss and significantly impact on wound healing and immunocompetence.

Where possible, the patient should be engaged in changes to their diet; they are the experts in their own dietary preferences and habits. Discussing the situation with the patient, including enquiry about their usual diet and whether they recognize that they have lost weight, maximizes the chances of any interventions being successful in preventing further weight loss and then promoting weight gain.

Nutrition support

Assessment of nutritional needs (energy, protein, fluid, and electrolyte requirements) based on basal energy needs

Table 7.5 Malnutrition Universal Screening Tool score

Score	BMI kg/m² score	Unplanned weight loss in past 3–6 months	Oral intake
0	>20	<5%	
1	18.5–20	5–10%	
2	<18.5	>10%	If patient is acutely ill and there has been or is likely to be no nutritional intake for >5 days

The scores for each column are added together. Those scoring 0 are at low risk of malnutrition, 1 denotes possible risk, and those scoring 2 or more are at high risk.

BAPEN. Malnutrition Universal Screening Tool (MUST) (www.bapen.org).

with addition of stress and activity factors provide a guide to current energy needs. It is worth noting that an increase in temperature of 1°C above normal will increase energy requirements by 10%. Protein needs vary with the patient's metabolic condition.

Example

A 72-year-old woman weighing 58 kg, BMI 22 kg/m^2 admitted with a stroke. Currently bed bound and immobile
- Energy requirements: basal metabolic rate = 1220
- Activity and stress factors = 15%
- Estimated energy requirement = 1400 kcal/day
- Protein requirements – normal (0.14–0.20 gN/day) = 51–72.5 g/day
- Fluid requirements (30 mL/kg) = 1740 mL/day

Strategies for managing patients in need of nutrition support are documented in the NICE guidance (2006). This describes the process of assessment and provides decision making tools. The application of this guidance is now commonplace in hospitals in the UK and supported by the National Patients Safety Agency.

Oral route available

Food fortification should be used where possible and there should be a focus on increasing the intake of nutrient dense foods.

Simple strategies include fortifying milk with milk powder and using in drinks and milk-based dishes such as sauces, custard, and milk puddings. Others include using energy-dense foods such as butter, cream, spreading fats and oils, or adding protein with eggs, meats, nut butters, or grated cheese. Protein foods should be eaten at all mealtimes and high-calorie snacks (e.g. cakes, buttered scones, fancy biscuits, cheese and crackers) between meals.

Where food fortification is insufficient to manage the patients need for nutritional support there is a range of products available to assist in providing protein and energy. Dietetic strategies to enhance intake with minimal impact on food intake build on the use of these supplements at times when food is unlikely to be consumed in quantity, e.g. between meals, after eating, in the evening prior to retiring. Commonly these supplements are presented in 200–250 mL bottles and supply 100–200 calories per 100 mL. Higher energy supplements supplying up to 450 calories per 100 mL are generally fat based and not well tolerated at doses above this. Using a combination of supplements to meet requirements is likely to prove more successful as there may be elements of taste fatigue associated with continuing the same supplement.

Although there may be compensation in normal weight patients (i.e. increasing the supplement decreases the intake of foods), for patients who are underweight this is not the case.

Patients with compromised gut function (e.g. short bowel syndrome) may need hydrolysed protein (peptides or amino acids preparations) to maintain nutritional status. The palatability of these products is poor and patient compliance may be affected. These are best served well flavoured and chilled and in a lidded cup or with a straw to reduce the bitter tastes and unpleasant odour. Overnight nasogastric tube feeding may be appropriate in the short term.

GI functioning but oral route not available/not sufficient

Nasogastric, percutaneous endoscopic gastrostomy (PEG) tube, jejunostomy tube can be considered, with nutrition being delivered directly into the gut. Nutritional needs are met by liquid feeds calculated by the dietician appropriate to the patient's condition. These feeds again supply 100–200 calories per 100 mL and are nutritionally complete (contain protein, energy, and micronutrients) according to the manufacturer's minimum dose.

The feed can be manipulated to meet the nutritional needs of clinical conditions such as diabetes or renal disease. The various methods of delivery such as continuous or intermittent feeding using an enteral feeding pump, bolus feeding, or a combination of pump and bolus feeding can be manipulated to meet the patient's environmental needs. In some cases this is used to support oral intake when oral intake alone is insufficient to meet nutritional needs.

Regular review is essential to ensure nutritional and hydration needs continue to be met. Anthropometry and biochemistry will indicate whether a change in the feed prescription is needed. Patients who are discharged from hospital on feed regimens require regular monitoring and follow up in the community.

GI route not available

Parenteral nutrition should be considered, with nutrition being delivered through intravenous pump directly into the bloodstream. Advice and support with this should be sought from the specialist nutrition team. Patients should be assessed on clinical need.

Dysphagia and diet

Chewing and swallowing problems associated with neurological disease can lead to a rapid decline in health as eating becomes more difficult. Progressive conditions such as motor neurone disease, Parkinson's disease, and multiple sclerosis, and acute events such as a stroke can leave patients unable to eat food without modification of texture and/or fluid consistency. Where the plan is to normalize food as much as possible, the concern is to maintain nutritional intake and minimize risk of choking and aspiration.

Easy chew diet – foods cooked until soft and easily crushed with a fork and can have a mixture of food and fluids (e.g. thin gravies or sauces). Often this option is used for patients who are able to eat but fatigue if eating becomes too effortful. Suitable dishes are, for example poached fish in sauce, chicken or sausage casserole, macaroni cheese or cannelloni, cottage pie with gravy.

Soft diet – may contain soft lumps that are easily crushed with a fork or by the tongue on the roof of the mouth. Examples include shepherds' pie, poached plaice in cheese sauce, and tuna mayonnaise with mashed potato. This is accompanied by thick sauces or gravies to prevent aspiration particularly in patients with delayed swallow. Foods to be avoided are peas/beans where the husk does not break down, stringy foods such as celery, pineapple or runner beans, and foods that form a solid bolus such as toffees or fresh bread.

Puree diet – smooth consistency that requires no chewing and forms a soft easily swallowed bolus in the mouth. These foods require fortification with protein and energy to enable the patient to meet their needs. Patients will need to eat regularly (five or six times a day) in order to meet their requirements.

Ideas to improve nutritional value of pureed diets.
- Add extra butter, cream, grated cheese, milk to improve the energy and protein content.

- Add pureed fruit to custards or smooth thick yoghurt.
- Thickened fluids (coffee, fruit juice) can be chilled and eaten as a pudding if there is difficulty drinking.

Polypharmacy and nutrition

With an aged population the need to manage clinical conditions using prescribed drugs is commonplace. The interaction **between** drugs and nutrients can influence both positively and negatively the efficacy of the pharmacological treatment. Examples include:

- The absorption of iron is positively influenced by the presence of vitamin C (commonly found in fruit juices), whereas the converse is true for tannins and polyphenols (commonly found in tea).
- Dietary proteins can reduce the absorption of some drugs to treat Parkinson's disease and adversely affect absorption of phenytoin, where food should not be consumed for two hours before and after oral administration.
- Grapefruit juice increases the plasma concentration of statins and concomitant use is recommended.
- Increased intake of foods containing vitamin K may affect clotting in patients taking warfarin.
- Metformin to control type 2 diabetes is implicated in vitamin B12 deficiency.

Side effects from drugs, such as reduced saliva production, gastrointestinal disturbance, nausea, appetite suppression and constipation, can lead to reduced oral intake and malnutrition. (See BNF Appendix 1 for details.)

Strategies to improve the dietary intake of older people in hospitals

On the hospital ward access to food is limited but a range of actions are recommended. Examples of these include:

- Age appropriate food: foods that currently form part of the patient's diet and are culturally appropriate and promote personal choice.
- Protected mealtimes: disruptions to eating such as ward rounds, tests, and investigations are kept to a minimum.
- Fortified menus: foods on the menu are fortified with extra protein/energy.
- Energy dense snacks: patients are offered foods and drinks that have a higher energy value, e.g. biscuits and cheese or cake rather than fruits, milk-based drinks rather than water.
- Red tray system: for patients who need assistance to eat a red tray helps staff to identify that they will need to spend time with this individual at mealtimes.
- Give drinks after meals and avoid unfortified soups as a starter, that are likely to prevent patients eating a more nutritious main meal.
- Ensure adequate hydration (6–8 drinks a day) to help prevent dehydration and constipation.
- Constipation should be treated early as this reduces appetite/oral intake.
- Adequate support and time for patients who need assistance and may take a long while to eat. Relatives and friends can be useful to help prompt patients with impaired cognition at mealtimes.

There is ongoing research addressing age-related deterioration in taste sensations, and the addition of natural flavour enhancers to improve oral intake.

Improving nutrition in the community

Older people are increasingly at risk of being isolated from their communities. Access to local services is affected by resource limitations and increased reliance on communication technologies that are developed by and for a younger population. These often require increased dexterity and complex technological instruction to gain access although the ageing population is becoming more familiar with these technologies.

Group education sessions for diabetes and weight management are available in most health communities and deliver programmes providing information, motivation, and support. Dieticians can provide domiciliary visits to support patients unable to travel.

Community dieticians are frequently involved in developing, implementing and evaluating community nutrition programmes. Community strategies to address some of the barriers to good nutrition require the involvement of a range of skills and organizations.

- Food delivery services that provide prepared meals that can be reheated or are delivered ready to eat are frequently used for patients unable to prepare their own foods easily.
- Care agencies may be commissioned to provide support to individuals to assist with their nutritional needs, helping to shop, prepare, and cook food.
- The use of lunch clubs and day centres where food is part of the service helps to prevent social isolation, can improve intake and may provide a monitoring function for at risk patients.
- Food delivery services such as those run by local cooperatives or by supermarkets help those patients who find carrying heavy items difficult.
- Residential and nursing home care is closely regulated and nutritional standards are part of the registration criteria.
- Education and training is available from community dieticians for individuals, groups, and organizations.

Further reading

BAPEN. Malnutrition Universal Screening Tool (MUST) (www. bapen.org)

British Dietetic Association and the Royal College of Speech and Language Therapists (2009). *National Descriptors for Texture Modification in Adults*. BDA and the Royal College of Speech and Language Therapists.

British Dietetic Association website – Nutrition Advisory Group for the Elderly (www.bda.uk.com).

Caroline Walker Trust (2004). *Eating Well for Older People – Practical and Nutritional Guidelines for Food in Residential and Nursing Homes and Community Meals*, 2nd edn. (www.cwt.org. uk).

Chernoff R (2006). *Geriatric Nutrition – The Health Professionals Handbook*, 3rd edn. New York, Aspen.

Cruz-Hentoft AJ, et al. (2009). Ageing Sarcopenia and Nutrition. Proceedings of the 2009 Hot Topics Meeting, Edinburgh, Abbott Laboratories.

DH (1990). *Dietary Reference Values for Food Energy and Nutrients in the United Kingdom*. Report on Health and Social Subjects No 41. London, HMSO.

DH (1992). *The Nutrition of Elderly People*. (Report on Health and Social Subjects No 43. London, HMSO.

DH (1998). *National Diet and Nutrition Survey. People Aged 65 years and Over*. Vols 1 & 2. London, HMSO.

Journal of Nutrition Health and Ageing

NICE (2006). *CG32 Nutrition Support in Adults: Oral Nutritional Support, Enteral Tube Feeding and Parenteral Nutrition*. London, NICE.

Thomas B, Bishop J (eds) (2007). *Manual of Dietetic Practice*, 4th edn. Oxford, Wiley Blackwell.

Coeliac disease in older people

Introduction

Coeliac disease (CD) is a unique autoimmune disease in that the genetic predisposition and environmental triggers are known. Once thought to be a rare syndrome of childhood, it is increasingly recognized as a common disease with an increased prevalence in older people. In a recent study in Finland, the prevalence in older people was shown to be increasing at a rate not simply accounted for by increased awareness and availability of screening. The rate of increase is too rapid to be accounted for by changes in genetic susceptibility, but neither are there known changes in the environmental triggers that could explain it.

Pathophysiology

In genetically predisposed individuals, those carrying HLA-DQ2 or HLA-DQ8 genes, the ingestion of gluten, a protein derived from wheat, barley, and rye, induces a T-cell-mediated immune response in the upper small bowel mucosa resulting in atrophy of the villi and increased lymphocytes. Gliaden, the alcohol soluble fragment of gluten, is the main source of toxicity.

Epidemiology

In UK, as in other populations of European ancestry, CD occurs in up to 1% of the population, although is often undiagnosed. The disease is becoming globalized but the epidemiology in much of Asia remains little known. The prevalence of symptomatic disease in older people appears to be increasing. In the Finnish study noted above, the prevalence was greater than 2%. In younger adults, it is commoner in women but older men are affected as commonly as older women.

Clinical Spectrum

CD presents with abdominal symptoms or those resulting from malabsorption or autoimmunity.

Abdominal symptoms

The commonest abdominal symptom is diarrhoea. Flatulence, abdominal pain, and reflux are also common, and some present with constipation. There is overlap with the symptoms of irritable bowel syndrome (IBS), which may delay CD diagnosis. It should be remembered that IBS rarely presents de novo in older people.

Consequences of malabsorption

Common features are weight loss, anaemia, and bone disease.

Haematological problems

Iron and folate are absorbed from the proximal small bowel, and deficiencies are common in CD. Microcytic anaemia is a common presentation but the anaemia may be normocytic due to combined deficiency. Red cell distribution width (RDW) may be increased in combined iron and folate deficiency due to dimorphism in the red cell population. Vitamin B12 deficiency has also been reported in CD, although the mechanism is unclear as it is absorbed from the terminal ileum, which is almost always spared. The extent of the deficiency of vitamin B12 is less than that of folate but sufficient to contribute to raised homocysteine levels, which may explain the increased prevalence of stroke and cardiac events in people with CD despite lower cholesterol levels. Hyposplenism also occurs and a twofold increase in pneumococcal infections has been reported.

Autoimmunity

Gluten sensitivity affects other organs, skin being the best understood causing dermatitis herpetiformis. Neurological syndromes have been described more recently. CD is associated with other autoimmune conditions, e.g. type I diabetes, thyroid, and liver disease.

The consensus is that CD tends to present more non-specifically in older people, e.g. with lethargy due to iron-deficient anaemia, rather than with specific abdominal symptoms. However, diarrhoea and abdominal discomfort are common in series reporting clinical findings in people with CD over 65 years of age and are often present for many years prior to the diagnosis being made.

Diagnosis

Duodenal biopsy obtained at oesophagogastroduodenoscopy (OGD) remains the definitive diagnostic test. However, autoimmune processes in the small intestine result in the formation of immunolubulin (Ig)A antibodies to gliaden, endomysium, and to tissue transglutaminase (tTGA)-2.

Antigliaden antibody tests are obsolete, being neither specific nor sensitive enough, and reporting antiendomysial antibody (EmA) is labour intensive. However, the automated ELISA test for circulating tTGA has increased potential for screening. In research facilities, the sensitivity and specificity of this test approaches 100% provided selective IgA deficiency, which affects 2.5 percent of people with CD, is excluded. Total IgA is measured routinely with coeliac antibodies in some centres. In people with selective IgA deficiency, EmA or IgG tTGA should be measured. In routine clinical practice both the sensitivity and specificity of IgA tTGA are lower and false negatives may occur in older people.

There is no evidence that the ageing immune system affects the serological tests, but the tTGA test is more likely to be negative in those with milder histological changes, which may be commoner at presentation in older people with CD. Conversely, false positives have been found in people with liver disease, end-stage heart failure and in patients attending a rheumatology unit.

Treatment

Gluten-free diet is the only treatment that reverses the small bowel changes. It is not easily complied with, especially when eating out. There is little variety to products available on prescription and gluten-free non-prescription items are expensive. Dietician follow-up should always be available for patients with CD and is especially relevant for older people who may be considerably underweight at time of diagnosis and who may have other comorbidities requiring competing dietary interventions. Despite these concerns, older people comply with gluten-free diets better than younger people.

Novel approaches, including genetic modification of cereals, recombinant enzymes that digest toxic gliaden fractions intraluminally, and therapies aimed at modifying immune responses, are at various levels of development.

Complications and associations

Many of the common complications and associations of CD occur more frequently in the general ageing population. These include osteoporosis, malignancy, and microscopic colitis.

Bone disease

Osteomalacia is now rare but bone mineral density (BMD) is commonly low at presentation of CD. Calcium, vitamin D, and magnesium malabsorption with secondary hyperparathyroidism are major factors in the bone disease associated with CD, but bone-specific antibodies have been described and improvements in BMD have been reported after gluten-free diet. Whether there is an increased risk of osteoporotic fractures in the CD population overall is controversial. However, calcium and vitamin D supplements are generally required to reverse secondary hyperparathyroidism. This is particularly relevant with age-related bone loss also occurring, and an increased prevalence of hip fracture in CD patients diagnosed over the age of 60 years has been reported. It is therefore reasonable to recommend DEXA scanning for older people diagnosed with CD.

Microscopic colitis

There is an increased incidence of microscopic colitis in CD. It should be excluded by colonoscopy and biopsy in those who have persistent diarrhoea, or who relapse despite adhering to a gluten-free diet. It is eminently treatable, although it has been reported that patients in whom it is associated with CD more frequently need steroids, such as budenoside, to control symptoms.

Dermatitis herpetiformis

An intensely itchy vesicular rash associated with antibodies to transglutaminase-3. It affects up to 10% of older people with CD compared with 2–3% of younger people. Treatment is with dapsone. Patients may be able to come off this after adhering to a gluten-free diet for 18 months.

Malignancy

An increased risk of malignancy in CD was first recognized about 50 years ago. The particular risk is for the rare enteropathy-associated T-cell lymphoma (EATL), which has a poor prognosis. There also appears to be a modest increase in the incidence of non-gut lymphoproliferative disease and carcinomas of small bowel, oesophagus, and oropharynx. Strict adherence to a gluten-free diet has seemed important in preventing EATL, and it would therefore be logical to expect higher rates in undiagnosed CD or those diagnosed in later life who have had symptoms for many years prior to diagnosis. However, this has not been found to be the case.

Neurological

A number of neurological syndromes have been associated with CD, including gluten ataxia and gluten neuropathy, with formation of antibodies to neural transglutaminase (tTG-6). There are case reports of clinical improvements with gluten free diet. Those with neurological manifestations of gluten sensitivity may have no gastrointestinal symptoms and it is reasonable to request tTGA in patients with neurological dysfunction, particularly ataxia and neuropathy, for whom there is no other convincing aetiology.

Refractory coeliac disease

The commonest causes of a poor response to a gluten-free diet are non-compliance and incorrect diagnosis. Once dietetic review has ruled out non-compliance, further investigations are indicated for pancreatic insufficiency and bacterial overgrowth, which are both common causes of persistent diarrhoea in older CD patients, as well as inflammatory bowel disease, malignancy, and microscopic colitis. Five per cent of CD patients are genuinely refractory. There is a higher incidence of progression to lymphoma in this group.

Conclusion

The increasing incidence and prevalence of coeliac disease in older people, in whom the diagnosis is often delayed, justifies increased awareness as its treatment, although arduous, reduces associated morbidity and possibly mortality.

Author's Tip

All patients with iron and/or folate deficiency should be screened for CD. A raised RDW should trigger measurement of iron, folate, and B12.

Investigation of iron-deficiency anaemia should included duodenal biopsies.

People with unexplained peripheral neuropathies or ataxia should be screened for CD.

People over 60 years who are diagnosed with CD should have DEXA scans.

Follow-up by dieticians should be routine and is especially important for older CD patients.

Further reading

Dickey W (2009). Symposium 1: Joint BAPEN and British Society of Gastroenterology Symposium on 'Coeliac disease: basics and controversies' Coeliac disease in the twenty-first century. *Proc Nutr Soc* **68**: 234–41.

Gasbarrini G, Ciccocioppo R, De Vitis I, *et al.* (2001). Coeliac disease in the elderly. A multicentre Italian study. *Gerontology* **47**: 306–10.

Green PH, Cellier C (2007). Celiac Disease. *N Engl J Med* **357**: 1731–43.

Green PHR, Stavropoulos SN, Panagi SG, *et al.* (2001). Characteristics of adult celiac disease in the USA: results of a national survey. *Am J Gastroenterol* **96**: 126–31.

Hadjivassiliou M, Sanders DS, Grünewald RA, *et al.* (2010). Gluten sensitivity: from gut to brain. *Lancet Neurol* **9**: 318–30.

Hankey GL, Holmes GKT (1994). Coeliac disease in the elderly. *Gut* **35**: 65–7.

Johnson MW, Ellis HJ, Asante MA, *et al.* (2008). Celiac disease in the elderly. *Nat Clin Pract Gastroenterol Hepatol* **5**: 697–706.

Logan RFA (2009). Malignancy in unrecognised coeliac disease: a nail in the coffin for mass screening? *Gut* **58**: 618–19.

Lurie Y, Landau D-A, Pfeffer J, *et al.* (2008). Coeliac disease diagnosed in the elderly. *J Clin Gastroenterol*, **42**: 59–61.

Schuppan D, Junker Y, Barisani D (2009). Celiac disease: from pathogenesis to novel therapies. *Gastroenterology* **137**: 1912–33.

Tilg H, Moschen AR, Kaser A, *et al.* (2008). Gut, inflammation and osteoporosis: basic and clinical concepts. *Gut* **57**: 684–94.

Vilppula A, Kaukinen K Luostarinen L, *et al.* (2009). Increasing prevalence and high incidence of celiac disease in elderly people: a population based study. *BMC Gastroenterol* **9**: 49.

Gastrointestinal bleeding

Upper gastrointestinal bleeding

Definition and clinical presentation
Upper gastrointestinal bleeding (UGIB) refers to haemorrhage arising from the oesophagus, stomach, or duodenum. The key symptoms of overt UGIB are haematemesis and/or melaena (>100 mL blood loss for melaena). The main causes of UGIB in adults are found in Table 7.6. Reports for older patients suggest a higher frequency of severe oesophagitis, non-steroidal anti-inflammatory drug (NSAID)-associated erosion/ulceration, and malignancy than in younger patients

Clinical assessment and risk scores
Assessment: Evidence of hypovolaemia; dyspeptic symptoms (often absent); drug history (antiplatelet agents, NSAIDs, anticoagulants, SSRIs, cholinesterase inhibitors); previous peptic ulceration; alcohol abuse; evidence of chronic liver disease (varices).

Acute management involves basic supportive care, including managing hypovolaemia/blood loss and clotting abnormalities. Treat comorbid illness and optimize cardiorespiratory status prior to intervention.

Risk stratification with a validated scoring system (e.g. Rockall (see Table 7.7 and Figure 7.5) or Blatchford) to estimate risk of mortality and guide timing of gastroscopy. Patients with suspected varices require early specialist input.

IV proton pump inhibitor commenced prior to gastroscopy is of uncertain benefit – it reduces the proportion of patients with stigmata of recent haemorrhage (SRH) at index endoscopy but an effect on mortality, re-bleeding or the need for surgery is not proven.

Gastroscopy. General anaesthetic may be required in high risk patients. Endoscopy helps confirm diagnosis, offers therapeutic options and guides risk stratification.

Endoscopic haemostatic therapy for non-variceal bleeding is targeted to high risk stigmata of recent haemorrhage (active spurting vessel, adherent fresh clot, visible non-bleeding vessel). Modalities include injection (e.g. adrenaline), thermal ablation and physical measures ('clips'). Dual modality therapy (e.g. adrenaline injection followed by heater probe) has been shown to be superior to single modality. Failure to secure haemostasis in active peptic ulcer bleeding requires consideration of surgery or interventional radiology (angiography with selective arterial

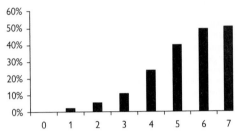

Figure 7.5 Mortality risk by Rockall Score Mortality (%, on vertical axis) versus pre-endoscopy Rockall score (on horizontal axis). Reproduced from 'Risk assessment following acute upper gastrointestinal haemorrhage' in *Gut*, Rockall T A, Logan R F A, Devlin H B, *et al.*, **38**, 3, pp. 316–21, 1996 with permission from BMJ Publishing Group Ltd.

embolization). A second attempt at endotherapy can reduce the need for surgery if re-bleeding occurs after initial haemostasis.

Bleeding oesophageal varices are treated by rubber band ligation ('banding') and/or injection of sclerosant. This is of limited benefit for gastric varices (glue injection can be used). If haemostasis of brisk bleeding is not possible, physical tamponade (e.g. Sengstaken-Blakemore tube) can stabilise the patient prior to repeat attempts at endotherapy or escalation to interventional radiology (transvenous intrahepatic portosystemic shunt, 'TIPSS', if the portal venous system is patent). Acute shunt surgery or oesophageal transection is available in specialist centres.

Specific therapy after endoscopy. For peptic ulcers requiring endoscopic haemostatic therapy, outcome is improved by omeprazole infusion, followed by oral proton pump inhibitor (PPI). Ulcers not requiring endotherapy are treated with standard dose PPI (intravenous initially, oral once eating). The duration of PPI therapy is tailored to the individual patient and endoscopic findings, but in severe bleeds treatment is often continued long term. *H. pylori* infection can be treated once normal diet is resumed and bleeding has stopped. Aspirin and NSAID use should be avoided where possible and the risk-benefit of any long term anticoagulation reassessed.

For bleeding varices, intravenous vasopressor agents (e.g. terlipressin) are used acutely. Patients with decompensated chronic liver disease are at risk of sepsis and broad spectrum antibiotics are recommended after endoscopic intervention. Beta-blockade with propranolol is established in secondary prophylaxis against re-bleeding. Oral nitrates are an alternative if there are contra-indications or side effects from propranolol.

Follow-up gastroscopy should be arranged to ensure healing of all gastric ulcers in order to exclude undiagnosed malignancy after 6–8 weeks. Patients with oesophageal varices require regular banding or sclerotherapy.

Table 7.6 Causes and frequency of upper gastrointestinal bleeding

Peptic ulcer (duodenal, gastric and stomal)	30–35%
Varices	5–10%
Oesophagitis	10–15%
Mallory–Weiss tear	5%
Erosions (gastric and duodenal)	10–15%
Tumours (benign and malignant)	2–4%
Vascular malformations	1–3%
Small bowel and colonic	5%
No source found	20–22%

Source: Palmer K (2006). Acute upper gastrointestinal bleeding. *Medicine* **35**: 3:b157. Elsevier Ltd.

> **Author's Tip**
>
> Use a scoring system to stratify mortality risk.
>
> Optimize condition before gastroscopy—liaise with anaesthetist if 'high risk' (e.g. shocked patient; hypoxia; high aspiration risk).
>
> Severe bleeds require access to multidisciplinary management (gastroenterology, intensivists, interventional radiology, and surgery).

Table 7.7 Rockall score

	Score (maximum additive score prior to endoscopy = 7; *maximum additive score following endoscopy = 11*)			
Variable	0	1	2	3
Age	<60 years	60–79 years	≥80 Years	
Shock	'No shock', systolic BP ≥100, pulse <100	'Tachycardia', systolic BP ≥100, pulse ≥100	'Hypotension', systolic BP <100	
Comorbidity	No major comorbidity		Cardiac failure, ischaemic heart disease, any major comorbidity	Renal failure, liver failure, disseminated malignancy
Diagnosis at endoscopy	Mallory-Weiss tear, no lesion identified and no stigmata of recent haemorrhage	All other diagnoses	Malignancy of upper GI tract	
Major stigmata of recent haemorrhage (SRH)	None or dark spot only		Blood in upper GI tract, adherent clot, visible or spurting vessel	

Reproduced from Rockall *et al.* (1996). *Gut* **38**: 316–21.

Lower gastrointestinal bleeding

Definition and clinical presentation
The term lower gastrointestinal bleeding (LGIB) tradition-ally refers to any bleed arising beyond the ligament of Treitz, but the main focus of this section is on acute or chronic blood loss from the colon or anorectum. The key symptom of clinically overt LGIB is passage of blood per rectum (haematochezia) but chronic bleeding may be occult (iron-deficiency anaemia or positive faecal occult blood test). The incidence of LGIB rises with age (more than 200-fold between age 20 and 80 years) and the average age at presentation of LGIB is over 60 years.

The key causes of LGIB are in Table 7.8. Two-thirds of people over 80 years have diverticulosis in the colon, but LGIB occurs in less than 5%. These common structures are easy to cite as a cause for bleeding when alternative lesions are not apparent. The presence of active bleeding or adherent clot is diagnostic.

Assessment and management
Assessment: hypovolaemia is less common than in UGIB. Acute LGIB stops spontaneously in 80–85%. Distinguish bright red or maroon blood (LGIB more likely) from melaena (UGIB more likely). Past history of inflammatory bowel disease; coagulopathy; cirrhosis; previous pelvic radiation therapy; recent colonoscopy/polypectomy; alarm symptoms suggestive of cancer; cardiovascular disease (risks factors for atheroma and gut ischaemia; angiodysplasia associated with aortic valve disease). Drug history (antiplatelet agents, NSAIDs, anticoagulants). *Per rectum* examination can confirm stool colour and detect anorectal pathology.

Acute management involves basic supportive care including correction of hypovolaemia/blood loss and clotting abnormalities. Treat comorbid illness and optimize cardiorespiratory status prior to intervention. Maintain haemoglobin concentration at 10 g/dL for high-risk patients (older patients with cardiovascular disease).

Investigation of LGIB is determined by the severity at presentation. In acute severe bleeds with haemodynamic instability, resuscitation is followed first by gastroscopy to exclude an upper gastrointestinal source. Otherwise, colonoscopy is the primary investigation for LGIB and should be performed wherever possible after purging of the colon (e.g. 3 L of polyethylene glycol-based solution, orally or via nasogastric tube) to improve visualization and diagnostic yield. Numerous studies have demonstrated the safety of colonoscopy in older subjects, but bowel prepa-ration requires care in those with renal impairment. Flexible sigmoidoscopy is less invasive and requires less invasive bowel preparation, although a significant number of lesions will be missed.

A range of endoscopic *haemostatic therapies* are availa-ble for active bleeding or high-risk lesions in the colon (e.g. injection of dilute adrenaline, metallic clips, thermal coagu-lation, argon plasma coagulation, rubber band ligation of piles, or varices) but the optimal approach has not been defined in trials. Colonic perforation is a risk with thermal methods, especially in the thin-walled right colon.

If the patient cannot be stabilized for colonoscopy or the procedure is unsuccessful (poor colonic visualization due to brisk bleeding, failed attempts at haemostasis) then active LGIB requires angiography (+/– selective arterial embolization). Reported detection rates for a bleeding site with angiography are around 50%.

A minority of patients with fulminant bleeding need prompt emergency surgery—the optimum approach is 'directed segmental resection' with the bleeding site local-ized by intraoperative endoscopy or angiography.

In stable cases with a negative colonoscopy, consider additional tests of the foregut and small intestine (gastros-copy; wireless capsule endoscopy; balloon enteroscopy).

Table 7.8 Causes of lower gastrointestinal bleeding

Diverticulum	17–40%
Angiodysplasia	9–21%
Colitis (ischaemic, infectious, inflammatory bowel disease, radiation)	2–30%
Neoplasia (including post-polypectomy)	11–14%
Anorectal disease (including piles and varices)	4–10%
Upper gastrointestinal source	0–11%
Small bowel source	2–9%

Source: Zuckerman GR, Prakash C. Acute lower intestinal bleeding. *Gastrointest Endosc* 1999;49:s228.

Bleeding stops spontaneously in most cases of LGIB: data for diverticular bleeding suggest over 80% of bleeds cease but there is a 25% risk of rebleeding over 4 years.

Pharmacotherapy has a limited role in acute LGIB except in the setting of portal hypertension (portal colopathy or varices) where octreotide/terlipressin are used. Thalidomide has been reported to reduce rebleeding in chronic LGIB secondary to angiodysplasia. The risk–benefit of ongoing medication (antiplatelet, NSAIDs, warfarin) should be reviewed.

Author's Tip

Overall mortality for LGIB is lower than for UGIB; most bleeding stops spontaneously.

Colonoscopy is the appropriate intervention in acute and chronic LGIB. Good bowel preparation is essential for success.

Visceral angiography is the key diagnostic and therapeutic approach for severe LGIB in the presence of major haemodynamic instability.

Diverticulae are very common in the distal colon of older subjects; if there is no evidence of active bleeding or stigmata of recent haemorrhage, it is wise to exclude more bleeding from more proximal sites.

Further reading

Barnert J, Messmann H (2009). Diagnosis and management of lower gastrointestinal bleeding. *Nat Rev Gastr Hepat* **6**: s637.

Edelman DA, Sugawa C (2007). Lower Gastrointestinal bleeding: A review. *Surg Endosc* **21**: s514.

Farrell JJ, Friedman LS (2000). Gastrointestinal bleeding in older people. *Gastroenterol Clin North Am* **29**: s1.

Yachimski PS, Friedman LS (2008). Gastrointestinal Bleeding in the Elderly. *Nat Clin Pract Gastroenterol Hepatol* CME **5**: s80.

Gastrointestinal cancer

Gastrointestinal (GI) cancers are common in the older population, and more than 50% of patients with a GI tract tumour are over 70 years of age at diagnosis. As tumours in the colon and rectum are the most common gastrointestinal tumours, colorectal cancer will be thoroughly discussed in this chapter. In general, the presentation of gastrointestinal tumours in older patients is similar to that observed in younger patients.

Oesophageal cancer

The incidence of oesophageal cancer increases with advancing age, and the median age at diagnosis is around 60 years. Dysphagia combined with severe weight loss or progressive dysphagia over a few weeks to a few months is highly suggestive of carcinoma. Difficulty in swallowing does not occur until approximately 60% of the circumference is infiltrated with cancer, and the disease is frequently incurable at the time of diagnosis.

Dysphagia in an older patient should lead to endoscopic examination of the oesophagus and ventricle, which allows for biopsy or cytological examination of the tumour and exclusion of other causes of dysphagia. A clinical examination before endoscopy may reveal enlarged supraclavicular lymph nodes or an enlarged liver. The malignant disease also spreads to bone and lungs. In addition to endoscopy, contrast radiographs may reveal tumours, but small, resectable tumours may be missed. A CT scan of the chest and abdomen is required if aggressive intervention is appropriate, to establish the extent of tumour spread to the mediastinum and para-aortic lymph nodes. Endoscopic ultrasound may be necessary for complete staging if this influences treatment decisions.

Two-year survival for oesophageal cancer is less than 5% for patients older than 80 years, about 10% for patients 70–79 years, and a little over 20% for patients between 50 and 70 years. Surgery is the primary curative option for oesophageal cancer, but fewer than 20% of patients with resectable tumours survive 5 years. Oesophagectomy is a high-risk procedure, and the postoperative mortality rate in general is about 2–6%. Even so, there are some reports that selected older patients may undergo this procedure with morbidity and mortality rates similar to younger patients. The majority of patients with oesophageal cancer will need palliative care support/input.

Maintaining the ability to swallow is one of the main focuses of palliative care for patients with incurable oesophageal cancer. Treatment options include endoscopic oesophageal dilation, intraluminal stenting, and laser therapy. Repeated treatments are often necessary. Chemotherapy is another palliative treatment option, but data regarding older patients is lacking. Maintaining an acceptable nutritional status is often difficult, and in some cases gastrostomy or jejunostomy may be considered.

Gastric cancer

Worldwide, gastric cancer is the second leading cause of cancer death. The incidence and mortality rates of gastric cancer increase with age. In the USA, the median age at diagnosis is 67 years for men and 72 years for women. The most common presentation of gastric cancer is a common symptom: upper abdominal discomfort. The physician should be alert to the following additional symptoms: progressive discomfort, weight loss, anorexia, nausea, acute GI bleeding, dysphagia, vomiting, and early satiety.

Clinical findings include iron-deficiency anaemia, and later in the course of the disease there may be hepatomegaly and ascites. These symptoms and findings should prompt an endoscopic investigation, with biopsy and cytological examination for pathological confirmation. An important clinical point is to take multiple biopsies of gastric ulcers in order to correctly identify malignant ulcers. Haemoglobin needs to be followed after treatment of ulcers in order to demonstrate ulcer healing and rule out bleeding from other GI sources that necessitates additional lower endoscopic investigation. CT scanning and endoscopic ultrasound is needed to determine tumour respectability and staging of disease.

Five-year relative survival with gastric cancer is about 13% in patients over 80 years, 22% in patients between 70 and 79 years, and 30% in patients younger than 70 years.

Surgery

Gastrectomy is the only curative treatment for gastric cancer. The long-term survival after complete resection of the tumour is approximately 35%, regardless of the patient's age. Survival after resection of the rare tumours that are limited to the mucosa approaches 90%. It has been shown that surgery can be safely performed in fit older patients with gastric cancer, and that outcome is similar to that of younger patients. However, only fit older patients were considered for surgery in these studies. Older patients tend to undergo less extensive lymph node dissections. It must be kept in mind that studies looking at surgery in older patients rarely include preoperative factors such as functional status, nutritional status, cognitive function, and depression. There is increasing evidence that such factors are of value in preoperative risk stratification of older surgical patients.

When deciding whether or not to perform surgery in older patients with gastric cancer, the risks of complications from the tumour must be considered. In gastric cancer, there is a risk of bleeding and perforation, both of which may lead to emergency surgery. Thus, the geriatrician needs to consult a surgeon who is an expert in this field.

Chemotherapy and radiotherapy

Recently, it has been suggested that patients with localized gastric cancer should be considered for pre- or postoperative chemotherapy, or even chemoradiotherapy, because randomized controlled trials have demonstrated an improvement in survival. In a trial by Cunningham et al, 5-year overall survival was 36% in the group randomly assigned to perioperative chemotherapy, compared with 23% in patients receiving surgery only (n = 503). Data specific to older patients are not extensive. A subgroup analysis of 105 patients in this trial showed a comparable benefit from perioperative chemotherapy for patients aged >70 years compared with younger patients. Chemotherapy is generally associated with an increase in toxicity in older patients, but the prognosis without chemotherapy is grim: gastric cancer recurs in more than 50% of patients within 2 years, and recurrence is usually incurable. When deciding whether to administer adjuvant treatment the remaining life expectancy should be taken into account, which depends on chronological age, comorbidity, and functional status.

Advanced gastric cancer: palliative care

The majority of older patients with gastric cancer will need palliative treatment. For highly selected older patients, chemotherapy may be a treatment option. Single agents that are commonly used in gastric cancer include capecitabine, 5-fluorouracil, taxanes, and irinotecan. Combination therapy is generally more toxic than single agents, but small, single-institution trials have shown a benefit of combination therapy for selected, fit older patients with advanced gastric cancer. Median survival in randomized trials for advanced gastric cancer is less than 12 months.

Gastric outlet obstruction is common in patients with advanced gastric cancer, and leads to vomiting, nausea, malnutrition, and dehydration. Invasive palliative procedures involve laparoscopic gastrojejunostomy and stent placement. Gastrostomy allows for a continuous decompression of the stomach that relieves the symptoms of obstruction. Nasogastric tubes may ease bloating and vomiting. Pharmacological treatment of bowel obstruction includes the use of analgesic (strong opioids), antiemetic and anti-secretory drugs. In addition, corticosteroids may be effective as they reduce oedema. A combination regimen is often necessary.

Pancreatic cancer

The prognosis for pancreatic cancer is extremely poor, with a 5-year survival of less than 5%. The majority of patients survive less than 9 months after diagnosis. A substantial proportion of the patients are older, and the median age at diagnosis is 72 years. Early-stage pancreatic cancer is more frequently seen in older patients than younger patients. Surgical resection is the only potentially curative treatment option. A pancreaticoduodenectomy (Whipple's procedure) can be performed in selected older patients, with morbidity and mortality rates approaching those observed in younger patients. It is crucial to carefully select older patients for surgical management, and surgical outcomes appear to be better in centres with a high volume of pancreatic cancers. In selected centres, the mortality rate following a pancreaticoduodenectomy has been reported below 10%. Other publications report post-operative mortality rates between 18% and 25% in older patients.

Palliative care

Approximately 85% of patients with pancreatic cancer are not candidates for resection. The main goals of palliative care are to relieve pain and icterus and maintain adequate nutritional status. Chemotherapy may be an option for some patients. Gemcitabine is the standard initial therapy. The 1-year survival rate of patients treated with gemcitabine is 20%. Patients up to 79 years have been included in a trial showing a benefit of gemcitabine for advanced pancreatic cancer. Patients with pancreatic cancer may experience a gastric outlet obstruction, and laparoscopic gastroenterostomy or stenting are invasive treatment options.

Colorectal cancer

Epidemiology

The peak incidence for colorectal cancer is between 70 and 80 years of age, with more than 50% of patients being older than 70 years at the time of diagnosis. In the first four decades of life, the probability of developing colorectal cancer is 0.07%, while it increases to 4.3% for females and 4.8% for males in the seventh decade. Most studies show that older patients present with disease stages similar to younger patients, but there is evidence suggesting that the older cohort is often under-staged. This may be related to competing treatment priorities in the most frail. Some studies have suggested that older patients more frequently have right-sided tumours, but as other studies have not confirmed this finding, it is still unclear whether patient age affects the distribution of colon cancer. Older patients have higher rates of obstruction and perforation. Prognosis of colorectal cancer is mainly dependent upon stage at diagnosis. Some studies have found that the relative survival of patients 65 years or older is poorer than younger patients, while other studies find no differences in cancer-specific survival. A French study found that survival rates after curative surgery increased for patients <75 years between 1976–1987 and 1988–1999, while they remained stable for patients aged 75 years and older. In the older group, the use of adjuvant or palliative chemotherapy was minimal.

Clinical presentation

Right-sided colon cancers may present with fatigue and dyspnoea secondary to iron-deficiency anaemia. Unfortunately, these symptoms may be interpreted as normal ageing both by patients and physicians, leading to delayed diagnosis. Left-sided colon cancers may present with change in bowel habits, bleeding, cramping abdominal pain, and signs of obstruction. Rectal cancers are frequently associated with urgency, a sense of incomplete evacuation, diarrhoea, bleeding, or constipation. Even though the presenting symptoms are similar in younger and older patients, symptoms in the latter are more difficult to interpret because of comorbidity and false expectations/limited knowledge about 'normal ageing'. Weight loss, changes in bowel function, abdominal pain, urgency, progressive dyspnoea, and fatigue must be carefully evaluated and should not be attributed to normal ageing.

Diagnostic studies

Further diagnostic studies include colonoscopy, sigmoidoscopy and CT scan of the thorax and abdomen (for staging). Sigmoidoscopy does not allow for investigation of the complete colon. If the symptoms or findings suggest a right-sided tumour (for example iron-deficiency anaemia), a negative sigmoidoscopy cannot rule out cancer. In addition, synchronous lesions may not be discovered when investigating only the left side of colon.

Surgery

Surgery is the most effective treatment modality for colorectal cancer. Patients with stage I or II colorectal cancer are mostly cured by surgery alone, although adjuvant chemotherapy has been proven beneficial for a small percentage of patients with stage II colon cancer. For stage III colon cancer, the standard treatment is surgery followed by adjuvant chemotherapy.

Surgery for colon cancer

Population based data provide evidence that in colorectal cancer, unlike lung cancer, the resection rate for stage I–III tumours remains high even in advanced age, despite the presence of comorbidities. This is probably because the risk of tumour complications, such as obstruction, bleeding or perforation, justifies the risks of undergoing a surgical procedure. A comparison of morbidity and mortality data between younger and older patients undergoing colorectal cancer surgery is complex as it involves confounders such as stage at diagnosis, emergency versus elective procedures, comorbidity and the type of treatment received. Because of higher rates of obstruction and perforation in older patients, they are more likely to undergo emergency procedures associated with substantially higher postoperative morbidity and mortality rates.

In 2000, the Colorectal Cancer Collaborative Group published a systematic review including 34 194 patients over the age of 65 who underwent surgery for colorectal cancer. They compared outcomes for the age groups 65–74 years, 75–84 years and 85+ years. Morbidity and mortality were found to increase with age, however, this could be attributed to higher rates of comorbidity, emergency operations, and advanced cancer stages in the older group. They also found that older patients were less likely to be operated upon with curative intent. Overall survival was poorer for the older patients, but the differences in cancer-specific survival were less noticeable. Examination of at least 12 lymph nodes is considered adequate lymph node evaluation in patients operated for colorectal cancer, and an inadequate evaluation correlates with inferior survival. It has been demonstrated that patients 71 years or older were half as likely to receive adequate lymph node evaluation.

Early postoperative discharge is feasible and useful in older and younger patients after colonic surgery. This entails early removal of nasogastric tubes, prompt removal of drains, the use of suprapubic catheters, physiotherapy, early mobilisation and any other mean that might facilitate quicker recovery. The role of laparoscopic-assisted colectomy in older patients needs to be elucidated, but some reports indicate that laparoscopic surgery may lessen surgical morbidity for frail, older individuals. Self-expanding metal stents appear to be a safe alternative to emergency surgery for obstructive colorectal cancer. They may be used as a bridge to surgery to avoid emergency surgery, as emergency surgery has a high mortality and morbidity. Stents may also be a suitable alternative in the palliative setting.

Surgery in rectal cancer

After the introduction of total mesorectal excision (TME) in the 1990s, the prognosis for patients with rectal cancer has improved. TME is now the standard for resectional treatment. However, in a study of older patients after the introduction of TME, no beneficial effect in older patients was demonstrated. In this study, the 30-day mortality in patients over 75 years was between 6.9% and 26% (highest in nonagenarians), while the 6-month mortality was between 13% and 39%. Surgical trauma was responsible for the increased mortality. The authors suggest that less invasive treatment options for rectal cancer in the older patients at high risk for complications after surgery may be suitable.

Local excision of rectal tumours is a well-described alternative to abdominoperineal resection or anterior resection in selected high-risk patients with early stage tumours. This technique results in reduced postoperative mortality and morbidity. Transanal endoscopic microsurgery was introduced into clinical practice in the 1980s. It is a minimally invasive technique allowing exposure of the distal part of the rectum, which is frequently affected by adenomas and adenocarcinomas. The technique is particularly indicated for large rectal adenomas, early-stage adenocarcinomas, and carcinoid tumours. The target is to provide a full-thickness excision of the tumour affecting the rectal wall without entering the peritoneal cavity. The excision is usually carried out as a same day procedure, and is associated with a low incidence of complications. Other treatment options for rectal cancer are chemoradiotherapy alone, radiotherapy in combination with local excision, and radiotherapy as a radical treatment option.

Chemotherapy and radiotherapy

For stage III colon cancer, surgery followed by adjuvant chemotherapy is the standard of care. Older patients are less frequently referred to oncologists for consideration of this treatment. Reasons may be lack of evidence from clinical trials, concerns of toxicity, comorbidities and concerns about death due to causes others than cancer. In the recommendations from the International Society of Geriatric Oncology, it is stated that although adjuvant therapy trials have included very few patients older than 80 years, the evidence for the older patient's ability to tolerate chemotherapy in general suggests that age alone should not exclude any stage III colon cancer patient from consideration for adjuvant therapy.

Clinical practice seems to be different in Europe compared with the USA. In one study from 2005, Jessup et al show that 40% of patients over 80 years with stage III colon cancer in the USA received adjuvant therapy. European practice is far more conservative. Recommended regimens are infusional 5-fluorouracil or capecitabine. For metastatic colon cancer, the superiority of 5-fluorouracil over best supportive care has been demonstrated in older patients. There are indications that combination therapy with irinotecan is also tolerated in fit older patients. Careful monitoring for toxicity and rapid intervention if it occurs is required.

In patients with T3 or T4 tumours or lymph node-positive rectal cancer, pre- and postoperative chemoradiotherapy reduces the rate of local recurrence, and increases disease-free survival. Preoperative chemotherapy also allows a 2- to 3-month window of opportunity to optimize the patient's general condition before surgery (i.e. nutritional support, treatment of depression, correction of anaemia, fluid corrections, and physiotherapy). The insufficient use of radiotherapy, either alone or in combination with surgery, has been documented in elderly patients. Radiotherapy is the treatment of choice in the management of inoperable patients with low rectal tumours.

Liver metastases

Five-year survival in patients with untreated metastatic colon cancer is between 0 and 4% even when receiving palliative chemotherapy. The only treatment offering long-term survival for patients with liver metastases is hepatic resection. The risks with liver resection are higher in older patients, and possible explanations are age-associated reductions in liver volume, hepatic blood flow, and regenerative capacity. However, several cohort studies with fit older patients failed to show that age is an independent risk factor for short-term and long-term mortality. One study reported on 178 patients over 70 years undergoing liver resections for colorectal metastases. 34 patients received chemotherapy prior to surgery. The measured postoperative morbidity and mortality rates were 39% and 5%, respectively. This is in accordance with previous series in both older and younger patients. It was concluded that resection of colorectal liver metastases in older patients could be performed with low mortality and acceptable morbidity rates. The overall and disease-free survival rates at 1, 3, and 5 years were 86%, 43%, and 32% and 66%, 26%, and 16%, respectively. Further research should focus on quality of life and functional status after major hepatic surgery in older adults.

The selection criteria for resectability is a fascinating and often contentious topic, especially since the introduction of neoadjuvant chemotherapy, which has proven to be very effective in rescuing non-resectable lesions. The number of liver metastases, the distance between them, and their location within 1-2-3 segments no longer guide their resectability. The research focus is thus on new chemotherapeutic agents and their role on older patients.

Authors' Tips

Carefully prepare patients for the surgical procedure: physiotherapy and correction of nutritional impairment, depression and anaemia may lead to better short-term outcomes.

Consider early postoperative mobilization and oral feeding.

Early removal of nasogastric tube is recommended; suprapubic urinary catheters are preferred in male patients when easily placed during laparotomy.

Surgery is the standard treatment for GI cancer, and older patients should only be excluded when too frail for surgery. Complications from the tumour when left untreated must be taken into account.

A geriatric assessment allows for tailoring the decision-making process as well as optimizing the patient preoperatively by treating comorbidities and correcting deranged functions such as anaemia, fluid, and electrolyte disturbances, malnutrition, and depression.

The diagnostic work-up should be as complete as possible, even when cure is not the aim of the treatment. Palliative care can only be targeted when the extent of the disease is known.

Oncologists and surgeons are the experts on cancer disease, and need to be consulted in order to make an informed decision. They have knowledge about treatment options, potential complications from tumour if not treated, and palliative options.

Changes in bowel habit, fatigue, weight loss and urgency should NOT be interpreted as normal ageing, but require further diagnostic work-up.

Radiation therapy is a palliative option that is underused in older people.

Further reading

Audisio RA, Pope D, Ramesh HS, et al. (2008). Shall we operate? Preoperative assessment in elderly patients (PACE) can help. A SIOG surgical task force prospective study. *Crit Rev Oncol Hematol* **65**: 156–63.

Colorectal Cancer Collaborative Group (2000). Surgery for colorectal cancer in elderly patients: a systematic review. *Lancet* **356**: 968–74.

Cunningham D, Allum WH, Stenning SP, et al. (2006). Perioperative chemotherapy versus surgery alone for resectable gastroesophageal cancer. *N Engl J Med* **355**: 11–20.

de Liguori CN, van Leeuwen BL, Ghaneh P, et al. (2008). Liver resection for colorectal liver metastases in older patients. *Crit Rev Oncol Hematol* **67**: 273–8.

di Sebastiano P, Festa L, Buchler MW, et al. (2009). Surgical aspects in management of hepato-pancreatico-biliary tumours in the elderly. *Best Pract Res Clin Gastroenterol* **23**: 919–23.

Janssen-Heijnen MLG, Houterman S, Lemmens VEPP, et al. (2005). Prognostic impact of increasing age and co-morbidity in cancer patients: A population-based approach. *Crit Rev Oncol Hematol* **55**: 231–40.

Kristjansson, SR, Nesbakken A, Jordhoy MS, et al. (2010). Comprehensive geriatric assessment can predict complications in elderly patients after elective surgery for colorectal cancer. A prospective observational cohort study. *Crit Rev Oncol Hematol* **76**: 208–17.

Kunitake H, Zingmond DS, Ryoo J, et al. (2010). Caring for octogenarian and nonagenarian patients with colorectal cancer: what should our standards and expectations be? *Dis Colon Rectum* **53**: 735–43.

Mazzoni G, Tocchi A, Miccini M, et al. (2007). Surgical treatment of liver metastases from colorectal cancer in elderly patients. *Int J Colorectal Dis* **22**: 77–83.

Papamichael D, Audisio R, Horiot JC, et al. (2009). Treatment of the elderly colorectal cancer patient: SIOG expert recommendations. *Ann Oncol* **20**: 5–16.

Rutten H, Dulk MD, Lemmens V, et al. (2007). Survival of elderly rectal cancer patients not improved: Analysis of population based data on the impact of TME. surgery. *Eur J Cancer* **43**: 2295–300.

Wagner AD, Wedding U (2009). Advances in the pharmacological treatment of gastro-oesophageal cancer. *Drugs Aging* **26**: 627–46.

Wind J, Polle SW, Fung Kon Jin PH, et al. (2006). Systematic review of enhanced recovery programmes in colonic surgery. *Br J Surg* **93**: 800–9.

Endocrine and metabolic

Endocrine physiology in old age

The clinical significance of changes in hormone secretion in ageing has been the subject of much recent research and the challenge of distinguishing 'normal' age-related changes from reversible pathological processes remains a clinical priority.

Growth hormone

Muscle mass falls by 1–1.5% per year from the age of 40 years onwards. By the age of 80, older individuals have lost 50% of the lean tissue they had as young adults. This change in lean mass is accompanied by a reduction in strength in healthy men and women of 1–2% per year. The changes in body composition seen in ageing are very similar to those changes seen in growth hormone (GH)-deficient adults. The secretion of GH is characteristically pulsatile and in older people the frequency of pulses remains the same as in young adults. However, the amplitude of the pulses is decreased and work has linked this to a reduction in growth hormone-releasing hormone (GHRH) secretion from the hypothalamus. A number of studies have explored the potential benefits of the anabolic properties of recombinant human growth hormone (rhGH) in healthy older people and, although there are favourable changes in body composition, there is little evidence to suggest that there is an improvement in function and much uncertainty as to the risks of malignancy in the higher insulin-like growth factor (IGF)-1 quartiles.

Melatonin

Studies have reported an age-related decrease in melatonin levels, which may have an aetiological role in sleep disturbance and there is some evidence that the use of melatonin as a therapeutic agent may improve sleep in some older patient groups. Further evaluation of the role of melatonin and factors including exposure to day time light is needed to provide an evidence base to guide management in treating sleep quality in older people.

Thyroid gland

Many features of thyroid disease may be attributed to 'normal ageing' or to other diagnoses, and hence there is a significant risk that treatable thyroid pathology may be overlooked with associated morbidity and mortality. Normal ageing is associated with a small decrease in thyroid-stimulating hormone (TSH) secretion from the pituitary. Studies have also confirmed a reduction in peripheral conversion of T4 to T3 with a subsequent minimal age-related decline in serum T3 concentration but no appreciable change in T4 levels. There is no evidence to support treatment of this age-associated decline in T3, and there is emerging evidence that subclinical hypothyroidism is associated with improved health and survival in the older population.

Parathyroid gland

The aetiology of changes in body composition seen in normal ageing is clearly multifactorial and much work has been done to investigate the roles of PTH and vitamin D. Higher PTH levels and lower 25 hydroxy vitamin D levels are associated with a loss of muscle mass and function in otherwise healthy older people. There is also evidence that ageing is associated with an increased sensitivity of bone to PTH and a reduced renal responsiveness to PTH, such that there is a decline in the conversion of 25 OH vitamin D to

1,25 dihroxy vitamin D. Therefore age-associated changes in PTH and vitamin D metabolism and function are causal aetiological factors in the changes in body composition seen with increasing age. As patients become frailer with less sun exposure and reduced dietary intake, vitamin D levels will fall further.

Adrenal gland

There is an age-related decline in the function of the cells in the zona reticularis of the adrenal cortex with a subsequent decline in the secretion of dehydroepiandrosterone (DHEA). Some studies have reported improved physical and psychological endpoints with DHEA replacement but conclusive studies are lacking, with concern regarding the risks of associated malignancy. With ageing there is an increase in both trough levels of cortisol and average levels of cortisol. Researchers have proposed a 'feed forward' mechanism to explain this phenomenon with subsequent pathological consequences such as cognitive decline (see Figure 8.1).

Pancreas

There is a clear increase in the prevalence of the metabolic syndrome with increasing age, with increased resistance to insulin and decreased peripheral glucose uptake. The greatest increase in the numbers of patients with diabetes mellitus is occurring in older people with the expectation that the majority of older patients with diabetes will be greater than 65 years in 25 years. The functional heterogeneity of this group demands that diabetic management focuses on individual needs and is governed by appropriate management decisions according to functional status. Management focusing on tight glycaemic control based on evidence from a younger population may not be appropriate in many older patients and care should be directed to minimizing symptoms and maximizing independence and quality of life.

Ovaries

The average age of the menopause is around 50 years and as life expectancy increases women can expect to spend a third of their life post-menopausal. Combination hormone replacement therapy has many proven benefits not only for the vasomotor symptoms of the menopause but also in preventing loss of bone mass and reducing atrophy of soft tissues including the urogenital tract and associated urinary incontinence. A Cochrane review (2002) does not support the claim that HRT protects against cognitive decline and the use of long-term combination HRT for longer than 5 years is associated with an increasing risk of venous thromboembolism, breast cancer, and stroke.

Testes

Studies confirm that the majority of older men have lower free testosterone levels than younger men. The 'andropause' is characterized by a decreasing number and function of testicular Leydig cells accompanying an age-related decline in the pituitary axis. Although there is an increase in erectile dysfunction in this age group, there is no evidence of a causal link with reduced testosterone secretion, and comorbidities such as atherosclerosis may be more significant aetiological factors. There is no evidence to support the use of testosterone in the treatment of erectile dysfunction. Although the anabolic effects of testosterone

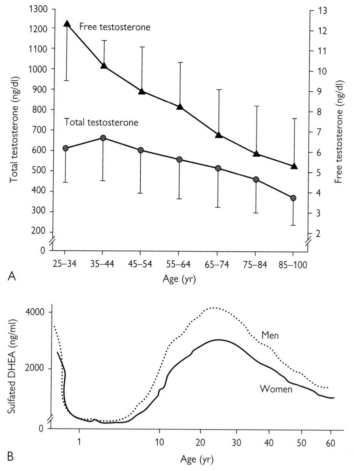

Figure 8.1 Changes in levels of serum testosterone in men (A) and sulphated DHEA in both men and women (B), according to age. Reproduced from Paul Steward, Age and Fountain of Youth Hormones, *NEJM*, 355, pp. 1724–6, Figure 1. Copyright 2006 Massachusetts Medical Society. All rights reserved.

may be considered favourable with respect to body composition in older men, there are few studies available which fully investigate the effects and risks of associated prostate malignancy and progression of coronary artery disease.

Author's Tip

It is a clinical priority to differentiate between normal physiological changes of ageing and endocrine pathology

Clinicians must be wary of industry driven research and balance clinical risks versus 'hard endpoint' benefits of treatment

---

Further reading

Agnusdei D, Gennari C (1994). Bone and renal responsiveness to parathyroid hormone with aging. *J Bone Miner Met* **12**: 55–9.

Brusco LI, Fainstein I, Márquez M, et al. (1999). Effect of melatonin in selected populations of sleep-disturbed patients. *Biol Signals Recept* **8**: 126–31.

Corpas E, Harman SM, Piñeyro MA, et al. (1992). Growth hormone (GH)- releasing hormone-(1-29) twice daily reverses the

decreased GH and insulin-like growth factor-1 levels in old men. *J Clin Endocrinol Metab* **75**: 530–5.

Engelgau MM, Geiss LS, Saaddine JB, et al. (2004). The evolving diabetes burden in the United States. *Ann Intern Med* **140**: 945–50.

Forbes GB, Reina JC (1970). Adult lean body mass declines with age: some longitudinal observations. *Metabolism* **19**: 653–63.

Garfinkel D, Laudon M, Nof D, et al. (1995). Improvement of sleep quality in elderly people by controlled-release melatonin. *Lancet* **346**: 541–4.

Gordon AL, Gladman JRF (2010). Sleep in Care Homes. *Rev Clin Gerontol* **20**): 309–16.

Grady D, Ruin SM, Petitti DB, et al. (1992). Hormone therapy to prevent disease and prolong life in postmenopausal women. *Ann Intern Med* **117**: 1016–37.

Gussekloo J, van Exel E, de Craen AJ, et al. (2004)Thyroid status, disability and cognitive function, and survival in old age. *JAMA* **292**: 2591–9.

Iguichi H, Kato K, Ibayashi H (1982). Age-dependent reduction in serum melatonin concentrations in healthy human subjects. *J Clin Endocrinol Metab* **55**: 27–9.

Lamberts SW, van den Beld AW, van der Lely AJ (1997). The endocrinology of aging. *Science* **278**: 419–24.

Ravaglia G, Forti P, Maioli F, *et al.* (1996). The relationship of dehydroepiandrosterone sulfate (DHEAS) to endocrine-metabolic parameters and functional status in the oldest-old. Results from an Italian study on healthy free-living over-ninety-years-old. *J Clin Endocrinol Metab* **81**: 1173–8.

Rudman D (1985). Growth hormone, body composition and aging. *J Am Geriatr Soc* **33**: 800–7.

Sack RL, Lewy AJ, Erb DL, *et al.* (1986). Human melatonin production decreases with age. *J Pineal Res* **3**: 379–88.

Sapolsky RM, Krey LC, McEwen BS (1986). The neuroendocrinology of stress and aging: the glucocorticoid cascade hypothesis. *Endocr Rev* **7**: 284–301.

Skelton DA, Greig CA, Davies JM, *et al.* (1994). Strength power and related functional ability of healthy people aged 65–89 years. *Age Ageing* **23**: 371–7.

Tenover JS (1994). Androgen administration to aging men. *Endocrinol Metab Clin North Am*, **23**(4): 877–92.

van Coevorden A, Mockel J, Laurent E, *et al.* (1991). Neuroendocrine rhythms and sleep in aging men. *Am J Physiol* **260**: E651–61.

Visser M, Deeg DJ, Lips P (2003). Low vitamin D and high parathyroid hormone levels as determinants of loss of muscle strength and muscle mass (sarcopenia): the Longitudinal Aging Study Amsterdam. *J Clin Endocrinol Metab* **88**: 5766–72.

Wald M, Meacham RB, Ross LS, *et al.* (2006). Testosterone replacement therapy for older men. *J Androl* **27**: 126–32.

Young A (1988). Muscle function in old age. *New Issues in Neuroscience* **1**: 141–56.

Endocrine investigations

Mrs A, an 84-year-old woman, was admitted in January, April, June and August of the same year. The history was of a general deterioration with weakness, fatigue, and lack of interest in day-to-day activities. During this time she had declined from living independently to being admitted to a nursing home. She did not like the nursing home at all and the staff found her a challenging patient to care for. She had a past medical history of sarcoidosis diagnosed nearly 40 years previously and was prescribed only senna and para-cetamol as required. Each previous admission was associat-ed with hyponatraemia, responding to fluid restriction for presumed syndrome of inappropriate antidiuretic hormone secretion (SIADH), although no formal diagnosis was made.

Syndrome of inappropriate ADH secretion

- Exclusion of: volume depletion, diuretics or ACE inhibitors
- Urine sodium >20 mmol/L and urine osmolaltiy >500 mosmol/kg
- Hyponatraemia Na<125 mmol/L and low plasma osmo-lality <260 mosmol/kg (for example heart failure, renal failure, liver failure)

In September she was admitted again with continued decline. Examination confirmed a lady who appeared depressed, heart rate 60 bpm, blood pressure 110/70 mmHg, body mass index 35 kg/m^2, but no other significant findings. ECG and chest radiograph were normal; urinalysis: protein + only.

Blood tests

- Sodium 120 mmol/L
- Potassium 4.4 mmol/L
- Urea 6.0 mmol/L
- Creatinine 98 μmol/L

Full blood count, liver function tests, random blood glu-cose, C-reactive protein, and corrected calcium were all normal

A 9.00 am cortisol was arranged to exclude adrenal fail-ure as a cause for this woman's symptoms, but the result was abnormal.

9 am cortisol 304 nmol/L

Adrenal failure is excluded by a 9.00 am cortisol >500 nmol/L

Author's Tip

Primary adrenal failure is associated with a high potassi-um due to a lack of glucocorticoid and mineralcorticoid. Secondary adrenal failure, for example from a pituitary cause, is associated with low sodium only as the miner-alcorticoid axis is maintained

---

Further analysis of baseline pituitary function suggested that the pathology was not adrenal in origin but more suggestive of a poorly functioning pituitary gland

- TSH 0.16 mu/L low
- Thyroxine 10.4 pmol/L

- LH low
- FSH low

The thyroid function tests are suggestive of secondary hypothyroidism with a differential diagnosis including sick euthyroid syndrome

The gonadotrophins are inappropriately low for a post-menopausal woman suggesting pituitary pathology, and a MRI scan was arranged (see Figure 8.2).

- MRI head: the sella was expanded and contained CSF signal with appearances suggestive of an empty sella
- Diagnosis: panhypopituitarism

The cause of the empty sella is speculative. An incidental non-functioning pituitary adenoma which had infarcted could explain these findings. The patient had no history of headache and had normal visual fields.

The possibility of neurosarcoid was discussed. Classically this condition presents with diabetes insipidus and this pat-tern of presentation with an empty sella is not typical but remains a possibility.

This case is a good example of how significant and reversible pathology may be overlooked in an older patient with global and non-specific decline. This patient's depres-sion, fatigue, and weakness responded well to glucocorti-coid and thyroxine replacement, and she was discharged to a rehabilitation facility with the goal of returning to her own home.

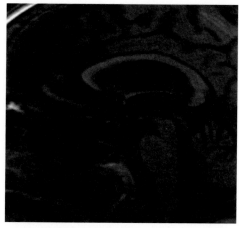

Figure 8.2 MRI of brain.

Diabetes in old age

Diabetes mellitus is a highly prevalent long-term illness often associated with comorbidities and complex clinical decision-making. Besides being a public health burden, it has a dramatic impact on the ageing population. Defining goals of care, organizing treatment plans and taking special notice of others involved in the care is paramount to achieving high-quality diabetes care.

Key areas to study in older subjects with diabetes include the evaluation of lower limb function. This is of particular importance in older patients who may have considerable but often unrecognized walking disabilities. The wide spectrum of vascular complications, acute metabolic decompensation, adverse effects of medication, and the effects of the condition on nutrition and lifestyle behaviour, may all create varying levels of impairment.

This chapter is aimed at health professionals and provides a scientific and clinical framework for managing older people with diabetes, which should be a basis for improving clinical effectiveness.

Key points

- Glucose tolerance worsens with age, the main factor being impairment of insulin-stimulated glucose uptake and glycogen synthesis in skeletal muscle.
- Diabetes can affect up 10–25% of older people (over 65 years) worldwide, with high rates in populations such as Pima Indians, Mexican-Americans and South Asians.
- Episodes of hypoglycaemia resulting from treatment with insulin or an insulin secretagogue may be severe and prolonged, particularly because there is an age-related decline in counter-regulatory responses
- High levels of disability and frailty are common in older people with diabetes and are often linked to higher healthcare expenditures.
- About 16% of older people with diabetes in the UK are registered blind or partially sighted (eight times more than the non-diabetic population), which suggests a role for regular screening for eye disease.
- Risk factors for foot ulceration affect 25% of older people with type 2 diabetes.
- Treatment strategies for many older people with diabetes are similar to those advocated for younger counterparts but when frailty or end of life scenarios emerge, then treatment targets are often modified with an emphasis on patient safety and quality of life.
- Effective delivery of diabetes care depends on close cooperation between hospital and community, the involvement of diabetes specialists and practice nurses, and attention to all causes of disability and ill-health.

Diabetes mellitus is a high-impact health disorder which imposes considerable economic, social, and health burdens. Associated medical comorbidities are common in this age group, and may influence treatment strategies.

Within Europe, type 2 diabetes affects 10–30% of subjects above pensionable age and in the USA, about 40% of all those with diabetes. Earlier studies suggest that older people with diabetes use primary care services two to three times more than their non-diabetic counterparts; in one Danish study, insulin-treated patients accounted for over half of the services provided, mainly because of macrovascular disease. The demands of hospital care is also increased two to three times in those with diabetes compared with an age-matched population, with more frequent clinic visits and a fivefold higher admission rate. Acute hospital admissions account for 60% of total expenditure in this group. Some 5–8% of general hospital beds in the UK are occupied by patients with diabetes aged 60 years or more, accounting for 60% of all inpatients with diabetes. Hospital admissions last twice as long for older patients with diabetes than for controls, averaging 7–8 days per year. By introducing insulin treatment, the costs increase fourfold, both in the community and in hospital, where bed occupancy rises to 24 days per year.

The management of type 2 diabetes is complicated in older subjects because of the added effects of ageing on metabolism and renal function, the use of potentially diabetogenic drugs, and low levels of physical activity. Cardiovascular risk is particularly high because many risk factors of the 'metabolic syndrome' can be present for up to a decade before type 2 diabetes is diagnosed.

Older people with diabetes, particularly those who are housebound or institutionalized, have special needs. Overall, there is increasing evidence that the quality of diabetes care for older patients appears to be improving in various countries.

Characteristics of older people with diabetes

High level of associated medical comorbidities

Varying evidence of impaired physical function and walking ability

Increased vulnerability to hypoglycaemia and increased risk of hospital admission

Increased risk of inpatient mortality

Increased risk of cognitive dysfunction and mood disorder causing more complex decision making

Increased need for spouses and informal carers to be involved in diabetes care

---

Epidemiology

Ageing is an important factor in the rapid worldwide rise of type 2 diabetes. The prevalence of diabetes begins to rise steadily from early adulthood, reaching a plateau in those aged 60 years or older; data from the Third National Health and Nutrition Examination Survey (NHANES III) in the US provides a clear account of these changes.

Overall prevalence rates of diabetes in older people are dominated by type 2 diabetes (see Figure 8.3), which accounts for 95% of all cases in the UK and European countries, and for virtually all in populations such as the Pimas and Mexican-Americans. Some older patients who present clinically with type 2 diabetes may have slowly evolving autoimmune β-cell destruction that requires insulin treatment, so-called late-onset autoimmune diabetes of adults (LADA). This condition is more prevalent in northern Europe but is rare in Asians and Africans.

There are marked ethnic and geographical differences in the prevalence rates of diabetes. In the UK and most developed countries, diabetes affects 9–17% of Caucasian subjects aged over 65 years and up to 25% of non-Caucasian people; the prevalence of diabetes in care homes in the UK is also 25%. Among subjects aged over 60 years from NHANES III, Mexican-Americans showed a consistently higher prevalence of diabetes than non-Hispanic white and black subjects.

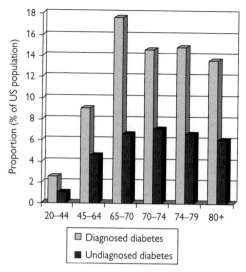

Figure 8.3 Prevalence rates of diabetes at different age cohorts (USA).

The aetiology of diabetes in old age

Various degrees of insulin resistance and impaired insulin secretion result in a progressive, age-related decline in glucose tolerance, which begins in the third decade and continues throughout adulthood. Plasma glucose levels at 1 and 2 hours after the standard 75-g oral glucose challenge rise by 0.3–0.7 mmol/L per decade, the increase being greater in women. Consistent with this, NHANES III found the prevalence of impaired glucose tolerance (IGT) to be 12% in subjects aged 40–49 years, rising to 21% in those aged 60–74 years

Several factors contribute to age-related glucose intolerance. An important change is impairment of insulin-mediated glucose disposal, especially in skeletal muscle, which is particularly marked in obese subjects. Post-receptor defects are likely to be responsible. Contributory factors in some cases may include increased body fat mass, physical inactivity and diabetogenic drugs such as thiazides. In contrast to younger people with type 2 diabetes, fasting hepatic glucose production does not appear to be increased in either lean or obese older people with type 2 diabetes.

Factors contributing to glucose intolerance in old age

Impaired glucose disposal and utilization
- Insulin-mediated uptake into skeletal muscle
- Insulin-mediated vasodilatation in muscle
- Non-insulin medicated glucose uptake (NIMGU)

Impaired glucose-induced insulin secretion

Other factors
- Obesity
- Physical inactivity
- Reduced dietary carbohydrate
- Diabetogenic drugs (e.g. thiazides, glucocorticoids)

Many older people with glucose intolerance show impairment of glucose-induced insulin secretion, especially

in response to oral rather than intravenous glucose. In addition, recent studies have shown that glucose effectiveness (i.e. the ability of glucose to stimulate its own uptake in the absence of insulin) is decreased in healthy older subjects. NIMGU accounts for 70% of glucose uptake under fasting conditions (primarily into the central nervous system) and for 50% of postprandial glucose uptake (especially into skeletal muscle). This is therefore a potentially important new target for therapeutic intervention, as exercise, anabolic steroids and decreased non-esterified fatty-acid (NEFA) levels can all enhance NIMGU and improve glucose tolerance, at least in younger patients.

Glucose-related metabolic complications

Hyperglycaemia

Older subjects with diabetes can develop diabetic ketoacidosis (DKA) and the hyperglycaemic hyperosmolar non-ketotic (HONK) state, which occurs predominantly in subjects aged over 50 years. In one study, 22% of admissions with DKA were in subjects aged 60 years or more, while in another study 13% of cases of hyperglycaemic coma in all ages were caused by HONK. Many people with type 2 diabetes maintain enough residual insulin secretion to suppress lipolysis and ketogenesis, and so develop HONK instead of DKA; hyperosmolarity can worsen insulin resistance and may also inhibit lipolysis. The tendency to hyperosmolarity may be worsened in older people, who lack thirst sensation and may not drink enough to compensate for the osmotic diuresis; they may also be taking diuretics.

Causes of hyperglycaemia include infection (55% of cases in one series of HONK), myocardial infarction, inadequate hypoglycaemic treatment or diabetogenic drug treatment. Thiazide diuretics and glucocorticoids can increase blood glucose levels and may precipitate DKA; thiazide diuretics, and furosemide appear particularly likely to cause HONK. A specific cause often cannot be identified. Residents of care homes are at increased risk of HONK coma, associated with appreciable mortality.

Compared with the young, older patients have higher mortality and longer stays in hospital; they are also less likely to have had diabetes diagnosed previously, and more likely to have renal impairment and to require higher insulin dosages. Death may occur from the metabolic disturbance or concomitant illnesses such as pneumonia or myocardial infarction.

The investigation and treatment of hyperglycaemic coma can be found in standard textbooks on diabetes but now most hospital units have protocols of management that provide guidance on fluid balance, potassium treatment, and initial insulin treatment.

The history and examination should pay special attention to previous diabetic symptoms, drug treatment, any precipitating infection, possible myocardial infarction or medication, evidence of heart failure and the degree of dehydration. Initial investigations are as for younger patients, including arterial blood gases and plasma osmolality.

In older patients, intravenous saline can often be given at a rate of 500 mL/h for 4 hours, then reducing to 250 mL/h; faster infusion is needed if the patient is shocked, when a central line may be helpful to monitor filling pressure, particularly in the presence of cardiac failure or recent myocardial infarction.

Some older subjects with HONK need very small doses of insulin to reduce plasma glucose levels, although hypercatabolic or severely insulin-resistant states require higher dosages.

Thrombotic complications may occur, especially in subjects with HONK coma; prophylactic anticoagulation with low-dose subcutaneous heparin is therefore recommended.

Hypoglycaemia

Older people may have little knowledge about the symptoms and signs of hypoglycaemia which increases their vulnerability to this complication of treatment. Even health professionals may misdiagnose hypoglycaemia as a stroke, transient ischaemic attack, unexplained confusion, or epilepsy.

Patients with cognitive impairment or loss of the warning symptoms of hypoglycaemia are at increased risk, as they may not recognize impending hypoglycaemia and/or fail to communicate their feelings to their carers. Multiple factors underlie the increased susceptibility to hypoglycaemia in this age group, including recent discharge from hospital with altered sulphonylurea dosages, renal or hepatic impairment, excess alcohol, and insulin therapy. In addition, older subjects mount a diminished counter-regulatory response to hypoglycaemia, and this may delay recovery.

Although the risk of hypoglycaemia is highest with insulin, prolonged hypoglycaemia can be an important clinical issue for older subjects taking certain drugs. Impaired renal function further prolongs hypoglycaemia secondary to sulphonylureas that are cleared through the kidneys. Shorter acting sulphonylureas are less likely to cause hypoglycaemia, although glipizide is considered by some to be unsafe in older people. Newer oral agents such as the thiazolidinediones, the DPP-IV inhibitors and GLP-1 agonists, and the longer acting insulin analogues may decrease the risk of hypoglycaemia in this group.

In older people, serious hypoglycaemia appears to carry a worse prognosis and higher mortality; permanent neurological damage may occur, presumably because of an already compromised cerebral circulation. Most sulphonylureas have caused fatal hypoglycaemia, most commonly glibenclamide. Other factors predisposing to fatal hypoglycaemia include alcohol consumption, poor food intake, renal impairment, and potentiation of hypoglycaemia by other drugs.

Some people cannot treat hypoglycaemia themselves; an educational programme should focus on detecting and treating hypoglycaemia, with advice to others about how to manage cases of unresponsive hypoglycaemia. In view of the additional vulnerability of older people to hypoglycaemia, extra caution is required when there is a history of recurrent symptoms, drowsiness is present, the patient is on relatively large doses of insulin, or when their diabetes care is delegated to an informal carer. This increased risk must be balanced by a lower threshold for admission to hospital when hypoglycaemia is suspected. In this setting, a glucose level less than 4 mmol/L may warrant admission.

Diabetic complications

In a 6-year study of 188 patients aged over 60 years in Oxford, the reported incidence rates of ischaemic heart disease, stroke, and peripheral vascular disease were 56, 22, and 146 cases per 1000 person years, respectively. These were slightly higher than the rates in the Framingham study, presumably because of the older age of the Oxford patients. Retinopathy occurred at a rate of 60 cases and cataract at 29 cases per 1000 person years, while proteinuria (urine albumin concentration greater than 300 mg/L) was 19 per 1000 person years. These incidence rates did not appear to be gender or duration of diabetes linked, but

stroke and peripheral vascular disease rose significantly with age.

In a cross-sectional study of patients with type 2 diabetes aged 53–80 years, a significant rise in the prevalence of retinopathy with ageing was seen, independent of the effects of metabolic control, duration of disease and other risk variables. Age also increased the prevalence of peripheral neuropathy, hypertension, and impotence.

Eye disease and visual loss

Cataract, age-related macular degeneration, and diabetic retinopathy remain the major causes of blindness and partial sight registration in most developed countries.

Cataract, the most frequent cause of deteriorating vision in the older population, is associated with premature death. Age-related macular degeneration is an important cause of central visual loss. Risk factors include atherosclerosis, diastolic blood pressure above 95 mmHg or antihypertensive medication, and elevated serum cholesterol. About 5% of older patients with diabetes show no evidence of retinal damage even after 15 years of the disease. The main sight-threatening consequence of diabetic retinopathy in this population is maculopathy and particularly macular oedema.

In one UK study, 16% of older people with diabetes were registered blind or partially sighted, which is approximately eight times more than among their non-diabetic counterparts. The Welsh Community Diabetes Study found that visual acuity was impaired in 40% of older subjects with diabetes, compared with 31% of non-diabetic controls (p = 0.007). Factors significantly associated with visual loss in people with diabetes included advanced age, duration of diabetes, female gender, a history of foot ulceration, and treatment with insulin. Reduced visual acuity was also significantly associated with poorer quality of life, as measured by the SF-36 questionnaire.

Screening for retinopathy

Older people with diabetes need annual measurements of visual acuity or retinal photography; where the latter may not be available or feasible, patients should undergo dilated pupil fundoscopy (or fundus photography) by experienced observers. Exudative maculopathy (hard exudates at or within one disc diameter of the macula) is easy to detect, but macular oedema is very difficult to detect by routine ophthalmoscopy; instead, slit-lamp stereoscopic fundoscopy is required to measure retinal thickness. Mydriasis is usually a short-term intervention and in the great majority of cases is not associated with any major problems, even in older people. It is always important to know whether patients have a history of glaucoma before mydriasis as this requires a different approach, often under specialist supervision. This highlights the importance of measuring the corrected visual acuity, which is decreased by maculopathy. Indications for referral to an ophthalmologist are generally identical to those in younger patients.

Management of diabetic retinopathy

Although new treatments such as the use of antibodies, cytokines, and fusion proteins to prevent diabetic retinopathy appear to be promising, currently the best way to prevent diabetic retinopathy is strict control of diabetes mellitus through the use of nutritional planning, exercise, and glucose and blood pressure control.

The benefits of tight glycaemic control in slowing the progression of diabetic retinopathy have been convincingly proven in both type 1 and type 2 diabetes in several trials. In the UKPDS, the risk of retinopathy progressing was reduced by 25% when HbA1c was maintained at <7.0% (53 mmol/mol), while improved blood pressure control also reduced risk by 37%.

Laser photocoagulation halves the risk of severe visual loss with macular oedema and exudative maculopathy (if visual acuity is 6/9 or better), which otherwise reaches 50–70% after 5 years.

Diabetes foot disease

Amputation is a major failure of detection and treatment of diabetes and often older people are affected. More recently, the National Institute of Clinical Excellence (NICE) has published guidelines on foot care for patients with type 2 diabetes. However, evidence is at last beginning to appear showing that structured diabetic foot care, performed in a multidisciplinary team, does eventually result in significant reductions in amputation rates among people with diabetes. One study identified increasing age and a higher level of amputation as important factors that increased both the duration and costs of hospitalization (estimated at over £10 000 (US$15 000) per hospitalization, lasting an average of 42 days). The 3-year survival following lower extremity amputation is about 50%, and in about 70% of cases amputation is precipitated by foot ulceration. The principal antecedents include peripheral vascular disease, sensorimotor and autonomic neuropathy, limited joint mobility (which especially prevents older people from inspecting their feet), and high foot pressures. Peripheral sensorimotor neuropathy, the primary cause or contributory factor in most cases, becomes commoner with increasing age, and affects 25% of patients with type 2 diabetes aged 80 years or above. As well as the common symptoms of numbness, neurogenic pain, 'pins and needles', and hyperaesthesia (all typically worse at night), peripheral neuropathy often causes gait disturbances, falls, and other foot injuries. Concomitant visual loss worsens the situation.

Risk factors for foot ulceration in older people

Peripheral sensorimotor neuropathy

Autonomic neuropathy

Peripheral vascular disease

Limited joint mobility

Foot pressure abnormalities, including deformity

Previous foot problems

Visual loss

History of alcohol misuse

Treatment of painful neuropathy associated with diabetes is often difficult. A thorough neurological evaluation with gait and walking tests, motor and sensory examination are essential. The finding of what appears to be a neuropathy affecting the limbs must trigger a search for other neuropathies, such as autonomic neuropathy. Recent-onset symptoms may remit with improved metabolic control, but pain associated with loss of sensation of more than 6 months' duration generally requires specific therapy. Localized pain may respond to topical application of capsaicin cream, which depletes pain fibres of the neurotransmitter, substance P. Other drugs include tricyclic antidepressants (e.g. amitriptyline), and antiepileptics, such as gabapentin. The SNRI (serotonin noradrenaline reuptake inhibitor), duloxetine, is licensed for treatment of painful diabetic neuropathy. Duloxetine is contraindicated in those with liver disease and nausea is a common side effect which is usually self-limiting.

Ischaemia secondary to peripheral vascular disease and perhaps microcirculatory disturbances is the other main contributor to diabetic foot ulceration. Many older people with diabetes may experience critical or worsening limb ischaemia or ischaemic ulcers that are slow to heal. These may benefit from surgical revascularization (angioplasty or arterial reconstruction). Appropriate cases should be referred early for surgery, ideally through joint protocols developed by the diabetes specialist and the vascular surgeon. A reasonable life expectancy is considered important by surgeons, as concomitant cardiac and cerebrovascular disease lead to death within 5 years in 50% of patients. Following proximal arterial reconstruction, the 5-year patency averages 70% and may exceed life expectancy in patients with major comorbidities; for distal reconstruction surgery, 5-year limb salvage rates approach 85%.

Prevention of diabetic foot ulceration is based on a multidisciplinary approach to identifying, educating and treating high risk patients. Many older patients have great difficulty in performing the most basic routine foot care, often because of poor vision and reduced mobility. In such cases, spouses and other carers must be involved to prevent and treat foot lesions. Education needs to be concise and repeated regularly.

Coronary heart disease and arterial disease

Angina, myocardial infarction, heart failure, stroke, and intermittent claudication are all more common in older subjects with diabetes than in age-matched, non-diabetic controls. Mortality is particularly high following myocardial infarction, especially because of acute pump failure and later onset of left ventricular failure.

Many older patients with diabetes present with atypical symptoms, including 'silent ischaemia' (which carries a worse prognosis than in the non-diabetic population); even myocardial infarction may be painless and present non-specifically as a fall, breathlessness, malaise, or hypotension.

Erectile dysfunction

Erectile dysfunction (ED) occurs earlier and more commonly in men with diabetes after 60 years of age; 55–95% of men with diabetes are affected, compared with 50% of their non-diabetic counterparts. According to a recent definition, ED is defined as the persistent inability to achieve or maintain an erection sufficient for satisfactory sexual intercourse. In the USA, ED is highly prevalent, affecting 20–30 million men (30–52% of men aged 40–70 years).

ED may be characterized by gradual onset, incremental progression, lack of erection during the night (organic causes), while psychogenic causes are characterized by sudden-onset immediate loss. Frequent organic causes are vascular diseases (40%) and diabetes (30%).

Investigation should begin with an interview with the patient and his partner, where appropriate. A thorough cardiovascular risk assessment is mandatory. Treatment today is generally via phosphodiesterase (PDE5) inhibitors: sildenafil (25–100 mg/day), tadalafil (10–20 mg/day), and vardanafil (10–20 mg/day), which are well tolerated and highly effective. Oral sildenafil achieved erections in 67% of older men in one study.

Other treatments have involved a vacuum tumescence device, misoprostol urethral pellets, and self-administered intracorporeal injection of vasoactive drugs (e.g. prostaglandin E1). The latter is relatively successful, but up to 50% of men eventually discontinue because of pain or loss of effect or interest.

Cognitive dysfunction

Diabetes and cognitive dysfunction are linked. Impaired cognitive function has been demonstrated in older subjects with diabetes, but these studies were mostly not population based, excluded subjects with dementia, and generally used a large battery of tests to show the deficit.

Impaired glucose tolerance has been shown to be associated with cognitive dysfunction. It has been suggested that certain components of the metabolic syndrome may each contribute to memory disturbance in type 2 diabetes abnormalities, and that hyperinsulinaemia is associated with decreased cognitive function and dementia in women. The overall risk of dementia is significantly increased for both men and women with type 2 diabetes; excess risk for Alzheimer's disease achieved significance in men only. Poor glucose control may be associated with cognitive impairment, which recovers following improvement in glycaemic control. Cognitive dysfunction in older subjects with diabetes is associated with a spectrum of adverse effects: increased hospitalization, less ability for self-care, reduced likelihood of specialist follow-up, and increased risk of institutionalization.

Background to relationship between diabetes and cognitive disorders

- Professional and public concern about the impact of diabetes on cognition.
- Long-term influence of hyperglycaemia and hypoglycaemia on cerebral function unknown.
- Pathophysiological mechanisms involved are uncertain, but may involve both vascular, inflammatory and neuronal mechanisms.
- No current agreement on the optimum method to detect or assess cognitive deficits in diabetes.
- Clinical relevance of the changes observed is uncertain.

Depression

A major depressive disorder increases significantly the risk of diabetes, this association being apparently independent of age, gender or coexistent chronic disease. Depression was the single most important indicator of subsequent death in a group of people with diabetes admitted into hospital. Failure to recognize depression can be serious and may be associated with worsening diabetic control and decreased treatment compliance.

Diabetes and depression may share similar symptomatology, for example, fatigue, irritability, and sexual dysfunction. This may delay or confuse the diagnosis, although the commonly used diagnostic assessment scales are unlikely to be invalidated. Enquiries about wellbeing, sleep, appetite, and weight loss should be part of the routine history, with a more comprehensive psychiatric evaluation if appropriate. A Geriatric Depression Scale (GDS) score >5 out of 15 can be regarded as indicative of probable depression. Although the GDS-15 may be the scale of choice for older people without cognitive impairment, it does not perform as well in those with dementia. Another scale to be considered is the WHO-5 Well-Being Index.

Depression in diabetes can be treated successfully with pharmacotherapy and/or psychological therapy, but blood glucose levels should be monitored closely, especially with pharmacotherapy. Goals for treating patients with depression and diabetes are two-fold: (1) remission or improvement of depressive symptoms; and (2) improvement of poor glycaemic control if present. The preferred first line treatment is a selective serotonin reuptake inhibitor (SSRI) or a serotonin noradrenaline reuptake inhibitor (SNRI) and psychotherapy. Treatment with SSRIs, such as fluoxetine, may improve symptoms and consequently metabolic control although close observation for side-effects and changes to glycaemic control are needed.

Disability

Diabetes is associated with both functional impairment and disability which are more clearly accounted for by vascular complications. However, metabolic disturbance, medication effects, and nutritional behaviour may superimpose themselves on a disabling state.

Several studies have identified diabetes as a predictor of functional decline, including studies in ageing subjects, which can be manifest as changes in activities of daily living (ADL), domestic and leisure abilities, or cognitive tests.

Enabling patients to take an active part in lifestyle modification including rehabilitation can foster their autonomy, improve their self-esteem and coping skills, and reduce their anxiety and depression associated with disability and functional decline. We need further research in the role of glycaemic control, untreated pain, and depression in modifying outcomes in those with diabetes-related functional impairments.

Falls and fall-related fractures are a source of enormous morbidity and resultant disability. In those over 65 years of age, falls are the most common cause of injury and hospital admission for trauma, and may account for more than 80% of fractures. In people with diabetes, the increased risk of falling is nearly threefold, and diabetic patients have a two-fold increase in having a significant injury, with fall-related fractures being more common in women. Factors contributing to falls include problems with gait and balance, as well as neurological and musculoskeletal disabilities. In addition, in people with diabetes, the high rate of cardiovascular disability, visual deficit, cognitive impairment, and treatment-related issues are likely to be contributory. For example, insulin treatment may increase significantly the risk of falling in older women with diabetes; factors that may be implicated are the duration and severity of the diabetes or possibly a higher rate of hypoglycaemia. Clinicians involved in managing older people with diabetes must directly question patients about the occurrence of falls and provide an estimate of risk.

Mortality in older people with diabetes

People with diabetes die prematurely, mostly from cardiovascular disease. Early reports suggested that excess rates among people with diabetes fell progressively with age, especially in those aged 65 years and over. This has been confirmed largely by the Verona Study, in which the standardized mortality ratio (SMR) declined from a range of 2–3.5 for middle-aged subjects with diabetes to 1.75 in those aged 65–74 and 1.3 in patients older than 75 years; at all ages, the impact of diabetes on the SMR was more pronounced in women. A recent systematic review has suggested a higher incidence of premature death in older subjects with diabetes. Cardiovascular mortality is primarily responsible, accounting for 42% of the overall mortality in the Verona Study. In the UK study, excess mortality rose substantially in subjects with diabetes aged >65 years, and impaired glucose tolerance was associated with a relative risk of death of 1.7.

Age remains the strongest predictor of mortality; the contributions of classical cardiovascular risk factors are uncertain in older subjects with diabetes. A Finnish study concluded that smoking, hypertension, low high-density lipoprotein (HDL) cholesterol and high total cholesterol did not affect overall mortality. In the Verona Study, long-term metabolic control was a better predictor of outcome, and subjects with more variable glycaemic control had lower survival rates, especially in those aged over 75 years.

Clinical features

The presentation of diabetes in older people is varied and often insidious, which may delay diagnosis. Many cases are detected by finding hyperglycaemia during investigation for comorbidities or acute illnesses.

Presentations of diabetes in older people
Asymptomatic (coincidental finding)
Classical osmotic symptoms

Metabolic disturbances
- Diabetic ketoacidosis
- Hyperosmolar non-ketotic coma
- 'Mixed' metabolic disturbance

Spectrum of vague symptoms
- Depressed mood
- Apathy
- Mental confusion

Development of 'geriatric' syndromes
- Falls or poor mobility: muscle weakness, poor vision, cognitive impairment
- Urinary incontinence
- Unexplained weight loss
- Memory disorder or cognitive impairment

Slow recovery from specific illnesses or increased vulnerability
- Impaired recovery from stroke
- Repeated infections
- Poor wound healing

Recognition of the diverse, atypical, and often cryptic symptom profile of hyperglycaemia in older people can be helpful in making an early diagnosis. Even when hyperglycaemia is recognized in hospital, about half of older people may receive no further evaluation or treatment of diabetes

Diagnosis of diabetes

Diagnostic criteria are as in younger people. In relation to the American Diabetes Association (ADA) criteria, diabetes can be diagnosed when a fasting glucose level exceeds 7.0 mmol/L. However, a single raised plasma glucose level does not make a diagnosis of diabetes, so confirmatory evidence is required in clinical practice, i.e. a further raised plasma glucose level at a different time, osmotic symptoms, or the presence of specific complications (retinopathy).

The latest WHO and International Diabetes Federation (IDF) criteria simplify matters greatly by introducing 'intermediate hyperglycaemia' as somewhere between normal glucose tolerance (venous plasma glucose fasting <6.1 mmol/L and 2 hours post challenge <7.8 mmol/L) and diabetes (venous plasma glucose fasting ≥7.0 mmol/L and 2 hours post challenge ≥11.1 mmol/L).

Mortality may be higher in those subjects diagnosed as diabetic with the 2-hour glucose value than with the new fasting criteria alone. Moreover, isolated postload hyperglycaemia with normal fasting glucose (<7.0 mmol/L) is associated with increased fatal cardiovascular disease and heart disease in older women.

Some older patients have hyperglycaemia secondary to acute illness, diabetogenic therapy or other stress-inducing disorders. This can be identified because the HbA1c is often normal, but the oral glucose tolerance test (OGTT) should be employed where doubt exists. Retesting following an acute illness may sometimes prevent a false diagnosis from being made. Particular difficulties may intrude. A true fasted sample may be difficult to obtain (and may be normal), while an OGTT may be declined because it is time consuming and inconvenient.

Management

A comprehensive set of evidenced based clinical guidelines for type 2 diabetes in older people has been developed, and these provide a logical pathway for clinical decision-making in older people.

An approach to management is indicated in the box below. It is important to identify 'frail' patients, i.e. those who are especially vulnerable to a wide range of diverse outcomes secondary to the effects of ageing, chronic diabetic complications, physical and cognitive decline, and the presence of other medical comorbidities. The Frailty Model of Diabetes can assist clinical decision-making by defining factors (e.g. recurrent hypoglycaemia, cardiac disease, and reduced recovery from metabolic decompensation), which may herald disability and often directly threaten independence, yet may have preventable or reversible components. In clinical practice, the presence of a mobility disorder or severe restriction of activities of daily living (ADL), or the presence of several comorbidities, and/or advanced age (>80 years) will increase the risk of becoming confined to a chair or bed by two- to threefold over 2 years.

An approach to diabetes care in older adults
1 Functional assessment, including cognitive testing and screening for depression
2 Vascular risk assessment, especially vascular prophylaxis and lifestyle modification
3 Metabolic targeting ('single disease' or 'frailty' models)
4 Devise appropriate interventions for diabetes related disabilities
5 Assess suitability for self care vs. carer assistance.

Glycaemia and blood pressure targets for older people with diabetes

A range of evidence-based values for glucose lowering has recently been developed based on the original set of European guidelines. In view of the concerns raised by recent trials of glucose lowering, the following recommendations for HbA1c have been proposed.

1 For older patients with type 2 diabetes, with single system involvement (free of other major comorbidities), a target HbA1c range of 7–7.5% should be aimed for (DCC T aligned). Evidence level 1+, grade of recommendation A. The precise target agreed will depend on

existing cardiovascular risk, presence of microvascular complications, and ability of individual to self manage

2 For frail (dependent; multisystem disease; care home residency including those with dementia) patients where the hypoglycaemia risk is high and symptom control and avoidance of metabolic decompensation is paramount, the target HbA1c range should be 7.5–8.5%. Evidence level 1+, grade of recommendation A

These address concerns about minimizing the risk of hypoglycaemia and provide some reduction in vascular risk.

The following are recommendations for blood pressure lowering in the non-frail.

1 The threshold for treatment of high blood pressure in older subjects with type 2 diabetes should be 140/80 mmHg or higher present for more >3 months and measured on at least three separate occasions during a period of lifestyle management advice (behavioural: exercise, weight reduction, smoking advice, nutrition/dietary advice). Evidence level 2++, grade of recommendation B.

2 In subjects with diabetes older than 80 years, a blood pressure threshold for treatment should be 160/90 mmHg or higher. Evidence level 1+, grade of recommendation B.

Modification of this guidance will be necessary for those with a history of frailty or those living in care home settings.

Thromboembolic prophylaxis, e.g. with aspirin (75 mg/day), or clopidogrel (75 mg/day) if aspirin is not tolerated, is appropriate in older subjects with diabetes and macrovascular disease or risk factors such as hypertension, obesity, albuminuria, or cigarette smoking. Atrial fibrillation is more common in older people with diabetes, but there is no specific evidence to support full warfarin anticoagulation in this population in the absence of other indications, such as hypertension.

The available methods which estimate cardiovascular risk (e.g. 10–20%) over a 5- or 10-year period, include the New Zealand tables and data from the Framingham and Seven European Countries studies; all are limited by the lack of data from people over 74 years of age. Reducing triglyceride levels may also help to reduce overall cardiovascular risk in older subjects. In a New Zealand study, subjects with type 2 diabetes aged over 70 years had an increased mortality if they had hyperlipidaemia, while the Veterans Affairs High Density Lipoprotein Cholesterol Intervention Trial (VA-HIT) study showed that treatment with gemfibrozil lowered cardiovascular mortality by over 20%; three-quarters of the latter population were aged 60–74 years, and 25% had diabetes. The Heart Protection Study included adults with diabetes aged 40–80 years treated with simvastatin 40 mg or placebo over a 5-year period. Treatment led to an average fall in LDL-cholesterol of 1.0 mmol/L and resulted in a 27% reduction in the incidence of first non-fatal myocardial infarction or coronary death, and a 25% reduction in first non-fatal stroke or fatal stroke. Evidence of benefit was observed as early as 12 months of treatment.

In a comparison of different antihypertensive regimens in the prevention of coronary heart disease and other cardiovascular events, the study was terminated early because of the obvious significant benefits on mortality being achieved with an amlodipine-based regimen. This study involved people up to age 79 years, and in those with type 2 diabetes benefits were similar. These included the incidence of the composite endpoint (total cardiovascular events and procedures) compared with the atenolol based regimen (hazard ratio 0.86, confidence interval 0.76–0.98, p = 0.026). In addition, fatal and nonfatal strokes were reduced by 25% (p = 0.017), peripheral arterial disease by 48% (p = 0.004) and non-coronary revascularization procedures by 57% (p<0.001).

The Micro-HOPE study investigated the effects of ramipril on macro- and microvascular disease in people aged over 55 years over a 4.5-year period. All subjects were at high cardiovascular risk or had diabetes together with another cardiovascular risk factor such as hypertension or dyslipidaemia. Primary endpoints were significantly reduced from 20% to 15%, while all-cause mortality fell by 24%.

Several recent studies have looked at the benefits of tighter glucose regulation with type 2 diabetes. Excess cardiovascular mortality was demonstrated in the Action to Control Cardiovascular Risk in Diabetes (ACCORD) in the intensive group where the average HbA1c was 6.4% (46 mmol/mol) whereas the Action in Diabetes and Vascular Disease: Preterax and Diamicron MR Controlled Evaluation (ADVANCE) study, excess mortality was not demonstrated. Neither study indicated any benefit in reducing cardiovascular outcomes despite similar reductions in HbA1c in the intensive groups. A further study in American veterans with type 2 diabetes (average HbA1c: 6.9% (52 mmol/mol) in the intensive group) also failed to show benefit at HbA1c level in the range usually aimed for by most clinicians. The rates of hypoglycaemia were significantly more common in the intensive groups in all studies. For older people, these results pose several dilemmas in management: first, they do not answer the important clinical question of how to reduce cardiovascular risk, and, second, what is the optimal level of blood glucose to aim for which substantially reduces microvascular risk and avoids severe hypoglycaemia. For now, we must continue to aim for realistic targets (similar to younger adults) for all those older patients who do not have marked evidence of frailty. Intensified treatment in this latter category is not justified at present on the basis of these recent intervention studies.

Principal aims in management

Medical

Freedom from hyperglycaemic symptoms

Prevent undesirable weight loss

Avoid hypoglycaemia and other adverse drug reactions

Screen for and prevent vascular complications

Detect cognitive impairment and depression at an early stage

Achieve a normal life expectancy for patients where possible

Patient orientated

Maintain general well being and good quality of life

Acquire skills and knowledge to adapt to lifestyle changes

Encourage diabetes self care

An initial diabetes care plan should be drawn up for the individual patient. The guidelines of the International Diabetes Federation for managing type 2 diabetes appear equally applicable to older subjects although more detailed specialist guidance is now available. Patients with type 1 diabetes are managed as in younger individuals.

Care plan for initial management of diabetes

1 Establish realistic glycaemic and blood pressure targets
2 Provide an estimate of cardiovascular risk over 5 years
3 Ensure consensus with patient, spouse or family, general practitioner, informal carer, community nurse or hospital specialist
4 Define the frequency and nature of diabetes follow up
5 Organize glycaemic monitoring by patient or carer
6 Refer to social or community services as necessary
7 Provide advice on stopping smoking, increasing exercise and decreasing alcohol intake

---

Lifestyle modification

Dietary and lifestyle advice are given as for middle-aged people, including an exercise programme if possible. Including a resistance training component may be important in minimizing the disability (by increasing muscle strength) associated with lower limb dysfunction. These measures may be sufficient for subjects with minimal symptoms, whose initial random glucose levels lie between 8 and 15 mmol/L. If metabolic targets are not reached by 6–8 weeks, oral therapy is required.

Active management of other cardiovascular risk factors, especially hypertension and dyslipidaemia, is necessary from the outset (see Principal aim in management).

Oral hypoglycaemic agents

Sulphonylureas

Sulphonylureas are often used initially in older people with diabetes failing on diet, because they are generally well tolerated. Their main hazard is hypoglycaemia. This is a particular problem with glibenclamide, which must be strictly avoided in older people. Glipizide can cause prolonged hypoglycaemia in older people and has been linked to hypoglycaemic deaths. Gliclazide has a relatively low risk of hypoglycaemia, and it is safer than glibenclamide from a hypoglycaemia risk perspective. Tolbutamide carries a low risk of hypoglycaemia and can be used in those with mild renal impairment (serum creatinine <150 µmol/L (eGFR <42 mL/min/1.73m^2 based on a 75-year-old non-black male).

With all sulphonylureas, the maximal glucose lowering effect is about 4–5 mmol/L. Patients with very high glucose levels will not therefore achieve adequate glycaemic control.

Metformin

Metformin is predictable and safe if it is used correctly and its contraindications are respected: these include renal impairment (serum creatinine >120 mol/L, eGFR <54 mL/min/1.73m^2 based on a 75-year-old non-black male), hepatic or cardiac failure, critical limb ischaemia, and severe acute illness.

Advantages of metformin are that it does not cause hypoglycaemia or weight gain on its own. Its glucose-lowering effect is similar to sulphonylureas, including in older individuals. The usual dose required is approximately 1.7g, and it is as effective in the lean as in the overweight. Metformin was the only antidiabetic drug shown to reduce macrovascular events in the UKPDS, and all-cause mortality and combined diabetes related endpoints were significantly lower with metformin than with insulin or sulphonylurea in obese people.

Thiazolidinediones

Thiazolidinediones (TZDs) reduce insulin resistance by activating the peroxisome proliferator activated receptor-(PPAR). They lower glucose by 3–4 mmol/L and as monotherapy they reduce HbA1c by 0.5–1.4% (5–15 mmol/mol). Although they do not cause hypoglycaemia, their main problems are mild oedema, dilutional anaemia (in 5% of people), and weight gain with a twofold increased risk of heart failure, in which they are contraindicated. TZDs can be given in combination with metformin or sulphonylureas, and pioglitazone can be given with insulin in the UK. Several meta-analyses suggest that rosiglitazone treatment may be associated with an increased cardiovascular risk and this is likely to limit its prescription in people with diabetes in the future. This increased risk has not been demonstrated for pioglitazone. Both TZDs are associated with an increased fracture risk, mainly in women, and this is an additional factor to consider when screening older people with osteoporosis for treatment with a TZD. They are safe in mild to moderate renal impairment. The liver damage associated with troglitazone (now withdrawn) does not appear to extend to rosiglitazone or pioglitazone, but frequent monitoring of liver function is required, especially during the first 12 months of treatment; this is a drawback for many older people.

Pioglitazone has comparable hypoglycaemic effects and shows a modest improvement in lipid profile; up to 6–8 weeks may elapse before the full beneficial actions are seen. This drug can be given as once daily, which is helpful for older patients.

Non-sulphonylurea insulin secretagogues (glinides)

Repaglinide predominantly lowers postprandial hyperglycaemia. It has a rapid onset of action and a lower risk of hypoglycaemia than the sulphonylureas, and achieves better postprandial glucose profiles. Repaglinide is predominantly metabolized in the liver to inactive metabolites and is safe in mild to moderate renal impairment. Tablets can be missed if meals are omitted, and it may be effectively combined with metformin and with thiazolidinediones (where licence permits).

Nateglinide is a recent meglitinide that has a faster and shorter duration of insulin secretory activity than repaglinide but is less effective as monotherapy or in combination than rapaglinide.

Incretin

Incretin therapies for type 2 diabetes provide a new and potentially valuable way of influencing the pathophysiology of diabetes and reducing risk. There are two main classes: dipeptidyl peptidase-4 (DPP-IV) inhibitors and glucagon-like polypeptide-1 (GLP-1) receptor agonists. By inhibiting the breakdown of the incretin hormones, DPP-IV inhibitors act by increasing the circulating level of incretin hormones, GLP-1 and glucose-dependent insulinotropic polypeptide (GIP). This can also be achieved by directly mimicking GLP-1 action by the use of GLP-1 agonists. Examples of DPP-IV inhibitors include sitagliptin and vildagliptin, although several new drugs are in development in this class. They can be considered as second-line therapy to metformin in those cases where hypoglycaemia is considered a major risk with a sulphonylurea. Weight neutrality and low risk of hypoglycaemia with both classes are valuable in managing diabetes in older people. Examples of GLP-1 agonists include exenatide and liraglutide, and may be considered as third-line therapy to metformin and a sulphonylurea in those with obesity (BMI >35 kg/m^2). These are given subcutaneously and have advantages similar to the DPP-IV inhibitor class with important reductions in HbA1c and relatively good tolerability.

Insulin

Recent improvements in the organization of care between hospital and primary care, and the expanding roles of diabetes specialist nurses and general practice nurses, have made it easier and safer to use insulin in the treatment of older people with diabetes. The main indications in older people are type 1 diabetes or type 2 diabetes, where metabolic targets have not been achieved with diet, exercise and oral agents. It should also be used following acute myocardial infarction, acute stroke, hyperglycaemic coma, and major surgery.

The main disadvantage of insulin is hypoglycaemia, although the UKPDS found that fewer than 2% of people treated with insulin suffered a major hypoglycaemic episode. Reported benefits include improvements in wellbeing and possibly quality of life and in cognitive function, partly following improved glycaemic control; however, others have found lower treatment satisfaction in insulin-treated patients.

Guidelines for insulin treatment in older patients are suggested in Table 8.1. Rapidly acting insulin analogues such as insulin lispro may cause less hypoglycaemia and weight gain, and can be given after eating where timing may be unpredictable, e.g. because of memory disorder. In patients with type 1 diabetes, premixed insulins given twice daily may achieve reasonable glycaemic control, although nocturnal hypoglycaemia may be troublesome because of the longer acting component of the pre-supper dose.

Table 8.1 Guidelines for insulin treatment in older people

	Indications	Advantages	Disadvantages
Once-daily insulin	Frail subjects Very old (>80 y) Symptomatic control	Single injection Can be given by carer or district nurse	Control usually poor Hypoglycaemia common
Twice-daily insulin	Preferred if good glycaemic control Suitable for type 1 diabetes	Low risk of hypoglycaemia Easily managed by most older diabetic people	Normoglycaemia difficult to achieve Fixed meal times reduce flexibility Expensive
Basal/bolus insulin	Well motivated individuals Can reduce microvascular complications	Enables tight control for acute illness in hospital Flexible meal times	Frequent monitoring required to avoid hypoglycaemia
Insulin plus oral agents	If glycaemic control is unsatisfactory with oral agents alone To limit weight gain in obese subjects	Limits weight gain Increased flexibility	May delay conversion to insulin reducing total daily insulin in thin or type 1 patients

In older patients with type 2 diabetes, a twice daily regimen of human isophane insulin can be used, adding short-acting insulin to cover meals if necessary. The newly introduced long-acting insulin analogues (e.g. glargine and detemir) have more reproducible pharmacokinetics and a 'peakless' action profile, and may prove safer in older people. Once daily insulin regimens alone are now little used, except where glycaemic control is not a priority or injections are impracticable.

Insulin can usefully be combined with an oral agent in patients failing to be controlled by diet and oral agents. A suitable regimen is a night time dose of intermediate acting insulin (e.g. isophane) together with metformin, which causes less weight gain and hypoglycaemia, and better glycaemic control than twice daily insulin or combinations of glibenclamide with insulin or metformin. The use of insulin in older people varies enormously even in developed countries. For frail older people, including those within care home settings, complex regimens should be avoided and the use of longer acting insulin analogues during the day often combined with oral agents is a feasible alternative.

Low vision aids are available to help to inject insulin, and some insulin pens have audible clicks for counting doses.

Managing diabetes in care homes

The numbers of care home residents are increasing, and the prevalence of diabetes in this setting will inevitably increase.

Between 7% and 27% of care home residents in the UK and US have diabetes. The wide range is partly because of differences in the diagnostic criteria used, the prevalence of IGT may be as high as 30%. People with diabetes in care homes should receive care commensurate with their health and social needs. The best possible quality of life and wellbeing should be maintained, without unnecessary or inappropriate interventions, while helping residents to manage their own diabetes wherever feasible and worthwhile.

Metabolic control should reduce both hyperglycaemic lethargy and hypoglycaemia with a well-balanced dietetic plan that prevents weight loss and maintains nutritional wellbeing. Foot care and vision require screening and preventive measures to maintain mobility and prevent falls and unnecessary hospital admissions.

> **Recommendations for improving diabetes management in care homes**
>
> - Screen on admission for diabetes and regularly thereafter
> - Policies must include strategies to minimize hospital admission, metabolic decompensation, pressure sore development, pain, diabetes-related complications, infections, and weight loss
> - All residents with diabetes must have an annual review and access to specialist services
> - Care home diabetes policies must be developed nationally, locally and at the level of the resident with diabetes
> - Research based on interventional strategies is needed
>
> Various strategies may improve diabetes care in this setting. The impact of these initiatives is being followed on outcomes including wellbeing, metabolic control, access to regular review, rates of hospitalization, and diabetic complications such as amputation and visual loss. Guidelines called 'Good clinical practice guidelines for care home residents with diabetes' are available at www. diabetes.org.uk.

At present, residents with diabetes in care homes appear to be generally vulnerable and neglected, with high prevalences of macrovascular complications and infections (especially skin and urinary tract), frequent hospitalization, and much physical and cognitive disability. Known deficiencies of diabetes care include lack of individual management care plans, and dietary supervision, infrequent review by specialist nurses, doctors and ophthalmologists, and poor knowledge and training for care staff.

Modern diabetes care for older people

Structured diabetes care is particularly important for older people who are often neglected at present, with the current shift in healthcare from hospitals to the community, general practitioners will play an increasingly important role. This will require considerable motivation by the general practitioner, effective screening and close liaison with diabetes specialist nurses. A shared care approach, with general practitioners working in partnership with hospital based diabetic and surgical specialists and based around agreed clinical protocols is particularly valuable for older people.

A modern geriatric diabetes service is based on a multi-dimensional intervention model. This emphasizes the importance of early intervention in diabetic complications and of establishing rehabilitation programmes for patients disabled by various complications, e.g. amputation, peripheral neuropathy, immobility, falls, stroke, and cognitive change. 'Critical event monitoring' denotes monitoring periods of ill-health or social care need where patient vulnerability is high and opportunity for intervention is paramount, e.g. admission to hospital, amputation or stroke, (see www.diabetes.nhs.uk).

Healthcare must be cost-effective, which presents a difficult challenge for diabetes, because of its high prevalence, long duration of impact, and wide spectrum of complications and emotional and psychological sequelae; in older people, the challenge is even more complex because of the many other confounding factors.

Further reading

Anonymous (2000). Effects of ramipril on cardiovascular and microvascular outcomes in people with diabetes mellitus: results of the HOPE and MICRO HOPE substudy. Heart Outcomes Prevention Evaluation Study Investigators. *Lancet* **355**: 253–9.

Collins R, Armitage J, Parish S, *et al.* (2004). Heart Protection Study Collaborative Group. Effects of cholesterol lowering with simvastatin on stroke and other major vascular events in 20536 people with cerebrovascular disease or other high risk conditions. *Lancet* **363**(9411): 757–67.

Diabetes Control and Complications Trial Research Group (1993). The effect of intensive treatment of diabetes on the development and progression of long term complications in insulin dependent diabetes mellitus. *N Engl J Med* **329**: 977–86.

Goyder EC, McNally PG, Drucquer M, *et al.* (1998). Shifting of care for diabetes from secondary to primary care, 1990–5: a review of general practices. *BMJ* **316**: 1505–6.

Kannel WB, McGee DL (1979). Diabetes and cardiovascular disease: the Framingham Study. *JAMA* **241**: 2035–8.

Krishhan S, Nash F, Baker N, *et al.* (2008). Reduction in diabetic amputations over 11 years in a defined UK population: benefits of multi disciplinary team work and continuous prospective audits. *Diabetes Care* **31**: 99–101.

Muggeo M, Verlato G, Bonora E, *et al.* (1995). Long-term instability of fasting plasma glucose predicts mortality in elderly NIDDM patients: the Verona Diabetes Study. *Diabetologia* **38**: 672–9.

Muggeo M, Verlato G, Bonora E, *et al.* (1995). The Verona Diabetes Study: a population-based survey on known diabetes mellitus prevalence and 5-year all cause mortality. *Diabetologia* **38**: 318–25.

Ostergren J, Poulter NR, Sever PS, *et al.* (2008). The Anglo- Scandinavian Cardiac Outcomes Trial: blood pressure lowering limb: effects in patients with type II diabetes. *J Hypertens*, **26**(11): 2103–11.

Sinclair AJ, Bayer AJ, Girling AJ, *et al.* (2000). Older adults, diabetes mellitus and visual acuity: a community based case control study. *Age Ageing* **29**: 335–9.

United Kingdom Prospective Diabetes Study (UKPDS) (1998). Effect of intensive blood glucose control with metformin on complications in overweight patients with type 2 diabetes. *Lancet* **352**: 854–65.

United Kingdom Prospective Diabetes Study (UKPDS) Group (1998). Intensive blood glucose control with sulphonylureas or insulin compared with conventional treatment and risk of complications in patients with type II diabetes. *Lancet* **352**: 837–53.

United Kingdom Prospective Diabetes Study (UKPDS) Group (1998). Tight blood pressure control and risk of macrovascular and microvascular complications in type II diabetes. *Br Med J* **317**: 703–13.

Thyroid disease

Investigating the thyroid
Thyroid function tests
Thyroid function tests are one of the most frequently requested endocrine investigations in general medical practice. Optimum assessment includes assay of free thyroxine levels (fT4) and serum thyroid stimulating hormone (TSH), but many laboratories will now perform TSH alone as a first-line screen of thyroid function, with automatic cascade of fT4 if TSH is outside the normal range. TSH above or below the normal range is indeed a sensitive marker of thyroid hypofunction and hyperfunction respectively, but can be normal in pituitary disorders despite over- or, most often under-activity, of the axis. Therefore, where TSH is normal but symptoms are strongly suggestive of thyroid dysfunction (or in the presence of known pituitary disease) a fT4 value is always essential. Free T3 (fT3) is essential when fT4 is normal but TSH suppressed, but otherwise is rarely contributory.

Thyroid antibodies
Thyroid antibodies, most commonly antithyroid peroxidase (TPO) antibodies, are a marker of autoimmune thyroid disease and useful in establishing the aetiology of thyrotoxicosis or goitre. Titre of TPO antibodies is rarely of clinical relevance and repeated measurement is rarely required. TSH receptor stimulating antibodies are available in some centres.

Imaging
Thyroid ultrasound is the simplest and most effective technique to image thyroid size and structure, but is very operator dependant. Isotope scans of the thyroid can help in the differential diagnosis of thyrotoxicosis, in particular to confirm the presence of a 'hot' thyroid nodule or thyroiditis (lack of uptake), and are essential in follow-up of treated thyroid cancer. The thyroid can be readily identified on computed tomography (CT) and magnetic resonance imaging (MRI) and incidental thyroid enlargement is often discovered this way, but they are rarely used as the primary imaging modality.

Hypothyroidism
Hypothyroidism is the most common endocrine deficiency and is increasingly common with advancing age (lifetime prevalence is 9% in women and 1% in men). Therefore patients undergoing assessment in a geriatric medicine service will often be treated with levothyroxine replacement, although the diagnosis and treatment of the condition is typically undertaken entirely in primary care.

Hypothyroidism may be suspected on the basis of typical symptoms listed below, but the diagnosis is dependent on biochemical results. An elevated TSH is the diagnostic marker, with treatment usually automatically indicated when TSH is >10 mIU/L; as hypothyroidism becomes more severe, the fT4 level falls below the normal range and may become undetectable in longstanding untreated cases. Minor elevations of TSH (<10) with normal fT4 usually do not require treatment (see below). Unless iatrogenic, the aetiology is almost always autoimmune and TPO antibodies may confirm this.

Examination may reveal typical physical signs, but these are neither specific nor sensitive in making the diagnosis.

Complications of untreated hypothyroidism may also be present, including carpal tunnel syndrome, worsening hypertension and heart failure, hypercholesterolaemia, and consequent increased incidence of ischaemic heart disease.

Symptoms and signs of hypothyroidism:
- Tiredness
- Weight gain
- Cold intolerance, rarely leading to hypothermia
- Constipation
- Dry skin and hair – loss of eyebrows
- Neck swelling or goitre
- Change in appearance – myxoedema facies
- General muscular weakness and pain, including cramps and stiffness
- Depression* (rarely psychosis 'myxoedema madness')
- Husky voice
- Unsteadiness*
- Oedema and worsening heart failure*
- Poor memory*
- Deafness*
- Anaemia

*Particular relevance in older population

Author's Tip

Screening for hypothyroidism is not considered clinically or cost-effective; having a low threshold to check thyroid function when suggestive symptoms are present is recommended.

Severe, untreated hypothyroidism may rarely lead to hypothyroid or 'myxoedema coma'. This is typically precipitated by an intercurrent illness, such as infection or infarction of different organs, and the patient presents with a reduced conscious level, clinical signs of hypothyroidism and usually hypothermia. Pericardial effusion is an important but rare complication of severe hypothyroidism.

Treatment
Treatment of hypothyroidism is almost always with levothyroxine replacement. The aim of treatment is a TSH in the middle to lower part of the normal range with a normal fT4 level.

Initiation of treatment depends on clinical context. A case with moderate elevation of TSH, normal fT4 and mild symptoms may be commenced directly on levothyroxine 50 µg once daily (or even 100 µg in younger patients). Patients with severe deficiency and associated comorbidities, particularly known ischaemic heart disease, are more safely started on 25 µg and increased to 50 µg after a couple of weeks. Dosage is increased up to 100 µg daily and then adjusted, usually in 25-µg increments, in the light of TSH levels, which should be checked 6–8 weeks after a dose change when steady state levels have been achieved (half-life of levothyroxine is about 1 week).

Parenteral thyroid replacement is rarely if ever necessary (and oral levothyroxine can be administered down a nasogastric tube or PEG if necessary). In suspected myxoedema coma, treat the hypothermia, fluid depletion, and electrolyte imbalance and infection conventionally first, check for hypoadrenalism (and replace if necessary) and leave the levothyroxine until later.

Author's Tip

Most cases of hypothermia are not due to hypothyroidism and thyroid function may be misleading during acute illness.

Hypothyroid symptoms with normal thyroid function tests

A substantial body of opinion on the internet and in the popular press asserts that symptoms of hypothyroidism can occur with normal thyroid function tests and may respond to thyroid replacement. This view is not supported by clinical trials nor by endocrine opinion worldwide. If fT4 and TSH are both normal then the patient is euthyroid and another cause should be sought for the symptoms, except in the presence of proven pituitary disease.

Author's Tip

Do not repeat thyroid function tests unnecessarily; if the TSH level was normal a few months ago (on or off levothyroxine) then it is unlikely to be abnormal now if symptoms are unchanged. TSH is normally simply checked annually on long-term levothyroxine replacement.

Thyrotoxicosis

Thyrotoxicosis (or hyperthyroidism) is the most common form of hormonal oversecretion affecting perhaps 2–5% of all females at some time and with a gender ratio of 5:1, most often between ages 20 and 40 years. Nodular thyroid disease becomes more common with increasing age.

Although thyrotoxicosis is typically suspected on the basis of symptoms, diagnosis is based on biochemistry with a very low TSH (typically undetectable, e.g. <0.05 mIU/L) with elevated fT4 and/or fT3 level. Individuals with suppressed TSH but normal fT4 and fT3 do not normally require treatment (see below).

Symptoms and signs of thyrotoxicosis:

- Weight loss despite increased appetite
- Tremor
- Palpitations (and frequently atrial fibrillation (AF) in older people)
- Heat intolerance and sweating
- Anxiety and agitation (sometimes depression)
- Neck swelling or goitre
- Diarrhoea
- Thirst and itching
- Breathlessness
- Muscle weakness, falls
- Worsening of heart failure
- Symptoms of thyroid-associated ophthalmopathy

Examination may reveal tachycardia, with or without AF, tremor, goitre and a typical 'toxic' affect as well as proptosis and other signs of thyroid eye disease.

Author's Tip

Thyrotoxicosis may present in older population without typical symptoms, for example as heart failure and AF or 'apathetic thyrotoxicosis'.

Aetiology of thyrotoxicosis:

- Autoimmune – Graves' disease
- Multinodular goitre
- Single 'hot' thyroid nodule
- Acute thyroiditis
- Drugs – particularly amiodarone
- Levothyroxine over-replacement

Graves' disease is the most common aetiology overall, but is more prevalent in younger age groups. Diagnosis is suggested by a personal or family history of autoimmune endocrine disease and a smooth regular goitre. It is confirmed by the presence of positive thyroid antibodies or thyroid-associated ophthalmopathy.

A nodular goitre is typically suspected clinically on examination and confirmed by thyroid ultrasound. In the presence of a single solid nodule, a thyroid isotope scan will confirm if the nodule is functioning ('hot') or non-functioning ('cold').

Acute thyroiditis may present with a smooth tender goitre, or with no palpable goitre, but will often be associated with a history of tenderness in the neck around the time of symptoms of an acute viral illness.

Amiodarone may cause thyrotoxicosis by precipitation of underlying Graves' disease by the associated iodine load (type I) or due to a drug-induced thyroiditis (type II).

Treatment

First-line treatment for thyrotoxicosis is usually with antithyroid drugs: carbimazole or propylthiouracil (PTU) in the case of allergy to the former. In Graves' disease, carbimazole may be continued for a standard course of 18 months in the hope that remission will occur (50% of cases). In nodular thyroid disease, a more permanent ablative treatment is usually indicated, radioactive iodine (RAI) or occasionally surgery.

Carbimazole is started initially at full dose. When fT4 is >30 pmol/L, 40 mg once daily reduced to 20 mg after 1 month will achieve biochemical control within a few weeks. Propranolol may be used to control symptoms in the interim (if there are no contraindications). For fT4 25–30 pmol/L, starting with 20 mg once daily is more appropriate to avoid hypothyroidism. Thyroid function tests are typically monitored every 6–8 weeks initially.

When TSH rises towards or above top of the normal range, then carbimazole dose can be slowly reduced, However, beware that in the early weeks of treatment TSH may remain suppressed when fT4 has fallen below normal: both fT4 and TSH levels are essential to monitor therapy at this stage.

Author's Tip

Do not monitor white cell count on carbimazole, as the neutropenia or agranulocytosis is idiosyncratic and sudden in onset. Rather, give written advice to every patient to attend urgently for full blood count if they get a severe sore throat or skin rash. Reactions typically occur in the first few weeks of treatment.

RAI is preferred treatment for nodular disease, after relapse or in case of patient preference. Antithyroid drugs are stopped 1–2 weeks before and RAI administered as a single oral dose. Strict radiation safety rules apply, which may be offputting to some patients and cause difficulties in the case of immobility or incontinence (although the radiation protection law makes allowances for 'comforters and carers'). RAI will usually control thyrotoxicosis within a few weeks, but the patient is at long-term risk of RAI-induced hypothyroidism (and requires lifelong monitoring for this).

Surgery rapidly controls thyrotoxicosis, but is rarely required except in the case of a large goitre, uncontrolled thyrotoxicosis despite drugs and/or patient preference.

T3 toxicosis
T3 toxicosis causes elevated fT3 and normal fT4 and must always be excluded (by measurement of fT3) when TSH is suppressed. It is more common in nodular thyroid disease, but the treatment is identical.

Thyroid-associated ophthalmopathy and dermopathy
These conditions are associated autoimmune manifestations of Graves' disease caused by interaction of the immune system with antigens related to the TSH receptor in orbital fibroblasts and in skin. Mild thyroid-associated ophthalmopathy (TAO) presents with watering eyes and irritation and inflammation of the conjunctivae, progressing to increasing proptosis or exophthalmos and limitation of eye movements (and diplopia) due to involvement of extra-occular muscles. In the most severe cases, compression of the optic nerve can lead to reduced visual acuity. In smokers, TAO is more common and more severe when it does occur. Lid lag and 'stare' may be simply caused by the sympathetic overactivity associated with the toxic state and do not in themselves confirm a diagnosis of TAO.

Mild TAO may require no treatment or simple management with 'artificial tears'. Severe TAO is treated with high-dose steroids and ultimately may require orbital decompression surgery; it always requires a specialist endocrine and ophthalmic opinion (preferably in a combined specialist service). An exacerbation of TAO is more frequent after RAI than on antithyroid drugs.

Dermopathy is rare but may present as pretibial myxoedema, a thickened and often tender eruption on the anterior aspect of the shin.

Borderline thyroid states
Borderline hypothyroidism
Borderline or subclinical hypothyroidism describe states where the TSH is elevated but fT4 remains normal (also described as 'compensated euthyroidism'). Where TSH is <10 mIU/L, this is rarely associated with symptoms and usually simply requires monitoring of thyroid function at increasing intervals. The main exception (when pregnancy is planned) is clearly not relevant to the geriatric clinic. Patients with unexplained symptoms which might be caused by hypothyroidism may be treated with levothyroxine as a therapeutic trial, but these symptoms will rarely improve with treatment. Unresolved hypercholesterolaemia is another reason to consider replacement. High levels of TPO antibodies makes progression to frank hypothyroidism more likely.

Most endocrinologists would give replacement to a patient with TSH >10 mIU/L whatever the fT4 value and whether or not symptoms are present.

Borderline hyperthyroidism
Borderline or subclinical hyperthyroidism describe the situation where TSH is below normal but fT4 and fT3 remain in the normal range (also known as 'autonomous thyroid function'). This is known to carry a significantly increased risk of atrial fibrillation, but randomized trials have never been undertaken to demonstrate overall benefits (or risks)

of treatment versus conservative management. There is therefore no consensus as to whether such patients should receive antithyroid treatment. Most endocrinologists would treat patients with suggestive symptoms or with unexplained or uncontrolled tachycardia or tachyarrhythmias and some advise more aggressive treatment to normalize thyroid function.

Drugs and thyroid function
Thyroid function may be influenced by numerous medications so a detailed drug history is important, particularly in the context of polypharmacy in older population. Amiodarone can cause either hypothyroidism or hyperthyroidism (see above) and reduces T4 to T3 conversion. Patients on lithium are at risk of hypothyroidism. Novel immunomodulatory drugs can cause thyroid dysfunction by activation of the immune system. Commonly prescribed drugs such as proton pump inhibitors, ferrous salts, and calcium can interfere with absorption of levothyroxine.

Pituitary–thyroid axis
Thyroid dysfunction as the result of pituitary disease is much less common than primary thyroid disease, but should not be forgotten.

In particular, in untreated hypopituitarism with TSH deficiency, the serum TSH may remain in the normal range even though fT4 levels are low. This is an important rare situation where the economically efficient use of TSH as a screening test fails to detect disease, and if unexplained hypothyroid symptoms and signs are clearly present when TSH is normal, then a fT4 level should always be checked.

TSH hypersecretion by a thyrotroph adenoma is extremely rare, but may result in symptoms and an elevated fT4 level whilst TSH remains in the reference range.

Sick euthyroid syndrome
Thyroid function tests are frequently misleading during acute intercurrent illness. fT4 levels are typically low during severe illness with altered de-iodination leading to increased levels of reverse T3 and lower levels of fT3. TSH may be normal, low or slightly elevated. It remains unclear whether this is an appropriate metabolic reaction to the stress of illness or whether it has adverse effects on the patient, but there is as yet no convincing evidence that thyroid replacement offers any benefit.

Overall, it is best to avoid checking thyroid function tests until the acute illness is controlled or resolved, and when tests have been performed, it is rarely appropriate to offer treatment without relevant specialist advice.

> **Author's Tip**
>
> A low free T4 with normal TSH may represent the sick euthyroid syndrome but is also consistent with pituitary TSH deficiency. If in doubt, further pituitary evaluation may be indicated.

Goitre and thyroid cancer
Goitre is common and is most often detected on inspection or palpation of the neck, often with no associated symptoms. When symptoms do occur they may be simply the presence of a swelling and associated cosmetic concerns, or pressure symptoms associated with neck movements or posture, swallowing or rarely breathing. Occasionally the patient is worried about the presence of a malignancy.

Thyroid function should always be checked, but if normal then investigation and treatment are initially guided by clinical assessment. A small, soft regular goitre can often be safely ignored. A larger goitre is typically best investigated by ultrasound, although a classic multinodular goitre can be diagnosed clinically. Isolated single nodules require investigation to exclude cyst or neoplasm (see below). Strongly positive TPO antibodies may confirm an autoimmune aetiology and if very high (>2000 IU/mL) may be labelled Hashimoto's thyroiditis.

If malignancy has been excluded, surgery is normally only indicated in cases of patient preference. RAI has also been advocated as a simpler treatment for euthyroid goitre.

Causes of goitre:
- Benign thyroid nodules (colloid; follicular adenoma)
- Thyroid cancer
- Iodine deficiency
- Multinodular goitre
- Autoimmune thyroiditis (Graves' and Hashimoto's)
- Thyroid cyst
- Physiological goitre (e.g. pregnancy)

Author's Tip

Goitre is common and often requires no treatment as long as thyroid function tests are normal and there are no red flag clinical features such as rapid enlargement or lymphadenopathy.

Nodules and thyroid cancer

The exclusion of thyroid cancer represents an important clinical challenge. A large majority of thyroid nodules (whether isolated or multinodular) are benign, but conversely differentiated thyroid cancer is a relatively common incidental finding histologically (e.g. in asymptomatic autopsy series or during thyroid surgery for another indication). Differentiated thyroid cancers (papillary and follicular thyroid carcinomas) usually have a very good prognosis with appropriate treatment, but the rarer medullary thyroid cancers and anaplastic thyroid carcinoma typically have a poor prognosis.

When a patient is found to have an isolated thyroid nodule (presenting symptomatically or discovered on examination) recommended investigation is to assess by fine needle aspiration cytology (FNA) either performed using simple palpation or optimally during ultrasound imaging. If an adequate FNA sample suggests benign disease then no further action is usually required. A result suggestive of a cellular lesion (or more rarely suspicious of malignancy) should normally lead to surgical excision of the nodule unless comorbidities contraindicate surgery. Most tumours excised surgically will, however, still prove to be adenomas rather than cancers.

National guidance on management of differentiated thyroid cancer suggests that appropriate treatment for a tumour >1 cm in diameter usually includes a total thyroidectomy followed by radioiodine ablation therapy. This management regime should always be discussed and agreed by the local thyroid cancer multidisciplinary team who will usually arrange long-term follow-up of the patient. Follow up will usually involve monitoring of serum thyroglobulin levels (to detect the presence of residual or recurrent thyroid disease following ablation of the normal gland), and often radioactive iodine uptake scans (particularly in the early stage following radioactive iodine ablation or when recurrence is suspected). Residual or recurrent tumour may be treated by high-dose radioactive iodine therapy and sometimes by external radiotherapy.

Patients in remission with differentiated thyroid cancer are usually treated with levothyroxine in doses aimed to suppress serum TSH below the normal range (although ideally not to undetectable levels). This is a particular situation where aiming to normalize TSH in a patient on levothyroxine is inappropriate.

When medullary thyroid carcinoma is diagnosed it is now usually appropriate to exclude an underlying genetic cause (such as multiple endocrine neoplasia type 2 (MEN2)). Specialist clinical genetic advice is indicated.

Further reading

BTA and RCP (2007) *Guidelines for the Management of Thyroid Cancer*, 2nd edn. London, British Thyroid Association and Royal College of Physicians (http://www.rcplondon.ac.uk/pubs/ or http://bookshop.rcplondon.ac.uk/details.aspx?e=223).

Cooper DS (2003). Hyperthyroidism. *Lancet* **362**: 459–68.

De Groot L, *et al. Thyroid Disease Manager* (http://www.thyroid-manager.org/ (online thyroid disease textbook).

Hegedüs L (2004). Clinical practice. The thyroid nodule. *N Engl J Med* **351**: 1764–71.

Howlett TA, Levy MJ (2009). Endocrinology. In (Kumar P, Clark M, eds) *Clinical Medicine*, 7th edn. Elsevier, pp. 963–1027.

Pearce EN, Farwell AP, Braverman LE (2003). Thyroiditis. *N Engl J Med* **348**: 2648–55.

Report of a Working Party (2007) Radioiodine in the management of benign thyroid disease: Clinical guidelines. Royal College of Physicians (London) (http://www.rcplondon.ac.uk/pubs/ or http://bookshop.rcplondon.ac.uk/details.aspx?e=208).

Roberts CG, Ladenson PW (2004). Hypothyroidism. *Lancet*, **363**: 793–803.

Sherman SI (2003). Thyroid carcinoma. *Lancet* **361**: 501–11.

Weetman AP (2000). Graves' disease. *N Engl J Med* **343**: 1236–48.

Hyponatraemia and hypernatraemia

Hypo- and hypernatraemia are common electrolyte disorders occurring in older people. Both are associated with high morbidity and mortality.

Changes in sodium and water metabolism in normal ageing

Sodium metabolism

Sodium metabolism is modified by ageing. Sodium reabsorption in the proximal tube is impaired by the higher levels of brain natriuretic peptide (BNP), but this effect on sodium excretion is counterbalanced by the influence of the renin–angiotensin–aldosterone system on the distal tube. However, a lesser reactivity of the renin–angiotensin system in most older people leads to insensible daily losses of sodium and more difficulties in coping with a poor salt diet or digestive sodium losses. This blunt response of renin–aldosterone system is the main factor in extracellular dehydration in older people.

Water metabolism

Water metabolism is also altered by ageing. In response to water restriction, the maximal urinary concentration (1200 mosmol/L) cannot be reached easily. In response to the osmotic stimulus, the arginine vasopressin (AVP) (also known as antidiuretic hormone) secretion threshold remains unchanged and the slope of secretion increases, so that AVP plasma levels are higher in older than in younger adults. However, two renal processes impair the normal water reabsorption in the collector duct:

- the osmotic concentration gradient created by sodium exchanges in loop of Henlé is often impaired by vascular alterations in the renal medullar
- the vasopressin V2 receptors of the collecting ducts have a lesser sensibility to AVP or an impaired transmission of the signal, so that in spite of significant AVP plasma levels, water reabsorption is decreased.

Furthermore, thirst threshold sensation becomes higher in normal ageing (298 vs 294 mosmol) and thirst sensation disappears with a smaller water intake than in younger adults predisposing the older person to intracellular dehydration.

Factors enhancing the physiological changes in sodium and water metabolism

- Diuretics modify sodium reabsorption in loop of Henlé and contribute to impairment of the osmotic corticopapillary gradient and increase urinary sodium losses.
- Sodium-restricted diets or long periods of anorexia lead to sodium deprivation.
- Drugs interacting with collecting duct V2 receptors: amphotericin B, lithium.

Hyponatraemia

Hyponatraemia is the more frequent electrolyte abnormality found in patients treated with diuretics and also in critically ill patients. Hyponatraemia is usually defined by a sodium plasma level of less than 135 mmol/L. Clinical symptoms are those of cellular overhydration: nausea, vomiting, headaches, seizures, coma, and non-specific symptoms, such as falls, weakness, and delirium. Hyponatraemia may also be asymptomatic when the disorder has occurred slowly.

Salt loss with dehydration

In geriatric clinical practice, hyponatraemia is often associated with low extracellular volume related to renal or extrarenal sodium losses. The major cause is treatment with thiazide diuretics. In this case, hyponatraemia is enhanced by AVP secretion in response to volumic stimulus and often by inadequate drinks (water) or hypotonic infusions (hypotonic saline or glucose).

Natriuresis is either low (<10 mmol/24 h) in of the case of extrarenal losses or high (>30 mmol/24 h) in the case of renal losses. Associated clinical symptoms are those of extracellular dehydration: loss of weight, hypotension, and falls. Clinical situations when this arises include digestive losses (diarrhoea, vomiting, fistulae), cutaneous losses (ulcers, heat stroke), or renal losses (diuretics, polycystic disease, interstitial nephritis). Correcting hyponatraemia requires intravenous normo- or hypertonic saline. The rate of infusion must be low to prevent centropontine myelinolysis to which older people are predisposed. The increase in sodium concentration must be less than 10 mmol/L/day.

Syndrome of inappropriate AVP secretion

In inappropriate AVP secretion, hyponatraemia is associated with normal extracellular volume: AVP secretion rate is high in spite of low plasma osmolarity and normal extracellular volume. Natriuresis reflects daily sodium intakes (>30 mmol/L). Many factors are able to enhance AVP secretion: malignancy (lung cancer, brain tumors), pulmonary conditions, brain trauma, drugs (SSRI, neuroleptics, carbamazepine), hypothyroidism. The treatment lies mainly on water restriction (<500 mL/day), treatment of the malignancy, and stopping the incriminated drugs. AVP antagonists (aquaretic agents) are promising drugs but very few older patients are included in clinical trials. Demeclocycline has many renal effects and must be used with caution in older patients.

Dilutional hyponatraemia

Dilution hyponatraemia is associated with high extracellular volume. High renin activity and high AVP plasma levels lead to an increased renal reabsorption of sodium and water. Natriuresis is low <10 mmol/L. Dilution hyponatraemia appears in congestive cardiac insufficiency, hepatic cirrhosis, nephrotic syndromes, and end-stage renal failure. Associated clinical symptoms are peripheral or pulmonary oedema. Treatment is based on loop diuretics (bumetamide, furosemide), water restriction, hemodialysis in the case of end-stage renal failure, and sometimes ultrafiltration in case of congestive cardiac failure with refractory oedema (see Figure 8.4).

Hypernatraemia

The prevalence of hypernatraemia or hyperosmolar state is reported from 1% to 30% varying with the type of hospital and patients. The prevalence increases in nursing homes or long-stay settings that admit frail older patients with cognitive impairment or stroke. In acute-stay settings, hypernatraemia is the first cause of hyperosmolar states. Hypernatraemia is associated with longer hospital stay and is a strong predictor of in-stay mortality and 1-year mortality. Renal, digestive, or cutaneous water losses associated with a decreased sensation of thirst and/or difficulties in accessing water lead rapidly to hypernatraemia.

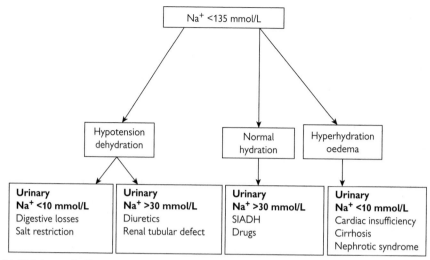

Figure 8.4 Clinical approach of hyponatraemia.

Various infections with fever are associated with hypernatraemia. Clinical symptoms are fatigue, hypotension, anorexia, fall, and delirium or coma. Thirst is an inconsistent finding.

The treatment is based on the compensation of water losses with a hypo-osmolar infusion with or without sodium (glucose 2.5%, glucose 5%, saline <9 g/L) and treatment of the cause. Most cases of hypernatraemia are easy to correct; however, the in-hospital mortality is about 40% and the 1-year mortality about 60%. Hypernatraemia is therefore more a witness of morbidity than a severe condition *per se*. Prevention is based on regular drinking or infusion of hypotonic solute by hypodermoclysis/subcutaneous infusion.

Further reading

Adrogué HJ, Madias NE (2000). Hypernatraemia. *New Engl J Med*, **342**: 1493–99.

Bourdel-Marchasson I, Proux S, Dehail P, *et al.* (2004). One-year incidence of hyperosmolar states and prognosis in geriatric acute care unit. *Gerontology* **50**: 171–6.

Miller M (2006). Hyponatraemia and arginin vasopressin dysregulation: mechanisms, clinical consequences and management. *J Am Geriatr Soc* **54**: 345–53.

Patel GP, Balk RA (2007). Recognition and treatment of hyponatraemia in acutely ill hospitalized patients. *Clin Ther*, **29**: 211–29.

Pavlevsky PM, Bhagrath R, Greenberg A (1996). Hypernatraemia in hospitalized patients. *Ann Intern Med* **124**: 197–203.

Hypercalcaemia

Calcium physiology

The elderly skeleton contains 99% of calcium in the body in the form of hydroxyapatite. The remainder is distributed in the soft tissues, teeth, and extracellular fluid (ECF). Cell and organ functions are dependent on the tight control of ECF calcium concentration. Plasma circulating total calcium concentration is tightly controlled between 2.2 and 2.60 mmol/L (8.8–10.4 mg/dL).

When the plasma protein concentration increases (in dehydration and after prolonged venous stasis), protein-bound calcium and total plasma calcium increase. If plasma proteins decrease (liver disease, nephrotic syndrome, malnutrition, cancer), the protein-bound calcium concentration is reduced, decreasing the total calcium, although ionized calcium can be maintained within the reference range 1.1–1.3 mmol/L (4.4–5.2 mg/dL). Many acute and chronic illnesses decrease plasma albumin concentration, which decreases plasma total calcium and can mask the existence of hypercalcaemia. It is therefore important to calculate the 'adjusted calcium': total plasma calcium adjusted for the patient's prevailing albumin concentration. This is achieved by means of a formula:

Adjusted Ca ACa (mmol/L) = measured total Ca (mmol/L) + 0.02 (40 − measured albumin [g/L])

Calcium absorption and excretion

Calcium is absorbed predominantly in the proximal small intestine; this is regulated through the quantity of calcium ingested in the diet, and two cellular calcium transport processes:

- active saturable transcellular absorption which is stimulated by 1,25(OH)$_2$D3;
- non-saturable paracellular absorption which is controlled by the concentration of calcium in the intestinal lumen relative to the plasma concentration.

In a normal adult, calcium balance is maintained: the amount of calcium intake and its deposition in bone are exactly matched by the excretion in urine and faeces. Reduced or increased calcium absorption reflects alterations in dietary calcium intake, intestinal calcium solubility, and vitamin D metabolism. As plasma calcium increases, calcium excretion in urine increases.

Hormonal control of circulating calcium

Hormonal control of circulating calcium involves the kidneys, bone and gastrointestinal tract. If plasma ionized calcium decreases, there is a change in binding at the calcium sensing receptor of the chief cells of the parathyroid gland resulting in parathyroid hormone (PTH) being released stimulating (1) reabsorption of calcium at the kidney, (2) osteoclast-mediated bone resorption releasing calcium from hydroxyapatite, and (3) absorption of calcium at the small intestine (mediated by 1,25(OH)$_2$D3). Increasing plasma calcium decreases PTH secretion reducing the three responses and stimulates calcitonin release from the thyroid (see Figure 8.5).

Vitamin D

Vitamin D2 (ergocalciferol) is synthesized by UV radiation of ergosterol (plant derived). Vitamin D3 (cholecalciferol) is produced by UV irradiation from 7-dehydrocholesterol in the skin of animals. Vitamin D3 and D2 are present in the diet and their absorption is associated with fats. They are released from chylomicrons in the liver and hydroxylated forming 25-hydroxycholecalciferol D3 and D2. The 25-hydroxylation is the rate-limiting step in conversion of vitamin D2/D3 to its active metabolite. Further hydroxylation to produce 1,25 dihydroxyvitamin D2/D3 (1,25(OH)$_2$D3:calcitriol) is accomplished mainly within the renal tubules, although bone and granuloma tissue can also perform this reaction. 1,25(OH)$_2$D3 is the most potent of the vitamin D metabolites and the only naturally occurring form of vitamin D that is active at physiological concentrations (see Figure 8.6).

1,25(OH)$_2$D3 increases the absorption of calcium and phosphate from the gut via active transport by calcium-binding proteins. Together with PTH, it stimulates bone resorption by osteoclasts. These effects increase plasma calcium and phosphate concentrations.

Other hormones affecting calcium homeostasis

Several hormones whose primary action is not related to calcium regulation directly or indirectly affect calcium homeostasis and skeletal metabolism.

Thyroid hormones stimulate osteoclast-mediated resorption of bone. Adrenal and gonadal steroids, particularly oestrogen in women and testosterone in men, have important regulatory effects, increasing osteoblast and decreasing osteoclast function. They also decrease renal calcium and phosphate excretion and intestinal calcium excretion. GH has anabolic effects on bone,

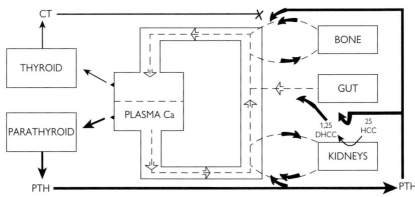

Figure 8.5 Plasma calcium regulation by parathyroid and thyroid glands via kidney, gut and bone. Reprinted from *The Lancet*, 374, William D. Fraser, Hyperparathyroidism, Figure 1, pp. 145–58. Copyright 2009, with permission from Elsevier.

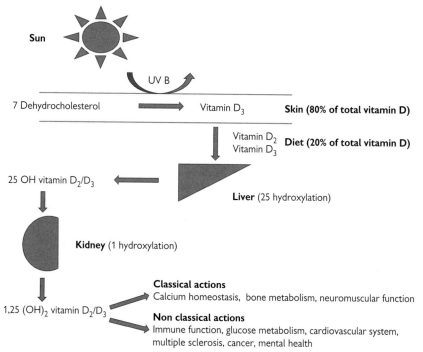

Figure 8.6 Vitamin D production and metabolism.

promoting remodelling of the skeleton. These effects of GH on bone are believed to be mediated by insulin-like growth factors (IGF-I and IGF-II) acting on cells of the osteoblast lineage. GH increases the urinary excretion of calcium whilst decreasing the urinary excretion of phosphate and decreasing GH in older individuals can alter bone and calcium metabolism.

Hypercalcaemia

There is considerable individual variation in the development of clinical symptoms in the older patient and signs of hypercalcemia (adjusted or ionized Ca above the reference range). The higher the adjusted calcium, and the more rapid the increase in plasma calcium, the more likely that symptoms will be present. In hospital practice the majority of cases are due to vitamin D excess, primary hyperparathyroidism (HPT) or malignancy. A greater diagnostic challenge is presented when attempting to differentiate occult malignancy from the less common causes of hypercalcaemia.

Symptoms of hypercalcaemia in older patients

Common
- Lethargy/weakness
- Confusion/impaired cognition
- Nausea/vomiting
- Abdominal pain
- Anorexia
- Constipation
- Polyuria/polydipsia

Variable
- Bone pain (fracture)
- Flank pain (renal stone)
- Impaired vision

Rare
- Depression/mental disturbance

Causes of hypercalcaemia in older patients

Common

Primary hyperparathyroid (1HPT)

Hypercalcaemia associated with malignancy (HCM)

Iatrogenic

Calcium with vitamin D supplementation or active vitamin D analogues in patients with:
- Chronic kidney disease (CKD)
- Metabolic bone disease especially osteoporosis (MBD)

Rare

Thyrotoxicosis

Sarcoidosis/other granulomatous disease

Atypical infection

Growth hormone excess

Lithium treatment

Excess vitamin A

Catecholamine excess

Addisonian crisis

Investigation of hypercalcaemia

In the majority of cases, the cause of hypercalcaemia will be identified by obtaining an accurate history, clinical examination, and appropriate biochemical tests. In some cases, however, additional valuable information on causation may be obtained from radiological investigations and tissue biopsies. Intact PTH measurement allows discrimination of primary HPT from non-parathyroid causes of hypercalcemia (particularly hypercalcaemia associated with malignancy (HCM)). An increased or inappropriately detectable intact PTH in the presence of hypercalcaemia is observed in primary HPT, whereas an intact PTH below the limit of detection of the assay (undetectable) is usually observed in non-parathyroid causes of hypercalcaemia (see Figure 8.7).

Primary hyperparathyroidism

Primary hyperparathyroidism (HPT) is a relatively common endocrine disease, particularly in post-menopausal women, characterized by hypercalcaemia associated with an increased or inappropriate intact PTH. The incidence rises with age ranging from 1 in 500 to 1 in 1000 of the population, demonstrates an ascertainment bias, with increasing adjusted calcium at the menopause and thiazide diuretic use in older people as possible contributing factors Most patients with primary HPT (70–80%) have no obvious symptomatology or signs of disease and are detected due to an incidental finding of hypercalcaemia. Symptoms and clinical signs often relate to chronic hypercalcaemia rather than elevated PTH. In 20–30% of symptomatic patients nephrolithiasis is common, overt skeletal disease is rare but osteoporosis with related fracture is increasingly recognized. Acute hypercalcaemic crisis with nephrogenic diabetes insipidus and dehydration is more likely in patients with an ACa >3.0 mmol/L. Acute pancreatitis is an uncommon but serious complication. Clinically evident neuromuscular disease is uncommon but proximal muscle weakness due to type II muscle fibre atrophy can be seen in association with severe bone disease (osteitis fibrosa cystica). Psychiatric symptoms include depression,

dementia, confusion, and stupor. Associations have been described with hypertension, diabetes, gastrointestinal ulceration, gout, increased weight and hyperlipidaemia. In 80–85% of patients, a solitary parathyroid gland adenoma is present, and the condition is curable by successful removal of the adenoma.

Non-parathyroid hypercalcaemia

Several laboratory tests may be required to differentiate non-parathyroid causes of hypercalcaemia. In a high percentage of cases, HCM is caused by tumours secreting parathyroid-hormone-related protein (PTHrP). Vitamin D excess or overdose may be obvious from the history, but sometimes only becomes apparent after measurement of the concentrations of vitamins D3 (cholecalciferol), D2 (ergocalciferol), and 1,25(OH)$_2$D3. The increasing therapeutic use of vitamin D2/D3 and potent vitamin D analogues to treat osteoporosis and renal disease makes this one of the commonest causes of hypercalcaemia seen in older people. Measurement of serum electrolytes, urea, and creatinine will confirm renal failure, and estimation of protein, albumin, and immunoglobulins may indicate the presence of myeloma, which should be investigated by both serum and urine electrophoresis. Thyroid function tests (measurement of thyroid-stimulating hormone, total or free thyroid hormones) can establish the diagnosis of thyrotoxic hypercalcaemia. Rare causes of hypercalcemia may be diagnosed by estimation of lithium (toxicity or overdose), growth hormone (acromegaly), vitamin A (toxicity), and urine catecholamines (phaeochromocytoma, MEN). In 15% of elderly patients malignancy and primary HPT may co-exist.

Hypercalcaemia associated with malignancy (HCM)

Hypercalcaemia tends to occur late in the course of malignant disease and is usually a poor prognostic sign.

Two major mechanisms of HCM are recognized. Calcium reabsorption by the kidney is often enhanced in HCM, interfering with the ability of the kidneys to limit the increased release of plasma calcium that results from

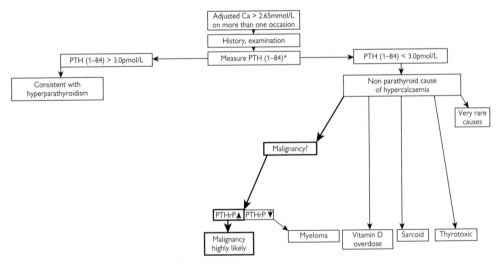

Figure 8.7 Biochemical investigation of hypercalcaemia.

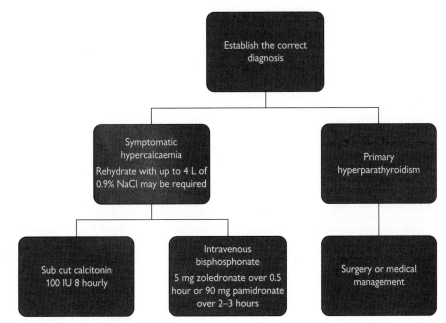

Figure 8.8 Management of hypercalcaemia.

increased osteoclast activity. There are two main sources of stimulation of the osteoclasts:
- a circulating humoral factor secreted by the tumour, parathyroid hormone related protein (PTHrP);
- locally active secretory factor(s) produced by the tumour or metastases in bone.

Parathyroid hormone-related protein

Parathyroid hormone-related protein (PTHrP) is synthesized as three isoforms containing 139, 141, and 173 amino acids, as a result of alternative differential splicing of RNA. There is amino terminal sequence homology with PTH with eight of the first 13 amino acids identical in PTHrP and PTH, three are identical within residues 14–34, and a further three are identical within residues 35–84. Activation of the classical PTH receptor is by the amino terminal portion of both PTH and PTHrP, and there is a common secondary structure in the binding domain of both peptides. As a result of this structural similarity, PTHrP possesses many of the biological actions of PTH.

There is, to date, little evidence to suggest that PTHrP has a role in normal adult calcium homeostasis. PTHrP is subject to post-translational processing, producing fragments with biological activities that have yet to be characterized

Current evidence indicates that the most common cause of HCM is the production, by tumours or their metastases, of PTHrP, that can circulate in blood and exert its effects on the skeleton and kidneys. Production of PTHrP is common in breast, lung, kidney, or other solid tumours, but is rarer in hematologic, gastrointestinal, and head and neck malignancies. The amino-terminal portion of PTHrP possesses PTH-like activity that results in hypercalcaemia, hypophosphatemia, phosphaturia, increased renal calcium reabsorption, and osteoclast activation. Osteoclast activation in HCM is mediated by PTHrP induced osteoblast production of Receptor Activator of NF Kappa Beta Ligand (RANKL) and reduction of binding of RANKL by the decoy receptor osteoprotegrin (OPG).

The second type of HCM is the result of increased bone resorption by osteoclasts stimulated by factors produced by the primary tumor or, more usually, by metastases, that stimulate osteoclasts via alteration of the RANKL/OPG balance. Mediators such as PTHrP, cytokines, prostaglandins, especially those of the E series (PGE2), and growth factors (e.g. IL-1, TNF, lymphotoxin, and TGF) have all been shown to possess osteoclast-stimulating activity that results in significant bone resorption.

Treatment of HCM

Treatment of hypercalcaemia can greatly improve the quality of life of patients. Symptomatic hypercalcaemia or plasma ACa concentrations exceeding 3.0 mmol/L (12 mg/dL) would merit emergency treatment. Dehydration results from hypercalcaemia-induced polyuria, reduced fluid and food intake, associated vomiting, decreased arginine-vasopressin, AVP (also known as anti diuretic hormone, ADH) activity at the distal tubule, and reduced renal perfusion. Fluid replacement with 0.9% NaCl corrects hypovolemia and provides a moderate sodium load, which will cause a concomitant increase in urinary calcium excretion. Bisphosphonates have improved the management of HCM, and are the most effective drugs available for treating hypercalcemia. This group of drugs have their major effects by inhibiting osteoclast activity immediately when infused, and then exert a more prolonged effect by being incorporated into bone matrix in a position normally occupied by pyrophosphate. Figure 8.8 outlines the approach to treatment of hypercalcaemia in older people.

Further reading

Fraser WD (2009). Hyperparathyroidism. *Lancet*, **11**; **374**: 145–58.

Ralston SH, Coleman R, Fraser WD, *et al.* (2004). Medical management of hypercalcemia. *Calcif Tissue Int* **74**: 1–11.

Santarpia L, Koch CA, Sarlis NJ (2010). Hypercalcemia in cancer patients: pathobiology and management. *Horm Metab Res* **42**: 153–64.

Sex hormones in older people

Background

The sex hormones, oestrogen, testosterone, and the adrenal androgens, decline in older people. Advocates of hormone replacement therapy have proposed them all as 'elixir of life' hormones. The female menopause is a familiar concept, but what about the 'andropause' and the 'adreno-pause'? Do they exist or are they a creation of pharmaceutical companies, keen to extend hormone replacement therapy beyond the tiny 'endocrine' market to a potentially enormous 'ageing' market?

Menopause

The female menopause results from ovarian failure. Premenopausal oestrogen levels in a cyclic fashion. Post-menopausal oestrogen levels vary are constant and very low with elevated luteinizing hormone (LH) and follicle-stimulating hormone (FSH) concentrations. The usual age of menopause is between 48 and 52 years. In two-thirds women the characteristic menopausal symptoms of hot flushes and night sweats resolve by 1 year, and in most women they resolve by 5 years, although they may recur later even in women who experienced few symptoms initially. Menopause also results in an increased risk of osteoporosis, coronary heart disease, and sexual dysfunction (loss of libido and vaginal dryness).

Post-menopausal hormone replacement therapy

Initial observational studies showed benefits of post-menopausal hormone replacement therapy (HRT), although these were subsequently attributed to 'healthy user bias'. Randomized controlled trials showed no benefits and increased risks, particularly with long-term HRT use (see Table 8.2). The reduction in osteoporosis and fracture risk only lasts for the duration of treatment and is inferior to specific anti-osteoporotic therapy such as the bisphosphonates. For women with troublesome and persistent menopausal symptoms, there is some evidence to support the use of non-hormonal treatment options to reduce the frequency of hot flushes. These include SSRIs (e.g. citalopram, fluoxetine, paroxetine), SNRIs (e.g. venlafaxine), and gabapentin.

Table 8.2 Absolute differences in major end points: post-menopausal women, HRT versus placebo, events per 1000 women

End point	First 2 years	5.2 year period
Coronary heart disease	3 more	4 more
Stroke	1 more	4 more
Venous thromboembolism	6 more	9 more
Breast cancer	No more	4 more
Hip fracture	1 fewer	2 fewer
Colon cancer	No difference	3 fewer
Death	No difference	No difference

Data from Women's Health Initiative randomized control trial in Solomon CG, Dluhy RG (2003). *NEJM* **348**: 579–80.

Table 8.3 Normal reference ranges for testosterone for healthy men

	Age (years)			
	40–49	50–59	60–69	70–79
Total testosterone (nmol/L)				
2.5th centile	8.7	7.5	6.8	5.4
97.5th centile	31.7	30.4	29.8	28.4

From Mohr BA, Guay AT, O'Donnell AB, McKinlay JB (2005). Normal, bound and non-bound testosterone levels in normally ageing men: results from the Massachusetts Male Ageing Study. *Clin Endocrinol* **62**: 64-73.

Male gonadal axis and age

In contrast to women, in men there is a gradual reduction in testosterone levels with increasing age. There is a wide range of normality at all ages (see Table 8.3). Additional variability is introduced by the testosterone assay (which is notoriously unreliable, particularly at low testosterone levels) and the diurnal variation (testosterone levels are highest in the morning). At 75 years, the mean male testosterone concentration is about two-thirds that of a 25-year-old man. However, there is a poor association between libido and erectile dysfunction and testosterone levels, at all ages. In older people, most erectile dysfunction is atherosclerotic. Despite this, there has been a marked increase in testosterone prescriptions over the past decade, much of which is for the treatment of 'ADAM' (androgen deficiency in the ageing male).

It has been proposed that the phenotype of the ageing male and the hypogonadal male is similar: both may develop an increased fat mass (particularly visceral fat), sarcopenia, a reduced bone mineral density, impaired quality of life or mood, an increased risk of atherosclerosis and sexual dysfunction (erectile dysfunction and loss of libido). However, such a phenotype is non-specific and has a high prevalence in the older man. The association with the decline in sex hormones with age does not imply causation.

Testosterone treatment in older men

In hypogonadal older men, testosterone treatment increases bone mineral density. The effect on fracture risk is uncertain. Bisphosphonates are effective independent of androgen status. Testosterone treatment in older men can also increase lean body mass and reduce fat mass, but no consistent or convincing functional benefits have been demonstrated unless supra-physiological doses are used. There is little or no evidence of benefit, or insufficient data, in relation to atherosclerosis and coronary artery disease, sexual function, cognitive function, mood, and quality of life. Risks of testosterone treatment include benign prostatic hypertrophy, prostate cancer, and enhanced erythropoiesis (an elevated haematocrit). There is also the 'hassle factor' of treatment: testosterone is not orally active; effective treatment is either delivered by intramuscular injection or daily application of testosterone gels.

Kaufman and Vermeulen concluded: 'The diagnosis of partial androgen deficiency in elderly males, and certainly the decision to implement any potentially harmful intervention, should be approached with pragmatism and appropriate reserve. ... As to the clinical picture, in view of its low specificity and the high prevalence of symptoms possibly associated with hypogonadism in the elderly population, one should avoid suggesting or soliciting symptoms.'

Male hypogonadism

Older men may develop 'pathological' hypogonadism, either primary or secondary. If this is suspected, and the testosterone concentration is low, an early-morning testosterone should be checked, together with the LH, FSH, prolactin, prostate-specific antigen (PSA), and full blood count. This is to confirm the initial testosterone value, and to determine whether the hypogonadism is primary (a testicular cause, associated with high LH and FSH concentrations) or secondary (a hypothalamic or pituitary cause, associated with low LH and FSH concentrations). It also establishes whether the hypogonadism is caused by hyperprolactinaemia and ensure whether the hypogonadism is caused by hyperprolactinaemia, and to ensure that the PSA and haematocrit are normal (before considering testosterone treatment). A DEXA scan should be considered to assess bone mineral density. If the biochemical results suggest secondary hypogonadism, with or without hyperprolactinaemia, the other anterior pituitary function tests should be checked (full thyroid function tests including free thyroxine (FT4) and/or free triiodothyronine (FT3) and a 9 am cortisol). An MRI scan of the hypothalamus and pituitary should be performed, and visual fields formally assessed if a pituitary macroadenoma or other suprasellar mass is found.

Adrenal androgens: DHEA and age

The final 'fountain of youth' sex hormone is the adrenal androgen dehydroepiandrosterone sulphate (DHEA). Levels of DHEA also decline with age, such that by 70–80 years of age concentrations are approximately 5–10% of their peak. Observational studies have suggested that higher DHEA levels are associated with better quality of life, higher bone mineral density, a slower cognitive decline, and less coronary heart disease. However, these associations may not be causal, and it is likely that a low DHEA concentration is a non-specific marker of ill-health, found in cancer, inflammatory diseases, type 2 diabetes and cardiovascular disease. In the US, DHEA is classified as a food supplement, not a drug. It is readily available through the Internet and unregulated. Claims for its benefits may be unsubstantiated by evidence, and preparations have been found to contain only 0–15% of the amount of DHEA stated on the packet.

DHEA probably acts via the androgen and/or the oestrogen receptors. DHEA treatment could therefore potentially result in adverse effects on prostate and breast tissues, though none have been demonstrated. In men, the contribution of DHEA to androgenic effects would be modest at most, compared with the more potent androgen testosterone. In the older person, there is no evidence of beneficial effects of DHEA treatment on body composition, physical performance, insulin sensitivity or quality of life. There may be small improvements in bone mineral density, but these are inconsistent, site and gender specific, less effective than bisphosphonate treatment, and unlikely to impact on risk of fracture. Stewart's review concluded that there is no convincing evidence of any benefit of DHEA treatment in the older population, and no evidence to support its use.

Conclusion

Any hormonal influence on ageing is probably dwarfed by genetic, environmental, and psychosocial factors, and comorbidities. The balance of benefit, harm and cost of proposed treatment must be carefully considered, avoiding an over-reliance on surrogate end points and undue influence by drug companies in research and clinical practice.

Further reading

Kaufman JM, Vermeulen A (2005). The decline of androgen levels in elderly men and its clinical and therapeutic implications. *Endocr Rev* **26**: 833–76.

Mohr BA, Guay AT, O'Donnell AB, McKinlay JB (2005). Normal, bound and non-bound testosterone levels in normally ageing men: results from the Massachusetts Male Ageing Study. *Clin Endocrinol* **62**: 64–73.

Nelson HD (2008). Menopause. *Lancet*, **371**: 760–70.

Solomon CG, Dluhy RG (2003). Rethinking postmenopausal hormone therapy. *NEJM* **348**: 579–80.

Sreekumaran Nair K, Rizza RA, O'Brien P *et al.* (2006). DHEA in elderly women and DHEA or testosterone in elderly men. *NEJM* **355**: 1647–59.

Stewart PM (2006). Aging and fountain-of-youth hormones. *NEJM* **355**: 1724–6.

Writing Group for the Women's Health Initiative Investigators (2002). Risks and benefits of estrogen plus progestin in healthy postmenopausal women. Principal results from the Women's Health Initiative randomized controlled trial. *JAMA* **288**: 321–33.

Hypokalaemia

Hypokalaemia (serum potassium <3.5 mmol/L) is a common electrolyte disturbance, particularly in patients admitted acutely to hospital. The majority of hypokalaemia is caused by diuretic use and diarrhoea.

Epidemiology

- In the community, the prevalence of hypokalaemia is <1%, but rises up to 7% in older patients taking diuretics.
- Patients admitted to hospital have a higher incidence of hypokalaemia (up to 3–5%), with older patients more likely to have more severe hypokalaemia (up to 5% have a K^+ <3.0).
- The majority of hypokalaemia (70%) is acquired in hospital
- Hypokalaemia is associated with longer hospital stay and increased mortality, particularly in those with pre-existing cardiac disease.
- The mortality rate of in-patients with hypokalaemia is as high as 20–34% in some series.

Complications associated with hypokalaemia

The majority of patients with hypokalaemia are asymptomatic and only identified following a screening blood test. Complications of hypokalaemia, such as cardiac arrhythmias, may be life-threatening and correlate poorly with the degree of hypokalaemia.

Cardiovascular complications

Cardiovascular complications are more common in elderly people, particularly in those with pre-existing ischaemic heart disease, cardiac failure, hepatic failure, or nephrotic syndrome. Features include

- ECG changes: prolonged Q-T interval, ST depression, T-wave depression and prominent U waves (see Figure 8.9).
- Cardiac arrhythmias - ventricular arrhythmias and premature atrial and ventricular ectopics.
- Increased digoxin toxicity.
- Hypertension.

Neuromuscular complications

- Muscle weakness and associated falls from hyperpolarised skeletal muscle cells, causing reduced muscle depolarisation and contraction.
- Reduced blood flow to muscles leading to cramps and rarely rhabdomyolysis.
- Gut dysmotility with constipation and ileus.

Acid–Base complications

Metabolic alkalosis due to enhanced proximal tubular absorption of HCO_3^- in the proximal tubule and increased $Na^+K^+ATPase$ activity in the distal collecting tubule with increased H^+ excretion.

Renal complications

Mild polyuria due to down-regulation of the water channel aquaporin-2 in the collecting duct.

Clinical approach to hypokalaemia (Figure 8.10)

Are there ECG changes or cardiac arrhythmias?

Treat first before investigating the cause.

Is hypokalaemia recent in onset (i.e. <24 hours)?

Indicates a transcellular redistribution of potassium into the cell. Causes include insulin therapy, beta-adrenergic agonists (e.g. salbutamol), refeeding syndrome (e.g. nasogastric feed following prolonged starvation), inappropriate intravenous fluids (typically 5% dextrose) and rarely familial periodic paralysis (onset usually age <20 years).

Is spot urine K^+/creatinine ratio <1.5- or 24-hour urine K^+ <20 mmol/24 hours, indicating a non-renal loss of potassium?

- With a hyperchloraemic metabolic acidosis (due to loss of bicarbonate) e.g. diarrhoea, enterocutaneous fistulae, villous adenoma and VIPoma.
- Excessive sweating or burns.
- Laxative use and misuse.
- Inadequate potassium in diet.
- Diuretics recently stopped.

Is spot urine K^+/creatinine ratio >1.5 or 24 hour urine K^+ >20 mmol/24 h indicating a renal loss of potassium?

Is the patient hypertensive?

Mineralocorticoid excess (regulates K^+ excretion from principal cell in cortical collecting duct)

- Primary aldosteronism (low renin and high aldosterone).
- Secondary aldosteronism (high renin and aldosterone) e.g. cardiac failure, hepatic failure, nephrotic syndrome.
- Cushings syndrome.
- Liddles syndrome. A rare autosomal dominant defect in apical Na+ channel (ENaC). Low renin–aldosterone, hypokalaemic metabolic alkalosis, and severe hypertension.

Is the patient normotensive or is the BP low?

- Hyperchloraemic metabolic acidosis with low bicarbonate
- Renal tubular acidosis type 1 and 2

Metabolic alkalosis with raised bicarbonate and increased urinary chloride (>10 mmol/L):

- Diuretic use
- Prolonged intravenous saline infusion
- Rare recessive mutations in the tubular cell transporters
  - Bartter syndrome: mutations in channels of the loop of Henlé. Presents at an early age with hypotension, hyper-reninaemia and hypercalcuria.

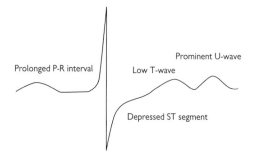

Prolonged P-R interval   Low T-wave   Prominent U-wave

Depressed ST segment

Figure 8.9 ECG changes in hypokalaemia.

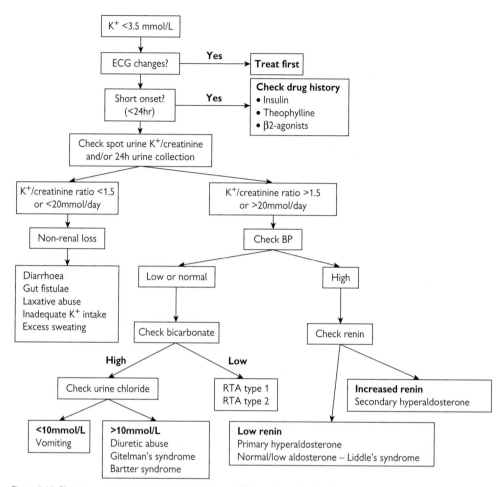

Figure 8.10 Clinical approach to hypokalaemia Monitor serum K$^+$ frequently, e.g. hourly after starting replacement.

- Gitelman's syndrome: mutation in the thiazide-sensitive NaCl cotransporter in distal tubule. Presents at a later age with hypokalaemia, hypomagnesaemia, hypocalcuria and hypotension.

Metabolic alkalosis with raised bicarbonate and reduced urinary chloride (<10 mmol/L):

- Vomiting – due to volume depletion causing secondary hyperaldosteronism and metabolic alkalosis causing increased tubular potassium loss.

Treatment of hypokalaemia

As a rule of thumb, a reduction in serum potassium of 1.0 mmol/L indicates a total deficit of ~200–400 mmol, e.g. a patient with K$^+$ 2.6 mmol/L needs approximately 300 mmol K$^+$ to correct the deficit to 3.5 mmol/L. Note, this is affected by pH, therefore the total deficit with pH 7.5 is *less* than if pH 7.2 due to transcellular potassium shift with increasing pH.

If K$^+$ >2.6 and no ECG changes or symptoms

- Oral replacement with potassium chloride 40–100 mmol K$^+$/day

- Monitor serum K$^+$ daily
- Caution in patients with chronic kidney disease: danger of hyperkalaemia

If ECG changes, symptoms or K$^+$ <2.6

- Intravenous potassium replacement with ECG monitoring.
- 20–40 mmol potassium chloride per litre of normal saline. Infuse at 10 mmol/hour
- If hypomagnesaemia with hypokalaemia, correct both simultaneously.
- If more rapid replacement necessary, 20–40 mmol/h can be given through a central venous catheter with ECG monitoring. 20 mmol/h increases serum K$^+$ by approximately 0.25 mmol/L/h.
- In severe hypokalaemic metabolic acidosis (e.g. from profound diarrhoea) replace K$^+$ first before giving sodium bicarbonate, to avoid worsening hypokalaemia due to transcellular shift of K$^+$.

Author's Tip

Retrospective studies show that hypokalaemia is poorly managed in 25% of patients in a hospital setting. Common pitfalls include
- failure to prevent hypokalaemia—e.g. when using high-dose diuretics
- failure to recognise and treat hypokalaemia
- insufficient monitoring of response to treatment (i.e. repeat blood tests).

Further reading

Groeneveld JH, Sijpkens YW, Lin SH, et al. (2005). An approach to the patient with severe hypokalaemia: the potassium quiz. *QJM* **98**: 305–16.

Paltiel O, Salakhov E, Ronen I, et al. (2001). Management of severe hypokalemia in hospitalized patients: a study of quality of care based on computerized databases. *Arch Intern Med* **161**: 1089–95.

Weiner ID, Wingo CS (1997). Hypokalaemia – consequences, causes and correction. *J Am Soc Nephrol* **8**: 1179–88.

Renal

Renal physiology in old age

Background

As an individual ages, the rate of adaptation by the kidney to changes in fluid or electrolyte status slows. Overall function is often reduced with a corresponding decrease in glomerular filtration rate (GFR), renal blood flow, and renal size. Functional changes often parallel structural or histological changes.

Histological features

Decrease in renal size and structure

Although individual renal size may vary, with larger individuals having larger kidneys, healthy kidneys are often around 10–11 cm in length with both the right and left kidney usually being symmetrical in size and appearance. In aged individuals:

- The kidneys reach their maximum size by the fourth decade of life. After this, the weight and length of each kidney decreases steadily, with losses approximating 10% per decade.
- Age-related changes are symmetrical. Renal asymmetry is usually associated with vascular disease or a long history of infective complications.
- Most of the tissue loss is due to cortical thinning, with minimal changes in corticomedullary and medullary thickness (see Figure 9.1).
- Cyst formation is common, with over 50% of those aged 65 years or over having one or more simple cysts within the kidney. Although malignant change can occur within these cysts, radiographic absence of solid material within the cyst is reassuring.

Microscopic changes in the glomerulus

At birth, the number of glomeruli seen in each kidney varies widely, from 200 000 to 1 800 000. The absolute number of glomeruli appears to be related to gestational events, particularly those occurring during weeks 32–36. After the first two decades, the number of glomeruli gradually decreases with each decade of life. Many become atrophied and sclerotic, with a differential increase in the size of glomeruli (particularly in the outer cortex and the juxtamedullary regions, probably because of compensatory hypertrophy of intact glomeruli. Additional changes seen in the glomerulus include

- a compensatory increase in glomerular size (due to hyperfiltration)
- thickening of the glomerular basement membrane
- increased mesangial and sclerotic tissue
- capillary tuft collapse.

Tubular changes

Unlike glomerular changes which occur largely in the cortex, tubular alterations are more prominent in the outer medulla. Changes include

- tubular atrophy and dilatation
- decline in size and number of tubules
- decreased length (proximal tubules)
- tubulointerstitial fibrosis
- thickening of the tubular basement membranes
- overall loss of tubular mass
- diverticulum formation: small diverticuli form within the tubules. These outpouchings are seen mostly in the distal tubules and the collecting system and may contribute to a higher risk of subclinical infections. Diverticuli are not consistently found in all aged kidneys.

It is postulated that some of the tubulointerstitial fibrotic changes are attributable to leucocyte infiltration, increased adhesive proteins, osteopontin, and high levels of intercellular adhesion molecule-1.

Vascular changes

Vascular changes are seen in the larger arteries and arterioles, the corticomedullary tissue and within the glomerulus tuft itself.

- The renal artery is prone to atherosclerotic narrowing, mostly arising close to the aortic orifice (although clinically significant stenoses would be considered pathological and not part of normal ageing). Renal blood flow declines significantly to 50–60% of peak perfusion at younger age, with a corresponding increase in the filtration fraction at the glomerular basement membrane.
- Tortuosity and spiralling of the interlobar arteries
- Angulation and irregularity of the arcuate arteries
- Loss of glomerular tuft capillaries
- 'Aglomerular glomeruli': in some areas of the kidney, particularly in the juxtamedullary region, a shunt between the afferent and efferent arterioles may form, allowing blood to be redirected away from the capillary loops in the glomerulus. This results in shunting of blood into the metabolically active areas within the medulla.
- The distinction between vascular changes due to normal ageing and that due to chronic age-associated disease, such as hypertension, is difficult as often these diseases coexist.

Changes in kidney function

Not all aspects of renal function are affected equally by ageing. Renal blood flow and, consequently, GFR together with the ability to respond rapidly to changes in fluid and electrolyte shifts are impaired with age. Little effect is seen on maintenance of acid–base balance or endocrine functions of the kidney.

Decrease in renal blood flow

- Renal blood flow falls at a rate of 10% per decade, such that octogenarians have renal blood flow rates of

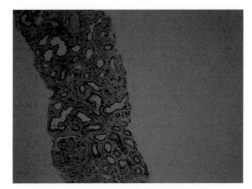

Figure 9.1 (colour plate 6) A&E stain taken from a biopsy from an older man. The large amount of green stain demonstrates widespread interstitial fibrosis.

~300 mL/min (compared to 600 mL/min in those aged 20–29 years).

- Blood flow to the medulla, rather than the cortex, is preferentially maintained.
- Vascular tone is higher, due to blunted responses to vasodilatory signals such as acetylcholine or nitric acid, resulting in a higher filtration fraction at the glomerulus.

Reduced glomerular filtration rate

- Most individuals have a gradual decline in GFR averaging 0.87 mL/min/1.73m^2 per year. However, longitudinal studies in humans have shown that each individual has a unique rate of change in GFR, with some individuals showing little or no change over time.
- The older kidney is less able to rapidly increase GFRs in response to a high load of toxins, e.g. from a large gastrointestinal bleed or large protein meal. This corresponds with the histological appearance of cortical glomerulosclerosis and may reflect an inability to recruit additional nephron units.
- Adaptive hyperfiltration, such as seen after surgical nephrectomy, still occurs and is similar to that seen in younger individuals.

Slowed renal tubular responses with age

- Sodium balance: baseline renin and aldosterone levels are lower in older individuals than younger controls. Compared with younger patients, sodium restriction leads to a blunted renin–angiotensin response, resulting in inappropriate sodium loss and a correspondingly higher risk of symptomatic dehydration. Conversely, urinary excretion of an excessive sodium load takes twice as long in healthy older than younger adults possibly as a result of impaired secretion of (and reduced sensitivity to) atrial natriuretic peptide (ANP). As a result both hyponatraemia and hypernatraemia are commonly seen with physiological stresses arising from even minor illnesses or changes in medication.
- Fluid balance: the kidneys' capacity to maximally dilute or concentrate urine is diminished with age. The ability to lower urinary osmolality and excrete free water is reduced and delayed with age resulting in a higher tendency to fluid retention, hypertension, and volume overload. The urinary concentrating ability is also diminished with age, independent of GFR. Maximal urinary osmolality is estimated at 600–800 mOsm/L in older patients (800–1200 mOsm/L in young adults). The risk of dehydration is compounded by the fact that older individuals also have impaired thirst sensation and are less likely to seek fluids when their plasma volume falls.

Inflammation and Oxidative Stress

Oxidative stress and inflammation are hallmarks of ageing kidneys. The inflammation process increases mesangial matrix secretion, basement membrane thickness, vascular permeability, production of collagens, and interstitial fibrosis.

Biomarkers linked with ageing of the kidneys are

- C-reactive protein
- interleukin-6
- tumour necrosis factor-alpha
- advanced glycation end products
- transforming growth factor-β
- angiotensin II
- cholesterol.

Deficiencies in nitric oxide synthesis, mitochondrial cytochrome C content and oxidative phosphorylation activity accelerate ageing in the kidneys. Nitric oxide deficiency is linked with oxidative stress, but it is seen later in women due to the protective effect of oestrogen, suggesting a delayed kidney ageing in women.

Genetics

Recent studies on the genetics of ageing have shed light on the molecular basis of the ageing process in the kidneys. However, most of the current knowledge is based on animal studies.

A polymorphism in the MMP20 gene is the only suggested genetic feature related to age-related reduction of GFR that is based on longitudinal studies in humans.

In animal studies, different sets of genes are shown to be upregulated or downregulated. These alterations impact cell integrity, proliferation, transport, and energy metabolism in the kidneys (see Table 9.1).

Putative modulators of the ageing process in the kidney

The mechanism for ageing continues to be an area of much research. Many factors have been studied, and continue to be studied. However, often the evidence is contradictory and confusing. Some of the putative factors are listed below.

Calorie intake

High calorie intake accelerates ageing of the kidneys. In an animal model, restriction of calorie intake attenuated

Table 9.1 Genes that may play a role in ageing kidneys based on animal models

Gene	Mechanism
Upregulated	
CSPG2	Tubular basement membrane thickening
ET-1	Vasoconstriction
COL1A2, TGF-beta	Fibrosis
RAGE	Advanced glycation end products deposition
VEGF	Tubular osteopontin and macrophage infiltration
MMP-7, KIM-1, Caudin-7	Extracellular matrix synthesis and tissue remodelling
HSP70	Stress response
Na+K+ATPase alpha2	Impairment of energy metabolism
FAF1, SAPK	Signal transduction
Zag	Inhibition of epithelial cell proliferation
PDEF, TSP-1	Inhibition of angiogenesis
Downregulated	
PMSR, SMP-30, Klotho	Impaired calcium/phosphate and vitamin D metabolism
Aqp-2	Impaired regulation of vasopressin 2 receptors and concentrating ability
COX1, GCS	Oxidative stress

glomerulosclerosis, tubular atrophy, interstitial fibrosis, vascular thickening, and mitochondrial enzyme abnormalities later in older ages. Interestingly, caloric restriction attenuates the overexpression of some genes in old rats.

Angiotensin II
Angiotensin II is recognized as a profibrotic agent. In rat studies, angiotensin-converting enzyme inhibitors appear to attenuate age-related proteinuria, glomerulosclerosis, and tubulointerstitial fibrosis.

Nitric oxide
Animal models suggest that decreased nitric oxide activity results in increased fibrosis. Administration of L-arginine (the substrate for nitric oxide) can reverse some of these changes.

Advanced glycation end products
Higher levels of advanced glycation end products are associated with normal and abnormal ageing. Their role in modulating age-related changes continues to be studied in detail. Substances such as aminoguanidine, an inhibitor of advanced glycation end product formation, may have a role in modification of age-related injuries.

Oxidative stress
High vitamin E diet in aged rats preserve renal blood flow and GFR. However, studies have not shown exogenous vitamin E to be effective in man.

Cholesterol
Age-related accumulation of cholesterol in the kidneys is documented but the beneficial effect of lowering plasma cholesterol remains unproven.

Further reading
Lerma EV (2009). Anatomic and physiologic changes of the aging kidney. *Clin Geriatr Med* **25**: 325–9.

Lindeman RD, Goldman R (1986). Anatomic and physiologic age changes in the kidney. *Exp Gerontol* **21**: 379–406.

Rowe JW, Andres R, Tobin JD, et al. (1976). The effect of age on creatinine clearance in men: a cross-sectional and longitudinal study. *J Gerontol* **31**: 155–63.

Zhou XJ, Rakheja D, Yu X, et al. (2008). The aging kidney. *Kidney Int* **74**: 710–20.

Renal investigations in older adults

The investigation and management of renal disease is heavily dependent on laboratory and radiological investigations. A detailed description is beyond the scope of this section, therefore only key investigations and those which may require different interpretation for older individuals are discussed (see Table 9.2).

Urinalysis and urine microscopy

Urine dipstick, followed where appropriate by urine microscopy, is one of the most useful and easily done renal investigations possible.

- In older individuals, the high prevalence of subclinical urinary or bladder infection may lead to overinterpretation of the dipstick analysis. Therefore, all patients with positive dipstick results should have urine culture performed.
- The presence of proteinuria and haematuria (in the absence of infection) are highly suggestive of glomerular disease. Other characteristic features, such as cellular casts or heme granular casts seen on urine microscopy, also aid diagnosis.
- Urine cytology samples are not useful in the investigation of microscopic haematuria. They may be used for the routine follow up of bladder cancer or for those with previous history of benzene dye or cyclophosphamide exposure.

The interpretation of serum creatinine and other measures of renal function

Serum creatinine is the most commonly used marker for renal function, as it is widely available and relatively inexpensive to measure.

- In older individuals, interpretation of a single value may be difficult as the absolute serum creatinine value is greatly dependent on the total body muscle mass, oral protein intake, and metabolism and intrinsic renal function (see Figure 9.2).
- Many national guidelines have suggested that physicians use conversion formulae to estimate glomerular filtration rate (or creatinine clearance) from the measured serum creatinine. The Modification of Diet in Renal Disease (MDRD) equation and the Cockroft–Gault equations are the most commonly used; however, each has limitations.
- Recently derived formulae may still be misleading in older individuals. Interpretation may vary depending on associated comorbidity and muscle mass.

Cystatin C is an alternative renal marker more commonly used in Europe than in N America.

- Although less influenced by age and muscle mass, it has some limitations with its interpretation in the older population.
- Currently, there does not appear to be sufficient evidence to suggest it is superior, or inferior, to the measurement of serum creatinine for the routine evaluation of a patient.

Based on recent concerns about the interpretation of renal function tests the following recommendations are made:

1 AVOID the use of estimating equations during acute illness.
2 Calculate the estimated glomerular filtration rate (eGFR) for any individual at any one time point and then follow changes over time rather than placing heavy emphasis on specific values.
3 Refer individuals for further assessment if the eGFR is:
   - below 30 mL/min (at any time point)
   - below 60 mL/min and the patient has persistent dipstick positive proteinuria or urinary proteinuria more than 1 g/day on a timed collection (see Figure 9.2)
   - reducing over time (it is unclear how much change over time is significant but a rough guide would be if the eGFR is falling at more than 3–5 mL/min/year)

Evaluation of proteinuria and albuminuria

The presence of proteinuria (or albuminuria) and a low eGFR is predictive of progressive renal disease. Therefore, it is important to both screen for and quantify protein losses.

- Both proteinuria and albuminuria may be measured by routine dipstick testing, on random urine samples sent to the laboratory for microalbumin/creatinine ratio or proteinuria/creatinine ratio or in timed urine samples.
- Screening for dipstick proteinuria:
   - false positives may occur in catheter specimens, in blood contaminated samples, and in very alkaline or decomposed urine.
   - false negatives are seen when urine is very dilute or acidic and when non-albumin proteinuria (such as seen with myeloma) is present.
- Patients with diabetes or hypertension and those with eGFR<60 mL/min should be screened at least yearly with a random sample of urine sent for microalbumin/creatinine ratio.

Table 9.2 Tests commonly used in the assessment of renal disease

Clinical	Urine dipstick analysis* and microscopy
	Urinary protein evaluation (random or timed collections)
	Renal biopsy
Laboratory	Serum creatinine*/cystatin C
	AKI markers – KIM-1/NGaL
	CKD profile: haemoglobin, potassium, bicarbonate, calcium, phosphate, albumin, parathyroid hormone, iron studies, lipid profile, glucose and PSA
	Myeloma screening: plasma protein electrophoresis*; Bence–Jones proteins
	Disease specific: vasculitis markers; hepatitis markers, urinary and plasma eosinophilia; complement levels
Radiology	Ultrasound scan* ± Doppler
	CT and MRI evaluation
	Nuclear scans

*Key investigations in the routine evaluation of renal function in an older individual.

AKI, acute kidney injury; CKD, chronic kidney disease.

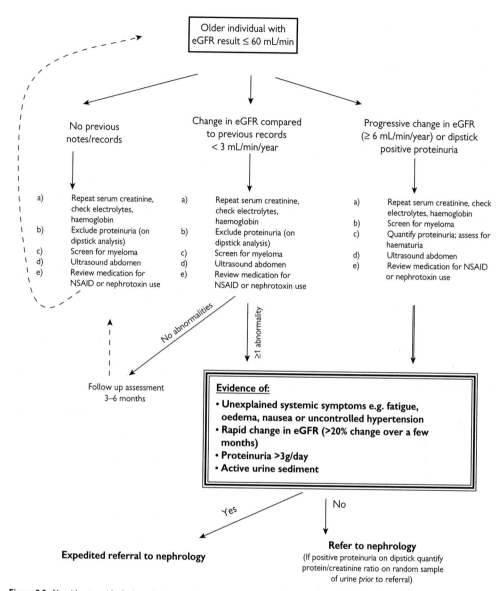

Figure 9.2 Algorithm to guide the investigations and management of older patients with low eGFR.

- The utility of routine screening in those with cardiac risk remains controversial despite clear evidence that the presence of microalbuminuria portends an increased mortality risk.
- Individuals with dipstick positive proteinuria should not have microalbumin/creatinine ratio measurement rather protein/creatinine ratio measurement. Interpretation of microalbumin/creatinine ratio and protein/creatinine ratio is similar regardless of age (see Table 9.3)
- Timed urine collections, such as the 24-hour urine collection, are not recommended for screening,

although they may be used by nephrologists for accurate measurement of heavy proteinuria. In older individuals, 6-hour timed collections may be equally useful.

Radiological investigation

- Ultrasonography, computerized tomography, magnetic resonance imaging, and nuclear scans all play an important role in the investigation of renal disease.
- Ultrasonography is often the easiest and first-line investigation for older patients with any evidence of renal disease. It is useful to exclude hydronephrosis and obstructive uropathy and to estimate renal size.

Table 9.3 British Renal Association Guidelines (CKD eGuide) for the interpretation of albumen/creatinine ratio (ACR) and the protein/creatinine ratio (PCR)

ACR (mg/mmol)	PCR (mg/mmol)	Implication
Males >2.5 Females >3.5	>15	Abnormal values consistent with CKD 1 or 2 even if normal renal function. Consider ACEI/ARB if diabetic
30	50	Consistent with proteinuria Consider ACE inhibitor/ARB particularly if hypertensive Suffix 'p' on CKD stage
70	100	Stricter BP limits apply. Refer for nephrology if non-diabetic
>250	>300	Approximates 'nephrotic range' proteinuria

Adapted from http://www.renal.org/whatwedo/ InformationResources/ CKDeGUIDE/Proteinuria.aspx

- Doppler studies may be useful in slender patients at high risk for renovascular disease. It is not useful in over-weight or obese patients.

Common abnormalities on ultrasound include:

1 Urinary obstruction: in males due to prostatic hypertrophy. Obstruction may occur insidiously and cause hydronephrosis and obstructive nephropathy, even in the absence of oligoanuria. Typical appearances on ultrasound include distended ureters and pelvicaliectasis, often referred to as the 'Mickey Mouse ears' appearance (see Figure 9.3).
2 Echogenicity, reduced renal size, and cortical thinning: seen in individuals with chronic kidney disease. Asymmetrical kidney size (>1.0 cm difference between left and right kidneys) in an aged individual is suggestive of renovascular disease. Less commonly renal asymmetry is due to repeated infections in association with chronic recurrent stone disease.
3 Renal cysts: frequently seen in ageing kidneys. Simple renal cysts with thin walls and no solid material are of little consequence. Prevalence is as high as 49% in those 60–79 years and 60% in those aged 80 years or above. Cysts seen more commonly in males and size and number of cysts tends to increase with age.

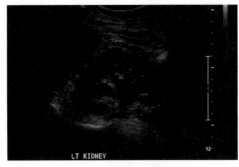

Figure 9.3 Ultrasound scan showing a left kidney with appearances consistent with hydronephrosis.

Computerized tomography and magnetic resonance imaging

- Used to clarify abnormal ultrasound findings (such as a complex renal cyst) or when assessing renal artery stenosis.
- May be useful in identification of extrarenal causes of obstruction and renal stones.
- Computed tomography (CT) angiograms and magnetic resonance (MR) angiograms are optimal for the assessment of clinically significant renal artery stenosis.
- Older patients must have eGFR assessment prior to either CT with contrast or MRI with gadolinium due to toxicity of these agents. In those with chronic kidney disease stage 4–5 (eGFR 30 mL/min), gadolinium use should be avoided as it may precipitate nephrogenic fibrosis or nephrogenic sclerosing dermopathy. Similarly, CT scanning without contrast or with carbon dioxide angiograms to visualize the renal artery is recommended for those undergoing CT. Under circumstances where CT contrast is required, prophylaxis with fluids and N-acetylcysteine is advisable and the use of low dose non-ionic, isosmotic contrast agents encouraged.

Nuclear renal tests

Technetium labelled nuclear scans (also known as DTPA, technetium-99m, or MAG3 scans) are useful in the assessment of renal blood flow and excretory function of the kidney. Results are often reported as a comparison between the left and right kidney. Therefore, in older individuals the clinical utility may be limited by the fact that disease occurs bilaterally. The role of captopril nuclear scans for the assessment of renal function and for renal artery stenosis is greatly diminished, particularly since MRI angiograms have become more widely available.

Renal biopsy

Age *per se* is not a contraindication for renal biopsy. Complications (bleeding and infection) are similar in all ages, though older patients are more likely to experience more consequences from the complications than younger individuals. Renal biopsy is warranted when patients present with atypical renal signs and symptoms, rapidly progressive renal failure and in situations where prognostic information will influence treatment (such as in individuals with a combination of acute tubular necrosis and myeloma, or those with nephrotic range proteinuria).

Author's Tip

Vasculitis is not uncommon and therefore in patients who present with an abnormal urine and systemic illness, ANCA and antiGBM serology is warranted. Routine screening for vasculitis is not appropriate in the otherwise healthy individual.

Patients with stable chronic kidney disease should undergo a comprehensive yearly assessment. This assessment should include blood pressure, urinalysis, cholesterol measurement, haemoglobin, potassium, bicarbonate, calcium, phosphate, albumin, parathormone, and iron studies.

Screening for myeloma with plasma protein electrophoresis is appropriate in undiagnosed renal impairment. Additional testing of urine for Bence–Jones proteins or bone marrow pathology may be warranted if the clinical suspicion is high.

New markers for acute kidney injury, such as Neutrophil Gelatinase-associated Lipocalin (NGaL) and Kidney Injury Molecule-1 (KIM-1) are emerging. These would allow for earlier detection of renal injury and hopefully allow preventative strategies to be used to modify health outcomes such as the need for dialysis or death. They may not be as predictive in older individuals and are currently not recommended for use in common practice.

Further reading

Hemmelgarn BR, Zhang J, Manns BJ, et al. (2006). Progression of kidney dysfunction in the community-dwelling elderly. *Kidney Int* **69**: 2155–61.

Jassal SV (2009). Clinical presentation of renal failure in the aged: chronic renal failure. *Clin Geriatr Med* **25**: 359–72.

Kellum JA, Bellomo R, Ronco C (2008). Definition and classification of acute kidney injury. *Nephron Clin Pract* **109**: c182-c87.

Munikrishnappa D (2009). Limitations of various formulae and other ways of assessing GFR in the elderly: is there a role for cystatin C? American Society of Nephrology On line Geriatric Curriculum (http://www.asn-online.org/education_and_meetings/geriatrics/Chapter6.pdf).

Riella MC (2005). Challenges in interventional nephrology. *Contrib Nephrol* **149**: 131–7.

Rodgers M, Nixon J, Hempel S, et al. (2006). Diagnostic tests and algorithms used in the investigation of haematuria: systematic reviews and economic evaluation. *Health Technol Assess* **10**: iii–259.

Shim RL, O'Hare AM (2009). Rate of decline in eGFR and clinical evaluation of the elderly with a low eGFR. American Society of Nephrology On line Geriatric Curriculum (http://www.asn-online.org/education_and_meetings/geriatrics/Chapter5.pdf).

Acute kidney injury

Acute kidney injury (AKI) occurs when the kidney is unable to maintain normal homeostasis. AKI results in a rapid change in renal function (within 48 hours) due to an insult that causes either structural or functional change in the kidney. It is a common clinical problem estimated to be present in up to 5% of hospital inpatients. It is a complex disorder which occurs in multiple clinical settings due to different aetiological factors. Sequelae include increased mortality, the progression of pre-existing renal disease, and the development of end-stage renal disease requiring renal replacement therapy.

In the past, studies of AKI have been limited by the differences in the way AKI has been defined and classified. Collaborative groups have therefore worked to produce consensus definitions of AKI (see Tables 9.4 and 9.5).

The National Confidential Enquiry into Patient Outcomes and Deaths (NCEPOD) investigated the care of patients with AKI in UK hospitals in 2009. They found that only 50% of patients received a standard of care that was considered to be good.

Acute kidney injury and the ageing kidney

In the absence of disease, the kidney undergoes age-related changes in both structure and function. Radiographically, the size of the kidney falls by 10% at age 40 and by 30% at age 80. Histological examination of the ageing kidney shows a reduction in the total number of glomeruli with many of those remaining being sclerosed. This may explain the linear relationship between age and renal function, with an overall decline in creatinine clearance of 0.87 mL/min/year beginning at the age of 40. However, there is a large amount of variation in glomerular filtration rate (GFR) with age and some individuals show no decline in GFR even in the ninth decade. Blood pressure is thought to be an important contributing factor.

With age, renal blood flow decreases by as much as 10% per decade. It is hypothesized that this may result from changes in the way the kidney responds to vasoactive substances. This makes older people more susceptible to AKI due to an attenuated response to vasodilators such as nitric oxide (NO) and an increased response to vasoconstrictors.

Tubular function also changes with age. The number and size of renal tubules fall. Deposition of connective tissue increases and there is more interstitial fibrosis in the ageing kidney. Elderly kidneys are therefore not able to dilute or

Table 9.5 AKIN Criteria for AKI

AKIN Stage	Serum Creatinine (Cr)	Urine Output
1	Cr ≥1.5–1.9× baseline or Cr increase by ≥ 26.2 µM	<0.5 mL/kg/h for ≥6 hours
2	Cr ≥2–2.9× baseline	<0.5 mL/kg/h for ≥12 hours
3	Cr ≥3× baseline or Cr ≥354 µM with a rise of at least 44 µM or initiation of renal replacement therapy	<0.3 mL/kg/h for ≥24 hours or anuria ≥12 hours

concentrate urine as effectively. This makes the older patient more susceptible to volume depletion, which is a significant risk factor for AKI.

In the healthy older person, the age-related changes in the kidney are matched by a change in renal haemodynamics which allows the GFR of the kidney to be maintained. However, in the context of illness and comorbidity, the physiological reserve of the kidney is less and therefore the elderly kidney is at increased risk of developing AKI.

Data from 2009 shows that 49.2% of all hospital admissions with acute renal failure occurred in patients aged 75 years or over. AKI can therefore be considered to be a geriatric disease. With an ageing population, the prevalence of this disease is set to increase.

Aetiology of Acute Kidney Injury

AKI in older people has the same spectrum of aetiologies as the general population; however, older patients are more likely to have multifactorial AKI.

The causes of AKI are outlined in Table 9.6.

Pre-renal AKI

Pre-renal AKI occurs as a result of poor perfusion to the kidneys. Age-related decreases in GFR and renal blood flow both contribute to the increased risk of pre-renal AKI.

Table 9.6 Causes of acute kidney injury in the older population

Pre-renal
Fluid loss: vomiting, diarrhoea, bleeding, inappropriate diuretics
Decreased cardiac output
Fluid redistribution: hypoproteinaemia, pancreatitis, burns
Drugs altering renal perfusion: ACE inhibitors, NSAIDs
Intrinsic renal failure
Prolonged pre-renal insult leading to acute tubular necrosis (ATN)
Nephrotoxics: aminoglycosides, radiocontrast agents, myoglobin
Interstitial nephritis
Glomerulonephritis
Post-renal (obstructive)
Prostatic hypertrophy or carcinoma
Pelvic neoplasms

Table 9.4 RIFLE Criteria for AKI

RIFLE category	Creatinine (Cr)/ glomerular filtration rate (GFR)	Urine output
Risk	Cr ≥1.5× baseline or decrease in GFR ≥25%	<0.5 mL/kg/h for ≥6 hours
Injury	Cr ≥2× baseline or decrease in GFR ≥50%	<0.5 mL/kg/h for ≥12 hours
Failure	Cr ≥3× baseline or Cr ≥354 µM with a rise of at least 44 µM or decrease in GFR ≥75%	<0.3 mL/kg/h for ≥24 hours or anuria ≥12 hours
Loss	Loss of kidney function for >4 weeks	
End Stage	Loss of kidney function for >3 months	

The most common cause of pre-renal AKI in older people is external fluid loss from vomiting, diarrhoea, sweating or bleeding accompanied by insufficient fluid replacement or inappropriate diuretic use. Dehydration is common and is estimated to affect 1% of older people in hospital. If hypernatraemia develops, the associated mortality is significant.

Drugs which interfere with the autoregulation of renal blood flow can exacerbate a pre-renal insult leading to AKI. Non-steroidal anti-inflammatory drugs (NSAIDs) are prescribed for musculoskeletal symptoms. In addition to their analgesic effect, NSAIDs will inhibit renal prostacyclin production thereby reducing renal blood flow and GFR.

Angiotensin-converting enzyme inhibitors (ACE-i) and angiotensin receptor blockers (ARBs) are used in the treatment of hypertension, congestive cardiac failure and in the secondary prevention of ischaemic cardiac disease. They are also widely prescribed to prevent progression of chronic kidney disease. By inhibiting the action of angiotensin, glomerular pressure is reduced - a desired effect in the stable kidney. However, the compensatory response to a pre-renal insult is to increase glomerular pressure and maintain perfusion. In the context of renal hypoperfusion, ACEi and ARBs prevent this physiological compensation, become nephrotoxic and contribute to AKI.

The diagnosis of pre-renal AKI may be more difficult in older people. Tachycardia and reduced skin turgor are not reliable signs. Age-related changes in urine concentrating mechanisms means that oliguria can be a late indictor of AKI.

The treatment of pre-renal AKI is to restore renal perfusion through appropriate fluid balance and the removal of nephrotoxic contributors. This can be complicated in older people due to a higher prevalence of cardiac dysfunction and a delay in the clinical response to volume expansion.

Intrinsic renal AKI

Acute tubular necrosis (ATN) is the most frequent cause of AKI in the older person. Prolonged ischaemic damage from pre-renal insults can lead to ATN. This represents established damage to the kidney which is no longer reversible by the correction of renal hypoperfusion.

ATN is a recognized complication of surgery in older patients who are more vulnerable to perioperative hypotension, postoperative fluid loss and cardiac dysfunction. In addition, sepsis will contribute to any hypotension. Cardiac and aortic aneurysm surgery carry a high risk of ATN and these operations are more likely to be required with increasing age. Careful fluid balance, nutrition, and the treatment and prevention of sepsis are important in the management of 'surgical ATN'.

Polypharmacy, including the use of nephrotoxic drugs, is a common problem in geriatric medicine. Age is known to be a risk factor for aminoglycoside nephrotoxicity. Pre-existing renal disease, volume depletion, and dosing contribute to the toxicity of both drugs and radiocontrast agents. Optimization of fluid balance and appropriate dosing will reduce the risk, although avoidance of nephrotoxic medication whenever possible is best practice.

Acute interstitial nephritis is an inflammation in the interstitium of the kidney resulting in AKI. This is most commonly due to drugs. NSAIDs and proton pump inhibitors are known to be precipitants and these drugs are more commonly prescribed with increasing age. Treatment is withdrawal of the offending agent.

Glomerulonephritis is a rare cause of AKI in older people, although rapidly progressive forms are more common in older populations. Diagnosis is made on renal biopsy. The higher risk of opportunistic infection with immunosuppressive treatment and complications due to co-morbidity both confer a significantly higher mortality in the older patient with glomerulonephritis.

Post-renal AKI

Post-renal AKI is due to obstruction at any level of the urinary tract. The most common cause in older men is prostatic hypertrophy. This is an age related disease affecting 50% of men at aged 50 and 90% of men by age 90. A proportion of these men will develop significant obstruction leading to AKI. Timely catheterization can improve or even reverse the AKI.

In addition, age increases the prevalence of pelvic and retroperitoneal carcinomas. Obstruction proximal to the bladder will not be relieved by bladder catheterisation. Ultrasound imaging can demonstrate dilatation of the collecting system proximal to the obstruction. Insertion of a nephrostomy tube to relieve pressure on the kidney should be considered.

Prognosis of acute kidney injury

It remains unclear whether age is an independent prognostic marker in AKI. Some studies suggest that recovery from AKI is less likely in older patients and that chronic kidney disease (CKD) is a more common outcome compared to younger patients. The age-related decrease in capacity for endothelial cell proliferation and tubular repair is cited as supporting evidence. However, other studies show no significant differences in mortality or renal recovery after AKI. Age should not therefore be used as a discriminating factor in therapeutic decisions in AKI.

Author's Tip

Older patients are at higher risk of AKI

Age-related changes in the kidney contribute to the risk of AKI.

Causes of AKI which are more prevalent in older people include pre-renal hypoperfusion and post-renal obstruction.

AKI may be multifactorial in older people.

Iatrogenic AKI should be considered in all cases and nephrotoxic drugs discontinued.

Age should not be a factor is determining how AKI is treated.

Further reading

Bellomo R, Ronco C, Kellum JA, et al. (2004). Acute renal failure – definition, outcomes, measures, animal models, fluid therapy and information technology needs: the second international consensus conference of the ADQI group. *Crit Care*, **8**: R204-R12.

Molitoris BA, Levin A, Warnock DG, et al. (2007). Improving outcomes of acute kidney injury: report of an initiative. *J Am Soc Nephrol* **18**: 1992–4.

Pascual J, Liaño F, Ortuño J (1995). The elderly patient with acute renal failure. *J Am Soc Nephrol* **6**: 144–53.

Rosner M (2009). Acute kidney injury in the elderly. In *Geriatric Nephrology Curriculum*. Washington DC, American Society of Nephrology, Chapter 18.

Rowe JW, Andres R, Tobin JD, et al. (1976). The effect of age on creatinine clearance in man: a cross sectional and longitudinal study. *J Gerontol* **31**: 155–63.

Stewart J, Findlay G, Smith N, et al. (2009). *Acute Kidney Injury: Adding Insult to Injury*. London, National Confidential Enquiry into Patient Outcomes and Deaths.

Chronic kidney disease

What is chronic kidney disease?

The five stages of chronic kidney disease (CKD) (see Table 9.7) are defined by reduced (estimated) glomerular filtration rate (eGFR, mL/min/1.73m^2) and/or a renal abnormality according to the current Kidney Disease Outcomes Quality Initiative guidelines.

CKD diagnosis requires >2 eGFR readings >3 months apart.

Prevalence of CKD in older people

In the UK, 8.8% of the population have CKD 3–5 (3.5 million) as defined above. The prevalence is greatest in people over 70 years for all stages, which is most marked for stage 3. The number of people over 65 years old with end-stage renal disease (ESRD) (requiring renal replacement therapy (RRT)) has doubled in the past 25 years. There is a higher incidence of ESRD in men.

However, despite the finding of a reduced eGFR in over a third of older people, only 1–2% progress to ESRD. Therefore, most of the otherwise healthy individuals with CKD stage 3 do not have a renal disease leading to an increased risk of ESRD. This appears most marked in females. Explanations for the majority not progressing from CKD 3 to CKD stage 5, and not seemingly of major clinical significance, are

- a reduced GFR is an expected part of the normal physiological ageing process
- the current definition in Table 1 does not take into account the influence of gender on eGFR
- the coexistence of comorbid conditions (e.g. hypertension (HT), diabetes mellitus (DM), ischaemic heart disease (IHD)) may have an additive effect on renal structure and function, amplifying the effect of age.

Establishing the cause of CKD

Age-related vascular changes and/or exacerbation by comorbidities of HT and atherosclerosis and polypharmacy may account for the decline in eGFR observed with ageing in the majority of older people. The challenge is to identify those patients at risk of an underlying renal disease which may progress to kidney failure.

Further investigations should be considered for

- Abnormal urinalysis (think of glomerulonephritis)
- Rapid unexplained fall in eGFR (think of obstructive uropathy, recent contrast or drug changes: NSAIDs, trimethoprim)
- eGFR falling by >10–15%/year (e.g. think of diuretic therapies and poorly controlled DM or HT)

Table 9.7 Stages of chronic kidney disease

Stage	GFR	Description
1 + 2	>60	Normal kidney function with a renal abnormality*
3	30–59	Moderately decreased GFR
4	15–29	Severely reduced GFR
5	<15	Kidney failure

*Must have documented renal damage, e.g. proteinuria, haematuria, micro-albuminuria, polycystic disease, or reflux nephropathy. eGFR >60 with no other abnormality is normal.

- Absence of an obvious diagnosis (think of multiple myeloma)
- Constitutional symptoms (think of vasculitis)
- Abnormal eGFR of sudden onset (think of acute kidney injury (AKI)).

Identifying and modifying CKD progression risk to kidney failure

The relative risk of ESRD increases with a decreasing eGFR and increasing albuminuria. Subdividing CKD3 to a smaller subgroup with either abnormal albuminuria and/or eGFR <45 may identify the patients with significant co-morbidity, at risk of functional impairment and/or high risk of potentially modifiable factors.

In practice, the target guidelines are

- *Proteinuria target:* urine protein–creatinine ratio (uPCR) <100; albumin–creatinine ratio (ACR) <70
- *Diabetes mellitus:* Target HbA1c <7.5%
- *Hypertension (HT):* Target BP <130/80 mmHg
  - Drugs of choice are angiotensin-converting enzyme inhibitors or angiotensin receptor blockers as first line treatment unless otherwise contraindicated
  - However in frail older people, rigid treatment of blood pressure may not be such a priority, as geriatric syndromes start to become more common, notably falls
- Remove/avoid nephrotoxins
- Avoid AKI: episodes of AKI can be a risk factor for a step-wise progression to ESRD.

Author's Tip

Referral to a nephrologist:

CKD 5: urgent referral (unless clinically inappropriate)

CKD 4: routine referral (if stable)

CKD 3: routine referral only if sustained fall in eGFR >5 mL over 12 months or other problems of PCR >100 or PCR >45 with microscopic haematuria, difficult HT or systemic disease, e.g. SLE

CKD1/2: routine referral if fall in eGFR >15 mL in 12 months or 5mL/year over 3 years or for other problems as in CKD 3 above

Otherwise monitoring of eGFR, BP and urine dipstick should continue in primary care

---

Optimizing management of complications

Mortality and cardiovascular events

Mortality and cardiovascular (CV) events are more common than progression to ESRD at all stages of CKD in older people. It has been estimated that the older person with CKD 3 will have a 1.1% risk of ESRD but mortality rate 24.3%, and those with CKD 4 have a 17.6% risk of progression to ESRD over 3 years but mortality rate of 45.7%.

The sharpest rise in CV risk is in subjects with eGFR less than 45 with albuminuria. Increased albuminuria is a strong independent risk factor and may be a reflection of underlying vascular changes and atherosclerosis rather than CKD in its own right.

There is an increased prevalence of both traditional and novel CV risk factors in older people with CKD (including anaemia, electrolyte disturbances, hyperparathyroidism, hyperphosphataemia, high C-reactive protein and metabolic acidosis). However, in the oldest group there is evidence of reversed causation of the traditional risk factors, HT and hypercholesterolaemia.

Management should be targeted at annual review of risk including lipids, BMI, smoking, exercise, and alcohol history with targeted interventions to reduce risk.

Functional ability

A decline in function and cognition associated with increased hospitalization, institutionalization, poor nutrition, and death is recognized in CKD. There is also an increased risk of falls, affecting 30% per year in patients over 75 years old with ESRD.

- Cognitive decline: 70% >55 year old with ESRD. Education of the patient and family is important.

Bone disease

- Less able to excrete phosphate, form vitamin D and control PTH
- Vitamin D supplementation may be indicated with raised PTH (>7.7 pmol/L); consider phosphate binders for phosphate >1.5 mmol/L.

Fluid and electrolyte disturbance

- Less able to excrete water, sodium, and potassium, or retain water or sodium when needed
- Careful attention to fluid balance is important. Sodium restriction 2 g/day benefits patients with HT, oedema, and cardiac failure.

Anaemia

- Less able to make erythropoietin (EPO); EPO treatment may be considered in those with eGFR <30.

Drug interactions & polypharmacy

- Less able to excrete drugs and/or their metabolites
- Care in dosing of drugs, especially nephrotoxics such as NSAIDs, and awareness of drug-drug interactions.

Key issues

- CKD in older people is common but the risk for progression to kidney failure is low
- The challenge is to identify which patients are at risk of CKD progression
- Treatment should be aimed at reducing cardiovascular risk and modifiable factors (e.g. HT, proteinuria, DM, polypharmacy) when clinically appropriate
- Aim for an individualised approach to care, identifying which patients would benefit from dialysis or conservative management.

Renal replacement therapy (RRT)

The rapid growth in people requiring dialysis may be explained by our ageing population and more liberal dialysis commencement criteria, in parallel with patients starting dialysis (haemodialysis or peritoneal dialysis) in better condition.

One year survival on dialysis in those aged over 75 years is approximately 50–84% to 2.5% at 5 years. The survival advantage on dialysis is lost in those patients with high comorbidity scores, especially where IHD is included but it

should be remembered that RRT may improve functioning and/or alleviate symptoms even if it does not extend life.

Older patients with CKD are heterogenous, so the decision for dialysis should be made on an individual basis. Timely, planned decision-making with the patient that would benefit from RRT is essential. The focus is on prolonging good quality life. Dialysis options have expanded to include assisted models of care such as assisted peritoneal dialysis for the more frail older patient.

Kidney transplantation is considered in selected older patients and patients over 65 years are an expanding proportion of the kidney transplant waiting list and successful recipients (approximately 15%).

Conservative management

An alternative to dialysis is non-dialysis care. The active decision to manage a patient conservatively should aim treatment at symptom control and disease management such as anaemia, involving multidisciplinary care in what can be increasingly complex issues.

This decision for non-dialysis care should be informed by the patient's overall prognosis, quality of life, treatment burden, and essentially informed patient preference to forgo dialysis.

The current recommendation is that a patient may benefit from a palliative care approach if there is more than one core and more than one disease specific indicators. Core indicators include

- loss of ADLs, dependency in >3 ADLs
- multiple comorbidities
- weight loss
- albumin <25 g/dL
- Karnofsky score <50.

Author's Tip

Many older people with a low GFR will never progress, especially in the absence of DM or proteinuria

Most will die with a low GFR, not because of it; cardiovascular risk should be addressed for all CKD patients

It is important to recognize the few that will progress to ESRD to plan RRT care in a timely fashion, taking into account patient preference

---

Further reading

CKD Guidelines (www.renal.org/clinical/guidelinessection and www.kidney.org/professionals/kdoqi/guidelines).

Glassock RJ, Winearls C (2008). An epidemic of chronic kidney disease: fact or fiction? *Nephral Dial Transplant* **23**: 1117–21.

Hallon S, Orth S (2010). The conundrum of chronic kidney disease classification and end-stage renal risk prediction in the elderly – what is the right approach. *Nephron Clin Practice* **116**: c307–c16.

Keith D, Nichols G, Gullion C, et al. (2004). longitudinal follow-up and outcomes among a population with chronic kidney disease in a large managed care organization. *Arch Intern Med* **164**: 659–63.

Roderick P, Atkins R, Smeeth l, et al. (2008). Detecting chronic kidney disease in older people: What are the implications? *Age Ageing* **37**: 179–86.

Urinary tract infections

Urinary tract infection (UTI) is a commonly seen condition in both elderly women and men. It has significant morbidity and results in up to 40% of hospital admissions. UTI may be divided into several categories:

- asymptomatic bacteriuria
- uncomplicated
- complicated.

Definitions

Asymptomatic bacteriuria: patients have a quantifiable number of different bacteria present when collected appropriately, but no symptoms.

Uncomplicated lower UTI: a symptomatic bladder infection in the presence of a normal genitourinary tract

Uncomplicated upper UTI: a renal infection in the presence of a normal genitourinary tract.

Complicated UTI is a symptomatic infection of any part of the whole urinary tract in a patient with genitourinary tract abnormalities.

Epidemiology

The true epidemiology of UTI is difficult to determine. Annually 50–60% of all women will have at least one UTI, and approximately 10% of all post-menopausal women have a UTI. Although UTIs are less common in younger men, the presence of prostatic enlargement increases the risk of UTI.

With increasing age, underlying diseases that predispose to UTI, such as diabetes mellitus, become more common.

Urinary tract instrumentation, either temporary or permanent, such as cystoscopy or bladder catheterization, increases the incidence and prevalence of UTI.

Microbiology

See Table 9.8 for causative organisms. Escherichia coli and other bacteria such as Proteus, Klebsiella, and Pseudomonas account for the majority of the organisms.

Candida species in the urine are most frequently seen in patients with indwelling urinary catheters. Although most patients with candiduria develop repeated infections, invasive candidiasis is rare.

Pathogenesis

The close proximity of the urethra to potential contamination from faecal flora accounts for the pathogenesis in most women. In younger men, UTI is less likely because of the anatomical differences and the presence of antibacterial substances in prostatic fluid; this protection is reduced with ageing.

Ascending infection from the lower urinary tract almost always accounts for upper tract UTI.

Complicated infections in older people are associated with urinary obstruction (faecal impaction in both genders, prostatic enlargement in males), altered host defences (immunosuppresion), increased incidence of predisposing conditions (diabetes mellitus), and the presence of foreign body (catheter).

Faecal soiling, as occurs with faecal incontinence, increases the risk of UTI in both genders.

Urine microscopy and dipstick

In older people there is much debate about the diagnosis of a UTI. Many individuals are admitted to hospital with a clinical diagnosis and receive treatment in the absence of

Table 9.8 Bacterial aetiology of urinary tract infections

Organism	Urinary tract infection (%)	
	Uncomplicated	Complicated
Gram-negative organisms		
Escherichia coli	70–95	20–55
Proteus mirabilis	1–2	1–10
Klebsiella pneumoniae	1–2	2–15
Citrobacter spp.	<1	5
Enterobacter spp.	<1	2–10
Pseudomonas aeruginosa	<1	2–20
Other	<1	5–20
Gram-positive organisms		
Coagulase-negative Staphylococci (S. saprophyticus)	5–20 or more	1–5
Enterococci	1–2	1–25
Group B streptococci	<1	1–5
Staphylococcus aureus	<1	1–2
Other	<1	2

confirmatory tests. Approximately 62% of women with a suspected UTI have confirmatory tests. Nitrite, leucocyte esterase, and blood in the urine independently predict the diagnosis of UTI. A dipstick positive for nitrite or both leucocytes and blood is moderately sensitive (77%) and specific (70%) positive predictive value (PPV) 81%, negative predictive value (NPV) 65%. Predictive values are better than the clinical rule of having two of the following: urine cloudiness, offensive smell, reported moderately severe dysuria, and moderately severe nocturia (sensitivity 65%, specificity 69%, PPV 77%, NPV 54%).

The identification of bacteriuria is required to confirm a UTI. However, in older individuals, collected urine is often contaminated with bacteria from the periurethral areas, particularly if faecal incontinence or poor hygiene is present. In addition, the presence of a urinary catheter prohibits a clean catch specimen, which is recommended to reduce the risk of contamination. A positive sample from a suprapubic aspirate is diagnostic, but should not be used unless other methodologies have failed. A bacterial count of 10^5 cfu/mL is considered to be significant bacteriuria.

Asymptomatic bacteriuria

This is a common problem encountered in clinical geriatric medicine. In women, it is defined as two consecutive voided urines, with isolation of the same bacterial strain, with a count of $\geq10^5$ cfu/mL and in men a single clean catch urine with isolation of a single bacterial strain with a quantitative count of $\geq 10^5$ cfu/mL. A single catheterized urine with isolation of a single bacterial strain, with a quantitative count of $\geq 10^2$ cfu/mL in men or women.

- Asymptomatic bacteriuria increases with age (20% in women ≥ 80 years 15% in men aged >75 years. It is associated with diabetes in women, impaired urinary voiding (due to drugs or prostatic enlargement, indwelling urinary devices, and in those resident in long-term care facilities.
- Asymptomatic bacteriuria increases the risk of symptomatic UTI
- Asymptomatic bacteriuria is important to diagnose in those about to undergo urological procedures. If detected, appropriate therapy should be given immediately prior to the procedure and then continued if an indwelling catheter remains in place.

Uncomplicated lower UTI treatments

Although many of the studies comparing short- and long-term antibiotics are of poor quality, there was an increased relative risk of persistent UTI when comparing single dose with both short course treatment and long course treatment (relative risk 2.01, 95% CI 1.9 to 3.84 vs RR 1.93, CI 1.01–3.7, 95%).

There is no evidence in differing efficacy for short versus longer treatments, and therefore 3–6 days should be sufficient for treating uncomplicated lower urinary tract infections. A study of the use of quinolones in treatment of acute cystitis in women of all ages found no significant differences in clinical or microbiological efficacy between different quinolones. Healthy older individuals can be managed with oral antimicrobials in the community. The antimicrobial choice should be guided by local antimicrobial sensitivity. Trimethoprim may cause nausea, vomiting, pruritus, or rash and is contraindicated in blood dyscrasias and severe renal impairment. Nitrofurantoin also causes anorexia and nausea. It can result in pulmonary reactions, peripheral neuropathy, and skin rashes. Amoxicillin and co-amoxiclav cause nausea, vomiting, and are contraindicated in penicillin hypersensitivity. They may causes pseudomembranous colitis, especially in older individuals. Cephalosporins should be avoided because of the increased incidence of pseudomembranous colitis. Unfortunately the widespread use of trimethoprim has resulted in 39% of E. coli isolates now being resistant. Trimethoprim has no activity against Pseudomonas and variable activity against Enterococci. Trimethoprim is absorbed readily from the GI tract and its peak serum level is found 1–4 hours after indigestion.

Uncomplicated upper UTI treatments

Although mild to moderate cases may be managed in the community, using oral antimicrobials, the inability of an older person to reliably take oral medication and the possibility of dehydration, should prompt hospitalization. Antibiotics should be guided by local antimicrobial sensitivity, in the knowledge that high concentrations of antibiotics are required in the renal medulla. Ciprofloxacin and levofloxacin are the oral drugs of choice. If an individual requires parenteral agents, either a third-generation cephalosporin or aminoglycoside should be given. In older patients, the onset of diarrhoea after such drugs, should be rapidly tested for Clostridium toxin

Mild cases should be treated for 5–7 days and in severe cases, there is no advantage of continuing therapy beyond 14 days.

Complicated urinary tract infection

This is the most common form of UTI seen in older individuals. The organisms implicated are from a wider range and many exhibit antimicrobial resistance. All suspected cases must have urine culture, the treatment with antimicrobial agents must be for at least 7 days and after initial empirical broad spectrum antibiotics microbial culture and sensitivity guide alterations in therapy.

Treatment

Standard therapy involves antibiotics given at least initially by injection. Whilst there is evidence that oral therapy is equally effective, once adequate drug levels are achieved, head to head studies are few, with varied outcome measures.

In elderly men, bladder scanning is essential to identify those with possible obstructive pathology and to look for residual post-voiding urine volumes. Ideally urine should be cultured 2 weeks after treatment in men to ensure that any nidus of infection in the prostatic bed has been cleared. Treatment of infections in this setting should be with antibiotics which penetrate the prostate gland (such as ciprofloxacin or trimethoprim) and continued for 28 days. The presence of recurrent UTI of the same organism should lead to the consideration of longer duration antibiotics.

Prevention of urinary tract infections

Cranberry juice has some antimicrobial properties, and there is limited evidence for its use in preventing UTIs in women, though the evidence in older men is less clear. It is not effective in people who require catheterization. Care should be taken owing to the interaction of cranberry juice with medication such as warfarin.

The use of antibiotics before or during catheter insertion reduces the incidence of infection and the number of bacteria or pus cells in the urine.

Although the evidence is limited, the use of antibiotics is recommended during the first 3 postoperative days or from postoperative day 2 until catheter removal in women with abdominal surgery and short-term catheterization.

Urinary catheters

Urinary catheters are often associated with problems. Most individuals with a long-term indwelling catheter will experience at least one catheter-related problem during an 8-month period, of which 70% report catheter-associated urinary tract infections, 74% blockage, 79% leakage, and 33% accidental dislodgement. Anecdotal evidence suggests that blockage predisposes to infection, although the debris associated with infection is often the underlying cause of the blockage! There is no evidence from systematic reviews that wash out with any solution in any clinical setting, with any type of catheter, resulted in reduced catheter blockage. Silver alloy catheters significantly reduce the incidence of asymptomatic bacteriuria in hospitalized adults who are catheterized for less than 1 week. Although a period of catheterization greater than 1 week also sees a reduction in asymptomatic bacteriuria with the use of silver alloy catheters, the risk ratio is diminished considerably. Antibiotic impregnated catheters reduce the rate of asymptomatic bacteriuria, although if catheterization is for greater than 1 week the results are not statistically significant. Urinary tract infections are also less likely to occur in patients with antibiotic-impregnated catheters, although the data for long-term catheterization is less robust.

Suprapubic catheters are less likely than indwelling catheters, to result in bacteriuria, recatheterization, and discomfort. However, not all bacteriuria results in a urinary tract infection and therefore data are difficult to extrapolate. Although intermittent catheterization is not ideal in the majority of older individuals, it does bring with it a lower risk of bacteriuria than an indwelling urethral catheter, and therefore despite it being more costly it should be considered as a strategy in certain time limited situations.

The key to the management of urinary catheters is to limit their use, recommend suprapubic catheterization in those where long-term usage is envisaged, and treat only evidence of systemic infection rather than randomly detected asymptomatic bacteriuria.

Further reading

Griffiths R, Fernandez R (2007). Strategies for removal of short-term indwelling urethral catheters in adults. *Cochrane Database Syst Rev* **18**;(2): CD004011.

Little P, Turner S, Rumsby K, *et al.* (2009). Dipsticks and diagnostic algorithms in urinary tract infection: development and validation, radomised trial, economic analysis, observational cohort and qualitative study. *Health Technol Assess* **13**: 1–73.

Lutters M, Vogt-Ferrier NB (2008). Antibiotic duration for treating uncomplicated, symptomatic lower urinary tract infections in elderly women. *Cochrane Database Syst Rev* **16**(3): CD001535.

Jepson RG, Craig JC (2008). Cranberries for preventing urinary tract infections. *Cochrane Database Syst Rev* **23**(1): CD001321.

Niël-Weise BS, van den Broek PJ (2005). Antibiotic policies for short-term catheter bladder drainage in adults. *Cochrane Database Syst Rev* **20**(3): CD005428.

Perrotta C, Aznar M, Mejia R *et al.* (2008). Oestrogens for preventing recurrent urinary tract infection in postmenopausal women. *Cochrane Database Syst Rev* **112**(3): 689–90.

Pohl A (2007). Modes of administration of antibiotics for symptomatic severe urinary tract infections. *Cochrane Database Syst Rev* **17**(4): CD003237.

Rafalsky VV, Andreeva IV, Rjabkova EL. (2006). Quinolones for uncomplicated acute cystitis in women. *Cochrane Database Syst Rev* **19**(3): CD003597.

Woodford HJ, George J (2011). Diagnosis and management of urinary infections in older people. *Clin Med* **11**: 80–3.

Lower urinary tract symptoms in elderly men

In order to understand voiding problems it is important to understand how and why the urinary tract is designed.

- Urine is made by filtration of blood through the kidneys. In so doing there is a marked pressure drop so that the pressure in the renal pelvis is low. It is akin to an espresso coffee machine with the high pressure of the steam driving the process but the coffee drips out at low pressure. It is vital to keep the pressure in the collecting system low, as a rise in pressure would stop the filtration process, resulting in renal failure, and this applies equally throughout the lower urinary tract including the bladder.
- As the bladder fills it has to relax to accommodate the delivered urine without a pressure rise. A trace plotting pressure against bladder volume for a normal bladder is a straight line. The only time the pressure rises significantly in the normal urinary tract is briefly during voiding. The whole design of the urinary tract is to transmit the urine to the bladder, store it, and expel it without a significant pressure rise.
- The bladder therefore is a complex organ requiring sensory receptors and both inhibitory and contractile motor pathways to maintain a low pressure while filling but allowing the detrusor muscle to contract at voiding to empty. Pathology of the sensory and motor pathways may result in lower urinary tract symptoms (LUTS).

Lower urinary tract symptoms may commonly be derived from pathology of:

Urine production

- If the rate of urine production is high then common sense dictates voiding will be more frequent.
  - diabetes mellitus
  - diabetes insipidus
  - nocturnal polyuria

Physical obstruction

- Benign
  - Benign prostatic hyperplasia
  - Urethral stricture
  - Phimosis, usually due to lichen sclerosus
- Malignant
  - Carcinoma of the prostate
  - Bladder cancer
  - External pressure from rectal cancer

Sensory and motor neuropathy

- Upper motor neurone
  - Stroke
  - Parkinson's disease
  - Multiple sclerosis
  - Trauma
  - Cord compression from tumour or benign spinal pathology e.g. prolapsed inter-vertebral disc.

Infection and inflammation

- Urinary tract infection

Differential diagnosis of LUTS

In Europe the prevalence of LUTS is >40% in men in their sixth decade. LUTS are divided into voiding symptoms and storage symptoms.

Voiding symptoms

- Poor and intermittent stream, hesitancy.
  - These are easy to understand in terms of physics. Flow is determined by the combination of detrusor pressure and outflow resistance. In the absence of other signs of peripheral neuropathy it is reasonable to presume obstruction (bearing in mind that elderly men frequently void with a lower detrusor pressure than younger men) if there is a major reduction in flow (see Figure 9.4).

Storage symptoms

- Urgency, frequency.
  - These symptoms are more bothersome to patients so they are more likely to complain of them. They are symptoms of detrusor overactivity and bladder outflow obstruction.

Nocturia

- This can be a sign of detrusor overactivity when associated with daytime frequency.
- In the absence of daytime frequency it can be due to loss or reverse diurnal rhythm. Nocturnal polyuria (passing more than a third of the urine produced after retiring and before rising) is common and easy to diagnose with an output chart. Unless present coincidentally, nocturnal polyuria is not associated with bladder outflow obstruction.
- Is associated with peripheral oedema especially due to CCF. The fluid collected in the legs re-enters the circulation on elevation leading to a nocturnal diuresis.
  - Is associated with sleep apnoea.

Incontinence

- An older man who becomes incontinent, especially at night, is in chronic retention of urine until proved otherwise.
- Urge incontinence may be associated with detrusor overactivity in the absence of retention.

Pneumaturia

- Usually a sign of an enterocolic fistula or due to a gas forming organism.

Common pathological conditions to consider in the diagnosis and treatment of LUTS.

Benign Prostatic Enlargement (BPE) and Bladder Outlet Obstruction

- BPE is a progressive disease commonly associated with LUTS when the enlargement causes obstruction.

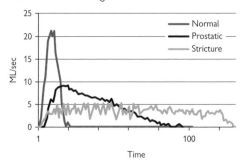

Figure 9.4 Normal and pathological flow rates.

- Associated with a smooth feeling prostate on DRE and a normal PSA.
- The level of PSA is, to some extent, related to the degree of enlargement. A PSA of <1 is unlikely to be associated with any significant degree of BPE. This does not exclude bladder neck muscle dyssynergia as a cause.

The aim of treating LUTS is to control symptoms and to prevent progression to acute or chronic urinary retention (AUR/CUR). The risk of AUR has been estimated at 23% for an average 60-year-old man if he survives another 10 years.

Management

- Lifestyle advice (LUTS not bothersome and at low risk of retention)
- Medical Management:
  - Alpha-blockers. Benign prostatic obstruction is caused in part by alpha-1-adrenoreceptor mediated prostatic smooth muscle contraction. Alpha-blockers promote relaxation of prostatic smooth muscle and the bladder neck. These have a rapid onset of action and improve symptom scores by 30–45% after 3 months treatment. Side-effects: (SE) dizziness, postural hypotension
  - 5-alpha-reductase inhibitors. Work by blocking the conversion of testosterone to dihydrotestosterone, the active metabolite which stimulates growth in BPE. The PLESS study showed treatment with finasteride for 4 years reduced the relative risk of AUR by 57% and surgery by 55%. These have a slow onset of action and should not be assessed for 6 months. SE: erectile dysfunction, reduce serum PSA by a median of 50% after 6 months

Surgical management:

- Indicated with failure of medical management, severely bothersome LUTS, recurrent acute urinary retention, chronic urinary retention. Options include a TURP, Laser vaporization and enucleation of the prostate and open prostatectomy. Laser enucleation and open surgery are suitable for larger glands.

Overactive Bladder (OAB) or detrusor instability

- Symptoms include urinary urgency, with or without incontinence, frequency and nocturia. These symptoms originate from spontaneous contractions of the detrusor during filling but before the bladder is full (see Figure 9.5).
- Prevalence: 16.6% in people >40 years.
- Aetiology can be idiopathic or secondary to bladder outflow obstruction or neuropathy. Common in patients after stroke.

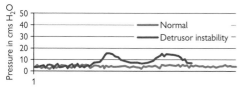

Figure 9.5 Bladder pressure and in normal and unstable bladders.

- Urge incontinence is associated with increase in the number of falls and fractures in the elderly population.
- Treatment is centred on inhibition of the overactive detrusor muscle through altering the parasympathetic system via cholineric muscarinic receptors with anticholinergic drugs. Side-effects: dry mouth, constipation indigestion.
- Surgical treatment: relief of bladder outflow obstruction, intravesical botox, neuromodulation, augmentation cystoplasty

Urinary tract infections

- Urinary tract infections are more common inwomen than men.
- In men, however, it is complicated by prostatic infection which nearly always accompanies a UTI in men.
- Acute bacterial prostatitis presents with feverand LUTS. If the prostate swells then it may cause retention of urine. Infection may also track down the vas to cause epididymitis.
- Causes include:
  - Indwelling catheters. It is impossible to eradicate infection under these circumstances and treatment should be limited to the systemic aspects of the infection. Continuing antibiotics after the patient is systemically well only encourages resistance.
  - After prostatic surgery or urethral instrumentation.
  - Poor bladder emptying and bladder stones. Quite frequently this can be a perpetuating triad where it is impossible to eradicate the infection without surgery to remove the stone and establish good bladder emptying.
- Investigations: MSU – typical pathogens include E. coli, Klebsiella, Pseudomonas, and Enterococcus.
- Treatment: UTIs associated with fever are complex and require a longer course of antibiotics than simple infections in women. Not all antibiotics penetrate well into the prostate. For prostatitis a 2–6 week course of a prostate-penetrating antibiotic is required. (E.g. Quinolones or Trimethoprim).
  - Progression to chronic bacterial prostatitis occurs in around 5%. Patients present with recurring infections. Rarely but increasingly as antibiotic resistance becomes more widespread, low dose suppression is all that is possible.

Prostate cancer

- Prostate cancer is the most common cancer in elderly men. Mean age at diagnosis is 69 years.
- Diagnosis is dependent on either
  - Biopsy—The indications for biopsy are an elevated PSA or abnormal digital rectal examination.
  - A grossly elevated PSA in the absence of UTI especially with evidence of dissemination (e.g. a positive bone scan).
- Management of prostate cancer depends on the stage, Gleeson score, comorbidities and the patient's wishes.
- At present there is no consensus about which therapeutic option is best for men with localized prostate cancer. There is no good evidence that hormone treatment gives a survival advantage in this group.

Treatment options for prostate cancer
Localized prostate cancer. T1/2 N0M0

For prostatitis a 2–6 week course of a prostate-penetrating antibiotic is required. (E.g. Quinolones or Trimethoprim). Treatment with curative intent is reasonable if life expectancy is predicted to be longer than 10 years. In addition elderly patients may be more inclined to avoid risk and less willing to sacrifice quality of life.

- Active surveillance (PSA is monitored for a significant rise every 6 months and treatment started according to PSA doubling time, progression on rebiopsy).
- Radiotherapy (external beam radiotherapy, brachytherapy)
- Surgical (open surgery, minimal access –laparoscopic/robotic).
- Hormones: there is no good evidence to say that patients with localized prostate cancer benefit from hormone treatment before it becomes extracapsular.

Locally advanced prostate cancer. T3N0M0

- There is good evidence that adjuvant hormonal treatment to radiotherapy gives a survival advantage.

Advanced prostate cancer. T4 and/or N1M1

The mainstay of treatment is hormonal—LHRH agonist or antagonist. Delaying treatment until the patient becomes symptomatic gives a higher rate of serious adverse events. Chemotherapy has also been shown to increase survival if the patient is robust enough to tolerate it. Usually it is reserved for patients where the PSA is rising despite castration but trials are ongoing to determine if it should be used earlier in the patient pathway.

Urinary retention

Incidence: 2.2 to 6.8 per 1000 men per year. As many as one in 10 men in their 70s may experience acute urinary retention within 5 years.

Acute Urinary Retention (AUR)

Definition: Painful inability to void, with relief of pain following drainage of bladder by catheterization. Residual volume usually between 500 and 800 mL.
Causes: BPE, Faecal impaction, clot retention, drugs (anticholinergic, sympathomimetic agents), neuropathy including neurotropic viruses, e.g. shingles.
   Management: Trial without Catheter (TWOC) is reasonable if the cause has been rectified (e.g. faecal impaction) or if no severe predating symptoms. However 50% will experience a further episode of retention within the next week, 70% within the next year.

AUR is associated with systemic disease and careful assessment of comorbidities should be made using a multidisciplinary approach. One study showed one in seven men admitted to hospital with spontaneous acute urinary retention and one in four with precipitated acute urinary retention die within a year.

Chronic Urinary Retention (CUR)

Definition: painless urinary retention which may be associated with

Classification: low pressure and high pressure

- *Low pressure chronic retention:* Large residual volume of urine within the bladder without associated renal dysfunction.
- *High-pressure chronic retention:* maintenance of voiding with a residual volume >800 mL, an intravesical pressure greater than 30 cmH$_2$O and hydronephrosis. In time this leads to renal failure.

- Patients tend to present with LUTS and especially complain of nocturnal enuresis. Abdominal examination reveals a markedly distended bladder. Blood should be tested to assess renal function.
- Following catheterization and drainage of a large residual, the patient should be admitted and monitored for a diuresis (>200 mL/h). This occurs with a salt losing nephropathy and an intravenous infusion should be administered to replace the lost fluid and electrolytes. Because of the electrolyte changes this is not suitable for primary care management.
- Haematuria may occur following catheterization in chronic retention as a consequence of decompression of prostatic and bladder veins.
- TWOC is not indicated for chronic retention which is managed by surgery or a permanent indwelling catheter or intermittent self-catheterization.

Assessment of the man with LUTS

History

- Is the oral fluid intake high?
  - Diabetes mellitus and insipidus
  - Is the patient just drinking excessively?
- Previous neurological disease
  - Consider various forms of neuropathy and detrusor instability
- Haematuria
  - Does the patient have cancer?
- Bowel symptoms
- Is the patient impacted or is there a large rectal carcinoma?
- Storage vs voiding symptoms
  - Is the patient obstructed or are the symptoms more of detrusor instability?
- Nocturia in isolation
  - Consider nocturnal polyuria

Examination

Abdominal examination

- Is the patient in retention?
- Is there a mass from a large pelvic cancer?

Penis

- Is there a significant phimosis or meatal stenosis?

DRE

- Does the patient have prostate cancer?
- Is there a large rectal cancer?
- Is the patient impacted?

Investigations

Urinalysis/MSSU

- Is the patient diabetic?
- Is there a UTI?
- Is there a major degree of microscopic haematuria?

Bloods

- U&E: Is the patient in renal failure?
- PSA: Does the patient have prostrate cancer? (PSA is also elevated in the presence of a UTI or retention or after catheterization).

Output chart

- What is the total volume passed in 24 hours?
- What proportion of the output is passed at night?

Flow rate and post micturition residue
- Is the patient obstructed and if so, how well is he emptying his bladder?

Urinary tract ultrasound
- Is there hydronephrosis secondary to retention?
- Might the patient have a ureteric stone causing the symptoms?
- Does the patient have a bladder stone or cancer?

Urine cytology

In patients with marked strangury or when the symptoms are not easily explainable, consider carcinoma *in situ* or cancer.

Further reading

Armitage JN, Sibanda N, Cathcart PJ, *et al.* (2007). Mortality in men admitted to hospital with acute urinary retention: database analysis. *Br Med J* **335**: 1199–202.

Brown JS, Vittinghoff E, Wyman JF, *et al.* (2000). Urinary Incontinence: does it increase risk of falls and fractures? Study of Osteoporotic Fractures Research Group. *J Am Geriatr Soc* **48**: 721–5.

Emberton M, Cornel EB, Bassi PF, *et al.* (2008). Benign Prostatic Hyperplasia as a progressive disease: a guide to the risk factors and options for medical management. *Int J Clin Pract* **62**: 1076–86.

McConnell JD, Bruskewitz R, Walsh P, *et al.* (1998). The effect of finasteride on the risk of acute urinary retention and the need for surgical treatment among men with benign prostatic hyperplasia. Finasteride long-term efficacy and study group. *N Engl J Med* **338**: 557–63.

Pfitzanmaier J, Altwein JE (2009). Hormonal therapy in the elderly prostate cancer patient. *Dtsch Arztebl Int* **106**: 242–7.

Sinibaldi V (2007). Docetaxel treatment in the elderly patient with hormone refractory prostate cancer. *Clin Interv Aging* **2**: 555–60.

Stangelberger MD, Waldert M, Djavan B (2008). Prostate cancer in elderly men. *Rev Urol* **10**: 111–19.

Musculoskeletal problems

Osteoarthritis

Osteoarthritis is the most prevalent joint disorder in the world today, and the incidence increases with age.

Definition

There are many definitions of osteoarthritis (OA), but perhaps the most useful in clinical practice is that of joint pain associated with characteristic radiographic findings of joint space narrowing and new bone formation, in the absence of another cause.

Pathologically, wear and damage to the articular cartilage causes a low-grade inflammation leading to pain and structural changes within the joint.

Another, widely quoted definition comes from the American Academy of Orthopaedic Surgeons (1995):

"Osteoarthritis diseases are a result of both mechanical and biologic events that destabilize the normal coupling of degradation and synthesis of articular cartilage chondrocytes, extracellular matrix and subchondral bone. Although they may be initiated by multiple factors, such as genetic, developmental, metabolic, and traumatic factors, osteoarthritis diseases are manifest by morphologic, biochemical, molecular and biomechanical changes of both cells and matrix which leads to a softening, fibrillation, ulceration and loss of articular cartilage, sclerosis, and eburnation of subchondral bone, osteophytes and subchondral cysts. When clinically evident, osteoarthritis diseases are characterized by joint pain, tenderness, limitation of movement and variable degrees of inflammation, without systemic effects."

ACR Classification Criteria for Osteoarthritis

Hand OA

Pain, aching or stiffness in the hand and three of the following:

Bony swelling of ≥2 distal interphalangeal (DIP) joints.

Bony swelling of 2 or more of 10 selected joints.

<3 swollen metacarpophalangeal (MCP) joints.

Deformity of 2 or more of 10 selected joints.

Knee OA (Clinical)

Knee pain and at least 3 of 6:

Age >50 years

Stiffness <30 minutes

Crepitus

Bony tenderness

Bony enlargement

No palpable warmth

Hip OA (Clinical and laboratory)

Hip pain and either:

Hip internal rotation ≤15° **and** ESR ≤45mm/h **or** hip flexion ≤115° if ESR unavailable

OR

Hip internal rotation >15° **and** pain on hip internal rotation **and** morning stiffness of the hip ≤60 minutes **and** age >50 years.

Epidemiology

Osteoarthritis is the most common joint disease in the Western world, and the prevalence increases with age, peaking around 70 years. Radiographic changes are present in a large number of people over the age of 50, hip 8%, hand 15%, knee 30%, and about 50% will have symptoms over 1 year. In 2007, 137 000 hip and knee operations were performed in England and Wales.

Caucasians have a higher rate of OA than other ethnic groups. This is thought to be primarily genetically determined. Environmental factors play a role in the prevalence of OA, for example in indigenous Chinese the tendency to squat may explain the higher incidence of knee OA.

Knee and hand OA are more common in females by a ratio of 2:1, but hip OA shows a less consistent difference (see Figures 10.1 and 10.2).

Occupational factors play a role: obesity and bending in knee OA; farming for hip; and extensive use of precision grip in hand OA.

Pathophysiology

Idiopathic (Primary) Osteoarthritis

There are several distinct patterns of idiopathic OA.

- Nodal generalized
  - fingers (Heberden's and Bouchard's nodes)
  - usually female
  - familial
  - distal joints more commonly involved, with proximal hand and wrist joints relatively spared
- Erosive or inflammatory
  - uncommon
  - ankylosis common, leading to impairment of function
  - episodes of inflammation
  - radiographic erosions visible
  - proximal involvement as common as distal

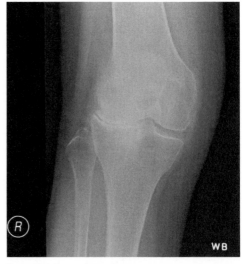

Figure 10.1 Osteoarthritis of knee.

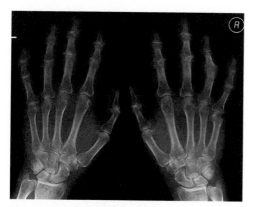

Figure 10.2 Nodal OA of hands.

- Large joints
  - hip (superior, axial, medial, diffuse)
  - knee (medial compartment, lateral compartment, patellofemoral)
- Spinal
- Other single sites (shoulder, temperomandibular joint, ankle, wrist, acromioclavicular joint)

Secondary osteoarthritis causes

- Trauma
- Inflammatory arthritis
  - metabolic/endocrine (e.g. haemochromatosis, parathyroid disturbance, alkaptonuria, acromegaly)
- Neuropathy
  - crystal deposition (Uric acid (gout), calcium pyrophosphate (pseudogout), hydroxyapatite (e.g. Milwaukee shoulder))
- Anatomical abnormalities

Histological changes

- Damage to cartilage and bony hypertrophy
- Biomechanical factors influence development of disease
  - trauma
  - muscle weakness and ligament factors
  - impairment of sensory function
- Inflammation plays a role in the pathogenesis, particularly, cytokines such as interleukin (IL)-1 and matrix metalloproteinase (MMP)-3
- Although associated with advancing age, the histological changes in OA are distinct from those of normal ageing
- Crystal deposition may mediate destructive changes
- Proteases activated in inflammatory processes may cause disintegration of the cartilage matrix.

Genetic

Genetic factors have a major influence in the development of OA, and are site and gender specific. First-degree relatives have a risk of two to three times that of the background population. There may be genetic influences both on structure of collagen, cartilage, bone metabolism, and in the inflammatory process, and mechanical stresses are linked to gene expression. Specific genes have been identified as being causal in OA, including collagen genes (COL2A1), vitamin D receptor and oestrogen receptor genes.

Clinical features

History

- Early disease: use-related pain
- Late disease: refractory or sleep disturbing pain
- Stiffness in the morning is usually of short duration, and confined to the affected joints rather than being generalized
- Impairment of function, particularly in the load-bearing joints
- Ask about
  - pain or stiffness in arms legs or spine
  - activities of daily living; effect on work/leisure
  - problems with steps or stairs
  - frequency of pain (most days in last month)
  - pain with use and after what duration of use
  - morning stiffness; night-time pain
- Consider risk factors in the history
  - obesity
  - previous injuries or surgery
  - repetitions of movements at work
  - family history (joint replacements, hand deformities)
  - hormonal status (menopause and HRT)
- Depression: a major factor in any chronically painful or debilitating condition
- Relevant past medical history to guide treatment, e.g. caution with NSAIDs in GI and cardiac problems).

Examination

Although a single joint may be the presenting problem, it is often useful to examine any other potential joints for involvement. The examination should be structured with the Regional Examination of the Musculoskeletal System (REMS) scheme: look, feel, move, function.

There are few signs specific to OA, but crepitus and pain on movement or weight bearing are typical. There may be wasting of surrounding muscles due to underuse.

Hands

- Heberden's (distal interphalangeal, DIP) or Bouchard's (proximalinter phalangeal, PIP) nodes present (bony enlargement of joint margins): nodal osteoarthritis
- OA of the thumb carpometacarpal joint (CMCJ) can cause squaring of the hand, and progressive hyperextension of the metacarpophalangeal joint (MCPJ) and loss of function
- Finger flexion can be reduced, and fixed deformities may occur
- Pain on movement
- Function, e.g. writing, fastening of clothing, grip.

Knees

- Cool effusions may be present
- Bony enlargement of the joint margins may be present
- Crepitus may be felt
- Pain on movement or palpation of joint line
- Assess ligaments
- Function: observe walking.

Hips

- Restriction of extension and internal rotation are early signs of hip OA
- Pain on movement
- Functional assessment of gait.

Cervical Spine
- Most common sites of involvement are C5-C7
- Particularly extension and lateral flexion may reproduce symptoms
- Pain with/without paraesthesiae in related nerve root distribution
- Tenderness over facet joints
- Paraspinal muscle spasm.

Lumbar spine
- Most commonly L3–L5
- Loss of lordosis with pain on extension
- Paraspinal muscle spasm
- **Individual vertebral tenderness should alert you to an alternative diagnosis**
- Pain of spinal stenosis may mimic claudication: 'spinal claudication' causes pain on standing, better with walking and relieved by flexing at the waist or sitting (e.g. cycling).

Red flags for spinal pain
Red flags are those symptoms or signs which indicate that more serious pathology may be present. It is important to consider further investigations should these be elicited.

History factors
- Previous history of malignancy (however long ago)
- Age <16 or >50 with new-onset pain
- Weight loss (unexplained)
- Previous longstanding steroid use
- Recent serious illness
- Recent significant infection.

Signs
- Saddle anaesthesia/reduced anal tone
- Hip or knee weakness
- Generalized neurological deficit
- Progressive spinal deformity
- Urinary retention.

Symptoms
- Non-mechanical pain (worse at rest)
- Thoracic pain
- Fevers/rigors
- General malaise.

Differential diagnoses
It is important to differentiate OA from inflammatory arthritis (although they may co-exist) such as rheumatoid arthritis (RA), gout, calcium pyrophosphate deposition disease (CPPDD or pseudogout), and psoriatic arthritis.

Investigations
In straightforward cases, where consideration for surgery would not be appropriate, investigation is not always required. However, it may be helpful in the exclusion of other possible diagnoses, such as CPPDD or RA.

Laboratory
- It is uncommon for inflammatory markers to be raised, though a slightly elevated ESR does not exclude OA
- Immunological tests such as rheumatoid factor and anti-CCP antibodies may assist in the differentiation of OA from inflammatory arthropathies

- If OA may be secondary, then further investigation may help, e.g. serum ferritin in haemochromatosis, parathyroid hormone levels in hyperparathyroidism
- Examination of synovial fluid in suspected gout or calcium pyrophosphate deposition disease

Imaging
Characteristic findings on plain radiograph include:
- subchondral bone cysts
- joint space narrowing
- osteophytosis
- subchondral sclerosis.

Magnetic resonance imaging
Although not specifically used for investigation of osteoarthritis, there are characteristic changes, which can be seen on magnetic resonance imaging (MRI). It is more sensitive in the detection of marginal and central osteophytes than plain radiographs:
- bone oedema – specifically associated with pain in OA
- cartilage defects
- signal changes associated with water concentration demonstrating cartilage density loss, a hallmark of OA.

It is also useful in the evaluation of spinal OA, specifically looking for evidence of spinal or foraminal stenosis, and in the assessment of disc degeneration.

Management
Management of osteoarthritis should be tailored to the requirements of the patient, their other conditions, and quality of life. Pharmacological and non-pharmacological interventions may be combined to provide optimal care.

The NICE guidelines for the management of OA advocate a holistic assessment, including:
- social assessment (e.g. effect on life; expectations)
- support network (e.g. effects on carers and their ideas, concerns and expectations)
- psychological (e.g. ideas; concerns; expectations; mood.)
- occupational (e.g. adjustments required to work)
- sleep quality
- attitude to exercise
- other musculoskeletal pain (e.g. other treatable causes of other pains; is there a chronic pain syndrome developing?)
- pain assessment (e.g. self-help; analgesia)
- comorbidity (e.g. fitness for surgery; assessment of drug therapy choices, interaction of modalities; falls).

Non-pharmacological Interventions
- Exercise—a core treatment for all patients with OA including both local muscle strengthening and general aerobic fitness
- Weight loss for those who are overweight or obese
- TENS, as an adjunct to other therapies
- Appropriate footwear advice
  - shock absorbing properties
  - support
- Assistive devices, often through occupational therapy services
  - sticks
  - jar-opening devices/kettle pouring aids
  - braces, supports, insoles
  - adaptive cutlery.

Referrals to, as appropriate, physiotherapy, occupational therapy, and podiatry/orthotics should be completed to provide a complete assessment of patient needs, and to provide the appropriate interventions.

Although glucosamine and chondroitin are not supported within the NICE guidance, there is some evidence to suggest that they are helpful in some cases. A trial of at least 3 months' duration may be considered, with subsequent reassessment to determine efficacy. There is an excellent side-effect profile; however, oral anticoagulants should be monitored due to reports of potentiation of warfarin.

Pharmacological interventions

Oral analgesics

- Paracetamol is an appropriate first-line analgesic in mild to moderate OA, and should be considered a baseline therapy to build upon.
- Opioids are often required, initially less potent, such as codeine or tramadol, then with progression to higher potency preparations depending upon efficacy.

Topical therapies

- NICE guidance suggests that topical NSAIDs should be offered before oral NSAIDs or opioids. Some preparations have more evidence of efficacy than others.
- Capsaicin cream can be helpful in hand OA, but some skin reactions may occur.

Oral NSAIDs and 'Coxibs'

- Considered where the combination of oral paracetamol and topical NSAIDs do not provide adequate pain relief, either as alternative or additive therapy
- It is important to consider both GI and cardiovascular risk factors before prescribing NSAIDs. Both COX-2 inhibitors and traditional non-selective NSAIDs have significant cardiovascular effects
- Both conventional NSAIDs and Coxibs should be used with gastro-protection in those with risk factors (e.g. previous peptic ulceration or gastritis; those taking aspirin) and other analgesics considered in preference
- Consideration of renal function is also appropriate prior to the prescription of NSAID/COX-2 inhibitors.

Intra-articular injection

- Intra-articular steroid injections are of benefit for the short-term relief of OA pain in both knees and hips. The duration of benefit is variable, and hip injection should only be performed under radiological guidance.
- Used for moderate to severe OA pain, sometimes as a bridge to arthroplasty, although surgeons often prefer patients to avoid intra-articular steroid for up to 6 months prior to joint replacement to aid in infection prevention.
- There is no strong evidence for intra-articular hyaluronic acid, though some patients do benefit. Their high cost and uncertain benefit led to NICE not recommending these agents for general use.

Surgical interventions

Arthroplasty can have a huge impact on the quality of life of patients with OA whose symptoms are refractory to conservative treatment strategies.

Hip resurfacing is becoming more widely available, and has advantages in younger patients as less bone is excised and revision to total arthroplasty is less technically demanding than a complete revision of a replaced joint.

Arthroscopy does not play a part in the standard management of OA, and should only be considered in those with meniscal or ligament pathology (locking or giving way, not gelling) or radiographic evidence of loose bodies.

Further reading

Altman RD, Hochberg MC, Moskowitz RW, et al. (2003). ACR Recommendations for the Medical Management of Osteoarthritis of the Hip and Knee: American College Subcommittee on Osteoarthritis Guidelines (http://www.rheumatology.org/practice/clinical/guidelines/oa-mgmt.asp)

Cooper C (2008). Osteoarthritis. In Mathieson P, ed. *Horizons in Medicine 20*. London, Royal College of Physicians of London.

Hakim A, Clunie G, Haq I (eds) (2006). *Oxford Handbook of Rheumatology*, 2nd edn. Oxford, Oxford University Press

Jordan JM (2008). Epidemiology and classification of osteoarthritis. In Hochberg MC, Silman AJ, Smolen JS, et al. (eds) *Rheumatology*, 4th edn. Philadelphia, Mosby.

Jordan KM, Arden NK, Doherty M, et al. (2003). EULAR recommendations 2003: an evidence based approach to the management of knee osteoarthritis: report of the Task Force of the standing committee for international clinical studies including clinical trials (ESCISIT). *Ann Rheum Dis* **62**: 1145–55.

NICE Guideline CG59. Osteoarthritis: the Care and Management of Adults with Osteoarthritis. London, HMSO, 2008. http://www.nice.org.uk/guidance/index.jsp?action=byID&o=11926

Watts R, Clunie G, Hall F, Marshall T (eds) (2009). Osteoarthritis. In *Oxford Desk Reference Rheumatology*. Oxford, Oxford University Press.

Wollheim FA, Lohmander LS (2008). Pathogenesis and pathology of osteoarthritis. In Hochberg MC, Silman AJ, Smolen JS, et al. (eds) *Rheumatology*, 4th edn. Philadelphia, Mosby.

Williams FMK, Zhai G, Spector TD (2008). The genetics of osteoarthritis. In Hochberg MC, Silman AJ, Smolen JS, Weinblatt ME, Wisman MH (eds) *Rheumatology*, 4th edn. Philadelphia, Mosby.

Zhang W, Doherty M, Leeb BF, et al. (2007). EULAR evidence based recommendations for the management of hand osteoarthritis: Report of Task Force of the EULAR Standing Committee for International Clinical Studies Including Therapeutics (ESCISIT). *Ann Rheum Dis* **66**: 377–88.

Gout

Introduction, definition and epidemiology

Gout is a curable form of inflammatory arthritis character-ized by self-limiting but excruciatingly painful attacks. These are a consequence of monosodium urate (MSU) crystals depositing within articular and periarticular tissue. After years of acute intermittent gout or polyarticular dis-ease, chronic tophaceous gout may develop. Tophi, nodu-lar masses of uric acid, can form anywhere but most commonly affect the soft tissues of the fingertips and the distal interphalangeal joints at the site of nodal osteoarthritis, particularly in older women.

It is one of the oldest recognized diseases, first identified by the Egyptians in 2640 BC. In 1848 Sir Alfred Garrod dis-covered the link between hyperuricaemia and gout, but not until the 1960s were MSU crystals identified in synovial fluid.

Gout has a UK prevalence of 1.4% on average but this increases with increasing age, with a rate approaching 7% in men over the age of 65. Rates then peak in men between the ages 75–84 years (7.3%), and in women prevalence continues to rise beyond 85 years (2.3%).

Recent discoveries including (i) the role of the inflamma-some and intracellular events demonstrating that pro-inflammatory cytokines promote neutrophil influx, and (ii) genetic advances with the identification of the URAT-1 transporter and genetic variation in SLC 2A9 as a key regu-lator of urate homeostasis have provided a deeper under-standing of the pathopyhsiology of gout and will allow the development of more targeted treatments.

Risk factors

Hyperuricaemia is the most important risk factor for gout. (see Table 10.1). Although not all subjects with raised serum uric acid (sUA) will develop gout, there is a strong positive correlation between sUA levels and frequency of gout flares. Compared with those whose sUA was <0.36 mmol/L, odds ratios were 1.3 with sUA 0.36–0.42 mmol/L (still in the normal range for UK laboratories) and 2.2 at sUA >0.53 mmol/L.

Gout can also occur with sUA levels within the normal laboratory range – sUA reflecting a balance between die-tary intake, synthesis, and rate of excretion of urate, with 90% of gout resulting from underexcretion of uric acid.

Table 10.1 Causes of hyperuricaemia

Urate underexcretion (90%)	Urate overproduction (10%)
Primary hyperuricaemia	**Primary hyperuricaemia**
SLC2A9 and URAT-1 polymorphisms	HPRT deficiency (Lesch Nyhan syndrome)
	Increased PRPP synthetase
	Glycogen storage disease
Secondary hyperuricaemia	**Secondary hyperuricaemia**
Renal impairment	Excess dietary purine intake
Hypertension	Haematological disorders
Drugs: aspirin; diuretics; ciclosporin; alcohol	Drugs: cytotoxics; Vitamin B12; alcohol
Hypothyroidism	Psoriasis
Lead nephropathy	

HPRT, hypoxanthine-guanine phosphoribosyltransferase; PRPP, 5-phosphoribosyl-1-pyrophosphate.

Table 10.2 Risk factors for gout

Male gender	Ageing
Hyperuricaemia	Family history
Genetic factors	Hypertension
Obesity	Alcohol
CKD	Trauma

Other risk factors particularly pertinent in the older population, include the use of drugs such as low-dose aspirin and diuretics (see Table 10.2).

Comorbidities

Hyperuricaemia should trigger assessment for commonly associated disease. These include obesity, hypertension, chronic kidney disease (CKD), type II diabetes mellitus, hyperlipidaemia, ischaemic heart disease, heart failure, and alcoholism. Additionally, with increasing sUA, there is trend for the prevalence of these comorbidities to be higher.

Complications

Longer term, if left untreated, gout can result in a chronic smouldering inflammatory arthritis, disability secondary to tophi and/or erosive joint disease, chronic kidney disease, and nephrolithiasis.

Management

Both the British Society of Rheumatology (BSR) and the European League against Rheumatism (EULAR) have pub-lished guidelines on optimum treatment of gout. They dif-fer in target sUA to attain (0.3 mmol/L for BSR and 0.36 mmol/L for EULAR) but share the same philosophy of keeping sUA lower than the saturation point of MSU, thereby preventing further crystal formation and encour-aging crystal dissolution.

Management can be divided into (i) lifestyle modifica-tion, (ii) treatment of acute gout flares, and (iii) treatment of chronic gout.

Lifestyle modification

Lifestyle factors confer around 10% of the morbidity of gout and therefore modification of adverse factors and optimization of protective factors are key to the overall management.

Adverse factors:
- high intake of red meat and shellfish
- high alcohol intake (especially beer)
- high intake of fructose-containing products (particularly sweetened fizzy drinks)
- dehydration
- obesity

Protective factors
- vitamin C (500 mg plus daily)
- cherries
- low-fat dairy products
- steady weight loss
- good hydration
- exercise in moderation.

Acute treatment

The aim of treating acute attacks is to treat promptly to safely resolve pain and inflammation. Delays in initiating treatment results in poorer treatment efficacy:

- exclude joint sepsis
- aspirate swollen joints and examine for urate crystals and organisms
- ice the affected joint regularly
- rest the affected joint for 1–2 days
- treat with acute pharmacological treatment immediately (NSAIDs; colchicine; steroid; IL-1) for 5–14 days dependent on response
- NSAIDs (non-steroidal anti-inflammatory drugs)
  - Full dose of any NSAID is indicated unless significant renal impairment, history of peptic ulceration or heart failure
  - All NSAIDs work as effectively as each other when given at full dose
  - Use with gastro-protection for 1–2 weeks
- Colchicine
  - Effective at reducing the severity of a flare but is slower to work than NSAIDs
  - 500 µg two–four times daily (lower dose for CKD) and assess renal function regularly
  - Can cause dose-limiting diarrhoea
  - Do **not** use intravenously
- Corticosteroids
  - Can be used orally (prednisolone 10–35 mg daily tapering over 2 weeks), intramuscularly, intra-articularly or intravenously.
  - In an acute monoarthritis, use intra-articular steroid as it rapidly terminates the attack.
  - Good alternative in patients who cannot tolerate NSAIDs or colchicine.
- Anti IL-1 receptor antagonists
  - Novel treatment.
  - Very expensive but rapidly effective.
  - Anakinra, rilonacept and canakinumab are currently unlicensed treatments in the UK.

Chronic management

Asymptomatic hyperuricaemia should not be treated; however, urate lowering therapy (ULT) is indicated as outlined in Table 10.3.

The aim of ULT is to suppress sUA <0.30 mmol/L and aid crystal dissolution. Sustained suppression below this level (the lower the better) provides good clinical outcomes and decreases flare frequency, although this may take a year following target urate levels being reached. Patients should be counselled accordingly and offered prophylaxis.

ULT can be divided into (i) uricostatic (allopurinol and febuxostat),(ii) uricosuric (benzbromarone, sulphinpyrazone, probenecid, losartan, and fenofibrate), and (iii) uricolytic agents.

Table 10.3 Indications for urate lowering therapy

Tophi	Erosive change on x-ray
Recurrent attacks of gout (>2 per year)	Disability secondary to gouty arthritis
CKD secondary to gout	Nephrolithiasis

Uricostatic drugs

Act by blocking the conversion of xanthine to uric acid thereby reducing sUA levels (xanthine oxidase inhibitors).

- Allopurinol
  - Commence at 50–100 mg daily and titrate upwards to reduce flare and risk of renal impairment (maximum dose 900 mg)
  - Titrate dose in CKD against creatinine clearance
  - In the UK, ~98% patients receive doses of ≤300 mg/day suggesting dosing is ineffective
  - Adverse effects include rash (2%); hypersensitivity reaction; acute hepatitis; interstitial nephritis
  - Avoid with azathioprine
- Febuxostat
  - New non-purine XO inhibitor approved by NICE if allopurinol fails or is contraindicated
  - Commence at 80 mg daily and increase to 120 mg daily if sUA remains >0.36 mmol/L at 4 weeks
  - No dose adjustment in moderate CKD
  - Can result in flare therefore use prophylaxis
- Prophylaxis
  - Given to avoid flare on initiation of ULT (occurs in up to 77% of patients)
  - Flare is a common cause of ULT non-concordance
  - Use low dose colchicine 500mcg once-twice daily for 6–26 weeks or low-dose NSAID for 6–12 weeks

Uricosuric agents

Enhance the renal clearance of uric acid. Used in <15% of patients with gout. Directly inhibit URAT-1.

- Sulfinpyrazone
  - Adverse effects similar to NSAIDs
  - Inefficacious in even mild CKD
  - 200–800 mg daily in divided doses
- Benzbromarone
  - Unlicensed in UK but available on a named patient basis at doses of 50–200 mg daily
  - Trialled in renal failure and patients with renal transplant effectively
  - Potential hepatotoxicity therefore need to monitor liver function
- Probenecid, losartan and fenofibrate
  - Probenecid is rarely used due to availability. Doses of 500 mg to 2 g in divided doses
  - Losartan (angiotensin I receptor antagaonist) and the lipid lowering agent fenofibrate are uricosuric; together they can decrease sUA by up to 40%

Uricolytics (uricase)

Uricase converts uric acid to allantoin which is 10 times more soluble and readily excreted via the kidney

- Rasburicase and pegylated uricase are available but expensive and given intravenously
- Dramatically reduces sUA but often results in significant flare

Summary

- Gout is a curable long-term condition with significant associated comorbidity.
- Optimize lifestyle factors and treat associated comorbid conditions.
- Current treatment options are highly effective but poorly utilized both in primary and secondary care.

- Aim for target sUA <0.30 mmol/L to ensure MSU crystal dissolution.
- Ensure sUA is assessed regularly when on ULT (6–12 monthly) and adjust treatment as needed.

Further reading

Annemans L, Spaepen E, Gaskin M, *et al.* (2008). Gout in the UK and Germany: prevalence, comorbidities and management in general practice 2000–2005. *Ann Rheum Dis* **67**: 906.

Jordan KM, Cameron JS, Snaith M, *et al.* (2007). British Society of Rheumatology & Professionals in Rheumatology guidelines for the management of gout. *Rheumatology* **46**: 1372–4.

Mikuls TR, Farrrar JT, Bilker WB, *et al.* (2005). Gout epidemiology: results from the UK General Practice Database, 1990–1999. *Ann Rheum Dis* **64**: 267–72.

Rider TG, Jordan KM, (2009). Treatment options for gout. *Rheum Practice* **7**: 4–7.

Rider TG, Jordan KM (2010). The modern management of gout. *Rheumatology* **49**: 5–14.

Zang W, Doherty M, Bardin T, *et al.* (2006). EULAR evidence based recommendations for gout. Part II: managment. Report task force of the EULAR standing committee for international clinical studies including therapeutics (ESCISIT). *Ann Rheum Dis* 65: 1312–24.

Rheumatoid arthritis

Background

Rheumatoid arthritis (RA) is a chronic systemic inflammatory disease characterized by symmetrical polyarthritis, morning stiffness and constitutional symptoms. In the last 20 years, major advances in translational research have led to the identification of new therapeutic targets. Development of newer biologic agents and the realization that early aggressive therapy can prevent joint damage has transformed our ability to improve the outlook and quality of life for nearly all patients with the disease.

Epidemiology

The prevalence of RA is 0.5–1% in European and North American populations with an incidence of 0.03%. The disease can occur at any age but peak incidence occurs in the fourth and fifth decades of life. Elderly onset RA (EORA) occurring over the age of 60, may represent a distinct subset of disease. EORA is said to have a more equal gender distribution, affect predominantly large joints, and have a milder clinical course, However, age as a determinant of clinical outcome remains controversial.

Aetiology

A number of genetic factors are associated with RA, the major one being the HLA-DR1 allele. Sex hormones clearly convey a risk. Women are two to three times more likely to be affected than men. Infectious agents have been implicated but none has been shown to cause RA. Tobacco smoking increases the severity of RA, and can stimulate anticyclical citrullinated peptide antibody (anti-CCP) production.

Pathogenesis

Virtually every cell type and cytokine has been implicated at some time in the pathogenesis of RA. The dominant theory of pathogenesis suggests an exogenous antigen targets the synovium leading to a chronic inflammatory response. Through the interaction between antigen-presenting cells (APC) and T cells an inflammatory cascade is initiated leading to secretion of proinflammatory cytokines and chemokines including interleukin (IL)-1, IL-6, IL-8 and tumour necrosis factor (TNF)-α. The resultant inflammation and proliferation of the synovium leads to permanent joint damage. B cells produce autoantibodies, e.g. rheumatoid factor (RF) and anti-CCP, which are associated with severe disease. Targeted therapy against B cells leads to clinical improvement.

Diagnosis and clinical features of RA

The diagnosis can be difficult especially in early disease, with signs and symptoms often waxing and waning. Development of the 2010 ACR-EULAR Classification criteria for RA should allow the earlier identification of patients with more severe disease. The new criteria cover four areas and establish a points value of 0 to 10. A patient with a score above 6 is classified as having RA.
- joint involvement (type and number)
- serology (RF and ACPA)
- acute-phase response (ESR and CRP)
- duration of disease (symptoms >6 weeks).

Following the diagnosis of RA treatment with synthetic DMARDS (disease-modifying antirheumatic drugs) should be initiated to induce disease remission. Comorbidities should be considered when choosing DMARDS and a careful assessment of infection risk made prior to treatment initiation or escalation.

Disease activity and treatment response is now routinely measured by the Disease Activity Score 28-joint count (DAS28). The score is based on the number of tender and swollen joints, ESR in mm/hour, and the patient's global health on a visual analogue scale. DAS28 does not include the ankles or toes, which are often affected in early disease. A DAS score above 5.1 is necessary to qualify for treatment with biologic therapies after failure of two synthetic DMARDS under NICE Guidelines TA 130.

Extra-articular features

These can affect up to 50% of patients, are commoner in men and in patients who have RF or anti-CCP antibodies. Older patients with longstanding disease where treatment initiation was delayed often have extra-articular features. They are a feature of severe disease not the age at onset.

Cutaneous: 25–30% of patients have rheumatoid nodules on the extensor surfaces and over pressure points. Nodules rarely occur in visceral organs. Histology reveals central fibrinoid necrosis surrounded by pallisading histiocytes. Leucocytoclastic vasculitis of the skin can be seen on extremities.

- Ocular: Keratoconjunctivitis sicca along with xerostomia occurs in 10–15% of RA due to secondary Sjogren's syndrome. Episcleritis and scleritis can also exist leading to scleromalacia perforans. The latter requires aggressive immunosuppressive treatment to prevent blindness.
- Cardiac: RA is an independent risk factor for cardiovascular disease. Chronic systemic inflammation leads to accelerated atherogenesis. Statins and aggressive control of the disease may reduce mortality. Pericarditis is less common with aggressive management and nodules in the myocardium leading to conduction abnormalities are now very rarely seen.
- Pulmonary: Pleurisy and pleural effusions occur in up to 70% of patients. RA pleural effusions are exudates with elevated protein and low glucose levels. Interstitial fibrosis is a common long-term complication and is commoner in smokers. Treatment can lead to pneumonitis and should be suspected in patients with acute dypsnoea on methotrexate, leflunomide or some biologics. Bronchiolitis obliterans and organizing pneumonia are rare, more difficult to treat and can be rapidly fatal. Caplan's syndrome (multiple nodules in coal miners' lungs) is rare.
- Others: Neurological manifestations include entrapment neuropathies, peripheral neuropathy and mononeuritis multiplex. Secondary AA-amyloid deposition can lead to renal failure. Infection risk is increased by fivefold. Cancer and lymphoproliferative malignancies occur in up to 14%.

Poor prognostic features

Poor prognositic factors in RA include the presence of RF or anti-CCP autoantibodies, high acute-phase response, female gender, HLA DRB1 0404, eosinophilia, family history and the presence of radiographic erosions.

Laboratory findings

Anaemia of chronic disease and thrombocytosis are common. Disease activity correlates with elevated acute phase reactants. RFs are antibodies, most commonly immunoglobulin (Ig)M, against the Fc portion of IgG. The sensitivity and specificity of RF for the diagnosis of RA is 70% and 82% respectively. RF is present in other conditions, such as systemic lupus erythematosus (SLE), hepatitis, Sjogren's syndrome, infection and sarcoidosis. Anticyclic citrullinated peptide (CCP) antibody is a more specific marker for RA with a similar sensitivity but higher specificity of 98%. Both antibodies can be present for up to 10 years prior to the onset of clinical RA. Antinuclear antibodies are found in 30% of patients with RA.

Imaging

Historically, radiographs have detected periarticular osteopenia, juxta-articular erosions and joint space narrowing. Subluxation and joint malalignment are seen in late disease. Their use is being superseded by more sensitive imaging modalities such as ultrasound and MRI. By detecting subclinical joint inflammation and erosions in early disease more aggressive treatment can be initiated this preventing joint damage occurring.

RA management and treatment

A holistic multidisciplinary approach is paramount for RA patients due to the chronicity of the disease and its physical and psychological impact. Early initiation of intensive treatment regimes and frequent specialist follow up result in better disease control and damage prevention.

The principles of modern medical management

- Early specialist referral
- Initiate treatment early, aiming for remission with validated outcome measures
- Initiate combination treatment
- Escalate the dose of methotrexate to 25mg/week (switch to subcutaneous route if intolerance.)
- Regular assessment 1–3 monthly until remission
- Early use of biologic agents for severe and unresponsive disease; use second biologic if the first fails.

Disease modifying anti-rheumatic drugs (DMARDs)

Combination therapy with DMARDs has been the initial therapy of choice for the last 15 years. Methotrexate (MTX) is currently the first choice DMARD owing to its favourable efficacy, acceptable toxicity profile, low cost, and patient convenience. The traditional treatment pyramid, starting cautiously before progressing to more potent drugs, for RA has been inverted. There is compelling evidence for using MTX in combination with other drugs such as hydroxychloroquine, sulfasalazine, cyclosporine, and leflunomide and with all the biologic agents. Unfortunately only a minority of patients will achieve lasting disease remission with MTX and many will still develop structural damage and disease progression while on the drug. DMARDs can take weeks to suppress inflammation so corticosteroids (either intramuscularly (e.g. depomedrone 40–80 mg), orally or intra-articularly) are used for more rapid disease control. In older people, infection is probably the greatest risk with combination therapy. Comorbidities, especially renal failure or lung disease may potentiate drug toxicity and limit target dosing of drugs like methotrexate.

Biological agents

The observation that TNF was an upstream dominant cytokine in the immune response ushered in a new era of treatment for patients with targeted therapy. Biologic agents target pro-inflammatory cytokines or target specific cell surface effector molecules of the immune response. They can all be used in older patients with active treatment-resistant disease. Age itself is not a contraindication to treatment with biologic agents; the principal risk is infection. This should be discussed with all patients prior to the initiation of therapy so prompt treatment can be sought if signs of infection develop.

The targets for these new biologic therapies include:

- TNF inhibition: Etanercept, adalumimab, infliximab, and certolizumab and golimumab inhibit TNF, either cell-bound or prior to receptor activation.
- B-cell inhibition: Rituximab, a chimeric anti-CD20 monoclonal antibody, causes long lasting B-cell depletion.
- Inhibition of T-B interaction: Abatacept is a CTLA4Ig fusion protein which inhibits T-cell costimulation.
- Il-6 blockade: Tocilizumab is an anti-IL6 receptor blocker.

Biologic therapies halt both clinical and radiological progression of the disease but probably only achieve true disease remission in a quarter of patients. They significantly improve functional status and lead to improvement in quality of life. The majority are safe with only a small increase in infections and lymphoproliferative disease. There use is restricted due to their high cost but rigorous clinical trials have shown additional benefits over traditional DMARDs when used early in severe disease in all age groups.

Future

It is encouraging that advances in translational research have led to the development of so many targeted therapies for RA in such a short period of time. Future advances in identifying specific patient characteristics and biomarkers will allow more appropriate tailoring of therapy to individual patients. The aspirational target of a cure, or 'drug-free' disease remission, is attainable in only a few patients. It remains the therapeutic goal for clinicians and scientists developing treatments and caring for patients with rheumatoid arthritis.

Further reading

Aletaha D, Neogi T, Silman AJ, et al. (2010). The 2010 ACR-EULAR classifiacation criteria for rheumatoid arthritis. *Ann Rheum Dis* **69**: 1580–8.

Dixon WG, Symmons DP, Lunt M, et al. (2007). Serious infection following anti-TNF alpha therapy in patients with rheumatoid arthritis: lessons from interpreting data from observational studies. *Arthritis Rheum* **56**: 2896–904.

Grigor C, Capell H, Stirling A, et al. (2004). Effect of a treatment strategy of tight control for rheumatoid arthritis (Ticora study): a single-blind randomised control trial. *Lancet* **364**: 263–9.

National Collaborating Centre for Chronic Conditions. (2009). *Rheumatoid Arthritis; National Clinical Guideline for Management and Treatment in Adults.* London, (Royal College of Physicians., London, 2009).

Van Hollenhoven RF (2009). Treatment of rheumatoid arthritis: state of the art 2009. *Nature Reviews* **5**: 531–41.

The swollen joint

Causes

Different causes of joint swelling predominate at different ages. In UK general hospitals, cases of joint swelling present in fairly equal numbers to medical or orthopaedic emergency departments.

The main causes (see Table 10.4) of joint swelling in the older population are:

- Osteoarthritis (OA)
- Crystal arthritis (gout or pyrophosphate arthritis)
- Unrecognized trauma including fracture
- Septic arthritis
- Single joint onset of polyarticular inflammatory arthritis (usually rheumatoid or psoriatic arthritis)
- Bursitis (olecranon and prepatellar) can resemble joint swelling and have the same causes with the exception of osteoarthritis.
- Haemarthrosis, e.g. anticoagulated patients, trauma.

Principles of diagnosis of joint swelling

- Septic arthritis can affect virtually any joint, including multiple joints in frail older patients.
- Systemic symptoms and signs (e.g. fever, rashes, limb pain, vomiting) point to possible infection yet all may be absent despite infection.
- Redness of the joint suggests septic arthritis or gout. Redness around the joint suggests cellulitis.
- Intense pain occurs with septic arthritis, fracture, gout or necrotizing fasciitis.
- Pain in a replaced joint requires immediate exclusion of sepsis, loosening or peri-prosthesis fracture.
- One joint may be the sentinel for other swollen joints so all peripheral joints should be examined.

Septic arthritis

Septic arthritis deserves early mention as it is so dangerous for older people. Its incidence is 2–10/100 000 in general and much higher in the older population and those with joint damage or replaced joints. It can be lethal even if recognized early; the overall mortality rate is 5–15% rising to 19–33% in older patients. The infecting organism can be seen on Gram stain in 50% of cases. Crystal arthritis and septic arthritis can coexist.

The key pointers to septic arthritis are rapid onset of pain, swelling, and immobility in the affected joint. Heat, redness fever, vomiting, leucocytosis, and a significantly elevated erythrocyte sedimentation rate (ESR) or C-reactive protein (CRP) are important indicators. Polyarticular septic arthritis is not uncommon so all peripheral joints should be examined where there is one suspected joint. An infective focus should be sought (e.g. heart, skin, chest).

Staphylococcus aureus followed by *Streptococcus pyogenes* are the commonest joint pathogens in the UK but Gram-negative organisms including *Escherichia coli* and *Pseudomonas aeruginosa* are comparatively common in older people. Environmental organisms, such as *Pantoea agglomerans*, suggest septic arthritis following a penetrating garden thorn injury. Rarely, tuberculosis or atypical mycobacterial infection cause chronic joint swelling; the latter can occur in immuno-suppressed patients and in joints previously injected with steroid.

Table 10.4 Pattern of joint involvement for each cause

Cause of limb swelling and pain	Usual pattern of musculoskeletal involvement
Joint swelling and pain	
Osteoarthritis	Polyarticular, often knees
Infection • bacterial including tuberculosis and brucella • fungal, mycobacterial (usually gradual onset) • viral (rarely if ever causes acute monoarthritis)	Single joint but polyarticular septic arthritis is not unusual in older people
Gout	Single joint, although polyarticular common in older people. Bursitis (especially olecranon or prepatellar) is common
Calcium pyrophosphate crystal arthritis	Single joint
Trauma (fracture alongside or through the joint line)	Single joint
Acute haemarthrosis (e.g. unrecognized trauma, coagulopathy)	Single joint
Loose bodies (osteochondral fragments)	Single joint
Rheumatoid or psoriatic arthritis	Polyarticular
Neuropathic [Charcot] joint (due to diabetes, rarely tertiary syphilis)	Single joint
Periarticular swelling and pain	
Cellulitis	Lower extremities, occasionally arms, e.g. intravenous cannula sites
Necrotizing fasciitis	Calves, forearms, thighs. Characteristically intense pain often with few signs other than some pinkness and mild swelling
Acute sarcoidosis	Erythema nodosum, 'periarthritis' of ankles
Osteogenic sarcoma and chondrosarcoma	Single ankle or knee

- *Gout/pseudogout:* see section Gout
- *Unrecognized trauma* should be actively excluded in patients who have single joint pain or swelling, particularly in people who have fallen. Most joints can be affected by trauma; a cool swollen joint which is exquisitely painful on pressure, movement or weight bearing should be radiographed immediately. Knee pain may be referred from impacted femoral neck fractures, so radiograph of the pelvis should be performed on patients with new intense knee pain and normal knee exam.
- *Late—onset rheumatoid arthritis (RA)* typically affects shoulders and often symmetrical involvement of hands,

wrists, knees, ankles, or feet. RA can be superimposed on OA, but the rapidity of onset and widespread joint pain distinguishes this condition from OA. Rheumatoid factor and high ESR and CRP are often absent in the early stages. Joints are often only mildly swollen in early RA.

- *Psoriatic arthritis* may present with a large painless effusion of a single joint, often a knee. A search reveals psoriasis, often hidden in the scalp margins or in the natal cleft.
- *Osteoarthritis* rarely presents as an emergency. A cool, swollen knee or ankle may be noted during an admission for another reason. Other joints may be painful, often a hip, the contralateral knee or ankle or the thumb bases. Pyrophosphate arthritis or gout may coexist.
- *Neuropathic (Charcot) joint* should be suspected in patients with diabetes, with peripheral neuropathy and a single painful, swollen, hot and deformed ankle or knee. Deep pain sensation (tested by squeezing the Achilles tendon) is often impaired. Radiographs show bone destruction. Osteomyelitis or septic arthritis can complicate the clinical picture of neuropathic arthropathy. Specialist help should be sought early.
- *Cancer (osteogenic sarcoma or chondrosarcoma)* affecting the joint or surrounding tissues may appear similar to infected neuropathic joints. The joint is swollen with a brawny appearance and texture. Symptoms tend to have developed gradually, but patients may give a short history. Investigation should be undertaken by specialists.
- *Cellulitis* affects the tissues around the joint rather than the joint itself. Aspiration of a joint through cellulitis risks introducing bacteria.
- *Acute sarcoidosis* may appear similar to cellulitis in the younger patient, often with swelling around the ankles resembling arthritis. The presence of erythema nodosum on the legs is characteristic.
- *Necrotizing fasciitis* is a potentially lethal infection of deep tissues due to a variety of organisms. It can be confused with septic arthritis when near a joint. Diabetic and other immunocompromised patients are at higher risk. Intense pain and tenderness are frequent, redness and swelling are often present, but joints are not directly involved. Immediate intravenous antibiotics, imaging (to define extent of muscle involvement) and tissue debridement may be life-saving.

Practical management of the acute joint

The key issues for the non-specialist are:

- Has joint swelling developed in the last two weeks or has pre-existing joint pain recently worsened?
- Is this swelling really in the joint or is it next to the joint, which would suggest cellulitis or fracture?
- Does it need immediate specialist attention or can it wait 24–48 hours? Orthopaedic or rheumatology specialist help should be sought at once if:
  - joint pain and swelling have developed or worsened in the previous fortnight; this must be assumed to be septic or a fracture.
  - joint pain is intense even if it is not warm.
  - systemic symptoms and signs (fever, rigors, malaise, vomiting) are present.

The following should be initiated in all patients with acutely painful, swollen and immobile joints:

1 Immediate aspiration, with fluid sent for microscopy for crystals and organisms and for culture.
2 Blood cultures, full blood count, ESR, CRP, renal and liver function, INR if anticoagulated.
3 Radiograph of affected joint(s) to exclude a fracture. In septic arthritis that is slow to improve despite apparently adequate treatment, an MRI scan is needed to exclude osteomyelitis.
4 Intravenous flucloxacillin 2 g qds immediately after cultures if purulent fluid is aspirated. Microbiologists should be involved at an early stage. There is no evidence to guide the duration of iv or oral antibiotics. Conventionally, they are given intravenously for up to 2 weeks or until signs improve, then orally for 4 weeks. Symptoms, signs and acute-phase responses are all helpful in guiding the decision to stop antibiotics.
5 Mobilization with physiotherapists starting with non-weight-bearing exercises as soon as the affected joint(s) are comfortable enough to move.

Joint aspiration

Immediate joint aspiration is needed if septic arthritis is a possibility. In the anticoagulated patient, firm pressure must be applied for several minutes afterwards. Full sterile draping is not required but a non-touch technique is, and the skin overlying the joint swabbed with alcohol before arthrocentesis. Joint fluid must be sent for culture, gram stain and microscopy for crystals.

- Milky joint fluid suggests intra-articular pus.
- High neutrophil counts, high lactate, and low glucose in the synovial fluid are typical for septic arthritis, although often not available. They can help where patients have received antibiotics and septic arthritis is a possibility.
- Frank blood (haemarthrosis) suggests over-anticoagulation, a bleeding disorder or a fracture through the joint line and a radiograph is required.
- Therapeutic joint drainage by repeat aspiration is favoured by rheumatologists while orthopaedic surgeons favour arthroscopic drainage. Both agree on arthroscopy for inaccessible joints, particularly the hip, and if infected joints fail to improve on repeat aspiration.

Further reading

Clarke JD, McCaffrey (2007). DD Case Report. Thorn injury mimicking a septic arthritis of the knee. *Ulster Med J* **76**: 164–5.

Coakley G, Mathews C, Field M, et al. (2006). BSR & BHPR, BOA, RCGP and BSAC guidelines for management of the hot swollen joint in adults. *Rheumatology* **45**: 1039–41.

Goldenberg D (1998). Septic arthritis. *Lancet* **351**: 197–202.

Shirtliff ME, Mader J (2002). Acute septic arthritis. *Clin Microbiol Rev* **15**: 527–44.

Pathology of polymyalgia rheumatica

Introduction

Polymyalgia rheumatica (PMR) is a chronic inflammatory disorder of unknown aetiology, which predominantly affects older people. Also, the pathophysiological mechanisms that drive the inflammatory process and the biological pathways underlying the age-related predisposition are not clear although both genetic and environmental factors have been implicated.

Pathophysiology

Muscles

Despite prominent symptoms of pain and stiffness in the neck, shoulder, and pelvic girdles in patients with PMR, biopsies of the affected muscle failed to demonstrate any significant abnormalities in the muscle fibres. Consistently, serum levels of muscle enzymes are normal in PMR. However, perivascular collections of inflammatory cells could be found in the muscular septa, fibroconnective tissue, and fat. Fassbender and colleagues examined the ultrastructure of skeletal muscle biopsies in patients with PMR and identified a profile of ultrastructural changes which may define it. They further suggest that these changes implicate neurogenic mechanisms playing a pathogenetic role in PMR. Finally, despite an initial report suggested a link between mitochondrial dysfunction and PMR pathogenesis, subsequent studies have shown that muscle energetics was normal and no significant molecular or biochemical abnormalities in mitochondria of skeletal muscles in PMR.

Articular and periarticular structures

Minor hyperplasia of the synovial endothelial cells, oedema with or without inflammatory changes of the synovium, subsynovium, bursa, joint capsules, and other periarticular tissue can be found on biopsies and arthroscopic examination. The inflammatory infiltrate is usually mild to moderate, and consists of macrophages and CD4$^+$ lymphocytes in a perivascular distribution. The paucity of neutrophils and the absence of B cells and $\gamma\delta$ T cells are said to be discriminatory between PMR and late-onset rheumatoid arthritis. The articular changes in PMR are generally considered to be non-erosive, although some earlier studies have reported that a variable proportion of PMR patients developed erosive arthropathy, most commonly affecting the sternoclavicular joints, symphysis pubis, and sacroiliac joints. Finally, whether peripheral joints are involved in PMR remains controversial.

The lack of consistent pathological changes in muscles and joints has prompted investigators to look for alternative pathological mechanisms underlying the classical symptoms of proximal pain and stiffness. Studies using ultrasonography and magnetic resonance imaging (MRI) demonstrated that bilateral subacromial–subdeltoid bursitis and trochanteric bursitis can often be detected in PMR. Similarly, by using fat-suppressed MRI, inflammation was most prominent outside the joint cavity leading to the postulation that PMR is primarily an inflammatory disease of the joint capsule and enthesis.

Vascular involvement and association with giant cell arteritis

The close association between PMR and GCA has led to the suggestion that these are the same condition with different manifestations and disease severity. The arguments for and against such hypothesis are beyond the scope of this section. Nevertheless, it has been reported that up to 60% of patients with giant cell arteritis (GCA) present with symptoms of PMR before, during, or after the onset of GCA. Conversely, 20% of patients with PMR have biopsy-proven GCA and can occur even in patients without symptoms suggestive of GCA. Asymptomatic vascular involvement can also be demonstrated by other imaging modalities such as positron emission tomography (PET). Histologically, the findings in temporal artery biopsies from PMR patients are similar to those with GCA. Endothelial proliferation and intimal thickening can also be identified in muscle and joint biopsies of the shoulder. More interestingly, regardless of histological evidence of arteritis, there is an increase in the mRNA expression of interleukin (IL)-6 and other inflammatory cytokines in temporal artery specimens from patients with PMR, with the exception of interferon (IFN)-γ. IFN-γ expression appears to be restricted to biopsies that revealed overt arteritis.

Immunopathology

A key clinical feature of PMR is the elevation of serum levels of C-reactive proteins (CRP) and erythrocyte sedimentation rate (ESR), both markers of systemic inflammation. Furthermore, the development of PMR is associated with certain alleles of major histocompatibility complex (MHC) class II molecules, the key role of which is to present antigens to CD4$^+$ helper T cells. These observations suggest that immune system dysfunction may play a key role in the pathogenesis of PMR.

Cellular immunity

It has been reported that circulating CD8$^+$ T cells are reduced in both percentages and absolute numbers in PMR and correlated with disease activity. However, subsequent studies by other investigators yielded conflicting results. Furthermore, the significance of reduced circulating CD8$^+$ T cells in the pathogenesis of PMR is unclear. Bacon and colleagues observed that circulating immunoblasts (activated leukocytes) were elevated in PMR. However, increased levels of immunoblasts are also found in other inflammatory conditions and therefore likely a reflection of an activated immune system rather than being specific to PMR.

Hazelman et al. measured the proliferative responses of peripheral blood leucocytes (PBL) from patients with PMR against arterial and muscle antigens using preparations of homogenates of arterial and muscle biopsy specimens. They showed that PBL from PMR patients proliferated in response to both arterial and muscle antigens. More interestingly, the response to arterial antigens appears to be specific to PMR PBL and to correlate with disease activity. The precise nature of the arterial antigen(s) that activate the PMR PBL is not known. These investigators postulated that intimal elastin, which is often damaged in age-related process, is a potential antigen that drives the autoimmune responses. It is also noteworthy that 10 of the 20 PMR patients studied had evidence of arteritis on temporal artery biopsy, and the data were not replicated in subsequent studies of different cohorts of patients.

Humoral immunity

Elevated serum levels of circulating immune complexes (IC) have been reported in active PMR and the levels reduced with treatment. However, raised serum levels of

IC are common in many different inflammatory conditions and the biological and clinical significance of IC in the aetiology of PMR is not known. Similarly, the role of autoantibodies in PMR pathogenesis is unclear despite early reports of the presence of various autoantibodies in PMR.

Cytokines and other molecules

With the advances in our understanding of the immune system and improved laboratory techniques, investigators have recently turned their attention from detecting abnormalities at cellular levels to identifying defects at molecular levels in PMR, particularly with regard to the role of cytokines.

IL-6 induces the production of CRP by hepatocytes. In PMR, serum levels of IL-6 are elevated and the levels reduce in response to steroid therapy. The correlation to other inflammatory markers, however, is more variable. The cellular source of IL-6 remains to be elucidated.

Vascular endothelial growth factor (VEGF) is another cytokine that may be important in PMR. Serum levels of VEGF and VEGF production by peripheral blood mononuclear cells are heightened in untreated PMR patients. Furthermore, mRNA expression of VEGF is raised in shoulder synovial tissue from patients with PMR.

Many different cytokines and chemokines have also been implicated in the pathogenesis of PMR. For instance, increased plasma levels of circulating cytokines such as IL-1β, IL-1 receptor antagonist, IL-2, soluble IL-2 receptor, IL-10, TNF-α, leukaemia inhibitory factor (LIF), RANTES, platelet-derived growth factor, and monocyte chemoattractant protein 1 have been demonstrated in patients with PMR. However, the sample sizes of these studies are often small and conflicting data have been reported. Therefore, the role of these cytokines, if any, remains to be defined.

The role of genes, environment and age-related physiological mechanisms

Genetic association

Many studies have been carried out to examine the genetic susceptibility loci in PMR, in particularly the MHC genes. HLA-DRB1*04 and *01 has been linked to PMR in white populations, these alleles are also associated with more severe disease and increased risk of relapse. HLA-DRB1 association varies with different populations which may reflect different genetic background of the populations studied and may explain some of the conflicting results. The role of MHC class I genes in the pathogenesis of PMR is less clear. Early reports suggested an association of PMR and the B8 and A10 alleles but conflicting data have also been reported.

Genetic polymorphisms of other genes may also be important factors in susceptibility to PMR. For instance, polymorphisms of ICAM-1, RANTES, TNF-α, IL-1 receptor antagonist (IL-Ra) genes have been associated with PMR.

Candidate physiological mechanisms of age-related predisposition

Age is the single most important risk factor for the development of PMR. Changes in the hypothalamic–pituitary–adrenal (HPA) axis have been thought to contribute to biological ageing. In addition, PMR is highly responsive to low-dose corticosteroid therapy. These observations have led to the hypothesis that HPA-dysfunction may predispose to PMR. Indeed, PMR patients have reduced basal plasma levels of androstenedione and DHEAS. Basal serum levels of cortisol were similar to age-matched healthy

controls, but the response to low dose ACTH was exaggerated in PMR. Since cortisol production increases in response to stress, these findings indicate that cortisol levels were inappropriately suppressed in PMR. However, the ability to synthesise and secrete cortisol in response to ACTH suggests that any potential defect is upstream to the adrenal glands in the HPA axis.

There is now increasing evidence suggesting that immunosenescence of the ageing immune system is associated with increased autoimmunity and inflammation, and could potentially account for the increasing incidence of PMR with age. Epigenetic mechanisms may also be important in age-related predisposition to PMR.

Role of infections and environmental factors

Several clinical features of PMR have been linked to an infective aetiology for PMR. For instance, during the acute onset of disease, prodromal flu-like symptoms are frequently described by patients with PMR. Also, there is a correlation between the incidence of PMR and latitude, as well as the seasonal and cyclic variation in the incidence of PMR. Many viral and microbial agents have been implicated including mycoplasma pneumoniae, chlamydia pneumonia, respiratory syncytial virus, parvovirus B19, and parainfluenza virus type I.

Evidence for these infective agents in the PMR pathogenesis was largely based on (i) increased prevalence of micro-specific antibodies in patients with PMR, or (ii) association between the incidence of PMR and epidemics of an infection. Furthermore, the occurrence of PMR in married couples has also been used as evidence supporting the importance of environmental factors in the pathogenesis of PMR. There is, however, no evidence for a common infectious or environmental agent for PMR. Furthermore, data from different studies on the prevalence of circulating IgG or IgM antibodies to various microorganisms are often conflicting. Finally, procalcitonin, an early marker of bacterial infections, is not elevated in PMR patients, arguing against bacterial triggers for PMR.

Conclusions

The pathophysiology of PMR remains poorly understood. The site(s) of tissue abnormality that are responsible for the cardinal symptoms of proximal pain and stiffness is not clear. The precise relationship between PMR and GCA is yet to be unravelled. Many immunological abnormalities have been described but their role in the pathogenesis of PMR remains to be determined. No satisfactory explanation has been identified for the age-related disposition of PMR, and the relative role of genetic and environmental factors in the development of PMR require further investigation.

A key difficulty in studying the underlying pathophysiological mechanisms is that the diagnosis of PMR remains largely clinical, and until recently, there is no consensus on the criteria for the diagnosis of PMR. Therefore, many of the studies may be carried out on a highly heterogeneous population making it difficult to identify distinct patterns and draw clear conclusions.

Author's Tip

The pathophysiology of PMR remains poorly understood.

The site(s) of tissue abnormality that are responsible for the cardinal symptoms of proximal pain and stiffness is not clear.

PMR is probably a polygenic disease in which multiple environmental and genetic factors influence susceptibility and severity.

Further reading

Alvarez-Rodr´guez L, Lopez-Hoyos M, Mata C, *et al.* (2010). Circulating cytokines in active polymyalgia rheumatica. *Ann Rheum Dis* **69**: 263–9.

Cimmino MA (1997). Genetic and environmental factors in polymyalgia rheumatica. *Ann Rheum Dis* **56**: 576–7.

Cutolo M, Straub RH (2000). Polymyalgia rheumatica: evidence for a hypothalamic-pituitary-adrenal axis-driven disease. *Clin Exp Rheumatol* **18**: 655–8.

Gordon I, Rennie AM, Branwood AW (1964). Polymyalgia rheumatica: biopsy studies. *Ann Rheum Dis* **23**: 447–55.

Kyle V, Tudor J, Wraight E, *et al.* (1990). Rarity of synovitis in polymyalgia rheumatica. *Ann Rheum Dis* **49**: 155–7.

Martinez-Taboada VM, Alvarez L, RuizSoto M, *et al.* (2008). Giant cell arteritis and polymyalgia rheumatica: role of cytokines in the pathogenesis and implications for treatment. *Cytokine* **44**: 207–20.

Miguel A Gonzalez-Gay (2001). Genetic epidemiology: Giant cell arteritis and polymyalgia rheumatic. *Arthritis Res* **3**: 154–7.

Roche NE, Fulbright JW, Wagner AD, *et al.* (1993). Correlation of interleukin-6 production and disease activity in polymyalgia rheumatica and giant cell arteritis. *Arthritis Rheum*, **36**: 1286–94.

Sakkas LI, Loqueman N, Panayi GS, *et al.* (1990). Immunogenetics of polymyalgia rheumatica. *Br J Rheumatol* **29**: 331–4.

Salvarani C, Cantini F, Hunder GG (2008). Polymyalgia rheumatica and giant-cell arteritis. *Lancet* **372**: 234–45.

Salvarani C, Cantini F, Olivieri I, *et al.* (1999). Polymyalgia rheumatica: a disorder of extraarticular synovial structures? *J Rheumatol* **26**: 517–21.

Clinical features, diagnosis, and management of polymyalgia rheumatica

Background

Polymyalgia rheumatica (PMR) is a common inflammatory rheumatic disease in older people and represents one of the commonest indications for long-term corticosteroid therapy in the community. It is characterized by proximal limb pain and stiffness, but systemic features are also common including constitutional upset, fatigue, and weight loss leading to a wide differential diagnosis at presentation. This necessitates a thorough and careful evaluation before committing a patient to the significant risks associated with long term steroid therapy, not to mention other pitfalls associated with the condition's tendency to relapse over time.

Epidemiology and overlap with giant cell arteritis

PMR is rare in patients less than 50 years of age and most common in those over 70 years of age. The age-adjusted incidence of PMR in England is 8.4 per 10 000 person years. It is most common in Caucasians of Northern European descent, particularly Scandinavians. PMR is three times as common in females, and women may go on to have a worse prognosis.

Since the 1960s, a relationship with giant cell arteritis has been recognized and symptoms of both conditions can be present at diagnosis, follow up or years later. GCA occurs in up to one-third of PMR patients, and PMR in up to two-thirds of GCA patients. PMR is more common than GCA.

Although the two conditions cannot be viewed in isolation of one another, this section will only consider the diagnosis and management of PMR in detail. Clarity of diagnosis is important as the need for referral to secondary care is higher in GCA and the steroid doses required for treatment are significantly different in the two conditions.

Investigation

Initial assessment of patients with suspected PMR should contain the following three elements:

1. Detailed assessment of symptoms and signs suggestive of a diagnosis of PMR, and meeting diagnostic criteria.
2. Exclusion of alternative diagnoses.
3. Assessment for the absence of features suggestive of GCA.

Diagnostic criteria

Bird described diagnostic criteria which, over 30 years later, remain the best validated set for clinical practice.

Other diagnostic criteria (e.g. Jones and Hazleman, Hunder) exist, but frequently these were developed purely by expert consensus or as inclusion criteria for clinical trials and not necessarily for use in clinical practice.

Bird diagnostic criteria (three required)
Age 65 years or over
Onset duration < 2 weeks
Bilateral shoulder pain and /or stiffness
ESR >40 mm/hour
Morning stiffness duration > 1 hour
Depression ± weight loss
Bilateral upper arm tenderness

Bird's criteria identified the seven most discriminatory features from clinical and investigative features and state 92% sensitivity and 78% specificity for the diagnosis of PMR if three criteria are satisfied. As age >65 years, weight loss, and an erythrocyte sedimentation rate (ESR) above 40 mm/hour may not be sufficiently discriminating for patients seen in geriatric medicine, inclusion of a fourth diagnostic criteria would ensure a myalgic component is present. In most cases, physicians should be wary of making the diagnosis without symptoms or signs of proximal pain, stiffness, or tenderness. One further advantage of Bird's criteria is that they do not include a positive response to steroid treatment, which, although important later, can only be confirmed retrospectively. Ultimately the most significant reflection of the physician's diagnostic certainty is to prescribe corticosteroid therapy and the design of these criteria offer support to this decision.

> **Authors' Tip**
>
> Be wary of making the diagnosis of PMR without myalgic symptoms or signs.

Clinical features

Symptoms of PMR frequently develop abruptly and usually present within days or weeks of onset. Some patients can recall the exact day their symptoms started.

Bilateral proximal limb girdle pains are the most predominant features with 70–95% experiencing symmetric pain and morning stiffness. These may lead to functional consequences, for example, difficulty getting dressed or rising from a chair. Only if chronically untreated will muscle weakness and atrophy be present. Peripheral synovitis is usually not seen, though pitting oedema of the hands and feet is recognized. Constitutional upset is common with symptoms including anorexia, weight loss, fatigue and fever.

Specific enquiry and examination should also be performed for symptoms or signs of GCA including:

- unilateral or bilateral headache - not necessarily temporal in origin
- scalp tenderness
- jaw claudication
- transient/persistent loss of vision or double vision
- tenderness, nodularity, thickening, or loss of pulsation in either temporal artery.

Any suggestion of the above, even if the myalgic or constitutional symptoms are of more concern to the patient, should lead to urgent investigation into GCA, which is outlined within this chapter. The diagnosis of GCA can be usefully thought of in clinical practice as 'trumping' the diagnosis of PMR.

In addition to the above, PMR frequently enters into the differential diagnosis of more non-specific presentations seen in geriatric medicine, including:

- general deterioration of mobility / activities of daily living
- pyrexia of unknown cause
- raised inflammatory markers 'query cause'

- low mood
- weight loss.

Differential diagnosis

The symptom complex at presentation combined with an assessment of the patient's specific general disease risk factors and past medical history determine the differential diagnosis, and frequently this can be very wide. Place of presentation, whether to primary care or inpatient/outpatient settings, are also important in determining the likelihood of differentials and plans for investigation.

A list of diagnoses which may mimic PMR is presented in Table 10.5. In geriatric medicine, frequently the two most difficult diagnostic groups to manoeuvre through are those of neoplastic disease and infective processes, including reactivation of tuberculosis and infective endocarditis. Not only here is an accurate diagnosis important for appropriate ongoing management but there is greater potential for harm if steroid treatment is instituted inappropriately.

Investigations

The following investigations should be regarded as essential:

- urinalysis
- inflammatory markers: ESR (or plasma viscosity) and CRP
- full blood count
- urea and electrolytes
- liver function tests
- bone profile
- protein electrophoresis
- thyroid function tests
- creatine kinase
- rheumatoid factor.

Table 10.5 Differential diagnosis of polymyalgia rheumatica

Infective	Acute viral illness
	Systemic or deep sepsis
	Tuberculosis
	Osteomyelitis
	Septic arthritis
	Infective endocarditis
Neoplastic	Bone metastases
	Myeloma
	Lymphoma
	Paraneoplastic manifestations of carcinoma e.g. dermatomyositis
Musculoskeletal	Rheumatoid arthritis
	Other inflammatory arthritides
	Vasculitis
	Connective tissue diseases
	Osteoarthritis
	Bilateral adhesive capsulitis
	Rotator cuff tear
	Inflammatory myopathy
	Osteomalacia
	Fibromyalgia
Endocrine	Hypothyroidism
Neurological	Depression
	Parkinson's disease

These investigations represent a thorough evaluation for conditions entering into the differential diagnosis for PMR. However, it is important to recognize that abnormalities may be seen in these results in PMR itself and there is a risk of embarking on a further set of unnecessary investigations. Specifically, a normochromic normocytic anaemia and abnormal liver function tests, particularly raised alkaline phosphatase, are commonly found in PMR which should go on to resolve with steroid treatment. The ESR may be significantly elevated above 40 mm/h, and above 100 mm/h in 20% of cases. Although patients can be diagnosed with PMR without a raised ESR, this may be over-recognized, and CRP can be elevated when the ESR is not. Creatine kinase should be normal in PMR and elevation suggests an inflammatory myopathy. A positive rheumatoid factor can cause diagnostic confusion with late onset rheumatoid arthritis, but may also be positive (usually weakly) in 5–20% of people over 65 years of age.

The following investigations should also be considered:

- chest radiograph (particularly in smokers or past history of tuberculosis)
- urine/sputum/stool/blood cultures (if sepsis suspected)
- ultrasound liver/abdomen (where malignancy or abdominal sepsis suspected)
- hand and feet radiographs (for erosions if positive rheumatoid factor)

Temporal artery biopsy has no place in the investigation of PMR in the absence of symptoms or signs of GCA.

Management of polymyalgia rheumatica

Corticosteroid regimen

The aim of corticosteroid treatment in PMR is primarily to render the patient symptom free. This is in contrast to GCA where higher doses of steroid are required and aim to prevent arteritic complications.

A starting dose of 15 mg of prednisolone is widely recommended and as few as 1% of patients require higher doses. This dose has been derived from mostly observational studies and a few small randomized controlled trials. Studies that have been conducted vary significantly in their quality, clinical settings, inclusion criteria, methods of assessing disease activity, and outcome measures.

The joint guidelines published in 2010 from the British Society for Rheumatology and British Health Professionals in Rheumatology suggest the following regimen:

- daily prednisolone 15 mg for 3 weeks
- then 12.5 mg for 3 weeks
- then 10 mg for 4–6 weeks
- followed by reduction of 1 mg every 4–8 weeks or alternated day reductions (e.g. 10/7.5 mg alternate days, etc.).

Side-effects of steroid therapy

Around 50% of patients treated with steroids for PMR will experience side-effects over the course of their disease. These include weight gain, impaired glucose tolerance, osteoporotic fractures, and hypertension. An increased likelihood of adverse events is associated with initial doses of prednisolone greater than 30 mg and a large cumulative dose.

Osteoporosis prophylaxis

Loss of bone mineral density (BMD) is greatest in the first few months of steroid use, and the risk of fractures particularly of the hip and spine are significantly increased.

The majority of patients will require bone protection, with a bisphosphonate and calcium/vitamin D supplementation commenced at onset of steroid therapy. This should follow local or national guidelines, for example, the Royal College of Physicians guidance on glucocorticoid-induced osteoporosis. These recommend all patients aged 65 or over and those of any age with a history of prior fragility fracture should commence bone protection without the need for measurement of bone mineral density. In other patients, where BMD should be measured, bone protection should be prescribed if the T score is −1.5 or lower, which represents a lower threshold for treatment than non-steroid-induced osteoporosis.

Peptic ulceration

Many physicians routinely co-prescribe proton pump inhibitors from the initiation of corticosteroid therapy, and this should certainly be considered in at least patients felt to be at high risk of peptic ulceration.

Authors' Tip

Regard corticosteroid therapy in PMR as a balance between relief of symptoms against the hazards of steroid-related side effects.

Steroid sparing and newer agents

Despite their high incidence of side effects, corticosteroids remain the cornerstone of management. Other agents (including deflazacort, azathioprine, infliximab, and NSAIDs) have undergone limited published investigation but have generally not demonstrated significant advantages over conventional corticosteroid treatment, or any lower cumulative steroid dose achieved was offset by the trialled agent's own side-effects.

Methotrexate's use as a steroid sparing agent is, however, supported by three randomized controlled trials demonstrating a reduction in cumulative steroid dosage and side-effects. Its use could be considered for patients thought to be at especially high risk for steroid-related side-effects. In practice though, its use is generally confined to a treatment adjunct later in patients who relapse twice or more at tapering steroid doses. Its main drawback is that its use necessitates expertise in secondary care from medical staff familiar with it, and systems in place to ensure safe patient usage and monitoring requirements. In the UK, this would generally require referral to a rheumatologist as most geriatricians are unaccustomed and unfamiliar with initiating and monitoring methotrexate.

The use of intramuscular methylprednisolone has been studied in two RCTs, with a lower cumulative steroid dose and side effects achieved. Its use could be consider in 'milder' cases of PMR, where adherence with oral treatment is difficult or for patients deemed at especially high risk of steroid related side effects. Again though, this would generally need to be under the supervision of a rheumatologist.

Follow-up and monitoring

Initial follow-up should be performed to ensure the patient's symptoms have resolved with steroid treatment. Frequently a response is dramatic and seen within 24 hours or within the first week and the timing of initial follow up should reflect this. Reduction in inflammatory markers usually takes longer with CRP reducing more rapidly and up to 4 weeks before the ESR. If a satisfactory symptom or laboratory response is not seen, then the diagnosis should be carefully reconsidered before increasing prednisolone dosage to 20 mg (or exceptionally 30 mg).

Following an initial successful reduction in steroid dosage, further follow up and monitoring should take place according to an agreed steroid reduction plan, either in primary or secondary care, at a frequency of around every three months. Each visit should include:

- an assessment of attributable symptoms and functional consequences
- a re-evaluation of the initial diagnosis
- monitoring of the full blood count, ESR and CRP
- an assessment for the development of symptoms or signs of GCA
- an assessment of complications of steroid therapy, including blood pressure, fragility fractures, and serum glucose.

Relapse

Relapse in patients with PMR is common, particularly in the first year after diagnosis, with relapse rates ranging from 25–60%. The most useful indication of a relapse of PMR is the patient's account of their symptoms, which may or may not be accompanied by an inflammatory response. Disease activity scores have been developed but are not in widespread use, nor recommended for use in clinical guidelines.

In the event of relapse, steroids should initially be increased in a stepwise fashion to the lowest dose that previously controlled symptoms and the frequency of follow up should be increased. After each relapse, the diagnosis of PMR should be reconsidered or any new intervening pathologies assessed. After the third relapse, consideration of the introduction of steroid sparing agents like methotrexate should ensue, and this will usually require rheumatology referral. Use of etanercept has also been subject to one small clinical trial for patients unable to reduce their dose of prednisolone.

Duration

Guidance for the duration of steroids originates from observational studies. A minimum duration of treatment appears to be 18 months, and around half of patients discontinue steroid therapy after 2 years. The majority of patients should be able to discontinue treatment by 4 years, and a minority need long-term low-dose steroids.

Multidisciplinary management

Patients particularly with functional problems as a result of their symptoms may benefit from a multidisciplinary assessment and intervention including physiotherapy and occupational therapy.

Patient education

- Patients should be provided with a steroid information/alert card.
- Patients should be counselled as to standard advice regarding common steroid-related side-effects, advised to avoid sudden discontinuation and the need to seek medical help if the event of vomiting/intercurrent illness.
- Patients should receive advice about maintaining good bone health through diet and lifestyle measures.
- Patients should know to seek urgent medical opinion if the event of developing symptoms suggestive of GCA, like headache or visual loss.

Prognosis

Unlike GCA, it is not thought that PMR is associated with higher mortality. High morbidity is associated with long-term steroid usage however. Greater age at diagnosis, female gender, frequent relapses, and higher inflammatory markers at presentation have been associated with lower rates of clinical remission and a requirement for a longer duration of steroid therapy.

Future research and developments

Much of our knowledge about the steroid regimen arises from observational studies and clinical convention. There is a need for high-quality research to better define an optimum initial dose, tapering method, and duration for steroid therapy.

Adjuvant and newer therapies like biologics and leflunomide have yet to find their place in the management of most patients with PMR.

Authors' Tip

A starting dose of prednisolone 15 mg should control the symptoms in the majority of patients.

Bone protection should be considered at onset of steroid therapy.

Both relapse and steroid-related side effects are common.

The diagnosis should be kept under review at all stages, particularly in the complex older patient with co-morbidity.

Further reading

Bird HA, Esselinckx W, Dixon A St J, et al. (1979). An evaluation of criteria for polymyalgia rheumatica. *Ann Rheum Dis* **38**: 434–9.

Bird HA, Leef BF, Montecucco CM, et al. (2005). A comparison of the sensitivity of diagnostic criteria for polymyalgia rheumatica. *Ann Rheum Dis* **64**: 626–9.

Dasgupta B, Borg FA, Hassan N, et al. (2010). *Rheumatology* **49**: 186–90.

Frearson R, Cassidy T, Newton J, (2003). Polymyalgia rheumatica and temporal arteritis: evidence and guidelines for diagnosis and management in older people. *Age Ageing* **32**: 370–4.

Hernandez-Rodriguez J, Cid MC, Lopez-Soto A, et al. (2009). Treatment of polymyalgia rheumatica: a systematic review. *Arch Int Med* **169**: 1839–50.

Jones JG, Hazleman BL (1981). Prognosis and management of polymyalgia rheumatica. *Ann Rheum Dis* **40**:1–5.

Kyle V, Hazleman BL (1989). Treatment of polymyalgia rheumatica and iant cell arteritis: steroid regimens in the first two months. *Ann Rheum Dis* **48**: 658–61.

Leeb BF, Bird HA, Nesher G, et al. (2003). EULAR response criteria for polymyalgia rheumatica: results of an initiative of the European collaborating polymyalgia group. *Ann Rheum Dis* **62**: 1189–94.

Royal College of Physicians (2002). Glucocorticoid-induced osteoporosis: guidelines for prevention and treatment.

Salvarani C, Cantini F, Hunder GG (2008). Polymyalgia rheumatica and giant-cell arteritis. *Lancet* **372**: 234–45.

Siebert S, Lawson TM, Wheeler MH, et al. (2001). Polymyalgia rheumatica: pitfalls in diagnosis. *J R Soc Med* **94**: 242–4.

Smeeth L, Cook C, Hall AJ (2006). Incidence of polymyalgia rheumatica and temporal arteritis in the United Kingdom, 1990–2001. *Ann Rheum Dis* **65**: 1093–8.

www.patient.co.uk/health/Polymyalgia-Rheumatica.htm

Pathology of giant cell arteritis

Introduction

Giant cell arteritis (GCA) is an inflammatory vasculopathy of unknown aetiology, which predominantly affects older people. It is also known as temporal arteritis because inflammation of the temporal arteries is a trademark feature of the condition. Similar to polymyalgia rheumatica (PMR), the underlying pathophysiological mechanisms have not been fully understood but both genetic and environmental factors are likely to play a part.

Pathophysiology

GCA is a primary vasculitis of the medium-sized to large arteries. GCA most commonly affects the cranial branches of aorta, but involvement of other vascular territories, such as subclavian and axillary arteries, is being increasingly recognized with improved non-invasive vascular imaging techniques. The reason for the predilection of certain vascular territories for the development of GCA is not clear.

Histologically, GCA is characterized by:

- cellular infiltrates consist of predominantly T cells and macrophages
- granuloma with/without multinucleated giant cells
- skip lesions
- disruption of the elastic lamina
- intimal hyperplasia.

Inflammation and the associated reparative process of the affected arteries lead to the increase in thickness of the vessel wall and hence reduces the luminal area of the vessels. In severe cases, the artery may be completely occluded. Diminished or interruption of blood supply in turn result in end organ ischaemia and damage.

In addition to vascular inflammation, GCA is usually accompanied by a systemic inflammatory response, manifested clinically with varying degrees of constitutional symptoms and elevated acute-phase proteins such as C-reactive protein (CRP). The systemic inflammatory process appears to be more than a mere overflow from the inflamed vascular lesions but involves additional mechanisms.

Immunopathology

In GCA, activated macrophages and CD4+ T cells are the predominant inflammatory infiltrates. The majority of the inflammatory cells are found in between the media and the elastic lamina of the affected vessels. Studies on T-cell clonalities of the lesion suggest that T cells have undergone clonal expansion, consistent with an antigen-specific driven process. However, to date, the identities of such putative antigens remain elusive. Activated macrophages secrete various growth factors, metalloproteinases, reactive oxygen species, and other molecules that further mediate the vascular pathology found in GCA.

Elevated levels of interferon (IFN)-γ are present in the inflamed arterial wall of the affected vessels. The production of IFN-γ by activated T cells is thought to play a key role in the activation of macrophages and correlates positively to intimal thickness and tissue ischaemia.

The underlying mechanisms that initiate the inflammatory process in GCA are less well understood. It has been proposed that dendritic cells located in the medial-adventitia border may be activated through their toll-like receptors (TLR), which in turn produce chemoattractants and costimulation signals that recruit and activate T cells to the affected vessels.

Serum levels of several cytokines (similar to those discussed in the earlier section Clinical features, diagnosis and management of polymyalgia rheumatica) have been reported to be elevated in GCA. Interleukin (IL)-6 is likely to be important in the systemic inflammatory responses in GCA. It has also been suggested that the angiogenic property of IL-6 may be protective against ischaemic complications of GCA because serum levels of IL-6 inversely correlate with the incidence of ischaemic events in GCA. However, the clinical and pathophysiological significance of other cytokines in GCA are not clear.

The role of genes and environment

Genetic association

Several human leucocyte antigen (HLA)-DR alleles have been linked to the development of GCA including HLA-DRB1*04 and HLA-DRB1*01, but similar to PMR, both the strength and the allele of the HLA association may differ between different populations.

Polymorphisms of other genes of the immune pathways have also been implicated, for instance, tumour necrosis factor (TNF)-α, IL-6 promoter, IFN-γ, and IL-1.

Environmental factors

Many infective agents have been implicated including mycoplasma, chlamydia, herpes virus, parvovirus B19, parainfluenza virus. However, these data were derived predominantly from association studies and no causal link has been demonstrated between these infective agents and GCA. Furthermore, conflicting data were often being reported. As in PMR, the levels of procalcitonin, an early marker of bacterial infections, are not elevated in GCA patients, arguing against bacterial triggers for GCA.

Traditional cardiovascular risk factors do not appear to be associated with the development of GCA with the exception of smoking in women.

Conclusions

GCA is a granulomatous vasculitis of the medium-sized to large arteries. Activated macrophages and IFN-γ-producing T cells play a key role in the vascular pathology. However, the cellular and molecular mechanisms which trigger the inflammatory process remain to be elucidated. Systemic inflammation in GCA may be more than a simple 'spillover' of vascular inflammation to the systemic circulation but involve additional aberrations of the immune pathways. Finally, the genetic and environmental factors that are important in the pathogenesis of GCA are only partially defined.

Authors' Tip

GCA is a medium-sized to large arterial vasculitis.

The vascular inflammation is driven by activated T cells and macrophages, while additional immune mechanisms may also be important in initiating the systemic inflammatory responses.

Both environmental and genetic factors may influence the susceptibility and severity of GCA.

Further reading

Duhaut P, Pinede L, Demolombe-Rague S, *et al.* (1998). Giant cell arteritis and cardiovascular risk factors: a multicenter, prospective case-control study. Groupe de Recherche sur l'Artérite à Cellules Géantes. *Arthritis Rheum* **41**: 1960–5.

Gonzalez-Gay MA, Vazquez-Rodriguez TR, Lopez-Diaz MJ, *et al.* (2009). Epidemiology of giant cell arteritis and polymyalgia rheumatica. *Arthritis Rheum* **61**: 1454–61.

Lie JT, (1990). Illustrated histopathologic classification criteria for selected vasculitis syndromes, *Arthritis Rheum* **33**: 1074–87.

Martinez-Taboada VM, Alvarez L, *et al.* (2008). Giant cell arteritis and polymyalgia rheumatica: role of cytokines in the pathogenesis and implications for treatment. *Cytokine* **44**: 207–20.

Miguel A Gonzalez-Gay (2001). Genetic epidemiology: Giant cell arteritis and polymyalgia rheumatic. *Arthritis Res* **3**: 154–7.

Roche NE, Fulbright JW, Wagner AD, *et al.* (1993). Correlation of interleukin-6 production and disease activity in polymyalgia rheumatica and giant cell arteritis. *Arthritis Rheum* **36**: 1286–94.

Salvarani C, Cantini F, Hunder GG (2008). Polymyalgia rheumatica and giant-cell arteritis. *Lancet* **372**: 234–45.

Diagnosis and management of giant cell arteritis

Introduction

The primary function of the geriatrician in giant cell arteritis (GCA) lies within the initial consideration of the diagnosis and instituting appropriate investigations. Although most geriatricians possess expertise in this area, close liaison with specialists in the diagnostic phase is important, but onward referral is paramount for the initial therapy and further management once the diagnosis is established. The most appropriate specialist to refer to will vary according to the severity of arteritic manifestations and local organization of services. In general terms however, this role would and should be coordinated by colleagues within rheumatology or ophthalmology. This chapter thereby describes the involvement of the geriatrician to what the authors consider an appropriate point prior to onward referral.

Epidemiology

The reported age-adjusted incidence of GCA in the UK is 2.2 cases per 10 000 person years. It is rare in patients aged less than 50 years old and reaches a peak of incidence in the seventh decade of life. GCA is at least twice as common in women as men.

Clinical features

The term temporal arteritis is inappropriate and underestimates the involvement of the extracranial vessels in GCA. The headache may not be localized to the temporal region. It may be unilateral or bilateral. The onset of the headache is frequently fairly abrupt and may be pinpointed in time to a particular day. Its character is usually different to any headache previously experienced by the patient. The patient may volunteer a suggestion of more widespread scalp tenderness, and this is frequently noticed during functional activities like washing or brushing the hair. Jaw claudication reflects ischaemia revealing itself during 'exercise' of the mandible while chewing.

Visual symptoms may be transient (amaurosis fugax) or persistent but are usually 'negative' in that vision is lost but may also be 'positive' with the perception of flashing lights, dots or lines. Diplopia may also be a presenting feature.

A minority of patients with involvement of the axillary/subclavian arteries present with arm claudication. Aortic arch involvement can even more rarely lead to cardiorespiratory symptoms. CT-PET scanning may demonstrate a more widespread arteritis than clinically anticipated however (see later).

As previously described within the section Clinical features, diagnosis, and management of polymyalgia rheumatica myalgic features of proximal limb pain, tenderness, and stiffness are common. Constitutional features including weight loss commonly coexist.

On clinical examination, the temporal artery or arteries may be tender, thickened, nodular, or non-pulsatile. Scalp tenderness may be elicited. Pupillary reflexes, eye movements, visual acuity, and fields should be examined. Fundoscopy should be performed to identify more gross ophthalmic manifestations like central retinal artery occlusion, but in practice the more subtle signs like the presence of micro-emboli may only be visible to the ophthalmologist with more specialized equipment and facilities. Particular attention should be paid to other clinically apparent signs of ischaemic manifestations including splinter haemorrhages, vascular bruits, and asymmetric pulses or blood pressure. A careful examination of the cardiovascular system should be vigilant for regurgitant murmurs or other signs of bacterial endocarditis as a potential disease mimic.

Differential diagnosis

A simple rule is that any older patient presenting with new-onset headache should be considered as suffering from GCA until proven otherwise. The differential diagnosis for such patients however is wide and laden with potential pitfalls. Other diagnostic possibilities include:

- transient ischaemic attack from thromboembolic disease related to carotid stenosis or atrial fibrillation
- acute glaucoma
- systemic sepsis from common sources of infection including the urinary tract and pneumonia
- acute shingles, particularly trigeminal/ophthalmic
- less common infections including tuberculosis, infective endocarditis, osteomyelitis, and cervical septic arthritis
- solid tumours including bony metastases
- multiple myeloma
- lymphoma
- other large vessel vasculitides, although Takayasu's arteritis generally only presents in young to middle age.

Although this is not well recognized in the literature, it is likely more atypical cases and those patients with multiple comorbidities gravitate towards geriatric and acute/general medicine giving the kinds of wide differential diagnoses listed above.

> **Authors' Tip**
>
> Infection and malignancy are two important mimics of GCA, requiring meticulous investigation and active exclusion.

Geriatricians and stroke physicians should remain alert to the possibility of GCA in patients presenting with stroke or transient ischaemic attack, particularly where visual symptoms or signs predominate. An ESR remains an essential investigation for all acute stroke patients.

Criteria for diagnosis are described in the box below. The presence of three or more of these criteria has been shown to yield sensitivity and specificity of above 90%. The control group in the original publication were patients suffering from 'other forms of vasculitis' making these conclusions less generalizable for the case mix seen within geriatric medical practice.

> **American College of Rheumatology diagnostic criteria, 1990: three or more criteria are required for a positive diagnosis of GCA**
>
> 1 Age at disease onset 50 years or above
> 2 New headache
> 3 Temporal artery abnormality (temporal artery tenderness to palpation or decreased pulsation, unrelated to arteriosclerosis)
> 4 Elevated erythrocyte sedimentation rate ≥ 50 mm/h by the Westergren method
> 5 Abnormal artery biopsy (biopsy specimen with artery showing vasculitis characterized by a predominance of mononuclear cell infiltration or granulomatous inflammation, usually with multinucleated giant cells)

Investigations

A similar set of baseline investigations should be performed as for polymyalgia rheumatica. An erythrocyte sedimentation rate (ESR) above 50 mm/h is suggested for use as a diagnostic criterion but frequently may be over 100. The acute-phase response is frequently also reflected in an elevated CRP, a normochromic normocytic anaemia and abnormal liver function tests (predominately raised alkaline phosphatase). Depending on the presenting symptom complex, brain imaging with CT or MRI may also need to be considered.

A number of case reports in the literature describe the use of CT-PET scanning for diagnosis, demonstrating increased uptake in the affected arteries. These cases have generally shown an unexpected arteritis or have confirmed the diagnosis where the clinical suspicion remained high after other negative investigations. CT-PET is an expensive investigation and should be reserved for the most challenging cases or when occult infections or malignancies are thought to be strong possibilities.

Temporal artery biopsy

Temporal artery biopsy (TAB) is not necessarily required in every case, and the physician should consider how a positive or negative result would change their clinical reasoning on a case by case basis. TAB is not therefore necessarily required for classical presentations but has greater diagnostic value in borderline or atypical cases. It should also be considered if an individual patient's characteristics suggest a high likelihood of corticosteroid-induced side-effects. A biopsy may also prove valuable when difficult decisions around relapse or poor response to steroid therapy ensue further down the line and a re-evaluation of the initial diagnosis needs to take place. False negative biopsy results are well recognized for a variety of reasons including the patchy nature of the inflammatory changes seen in GCA. Overall, opinion and practice varies as to whether or not a TAB should be preformed in every case.

A decision to proceed with TAB should not delay the administration of corticosteroids. It is, however, recognised that the positive yield from TAB decreases rapidly following the initiation of steroids but it may still have some utility up to 6 weeks. In one study of 132 cases of GCA, 82% of biopsies were present prior to the initiation of corticosteroids, decreasing to 60% and 10% after 1 and 2 weeks of treatment respectively. The symptomatic or most symptomatic temporal artery should be biopsied with a specimen of around 1 cm in length. Who performs the procedure varies according to local agreed provision of services and this may be ophthalmologists, general or vascular surgeons.

Temporal artery ultrasound is currently mainly a promising research tool and may provide an alternative to TAB in the future or presently if already locally available.

Treatment and prognosis

The aim of treatment in GCA is different to that in polymyalgia rheumatica. As well as leading to a symptomatic improvement for the patient, corticosteroids should induce remission from the arteritic process and risk of ischaemic complications. Steroid treatment should be initiated urgently to prevent permanent visual loss which could affect up to 60% of patients with untreated GCA.

Guidelines from the British Society for Rheumatology and British Health Professionals in Rheumatology published in 2010 recommend initial corticosteroid doses of:
- uncomplicated GCA (no jaw claudication or visual disturbance): 40–60 mg prednisolone daily
- complicated GCA (evolving visual loss or amaurosis fugax): 500 mg to 1 g of iv methylprednisolone for 3 days before oral glucocorticoids
- established visual loss: 60 mg prednisolone daily to protect the contralateral eye

As stated within the PMR chapter, measures to reduce the risk and consequence of steroid-induced side-effects, including osteoporosis, upper GI effects, hypertension, and diabetes should be instituted.

Ongoing steroid therapy and disease monitoring should be under the supervision of the appropriate specialist as stressed earlier. As in PMR, relapse is common. The use of methotrexate as a steroid-sparing agent may be considered after the third relapse, or sooner in the event of troublesome steroid-related side-effects, but this requires initiation and monitoring from specialists familiar with its use, generally rheumatologists. Patients generally require treatment with steroids for a minimum of 2 years.

Patients are at risk of death in the event of ischaemic complications, particularly stroke. Whether overall GCA is associated with excess mortality is not clear from the literature with studies yielding conflicting results. The picture is made more complex when the sequelae of serious steroid induced side effects are considered alongside the risk of fatal ischaemic events.

Authors' Tip

Acute onset headache and/or visual symptoms within an older patient requires urgent medical attention and thorough investigation for GCA.

Initial and ongoing management should be within close liaison or referral to appropriate specialists, usually ophthalmology or rheumatology.

Further reading

Allison MC, Gallagher PJ (1984). Temporal artery biopsy and corticosteroid treatment. *Ann Rheum Dis* **43**: 416–17.

Dasgupta B, Borg FA, Hassan N, et al. (2010). BSR and BHPR guidelines for the management of giant cell arteritis. *Rheumatology* **49**: 1594–7.

Dasgupta B, Hassan N (2007). Giant cell arteritis: recent advances and guidelines for management. *Clin Exp Rheumatol* **25**: 62–5.

Hunder GG (2002). The epidemiology of giant-cell arteritis. *Cleve Clin J Med* **69**: SII 79–82.

Hunder GG, Bloch DA, Michel BA, et al. (1990). The American College of Rheumatology 1990 criteria for the classification of giant cell arteritis. *Arthritis Rheum* **33**: 1122–8.

Smeeth L, Cook C, Hall AJ (2006). Incidence of diagnosed polymyalgia rheumatica and temporal arteritis in the United Kingdom, 1990 to 2001. *Ann Rheum Dis* **65**: 1093–8.

Feet

Foot problems are very common in older people and affect independence and quality of life, especially with regard to mobility and falls risk. Age-related changes of the foot can predispose the older adult to discomfort, pain, fungal infection, reduced range of joint motion, and itchy dry skin.

Foot problems, such as pain from corns, callosities (hard skin), bunions, and foot deformities, such as hammer toes, and nail conditions, are associated with increased falls risk. Falls risk rises as the number of foot problems increases.

Reduced sensation in the feet increases the risk of falls in people with diabetes. Reduced somatosensory feedback from the feet about the supporting surface can impair postural stability, particularly when walking on irregular surfaces. Podiatric interventions can help manage these conditions.

A major issue is that many older adults cannot see their feet, reach them, or care for them properly. Foot problems can be exacerbated by poor footwear, with shoe size and fit being contributing factors to mobility, falls, and fractures. Many older people wear inappropriate or poor-fitting footwear believing them to be adequate. Studies have reported that many community-dwelling older adults wore shoes that were too narrow, and approximately half of older people on a rehabilitation ward wore shoes that were too loose. People who have fallen are four times more likely to have been wearing socks or slippers without a proper sole. Going barefoot or wearing stockings is associated with a 10-fold increased risk of falling, while athletic shoes have the lowest risk.

The expected growth of the older population will have an unprecedented impact on the NHS, especially in terms of supply of and demand for podiatrists. The demand for podiatric services will grow. These population changes will also affect the nature of the skills and services podiatrists must provide and the settings in which these are done. The provision of foot health services is primarily (though not exclusively) the domain of the podiatry profession, and whether this is able to meet these future demands is uncertain.

Foot pain

Foot pain has long been recognized as highly prevalent in older people, affecting approximately one in three people aged over 65 years. In one study 17.4% of 3206 participants reported foot pain, aching, or stiffness, especially in females, those over 50 years, and obese patients.

The origin of foot pain can be multifactorial, yet commonly manifest through suboptimal biomechanics of the hallux or lesser toes, both having significant functional implications. Poor fitting footwear is also a major factor. Chronic and severe foot pain is associated with disability in older females; balance; poor walking performance; and falls risk. Foot pain may lead to antalgic gait patterns, increasing instability. Common clinical features observed in older people are calluses and corns (see Figure 10.3).

Common foot problems

Foot calluses and corns develop due to changes in lower limb and foot biomechanics, soft tissues including atrophy of the plantar fat pad and arthritic changes (e.g. osteoarthritis) or inflammatory arthritis (e.g. rheumatoid arthritis.)

Osteoarthritis of the first metatarsophalangeal joint leading to hallux rigidus (no motion) or limitus (limited

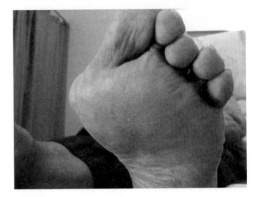

Figure 10.3 Calluses and corns.

motion) is often observed. Another common observation is the presence of hallux valgus (see Figure 10.4).

Hallux valgus (bunions) can lead to widening of the forefoot. Pain can arise from irritation of soft tissue surrounding the medial prominence of the first metatarsal head, the 'bunion', posing a risk of bursitis. Secondary complications can include hammer toe deformity of the second toe, hyperkerotic lesions under the lesser toes, and metatarsalgia due to altered foot loading. Hallux valgus has been associated with gait instability and a risk of falling in older people. Associated with lesser toe deformities (see Figure 10.5) are a range of nail conditions that could lead to fungal or bacterial infections.

Nail problems

Dermatological conditions commonly found in older adults include thickened, elongated, and ingrown nails. Many older people suffer with fungal and related symptoms. Thickened toenails, cracks, and fissures, maceration, and ulcers or lacerations are more commonly seen in men, while corns and calluses are more common in women. Thickened toenails can be painful and may impede personal hygiene, and fungal infection may indicate a compromised immune system. Any nail condition resulting in discomfort or creating barriers to obtaining well-fitting, comfortable shoes may increase the risk of activity limitation, falls, and decreased quality of life.

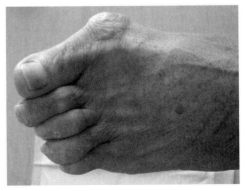

Figure 10.4 Hallux valgus.

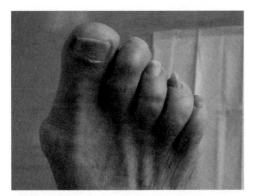

Figure 10.5 Lesser toe deformity.

Clinical assessment

The foot should not be assessed independently of the lower limb. Essential aspects of podiatric assessment, with commonly used clinical measurement tools, include:

- Foot type—Foot Posture Index. This is an index that allows clinicians to identify foot type into high-arched, low-arched, or normal feet based upon a criteria of six clinical foot observations, with three items each, specific to the rearfoot and forefoot
- Structural deformities – rearfoot, midfoot, forefoot
- Ankle and foot joint movement
- Plantar pressure measurements
- Lower limb, foot and toe muscle strength, tone and bulk
- Nail and skin inspection (lesions, ulceration, bacterial and fungal infection, skin hydration, appearance)
- Foot Pain – Manchester Foot Pain and Disability Index. The 19 item questionnaire is used to assess the impact of foot pain on functional, work and leisure activities, pain severity, and foot appearance
- Foot Sensitivity Testing (tactile sensitivity, temperature, vibration, pressure and pain perception, proprioception, ankle reflex)
- Vascular assessment (arterial disease, claudication, deep vein thrombosis and ankle–brachial pressure index)
- Footwear (size, style, suitability, patient preference): Based on a systematic literature review, older people should wear shoes with low heels and firm slip-resistant soles both indoors and outdoors. High-heeled shoes can impair posture, balance, and gait and can increase falls risk. A softer sole can alter balance control, so older people should wear thin, hard-soled shoes to optimize foot position and prevent dampening of sensory information. Treads on the sole and bevelled heel may prevent slips on wet and slippery surfaces. Shoes fitting too tightly can impair mechanical loading transmission between the foot and shoe, leading to problems including corns, calluses, and hallux valgus. Loose-fitting shoes can cause excessive foot slippage within the shoe during walking, altered contact area between the foot and shoe, impairing foot stability and walking parameters
- Functional testing (gait assessment, including either a 6- or 10-metre walking test; evaluation of activities of daily living)

- Blood sugar level: diabetes can lead to infections, ulceration, gangrene, or amputation.

Non-surgical management

Healthcare professionals have a prominent role to play in symptom relief and improving overall quality of life through specific interventions, providing foot health advice and education, and also in certain health behaviours and other aspects of the condition. There is a broad range of devices which are employed to modify foot and lower limb structure and function, such as foot orthoses. Foot orthoses fall into one of three main groups:

- simple cushioning insoles
- insoles to which additional padding/additions can be applied (known as accommodative foot orthoses)
- contoured insoles intended to change the function of leg and foot joints, either custom made to a cast of the patient's foot or supplied off the shelf (referred to as functional foot orthoses).

Inappropriate footwear can be a major contributing factor to foot impairment. However, when older people wear suitable footwear, it has the potential to alleviate pain, increase mobility and independence (with or without foot orthoses). The role of the podiatrist is to assess and advice the type of footwear.

Conclusions

Podiatry management can relieve pain, maintain function and mobility, prevent or minimize deformity, prevent falls, and reduce the risk of ulceration, and so maintain or improve the individuals' independence and quality of life.

Further reading

Chaiwanichsiri D, Janchai S, Tantisiriwat N (2009). Foot disorders and falls in older people. *Gerontology* **55**: 296–302.

Dunn J, Link C, Felson D, *et al.* (2004). Prevalence of foot and ankle conditions in a multiethnic community sample of older adults. *Am J Epidemiol* **159**: 491–8.

Garrow A, Papageorgiou A, Silman A, *et al.* (2000). Development and validation of a questionnaire to assess disabling foot pain. *Pain* **85**: 107–13.

Menant J, Steele J, Menz H, *et al.* (2008). Optimizing footwear for older people at risk of falls. *J Rehabil Res Dev* **45**: 1167–82.

Menz H (2008). *Foot Problems in Older People: Assessment and Management*. Philadelphia, Churchill Livingstone Elsevier.

Menz H, Sherrington C (2000). The footwear assessment form: a reliable clinical tool for the evaluation of footwear characteristics of relevance to postural stability in older adults. *Clin Rehabil* **14**: 657–64.

Menz H, Lord S (2001). Foot pain impairs balance and functional ability in community-dwelling older people. *J Am Podiatr Med Assoc* **91**: 222–9.

Menz H, Morris M (2005). Footwear characteristics and foot problems in older people. *Gerontology* **51**: 346–51.

Menz H, Morris M, Lord S (2006). Foot and ankle risk factors for falls in older people: a prospective study. *J Gerontol A Bio Sci Med Sci* **61**: 866–70.

Redmond A, Crosbie J, Ouvrier R (2006). Development and validation of a novel rating system for scoring foot posture: the Foot Posture Index. *Clin Biomech* **21**: 89–98.

Tyrrell W (2002). Podiatric management of the elderly. In: Lorimer D, *et al.* (eds) *Neale's Disorders of the Foot*, 6th edn. Churchill Livingstone, Edinburgh, pp.181–96.

Infections

Fever of unknown origin

Fever of unknown origin (FUO) was first defined in 1961 by Petersdorf and Beeson as persistent fever greater than 38.3°C (101°F) that evades diagnosis despite more than 3 weeks of investigation, including at least 1 week in hospital. This has been refined to include four different groupings, each requiring different investigative strategies: classical, nosocomial, neutropenic, and HIV-related FUO. FUO in older people tends to be considered under the classical heading, but the presentation, underlying conditions, and subsequent treatment differ considerably from FUO in a younger adult age group, and FUO in the over 65s could be considered a fifth category.

One of the major differences in presentation is a relative reduction in the frequency and severity of fever. Physiological changes associated with ageing mean that baseline temperature tends to be lower than that of healthy young adults. Even in the presence of infection, there is a blunted or absent fever response in 20–30% of cases. Studies of care home residents suggest that a single oral temperature >37.8°C, persistent temperature >37.2°C, or an increase in 1.1°C from baseline are all significant in this population and should trigger further investigations. Clinical presentation is often atypical, with a lack of localizing symptoms.

Compared with younger patients, those over 65 have a greater likelihood of the underlying condition being diagnosed. Infections account for 25–35% of FUO in older populations, although this is higher in developing country settings. Non-infectious inflammatory conditions account for an increasing proportion of FUO cases (21–31%), with malignancy identified in up to 21% of patients. The rest are a mix of miscellaneous conditions, drug reactions, and thromboembolic disease. Factitious fever, familial and benign periodic fevers are very uncommon as a new presentation in older people. Detailed lists of potential causes can be found in the further reading, but some of the more common diagnoses are discussed below.

Infection

Older patients are predisposed to infection for a variety of reasons, including the physiological effects of ageing, multiple comorbidities and more frequent contact with healthcare settings. Infective processes presenting as FUO can include common infections presenting in an uncommon way, infections with long latent periods, and infections in occult locations. Tuberculosis remains a clinical problem in this group, often without a prior history of exposure or treatment, and should be considered in all cases. Recent hospital attendance should prompt searches for sites of haematogenous spread of infections related to intravenous lines and invasive procedures such as urinary catheterization and endoscopy. All implanted medical devices including heart valves, pacemakers, and prosthetic joints should be considered a potential source of an FUO. However, not all older patients are frequent hospital attendees and a travel and sexual history may be more revealing than past medical history. HIV should not be discounted on the basis of age alone.

Non-infectious inflammatory

Non-infectious inflammatory conditions encompass a range of rheumatological and vasculitic conditions. Giant cell arteritis (including temporal arteritis) is the main cause of FUO in this group of conditions in the over 65s (up to 65% of cases). Onset is typically insidious and associated with anaemia and weight loss. Delays in diagnosis because of searches for infections or malignancy can lead to loss of vision, so high clinical suspicion and early consideration of treatment is important. Although temporal artery biopsy is the gold standard investigation, it does have a significant false-negative rate and modern imaging techniques (including positron emission tomography–computed tomography (PET-CT) scanning) are proving useful in this group. Other common diagnoses include polymyalgia rheumatica. As there is a blunted response of the erythrocyte sedimentation rate (ESR) in up to 20% of these patients, diagnostic suspicion must be maintained.

Malignancy

An underlying malignancy is identified in 12–21% of patients with an FUO. This may be due to a paraneoplastic effect of the tumour or result from infective complications such as infective endocarditis and liver abscesses. Haematological malignancies account for a relatively high proportion of underlying malignancies, but colonic and renal tumours and atrial myxomas remain important and common differential diagnoses. With earlier diagnosis due to the increased availability of cross-sectional imaging, malignancies are becoming a less common cause of true FUO.

Drugs

Because of polypharmacy, drugs remain an important (and readily reversible) cause of FUO. The typical onset of drug fever is 7–10 days after commencing the medication but can be earlier or later than this. Patients often have a relative lack of systemic symptoms despite high swinging fevers. A rash and/or eosinophilia may be present but is uncommon. Antibiotics are common culprits along with non-steroidal anti-inflammatory and cardiovascular drugs. Specific drug-related syndromes to consider include the neuroleptic malignant syndrome (typical and atypical antipsychotics, metoclopramide, lithium) and serotonin syndrome (SSRIs, anticonvulsants, dopaminergic drugs, St John's Wort). It may be necessary to withdraw each drug in turn until the offending drug is identified; the fever typically abates within 48–72 hours and will return if rechallenged.

Clinical approach

As with all patients presenting with an FUO, the starting point is a thorough history and examination. As well as providing important clues to diagnosis it is important to have an idea of premorbid function. Although many of the causes are treatable, not all older patients will be able to undergo rigorous invasive investigation and in some patients it may be inappropriate to investigate at all. The concept of 'first do no harm' applies equally well to FUO and the investigation and management should not cause more distress than the clinical symptoms.

Common omissions in the physical examination include pressure areas, teeth, prostate, spine, joints, and implanted medical devices, including heart valves. The examining clinician should be careful not to miss infection in these areas as well looking in the common sites. First-line investigations such as chest radiograph, urinalysis, relevant wound swabs, and initial blood tests should already have been performed before the diagnosis of FUO is made. Further assessment should be guided by the findings of these preliminary investigations, history and examination.

Common pitfalls and good practice points

- Failures to consider the diagnosis: symptoms are often vague, with an insidious onset. Temperature is lower than in younger patients, consider diagnosis in those with temperature persistently higher than 37.2 °C.
- Failure to take an adequate history.
- Failure to elicit history of invasive procedures up to 6 months prior to onset of FUO, as a clue to presence of deep tissue infection such as endocarditis or discitis.
- Failure to examine the patient fully, including oropharynx and teeth, optic fundi, temporal arteries, pressure areas, prostate, spine, joints, and implanted medical devices.
- Failure to consider:
  - discitis in a patient with back pain/tenderness
  - empyema in slowly resolving pneumonia
  - peritonitis in a patient with ascites
  - TB in a patient with sterile pyuria
  - endocarditis in patients with 'skin commensals' in blood cultures (including coagulase negative Staphylococci)
  - chronic prostatitis in patients with lower urinary tract symptoms
- Sensitivity of transthoracic echo in older people is reduced so consider a transoesophageal echocardiogram
- Tuberculin skin test and TB interferon-γ release assays are often negative in disseminated mycobacterial disease. A negative result does not rule out the diagnosis and a positive result only indicates past TB exposure (not necessarily current disease)
- Inappropriately enthusiastic investigation. Treat the individual rather than the symptoms. Not all patients will be well enough for invasive investigations
- Early initiation of empirical antibiotic, which can impede microbiological diagnosis and sometimes cause fever
- Failure to look for a further diagnosis if fever persists after treatment for the first diagnosis considered

---

A fixed diagnostic algorithm is not necessarily helpful but suggested approaches can be found in the further reading section.

It is essential to take a logical and stepwise approach to requesting specialised investigations. This reduces unnecessary discomfort and possible side-effects for the patient and allows the health care team time to re-evaluate the patient at successive stages. It also reduces the very common problem of failing to recognize or discount 'red herrings' thrown up by multiple concurrent investigations. Patients should be re-examined clinically at least twice a week, including fundoscopy.

Samples such as sputum, early morning urine and relevant tissue biopsies should be submitted for staining and culture for mycobacterial disease in all older patients. If liver function is abnormal, the yield of liver biopsy is usually better than bone marrow (which must include trephine) for occult TB. The value of tuberculin skin tests and serum interferon-γ release (IGRA) tests for detecting prior TB exposure varies with the clinical setting, but is generally less helpful in older than younger patients with FUO. If miliary TB is still suspected, the chest radiograph should be repeated after 2 weeks, as it may be normal at initial presentation.

Once the first wave of special investigations has been completed without an obvious diagnosis, including CT screening for lymphomas, it is likely that PET scanning will be increasingly used in future to direct further investigation of patients with FUO.

Treatment

Specific treatment of a patient with FUO should be avoided as much as possible until a firm (or strongly suspected) diagnosis is made. Empirical antibiotics should be avoided at the investigative stage unless there is a clear sign of deterioration and/or sepsis syndrome, as microbiological investigations are rarely positive while taking antimicrobials. If there is no diagnosis after all appropriate investigations have been performed, a therapeutic trial of either broad spectrum antibiotics, tuberculosis treatment, and/or steroids may be necessary. A therapeutic trial must have a pre-specified end point (normally 2 weeks) and preferably a pre-specified target symptom or sign (e.g. resolution of fever), and if there is no improvement at this stage then the treatment strategy should be reassessed.

In most older patients with a FUO, a cause is eventually identified. In those for whom no diagnosis is made, follow-up studies suggest that the majority become asymptomatic and have a good long-term prognosis, even if symptoms recur occasionally. It is important to convey this prognostic information to patients and their families, who are frequently as frustrated as their physicians by the failure of a prolonged period of intensive investigation to provide a clear diagnosis.

FUO remains a diagnostic challenge, but the route to identifying the underlying cause is via the basics of medicine, using a good history and examination to guide further investigation and treatment.

Further reading

Bleekers-Rover CP, van der Meer JWM, Beeching NJ (2009). Fever. *Medicine* **37:1**: 28–34.

Durack D (2005). Fever of unknown origin. In (Warrell DA, Cox T, Firth J, eds) *Oxford Textbook of Medicine*, 4th edn. Oxford, Oxford University Press, pp. 271–5.

Infectious Diseases Society of America (2008). Clinical practice guideline for evaluation of fever and infection of older adult residents of long term care homes. *Clin Infect Dis* **48**; 149–71.

Nguyen C, Cross A (2010). Fever of unknown origin. In (Cohen J, Powderly W, Opal S, eds) *Infectious Diseases*, 3rd edn. Mosby Elsevier, pp. 688–95.

Tal S, Guller V, Guervich A (2007). Fever of unknown origin in older adults. *Clin Geriatr Med* **23**: 649–68.

HIV in older people

Background

HIV infection has typically been seen as a disease of younger people. However, due to the success of anti-HIV therapies, the epidemiology is shifting and a significant proportion of HIV-infected persons are entering older life (defined here as patients over 50 years). It has been postulated that these patients exhibit premature ageing, with more comorbidities being recognized over time. Consequently, geriatricians are likely to be increasingly involved in the management of patients with HIV. Furthermore, they have a role in detecting undiagnosed infection, particularly as late diagnosis occurs more frequently in older individuals. This chapter focuses on the role of the geriatrician in caring for HIV-infected patients.

Epidemiology of HIV

As a result of ongoing transmission of HIV, improved survival of those with diagnosed infection and access to effective treatment, the numbers of individuals with HIV continues to rise.

- Globally, at the end of 2008 there were an estimated 33.4 million adults and children living with HIV, of whom 22.4 million were in sub-Saharan Africa
- There were an estimated 2.7 million new infections in 2008, mostly in sub-Saharan Africa (1.9 million), though others were from places including Eastern Europe (110 000), whence migration may occur into the UK
- In the UK in 2008, there were an estimated 83 000 adults and children with HIV, of whom approximately 24% were unaware of their infection (i.e. undiagnosed)
- In the UK during 2008, there were approximately 7300 new diagnoses of HIV. This is slightly fewer than in the mid-2000s, but significantly more than in the 1980s and 1990s. The proportion of new diagnoses in heterosexuals outnumbered those in men who have sex with men (MSM) from 2000 onwards, largely due to 'imported' HIV infection from high-prevalence countries, but this trend may now be reversing due to increasing infections in MSM and changing immigration patterns and policies

The number of new cases of AIDS and number of deaths in individuals with HIV has decreased significantly in proportional terms, but has remained essentially static in numerical terms. This is largely driven by late diagnosis of HIV, i.e. individuals being diagnosed too late for effective anti-HIV therapy and immune restoration. Of note, multiple studies show that the majority of these individuals have accessed healthcare relatively recently, often with HIV associated conditions, but infection has gone unrecognized and undiagnosed.

Epidemiology of ageing and HIV

As a result of improved life expectancy associated with highly active antiretroviral therapy (HAART), along with new infections, including those at an older age, the number and proportion of older individuals with HIV is increasing year on year.

- In the USA, it has been estimated that by 2015, 50% of individuals with HIV will be over 50 years
- In the UK, the proportion of individuals with HIV accessing care aged over 50 has increased from 1 in 10 (1999) to 1 in 6 (2008)
- Both the number and proportion of older individuals with HIV is higher in certain locations due to a variety of migrational and behavioural factors, e.g. cohorts in Amsterdam, Switzerland and Brighton report proportions of ~30% of HIV-infected individuals being aged over 50 years
- With regard to undiagnosed infection and those who are diagnosed or present 'late', every study has shown that older individuals are disproportionately represented. It is likely that this is due to a combination of factors including: less willingness of older individuals to disclose risk behaviour, less willingness of healthcare providers to enquire about risk behaviour, less clinical suspicion of underlying HIV infection, wider differential diagnosis.

Effect of ageing on HIV

It is clear from multiple large cohort studies that age has an impact on the natural history of HIV (in the absence of HAART). Older age is associated with

- significant increase in the risk of progression to AIDS or death after seroconversion
- more rapid rate of CD4 decline
- opportunistic complications occurring at higher CD4 counts
- increased risk of death after diagnosis of an opportunistic complication.

In the post-HAART era, however, the picture becomes less clear. Older individuals appear to experience

- less immunological recovery with HAART (i.e. CD4 count rise) than younger individuals
- greater rates of virological response to HAART (likely mediated through greater adherence).

The overall consensus is that older age does not reduce the benefits of HAART. However, potential toxicity and tolerability are of greater importance, particularly considering polypharmacy, potential drug interactions, and the possibility of accelerated ageing.

Effect of HIV on ageing

The effects of HIV on the immune system have been described as similar to those of natural ageing. In addition, it has been postulated that HIV infected individuals may be predisposed to some of the common conditions of ageing due to higher rates of risk behaviour (e.g. smoking, alcohol, drug use), the potential adverse effects of HAART and the potential of chronic inflammation and immune activation to accelerate the ageing process. HIV infected individuals have higher rates of

- cardiovascular disease
- reduced bone mineral density
- renal and hepatic impairment
- cognitive impairment
- all malignancy (as well as those typically associated with AIDS) with the possible exceptions of breast and prostate

Principles of HIV management

The current paradigm of management of HIV infection is to initiate HAART at a time to minimize the risk of opportunistic complications. HAART is then continued lifelong, but potentially altered depending on tolerability or potency, based on clinical and laboratory monitoring. Given the success of most HAART regimens and the increasing availability of alternative options, it is anticipated that the lifespan of an HIV infected individual will approximate that of the general population, albeit with increased comorbidities due to accelerated ageing, if the diagnosis is made in time to allow intervention.

Guidelines are systematically developed and updated by a number of international societies, including the International AIDS Society (IAS), and British HIV Association (BHIVA). These differ intermittently but broadly currently advise:

- all HIV-infected individuals with a CD4 count of <350 cells/mm^3 should receive HAART
- individuals with a higher CD4 count (usually 350–500 cells/mm^3) may be considered for earlier initiation of HAART if they have a significant co-morbidity (e.g. hepatitis B or C co-infection, higher cardiovascular disease risk or are of an older age (usually >50 years)

The aim of HAART is to achieve and maintain virological suppression (i.e. an undetectable viral load) and thereby optimize immune function (i.e. higher CD4 counts). Specific HAART regimens vary according to the latest clinical trial data and individual patient circumstances, and will be modified according to treatment response, tolerability, drug resistance, etc.

Key clinical issues for the geriatrician

Spotting undiagnosed HIV
Undiagnosed HIV infection is of concern for both individual (morbidity and mortality) and public (onward transmission) health. The older patient is more likely to be diagnosed late and geriatricians need to be as attuned as other physicians.

Recent guidance has advocated a shift towards normalization of HIV testing without specialist pre-test counselling. The recent UK guidelines identify a number of 'clinical indicator diseases' for which all patients, irrespective of age, should be offered an HIV test. These include bacterial pneumonia, space-occupying lesion of unknown cause, dementia, peripheral neuropathy, chronic diarrhoea, or weight loss of unknown cause, lung cancer, and any unexplained blood dyscrasia.

If underlying HIV infection is considered and the clinician feels unable to raise this issue with the patient, discussion with the local HIV/GUM team is advised.

Coprescribing
For patients receiving HAART, there are heightened concerns regarding co-prescribing of other medication. Many HAART agents (particularly protease inhibitors and non-nucleoside reverse transcriptase inhibitors) are either metabolized by, or induce or inhibit, the cytochrome P450 system as well as a number of other metabolic pathways. (See the British National Formulary, or for more detail, the Liverpool University website (http://www.hiv-druginteractions.org/). There is a risk that some coprescribed drugs may reduce the levels of anti-HIV drugs (thereby increasing the risk of virological failure) or that anti-HIV drugs may increase or decrease the levels of concomitant drugs thereby either reducing efficacy or increasing toxicity. This can usually be managed by using an alternative concomitant medication, dose adjustment or careful monitoring. The commonest significant coprescribing errors are:

1 Statins – ritonavir (an HIV protease inhibitor used as a 'booster' due to its strong inhibition effect on CYP450) can increase statin levels. This is particularly significant for simvastatin (absolutely contraindicated). Atorvastatin and rosuvastatin should be given at lower doses.

2 Proton-pump inhibitors (PPIs)—the HIV protease inhibitor atazanavir requires an acid environment for absorption and co-administration with PPIs is contraindicated.

3 Fluticasone – although usually administered via inhalation, co-administration with ritonavir results with significant systemic corticosteroid absorption and many cases of Cushing's and Addison's syndromes have been described. These agents should not be co-administered.

Emergency presentations
The older HIV-infected individual may present as an emergency for a number of reasons:

- Opportunistic complication with previously undiagnosed HIV. The commonest opportunistic presentations of advanced HIV in the UK are *Pneumocystis jirovecii* pneumonia (PCP), with gradual onset of exertional dyspnoea and a dry cough, and tuberculosis, which may frequently present as extrapulmonary disease.

- Opportunistic complication with known underlying HIV infection. Such presentations are now rare due to the success of HAART. However, the effect on malignancies, not previously thought to be related to HIV infection, may be increasing in the HAART era.

Healthcare issue unrelated to HIV infection.
The latter is likely to be the commonest reason for hospital admission. It may be more appropriate for an older patient with HIV presenting with a non-HIV-related condition to be primarily cared for by a generalist team, but with close liaison with the HIV team. BHIVA guidelines (accessible at www.bhiva.org) are also available to support generalists involved in the management of patients with opportunistic infections or malignancies.

Palliative care
As previously outlined, it is increasingly likely that patients with HIV will in the future die with, rather than from, HIV. Many malignancies not typically considered to be HIV related appear to be occurring with increased frequency and at an earlier age than in the general population. After the successful introduction of HAART, specialist palliative care facilities for patients with HIV have been largely disbanded, and so generic palliative care facilities are likely to be utilized. Caution should be taken with drug dosing due to interactions. HAART is often continued (unless specifically declined by the patient) until the very end of life, as patients usually feel worse without this.

Further reading

Deeks SG, Phillips AN (2009). HIV infection, antiretroviral treatment, ageing, and non-AIDS morbidity. *Br Med J* 338:a3172.

European AIDS Clinical Society (EACS) guidelines for the prevention and management of management of non-infectious co morbidities in HIV 2009. (http:// www.europeanaidsclinicalsociety.org/guidelinespdf/2_Non_Infectious_Co_Morbidities_in_HIV.pdf).

Health Protection Agency. HIV in the UK: Annual report. (www.hpa.org.uk).

Guaraldi G, Zona S, Alexopoulos N, et al. (2009). Coronary Aging in HIV-infected patients. *Clin Infect Dis* 49: 1756–62.

Kirk JB, Goetz MB (2009). Human Immunodeficiency Virus in an aging population, a complication of success. *J Am Geriatr Soc* 57: 2129–38.

Onen NT, Overton ET, Seyfried W, et al. (2010). Aging and HIV Infection: a comparison between older HIV-infected persons and the general population. *HIV Clin Trials* 11: 100–9.

Palfreeman A, Fisher M, Ong E, et al. (2009). Testing for HIV: concise guidance. *Clin Med* 9: 471–6.

Smith RD, Delpech VC, Brown AE, et al. (2010). HIV transmission and high rates of late diagnoses among adults aged 50 years and over. *AIDS* 24: 2109–15.

UK National Guidelines for HIV Testing 2008. (http://www.bhiva.org/documents/Guidelines/Testing/GlinesHIVTest08.pdf).

Clostridium difficile diarrhoea: a geriatric syndrome

Background

Clostridium difficile is a spore-forming, anaerobic, toxin-producing, Gram-positive bacterium. Intriguingly *C. difficile* is frequently a harmless commensal of the infant gut but is rarely found in the faecal flora of healthy adults. With advancing age and illness, *C. difficile* is found again in the bowel flora. Between 10% and 50% of older people who are debilitated or have extensive healthcare contact have *C. difficile* in their stools, but it is not clear whether it can ever be considered a harmless commensal in this population or a prelude to clinically active *C. difficile* infection (CDI).

Epidemiology

C. difficile was first recognized as a cause of antibiotic-associated diarrhoea in 1978. Rates increased gradually during the 1990s but rose more dramatically after 2000. Mandatory reporting to the Health Protection Agency was introduced in 2005 and the number of cases peaked in the UK in 2006 at around 60 000, with 80% being in those over the age of 65 years. Not only has CDI become more common but the severity of CDI also seems to have increased. Historically CDI was associated with an additional mortality of only 1–2%. First reports of changes in severity came from the USA and Canada in 2002. A new 'hypervirulent' type was identified, which most commonly is termed ribotype 027. Infections caused by ribotype 027 strains have been associated with more severe disease and a higher mortality. In the UK ribotype 027 strains were involved in notorious outbreaks of *C. difficile* at Stoke Mandeville, Maidstone, and Tunbridge Wells Hospitals, where attributable mortality rates of over 10% were identified. At the peak of the ribotype 027 epidemic in the UK, in around 2006, this strain accounted for 30% of all cases. The all cause mortality in patients following a diagnosis of CDI was around 30%, approximately double that of other hospitalized frail older patients.

Since 2006, the rate of *C. difficile* infections in the NHS has fallen; there were just over 25,000 cases reported in 2010 and ribotype 027 strains have become uncommon in many regions. However, the rate of decline has slowed markedly. *C. difficile* strains of ribotypes 017 and 078 are now being reported as associated with more severe disease. A further change in epidemiology has been an increase in the proportion of cases having their onset outside hospitals. Community-onset cases comprise almost 50% of cases in 2010. In North America, community onset cases have been described in patient groups previously regarded as low risk but in the UK community onset CDI generally remains a disease of frail older people.

Pathophysiology

Symptomatic CDI is thought to result when a person who is colonized with *C. difficile* receives antibiotics which disrupt the healthy gut flora and trigger toxin production. Symptoms range from mild diarrhoea to severe colitis, ileus, and toxic megacolon. They can be largely explained by the actions of two cytotoxins which cause disruption of the actin cytoskeleton and tight junctions resulting in fluid leak and destruction of the intestinal epithelium. Ribotype 027 strains have mutations in the genes regulating toxin production and produce much larger quantities of these toxins *in vitro* than other strains. They also synthesize a third 'binary toxin', the clinical significance of which is not clear.

Prevention

The Department of Health Saving Lives Campaign proposes a five-pronged approach to preventing CDI:
* prudent antibiotic use
* hand hygiene
* use of personal protective equipment
* environmental contamination and
* isolation or cohort nursing.

The antibiotics most closely linked with risk of CDI since the advent of ribotype 027 strains are cephalosporins and quinolones. Most hospitals have introduced policies which try to minimize use of these classes of drug, replacing them with aminoglycosides and penicillins. The 'Saving Lives Campaign' also aims to minimize unnecessary and inappropriate antibiotic use by ensuring indications for antibiotic use are clearly recorded with a stop or review date, intravenous antibiotics are avoided where possible, and surgical prophylaxis is restricted to single doses where possible. Alcohol hand gels are less effective at removing *C. difficile* spores from the hands than washing with soap and water. Infection control measures to reduce CDI have focused on staff wearing gloves and aprons when looking after patients with diarrhoea, use of chlorine releasing disinfectants to clean affected areas and isolation or cohorting of patients with diarrhoea. Patients who may be colonized by *C. difficile* but not have active disease also shed *C. difficile* into their environment and good infection control practice should be maintained for all people at risk of *C. difficile*.

Proton pump inhibitors (PPIs) are associated with an approximately twofold increased risk of CDI. Careful consideration to this should be given when starting frail older people on PPIs.

Probiotics have been proposed for the prevention of CDI particularly in 'at-risk' patients starting antibiotics. One small double-blind trial found a beneficial effect of one but a recent meta-analysis concluded there was insufficient evidence to support routine use. A large, double-blind RCT of probiotic primary prevention is underway in the UK.

Assessment

The gold-standard approaches for CDI diagnosis depend on demonstrating the cytoxic effects and neutralization with antitoxin. These techniques are slow, laborious and expensive, so that most diagnostic laboratories now rely on ELISA tests for toxins A and/or B in diarrhoeal stool. Commercial ELISAs have specificities of over 90%, but since most patients with diarrhoea do not have CDI, this can result in an unacceptably high number of false positive tests. This becomes particularly problematic as the rate of CDI falls. In most settings a negative ELISA has a negative predictive value of >90%; however, if clinical suspicion is high, repeat testing should be performed. Two or three-step testing algorithms may be introduced by diagnostic laboratories in the near future to reduce the number of false positives.

A small proportion of people with CDI present without diarrhoea, but with abdominal distension, ileus and sepsis, representing severe disease. In such cases abdominal radiograph, or abdominal CT to look for thickening of the colonic mucosa, or endoscopy to detect pseudomembrane formation can help if readily available.

There is no currently accepted approach to severity assessment of CDI. Current European guidelines recommend that patients be identified as having severe colitis if they have a range of physical signs including abdominal tenderness or ileus, laboratory abnormalities including a white blood count over 15, a rising creatinine or an elevated lactate or radiological evidence of colonic wall thickening. Stool frequency and hypoalbuminaemia are no longer recommended as markers of severe disease.

Pharmacological management

Patients developing CDI should have any on-going antibiotic treatment reviewed and where possible stopped. Two drugs are currently in general use to treat CDI; metronidazole and vancomycin. Resistance to either drug is not currently a clinically significant problem.

Metronidazole is active orally and intravenously and has long been considered the drug of first choice. However, the concentration of metronidazole achieved in liquid stool is frequently very close to the concentration required to inhibit *C. difficile* growth. A series of studies confirm that metronidazole is inferior to vancomycin, particularly in patients with severe disease, in terms of treatment response, relapse and mortality.

Vancomycin is active orally but not intravenously. A dose of 125 mg 6 hourly usually achieves a faecal concentration vastly above the concentration required to inhibit *C. difficile* growth. In some settings, doses up to 500 mg 6 hourly are advocated on the basis of anecdotal evidence. At such doses systemic absorption occurs and blood levels should be checked in the context of renal impairment.

In refractory disease instillation of vancomycin directly into the rectum has been described and UK guidelines suggest consideration of rifampicin or immunoglobulin but there is no good evidence for any of these approaches.

Up to 30% of patients treated for a first episode of CDI will experience at least one relapse of symptoms, usually between 1–3 weeks after stopping treatment. The diagnosis of relapse is usually on clinical grounds alone, as toxin persists in stool after successful treatment and most laboratories will not re-test stool within 28 days of a previous positive stool. Recurrences should be treated with the antibiotic used for the first episode unless greater severity indicates otherwise. Observational studies support the use of tapering courses of vancomycin and a single small series described the successful use of immunoglobulin. The approach with the best evidence base is faecal transplantation but use is limited by acceptability and safety concerns.

Non-pharmacological management

High level inquests in England highlighted that doctors often fail to manage CDI as a disease in its own right, pay insufficient attention to fluid balance or nutrition and do not undertake multidisciplinary assessments. Many hospitals have found it helpful to identify a consultant or team to lead on the management of CDI cases and ensure close involvement of infectious disease specialists, geriatricians and surgeons.

Future developments

Fidoxomicin is a new drug developed specifically for the treatment of CDI which recently completed two phase III trials in Europe and North America. It was granted regulatory approval for treatment of adults with CDI in the USA and Europe in late 2011 and will be available in the UK in 2012. Successful use of tigicycline in refractory disease has recently been reported. Other promising interventions in development include both passive and active immunization against toxins A and B.

Further reading

Saving Lives: Reducing Infection, Delivering Clean and Safe Care. London, Department of Health, 2007 Gateway ref: 8331.

Clostridium difficile Infection: How to Deal with the Problem. London, Department of Health, 2008 Gateway ref: 9833.

Shannon-Lowe J, Matheson NJ, Cooke FJ, *et al.* (2010). Prevention and medical management of *Clostridium difficile* infection. *Br Med J* **340**:c1296.

Wilcox MH, Freeman J (2006). Epidemic *Clostridium difficile*. *N Eng J Med* **354**: 1199–203.

Bauer MP, Kuijper EJ, van Dissel JT (2009). European Society of Clinical Microbiology and Infectious Diseases (ESCMID): treatment guidance document for *Clostridium difficile* infecion (CDI). *Clin Mlcrobiol Infect* **15**:1067–1079.

Psychiatric

Dementia

What it is

Dementia is a syndrome caused by a variety of brain diseases, and comprising a loss of cognitive functions.

Dementia

- is acquired
- is global (usually memory plus at least one other domain)
- is progressive
- impacts on daily functioning
- does not impair consciousness
- does not occur solely during delirium
- is not better explained by another diagnosis
- persists more than 6 months.

Cognition is the ability to think, understand, and reason. Cognitive functions include memory, orientation, language (verbal fluency, receptive, and expressive communication), praxis (doing things), recognition, visuospatial ability, abstract thought, executive function (decision-making, planning, judgement), and insight.

Ambiguities abound, however. There is no sharp cut-point between 'normal' cognition and dementia, rather a continuum. Onset of cognitive impairment may be sudden following a stroke or head injury. Impact on daily function depends on culture, education, background, and expectations. Conscious level may be impaired in dementia with Lewy bodies (DLB) and the very advanced stages of all dementias. Delirium is common in dementia, dementia may present with delirium, and cognitive function does not always recover after delirium. Confirmation of dementia requires that delirium is not present (although a carefully taken history may be suggestive); hence the ICD-10 criteria require that symptoms be present for at least 6 months.

In the later stages, physical functions are affected, including gait, balance, continence, appetite, and swallowing.

Mild cognitive impairment is a demonstrable loss of cognitive function that does not interfere with everyday function. Half eventually go on to develop overt dementia.

People with learning disabilities are at especial risk of developing dementia at a young age.

Different types

Alzheimer's disease (AD) is the most common type in the population (55%). It is characterized by early memory loss and relentless, gradual, progression.

Vascular dementia (VaD; 15%) has a stepwise and irregular progression, meaning that it often presents with crises: sudden worsening of confusion, often associated with falls, immobility, or incontinence. A history of stroke or other vascular disease, pseudobulbar or upper motor neurone neurological signs, and imaging evidence of ischaemia, support the diagnosis. Three subtypes can be described:

- sudden onset of cognitive impairment affecting about 25% of acute stroke patients
- multi-infarct dementia
- dementia associated with subcortical white matter ischaemia (associated with gait abnormalities, executive and information processing problems).

Mixed Alzheimer's and vascular is seen in a further 20–30%.

Dementia with Lewy bodies (DLB, 5%) is a syndrome of:

- cognitive impairment
- Parkinsonism
- fluctuation in alertness or cognition
- delusions and hallucinations
- increased sensitivity to neuroleptic drugs.

The term Parkinson's disease dementia (PDD) is used when motor symptoms precede cognitive impairment by more than 12 months.

Other dementias include frontotemporal dementia (characterized by problems with initiative and planning, disinhibition and poor language), and dementia associated with neurodegenerative diseases including Huntingdon's disease, Creutzfeld–Jakob disease, multiple sclerosis, motor neurone disease, corticobasilar degeneration, alcohol excess, and HIV infection.

Research diagnostic criteria exist for subtypes. In clinical practice, subtyping has some role: patients with AD and DLB may respond to cholinesterase inhibitors; patients with DLB should avoid neuroleptic drugs; those with VaD may be offered vascular prevention drugs or advice.

However, in practice differentiating them is neither easy, nor reliable. For example, aphasia may be prominent in AD, giving the appearance of a 'focal' neurological sign. Parkinsonism and gait abnormalities are common in AD and VaD as well as DLB. Patients fulfilling the diagnostic criteria are highly likely to have appropriate pathological changes, but the sensitivity of these criteria is low (i.e. they miss a lot of cases). Up to a third of patients have mixed pathology and diagnostic criteria are poor at detecting these.

The summarized research diagnostic criteria for dementia subtypes are below.

General criteria for diagnosing Dementia

- Cognitive decline from a previously higher level of functioning, with impaired memory and at least one other cognitive domain.
- Deficits are severe enough to interfere with activities of daily living, not due to the physical effects of comorbid disease alone.
- No other neurological disease, or delirium, accounts for impairment better.

DSM-IV criteria for Alzheimer's disease

Memory impairment demonstrated on cognitive testing.

At least one other cognitive deficit such as orientation, aphasia, impaired executive function (difficulty with planning, judgement, set-shifting, abstraction, problem solving), agnosia, or apraxia. The onset is gradual onset and there is progressive decline.

NINCDS-ADRDA criteria for AD

These are similar to the DSM-IV criteria, but also require histopathological evidence on biopsy or autopsy to diagnose definite AD. 'Probably AD' is diagnosed on clinical grounds alone. 'Possible AD' is dementia with atypical onset, presentation or progression; and without known aetiology, but no alternative diagnosis better explains symptoms.

NINDS-AIREN criteria for vascular dementia

Cerebrovascular disease defined by the presence of focal signs on neurological examination consistent with stroke and evidence of cerebrovascular disease on brain imaging.

The criteria require one or more of

a onset of dementia within 3 months of a diagnosed stroke

b abrupt deterioration in cognitive function

c fluctuating, stepwise progression of cognitive deficits.

Clinical features consistent with a diagnosis of probably vascular dementia include

a early gait disturbance

b unsteadiness or frequent, unprovoked falls

c early urinary frequency, urgency, or other symptoms not otherwise explained

d pseudobulbar palsy

e personality and mood changes, abulia (inability to take decisions), depression, emotional lability, or subcortical deficits including psychomotor retardation and abnormal executive functions.

International consensus criteria for dementia with Lewy Bodies

1 Progressive cognitive decline. Prominent memory impairment may not necessarily occur in the early stages but is usually evident with progression. Deficits on tests of attention and frontal-subcortical skills and visuospatial ability may be prominent.

2 In addition, two of the following are required for probable DLB:

• fluctuating cognition with variations in attention and alertness

• recurrent visual hallucinations, typically well-formed and detailed

• motor features of Parkinsonism.

3 Features supporting the diagnosis are:

• recurrent falls

• syncope or transient loss of consciousness

• neuroleptic sensitivity

• systematized delusions

• hallucinations in other modalities.

LUND-Manchester criteria for fronto-temporal dementia

All core components must be present:

1 Insidious onset and gradual progression

2 Early decline in social interpersonal conduct

3 Early impairment in regulation of personal conduct

4 Early emotional blunting

5 Early loss of insight

Supportive features include:

A Behavioural disorder

• decline in personal hygiene or grooming

• mental rigidity and inflexibility

• distractibility and impersistence

• hyperorality and dietary change

• utilization behaviour

B Speech and language: altered speech output (lack of spontaneity and economy of speech, pressure of speech), stereotypy of speech, echolalia, perseveration, mutism

C Physical signs: primitive reflexes, incontinence, akinesia, rigidity, tremor, low/labile blood pressure

D Investigations

• impaired frontal lobe tests; without amnesia or perceptual deficits

• normal EEG

• frontal or anterior temporal abnormalities on brain imaging.

Assessment and diagnosis

Diagnosis is primarily clinical and depends on:

1 a collateral cognitive history

2 examination of the mental state

3 cognitive testing

4 physical examination

5 observation of abilities and behaviour

6 follow-up

Dementia may present as memory loss. However, it is normal for memory and other cognitive functions to deteriorate with age, and memory loss alone is insufficient to make a diagnosis. Normal adaptation, compensation, and social reciprocity will mean that sometimes declining cognition will not be noticed, not cause problems, be dismissed as 'normal ageing', denied or suppressed, until a crisis emerges.

A crisis may be related to dementia (such as onset of difficult behaviour or problems related to poor judgement), social (death or illness of a key carer), environmental (going on holiday or into hospital) or a comorbid health problem, such as a physical illness, loss of function, or the onset of delirium.

This means that enquiry must probe, and look for hints that cognition was declining prior to the problem becoming overt. Where hospital admission is with a comorbid condition, the opportunity should be taken to review the dementia diagnosis, its progression and the problems that it is causing.

Ask:

• When were problems first noticed?

• How have things changed over time?

• What are the current problems? (forgetfulness, repetition, accusations?)

• What is the impact on function? Including falls, continence, driving and safety awareness.

• What support and care arrangements are in place: professional and family or informal care?

Mental state examination is a combination of questioning and observing (much is embedded within a good 'geriatric medical clerking'). This includes:

• Record appearance, behaviour, speech, mood, and cognition.

• Specifically ask about delusions and hallucinations (has anything been happening to you that you can't explain? has anyone being trying to harm you? Do you see visions that other people don't seem to see?).

Assess insight, judgement and planning, and, if interventions are planned, capacity to consent.

Both receptive and expressive language function can be affected in dementia, but look out for 'pure' aphasia (due to stroke or tumour) being mistaken for dementia.

For formal cognitive testing, the Abbreviated Mental Test Score is reasonable for use in acute or general medical settings, but otherwise use the Folstein Mini Mental State Examination. The revised Addenbrooke's Cognitive Examination (ACE-R) is better still, with more domain coverage, but longer. Get a formal neuropsychological assessment where there is diagnostic doubt or where there is a specific problem to address (such as work performance).

Ask professional staff (care home staff, ward nurses, or therapists) for details of observed function, or specific functional assessments.

Carefully consider the possibility of super-added delirium and the role of any drugs taken (anticholinergic drugs worsen cognition, these and others may cause delirium).

Early diagnosis is beneficial because it allows time for planning the future while mental capacity is preserved, and the early institution of support, which may prevent or delay crises and the need for care home placement. However, the earlier the diagnosis is made, the more uncertain it is. In these cases, follow up over 6 months to a year or more may be required to monitor for progression.

Investigation

Investigation plays relatively little part in the diagnosis of dementia, although many patients and carers have high expectations of 'brain scans'. Current NICE guidance is that people with dementia should have structural imaging (CT or MRI). There are definable changes associated with AD. Visible infarcts or subcortical white matter ischaemic changes are required to diagnose vascular dementia, but imaging lacks specificity (abnormalities are common among people without dementia as well). Dementia cannot be diagnosed or excluded by a scan.

SPECT scanning may help in the diagnosis of AD where it is important to make this diagnosis. Ioflupane (DaT) scanning can fairly reliably diagnose or rule out DLB.

One purpose of a head scan is to rule out mimics, such as normal pressure hydrocephalus, subdural haematoma, or tumours. These are diagnosed in about 1% of cases where there is no clinical suspicion of an abnormality. Another is to contribute to making a diagnosis of vascular dementia.

Some tests of metabolic function and inflammation should be done to investigate the possibility of a coexisting delirium (U&E, FBC, CRP, calcium, glucose, LFT). Other commonly recommended tests include vitamin B12 and folate, thyroid function, and syphilis serology. It is sensible to exclude easily treatable comorbid conditions, but only rarely, if ever, will these be the cause of a 'treatable dementia'.

Family and carers

Family members and other informal carers, or networks of professional and informal care, have a special role in the lives of people with dementia. Relationships vary from overseeing and help with more difficult or demanding tasks, to very intensive hands-on supervision and care. Carers act as informants and advocates; health professionals must recognize and respect this role, and the insights carers may have into the life of someone with dementia.

Carers provide an indispensable source of information to guide assessment and decision-making. In most cases, it is in the interests of both the person with dementia and statutory services that this care is supported and maintained, often in the face of considerable carer strain. However, they may be tired, anxious or angry, and need considerable explanation and information about what is happening to the person with dementia. They have statutory rights of consultation on decisions under the Mental Capacity Act 2005. A partnership approach is necessary.

Treatment and care

Objectives of treatment:
- maximize and maintain function
- minimize distress and disability
- support families and carers.

Approaches to treatment

Dementia is incurable and is sometimes described (perhaps unhelpfully) as a 'terminal condition'. The emphasis is on living well with dementia, maintaining activity, control, choice, and relationships to an extent compatible with the severity of the disease.

Much of this approach is familiar to geriatricians from rehabilitation practice, but as the disease is progressive and impairs learning ability, the philosophy differs from that familiar in physical diseases.

In common with other long-term neurological and psychiatric conditions, a number of 'phases' can be distinguished:
- early: goals are diagnosis (and excluding other explanations for problems), information, education and support, advance planning
- middle: disability and dependency increase, increasing help and support is required, and poor management is prone to making matters worse
- late: associated with severe disability, and intensive care needs provided at home or in a care home
- end of life care.

Provision of information (diagnosis, explanation and prognostication) has value. Early stage planning might include retirement from work, deciding about continuing driving, making a will, discussing future care options (such as an Advance Decision to Refuse Treatment or a Statement of Wishes and Preferences), arranging a Lasting Power of Attorney and considering a move to sheltered accommodation. Use of cognitive enhancing drugs and non-pharmacological means of supporting cognition should be considered.

The middle phase requires maintenance of function and morale. 'Decompensation' is a major risk, due to illness or disruption of familiar environment and routine. Crises can develop quickly, so mechanisms for surveillance and ready access to support are necessary to anticipate and react to problems if they occur. Intercurrent physical illness brings a high risk of losing abilities; especial effort should be directed at preserving these, and on recovery, attempts made at restoration. However, abilities will also be lost with disease progression and ultimately, 'restorative' rehabilitation will inevitably fail. Instead, 'adaptive rehabilitation' aims to identify and provide support in continuing to perform tasks (shopping, kitchen, basic activities of daily living) where independence is no longer possible. In this phase, it is easy for a person with dementia to be ignored, lose social contact, be deprived of choice and the chance to make decisions: so-called loss of 'personhood'. The result is often distress, which may be communicated through disturbed behaviours. The philosophy of 'person centred care' aims to avert this.

The late phase sees progressive loss of communication and function, often with falls or immobility, incontinence, and poor nutrition. The person with dementia is frail (prone to crises and deteriorations) and may suffer frequent intercurrent physical illnesses and complications, including infections, pressure sores and fractures.

The approach of the end of life can be difficult to predict, but as increasing disability and frailty progress the focus of medical management shifts towards comfort and dignity, rather than the prevention or aggressive management of physical illness.

Swallowing and appetite may fail. If the patient's swallow is deemed 'unsafe' (due to the risk of aspiration), the approach is different from that familiar in stroke, unless there is a short-term intercurrent illness that may account for the swallowing failure. Emphasis is given to maintaining oral feeding, using the safest possible consistencies (often, thickened fluids, and a soft or pureed diet). Tube feeding is rarely tolerated well, nor makes much difference to outcome. Short-term corticosteroids (prednisolone 15 mg/day for 2 weeks) sometimes helps with appetite failure.

Self-fulfilling prophesy is a potential problem. Many people with dementia who are acutely ill may appear to be dying, but recover with treatment. Admission to hospital should not be excluded but requires clear consideration of its purpose and of possible alternatives.

Person-centred dementia care

Current best practice dementia care attempts to respect the person with dementia as an individual, with a history (biography), values, preferences, and the right to make choices. This aims to enhance engagement and enjoyment of life, preserve abilities, and avoid or defuse distress or disturbed behaviour.

How we see a person with dementia depends on five factors. All are important:

- neurological impairment
- biography
- personality
- social psychology (how other people interact with them)
- physical health.

The approach can be counterintuitive. People usually respond to unusual behaviour by confronting, correcting, or admonishing. This is unlikely to be understood by someone with poor language, reasoning, and abstract thought skills and invariably makes matters worse. Person-centred care seeks to maximize positive interactions and experiences ('personal enhancers'), such as comforting or including, while avoiding negative ones ('personal detractors') such as ignoring, outpacing, threats, or mocking.

This can be demanding for carers when behaviours are persistent or repeated, and the usual rules of response and reciprocity don't apply. Purposeful activity is used to enable engagement and a give sense of achievement. This provides a diversion and distraction, both to avoid distress behaviours and as a 'treatment' for them. The aim is to make 'connections' with retained abilities. These can include talking (often using the biography as a source of relevant personal information), games, personal care, or domestic tasks.

Person-centred care is best delivered proactively and consistently, by the whole team (be it in a care home, acute hospital, or other setting). This requires training and supervision, as it can be emotionally draining. It requires the development and sustaining of a three-way relationship between patient, staff, and family caregivers, with some

thinkers emphasizing 'relationship-centred care' focusing on senses of security, continuity, belonging, purpose, achievement, and significance.

Cognitive enhancement

Drugs (donepezil, rivastigmine, galantamine) are effective in AD and DLB but the size of the effect is small (in trials a mean difference from placebo of only 1 MMSE point) and they are not side-effect free (including gastrointestinal, cardiac conduction, and urinary symptoms). The impact on important higher level outcomes such as quality of life, disability, and institutional placement is more uncertain (but probably mirrors that for cognitive function). However, there is variation in response to drugs for different individuals. Fifteen per cent to 20% are 'super-responders' with an improvement of 4 or more MMSE points. NICE guidance restricts prescription to those with mild to moderate disease (MMSE of >10, with caveats about its interpretation with language, sensory impairment, education, and learning disability) and the need for regular reassessment of response. Memantine has a similar small effect on patients with moderate to severe disease. The effect is a step change without any impact on the rate of deterioration.

Systems, such as a memory service, are required to assess, deliver and monitor treatment, and shared care protocols for primary care need to be in place.

How to communicate to someone with dementia

Implicit memory may be preserved even when explicit memory is poor. This is responsible for many motor behaviours (e.g. walking), but also in recognizing emotions and threats. Friendliness, courteousness, and non-confrontation count for a lot. Engaging the person in conversation, listening, and talking to them may be a relatively rare event and can help establish a relationship even when language content is weak. A handshake, smile, and a calm friendly voice can be disarming in difficult situations.

Conversation will change for everyone with dementia. Some people will have aphasia, both receptive, or expressive, as well as memory and other cognitive problems impacting on communication.

Be clear about the purpose of the conversation. If it is to gain specific information, you will probably need to speak to a family carer or other informant. If it is to engage or comfort, take it slowly. Avoid direct questioning; instead, make a comment and wait for a response. Use your knowledge of the person's past to raise a topic of mutual interest. Find something in the environment to comment on or discuss.

Additional strategies that can be helpful to support those with language difficulties include

- speaking simply in short sentences
- avoiding jargon, complex, or abstract ideas
- repeat if necessary
- give time to respond
- make use of gesture, or pictures
- speak as if speaking to a competent, but non-fluent, second-language English-speaker.

Do not get angry or try to argue or reason. Challenging misperceptions or mistaken reality is unlikely to be helpful (e.g. someone 'living in the past' asking for a dead husband or mother). Instead, use the opportunity to ask about the people involved or to explore the emotional content behind requests. For example, someone asking for their mother may feel abandoned and afraid; the resolution will be to find a way to offer reassurance and comfort.

People with dementia may not be able to communicate well verbally, but they may be better at communicating on an emotional level. Be aware of:

- facial expression
- eye contact
- touch and bodily contact
- voice characteristics: loud, annoyed, happy
- non-verbal vocalization: humming, groaning
- gesture and body movement.

Family members may be able to understand more. Dementia specialist speech and language therapists may also be able to help but are few and far between.

Distress responses

These are also called behaviours that challenge, difficult, or disturbed behaviour, non-cognitive symptoms or behavioural, and psychological symptoms of dementia (BPSD).

There is a high premium on making non-drug approaches work (such as person-centred care).

Psychological responses include depression and anxiety. In the person-centred care philosophy behaviours represent communication of an unmet need. Difficult behaviour represents distress that has to be understood and addressed. Person-centred care aims to prevent or minimize distress.

Response to drugs is generally disappointing. No drug is markedly successful for any symptom or behaviour. There is evidence that risperidone (0.5–1 mg/day) has a small effect in relieving 'aggressive agitation'. But antipsychotic drugs are associated with shorter survival and carry an increased risk of stroke. They are particularly poorly tolerate in DLB, where quetiapine (starting at 25 mg at night) is the best choice if absolutely necessary.

Antipsychotic drugs may relieve psychosis, anxiety, or, more uncertainly, delirium. If these are driving distress, and if, as 'palliative drugs', one is found to be genuinely effective for relieving distress in a given individual, the risks may be acceptable. SSRIs are disappointing in managing depression. Mirtazepine and trazodone may be tried for anxiety. Long-acting benzodiazepines are also disappointing and may accumulate or cause paradoxical agitation. Short-acting benzodiazepines or clomethiazole can be justified for night sedation. All increase the risk of falling.

The key is to try things, but to follow up assiduously and critically to judge if any effect is beneficial or not. Rating scales may help in deciding. However, symptoms often fluctuate with time and apparently beneficial changes may not be casually related to starting a drug. In any case, antipsychotic or other psychotropic drugs should be reviewed at least every 3 months and a trial of stopping considered.

Decision-making

Western culture values and respects autonomy. Cognitive impairment challenges the presumptions behind the exercise of autonomy; reasoning and judgement may be impaired, making decision-making difficult, and people with dementia open to exploitation or risk. English and Scottish law is well developed in this field (in England, the Mental Capacity Act 2005).

Assessment of capacity requires examination of abilities to

- understand information relevant to the decision
- retain it for long enough

- use it to weight up options
- communicate a decision.

Relevant information includes the nature, purpose, and consequences of an intervention, any alternatives and the likely consequences of refusal. Understanding need only be in broad terms and the degree of understanding can vary with the gravity or complexity of the decision.

For someone lacking capacity, English law makes provision for a proxy to be involved (if appointed in advance or by a Court: a health and welfare Lasting Power of Attorney, or a court-appointed deputy), or for a decision-maker to assess best interests and act accordingly.

Assessing best interests is not always easy. It requires involvement of the person lacking capacity, using any means possible to help aid understanding, and respecting any values and preferences, previously, or currently expressed. Family or other carers have a statutory right to be consulted and have their opinion heard. The least restrictive alternative is to be favoured. All this presumes that a feasible, effective, and reasonably safe intervention is proposed, although judging this may also be open to discussion. Balancing different viewpoints can be difficult. Sometimes a trial of one option (such as living alone at home) is necessary to establish feasibility, in the face of strongly expressed views, even when success is unlikely.

Dementia in hospital

About 25% of adult acute hospital beds are occupied by people with dementia. As many as half of these cases are diagnosed for the first time in hospital.

The great majority of people with dementia who are admitted to general hospitals are admitted appropriately. On average, people with dementia admitted to hospital are more severely ill (on the basis of physiological scores) and are often very dependent (25% have a Barthel Index worse than 5/20, often representing a rapid decline from baseline function).

Dementia in hospital is very different from that seen in community settings. Acute hospitals see patients in crisis:

- with comorbid delirium
- with comorbid physical illness or injury
- with a functional problem such as a fall or inability to cope.

Dementia and delirium

Half to two-thirds of people with dementia in hospital have superadded delirium. History is key in detecting a sudden change in cognition, behaviour or function, night-time disturbance, and fluctuation. Family members and carers tend to be better at detecting these changes than healthcare staff. Nurse reports may be useful, but continuity is often poor, and many staff will not recognize what they are seeing.

Preponderence of vascular dementia

Most dementia cases in hospital (60%) are vascular. This is because of associated falls or physical disability, and because the steps in a stepwise decline look like delirium (and in many cases will be diagnosable as delirium). Most cases of 'delirium' where a physical cause remains elusive are presumed to be due to cerebrovascular disease.

Environment

Acute hospital processes and environment are not well suited to people with dementia and often serve to make their symptoms and behaviour worse. Much 'difficult' behaviour can be explained by fear or misinterpretation in someone who cannot make sense of an environment they do not understand, and who cannot communicate effectively; they have 'decompensated'.

Emergency Departments and Medical Admissions Units are busy, noisy, uncomfortable, and lack continuity of staff, and are the source of much unhappiness. There are many strange faces and repeated intensive questioning. Location may be changed rapidly and repeatedly as the admission pathway is followed. Wards and bed spaces are often bland, with identical bays mitigating against correct orientation. Lack of personal space can lead to conflict with other patients and an exaggerated impact of noise. Radios are arousing and altering. Night time noise contributes to already difficult sleeping conditions. Signage and contrast need to take account of agnosia (pictures and words) and comorbid visual problems.

Activity

Modern hospitals assume a narrow biomedical care model and short lengths of stay. You sort the physical problem and discharge. In practice, of course, life is not so simple. Multiple comorbidities, complications, and disabilities contribute to a range of lengths of stay. Provision must therefore be made for those who stay longer. Structured activity serves two purposes: maintenance of skills (dressing, kitchen) and diversion of attention to avert boredom and distress behaviours. This can be difficult to provide when staff are busy. One solution is to make the most of routine care tasks, such as getting washed and dressed, or eating a meal. Unregistered staff (healthcare assistants) and volunteers can lead on leisure activities, if possible directed by an occupational therapist or interested registered nurse.

Discharge

Discharge requires a lot of information and careful planning. It may be easy if the person with dementia was previously resident in a care home or had well-established home care support and function had not changed from previously. However, loss of function during times of intercurrent illness, presentation with a crisis when no previous formal care arrangements were in place, or where progression of disease has led to a collapse in care arrangements, all require considerable effort to make it safe and sustainable. Multidisciplinary functional and risk assessments, and close liaison with family, other informal carers and adult social care are required. Sometimes a 'trial of discharge' is needed, where the best future arrangements are uncertain, or the patient or family contest an apparent need for care home placement (as part of a formal assessment of best interests under the MCA 2005). Specialist mental health intermediate care or community mental health teams may provide additional support.

Long-term support

In the UK, long-term support is based in primary care, although patients and their families would prefer specialist follow up. Community mental health teams, and in particular, community psychiatric nurses supported by old age psychiatrists, provide most long-term surveillance and advice where there are behavioural or psychological problems, including supporting care homes. However, they usually lack the capacity to follow up all people with dementia. Other models of community nursing support focus on the needs of carers (such as 'Admiral nurses' in the UK).

This approach can be controversial, but services are popular with clients.

Specialist adult social care (social services) support for people with dementia, typically providing more flexibility, better staff continuity, additional training and liaison with community mental health teams is preferable to standard service models.

'Telecare' uses remotely monitored electronic devices to enable emergency assistance to be summoned (e.g. pendent alarms). Most telecare mitigates harm by alerting family or other carers to events, but can potentially play a more proactive monitoring or preventative role. Systems can detect falls, environmental changes such as floods, fire and gas leaks, and give an alert if someone enters or leaves the house (see Chapter 26, Gerotechnology). Supporting people with dementia is a key goal, but taking full advantage requires sufficient cognitive ability. Repeated 'false alarms' quickly make response untenable.

Care homes

In the UK, 70% of care home residents have dementia. Care homes both with and without nursing can be registered to look after people with dementia.

At least a quarter of people with dementia in care homes take anti-psychotic medication, a cause of considerable concern. Poor staffing numbers and training likely contribute to lack of non-pharmacological management regimens such as person-centred care.

The decision as to when a care home is necessary for a person with dementia can be difficult and will vary greatly between individuals. Factors include the degree of physical and mental disability, available support and degree of carer strain, previously expressed wishes, and family views. Safety awareness and tolerance of risk are key variables. Falling at night, wandering outside and unsafe use of cooking and heating appliances are particular problems. When things go wrong, the result is often unpleasant and inconvenient (e.g. spending the night on the floor, or being found wandering by the police), rather than catastrophic (e.g. causing an accident or breaking a hip); some people and their families will be willing to tolerate such risk, others not.

Care homes are not without problems but can provide for social contact and activities that would be impossible for a very disabled older person living alone in their own home. In some cases, making this move earlier rather than later can enable someone to establish friendships and routines while they still have the ability to do so. However, any change in residence is disruptive, and it can take several weeks for a person with dementia to 'settle', during which time distress and difficult behaviour may be evident. Care must be taken to support this period, not to make a premature decision about further relocation, and to minimize the temptation to use antipsychotic drugs (or to make sure they are reviewed within 3 months if they are used).

Medical care is the responsibility of general practitioners and there are a wide variety of models of providing this, often fragmented and inconsistent. There may in addition be support from community psychiatric nurses. The role of the care home manager is crucial in planning, decision-making and access to healthcare.

Prognosis

Survival with dementia varies with age at diagnosis, and comorbidity:

• 11 years at age 60–69 years

- 5 years at age 70–79 years
- 4 years at age 80–89 years.

Four years after diagnosis of dementia, severity will be moderate in 70% and half will be in institutional care.

Difficult behaviours may remit over a period of 3–6 months. Drug treatments should be reviewed regularly and withdrawn if ineffective or no longer clearly needed. As the disease progresses, the onset of immobility may make some symptoms (such as wandering and falling) easier to manage. A palliative (or 'supportive') philosophy, seeking to maximize dignity and comfort above investigation and cure, are the order of the day in late stage dementia.

Further reading

National Institute for Health and Clinical Excellence; Social Care Institute for Excellence (2006). *Guideline on supporting people with dementia and their carers in health and social care*. National Clinical Practice Guideline Number 42. London, British Psychological Society/Gaskell (www.nice.org.uk).

Office of the Public Guardian (2009). Making decisions A guide for family, friends and other unpaid carers. OPG 602. Office of the Public Guardian, London (http://www.publicguardian.gov.uk/docs/opg-602–0409.pdf).

Waite J, Harwood RH, Morton IR, *et al.* (2008). *Dementia Care: a Practical Manual*. Oxford Care Manuals. Oxford, OUP.

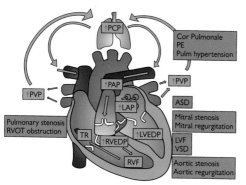

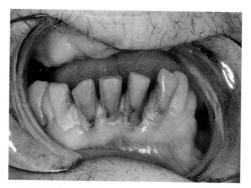

Plate 1 (see Figure 5.12) Backward pressure paradigm; increased pressures from any area of cardiopulmonary circulation can lead to back pressure on the right ventricle, subsequent pressure overload and ultimately RV dysfunction. Stages in backward pressure with pathologies are highlighted. LVEDP, left ventricular end diastolic pressure; LAP, left atrial pressure; PVP, pulmonary venous pressure; PCP, pulmonary capillary pressure; PAP, pulmonary artery pressure; RVEDP, right ventricular end diastolic pressure; RVF, right ventricular failure; TR, tricuspid regurgitation.

Plate 3 (see Figure 7.1) Plaque on teeth. Victoria Ewan and Konrad Staines, Diagnosis and management of oral mucosal lesions in older people: a review, *Reviews in Clinical Gerontology*, **18**, 2, pp. 115–28, reproduced with permission. Copyright Cambridge University Press.

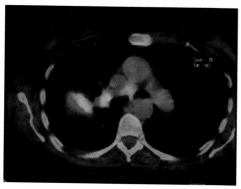

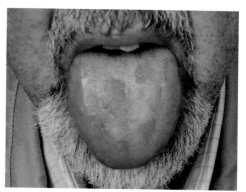

Plate 4 (see Figure 7.2) Geographic tongue. Victoria Ewan and Konrad Staines, Diagnosis and management of oral mucosal lesions in older people: a review, *Reviews in Clinical Gerontology*, **18**, 2, pp. 115–28, reproduced with permission. Copyright Cambridge University Press.

Plate 2 (see Figure 6.5) Fluorodeoxyglucose (FDG) positron emission tomography–computed tomography scan showing high FDG uptake in right mid zone tumour, right hilar and subcarinal lymph glands.

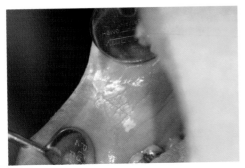

Plate 5 (see Figure 7.3) Chronic hyperplastic candidosis. Victoria Ewan and Konrad Staines, Diagnosis and management of oral mucosal lesions in older people: a review, *Reviews in Clinical Gerontology*, **18**, 2, pp. 115–28, reproduced with permission. Copyright Cambridge University Press.

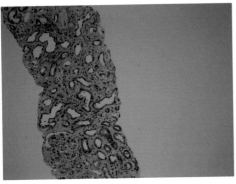

Plate 6 (see Figure 9.1) A&E stain taken from a biopsy from an older man. The large amount of green stain demonstrates widespread interstitial fibrosis.

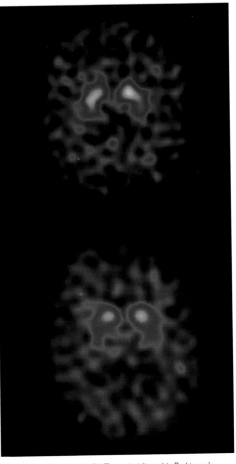

Plate 7 (see Figure 13.1) DAT scan in idiopathic Parkinson's disease.

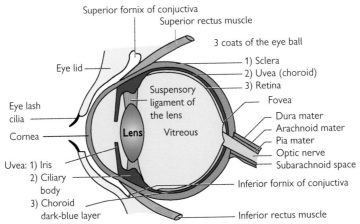

Plate 8 (see Figure 14.3) Anatomy and physiology of vision. Reproduced from Judith Collier, Murray Longmore, and Mark Brinsden, *Oxford Handbook of Clinical Specialties* (7th edition), 2007, figure on page 433, with permission from Oxford University Press.

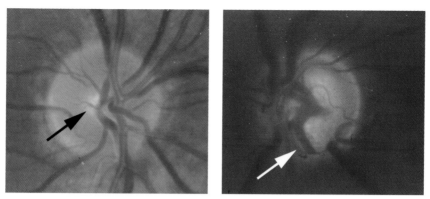

Plate 9 (see Figure 14.6) Normal optic disc (left). The black arrow points to the edge of the optic disc cup which occupies <30% of the disc area. Compare this with the glaucomatous optic disc (right) where the cup occupies around 80% of the disc area and the surrounding rim is pathologically thin. The white arrow points to a very thin area of optic disc rim (notch). Reproduced from Moorfields Eye Hospital with permission.

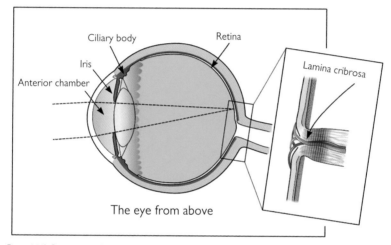

Plate 10 (see Figure 14.8) Cross-sectional drawing of the eye showing the position of the *lamina cribrosa* and the optic nerve in relation to the other major structures. Reproduced from Moorfields Eye Hospital with permission. Figure kindly drawn by Alan Lacey.

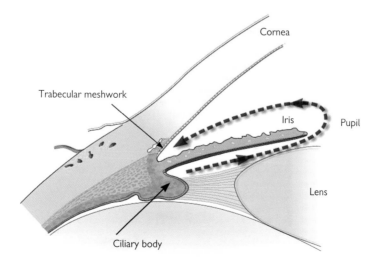

Plate 11 (see Figure 14.9) Cross-section of the anterior chamber periphery demonstrating the normal pathway of aqueous humour flow. Reproduced from Moorfields Eye Hospital with permission. Figure kindly drawn by Alan Lacey.

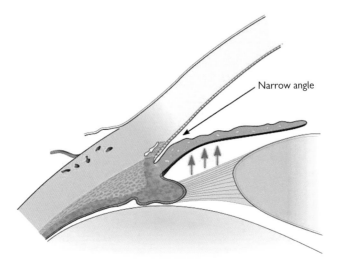

Narrow angle

Plate 12 (see Figure 14.10) Cross-section of the anterior chamber periphery showing the anatomical changes that occur in angle closure secondary to pupillary block. Reproduced from Moorfields Eye Hospital with permission. Figure kindly drawn by Alan Lacey.

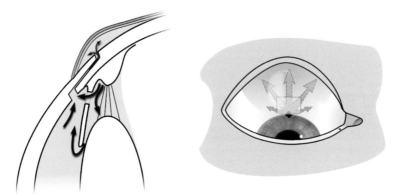

Plate 13 (see Figure 14.11) In a trabeculectomy operation, aqueous exits the anterior chamber through a guarded sclerostomy (a partial thickness flap in the sclera) to a drainage bleb at the superior conjunctival limbus, from whence it is reabsorbed via the venous system. Reproduced from Moorfields Eye Hospital with permission. Figure kindly drawn by Alan Lacey.

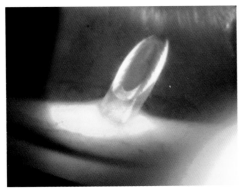

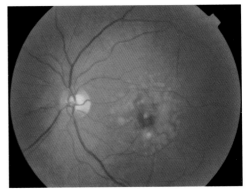

Plate 14 (see Figure 14.12) Aqueous shunts (commonly called *tubes* or *glaucoma drainage devices*) usually involve insertion of a small silicone tube of approximately 600 µm diameter into the anterior chamber (illustrated), which drains aqueous to a conjunctival bleb over an external plate. Reproduced from Moorfields Eye Hospital with permission.

Plate 15 (see Figure 14.13) Colour fundus photo of left macular showing soft drusen. Reproduced from Venki Sundaram, Allon Barsam, Amar Alwitry, and Peng T. Khaw, *Training in Ophthalmology*, 2009, Figure 4.31, p. 170, with permission from Oxford University Press.

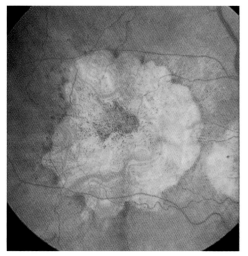

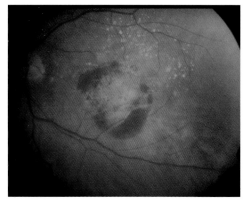

Plate 17 (see Figure 14.15) Colour fundus photo of macular haemorrhage due to choroidal neovascular membrane

Plate 16 (see Figure 14.14) Colour fundus photo of right macular showing large area of geographic atrophy. Reproduced from Venki Sundaram, Allon Barsam, Amar Alwitry, and Peng T. Khaw, *Training in Ophthalmology*, 2009, Figure 4.32, p. 171, with permission from Oxford University Press.

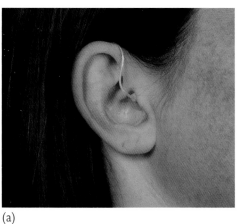

(a)

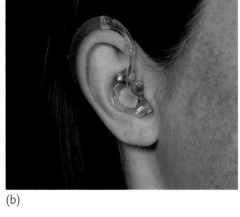

(b)

Plate 18 (see Figure 14.23) Inserting the earmould.

Plate 19 (see Figure 22.1) Crusted scabies.

Plate 20 (see Figure 22.2) Multiple lesions of nodular prurigo on lower legs.

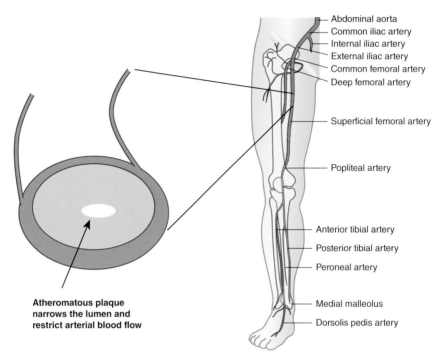

- Abdominal aorta
- Common iliac artery
- Internal iliac artery
- External iliac artery
- Common femoral artery
- Deep femoral artery
- Superficial femoral artery
- Popliteal artery
- Anterior tibial artery
- Posterior tibial artery
- Peroneal artery
- Medial malleolus
- Dorsolis pedis artery

Atheromatous plaque narrows the lumen and restrict arterial blood flow

Plate 21 (see Figure 23.2) Pathogenesis of arterial ulcers. Is associated most commonly with atheroma formation from atherosclerosis. The large artery walls accumulate lipid that induces local inflammation and intimal proliferation; progressively leading to narrowing of the lumen. The distal blood supply gradually reduces and as the lumen narrows, beyond the watershed tissues undergo atrophy. Occasionally, the atheromatous plaque will rupture and either embolize or thrombose, whereupon the affected distal tissues suddenly become necrotic. The distribution of tissue atrophy and necrosis follows the distribution of the arterial branches that are involved. Arterial flow duplex scan can be used to determine the size, location and blood flow; thus provide useful information regarding the need for surgical intervention.

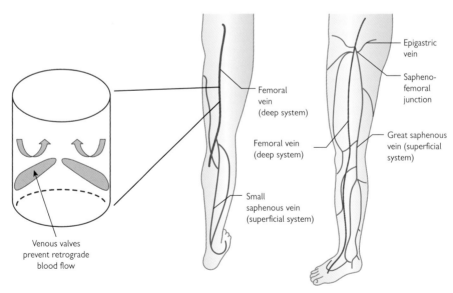

- Epigastric vein
- Sapheno-femoral junction
- Femoral vein (deep system)
- Great saphenous vein (superficial system)
- Femoral vein (deep system)
- Small saphenous vein (superficial system)

Venous valves prevent retrograde blood flow

Plate 22 (see Figure 23.3) Anatomy of venous valves. Venous valves maintain blood flow back to the heart. When these valves are absent or destroyed by thrombosis, there is increased venous pressure. In such cases, contraction of the calf muscle pump results in retrograde flow, which is normally prevented by the presence of the venous valve, thus further increasing venous pressures at the ankle. This in turn leads to varicosities and local tissue oedema, a prelude to venous ulceration.

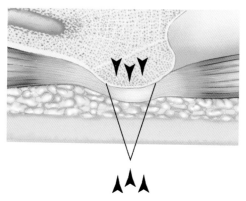

Plate 23 (see Figure 23.6) Distribution of external pressure at the bone/muscle interface.

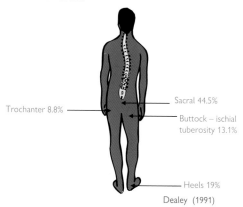

Trochanter 8.8%

Sacral 44.5%

Buttock – ischial tuberosity 13.1%

Heels 19%

Dealey (1991)

Plate 24 (see Figure 23.7) Common sites of pressure ulceration. Reproduced from Dealey, C., The size of the pressure-sore problem in a teaching hospital, *Journal of Advanced Nursing*, **16**, 6, pp. 663-70, Copyright Wiley 1991, with permission.

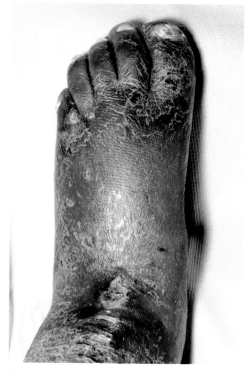

Plate 25 (see Figure 23.9) Feet and toe pressure ulcers.

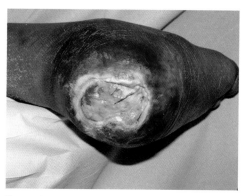

Plate 26 (see Figure 23.10) Heel pressure ulcer.

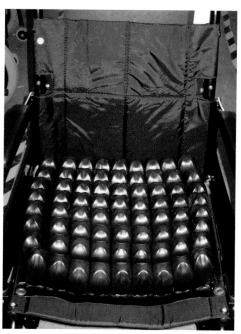

Plate 27 (see Figure 23.11) ROHO cushion.

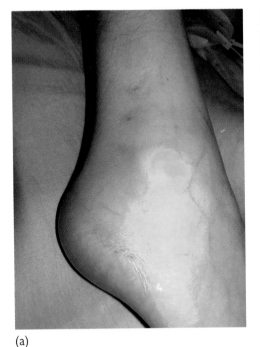

(a)

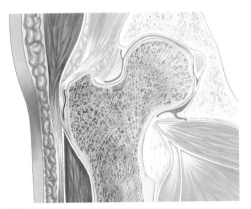

(b)

Plate 28a and b (see Figure 23.12a and b) *Category/stage I: non-blanchable redness of intact skin*. Intact skin with non-blanchable erythema of a localized area usually over a bony prominence. Discoloration of the skin, warmth, oedema, hardness or pain may also be present. Darkly pigmented skin may not have visible blanching. Further description: the area may be painful, firm, soft, warmer, or cooler than adjacent tissue. Category/Stage it may be difficult to detect in individuals with dark skin tones. May indicate 'at risk' persons.

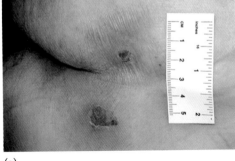

(a)

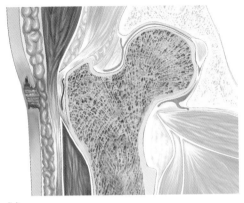

(b)

Plate 29a and b (see Figure 23.13a and b) *Category/stage II: partial thickness skin loss or blister*. Partial thickness loss of dermis presenting as a shallow open ulcer with a red/pink wound bed, without slough. May also present as an intact or open/ruptured serumfilled or sero-sanginous filled blister. Further description: presents as a shiny or dry shallow ulcer without slough or bruising. This category/stage should not be used to describe skin tears, tape burns, incontinence associated dermatitis, maceration or excoriation.

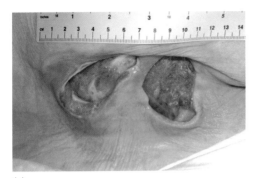

(a)

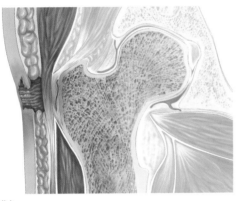

(b)

Plate 30a and b (see Figure 23.14a and b) *Category/stage III: full thickness skin loss (fat visible).* Full thickness tissue loss. Subcutaneous fat may be visible but bone, tendon or muscle are not exposed. Some slough may be present. May include undermining and tunnelling. Further description: the depth of a Category/Stage III pressure ulcer varies by anatomical location. The bridge of the nose, ear, occiput and malleolus do not have (adipose) subcutaneous tissue and Category/Stage III ulcers can be shallow. In contrast, areas of significant adiposity can develop extremely deep Category/Stage III pressure ulcers. Bone/tendon is not visible or directly palpable.

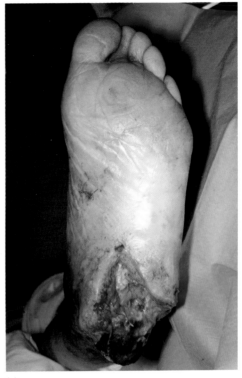

(a)

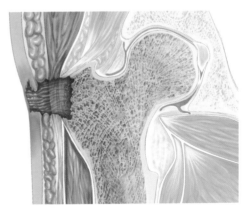

(b)

Plate 31a and b (see Figure 23.15a and b) *Category/stage IV: full thickness tissue loss (muscle/bone visible).* Full thickness tissue loss with exposed bone, tendon or muscle. Slough or eschar may be present. Often include undermining and tunnelling. Further description: the depth of a Category/Stage IV pressure ulcer varies by anatomical location. The bridge of the nose, ear, occiput and malleolus do not have (adipose) subcutaneous tissue and these ulcers can be shallow. Category/Stage IV ulcers can extend into muscle and/or supporting structures (e.g., fascia, tendon or joint capsule) making osteomyelitis or osteitis likely to occur. Exposed bone/muscle is visible or directly palpable.

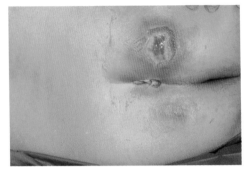

Plate 32 (see Figure 23.16) Slough on buttock pressure ulcer.

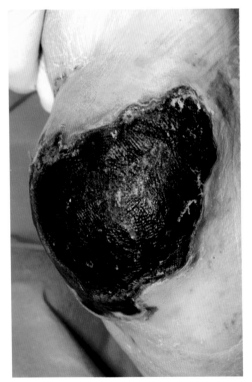

Plate 33 (see Figure 23.17) Eschar on heel pressure ulcer.

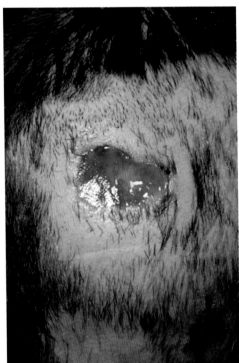

Plate 34 (see Figure 23.18) Locally infected scalp pressure ulcer.

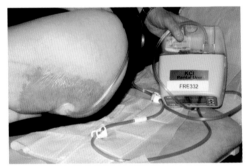

Plate 35 (see Figure 23.19) Negative pressure device *in situ*.

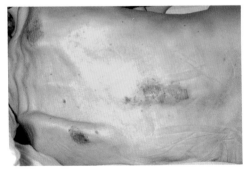

Plate 36 (see Figure 23.20) Pressure ulcers in cachectic patient with terminal illness.

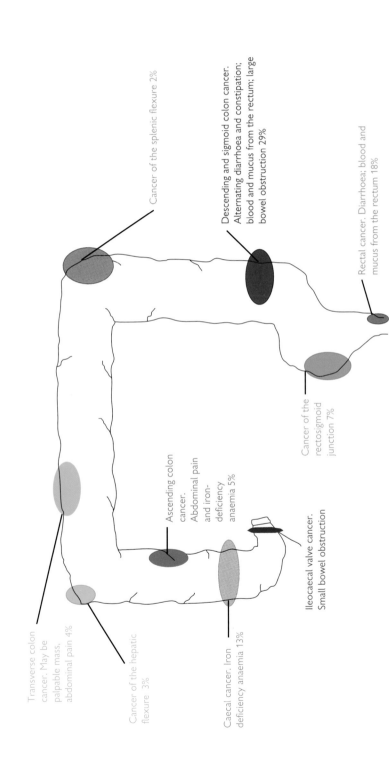

Cancer of the splenic flexure 2%

Descending and sigmoid colon cancer. Alternating diarrhoea and constipation; blood and mucus from the rectum; large bowel obstruction 29%

Rectal cancer. Diarrhoea; blood and mucus from the rectum 18%

Cancer of the rectosigmoid junction 7%

Ascending colon cancer. Abdominal pain and iron-deficiency anaemia 5%

Ileocaecal valve cancer. Small bowel obstruction

Caecal cancer. Iron deficiency anaemia 13%

Transverse colon cancer. May be palpable mass, abdominal pain 4%

Cancer of the hepatic flexure 3%

Plate 37 (see Figure 24.1) Clinical presentation of colorectal cancers by site and the percentages that occur at each site. Data from Cancer Research UK figures for distribution of cases by site within the large bowel. Data relate to diagnoses in England 1997–2000

Delirium

Background

Delirium is an organic psychiatric syndrome: a psychological response to a physical illness. It is a syndrome and not a disease and there can be many underlying medical causes. The main reason it is often poorly managed is that doctors and nurses either fail to recognize the psychological symptoms or, even worse, they wrongly attribute the symptoms to a primary psychiatric illness, such as schizophrenia, depression, or dementia. Early recognition and correct diagnosis is crucial and improves outcome. The standard criteria for diagnosis of delirium are described in the Diagnostic and Statistical Manual of Mental Disorders (DSM IV) (1994) and are:

1 Disturbance of consciousness (i.e. reduced clarity of awareness of the environment) with reduced ability to focus, sustain or shift attention.

2 A change in cognition (such as memory deficit, disorientation, language disturbance) or the development of a perceptual disturbance that is not better accounted for by a pre-existing, established or evolving dementia.

3 The disturbance develops over a short period of time (usually hours to days) and tends to fluctuate during the course of the day.

4 There is evidence from the history, physical examination and laboratory findings that the disturbance is caused by the direct physiological consequence of a general medical condition.

The main symptoms of delirium are recent onset of fluctuating awareness, impairment of memory and attention, and disorganized thinking. There may also be hallucinations (especially visual) and disturbance of the sleep–wake cycle. There are three clinical subtypes of delirium: (a) hyperactive (characterized by agitation, delusions and hallucinations); (b) hypoactive (characterized by a sleepy state, lethargy and sometimes misdiagnosed as depression); (c) mixed (patients can move between the two subtypes (a) and (b).

Delirium can be due to any medical illness, but especially infection, electrolyte disturbances, and respiratory, cardiac, or renal failure. Delirium may also be due to drugs or drug withdrawal, for example benzodiazepine withdrawal. Delirium due to alcohol withdrawal (delirium tremens) is very common and requires special management and is not considered in this section.

Table 12.1 Confusion Assessment Method (CAM)

	Score
1. Is there a history of recent onset of confusion that has fluctuated?	0 or 1
And:	
2. Attention impaired (count backwards from 20)?	0 or 1
And either:	
3. Is there disorganized thinking or incoherent speech?	0 or 1
Or:	
4. Is the patient sleepy, lethargic or stuporose?	0 or 1
Score 3 or more = consider delirium	

Delirium is a very common problem in modern hospitals. Roughly 15% of all medical and surgical inpatients are or become delirious (up to 30% on geriatric medicine wards and 50% post hip fracture patients). Despite its frequency, delirium is missed in at least one third of older inpatients by clinical teams. The development of delirium is associated with mortality rates of 25–30%, increased morbidity, functional decline, considerably extended length of stay, and an increased requirement for institutional care. At least half of patients with delirium will have an underlying dementia.

Pathophysiology

There are two main theories as to the pathophysiology of delirium. The first is the 'cholinergic hypothesis' and that the symptoms of delirium are due to reduced cholinergic transmission in the brain. This is supported by the observation that serum levels of anticholinergic activity are elevated in patients with post-operative delirium and correlate with the severity of cognitive impairment. Thiamine deficiency, hypoxia and hypoglycaemia, all of which can cause delirium, are known to reduce the amount of acetylcholine in the brain. Dopamine activity is increased as a result of reduced cholinergic activity and excess levels of dopamine in the brain are known to cause florid visual hallucinations and delusions. Acetylcholinesterase inhibitor drugs should theoretically be useful in the treatment of delirium but, so far at least, results of randomized controlled trials have been disappointing.

A second proposed mechanism for delirium is that delirium is a result of increased inflammatory activity in the vulnerable brain as a result of an increase of proinflammatory cytokines which arise particularly in systemic infection. Although cytokines are not themselves neurotransmitters, it may also be that they exert their effect by causing increased levels of dopamine and reduction of acetylcholine levels in the brain. It is possible that although many physiological insults can result in delirium that there is a final common pathway which involves an imbalance of neurotransmitters, especially dopamine and acetylcholine. In many cases the process is reversible, but it is now being increasingly recognized that sometimes an episode of delirium may represent a progression or acceleration of a pre-existing cognitive decline.

Clinical assessment of older patients at risk or with potential delirium

Delirium should always be suspected in any older patient with a recent change in cognitive state or behaviour. The Confusion Assessment Method (CAM) is based on DSM IV and is a useful checklist (see Table 12.1).

The main risk factors for developing delirium are: (1) increasing age; (2) dementia; (3) severity of illness; (4) fracture of the neck of femur. Patients at risk and patients with suspected delirium should receive a multicomponent care package (see Table 4). This multicomponent care intervention has been shown to prevent delirium in up to a third of older patients at risk, and also improves outcomes in patients with delirium. All older patients (over 65) should have a routine cognitive assessment, such as the abbreviated mental test score (AMT) or six-item screener (SIS), or the Mini Mental State Examination (MMSE) (see Chapter 2, Comprehensive geriatric assessment) in order to detect patients with, or at risk of delirium.

Assessment of attention is particularly important in delirium recognition, and tests such as serial sevens or counting backwards from 20 to 1 can be used to detect inattention. A careful drug history should be taken in all patients with delirium (including any recent changes and 'over-the-counter drugs'). Patients should always be asked about alcohol intake. Drugs or alcohol withdrawal can cause a particularly severe hyperactive delirium. A collateral history should be taken from relatives and carers about any pre-existing cognitive problems. Carers and relatives are often over-protective and many underplay previous problems. Always ask about instrumental activities of daily living to get an idea of premorbid cognitive function. A full physical examination should be carried out looking for possible causes of delirium. The investigations required are listed below. A mid-stream specimen of urine for culture should be only taken if clinically indicated as asymptomatic bacteriuria is very common in this group of patients and unnecessary antibiotics may lead to *Clostridium difficile* infections in vulnerable patients.

Investigations for delirium

Essential

- Full blood count
- Urea and electrolytes
- Liver function tests and calcium
- Blood glucose
- Thyroid function Tests
- C-reactive protein
- ECG
- Chest radiograph

May be required

- Blood cultures
- Blood gases
- CT Head
- EEG
- MSSU for culture and sensitivity
- Sputum culture
- Lumbar puncture if meningitis suspected

Author's Tip

Always suspect delirium if there has been any sudden change in behaviour or mental state. If not sure, always investigate and treat as delirium first and review the diagnosis later.

Differential diagnosis

It is not surprising that delirium is sometimes mistaken for dementia. It is safer to assume delirium and manage appropriately if there is any doubt until the history becomes clearer. Dementia with Lewy bodies can be particularly difficult to distinguish from delirium, as attention in this condition is often poor and the confusion often fluctuates, often with visual hallucinations. The presence of parkinsonism makes dementia with Lewy bodies more likely. A collateral history from carers of previous symptoms may be helpful in making the distinction. Stroke can cause delirium, particularly lesions in the non-dominant hemisphere and anterior thalamus. However, sometimes stroke causing focal deficits, such as receptive dysphasia or apraxia, is sometimes mistaken for global cognitive impairment

and delirium. Hypoactive delirium may sometimes be mistaken for depression, but any sudden mood change in a patient with a physical illness should alert the clinician to the possibility of delirium.

Author's Tip

Always take a good collateral history from relatives and carers, but remember relatives often 'cover up' intellectual problems. Ask particularly about instrumental activities of daily living to assess premorbid cognitive function, e.g. use of telephone, paying bills, transport use (including driving), and compliance with medication. A crucial question to relatives is 'Can the person be left safely to care for themselves on their own overnight?' At least half of patients with delirium have a background of dementia.

Causes of delirium

Almost any physical illness or drug can cause delirium, as well as other factors such as sleep disturbance or change of routine. There may be several contributing causes in vulnerable patients. However, there are several common causes including infections, electrolyte disturbances, drugs, and drug withdrawal.

Common causes of delirium

- Drugs and drug withdrawal: especially opiates, tramadol, sedatives, antiparkinsonian drugs, anticholinergic drugs, and antidepressants
- Infection: especially chest, urinary and biliary
- Dehydration and electrolyte disturbances: especially hyponatraemia
- Hypercalcaemia
- Respiratory failure which may be due to chronic obstructive pulmonary disease,
- Pneumonia or pulmonary embolus
- Cardiac failure
- Renal failure
- Sensory impairment—vision and hearing
- Constipation
- Sleep deprivation
- Multiple contributing causes

Author's Tip

In severe hyperactive delirium, always suspect a drug cause or drug or alcohol withdrawal

---

Prevention of delirium

Delirium is not an inevitable consequence of hospitalization, and can be prevented in at least a third of cases by instituting a multicomponent intervention (see Table 4). This is desirable for all patients at risk, i.e. older patients (over 75 years), admitted to hospital with cognitive impairment, severe illness, or fracture neck of femur. The multicomponent intervention consists of providing a stable orientating rehabilitation environment, avoiding and treating hypoxia, dehydration, immobility and pain, optimizing vision and hearing, reviewing medication, and restoring a good sleep pattern. Frequent unnecessary ward moves should be avoided. These interventions are most easily applied on a ward delivering comprehensive geriatric assessment (CGA).

Management of delirium

The aim of management of delirium is to find and treat the underlying cause, to treat the symptoms, to avoid complications and to arrange discharge and follow-up. Treatment of the underlying cause may involve stopping culprit medications, treating infection with antibiotics, and treating dehydration, constipation, and electrolyte disturbances. Patients with delirium are often dehydrated and need fluid replacement; this may be difficult in a confused, uncooperative patient and subcutaneous fluids may be the best option. It may not be possible to complete all the necessary investigations in a very disturbed patient, in which case the clinician may have to treat on clinical suspicion, e.g. antibiotics for a presumed chest infection. Complications are common in delirium, including falls, pressure sores and over sedation. Using the same multicomponent interventions as in prevention has been shown to improve outcomes in delirium.

An important part of management is to explain to the relatives and carers the diagnosis of delirium and the proposed management plan and how they can help with recovery. Often relatives may be able to stay with the patient to help reorientate and reassure. In severely ill patients with delirium and without mental capacity it may be necessary to treat patients with delirium in their 'best interests' under the Mental Capacity Act. If a patient is severely distressed or severely agitated and at risk to themselves or others then they may need to be sedated. No drug is licensed for treatment of symptoms of delirium but haloperidol in small doses (0.5–1.0 mg.) orally or intramuscularly is an option. Olanzapine is an alternative. In patients with parkinsonism, lorazepam in similar low doses is a reasonable alternative. Use of sedation should be regularly reviewed (every 24 hours) and should not be continued for longer than a week, and only if absolutely necessary. One-to-one nursing is a far better option if available for acutely disturbed patients with delirium.

Multicomponent intervention for managing and preventing delirium

1. Orientation
- reorientate person by explaining where they are and what your role is
- facilitate regular visits from family and friends
- provide adequate lighting, a clock and a calendar
- avoid unnecessary ward moves.

2. Hydration
- encourage the person to drink (at least one and a half litres of water per day)
- consider subcutaneous or intravenous fluids.

3. Infection
- look for and treat infection
- avoid catheters

4. Pain
- assess for pain. Look for non verbal signs of pain. Treat with appropriate analgesia

5. Sensory impairment
- ensure hearing aids and spectacles are available, if appropriate and working

6. Medication review
- review all medications;
- stop any unnecessary medication;

- reduce or stop any anticholinergic medication/sedatives if possible

7. Hypoxia
- assess for hypoxia and optimize oxygen saturation if necessary

8. Mobility
- encourage mobility, or if not mobile encourage range of motion exercises;
- consider thromboprophylaxis

9. Sleep hygiene
- promote good sleep patterns and sleep hygiene

10. Nutrition
- complete nutritional assessment and encourage adequate food intake;
- avoid constipation

Key issue

Modern management of medical emergencies in acute hospitals often makes proper management of delirium difficult because of frequent patient moves and multiple handovers. Early recognition of delirium and patients at risk is needed to facilitate immediate transfer to specialist wards for comprehensive geriatric assessment to improve outcomes.

Follow up and referral

Delirium may be the first presentation of dementia and patients should be followed up after discharge to reassess their cognition. Referral to psychiatry is appropriate for a second opinion about diagnosis, for advice concerning management of severe psychiatric symptoms and to consider follow up in patients with underlying dementia.

Prognosis of delirium

Delirium is a serious condition with a 25% mortality and a high morbidity. Complications of delirium are common and include pressure sores, venous thromboembolism, falls and fractures, and hospital-acquired pneumonia. Many of these complications are secondary to immobility and oversedation and are preventable with good care. Unfortunately, delirium may persist in 25% of patients at 3 months and 20% after 6 months. If a patient still has delirium after a comprehensive assessment and treatment then the following possibilities need to be considered:

1 The underlying cause or causes of the delirium have not yet been discovered and treated. Consider again possible drug causes and look again for any possible underlying infection or neoplastic cause. A persistently raised C reactive protein would suggest this;

2 The diagnosis of delirium is incorrect and the problem is dementia, especially dementia of the Lewy body type which can closely mimic delirium. Check the premorbid history again for any evidence of pre-existing cognitive impairment, especially executive or visuospatial problems;

3 This is 'persistent delirium' and may be part of an irreversible progressive decline into a dementing illness.

Summary

Delirium is common and frequently overlooked in older people and has a high mortality and morbidity. Good management depends on early recognition of patients with delirium, or at risk of delirium, and comprehensive geriatric assessment and care. This can prevent delirium in a third and considerably improve outcomes in the remaining two-thirds.

Further reading

British Geriatrics Society (2006). *Guidelines for the Prevention, Diagnosis and Management of Delirium in Older People in Hospital*. (www.bgs.org.uk).

Inouye SK, van Dyck C, Alessi CA, et al. (1990). Clarifying confusion: the confusion assessment method. A new method for detection of delirium. *Ann Intern Med* **113**: 941–8.

NICE (2010). Guidelines on Delirium (www.nice.org.uk).

Trzepacz PT, Meagher DJ (2008). Neuropsychiatric aspects of delirium. In Yudofsky SC and Hales RE, eds. *Neuropsychiatry and Behavioural Neurosciences*, 5th edn. Arlington, American Psychiatric Publishing.

Young J Inouye SK (2007). Delirium in older people. *Br Med J* **334**: 842–6.

Anxiety

Neurotic disorders

The term neurotic disorders include generalized anxiety disorder (GAD), panic disorder, phobic disorder, obsessive compulsive disorder (OCD), acute stress disorder, post-traumatic stress disorder (PTSD), dissociative states, and somatoform disorder. Though they are considered to be at the milder end of the mental health spectrum, they can be severe and disabling. They are much less common in older people than younger adults. Indeed, onset in later life is rare with some (OCD, panic disorder, GAD in particular). However, they frequently accompany other mental disorders. In depression for example, 74% of people also have anxiety symptoms. Late-onset neurosis should first make one suspect that it is not the primary condition.

Most neurotic disorders have their onset well before the age of 65, and those which present in late life are usually secondary to another mental or physical disorder. The epidemiological catchment area study in the USA found 90% of all neurotic disorders occurred by the early 50's.

Generalized anxiety disorder and panic disorder

- GAD is characterized by excessive anxiousness or worry which is free floating in nature on most of the days for at least six months and includes restlessness, fatigability, poor concentration, irritability, muscle tension, and disturbed sleep.
- Panic disorder consists of panic attacks which are episodes of intense anxiety associated with physical symptoms of palpitations, sweating, tremulousness, shortness of breath, chocking sensation, chest pain, nausea, light-headedness, numbness. They are typically accompanied by the fear of dying or going crazy, with each episode lasting between 5–30 minutes.
- Episodes are often recurrent and lead to avoidance and anticipatory anxiety.
- May develop agoraphobia, a fear of public and open spaces, where escape or immediate availability of help is thought to be difficult.
- 97% of GAD has its onset before the age of 65.
- Panic disorder is rare after 65 years of age.
- GAD and panic disorders are more common in females, those with poor social support network, lower education, and chronic physical illnesses.
- It is often precipitated by a life-threatening (acute medical illness) or loss event.

Diagnosis

- exclude undiagnosed physical health problem and depression.
- the medical work up needs to take into consideration
  1 onset
  2 duration
  3 length of episode
  4 cluster of symptoms
  5 past medical history
  6 current medications

Physical conditions that needs to be considered in diagnosing panic disorder or GAD

1. Cardiac
Angina, dysrythmia, mitral valve prolapse, myocardial infarction

2. Endocrine
Hypo or hyperthyroidism, hypo or hyperparathyroidism, hypoglycaemia

3. Neurological
Complex partial seizures, Huntington's disease, migraine, Meniere's disease

4. Neoplasm
Carcinoid syndrome, phaeochromocytoma

5. Others
COPD, hypoxic state, asthma, porphyria

6. Medications
Anticholinergics, sympathomimetics, psychostimulants, caffeine, drug withdrawal (benzodiazepines, sedatives, antidepressants)

7. Alcohol withdrawal, illicit substances

Treatment
- First-line treatment is psychological therapy: anxiety management, behavioural therapy, self-help.
- Pharmacological management may include SSRIs, venlafaxine, and pregabalin.
- Short-term use of benzodiazepines (2–4 weeks).

Obsessive compulsive disorder (OCD)

- Obsessions are ideas, thoughts, impulses, or images which are experienced as intrusive, and when resisted provoke mounting anxiety.
- Compulsions are rituals performed in order to reduce or prevent anxiety in relation to obsessions.
- Common form of obsessional ideas includes contamination, doubting, ordering, aggression, and sexual imagery
- Compulsions include washing, checking, ordering, counting, hoarding, and repeating words.
- Late life onset of OCD is extremely rare and likely to be symptomatic of depression or organic brain disorders including cerebral tumours
- Less than 5% of patients in tertiary OCD clinics are >60 and less than 5% have onset after age 40
- Some people will present with OCD in later life with a condition that began many years earlier because their circumstances change, for example a spouse dies, leading to decompensation
- OCD is equally prevalent in either gender, more likely to have family history; often symptoms are exacerbated by life stressors.

Treatment
- First-line treatment is cognitive behaviour therapy and response prevention (patient is exposed to their obsessions and learn how to manage mounting anxiety allowing them to resist performing rituals).
- Often a combination of SSRI and cognitive behavioural therapy (CBT) is more effective than either alone, particularly those with obsessional thoughts without rituals.
- when using SSRIs for OCD, the dose range is higher than the dose used for depression (e.g. up to 60 mg of fluoxetine).

Phobias

- Phobias are specific, social or agoraphobia.
- Specific phobias like fear of heights, enclosed places usually has onset in childhood and rarely require treatment.

- Social phobia is a fear of performance in social situations including avoiding eating and drinking in public, usually develops in young people and fluctuates in severity.
- Agoraphobia is the most common with onset in later life and often disabling especially if living alone.
- Agoraphobia typically begins following a traumatic event such as an acute illness, falls, mugging or robbery that affect the person's confidence or fear of leaving the home.
- The prevalence is 1.4–7.9% in community samples.
- Underlying depression is to be considered in all late onset cases.

Treatment (see Table 12.2)
- Rehabilitation following an incident of acute medical illness or a traumatic event is essential to prevent onset of agoraphobic symptoms.
- Treatment is mainly behavioural in the form of graded exposure from the least anxiety provoking to most anxiety provoking situation.
- This needs to be supplemented by psychological support, anxiety management and occasionally short-term use of anxiolytics or antidepressants.
- If significant symptoms of depression are present, this needs to be actively treated along with the behavioural management.

Post-traumatic stress disorder
- Symptoms consists of recurrent intrusive memories; avoidance of thoughts, feelings and conversation about the trauma; hyperarousal, difficulty falling asleep; hyper vigilance, startle response; poor concentration; anger outbursts.
- Post-traumatic stress disorder (PTSD) develops after exposure to a significant trauma which is experienced directly or indirectly.
- This includes incidents such as road traffic accident, mugging, or a violent event.
- Prevalence of PTSD ranges between 0.9% and 13% for syndromal and subsyndromal PTSD.
- Early childhood adverse events and neuroticism are the strongest predictors for development of PTSD.
- Mainstay of treatment is trauma focused CBT which includes self-monitoring of symptoms, anxiety management and cognitive restructuring.
- Eye movement desensitization and reprocessing (EMDR) is a novel treatment which is useful in PTSD where saccadic eye movements are used to reduce the anxiety and replacing adaptive cognitions.
- Pharmacological management includes SSRIs, phenelzine (MAOI); there is some evidence for tricyclic antidepressants.
- Recovery is aided by good social support and the absence of avoidance and further traumatic events.

Dissociative states
- Used to be called hysteria.
- Refers to physical or behavioural symptoms thought to arise from subconscious conflict.
- Extremely rare in later life.
- Very dangerous diagnosis to make in older people where symptoms will almost certainly arise from a physical disease or other major mental illness and not subconscious mechanisms.

Somatoform disorder
- Includes somatization (people with multiple physical symptoms constantly seeking investigation) and hypochondriasis (preoccupation that one has a particular medical condition).
- Is much less common in later life as a primary disorder though often accompanies depression.
- Is now usually referred to as medically unexplained symptoms.
- May present in about 5% of older people attending primary care. Is commonly transient. More often it is associated with high rates of depression, physical illness, and perceived lack of social support.
- Once all reasonable medical investigation is complete further investigation should be avoided and the patient confidently reassured.
- Treatment with antidepressants, cognitive behavioural therapy, and improved social support show some benefit suggesting depression is an important part of these presentations.

Table 12.2 Treatment options for neuroses

	First line	Second line	Others
GAD	SSRI Anxiety management Relaxation training CBT	Venlafaxine Mirtazapine Duloxetine Pregabalin	Buspirone Beta-blockers (for somatic symptoms)
Panic Disorder	SSRIs Anxiety Management CBT	Mirtazapine MAOIs	Venlafaxine
OCD	SSRI Clomipramine Exposure and response prevention Behavioural therapy	Combined treatment Clonazepam	Antipsychotic as augmentation for antidepressants Mirtazapine + SSRI
PTSD	Trauma focused CBT EMDR Anxiety management augmentation	SSRIs Phenelzine Mirtazapine Antipsychotic	Clonidine Carbamzepine Counselling
Social Phobia	Behaviour therapy Systematic desensitization	SSRI Buspirone Clonazepam	Venlafaxine Propranolol MAOI
Somatoform disorder	Antidepressants CBT Improve social support		

Further reading

Age Concern. UK Inquiry into Mental Health and Well-being in Later Life. London: Age Concern, 2007.

Alexopoulos GS (2005). Depression in the elderly. *Lancet*; **365**(9475): 1961–70.

Copeland J, Dewey M, Wood N, *et al.* (1987). Range of mental illness among the elderly in the community: prevalence in Liverpool using the GMS-AGECAT package. *Br J Psychiatry* **150**: 815–22.

Kohn R, Westlake RJ, Rasmussen SA, *et al.* (1997). Clinical features of obsessive-compulsive disorder in elderly patients. *Am J Geriatr Psychiatry* **5**: 211–15.

Manela M, Katona C, Livingston G (1996). How common are the anxiety disorders in old age? *Int J Geriatr Psychiatry* **11**: 65–70.

Moussavi S, Chatterji S, Verdes E *et al.* (2007). Depression, chronic diseases, and decrements in health: results from the World Health Surveys. *Lancet* **370**: 851–8.

Depression

Depression is the commonest mental health problem affecting older people, although only 15–20% receive any treatment. It is the commonest cause of suicide and self-harm, a major cause of poor quality of life, and doubles mortality from natural causes. Ten per cent to 15% of older people have diagnosable depression and the incidence of new cases in the UK is 24 per 1000 people per year, in those aged over 65 years. Consequently, a general practitioner in the UK with 2000 patients would expect around 320 (16%) to be over age 65 producing 30–40 prevalent cases of depression and 8–10 new cases per year in that age group. Women are affected twice as frequently as men and the prevalence of major depression increases with age after 65.

Depression can also have an adverse effect on a person's physical health by causing biological symptoms and disengagement, apathy, self-neglect, non-compliance, and neglect of coexisting physical illness. Depression substantially increases the burden of illness in long-term conditions like angina, asthma, and diabetes and is more common in people with long-term conditions, disability, or handicap (see Table 12.3).

Risk factors include female gender, past or family history of depression, bereavement, loss events, physical illness, disability, handicap, and psychosocial adversity. Protective factors include marriage, good physical health, and religious faith.

Diagnosis

Diagnosis requires the presence of at least one of the core symptoms of depressed mood, loss of interest or enjoyment, or reduced energy (fatigability) with at least two of the common symptoms listed below. Severe depression requires all three core symptoms and at least four of the common symptoms.

ICD-10 criteria for major depressive episode

Depressed mood, loss of interest and enjoyment, and increased fatigability are usually regarded as the most typical symptoms of depression.

Other common symptoms are
- reduced concentration and attention
- reduced self-esteem and self-confidence
- ideas of guilt and unworthiness (even in a mild type of episode)
- bleak and pessimistic views of the future
- ideas or acts of self-harm or suicide
- disturbed sleep
- diminished appetite.

A duration of at least 2 weeks is usually required for diagnosis, but shorter periods may be reasonable if symptoms are unusually severe and of rapid onset.

Older people with depression tend to present with more somatic or hypochondriacal symptoms, cognitive impairment, or poor insight compared with younger people. Screening in primary care might involve the two questions recommended by NICE in people with chronic physical health problems or an instrument such as the four-item Geriatric Depression Scale validated for use with older people (see Table 12.4).

With a good history and mental state examination it is not difficult to detect depression, though it can be more difficult in people with comorbid physical illnesses when it can be challenging to determine the cause of physical symptoms. In this situation the presence of psychological symptoms (negative thoughts, hopelessness, suicidal ideas) may give a better clue to diagnosis. It is always important to be sure there is no underlying physical disease masquerading as depression. The view of a relative or friend can be very helpful in uncertain cases.

A less common but very serious form of depression is psychotic depression. In addition to the syndrome already described there are delusions and/or hallucinations. Delusions are typically mood congruent that is in keeping with the misery and negative thought processes of depression, usually in the form of irrational guilt, hypochondriasis (having terminal or infectious disease) or persecution. Hallucinations are less common, and typically auditory (voices making derogatory remarks, accusations, or threats), olfactory (bad smells), gustatory (bad tastes), or somatic (physical sensations implying disease). Psychotic depression, regardless of the psychosocial circumstance, should be referred urgently to mental health services and usually requires inpatient treatment. The risk of suicide and serious self-neglect is high.

A variety of common situations including help-seeking behaviour, repeated reassurance seeking, revolving presentations, preoccupation with physical symptoms, and self-critical thoughts should raise the possibility of depression.

Table 12.3 Depression prevalence with physical comorbidity

	%
Parkinson's disease	50
Huntington's disease	40
Neurological disorders	24
Stroke at 12 months	16
Myocardial infarction at 12 months	15–30
Coronary heart disease	
Major depression	20
Minor depression	27
Cancer	20
COPD Clinic	42

Table 12.4 Screening for depression

Item geriatric depression scale		
Are you basically satisfied with your life?	Yes	No
Do you feel that life is empty?	Yes	No
Are you afraid that something bad is going to happen to you?	Yes	No
Do you feel happy most of the time?	Yes	No

Cut off score of 1/2 suggests depression.

Situations to consider the diagnosis of depression
Cognitive impairment
Self-harm
Increased use of analgesics, tranquilizers, hypnotics
Non-compliance
Repeated presentations
Failure to attend appointments
Frequent attendance
Increased withdrawal and isolation
Anorexia, weight loss, insomnia
Increased alcohol use
Unexplained deterioration of physical health
Medically unexplained symptoms

Recognizing depression in chronic health problem
1 During the last month, have you often been bothered by feeling down, depressed or hopeless?
2 During the last month, have you often been bothered by having little interest or pleasure in doing things?

If YES to any of the above ask three further questions
1 During the last month, have you often been bothered by feelings of worthlessness?
2 During the last month, have you often been bothered by poor concentration?
3 During the last month, have you often been bothered by thoughts of death?

http://www.nice.org.uk/nicemedia/pdf/CG91 NICE Guideline.pdf

Assessment of self-harm
Enquiring about thoughts of self-harm should be a routine part of assessment. Eighty per cent of suicides in older people are associated with depression and nearly half of older people who commit suicide visit their general practitioner in the preceding month.

Age is a major risk factor for suicide and the risk of completed suicide after self-harm is much higher with older people. Over a 20-year period following an episode of self-harm in older people, death by suicide and open verdicts are 49 and 33 times respectively higher than expected. Common accompaniments in older people with self-harm include coexisting physical morbidity (46.1%), social isolation (33.5%), relationship difficulties (29.4%), and bereavement or loss (16.7%). Seventy-five per cent of self-harm episodes involved high suicidal intent, only 15.3% were under psychiatric treatment, 23.7% had a history of self-harm, and 41.3% previous psychiatric treatment.

Ideas of self-harm or suicidal thoughts should be evaluated in all patients with depression. Suicidal thinking, even fleeting suicidal thoughts, should be probed further. Usually patients are relieved to discuss these thoughts which are distressing to them.

Any suicidal thinking should be assessed in terms of several characteristics to determine level of risk:
- fleeting or persistent thoughts
- actual ideas of self-harm
- any plans on methods or means
- formed intent
- attitude to suicide

- degree of hopelessness and helplessness
- degree of subjective distress
- severity of depression/presence of psychosis
- history of self-harm
- impact of recent stressor/life event
- protective factors: family ties, support network, religious objection
- any older person presenting with suicidal thoughts or self-harm should be promptly referred for specialist assessment.

Treating depression
Most depression will be treated in primary care and it is essential that primary care physicians identify and treat depression vigorously: the better the initial recovery, the better the long-term prognosis. Antidepressants and psychological approaches are as effective in older adults as in younger people.

With mild depression it may be worthwhile waiting for at least 2 weeks and review before commencing any form of treatment. If symptoms persist or become distressing treatment should be started in the form of either pharmacotherapy or psychotherapy. If bereavement or an acute stressor precipitates depression focused psychosocial intervention such as bereavement counselling or social help may be appropriate. Problem-solving therapy, cognitive behaviour therapy (CBT), self-help guides, or computerized CBT are appropriate.

Moderate depression usually requires a combination of antidepressants and psychotherapy though the patient may have a preferred approach. Greatest sustained benefits are derived from the combination as it helps to develop coping skills which are useful in relapse prevention.

Severe depression and psychotic depression are to be treated with urgent attention and need specialist treatment. Biological treatments are the mainstay of acute treatment in the management of these more severe depressions

Antidepressants
SSRIs or mirtazapine are used as first-line agents, the latter if sedation is preferred (see Table 4). Sertraline and citalopram are least likely to cause drug interactions and have been shown to be safe in people with ischaemic heart disease. Mirtazapine is least likely to impair sexual function, and fluoxetine has an advantage if compliance is an issue because of its long half-life. When choosing an antidepressant consider:
- comorbid physical disorders
- concurrent medication and risk of interactions
- side-effect profile
- toxicity in overdose
- past history of response to a particular drug.

Things to consider when using SSRIs
- Increased risk of gastrointestinal bleeding, particularly, with other drugs carrying similar risk e.g. NSAID, aspirin, warfarin, heparin, due to effect on platelets
- Consider adding a PPI when used in people at risk of GI bleeding
- Do not use with 'triptan' drugs used for migraine
- Consider mirtazapine in patients taking heparin, Warfarin, aspirin
- Hyponatraemia especially when used with diuretics
- Increased risk of falls, address falls risk factors

Treatment issues

dosing: start low, go slow'

- final therapeutic dose would be expected to be similar to that for younger adults
- educate about possible side-effects and withdrawal symptoms
- 60% of people will respond to monotherapy
- Response usually takes 2–3 weeks to start
- maintain the therapeutic dose at least for 4 weeks before considering change of medications.

Treatment non-response

- check compliance (introduce compliance aids)
- reassess diagnosis
- treat comorbid disorders, painful conditions
- address disabilities and psychosocial factors
- address alcohol misuse (if relevant)
- swap to another class of antidepressant
- referral to specialist service if failed treatment with two antidepressants in succession or deteriorating

Referral to mental health service

- all severe depression
- all psychotic depression
- significant suicide risk or self-harm
- treatment resistant
- condition deteriorating
- significant self-neglect
- persistent non-compliance
- complex psychosocial circumstances
- complicated physical comorbidities

Duration of treatment

- 90% will relapse without prophylaxis at three years.
- Continued treatment will reduce this to 50–60%
- Maintenance dose should be the same as used for recovery.
- Single episode treatment should continue for 1–2 years from the point of remission.
- Three lifetime episodes – treatment should continue for at least three years or longer.
- If antipsychotic used for psychotic depression it can be withdrawn slowly 6 months following remission.

Treatment Resistant Depression (TRD)

Treatment resistance is defined as failure to respond to treatment with two antidepressants (in series) in a therapeutic dosage after 6 weeks of treatment. Further treatment would depend on the severity, past response to treatment and associated medical illnesses. For severe and psychotic depression Electroconvulsive therapy (ECT) is effective. ECT is recommended in life-threatening conditions (food or fluid refusal, serious suicide risk) or when other treatment options have failed.

Other evidence-based treatments include venlafaxine, lithium augmentation (lithium combined with other antidepressants), atypical antipsychotic augmentation, and combination antidepressants. Less robust evidence exists for MAOIs, anticonvulsant augmentation, and thyroid hormone augmentation. Though tricyclic antidepressants are avoided in uncomplicated depression because of their side-effect profile and toxicity, they are a consideration for treatment resistance.

Comorbid depression

Depression can be a challenge when it presents with multiple medical comorbidities and this is common in later life. Clinicians prescribing antidepressants should consider drug interactions, the influence of antidepressants on the physical condition (positive and negative), hepatic and renal clearance, possible causal mechanism between depression and physical illness. There is evidence in some comorbidities that might be clinically useful:

Ischaemic heart disease

Sertraline and citalopram shown to be safe and effective even with unstable angina and 10 days post myocardial infarction.

SSRIs

Reduce risk of subsequent fatal and non-fatal cardiac ischemic events after myocardial infarction over a period of time (probably by reducing platelet coagulability). There may be some benefit on frontal executive function following stroke, over and above any direct antidepressant effect. Sertraline and citalopram are probably the least likely to cause drug interactions.

Parkinson's disease

The best evidence is for nortriptyline but pramipexole, a dopamine agonist has also been shown to have a greater antidepressant effect than sertraline.

Vascular depression

The concept of vascular depression was developed after white matter hyperintensities were noticed on magnetic resonance imaging of the brain in some people with depressive symptoms. Vascular depression is associated with vascular risk factors, history of transient ischaemic attack or stroke. People with vascular depression tend to have greater disability, cognitive impairment, apathy, and psychomotor retardation. They respond less well to antidepressants resulting in a poorer prognosis. Anterior frontal and basal ganglia lesions are most significant lesions contributing to depression. Though it is thought that vascular brain disease is the underlying cause of the depression the relationship between vascular disease and depression is complex. Management is essentially managing vascular risk factors, trial of antidepressant, augmenting anti depressant with lithium and ECT in some situations.

Further reading

Age Concern (2007). *UK Inquiry into Mental Health and Well-being in Later Life*. London: Age Concern.

Alexopoulos GS (2005). Depression in the elderly. *Lancet* **365**: 70.

Beekman ATF, Copeland JRM, Prince MJ (1999). Review of community prevalence of depression in later life. *Br J Psychiatry* **174**: 307–11.

Copeland J, Dewey M, Wood N, et al. (1987). Range of mental illness among the elderly in the community: prevalence in Liverpool using the GMS-AGECAT package. *Br J Psychiatry* **150**: 815–22.

Copeland JR, Davidson IA, Dewey ME, et al. (1992). Alzheimer's disease, other dementias, depression and pseudodepression: prevalence, incidence and three-year outcome. *Br J Psychiatry* **161**: 230–9.

Moussavi S, Chatterji S, Verdes E, et al. (2007). Depression, chronic diseases, and decrements in health: results from the World Health Surveys. *Lancet* **370**: 851–8.

Teper E, O'Brien JT (2008). Vascular factors and depression. *Int J Geriatr Psychiatry* **23**: 993–1000.

Van der Kooy K, van Hout H, Marwijk H, et al. (2007). Depression and the risk for cardiovascular diseases: systematic review and meta analysis. *Int J Geriatr Psychiatry* **22**: 613–26.

Sleep problems

Sleep problems are common in later life, with up to 42% of those over 65 years reporting problems in initiating and maintaining sleep, compared with 25% of 21–30 year olds. For many, these problems are short-lived, with approximately 50% showing resolution of symptoms at 3-year follow-up. The prevalence of excessive daytime sleepiness decreases for much of adult life from a peak in the 20s, but increases rapidly over the age of 75 years. Although it is often assumed to be the correlate of night-time sleeplessness, not all patients with such daytime hypersomnia have sleep disruption.

Sleep disruption is associated with decreased health-related quality of life and a higher prevalence of self-reported anxiety and depression compared with the general population, whilst resolution of sleep disturbance results in an improvement in self-rated health status. Impaired sleep is also associated with cognitive impairment and is an independent risk factor for falls. Several population-based studies have demonstrated sleep disturbance to be an independent predictor of all-cause mortality, although the precise nature and causality of this association is unclear.

Sleep problems are common in later life because of age-related changes in circadian rhythm and sleep architecture, coupled to an increased prevalence of sleep-specific disorders and comorbid conditions. Comorbid conditions with a particular effect on sleep are heart failure, Parkinson's disease, depression, and dementia.

Changes in circadian rhythm in later life

Circadian rhythm describes the natural diurnal rhythm seen in many body functions, including core temperature, heart rate, secretion of some hormones, red blood cell production, levels of arousal, and the sleep–wake cycle. It is mediated, in part, by responses to external stimuli (zeitgebers), particularly bright-light exposure.

The suprachiasmatic nucleus (SCN) of the hypothalamus plays an instrumental part in synchronizing circadian rhythm to external stimuli and is affected by age-related degenerative changes. The SCN undergoes particularly marked degeneration in Alzheimer's disease.

Healthy older subjects characteristically demonstrate phase-advancement of the sleep wake cycle. This means that they tend to wake earlier and feel ready for sleep earlier in the evening. Two maladaptive responses, undertaken to try and synchronize sleep patterns with societal norms, have been described. In the first of these, the subject stays awake until a more normal time but, despite going to bed later, still wakes early. In the second, the patient naps in the early evening before waking up and moving to bed, where they find it difficult to resume sleep. In both instances, sleep deprivation results.

Patients with Alzheimer's disease demonstrate greater variability in circadian rhythm than other groups and demonstrate a particular dissociation between temperature rhythm and the sleep-wake cycle. A common phenomenon amongst those with Alzheimer's is the phase-delayed sleep–wake cycle, where patients have peak activity and temperature levels later in the day than age-matched controls. An association between phase-delayed rhythms and 'sundowning' behaviour – where patients with dementia become particularly agitated in the evenings—has been demonstrated.

Changes in sleep architecture in later life

Older patients display the same range of sleep patterns seen in the younger population but certain patterns become more prevalent in later life, particularly:

- Shorter duration of slow-wave sleep, thought to be the restorative component of sleep.
- Shorter duration of rapid eye movement (REM) sleep, where dreaming occurs, with less intense eye movements during this sleep, suggesting the sleep is less intense.
- Lower sleep efficiency, defined as the amount of time in bed spent asleep.
- More frequent night-time awakenings and a lower arousal threshold for noise while asleep.

The net effect of these changes is to render older patients more rousable and therefore vulnerable to sleep disorders.

Sleep specific disorders in later life

Snoring and obstructive sleep apnoea

Snoring and obstructive sleep apnoea–hypopnoea syndrome (OSAHS) represent different ends of a continuum of sleep disordered breathing characterized by increased airways resistance due to pharyngeal collapse during inspiration. During airway collapse, patients stop breathing until they partially waken, resuming respiration with increased arousal. The patient is usually unaware that they have awoken but the disturbance to sleep quality is such that they suffer daytime hypersomnolence as a consequence. The association of OSAHS with obesity and snoring is less robust in older people than in other population groups and it has been suggested that older patients may suffer quiet apnoeic or hypopnoeic episodes more frequently.

The severity of sleep apnoea is quantified using the apnoea–hypopnoea index (AHI), which is a measure of the number of awakenings related to disordered breathing per hour and is recorded using polysomnography. The level of AHI at which sleep apnoea is diagnosed is, to an extent, arbitrary and varies depending on the diagnostic criteria used – therefore estimates of prevalence of OSAHS in population studies of older people are highly variable, ranging from 5.6% to 70%. The most robust data, however, suggest a prevalence of around 10% in over 65s when conservative diagnostic criteria are used and 24% when more liberal ones are applied. This compares with 0.3–4% in middle-aged men and 0.5–1% in middle-aged women. All data suggest that the prevalence of the condition increases continuously with advancing age and that the male predominance continues into later life.

OSAHS is problematic because the daytime hypersomnolence results in a greater incidence of accidental injury and because of haemodynamic sequelae from recurrent episodes of obstructed respiration. Most of the data on injuries relates to road-traffic accidents, which are particularly sensitive to OSAHS because of the high level of arousal required for maintained concentration in this context. It is not clear how it impacts on the risk of falls, which are the most common cause of serious injury in the older population. The haemodynamic effects of OSAHS are well documented and include hypertension, cardiac failure, and nocturia. Patients with the condition are also more likely to suffer a stroke.

OSAHS is associated with impairment of cognitive function, with particular effects on attention, memory, learning and executive performance. These effects are small across the cohort as a whole but become more marked as the AHI rises. They improve when apnoea is treated. A separate phenomenon seems to be the higher incidence of snoring and obstructive sleep apnoea in patients with vascular and Alzheimer's type dementia. The causality of this association is, as yet, unexplored.

Nocturnal continuous positive airway pressure (CPAP) has been well documented to reduce night-time sleep disturbance in OSAHS and the haemodynamic, cardiac and cognitive dysfunction seen as a consequence. When patients over 65 are considered as a whole, they tolerate and comply with CPAP therapy as well as younger ones. The treatment, however, involves wearing a tight-fitting mask and is associated with sensations of claustrophobia – it is not, therefore, likely that it would be well tolerated or appropriate in patients with more than mild cognitive impairment.

REM sleep behaviour disorder

The prevalence of REM sleep behaviour disorder is uncertain but it is probably about four in every 10 000 over 75s. Dreaming occurs during REM sleep, with electroencephalographic recordings resembling those seen during wakefulness. Patients remain inactive in bed despite these high levels of brain activity because of muscle atonia mediated by active suppression of spinal level motor activity by a number of midbrain loci. Higher centres in the motor neuraxis remain very active and relatively minor changes in the midbrain can result in termination of the suppression of movement.

In REM sleep behaviour disorder, patients manifest motor behaviours ranging from simple jerks to more complex behaviours such as kicking, punching, pulling hair, swearing, and running or jumping out of bed. Patients can often recall performing similar manoeuvres within their dreams once awakened, leading to the suggestion that they may be 'acting out' their dreams in the real world. Problems tend to occur towards the end of the night, when REM forms a greater proportion of sleep. This is distinct from the non-REM parasomnias, such as somnambulation, which occur during deep sleep and therefore take place earlier in the night – these rarely present in late life, as opposed to REM sleep behaviour disorder, which does so commonly.

REM sleep behaviour disorder is particularly important in geriatric practice because up to 25% of those affected go on to develop Parkinson's disease, multisystem atrophy, or dementia with Lewy bodies. The diagnosis therefore may prove useful in selecting patients for treatment should neuroprotective agents, delaying the onset of these conditions, become available.

The condition has been shown to respond well to treatment with clonazepam.

Restless legs syndrome

Prevalence of restless legs syndrome (RLS) increases steadily through the first seven decades of life, rising from 2.7% in the teenage years to 8.2% by age 70–79. Some of this late peak may be explained by a long latency from onset to diagnosis. The condition is characterized by the recurrent and overwhelming urge to move ones legs, often associated with an uncomfortable sensation in the legs. It is worse when patients are resting, is totally relieved by movement and shows a diurnal variation, with symptoms more manifest in the evening and at night. It is usually a primary condition but can be secondary to iron deficiency or end-stage renal failure.

RLS, because it manifests when patients rest, causes problems with both the initiation and maintenance of sleep, with some studies reporting sufferers to get up to five hours less sleep per night. It can also cause sleeplessness in bed partners.

It is treated using dopaminergic medications, most of which have been shown to be effective in treating RLS. However, only pramipexole, ropinorole, and rotigotine are licensed for treatment of the condition in the UK at the time of going to press.

Although it is treated with dopamine agonists and has been suggested by some studies to have a higher incidence in patients with Parkinson's disease, no convincing pathophysiological or epidemiological association between the two conditions has thus far been demonstrated.

Pharmacological treatment of insomnia

The temptation for clinicians to treat insomnia with hypnotic medications is considerable. Of these, the benzodiazepines, zopiclone and zolpidem are doubtlessly effective in terms of improving both the quality and quantity of sleep. However, most recommendations suggest that these only be used short-term in older patients and even then with caution. A meta-analysis of 2414 participants with a mean age of 60 across 24 studies comparing sedative medications with placebo revealed a number needed to treat of 13, versus a number needed to harm of six, i.e. a sedative drug is twice as likely to be harmful than it is beneficial. The evidence for sedative antihistamines, antidepressants, and antipsychotic medications when used as hypnotics is even less compelling.

Melatonin is an endogenous hormone produced in the pineal gland, with its secretion mediated by stimulation from the suprachiasmatic nucleus in response to light. Exogenous melatonin, administered orally, has been shown to be effective in promoting shifts in circadian rhythms. Despite this, evidence of its efficacy as a hypnotic in older patients, especially those with Alzheimer's disease, is not overwhelming. This may be because of the timing or dose of drug used in studies to date. A melatonin agonist, ramelteon, has been shown to be well-tolerated and to reduce the time to onset of sleep in healthy older adults with insomnia. It has not, however, been tested in frail older adults, nor is it at present licensed in the UK.

Non-pharmacological treatment of insomnia

Cognitive behavioural therapy for insomnia (CBT-I) has been shown both to have a greater magnitude treatment effect and produce more lasting benefits than pharmacological therapies in older adults with insomnia. CBT-I programmes incorporate aspects of sleep hygiene, stimulus control, sleep education and sleep restriction. Although such programmes are clearly of limited benefit in patients with moderate to severe cognitive impairment, some lessons can be taken from them—particularly the sleep hygiene, sleep restriction, and stimulus control components.

Sleep hygiene involves ensuring that factors which might interfere with sleep are minimized. Bedrooms must be free from noise, light, and interruption, and patients must avoid caffeine or exercise before bed and minimize daytime napping.

Sleep restriction suggests minimizing the amount of time spent in bed, such that most of that time is spent asleep.

Stimulus-control involves avoiding the maladaptive responses commonly developed by insomniacs to fill their time awake. At its core is the assertion that the bedroom should only be for sleeping and sex.

Sleep problems in institutionalized patients

Older people living in long-term institutional care are at particular risk of sleep problems. This is, in part, due to the greater prevalence of dementia and physical illness in this cohort but also reflects institutional factors which influence sleep, particularly lack of exercise, lack of exposure to bright light, and night-time noise.

Exercise and exposure to bright-light are potent zeitgebers and there is evidence that both are less effectively delivered in the care home population. Data gathered from 95 care home residents using motion sensors to measure activity levels found that unrestrained residents spend most of their time immobile, with 84% of measurements recording participants sitting or lying flat. With regard to bright light, data recorded using wrist worn photosensors from 66 care home residents recorded a median exposure of only 10 minutes per day, compared with average exposures amongst young adults of 58 minutes and healthy older people of 60 minutes per day.

Disruption of sleep can also be institutionalised. One study of care homes residents, using bedside monitors to record night-time noise and light levels, recorded 32 noises per resident per night at the volume of loud speech (60 decibels) or louder. Another study using similar technology revealed 22% of waking episodes to be associated with noise alone, 10% with light or light and noise and 10% with incontinence care routines. Seventy-six per cent of all incontinence care practices resulted in awakenings.

A number of interventions have been developed to address these issues and subsequently evaluated using randomized controlled trials, including exercise programmes, artificial or man-made bright light exposure and noise and disruption minimization. These have met with limited success. Only when multiple interventions are combined (for example exercise, plus noise minimization plus bright light) do they have any meaningful effect on sleep patterns and this effect is more marked for the reduction of daytime sleepiness than it is for improvement in continuity of sleep at night.

Further work is clearly needed to understand the interaction of institutional and individual factors in order to identify strategies to improve sleep in this population.

Further reading

Ancoli-Israel S, Ayalon L (2009). Diagnosis and Treatment of Sleep Disorders in Older Adults. *Focus* **7**: 98–105.

Avidan AY (2002). Sleep changes and disorders in the elderly patient. *Curr Neurol Neurosci Rep* **2**: 178–85.

Gordon AL, Gladman JR (2010). Sleep in care homes. *Reviews in Clinical Gerontology* **20**: 309–16.

Swift CG, Shapiro CM (1993). ABC of sleep disorders. Sleep and sleep problems in elderly people. *Br Med J* **306**: 1468–71.

Capacity assessment

Background

Illness will often impair people's capacity to make decisions for themselves. In these circumstances there needs to be a legal mechanism to make decisions on their behalf. The assessment of capacity is both a legal and a clinical matter. The legal details will vary according to the jurisdiction in which the assessment is made. This account is based on the England and Wales Mental Capacity Act 2005 (MCA). You should always refer to the Code of Practice to the Act (or other relevant documents).

Where a person has been shown to lack capacity, relatives, carers, professionals, and others close to the person should try and ascertain their best interests. The aim is to determine what the person would have wanted in a given situation, not what others think is best for them – a subtle but important distinction. People may make advanced decisions when they have capacity, about treatments they do not wish to have when they lack capacity; they may appoint other people to make decisions for them, or decision-makers may be appointed by courts of law, such information may also inform a best interests decision.

People are presumed to have capacity unless it can be shown they have not; all practicable help must be given to assist them in reaching a decision. They should not be regarded as incapable because they make an unwise decision. Where action needs to be taken, always consider whether a less restrictive course of action might be preferable.

Definition (from England and Wales MCA 2005. Crown copyright)

A person is unable to make a decision for himself if he is unable

(a) to understand the information relevant to the decision

(b) to retain that information

(c) to use or weigh that information as part of the process of making the decision, or

(d) to communicate his decision (whether by talking, using sign language or any other means).

The fact that a person is able to retain the information relevant to a decision for a short period only does not prevent him from being regarded as able to make the decision.

The information relevant to a decision includes information about the reasonably foreseeable consequences of

(a) deciding one way or the other, or

(b) failing to make the decision

Capacity is specific to a particular time and decision.

Best interests

Any decision made on behalf of an incapacitated person must be in their best interests; this is not necessarily the decision which the doctor (or the family) thinks would be best for the patient. The law does not define 'best interests' but gives guidance as to how best interests should be determined. The process is based on establishing which decision the person would make for themselves, if they had capacity.

People often have values and feelings which are not entirely consistent and it is often helpful to draw up a balance sheet of pros and cons for a particular decision.

Advance decisions to refuse treatment

There is no requirement for an advance decision to be in a particular format (or even made in writing) unless it is to refuse life-sustaining treatment. In this case it must be verified by a statement confirming that the decision is to apply even if life is at risk. Both the decision and the statement verifying it must be in writing, and be signed, and the signature must be witnessed. The person making the advance decision may instruct another person to sign it on his behalf in his presence, if he is unable to write himself. Advance decisions recorded in medical notes are considered to be in writing, which can also include electronic records.

A person must have capacity at the time they make an advance decision; they must specify the treatment that is being refused, although this can be in lay terms. It may specify particular circumstances when the refusal will apply. They may change or completely withdraw the advance decision, so long as they have capacity to do so – this does not need to be in writing.

An advance refusal is not valid if they subsequently make a welfare Lasting Power of Attorney appointing someone else to make the same decision, or if they do anything clearly inconsistent with the advance decision remaining their fixed decision.

It is not applicable except for the treatment specified in the advance decision or if any circumstances specified in the advance decision are absent. It may be invalid if there are reasonable grounds for believing that circumstances exist, which the person did not anticipate at the time of the advance decision and which would have affected their decision had they considered them.

A practitioner is not liable if he does not give a patient a treatment which he reasonably believes the patient has refused, or if he treats a patient when he reasonably believes there is no valid and applicable advance refusal.

Wishes and feelings

It is not possible to make binding advance requests for treatment, mainly because there is no requirement for a doctor to provide treatment for a patient which would not – in the doctor's opinion – be appropriate for the patient. It is helpful as part of the process of advance care planning to get an idea of the types of treatments which patients may wish to have in the future if they lose capacity to express their feelings.

Practical aspects

It is generally helpful for assessments to be conducted by a doctor who has previous knowledge of the patient. They will need to consider the patient's general intellectual ability, their memory, reasoning, attention, and concentration. They will need to assess the patient's ability to reason and express themselves and also bear in mind cultural influences and the social context in which the assessment is being undertaken.

The more complex the decision which is being made, the greater the level of cognitive ability that will be required. A person's capacity must not be judged simply on the basis of their age, appearance, condition, or an aspect of their behaviour. It is always important to try to involve the patient as much as possible in the process of assessment, but they cannot be forced to undergo an assessment of capacity. In the end the assessor has to make a decision on the best available evidence

Preparation

* Read any available background documents.
* Speak to family and close friends, find out the best way of communicating with the patient.
* Explain to the relevant person in the most appropriate way what is required.
* Check understanding after a few minutes.
* Avoid questions which can answered 'yes' or 'no'.
* Don't be misled by maintained social façade or preserved skills.
* It may necessary to repeat the procedure to confirm the result.

Understanding

* Is someone that they trust present to reassure them?
* Do they need a translator?
* Are they physically as well as they can be?
* Has the process of establishing a diagnosis upset them?
* Have you chosen the best time, day, and place to undertake the assessment?
* Do they have their glasses? Are the glasses clean?
* Is their hearing aid working?
* Is the television/radio turned off?
* Would it help for the information to be presented in a different format (writing, pictures, audio tape or video?)

Communication

* Have you communicated with the person in the most effective way?
* Use simple language, speak at the right volume and speed.
* Reduce difficult information into simpler concepts.
* It may be necessary to repeat information several times.
* Would pictures or written information help?
* If using pictures to help communication, make sure they are relevant and the person can understand them easily.

It may be necessary to involve speech and language therapists, specialists in non-verbal communication or other professionals to establish that all practical steps have been taken to help the patient communicate.

Specific decisions

Deciding where to live

There is no specific legal test for this: the practitioner may find it helpful to consider the following questions. An occupational therapy assessment in the patient's home will often clarify whether their wish to return is realistic.

* Where do they think they are?
* Where do they wish to be?
* Are they able to care for themselves?
* Do they recognize their disabilities and limitations?
* What degree of support would they require?
* Are the expectations they have of others realistic?

Making a will

Traditionally this has been assessed on the basis of the common law test:

* Do they understand the act of making a will?
* Are they aware of the extent of their assets?
* Do they realize who might have a claim on their estate?
* Are their decisions affected by psychotic beliefs?

At the time of writing it is not clear whether this test or the MCA definition of capacity (which would require an understanding of intestacy – the effect of not making a will) should apply.

Managing property and affairs

Many people choose to create a Lasting Power of Attorney appointing someone to manage their finances if they should later become incapable. If they have not done so and they have significant assets an approach may be made to the Court of Protection to appoint a financial deputy to act. The application needs to be supported by a medical certificate of capacity (COP3). When completing the certificate the following questions may be useful:

* Can they recognize coins and bank notes?
* Can they perform simple arithmetic?
* Do they know how to use their bank account?
* Do they have some idea of their income and necessary expenditure?
* Do they know the extent of their assets?

Summary

There are legal mechanisms for making decisions for people without capacity. Before concluding that a person lacks capacity thorough assessment is necessary; further guidance on how this should be undertaken is available in government publications.

Further reading

Bartlett P (2008). *Blackstone's Guide to The Mental Capacity Act 2005*, 2nd edn. Oxford, OUP.

Conroy S, Fade P, Fraser A, Schiff R (2009) *Advance Care Planning: Concise Guidance to Good Practice Series, number 12*. London: RCP.

Mental Capacity Act 2005. Code of Practice (2007) London, TSO.

Neurology

Epilepsy in older people

Epilepsy is the third most common neurological disorder in older people following dementia and cerebrovascular disease. Within the general population the prevalence is highest in older people. However the clinical features differ in younger compared with older people. In older people, epilepsy may present atypically often leading to misdiagnosis, or delayed diagnosis.

Incidence and Prevalence of seizures in old age

Epidemiological data shows that by the age of 70 years the incidence of epilepsy is twice as common as children. Data from primary care practices, including 62 000 patients over the age of 65 years, showed an prevalence of 12 per 1000 and incidence of 147 per 100 000 in over 75 years (compared with 9 and 69 respectively in the general population). These figures increase with increasing age and are expected to rise further as the proportion of older people in the population grows. If under-diagnosis is taken into account, the incidence of epilepsy in older people may be two to three times higher than that suggested and possibly six- to 10-fold greater than among younger people.

Causes

Epilepsy is conventionally defined as two or more unprovoked seizures and therefore theoretically the diagnosis cannot be made based on a single seizure. However, this arbitrary separation is not clear cut at least in older individuals since the majority who present with a single seizure go on to develop further events.

New-onset epilepsy in old age is due to underlying brain disease. Despite the wide variability among the studies, the common causes are cerebrovascular disease (30–65%), dementia (10–15%), and primary or metastatic brain tumours (5–15%). Other causes include trauma (1–3%) with resultant intracerebral, subarachnoid haemorrhage, or subdural hematoma, central nervous system (CNS) infections, hypertensive encephalopathy, and cerebral vasculitis.

Cerebrovascular disease is by far the most common underlying aetiology. Compared with the general population, individuals with stroke are 20 times more likely to develop epilepsy. The incidence increases over time. In the Minnesota study, the incidence of late seizures was 2.9% at 1 year, 6.8% at 5 years, and 8.1% by 10 years. Higher figures have been reported in other studies. The disorder is also the leading cause of status epilepticus, occurring in about a third of these patients. Epileptic seizures in old age may be the first sign of cerebrovascular disease, usually the result of a 'silent' infarct.

Alzheimer's disease (AD) is associated with a six- to 10-fold increase in risk of epilepsy. A similar risk occurs in patients with other forms of dementia.

In 25–40% of older people, the aetiology remains unknown (cryptogenic). However, in many of these individuals the underlying pathology is thought to be cerebrovascular or micro-infarcts since they have been shown to have significant vascular risk factors (hypertension, myocardial infarction, peripheral vascular disease, raised cholesterol).

Metabolic and electrolyte abnormalities may precipitate seizures but do not cause epilepsy.

Clinical features

The majority of new onset seizures are focal presenting as complex partial seizures with or without secondary generalization whereas the classical tonic–clonic seizures occur in only 25%. In contrast to younger people, auras are infrequent and non-specific, automatisms (lip smacking, recurrent movements) are fewer but the duration of the post-ictal period can be prolonged, at times lasting for days or even up to 2 weeks, compared with minutes to hours in younger adults. The variation in the clinical presentation is probably due to involvement of frontoparietal regions rather than temporal lobes.

The symptoms are often non-specific and the patient or carer may report a variety of complaints ranging from lapse in memory, periods of inattention or confusion, brief unresponsiveness, blank staring, or simply loss of time which cannot be accounted for. Dizzy spells, syncope and blackouts are among the other presenting complaints. In the post-ictal stage the patient may develop stupor, confusion, disorientation, hyperactivity wandering, incontinence, and persistent headache, raising the possibility of delirium. Todd's paresis may persist for days and can be misinterpreted as a new stroke.

The paucity of specific clinical signs often leads to misdiagnosis and in one study the delay to diagnosis was 1.7 years.

Diagnosis

Regardless of age, the diagnosis of epilepsy is clinical. Many older patients are unaware of their seizures. They live on their own, with no witness to provide a collaborative history. Nonetheless, diagnosis relies heavily on a comprehensive history and importantly, an increased awareness by the clinician. A detailed history of the circumstances and description of the event(s) through a witness when possible is the mainstay in making the diagnosis.

> **Author's Tip**
>
> Diagnosis of epilepsy in older people relies on history taking and increased awareness by the clinician of the atypical presentation.

Investigations:

Routine investigations only aid in identifying comorbidities and in tailoring antiepileptic treatment rather than confirming the diagnosis. MRI is the imaging modality of choice if available. Otherwise a CT head scan should be used, although it may not identify smaller structural lesions. Imaging aids in identifying an underlying pathology that may be responsible for the seizures rather than establishing the diagnosis of epilepsy. Therefore demonstrating a structural lesion on brain imaging, although helpful, does not necessarily establish a cause and effect relationship.

Electroencephalography (EEG) lacks specificity in older people and should be interpreted with caution. Up to 38% of this age group have abnormalities on EEG and a normal recording does not exclude the diagnosis. The pattern and periodicity of wave abnormalities may be useful, as is a recording during non-convulsive epileptiform activity. A more reliable investigation is video-EEG monitoring conducted in specialist centres. This test has proven invaluable in the diagnosis and classification of epileptic syndromes in younger patients, but tends to be under-used in older people. Inpatient video-EEG monitoring can provide a definitive diagnosis.

It is important to consider cardiac problems in patients with unexplained blackouts; a baseline ECG is important followed by a 24-hour or 7-day ambulatory ECG if the 12-lead ECG is abnormal, and possibly carotid sinus studies if the history suggests otherwise unexplained syncope.

Treatment

Establishing a diagnosis and starting treatment early is important since the chance of recurrence following a single seizure in older people is around 80%. Whether treatment should be started after a single unprovoked seizure remains controversial.

The mainstay of treatment is drug therapy. Epilepsy in older people generally responds well to treatment; between 65% and 80% of these patients with new-onset epilepsy remain seizure-free with monotherapy compared with 30% of patients aged 40 or younger. Unlike young patients where the choice of antiepileptic drug (AED) is determined by the type of epilepsy, treatment in older patients should take into account other factors including age related changes in pharmacokinetics, associated comorbidities and the fact that these patients are often on multiple drugs which may interfere with AEDs. Among the other special adverse effects that AED may pose in older people are the risk of unsteadiness and falls, effect on bone health, and worsening cognition.

Practical considerations in older people when prescribing AEDs

1 Effective
2 Low side-effect profile
3 Effect on cognition
4 Few (or no) interactions with other drugs
5 Taken infrequently - prolonged action

Older patients respond to therapy with smaller doses of AEDs and lower serum drug concentrations. They are more sensitive to the central and systemic side-effects of AEDs including cognitive adverse effects. Slow titration and low target doses should help reduce the side-effects. A good rule is to start with about half the recommended dose for young adults and titrated slowly upwards if needed.

Author's Tip

Since older patients respond to smaller doses of AEDs with lower serum drug concentrations, and are more susceptible to concentration-dependent adverse effects: **Start LOW and go SLOW**

Choice of AED

The last two decades has seen an abundance of new AEDs offering better pharmacokinetic properties compared to the older AEDs (phenytoin, phenobarbitone, primidone, valproate, and carbamezapine). Unfortunately, only a few controlled drug trials targeting older people are available. The studies to date show that lamotrigine and gabapentin are better tolerated than carbamazepine, although they all provide comparable effectiveness.

Further recommendations are based on 'best evidence' following the special considerations for older people outlined above. Table 13.1 shows the interactions of AEDs

Table 13.1 Interaction of AEDs with commonly prescribed drugs

Medication	Gabapentin	Lamotrigine	Levetiracetam	Vigabatrin	Topiramate	Tiagabine	Phenytoin, carbamazepine, valproat, primidone, oxycarbazepine*
Warfarin	-	-	-	-	-	-	+
Digoxin	-	-	-	-	±	-	+
Neuroleptics	-	-	-	-	-	?	+
Antibiotics	-	-	-	-	-	?	+

with other commonly prescribed drugs and demonstrates the possible advantages of newer AEDs.

The few available studies on the effect of AEDs on bone health are controversial. Even the newer AEDs are associated with increased rates of bone loss. Although no guidelines exist, it may be reasonable to start supplemental vitamin D and calcium when initiating AEDs, but this remains speculative.

Table 13.2 shows important properties of individual AEDs, in relation to use in older patients.

On the basis of the evidence from the limited comparative studies of AEDs conducted to date in older patients with epilepsy, it appears that Lamotrigine has the most favourable profile when considering adverse effects on cognition and drug-drug interactions. Alternative drugs are levetiracetam, gabapentin or valproate. If the initial AED fails to achieve adequate control, the recommendation is to substitute a second drug before instituting polytherapy.

Epilepsy and quality of life issues

Compared with the general population, older patients with epilepsy report significantly lower quality of life (QoL) across all domains. The unpredictable nature of seizures can lead to social withdrawal, loss of confidence, and reduced independence. They are particularly vulnerable to injuries during seizures and the situation is complicated further by the underlying aetiology and associated comorbidities. Though seizures are generally easily controlled, it is possible that AED side-effects and depression indirectly affect their QoL. Education of both patients and carers about the nature of disorder and adherence to treatment is therefore essential. The objective of care should be complete control of seizures with no adverse effects and enhanced QoL.

Conclusion

Epilepsy in older people is a common problem of increasing proportion. Seizures and epilepsy can impact adversely on the quality of life through falls and injuries resulting in depression, loss of independence or social isolation. Awareness of the atypical presentation in this age group improves the chances of accurate diagnosis. Since there is high risk of recurrence early diagnosis is crucial for prompt and appropriate drug therapy. AEDs provide good control frequently achieved by monotherapy but should be

Table 13.2 Comparative properties of AEDs and relevant characteristics related to older patients

Drug	Protein binding (%)	Hepatic clearance (%)	General pharmacodynamic effects	Adverse effects and safety issues in older people	Cognitive impairment	Frequency of maintenance daily administration	Rating according to available evidence
Phenytoin	90	10	Hepatic enzyme inducer	Adverse effects usually dose-related Osteoporosis 3× increased risk of falls. Ataxia	Mild–moderate. CNS effects usually dose-related	Once–twice	Low
Carbamazepine	75–85	100	Hepatic enzyme inducer	Hyponatraemia (especially in patients on diuretics), tremor, myoclonus, conduction defects Osteopenia – Osteoporosis Gait impairment. Increased risk of falls. Caution in pre-existing cardiac disease	Mild–moderate	Twice	Medium
Valproic acid	75–95	100	Hepatic enzyme inhibitor	Neurotoxicity in hypoalbuminaemic states despite therapeutic levels Osteopenia–osteoporosis Gait impairment	Mild–moderate	Twice–tds	Medium
Oxycarbazepin	40	60–70	Needs dose adjustment in renal failure. Reduced idiosyncratic reactions	Similar to CZB but fewer interactions Hyponatraemia remains a problem in older people.*	Mild	Twice	Medium
Topiramate	15	20	80% excreted by kidneys— dose adjustment in renal failure	decreased clearance in older people (8% per decade). Reduce dose by 50% in CrCl <70 mL/min	Cognitive impairment, mental slowing, word finding difficulty	Twice	Medium–low
Lamotrigine	55–60	100	Needs slow titration to minimize risk of rash	Rash especially when coadministered with valproate Better QoL scores than CBZ (SANAD)	None. May have mood stabilizing properties. Improves neuropsychological performance	Twice (since t$_{1/2}$ of 30 h – once daily dosage may be appropriate in readily controlled seizures	High
Gabapentin	0–5	0	Does not induce hepatic enzymes. Excreted fully by kidneys, dosage can be calculated from Cr clearance.	Pedal oedema Favourable *but not very effective* (SANAD)	None	Twice – tds (short t$_{1/2}$)	High
Pregabalin	5–10	0		Somnolence, dizziness, may cause motor and cognitive slowing, weight gain	Cognitive slowing	Twice	High

Levetiracetam	0	33	Renal excretion (66%)— requires adjustment in renal failure	Behavioural SEs, agitation, hostility, anxiety, emotional lability, depression depersonalization, Care in patients with mood and cognitive problems Add-on, responder rate 32–48%	few mood and cognitive problems reported in some studies	Twice	High
Vigabatrin	0	0	Renal excretion of 70%. Requires adjustment in renal impairment	Concentric visual field defects >40%	None	Once–twice	High
Felbamate	50–60	55	Clearance reduced in elderly	Reserved for refractory epilepsy. Serious side-effects - aplastic anaemia and hepatotoxicty limit its use Adverse effects more common in older people	None	tds	Low
Zonisamide	40–60	50–70	Decreased clearance in elderly	Dizziness, somnolence, weight gain, psychiatric symptoms – depression, hallucinations and psychosis Should be titrated slowly. Risk of kidney stones – ensure adequate hydration	Attention, memory, and language function may be affected	Once or twice (Long $t_{1/2}$ 63 h)	Medium
Tiagbine	95	100	No dose adjustment necessary in renal disease	Knee buckling and falls encephalopathy, altered cognition and coordination Adverse effects tend to be dose dependent	Encephalopathy, altered cognition and coordination Adverse effects tend to be dose dependent.	Twice	Low
Locasamide	15	–	40% renal clearance	Visual blurring, somnolence Adverse effects tend to be dose dependent	Early studies show memory impairment, cognitive disorders, confusion, disruptions in attention, and mental difficulties (8.5% on 400 mg/day)	Twice	Medium

*Drug interactions are minor, no interaction with warfarin.

introduced at low dose and stepped up slowly. The newer AEDs offer significant advantages over the older AEDs through lower adverse effect profile and drug interactions.

Further reading

Bagshaw J, Crawford P, Chappell B (2009). Care in people 60 years of age and over with chronic or recently diagnosed epilepsy: a note review in United Kingdom general practice. *Seizure*, **18**: 57–60.

Tebartz van Elst L, Baker G, Kerr M (2009). The psychosocial impact of epilepsy in older people. *Epilepsy Behav* **15**: S17–9.

Functional neurological syndromes

Background

Functional symptoms and syndromes in neurology are somatic symptoms that appear similar to those in diagnosable neurological conditions but for which no physiologic explanation is found. They may be classified under 'somatoform disorders' and include conversion and dissociative disorders. They may represent up to 15% of presentations in neurology clinics and may be as disabling as neurological symptoms with known causes. Such syndromes most often occur in younger females, but are increasingly recognized in the older population.

Diagnosis may be complicated since they may occur in the context of existing neurologic disorders. For example, non-epileptiform seizures (NES) may occur in someone with diagnosed epilepsy. The onset of such syndromes may be gradual, in the case of somatization disorders (involving several, more diffuse symptoms in more than one body system), or sudden, in the case of conversion disorders (usually involving one specific symptom). In older patients, caution must be taken in diagnosing functional neurological syndromes since non-functional conditions may often be present. For example, in a case series of NES in people over the age of 60, physiologic (e.g. idiopathic thrombocytopenic purpura, syncope, atypical movement disorders) and psychogenic NES may be equally prevalent, whereas in younger populations NES are most commonly psychogenic in origin.

Range of clinical symptoms (Table 13.3)

- Weakness/hemiplegia
- Numbness/anaesthesia
- Dizzy spells
- Headache
- Ataxic gait
- Deafness
- Blindness/diplopia/blurring of vision
- Aphonia
- Dysphagia/globus
- non-epileptiform seizures

Clinical features

- Onset often after major life event, e.g. bereavement
- Onset may be abrupt (conversion disorder) or gradual (somatization disorder)
- History may be exaggerated or vague and inconsistent
- The patient has often seen several doctors about the same complaint already
- If told that all tests are negative, the patient may become upset or angry
- Often coexists with depression and/or anxiety
- The patient may demand complex interventions, even if they are invasive
- Review of systems may be complex and involve several body systems (somatization disorder)

Author's Tip

Hoover's sign: In conversion paralysis, the examiner does not feel the expected downward pressure in the palm of their hand underneath the unaffected leg's heel when asking the patient to lift the affected leg from the recumbent position (face up).

Table 13.3 Findings on examination or laboratory study

Conversion symptom	Anomalous finding on examination
Blindness	Intact papillary light reflex
	Normal cortical visual evoked potential May not bump into things
Anaesthesia	Non-anatomical distribution with abrupt boundaries; Complains of diminished/absent sensation in all other sensory modalities as well despite normal position sense in big toe May affect one half of the body
Weakness/ paralysis	Non-anatomical distribution Weak limb may lack expected flexed posture if chronic Intact deep tendon reflexes on exam Absent Babinski sign Weak leg may be dragged, not circumabucted
Deafness	Positive blink reflex to sudden, unexpected noise Normal brainstem auditory evoked potential
Tremor	Irregular, slow, coarse and will vary according to when patient is not concentrating on it
Seizures	Atypical pattern with lack of tonic-clonic rhythm Patient may remain responsive No urinary incontinence Patient rarely hurts themselves; Minimal or no post-ictal somnolence or confusion Serum prolactin within 15 minutes post-ictal is normal May start and stop abruptly
Parkinsonism	Abrupt onset; lacks typical progressive deteriorating course Atypical tremor; not pill-rolling Cogwheel rigidity absent No masked facies or change in voice quality
Ataxia ('astasia–abasia')	Atypical staggering and swaying, often in a dramatic manner No abnormalities on finger-nose and heel-shin testing Patient rarely hurts themselves or falls
Dysphagia ('globus')	No problem swallowing solids Normal oesophageal manometry

Aetiology

There is no clear aetiology for conversion syndromes, however there are certain associated factors which can be considered. These may be classified into predisposing, precipitating and perpetuating factors.

- Predisposing factors include a history of depression, certain personality vulnerabilities, a pre-existing diagnosis of epilepsy, low education, and certain cultural attitudes or culturally based gender roles.
- Precipitating factors which may trigger the onset of the syndrome include bereavements, trauma (sexual and non-sexual), change in health status and change in social or family circumstances leading to loneliness or a sense of abandonment. At times, declining health status in a spouse or carer may precipitate symptoms, or withdrawal of a chronically ill spouse's care package due to death or institutionalization.

- Perpetuating factors in the older patient often include untreated depression, loneliness, social isolation, and loss of confidence due to declining general health and cognitive status. Financial gain or legal implications are less common factors in older compared to than younger cohorts with conversion syndromes.

A physiological basis of conversion disorders has been suggested by functional neuroimaging studies which point to disruptions in neural pathways underlying perception, movement and volition. For example, frontosubcortical pathways as well as the anterior cingulate cortex, which has a role in the control of consciousness, may be involved.

Approach and management

- A clear and detailed history of the symptom(s) including onset, and ameliorating/exacerbating factors should be sought.
- Search for possible trigger factors such as significant life events.
- Consider the impact of the symptoms on the patient's life and put supports in place to manage this.
- Assess carefully for symptoms of depression and anxiety and treat accordingly.
- Undertake enough investigations to ensure that key diagnoses have been ruled out.
- Try to avoid being pressured into undertaking dangerous or invasive procedures.
- Once the diagnosis is clear, it should be discussed with the patient in a clear way acknowledging that their distress may be as great as if a physiological cause had been found.
- Negative findings on investigations can be framed in a positive light suggesting that the patient does not have to worry about life-threatening conditions.
- The strong chance of a positive outcome with spontaneous remission can be discussed, giving the patient 'permission' to get better.
- Physical or occupational therapy may be put in place in order to facilitate recovery and further acknowledge that the patient's symptoms are being taken seriously, however the therapists should be familiar with the diagnosis and how to manage it.

- If depression or anxiety are prominent, talking therapies such as cognitive behaviour therapy or hypnosis may be helpful, as well as therapies focused on improving self-esteem, coping, and problem-solving.

Pitfalls in diagnosis

Extra care should be taken when diagnosing conversion or somatization disorders in an older person due to clinical presentations in this group often being atypical, subsyndromal or masked. A balance should be struck between ensuring that all potential differential diagnoses have been ruled out and not exposing the patient to excessive and possibly dangerous invasive procedures. Lack of an explanation for a symptom or syndrome is not sufficient to make the diagnosis. Rather, the anomalous presentation and physiologic or anatomical impossibility of the presentation needs to be clearly demonstrated.

Differential diagnosis

- Transient ischaemic attack
- Syncope
- Late-onset Huntington's disease
- Multiple sclerosis
- Sarcoidosis
- Unusual seizures (supplementary motor seizures, akinetic seizures)
- Torsion dystonia
- Sleep disorder
- Malingering
- Factitious disorder

Further reading

Black DN, Seritan AL, Taber KH, *et al.* (2004). Conversion hysteria: lessons from functional imaging. *J Neuropsych Clin Neurosci* **16**: 245–51.

Kellinghaus C, Loddenkemper T, Dinner DS, *et al.* (2004). Non-epileptic seizures of the elderly. *J Neurol* **251**: 9.

Stonnington CM, Barry JJ, Fisher RS (2006). Conversion disorder. *Am J Psych* **163**: 1510–17.

Parkinson's disease: diagnosis, differential diagnosis, and prognosis

Incidence and prevalence

Parkinson's disease (PD) is a chronic neurodegenerative condition. The incidence of new cases is 4–20/100 000 population in the UK with a prevalence of 100–180/100 000 population, such that most general practitioners see few patients with the condition. The incidence and prevalence rise dramatically with age, and the vast majority of patients are older than 60 years at diagnosis. The prevalence of PD rises from 0.6 % of the population aged 65–69 years to 3.5% of those aged 85–89 years, when the prevalence of parkinsonism is estimated to be as high as 52%.

Pathogenesis

Age

Increasing age is the main known risk factor for PD and also the most important determinant of the rate of clinical progression of PD. Older age at diagnosis is associated with a faster rate of progression of motor features, reduced levodopa responsiveness, and more severe gait and posture impairment, while increased current age is associated with more severe cognitive impairment and the development of dementia.

Environmental risk factors

Never smokers are twice as likely to develop PD, and non/very low caffeine intake confers 25% additional risk. Weak associations are reported between PD and rural living, well water ingestion, herbicide and insecticide exposure, middle age obesity, lack of exercise, and head injury.

Genetic risk factors

Genetic studies reveal mutations in leucine rich repeat kinase 2 (LRRK-2) in 1% sporadic cases of PD worldwide but in almost one-third North African Arabs and 28% Ashkenazi Jews with hereditary parkinsonism. Genetic mutations have been identified in early onset recessive parkinsonism (<40 years). Glucocerebrosidase (GBA) mutation is found in about 4% UK PD patients, particularly Jewish patients.

Neuropathological findings in PD

A selective loss of dopaminergic neuromelanin-containing neurones from the pars compacta of the substantia nigra is accompanied by Lewy bodies in the substantia nigra and the cortex. Lewy bodies are intraneuronal inclusions and consist largely of abnormal aggregated alpha-synuclein. Lewy bodies are also found at post-mortem in 10% people over 60 years without PD.

Diagnosis

PD has an insidious onset over several years and early symptoms and signs may be ascribed to increasing age, low mood, or arthritis. After diagnosis patients and their family may recall a gradual impairment of dexterity, changes in writing, fatigue, or constipation for some years. The diagnosis of PD is made using the UKPDS Brain Bank Criteria, which is based on motor symptoms and requires unequivocal bradykinesia with at least one of resting tremor, muscular rigidity, or postural instability.

Motor symptoms

Bradykinesia

During a consultation, the following may be observed and elicited: hypomimia (reduction of facial expression, slow to smile, infrequent blinking) and quiet and monotonous speech. Formal testing of repetitive finger movements reveal increasing and asymmetric difficulty maintaining the rhythm and/or range of movement when finger tapping index finger on thumb of each hand for 20 seconds, similarly with piano playing movements and sequentially tapping each finger on the thumb. When asked to write the size of the letters may diminish while writing their address, and episodes of freezing may be noted.

Repetitive foot tapping may show increasing asymmetric difficulty maintaining the rhythm and/or range of lifting the heel 10 cm on and off the ground repetitively for 20 seconds. Posture may be stooped with flexed knees and ankles, which may be difficult to distinguish from 'normal for older person'. Walking may reveal reduced arm swing on one side with mild elbow flexion, reduced foot clearance, and/or shuffle. Gait may be reported as slow but often better when seen in clinic. It may be possible to observe or elicit reports of freezing of gait (feet feel as though stuck to the floor for a moment without warning) on starting to walk, going through a doorway/over the edge of a carpet or on turning especially in small spaces. Patients may take five or more steps to turn through 180°, with truncal rigidity.

Tremor

Typically a resting 'pill rolling' tremor of 4–6 Hz starting in one hand, best seen with hands relaxed in the lap or when walking. The patient may be able to suppress the tremor initially, which may be worse when anxious. The tremor may have a postural component but is absent initially on movement, e.g. holding hands out (unlike essential tremor), before quickly returning. Patients may complain of difficulty managing buttons or drinking from a cup. The tremor spreads first to the ipsilateral leg and later to the opposite limbs. An older patient may also have a tremor of the jaw, chin, lips, and tongue. While tremor is the first symptom in about 75% of patients with PD up to 20% never develop tremor. Tremor dominant PD is associated with a less aggressive disease course, lower age at onset and lower incidence of dementia.

Rigidity

Asymmetrically increased tone felt on passive limb movement, enhanced by similar passive movement of the opposite limb. Rigidity is constant lead-pipe in PD rather than 'clasp-knife', and 'cogwheeling' may be felt from tremor superimposed on the increased tone even if no tremor is visible. Patients may experience rigidity as stiffness.

Postural instability

This important feature of PD develops later in the disease. Falls in the first year of diagnosis make a diagnosis of PD unlikely.

Non-motor symptoms supporting the diagnosis

Direct questioning may reveal a reduced sense of smell (hyposmia), a history of constipation, change in micturition (urgency or retention), pain, e.g. in limbs, altered temperature sensation, sweating, a poor sleep pattern including violent movements, or shouting while dreaming

(REM sleep behaviour disorder), fatigue, apathy, poor concentration, and slowness of thought.

Early supportive prospective positive PD Brain Bank Criteria

Three or more of the following required: unilateral onset, resting tremor present, progressive disorder, persistent asymmetry affecting the side of onset most, excellent (70–100%) response to levodopa.

Differential diagnosis

Essential tremor
Unlike PD this symmetrical postural tremor is worse on action, e.g. signing a cheque and managing buttons is less difficult. Tremor of the head and/or voice may be seen, and a family history of tremor elicited. The tremor may improve after an alcoholic drink, and sense of smell is normal.

Cerebrovascular disease
Difficult to differentiate in older patients with vascular risk factors who may have coexistent cerebrovascular disease and PD. This presents as lower body parkinsonism, with normal facial expression and no reduction in sense of smell. There may be severe gait initiation difficulty with a broad based shuffling gait, no tremor and poor response to levodopa.

Drug induced parkinsonism
Dopamine antagonists, e.g. metaclopramide and prochlorperazine, calcium channel blockers, e.g. cinnarizine, atypical antipsychotics, e.g. amisulpiride and olanzapine, and sodium valproate may precipitate parkinsonism which can take several months to subside after stopping the medication, if ever.

Lewy body dementia
Prominent hallucinations (usually visual, can be auditory) and fluctuating confusion in the first year of presentation (PD dementia presents in a similar way but after several years of physical symptoms). Levodopa is drug of choice for Parkinsonism in small doses with close monitoring as it may aggravate dementia.

Parkinson's plus syndromes
Progressive supranuclear palsy (PSP), multiple system atrophy (MSA), and corticobasal degeneration are described in section 14.2. Differentiation from PD can be difficult in the early stages but falls within the first few years, poor response to levodopa, ophthalmoplegia (PSP), autonomic disturbance, and cerebellar signs (MSA) and rapid progression should alert the physician to reassess the diagnosis.

Red Flags making diagnosis of PD unlikely
- Good sense of smell
- Symmetrical tremor
- History of stroke, anti-dopaminergic agents
- Falls in first year
- Hallucinations and cognitive impairment in first year
- Rapid disease progression/poor response to levodopa

Diagnostic tools

Functional Imaging
Striatal dopamine terminal function can be demonstrated with PET or SPECT scans as an aid to clinical diagnosis, but are not required routinely to make a firm diagnosis. Scan is normal in essential tremor and drug-induced Parkinsonism.

It will not differentiate idiopathic PD from the Parkinson's plus syndromes or Lewy Body dementia as all will have abnormal scans. In vascular Parkinsonism, cerebrovascular disease can give a false positive scan and an MRI may be required. A trial of medication is often indicated as patients may still respond to dopamine replacement.

Structural imaging
MRI shows normal nigral structure in PD but can exclude structural causes of Parkinsonism, e.g. normal pressure hydrocephalus, and can identify the extent of cerebrovascular disease in the basal ganglia. Diffusion-weighted MRI may have a role in discrimination of PD from PSP or MSA. Transcranial sonography is not currently recommended for the investigation of Parkinsonism.

Olfactory testing
Commercially available kits for olfactory testing are being evaluated in research studies and their use in clinical settings is unclear and not currently recommended.

Medication challenge
Acute challenge testing with levodopa is no longer recommended because of the possibility of increasing the risk of future dyskinesia. A trial of medication, increasing the dose gradually to that recommended, will lead to a response in idiopathic PD. Failure to respond raises the possibility of one of the differential diagnoses above and imaging may be indicated

Who should make the diagnosis?
In accordance with the NICE guidelines in England and the SIGN guidelines in Scotland patients with suspected PD should be referred untreated to a specialist, defined as someone who regularly manages people with this condition. Evidence suggests that when specialists diagnose PD using the Brain Bank criteria there is a 90% concordance with the presence of nigral Lewy bodies at autopsy, while the diagnostic error of parkinsonian syndromes diagnosed by non-specialists may be 50%.

Prognosis of Parkinson's disease
People with PD have a standardized mortality ratio of 1.5–2.0 compared with age-matched controls. The mean duration of disease from diagnosis to death is 15 years, although symptoms may have been present for some years prior to diagnosis. Pneumonia is the most common cause of death recorded on the death certificate. Executive dysfunction occurs early in the disease and is present in 85% patients after 15 years of disease, when 48% have dementia.

Further reading
Lees AJ, Hardy J, Revesz T (2009). Parkinson's disease. *Lancet* **373**: 2055–66.

MacPhee G (2008). Diagnosis and differential diagnosis of Parkinson's disease. In Playfer J and Hindle J (eds) *Parkinson's Disease in the Older Patient*, 2nd edn. Oxford, Radcliffe, pp. 41–75.

National Institute for Health and Clinical Excellence (2006). *Parkinson's Disease: Diagnosis and Management in Primary and Secondary care.* NICE Clinical Guideline CG035 (www.nice.org.uk).

Scottish Intercollegiate Guidelines Network (2010). *Diagnosis and pharmacological Management of Parkinson's Disease.* SIGN Guideline 113 (www.SIGN.ac.uk).

Parkinson's disease: treatment

The needs of the Parkinson's patient will vary throughout their journey with the disease. At *diagnosis* they may just need the support of the Parkinson's Disease Specialist Nurse (PDSN) and advice from the physiotherapist; many will ask about neuroprotection. In the *maintenance phase* drug treatment will be initiated and support of occupational and speech and language therapists will become important. As Parkinson's disease (PD) becomes more *complex,* so too do the management strategies with involvement of all the PD team. In the *palliative* stage, management of the neuropsychiatry and carer support generally comes to the fore.

Drugs do not alter the natural history of PD. Initiation of treatment depends upon

- patient preference
- disease severity and functional status
- phenotype
- tremor dominant
- postural instability: gait difficulty
- biological fitness and comorbidities.

The aim is to minimize the substantial burden of PD on individuals, their families, medical services, and society as a whole. Regular review of PD patients and their carers allows each individual's trajectory of disease to be assessed; treatment to be adjusted to minimize symptoms, avoid side-effects and reduce complications as PD progresses. When response to drug treatment is poor, non-existent, or fraught with side-effects, consider alternative diagnoses and that comorbidities may be limiting drug dosage or the cause of residual disability. The treating clinician must have a keen understanding of the pharmacokinetic and pharmacodynamic changes of ageing as well as the treatment options for PD. The treatment of PD frequently necessitates multiple doses of multiple drugs, thus the potential for drug–drug interactions is extremely high, especially in those with comorbidities. There is rarely a need to rapidly escalate drug dosing, as dopaminergic therapies are generally better tolerated and their effect easier to assess if one 'starts low and goes slow'.

Treatment of non-motor problems such as sleep disturbance, constipation, urinary incontinence, drooling, dysphagia, depression, psychosis, dementia, and orthostatic hypotension are dealt with in a separate chapter.

Parkinson's disease specialist nurse

Regular access to a Parkinson's disease specialist nurse will help:

- with clinical monitoring and medication adjustment
- provide a continuing point of contact for support, including home visits, when appropriate
- provide a reliable source of information about clinical and social matters of concern for people with PD and their carers (including concerns regarding driving).

Non-drug treatments

At the time of diagnosis, drug treatment may not be necessary; the impact of non-pharmacological interventions, i.e. physiotherapy and occupational therapy, should be assessed first.

Physiotherapy

Physiotherapy may be useful throughout the course of PD to improve or maintain functional independence by:

- maintaining current physical function

- specific exercises to regain movement (gait re-education and initiation), prevent falls (balance and flexibility), maximize respiratory function (aerobic capacity), or reduce pain
- provision of advice regarding safety in the home
- to enhance the beneficial effects of medical or surgical interventions

The Alexander technique, yoga, conductive education, or Pilates can also promote movement and are linked with social well-being. The Alexander technique in particular may help the individual make lifestyle adjustments that affect both their attitude to and the physical nature of their PD.

Occupational therapy

Occupational therapy, at any stage of PD, may help to

- maintain work and family roles, home care and leisure activities
- improve and maintain transfers and mobility
- improve personal self-care activities such as eating, drinking, washing and dressing
- improve environmental safety, both from a motor and cognitive perspective.

Speech and language therapy

Speech and language therapy is more likely to be required in the later stages of PD, and can

- improve vocal loudness and pitch range, including speech therapy (Lee Silverman voice treatment)
- teach strategies to optimize speech intelligibility
- ensure an effective means of communication is maintained throughout the course of the disease, including use of assistive technologies
- support the safety and efficiency of swallowing to minimize the risk of aspiration.

Drug treatments

Some important considerations at all stages:

- orange tongue and lips mean entacapone is being chewed and may not be effective
- salt and base dosings for pramipexole can be confusing to patient and doctor
- complex dosing regimens are for a purpose and should be adhered to when the individual is hospitalized
- nil by mouth SHOULD NOT mean nil medication
- modern anaesthetic agents allow dosing with oral medication to within 30 minutes of anaesthetic
- PD patients should be given similar consideration as diabetic patients on operating lists.

Neuroprotection

Neuroprotection is one of the 'holy grails' of Parkinson's management but, to date, there is no definite evidence that any drugs are neuroprotective in PD. Putative candidates have included:

Monoamine oxidase-B inhibitors (MAOB-I)

Selegiline and rasagiline. MAOB-I increases striatal dopamine by partially blocking dopamine metabolism, and therefore the production of free hydroxyl radicals. MAOB-I may also stimulate dopamine synthesis and inhibit dopamine reuptake.

In vitro, rasagiline's possible neuroprotective effects appear to be independent of MAOB-I.

Selegiline should be taken before midday to reduce the risk of insomnia induced by its amphetamine metabolites.

The therapeutic effects of MAOB-I may persist for several months after stopping the drug, as loss of activity is dependent upon the generation of new cerebral MAOB. Rapid cessation of treatment may result in rapid deterioration in symptom control.

Coenzyme Q

This is a powerful antioxidant involved in the mitochondrial respiratory chain. In a small pilot study, most benefit was seen in the activities of daily living (ADL) (II) section of the Unified Parkinson's Disease Rating Scale (UPDRS), with no benefit in delaying introduction of L-DOPA. CoQ-10 is supplied by a variety of manufacturers in differing doses.

Riluzole

This is a glutamate inhibitor, has not been shown to effect clinical staging, motor function, or delay time to commencing levodopa.

Dopamine agonists

The oxidation of dopamine in the brain to DOPAC and hydrogen peroxide by MAOB is a potential source of additional oxidative stress and neuronal damage. By suppressing dopamine release, dopamine agonists (DAs) might be expected to reduce the production of reactive oxidative species, such as hydroxyl radicals, offering some neuroprotective benefit. *In vitro*, DAs have also been demonstrated to be free radical scavengers and to be capable of protecting against MPP$^+$ neurotoxicity.

DAs as monotherapy in early PD all delay later motor complications and dyskinesias. Follow on studies with ropinirole (using beta-CIT PET) and with pramipexole (using beta-CIT SPECT) show a reduction in dopaminergic neuronal degeneration, suggesting an *in vivo* neuroprotective role for DAs. The apparent reduction in loss of dopaminergic neurones with pramipexole (44% at 34 months and 37% at 46 months) did not translate in to clinically detectable benefit.

Motor symptoms

Most will require symptomatic treatment within 1–2 years of diagnosis. Which treatment to initiate will largely be determined by whether tremor alone or bradykinesia with or without tremor is the problem; life expectancy (is delaying levodopa relevant?); comorbidities (avoid DAs if cognition impaired) and impact of symptoms on quality of life, i.e. urgency of need for symptom relief (levodopa gives benefit quickly; MAOB-I have weak therapeutic effect; DAs take time to titrate to effect). Although the patient may be worried about the possibility of levodopa-related motor complications and dyskinesias, the geriatrician is worried about drug-induced psychosis and cognitive impairment! Early results of the PD-Med trial suggest levodopa is associated with a better quality of life at the expense of slight excess of dyskinesia and that MAO-I may be preferable to DA due to a lower incidence of non-motor side-effects.

All motor symptoms of PD may be exacerbated by stress (emotional and/or physical).

Tremor

Tremor rarely disappears; at best treatment may only dampen down tremor. Troublesome tremor may respond (30–50% reduction) to levodopa or DAs; however the response to anticholinergics is usually greater.

Anticholinergics (antimuscarinics)

These should be avoided if there is any suggestion of cognitive impairment. They have minimal effect on bradykinesia. Side-effects are not infrequent and limit either their use

completely or restrict dose escalation. Common side-effects include: confusion; hallucinations; altered cognition; xerostomia (may cause problems retaining dentures); urinary retention; constipation; blurring of vision (BEWARE closed angle glaucoma); and delayed gastric emptying affecting levodopa absorption. Perversely, one might use the side-effect profile of low dose anticholinergic to reduce both tremor and detrusor instability.

Beta-blockers

These may be useful alternatives to anticholinergics by reducing the adrenergic response that exacerbates tremor. Low dose propanolol may be particularly useful taken 30–60 minutes before an important stressful event to reduce distressing tremor.

Clozapine

This may be worth trying before resorting to neurosurgical techniques for severe disabling tremor, or if neurosurgery is out of the question. Use of clozapine is limited by the necessity for frequent monitoring of blood count and, in some parts of the UK, is further restricted to being prescribed only by a psychiatrist.

Bradykinesia and gait disturbance

The decision whether to initiate levodopa or DA will be determined by

• level of disability

• any desire to delay possible long-term problems

• immediacy of need

• cognition.

If the need is for immediate symptomatic benefit then levodopa should be initiated. Once the older person, living alone can manage their personal activities of daily living again and is not at risk of getting stuck in the bath, then levodopa dosage can be minimized by judicious introduction of a DA as early adjunctive therapy; thereby dealing with the here and now whilst also paying attention to the long-term. If there is any evidence of cognitive impairment then DAs should not be used. Levodopa and DAs have limited effect on tremor.

Dopamine agonists (ropinirole, pramipexole, rotigotine)

These provide comparable symptomatic benefit to levodopa in early PD, and delay the onset of motor fluctuations and dyskinesias. However, there is a higher incidence of hallucinations and somnolence in those patients treated with DA monotherapy. Initial problems with nausea may be circumvented by slow titration of the DA or coadministration of, the peripheral dopamine antagonist, domperidone (short term, as long-term administration may cause anorexia and weight loss). The correct dose of DA is that which adequately controls symptoms, without causing side-effects. As PD progresses increasing numbers of patients will need to start levodopa (one third after 2 years; one half after 3–4 years; two-thirds by 5 years; all by 10 years).

Pramipexole may be particularly useful in those with concomitant depression.

Rotigotine patches offer a once daily formulation of DA, although their use may be limited by local skin reactions.

Ergot derived DAs (pergolide, cabergoline, lysuride and bromocriptine) are no longer used because of fibrotic complications (pulmonary, cardiac valve and retroperitoneal fibrosis).

Levodopa

This still offers best symptomatic relief and has been the 'gold standard' of PD treatment since 1968. Traditionally when one refers to levodopa this is short form for levodopa in combination with a peripheral dopa-decarboxylase inhibitor (DDI). Carbidopa, the DDI in Sinemet, and benserazide, the DDI in Madopar, increase the amount of a given dose of levodopa that crosses the blood brain barrier from around 1% to 10%.

Levodopa should be taken 30 minutes before or 60 minutes after a meal. Response to levodopa may be unpredictable due to

- delayed absorption (meals, coadministration of an anticholinergic)
- other large neutral amino acids competing for absorption leading to unpredictable response
- delayed gastric emptying (old age, diabetic gastroparesis)
- reduced hepatic metabolism (old age, delirium, disease).

This unpredictability becomes more important as PD progresses and motor fluctuations occur.

Nausea, the commonest side effect of levodopa, may be avoided by taking the dose shortly after a meal or with a light snack, or by the coadministration of domperidone. Domperidone also promotes gastric emptying, thereby facilitating levodopa absorption. Other antiemetics, such as metoclopramide or prochlorperazine, should be avoided because of their central dopamine blocking properties and potential for extrapyramidal side-effects. Other side-effects of levodopa include: anorexia, somnolence, worsening of closed angle glaucoma, postural hypotension, delusions, hallucinations, and altered cognition.

Response to levodopa may be dramatic and evident within 24 hours of dosing. In older people, failure to respond to levodopa (600mg equivalent per day) should lead to the diagnosis being questioned. In the early stages of PD response to levodopa lasts several hours. As the disease progresses, there is a narrowing of the therapeutic window, with therapeutic response more closely matching the short plasma half-life of levodopa, the development of motor fluctuations, and dose failures. Patients may then also complain of diaphoresis, anxiety or mood disturbance.

Shortness of breath in the Parkinson's patient may be a symptom of PD, an indicator of ergot induced pulmonary fibrosis, or an indicator of other comorbidities (anaemia, cardiac failure, intrathoracic malignancy). Impaired respiratory function with upper airways obstruction in PD may respond to levodopa.

There is a theoretical risk that levodopa may be toxic to dopaminergic neurones by increasing oxidative stress. However, there is no evidence that this is so *in vivo*. Nevertheless, this concern has tended to drive down the doses of levodopa used, with resultant lower incidence of motor fluctuations. Motor fluctuations relate to

- disease duration
- duration of treatment with levodopa
- cumulative dose of levodopa exposed to
- current daily dose of levodopa.

The prevalence of motor fluctuations and dyskinesias is probably not as high as the frequently quoted 50% at five years, with rates possibly being as low as 22% or even 10% due to the lower doses of levodopa currently used. As Parkinson's symptoms progress most specialists rarely escalate the dose of levodopa above 400–600 mg equivalent of levodopa without first trying adjunctive therapy.

'On–off' fluctuations and 'peak-dose' dyskinesias seem to be related to pulsatile stimulation of the dopaminergic system and are less likely to occur with continuous stimulation with the same dopaminergic agent. 'Wearing-off' tends to be the first and most common motor fluctuation, characterized by end-of-dose deterioration and recurrence of PD symptoms, due to a shortening of the response to a dose of levodopa. 'Wearing-off' may not be experienced with every dose of levodopa. A variety of treatment strategies may be tried to limit the development of motor fluctuations or to reduce their frequency and severity once they emerge:

- controlled-release levodopa (delay? and treat)
- catechol-O-methyl transferase inhibitor (COMT-I) (treat/? delay)
- dopamine agonists (delay and treat)
- frequent smaller doses of levodopa (treat)
- MAOB-I (treat)
- diet (minimize)
- amantadine (treat)
- botulinum toxin (treat).

Patient diaries will help identify any pattern to motor fluctuations and dyskinesias, guiding management and enabling assessment of the impact of any medication changes.

Theoretically, controlled release (CR) levodopa offers a less pulsatile delivery of levodopa which should result in a reduced incidence of dyskinesias, although this has not been shown in clinical trials. CR-levodopa is as effective as immediate release (IR) levodopa and gives better nocturnal control of symptoms, with improved quality of life.

If changing from IR to CR, the daily levodopa dosage may need to rise by around 20%, although the overall number of doses will fall by around 30–50%. The slow rise to peak levels of CR levodopa may necessitate the use of a 'kick-start' of IR levodopa first thing in the morning and often at other times during the day. Unfortunately, CR formulations may worsen peak dose dyskinesias especially later in the day and, when given at night, may cause nightmares and vivid dreams.

Fractionating the total daily dose of levodopa, so that smaller doses are taken more frequently, perhaps with a CR preparation for nocturnal control, may improve control when motor fluctuations occur. The dose of levodopa is lowered until it causes only mild dyskinesias and the dosing interval is determined by how quickly each dose 'wears off'. The ability of Parkinson's patients to adhere to their complex regimens is testimony to the horrors of being undermedicated or 'off'. However, this strategy has the potential disadvantages of increasing pulsatility of levodopa delivery to the brain potentially 'driving' dyskinesias, and increasing the complexity of dose scheduling, thereby rendering the patient 'tied' to the clock. The more complex the drug regime, the less able institutions (hospitals and care homes) seem able to adhere to it, with resultant loss of quality of life for the patient and increased complication rates, e.g. pressure sores, infection, confusion, anxiety.

Eventually, almost all patients develop 'wearing off' or end of dose deterioration with levodopa, where Parkinson's motor, sensory (paraesthesias and pain), autonomic (breathlessness, tachycardia, sweating), and neuropsychiatric (predominantly bradyphrenia, depression, panic, and anxiety) symptoms increase. Generally these are easy to treat with either more frequent levodopa dosing or extending the duration of action of levodopa by using CR preparations or delaying levodopa metabolism with either a COMT-I or MAOB-I.

Catechol-O-methyl transferase inhibitors (COMT-I)
Once peripheral decarboxylation is inhibited by a DDI, then COMT accounts for most peripheral levodopa metabolism. Entacapone, is a selective, reversible, peripheral COMT-I, tolcapone is a partially reversible peripheral and centrally acting COMT-I (which, due to risk of hepatotoxicity, should only be used if entacapone can not be tolerated).

By prolonging the duration of action of each levodopa dose COMT-I may reduce the daily levodopa requirement (by around 100mg), by enabling a reduction of each dose or an increase in dose intervals (approximate reduction of one dosing interval).

Adjunctive therapy with a COMT-I is more likely to benefit predictable fluctuations than unpredictable ones and should be particularly considered for end of dose 'wearing-off'. Addition of a COMT-I will not benefit dose failures. COMT-I in the absence of levodopa is ineffective; to ensure that IR levodopa and COMT-I are taken simultaneously, it may be better to prescribe them in combination (Stalevo) rather than separately.

Diarrhoea is the most frequent non-dopaminergic adverse events with COMT-I, and liver function must be monitored with tolcapone.

As apomorphine is a potential substrate for O-methylation, caution is advised in the coadministration with a COMT-I. COMT-I should not be taken within 3 hours of taking iron. Entacapone should not be given to patients with liver impairment.

Further options in the treatment of troublesome motor fluctuations and dyskinesias
All adjunctive agents may exacerbate dopaminergic side-effects (e.g. dyskinesias); this means they are working! Dyskinesias are more likely with higher doses of adjunctive therapy – the correct response is to reduce the dose of levodopa. This may be targeted at particular doses that cause dyskinesia or a reduction in total daily dose. Pre-emptive reduction in levodopa dosage should be avoided as this may cause deterioration in symptom control, undermining patient confidence, and quality of life, before the effects of the adjunct 'kick-in' or the effective dose is reached. Dyskinesias that are non-troublesome, and do not cause functional difficulty or distress may not require any reduction in dopaminergic therapy. Most PD patients prefer being 'on' with mild dyskinesia (slightly over-medicated) than being 'off' (under-medicated).

The aim of treatment for patients with motor fluctuations and dyskinesias is to maximize time 'on' without dyskinesia and minimize time 'off'. Patient diaries can delineate problem periods guiding treatment strategies and aiding assessment of the impact of any medication changes. Peak dose dyskinesias generally respond to strategies to reduce dopaminergic peaks and troughs' i.e. to smoothing out the delivery of levodopa to the brain:

- CR levodopa
- COMT-I
- MAOB-I
- DA
- lower doses of levodopa
- amantadine.

'Wearing-off' dystonia generally responds to strategies to provide more sustained dopaminergic stimulation:

- COMT-I
- DA

- MAOB-I
- more frequent dosing with levodopa.

Diphasic dyskinesias often occur randomly with no fixed pattern on a day-to-day basis and prove difficult to treat. Freezing attacks whilst 'off' generally respond to elimination or reduction of 'off' time. Freezing while 'on' is more disappointing to treat.

In this complex phase of PD, much time and effort will be spent tailoring a complex polypharmacy of dopaminergic agents to provide optimal symptom control. Every opportunity should be taken to minimize other drugs, e.g. the hypotensive effects of dopaminergic therapy may allow reduction in antihypertensives.

Dopamine agonists
All DAs are potentially useful adjuncts when motor complications do occur with levodopa. When adding a DA in such circumstances, the total daily dose of levodopa may need to be reduced by around one-fifth to one-quarter.

Apomorphine is highly effective in treating the motor complications of advanced PD, reducing 'off' time by around 50%. Owing to its extensive hepatic first-pass metabolism, it can only be administered by intermittent subcutaneous injections (Apo-Pen) or continuous subcutaneous infusion (ApoGo pump). Its use is often limited in older PD patients due to

- reduced awareness of entering the 'off' phase
- reduced manual dexterity
- absence of someone to administer injections
- reluctance to have someone else determine their daily routine
- needle phobia
- cognitive impairment
- panniculitis (inflammation of the subcutaneous adipose tissue) and subcutaneous nodule formation
- limited availability of PD nurses to supervise apomorphine use.

Intermittent injections rescue the patient from the 'off' state usually within 10 minutes and last around one hour. Where 10 or more injections are needed each day then continuous daily infusion using an ambulatory syringe driver may be used. A nocturnal dose of an oral DA, or low dose rotigotine patch, in conjunction with daytime apomorphine can provide 24-hour control of symptoms. Most patients who start on intermittent injections progress to subcutaneous infusion of apomorphine.

Initiation of apomorphine therapy requires pre-treatment for at least 3 days with domperidone (20 mg tds), to block the emetic and hypotensive effects of apomorphine, before undertaking an 'apomorphine challenge' to determine patient response to the drug and threshold dose. The threshold dose can be used to determine the hourly infusion rate for initiating continuous infusion of apomorphine. Apomorphine can enable significant reductions in other dopaminergic therapies.

Apomorphine may be a useful temporary measure in dysphagic PD patients, e.g. where nasogastric tube can not be tolerated, while awaiting PEG insertion, or those nil by mouth after bowel surgery.

Non-dopaminergic side-effects of apomorphine include panniculitis and nodule formation, eosinophilic myalgia, and haemolytic anaemia. Blood count and Coombe's test should be performed 6 monthly whilst on apomorphine.

MAOB-I

This may be used as adjunctive therapy to reduce 'off' time and improve motor symptoms. Evidence of benefit should be seen within 2–4 weeks.

It has been suggested that long-term use of selegiline with levodopa leads to an excess mortality, more apparent in older patients with a history of falls and dementia. The melt preparation (Zydis Selegiline) may potentially be a safer alternative, as it is one eighth the dose and so has equal reduction in amphetamine metabolites. The absence of amphetamine metabolites with rasagiline may also be of advantage in those with significant cardiovascular disease.

Diet

When motor fluctuations occur, a dietary history should be taken to ascertain whether ingestion of large protein meals are competing with levodopa for absorption (patient switches 'off' after meals or experiences dose failures after certain meals), and appropriate adjustments made in dietary intake if necessary. In general, protein restriction is not necessary and may even be deleterious in older people where poor nutrition and weight loss may reflect advancing disease.

Amantadine

This increases dopamine release, blocks dopamine reuptake, stimulates dopamine receptors, blocks N-methyl D-aspartate (NMDA) receptors and has anticholinergic properties. Drugs with multiple actions usually have poor side-effect profiles; so it is no surprise that amantadine is often poorly tolerated in older people. The propensity for adverse effects in older age is heightened by the prolongation of amantadine's half-life as creatinine clearance falls. The long half-life of amantadine may enable single daily dosing, if the drug is tolerated (remember: 'start low and go slow').

When used as adjunctive therapy to levodopa, amantadine's beneficial effect in reducing dyskinesias and motor fluctuations may be due to its effects as an NMDA antagonist.

Botulinum toxin

This may benefit severe focal dystonias, unresponsive to dopaminergic therapy. Beneficial effects may be seen within days and can last several months. The use of botulinum toxin should be reserved for experienced users only.

Other drugs

Clozapine, fluoxetine, and propanolol have all been shown to reduce levodopa induced dyskinesias and motor fluctuations.

Complementary and alternative therapies

Complementary and alternative therapies (CAM) are used by more than one-third of PD patients. The potential for interaction of CAM with conventional Western therapies should not be forgotten. There is very little evidence to either refute or support their use.

Neurosurgery

May benefit the patient who is
- biologically young
- otherwise healthy
- psychologically motivated
- free of psychiatric disease (depression, dementia)
- who remains levodopa responsive
- with disabling symptoms refractory to optimal drug therapy.

Options include subthalamic deep brain stimulation (DBS), globus pallidus interna DBS, and thalamic DBS. It is not possible to say if one type of DBS is better than another, although thalamic DBS is generally only recommended for those who predominantly have severe disabling tremor.

Palliative care

Palliative care needs should be considered throughout the course of the disease, with opportunity for the PD sufferer and their carers to discuss end-of-life issues as they feel appropriate and to be given advice on Advance Care Planning.

There tends to be a subtle shift of emphasis (of care and support) from the PD sufferer to their carer as PD moves from complex to palliative care.

It is not always easy to predict which episode of aspiration pneumonia or which fall and fracture will be the terminal event. However, the following pointers may help identify those in whom the Gold Standards Framework and Preferred Priorities of Care should be utilized:
- more than three unplanned hospital admissions in the last year
- admission to a care home as a resident (not respite)
- continued weight loss that can only be attributed to the PD
- dementia and/or autonomic dysfunction with multiple, daily falls.

A balance will need to be struck between maintaining mobility, minimizing psychosis (hallucinations and delusions), minimizing falls risk, managing dementia and depression, minimizing non-motor symptoms, maintaining nutrition, and 'preserving the carer,' who often feels they have 'failed' if institutional care is needed.

Minimizing the neuropsychiatry usually trumps maintaining mobility. This usually entails a systematic unpicking of a previously carefully crafted drug regime. The order of drug withdrawal is usually
- anticholinergics
- tricyclics
- MAOB-I
- amantadine
- other antidepressants
- DAs
- apomorphine
- levodopa.

Carer support

The educational needs of carers mirror those of the PD sufferer throughout the progression of PD. Carers require recognition of their role and access to social care and benefits. Respite care will need to be considered as will the health needs of the carer (many of whom will also be old and have their own health problems). The PD team need to be vigilant for signs of carer strain and depression (increasingly common as carer burden increases) and consider the possibility of insipient dementia in the older carer who is struggling to cope.

What does the future have in store?

The pharmacological treatment of PD has come a long way since the introduction of levodopa in the 1960s and has become far more complicated (Table 13.4 summarizes the place of current drug treatments). The immediate future promises even more complexity of choice and

Table 13.4 Indications and cautions for drugs used in Parkinson's disease

Drug	Indications	Cautions *(see also BNF)*
Levodopa Madopar Sinemet	*De novo* (biologically frail) Motor fluctuations	Postural hypotension Closed angle glaucoma History of malignant melanoma
Dopamine agonists Ropinirole Pramipexole Rotigotine	*De novo* (biologically sound) Motor fluctuations	Cognitive impairment Psychosis Postural hypotension
MAOB-I Selegiline Zydis selegiline Rasagiline	Very mild early disease Motor fluctuations	Cognitive impairment Cardiovascular disease Postural hypotension Co-prescribing with antidepressants
COMT-I Entacapone Tolcapone	End of dose wearing-off	Tolcapone is only licensed for use where entacapone has failed and there is no evidence of hepatic dysfunction; it requires frequent liver monitoring.
Amantadine	Dyskinesias Motor fluctuations	Cognitive impairment Ischaemic heart disease Postural hypotension
Apomorphine	Resistant motor fluctuations and/or dyskinesias	Cognitive impairment Psychosis
Anticholinergics	Tremor	Cognitive impairment Closed angle glaucoma Severe prostatism Postural hypotension

decision making. The complexity of the disease and its treatment strategies should dictate that all Parkinson's patients are managed within a specialist service.

As well as novel drug delivery systems (e.g. transdermal patches), modulators of other neurotransmitter pathways will enter in to our armamentarium:

- cannabinoid agonists and antagonists may have beneficial effects on drug induced dyskinesias, mediated through their effects on gamma-aminobutyric acid receptors
- alpha-2-adrenoreceptor blockade (e.g. idazoxan) reduces levodopa induced dyskinesias
- adenosine receptor antagonists may be beneficial in PD
- manipulation of 5-hydroxytryptamine (serotonin) pathways may improve motor functioning in PD.

Conclusion

The pharmacological management of PD in older age requires an in depth understanding of the complexities of both the disease and age related changes in pharmacokinetics and pharmacodynamics. There is an ever increasing armamentarium at our disposal, but the results of clinical trials have to be extrapolated in to a population rarely included in them (older people with comorbidities).

A pragmatic approach to minimizing the symptoms of PD, whilst not causing untoward drug induced side-effects, is necessary. This can best be achieved by attending to detail:

- understand your patient's problems
- know the limitations of drug treatment
- consider non-pharmacological options
- keep the patient informed of the options
- monitor the effects of treatments (beneficial and negative).

There is rarely a need to rush, so start low and go slow with dose titrations. Know the limitations of your expertise and call in an expert when necessary.

Further reading

Forsyth DR (2004). CME drug treatment of Parkinson's disease. *J Geriatric Med* **6**: 47–63.

Gold Standards Framework (www.goldstandardsframework.nhs.uk).

Preferred Priorities of Care (www.endoflifecare.nhs.uk)

NICE (2006). *Parkinson's Disease: Diagnosis and Management in Primary and Secondary Care.* NICE Clinical Guideline 35. London, National Institute for Health and Clinical Excellence.

RCP (2006). *Parkinson's Disease.* National clinical guideline for diagnosis and management in primary and secondary care. London, Royal College of Physicians.

Parkinson's disease: non motor symptoms

The non-motor symptoms of Parkinson's disease (PD) result in as much of the disease burden as the motor aspects. Many are amenable to specific treatments, though with all, treating any concurrent conditions and optimizing the medication are important. This section concentrates on other specific approaches to reducing symptoms with the older population in mind. The next section addresses some of the important aspects of the condition not covered elsewhere. Many of the treatment options suggested are not licensed for use in the setting described.

Autonomic symptoms

These are features in many PD patients, though multisystem atrophy should be considered when they are significant clinical features at or soon after presentation.

Constipation: should be managed as normal with a high-fibre diet, high fluid intake, and laxatives as required. This common symptom causes reduced appetite and nausea, and has been associated with reduced efficacy off medication owing to reduced absorption. Entacapone can cause diarrhoea and so can be useful where medication needs increasing and constipation has been a problem.

Postural hypotension. This is typically associated with medication, dehydration, and autonomic dysfunction; it can be aggravated by infection, warm temperatures, and alcohol. The mainstay of treatment is to avoid sudden postural changes, increase fluid intake, often with small amounts taken regularly, combined with increased salt intake (e.g. crisps). Medications, such as antihypertensives should be reviewed. Fludrocortisone and midodrine can help. Compression stockings can be tried, but need to be full length, and are often poorly tolerated.

Abnormal sweating. An autonomic feature in its own right, this can also be seen as a feature of the PD medications wearing off. Rule out treatable causes such as infection, hormonal imbalance, or medication. Otherwise this will reflect autonomic dysfunction, treatment can be difficult, and includes wearing breathable fabric such as cotton, ensuring good fluid intake. Where sweating is excessive, patients can be considered for Botox injections.

Sialorrhoea. This does not result from excessive saliva production but from reduced swallowing. Poor lip closure and poor posture with a tendency to lean forwards can aggravate drooling. It can be exacerbated by cholinesterase inhibitors. Conservative treatment options include stimulating conscious swallowing, such as with a glass of water or sugar-free sweets, or optimizing posture with lifting the chin up. Topical options include atropine 1% drops sublingually (up to 2 drops tds; the same drops as used in glaucoma) or Ipratropium inhaler sprayed around the mouth. Both work best with a drier mouth; the atropine drops tend to last for a longer time period, while the Ipratropium can be helpful for short term use, with benefits lasting around 1 hour. Other options include hyoscine patches, although these will have systemic side-effects including confusion and hallucinations, and botulinum toxin injections.

Erectile dysfunction. This can be treated with phosphodiesterase inhibitors such as sildenafil, but these may aggravate postural hypotension. Prescribing medication here should take into account issues such as the psychological side-effects from dopamine agonists (see below), and also the effects they may have it on a partner. Be aware of other coexisting problems such as depression.

Urinary symptoms

Retention: This sometimes responds to medication, such as tamsulosin, where there are concomitant problem such as benign prostatic hyperplasia, and is better when constipation is treated. Otherwise it may require an indwelling catheter. Alpha-adrenoceptor blocking drugs can aggravate Parkinsonism, depression and postural hypotension. Most patients with idiopathic PD who have this degree of autonomic dysfunction will not be suitable for intermittent self-catheterization.

Urinary urgency: As always, urinary infections should be excluded and the patient should be advised to optimize fluid intake to avoid concentrated urine (which is irritant to the bladder and can increase frequency albeit with smaller volumes) and aggravate incontinence. Trospium does not cross the blood brain barrier, and so is less likely to cause confusion, whereas solifenacin is the most selective agent in this class. All these medications can precipitate urinary retention.

Nocturia: Some studies have shown this to be one of the features linked most closely with reduced quality of life. Optimizing overnight PD control, such as with long acting dopamine agonists, and ensuring fluid intake is maximized earlier in the day so it is safe to reduce in the evening, can both help. Desmopressin can be tried.

> **Author's Tip**
>
> It is not uncommon to see older men with PD labelled with 'prostatism', when their symptoms actually reflect autonomic dysfunction and PD. Formal urodynamic studies can help guide interventions and potentially avoid unnecessary operations.

Sleep problems and Parkinson's disease

Increasing recognition is recently being given to the various sleep disturbances associated with PD. Symptoms can pre-date the onset of PD by a number of years. Generic treatment should include:

- Optimizing sleep hygiene (regular sleep pattern, avoid caffeine pre-bed, blackout curtains).
- Ensuring adequate motor control of PD overnight, through the use of long-acting dopamine agonist or addition of COMTi to night time levodopa.) Controlled-release formulations are erratically absorbed and so no longer recommended.

Restless legs syndrome (RLS). This is the irresistible urge to move ones legs when at rest, particularly in the evenings and overnight. This is distinct from the dopamine agonist withdrawal syndrome (DAWS), with akathisia and often associated with an overwhelming sense of anxiety, though without any diurnal variation. Treatment for RLS includes optimizing overnight dopaminergic stimulation, and excluding and treating other pathologies, such as iron deficiency (with or without anaemia) and peripheral vascular disease. Clonazepam can help. Sometimes 'augmentation' can be seen, whereby after reduction in dopaminergic treatment, the restless leg syndrome returns at greater severity.

REM sleep behaviour disorder. Patients are occasionally aware of having vivid dreams at night, though more commonly it is the partner who comments on restless sleeping patterns and calling out. Where treatment is required, clonazepam can be used.

Obstructive sleep apnoea. This is relatively common in patients with PD, though typically mild with oxygen saturations not dropping below 90%. Treatments such as CPAP are usually poorly tolerated.

Excessive daytime somnolence. Patients describe sleeping reasonably well overnight, but then dropping off frequently throughout the day, which in turn can interfere with daily activities. It can be exacerbated by PD medication, particularly dopamine agonists. Modafinil can help, though side-effects include anxiety and confusion.

Blepharospasm. Some patients complain of an inability to keep their eyes open, distinct from excessive daytime sleepiness. Blepharospasm is treatable with botulinum toxin.

Oropharyngeal problems

Hypophonia: Patients with PD often have soft voices, though may not always be aware of this. Typically, it is partners and families who complain that the patient is 'always mumbling' and the patient is frequently asked to repeat themselves. After medication optimization, patients should be referred to the speech therapists. The Lee Silverman Voice Technique involves encouraging the patient to 'Think loud; shout loud.' In turn, this brings the patients voice up to more audible levels, with benefits being evident up to 2 years after starting the intervention. Some patients describe mentally using a similar technique to aid their writing.

Dysphagia: This is common in advanced PD and should be suspected where hypophonia is present. Dysphagia is associated with weight loss, which can be aggravated by reduced enjoyment of food through loss of olfaction (frequently pre-dating the onset of PD by several years) and reduced sense of taste. Management includes:

1 Optimize posture when eating.
2 Opportunistic approach to feeding, from small amounts frequently (patients often fatigue) to feeding when the patient is 'on' and awake, rather than sticking to set mealtimes.
3 SALT and dietician referrals.
4 Consider liquid medications (e.g. soluble co-beneldopa) or patches (e.g. rotigotine).
5 Soft moist mashable diet; good nutrition and fluid with yoghurts or smoothies; dietitians can guide on keeping diet palatable and varied.
6 Patients with advanced progressive supranuclear palsy sometimes have trismus and are unable to seal their lips when swallowing. Anecdotally, low doses of clonazepam 0.5 mg nocte may help (may need to be given subcutaneously.)

Psychiatric

Depression

Reported prevalence rates for depression in PD are very variable, though around 30–40% of PD patients will have significant depressive features at some stage, albeit without necessarily being formally diagnosed with depression or treated for it. It can be difficult to recognize depression as the cause for the patient's symptoms rather than PD itself. Presenting features include anhedonia; apathy; psychomotor retardation, and cognitive impairment (pseudo-dementia); dropping of hobbies and interests (in excess of that attributable to the patient's Parkinsonism); reduced level of functioning; a sense of pessimism with generally 'negative' comments; increased carer strain; and a feeling that the PD is never adequately controlled. Depression is usually treatable.

Biochemically, dopamine is involved in 'reward' systems in the brain, and without this it is postulated that patients do not feel the same sensation when they have done something well or are complemented on something. In turn, dopaminergic stimulation can in itself improve mood with optimization of the PD medication often being sufficient.

Cerebral imaging in PD patients with depression has shown proportionately more noradrenergic than serotonin deficits. However, medications such as tricyclic antidepressants may aggravate autonomic features and increase confusion. In practice, SSRIs tend to be used as first-line agents to treat depression as they are better tolerated. Mirtazepine can be helpful for depressed patients with anxiety and sleep problems, though its sedative properties increase falls risk and daytime somnolence.

Non-pharmacological interventions include simple measures such as having regular meals with family and friends to get the patient and their carer out of the house more. Depression puts an increased strain on the carer and respite should be considered.

Cognitive impairment

This will affect most older PD patients at some stage, and often the cognitive decline will be associated with visual hallucinations. Visuoperceptual problems appear early and may be missed if screening is done via the Abbreviated Mental Test Score, and only start to become apparent with the MMSE. SCOPA-COG (SCales for Outcomes of PArkinson's disease–cognition) was designed specifically for PD patients, and consists of 10 items with a maximum score of 43, with higher scores reflecting better performance. More constructional based tests are likely to pick up problems sooner, such as clock drawing tasks.

Non-pharmacological interventions are the same as for other patients with cognitive problems. Minimizing medication where possible can help, initially withdrawing anticholinergic agents, then amantadine, then dopamine agonists. The mainstay of motor PD control here is with levodopa and COMT inhibitors, as these are the least likely to aggravate confusion. Other aggravating non-PD medication should also be reviewed. Cholinesterase inhibitors, such as rivastigmine, have a role in treatment; there are some reports of memantine improving symptom control. Often the development of cognitive problems significantly increases strain on the carer, and support for them should be reviewed at this stage.

Hallucinations

These are common especially in advanced PD. Hallucinations occurring within the first 2 years of disease onset suggest Lewy Body Disease. The hallucinations are typically extracampine (i.e. outside the body) and complex (i.e. seeing cats or children, rather than just flashing lights). They often start with vivid dreams overnight or an awareness of people at the peripheries of vision, and tend to progress with time. Sometimes delusions can be present, such as Capgras syndrome or Othello syndrome. Treatment for these is the same.

The management for hallucinations includes:
• check cognition
• rule out infection/other acute reversible causes
• ascertain impact on patient: often minimal at first and risks of medication outweigh benefits, though this balance often changes with time

- reduce medication: dopamine agonists are particularly likely to cause hallucinations
- consider cholinesterase inhibitors e.g. rivastigmine, or atypical antipsychotic e.g. quetiapine (fewest extrapyramidal side-effects), although the evidence base is limited.

Impulsive–compulsive disorders

This range of disorders are most commonly associated with dopamine agonist therapy, though can occur with other dopaminergic treatments. There are a number of recognized patterns and patients may show features of several, including:

Impulse control disorders

The patient has an urge to do something, with pleasure being derived afterwards. Variants include pathological gambling or shopping (with the potential for bankruptcy), sexual disinhibition (including hypersexuality and paraphilias), and binge eating.

Compulsive disorders

Here the patient has an urge to do something, with relief being derived afterwards. Features include repeated hand washing or double-checking everything.

Punding

This describes the purposeless repeated behaviours. Sometimes this involves constant reorganization of, for example, books or videos, while other times it is the constant repainting of the sky on a drawing, despite satisfaction with the original version. Often the behaviour reflects pre-morbid interests. The patient typically gets no emotional benefit from the behaviour, though can be irritable if interrupted. The issues can result in the patient neglecting their basic needs, such as personal hygiene, sleep, or meals.

Dopamine dysregulation syndrome

Here the patient exhibits an addictive attitude towards their medication and their usage of it. There can be features such as hoarding, followed by taking excessive quantities (more than required for clinically adequate control) for the 'high' from this. It can be very difficult to recognize, and should be suspected in patients requiring unusually rapid dose escalations or where there are significant discrepancies between subjective and objective states of the patient. Diagnosis can be aided through review of GP prescribing records, and PD nurses seeing how many tablets are taken and the dates on the packaging.

Detecting any of these features can be a problem, not least as people do not associate medication or disease with this behaviour and look for other causes. The Questionnaire for Impulsive-Compulsive Disorders in Parkinson's Disease (QUIP) is a screening tool that can help. Often the patient has poor insight into their behaviour or that it is abnormal, while at other times they wish to conceal it, either because they do not want to lose the pleasure they gain from it, or wish to cover up its consequences (such as gambling debts). Diagnosis is through vigilance for the condition, education of patients, families, carers, and GPs of their

existence (e.g. through clinic letters to GPs which can be copied to the patient) and ensuring the topic is mentioned when initiating or increasing dopamine agonist medication.

Pain

Dopamine is thought to be related to perceived pain thresholds, with reduced dopamine lowering these. In turn, optimizing dopaminergic stimulation can alleviate symptoms. Pain or discomfort related to PD affects about 40% of patients. Other causes of pain clearly should also be considered, such as pain due to osteoarthritis, polymyalgia rheumatic, or osteomalacia. Ford classified pain related to PD into five main categories:

Musculoskeletal: This is aching in nature with muscle tenderness; it may relate to Parkinsonian posture. Treatment is with simple analgesia and physiotherapy.

Radicular/neuropathic: This is associated with poor posture combined with age-related changes. Treatment is with physiotherapy to optimise posture, neurosurgery if appropriate, and medication for neuropathic pain.

Dystonic: This can affect any limb or facial/pharyngeal muscles and cause quite severe pain. It often correlates with medication timing and diary cards be helpful. Types include early morning dystonia, beginning and end of dose dystonia, peak-dose dystonia and off-periods. Treatment is to optimise continuous dopaminergic stimulation. Anticholinergics and amantadine can be considered, though may aggravate confusion. Baclofen or Botulinum toxin can also be used.

Central: This is variable in character, including burning/typical neuropathic qualities, formication, sometimes with autonomic features, e.g. abdominal pains or dyspnoea. It can be difficult to treat; if optimizing dopaminergic therapy and simple analgesia are unsuccessful, agents such as tricyclics and gabapentin can be tried.

Akathisia: Patients complain of a sense of restlessness with an irresistible urge to move and sometimes marked anxiety. It can affect daily activities, e.g. driving, sitting for mealtimes. It can occur as a feature of medication wearing off or with reductions in dopaminergic medication. It improves with dopaminergic medication.

Further reading

Evans AH, Strafella AP, Weintraub D, et al (2009). Impulsive and compulsive behaviors in Parkinson's disease. *Mov Disord* **24**: 1561–70.

Ford B. (2010), Pain in Parkinson's disease. *Mov Disord* **21**: S98–S103.

Mostile G, Jankovic J (2009). Treatment of dysautonomia associated with Parkinson's disease. *Parkinsonism Relat Disord* **15**: S224–S32.

NICE (2002). Parkinson's disease: diagnosis and management in primary and secondary care. NICE clinical guideline 35. London, NICE (www.nice.org.uk/CG035).

Scottish Intercollegiate Guidelines Network (2010) Diagnosis and pharmacological management of Parkinson's disease. Edinburgh, SIGN (www.sign.ac.uk/guidelines/fulltext/113/index.html).

Weintraub D, Hoops S, Shea JA, et al (2009). Validation of the questionnaire for impulsive-compulsive disorders in Parkinson's disease. *Mov Disord* **24**: 1461–7.

Living with Parkinson's disease

Falls

Postural instability is in one of the key features of parkinsonism. Frequent falls early in the disease suggests alternative pathology, including vascular parkinsonism or a Parkinson's disease (PD)-plus syndrome. The medical management of falls adopts the standard approaches, including minimizing medication, checking for orthostatic hypotension or other causes of syncope, and starting appropriate bone protection (many patients have relatively poor intakes of calcium and vitamin D; consider either strontium or intravenous zoledronate in dysphagic patients.)

Physiotherapists and occupational therapists should be involved, and there is good evidence for interventions such as tai chi, which encourage making slow purposeful movements with a low centre of gravity.

Freezing

- Optimize continuous dopaminergic stimulation (e.g. long-acting dopamine agonists or COMT inhibitors) Some authors suggest rasagiline and amantadine can be helpful.
- Refer to the physiotherapists for gait review. Cueing techniques prompt raising of the feet with walking (such as counting 'One, two, one, two...' or music).

Sometimes patients are worse with anxiety, which can be precipitated by being in crowds or other busy and stressful situations, for which avoidance is the best cure

Bed mobility and overnight PD control

Many patients have poor PD control overnight, such as with turning in bed or getting to the toilet, and into the following morning. Often adjustment of medication timings can be sufficient (some patients have their last medication at 6 pm and none until the following morning.) Once-daily medications, such as the long-acting dopamine agonists, may be helpful. To help achieve rapid control for the early morning, soluble co-beneldopa (62.5–125 mg) is rapidly absorbed.

Other ways to facilitate turning over in bed include having a grab rail adjacent to the bed, or having satin sheets or night clothes.

Dressing

Many simple things can ease this, such as choosing clothes with larger buttons or zips, shoes with Velcro straps, stretchy fabrics, 'clip-on ties, bras that fasten at the front; sitting down while dressing. Avoid distractions while dressing as this can affect the flow. Lighter shoes may reduce shuffling. Choice of sole can either be to facilitate movement (the more slippery leather soles) or enhance grip (such as with rubber soles.)

Choose clothes that make going to the toilet easier, especially if urgency is an issue. Adding tabs to zips or thumb straps to underwear can facilitate dressing.

Loose skirts that can be tucked into underwear can ensure that both hands are free to help when standing, and without risking the skirt getting wet with falling into the toilet bowl.

Writing

Patients' writing tends to get smaller and increasingly spidery as the sentence goes on. Different types of pen can help, such as felt tip pens. Weights around the wrist (such as those available from sports shops) may help reduce the amplitude of the tremor, but are not always well tolerated. Using a clipboard or a non-slip mat prevents the page moving with the tremor. Having a pause and a stretch after each sentence, or whenever the writing starts to get a bit smaller, can keep the writing at a better size. Alternatives include the use of a Dictaphone. Some patients report that speaking out loud while writing helps improve their micrographia. Alternatives include use of a computer, although this can be limited by cognitive impairment.

Driving

People with PD have to inform the DVLA of their condition. Most will be able to continue driving for a number of years after their diagnosis, with issues such as their motor control, the presence of hallucinations and cognitive impairment determining whether this is safe in the longer term.

Disability badges ('Blue badges') can help (with the main criterion being the ability to walk 50 metres), and mobility scooters can make the difference between being stuck indoors all the time and being able to get out a little.

Carer strain

As the disease progresses, there are increasing demands on the carer: physically, psychologically, and financially. One survey found that 75% of carers (including non-PD patients) felt they did not have their own life, and had lost touch with family and friends. Support through the medical team, PD specialist nurses, social services, and community matrons are invaluable. Carer strain can be improved through attention to treating any depression in the patient and optimizing control overnight to ensure a good night's sleep for both. Some carers benefit from the group support through regional Parkinson's UK (PD UK) meetings.

Regular respite is often required, either through Day Centres, sitting services or intermittent admission to a care home, and can prolong the overall length of time that the patient is able to stay at home. Holidays which cater for those with chronic disease and their carers also help, though can be quite expensive.

Finances

Although most older people with PD will no longer be working, there are significant costs from PD through the need for providing care, either at home or in residential care. Various allowances are available, and help going through the forms can be through social services. PD UK has a helpline and funds posts to help with these issues.

Legal issues

PD is a slowly progressive disease associated with significant cognitive impairment and dependency. While never easy topics to raise, issues such as Power of Attorney, advanced care planning and financial wills should be addressed early on and reviewed regularly.

Further reading

Schrag A, Hovris A, Morley D, et al. (2006). Caregiver-burden in Parkinson's disease is closely associated with psychiatric symptoms, falls, and disability. *Parkinsonism Relat Disord* **12**: 35–41.

www.parkinsons.org.uk
www.enableholidays.com

Parkinson's plus syndromes

Introduction
'Parkinson's plus syndromes' is the name giving to a heterogeneous group of progressive neurodegenerative disorders including progressive supranuclear palsy (PSP), multisystem atrophy (MSA) and cortical basal ganglionic degeneration (CBGD). These disorders share parkinsonism as a common feature but have their own unique characteristics and are very distinct from idiopathic Parkinson's disease (PD), with a worse prognosis and poorer response to treatment.

Progressive supranuclear palsy
Definition and epidemiology
PSP was first described in 1964 by Steele *et al.* The prevalence is approximately 6 per 100 000, with symptoms typically beginning in the sixth or seventh decades. Men are more commonly affected.

Aetiology and pathology
The aetiology of PSP is unknown. A few familial clusters have been reported. Pathologically, PSP causes neuronal loss and gliosis with atrophy of the midbrain tegentum, frontal lobe, superior cerebellar peduncle, and subthalamic nucleus. The substantia nigra is depigmented. Histologically, the key feature is the deposition of Tau protein containing neurofibrillary tangles.

Clinical features
The most striking features are early postural instability with falls and supranuclear gaze palsy. These backward falls tend to occur within 12 months of disease onset. The gaze palsy is classically downward, although eventually both upward and horizontal gaze are impaired. Doll's eye manoeuvre is normal, indicating its supranuclear origin. Other features are a characteristic facial expression (wide-eyed Mona Lisa stare with decreased blink rate), distinctive slurred growling voice and early, frontal type dementia with executive dysfunction, bradyphrenia, and personality changes.

Unlike PD, PSP rarely causes tremor, and rigidity tends to be axial with relative sparing of the limbs. The classic stooped posture of PD is also absent. Instead, patients tend to display a hyperextended, retrocollic stance.

Investigations
The diagnosis is principally clinical. The recently devised National Institute of Neurological Disorders and the Society for Progressive Supranuclear Palsy criteria are found to have high diagnostic sensitivity and specificity. The classic brain magnetic resonance imaging (MRI) findings (70% sensitivity) include atrophy and high signal in the midbrain and red nucleus as well as frontal and temporal lobes. However, these findings are non-specific and can be seen in other neurodegenerative conditions, including MSA. The role of cerebrospinal fluid analysis for biomarkers is not established.

Management and prognosis
Drug therapies are largely ineffective and give rise to frequent side effects. Levodopa response is often modest and short-lived with benefit seen in <30% of patients. The course tends to be unremitting with a median survival of approximately 6-8 years. Treatments should therefore be symptomatic with emphasis on quality-of-life improvement. Therapies including botulinium toxin for blephorospasm and neck rigidity, antidepressants for emotional disturbances, speech therapy for dysarthria and dysphagia, as well as physiotherapy and occupational therapy can all be helpful.

Multisystem atrophy
Definition and epidemiology
MSA encompasses striatonigral degeneration (snd), olivopontocerebellar atrophy (OPCA) and Shy–Drager syndrome (SDS). These alpha-synucleinopathies cause parkinsonism, cerebellar dysfunction, pyramidal signs, and autonomic failure in varying combinations. The names SND, OPCA, and SDS are now being replaced by 'MSA-P', which refers to a parkinsonism dominant phenotype and 'MSA-C' for the predominantly cerebellar type. The prevalence is approximately 4 per 100 000 with a mean onset age of 54 years.

Aetiology and pathology
The aetiology of MSA is unknown with no reported genetic links. It is typified by neuronal loss, atrophy, and gliosis in the substantia nigra, putamen, pontine nuclei, cerebellum, and intermediolateral columns of the spinal cord. The histological finding of glial cytoplasmic inclusions containing α-synuclein links the subtypes of MSA.

Clinical features
In order of frequency, the most common signs are parkinsonism, autonomic dysfunction, cerebellar ataxia, and pyramidal signs. MSA-P usually presents with symmetrical parkinsonism (often without tremor), early postural instability, and an exaggerated antecollis posture. MSA-C patients have Parkinsonism with prominent cerebellar signs.

Autonomic failure including postural hypotension, urinary incontinence, and impotence develops in the majority of patients and may precede the onset of motor symptoms. Other features include irregular myoclonic jerks, sleep disturbances, and laryngeal dystonia. Cognitive function is relatively well preserved. Exclusion criteria for diagnosis include onset age less than 30, familial history, and early dementia.

Investigations
There is no definitive investigation and validity of brain imaging (structural and functional), autonomic testing, sphincter EMG, and sleep studies is not established. MRI may reveal atrophy, striatal hypointensity and infratentorial signal changes. Occasionally the 'hot cross bun sign', thought to be due to selective degeneration of pontine fibres, is seen.

Management and prognosis
Prognosis is poor with a mean survival of just 7 years. Just like PSP, drug therapies are disappointing and allied health professionals have a crucial role in relieving symptoms and improving quality of life.

Cerebellar symptoms tend to be refractory; though MSA-P shows a better response to levodopa with occasional help derived from additional dopamine agonists and/or amantadine.

Autonomic features are most amenable to interventions. Urinary symptoms may be improved by anticholinergics and postural hypotension by non-pharmacological measures as well as fludrocortisone or midodrine.

Corticalbasal ganglionic degeneration

Definition and epidemiology

Corticalbasal ganglionic degeneration is extremely rare and is characterized by an asymmetrical and akinetic rigid syndrome with localized cortical deficits. The mean age of onset is 64 years. Male and female are equally affected.

Aetiology and pathology

The aetiology is unknown. Pathologically, there is asymmetrical focal frontoparietal atrophy, depigmentation of the substantia nigra with Lewy bodies, and diffuse neuronal loss. Like PSP, it is a tauopathy with tau-positive neuronal and glial inclusions seen in the cortex and substantia nigra.

Clinical features

CBGD is characterized by asymmetrical rigidity and brady-kinesia affecting typically one limb which is often described as 'useless' or 'dead'. Apraxia occurs in both affected and unaffected limbs. 'Alien-limb phenomena' with intermanual conflict occurs in 50%. Cognitive impairment is common. Other features include dystonia, myoclonus, cortical sensory loss and abnormal eye signs (horizontal saccades impairment). Rest tremor is rare, but when present is usually faster and more irregular than in PD.

Investigations

There is no diagnostic test. Neither structural nor functional brain imaging reveal any characteristic features.

Management and prognosis

Drug therapies are ineffective. Parkinsonism is particularly resistant to levodopa. Clonazepam and botulinium toxin may improve myoclonus and dystonia respectively. The prognosis is poor with death usually occurring within 10 years of diagnosis.

Further reading

Gilman S, Wenning GK, Low PA, et al. (2008). Second consensus statement in the diagnosis of multiple system atrophy. *Neurology* **71**: 670–6.

Litvan I, Agid Y, Lalue D, et al. (1996). Clinical research criteria for the diagnosis of Progressive Supernuclear Palsy (Steele-Richardson-Oleszwski syndrome): report of the NINDS-SPSP International workshop. *Neurology* **47**: 1–9.

Litvan I, Bhatia K, Burns D, et al. (2003). SIC task force appraisal of clinical diagnostic criteria for parkinsonian disorders. *Movement Disorders* **18**: 467–86.

Mahaptra R, Edwards MJ, Schott JM, et al. (2004). Corticobasal degeneration, *Lancet Neurology* **3**: 736–43.

Nath U, Ben-Shlomo Y, Thomson R, et al. (2003). Clinical features and natural history of Progressive Supranuclear Palsy. *Neurology* **60**: 910–16.

Quinn NP (2004). Multi-system atrophy. In Marsden CD, Fahn S (eds). *Movement Disorders*, **3**: 262–81.

Other useful information can be found on the PSP website (www.psp.org).

Benign essential tremor

Also known as essential tremor, familial tremor or hereditary essential tremor

Epidemiology

Benign essential tremor (ET) is probably the most common adult-onset movement disorder, although others may argue that restless legs syndrome is more common. Although ET can start at any age, its prevalence clearly increases with age. The exact prevalence of ET is not known, as various epidemiological studies show a wide variability, with prevalence rates varying from 0.01% to 21%. In a meta-analysis of pooled worldwide studies, the prevalence of ET was reported to be 0.9% for all ages, and 4.6% for those above the age of 65 years. This marked variability is probably more related to different methodology rather than a true difference in population prevalence. ET is markedly underdiagnosed and at least 75% of cases identified through epidemiological studies have not been diagnosed before. There is no significant gender difference in ET, although some studies show a slightly higher prevalence in males.

Pathophysiology:

Electrophysiological studies point to a central tremorgenic oscillation. This results in a disturbance of rhythmic activity of neuronal network involving the thalamus, sensorimotor cortex, inferior olivary nuclei and the cerebellum. In the harmaline (a reversible monoamine oxidase inhibitor) animal model of ET, tremorgenic oscillations of the olivocerebellar pathway were identified. It was also noted that lesions in the ventrointermedial (VIM) nucleus of thalamus or cerebellum could reduce or even abolish the tremor.

Pathology:

Recent pathological post-mortem studies show different patterns of pathology in different patients. Cerebellar damage can be seen in some patients with a reduction in the number of Purkinje cells, together with an increased number of swollen Purkinje neurons named 'torpedoes', which are thought to be a sign of Purkinje cells damage. An alpha-synclein positive brainstem Lewy body pathology can be seen in others, but is generally less common.

Clinical picture:

The tremor most commonly affects the upper limbs followed in frequency by the head, jaw, voice, legs, and finally the trunk. The tremor is usually both postural and kinetic, occurring during action, and a mild degree of asymmetry is common. Essential tremor has a frequency of 4–12 Hz, and the frequency appears to be inversely related to age. The tremor is most evident on holding or carrying things like cups, trays and books, and with performing fine dextrous hand movements. Handwriting becomes scrawly and untidy, but not small. Head tremor usually results in a rhythmic nodding (yes, yes), or a horizontal (no, no,) tremor, while voice tremor results in quivering speech. Resting tremor can be seen in some patients with ET, especially in those with a severe tremor. The examiner however needs to be aware that a postural tremor may be misinterpreted as a resting tremor if the affected limb is not fully supported to eliminate the effect of gravity. Patients with ET should have no parkinsonian features, particularly bradykinesia. It does however appear that patients with ET have a slightly higher risk of developing Parkinson's disease. ET is a very slowly progressive disorder. Approximately half the patients have a positive family history, usually with an autosomal dominant mode of inheritance. Some patients with ET report a significant improvement in the tremor with alcohol. In recent years some investigators have identified subtle impairment of cerebellar and cognitive functions, suggesting that ET patients may have a mixture of motor and non-motor features and is not simply a monosymptomatic disorder.

Investigations:

The diagnosis of ET is a clinical one relying on a good comprehensive history, and a careful clinical examination. Checking thyroid function tests may be necessary in some patients with suspected thyroid disease. Occasionally, a dopamine transporter (DAT-SPECT) scan can be helpful to differentiate ET from Parkinson's disease. A preserved sense of smell can also help to point more to ET, rather than Parkinson's disease. Rarely, recording the amplitude and frequency of the tremor with an accelerometer is necessary. This can be useful in diagnosing psychogenic tremor, and in differentiating ET from enhanced physiological tremor.

Differential diagnosis:

Enhanced physiological tremor

A benign high frequency low amplitude tremor that can occur in any person in the absence of neurological disease. It can be precipitated by thyrotoxicosis, hypoglycaemia, excess caffeine or drugs such as beta-adrenergic agonists.

Parkinson's disease

Tremor is predominantly a resting tremor that usually improves with action. Other features such as bradykinesia and rigidity are present.

Drug induced tremor

Common examples include neuroleptics, lithium, amiodarone, theophylline, and beta-adrenergic agonists like salbutamol. Withdrawal from drugs such as alcohol can also result in a tremor.

Cerebellar tremor

A predominantly goal-directed tremor. Other cerebellar features such as nystagmus, ataxia and incoordination may be present.

Task-specific tremor

Tremor occurs only during certain repetitive tasks such as in writer's tremor.

Dystonic tremor

Tremor in association with dystonia is usually jerky, irregular, asymmetrical and variable depending on posture. Dystonic head tremor is the most common example.

Psychogenic tremor

Tremor may have a sudden onset and unusual neurological signs. It varies in frequency and improves with distraction.

Clinical diagnosis criteria

One of the most widely accepted are those proposed by the tremor investigation group (TRIG) of the Movement Disorders Society.

Definite essential tremor

Inclusion criteria

- Bilateral postural tremor with or without kinetic tremor, involving hands and forearms, that is visible and persistent.
- Duration greater than five years.

Exclusion criteria

- Other abnormal neurological signs (except Froment's sign).
- Presence of known causes of increased physiological tremor.
- Concurrent or recent exposure to tremorogenic drugs or a drug withdrawal state.
- Direct or indirect trauma to the nervous system within three months before the onset of tremor.
- Historical or clinical evidence of psychogenic origins.
- Sudden onset or stepwise deterioration.

Probable essential tremor

Same as in definite ET, except
- tremor may be confined to body parts other than the hands
- duration greater than 3 years
- exclusions also include primary orthostatic tremor, isolated voice tremor, isolated task or position specific tremor, isolated tongue or chin tremor.

Management:

Explanation and reassurance that the tremor is not caused by Parkinson's disease is frequently sufficient in those with mild tremor. Some patients find benefit in using wrist weights, weighted cups, and straws. Alcohol can be effective in some patients, but the risk of intoxication and addiction limits its usefulness. In those with moderate or severe symptoms, drug treatment is frequently necessary.

The two main drugs that have been proven to be of benefit are beta-blockers, such as propranolol, and the barbiturate primidone. The dose of each drug needs to be gradually increased, in order to minimize adverse reactions. Both drugs can also be combined together if necessary. Other drugs include benzodiazepines, topiramate and gabapentin. Botulinum toxin injections can be helpful in selected patients especially in head tremor. Stereotactic surgery with thalamic deep brain stimulation can be very effective in patients with severe ET that is resistant to medical treatment.

Further reading

Axelrad JE, Louis ED, Honig LS, *et al.* (2008). Reduced Purkinje cells number in essential tremor: a postmortem study. *Arch Neurol* **65**: 101–7.

Deuschl G, Bain P, Brin M (1998). Consensus statement of the Movement Disorder Society on Tremor. *Mov Disord* **13**: 2–23.

Deuschl G, Elble RJ. (2000) The pathophysiology of essential tremor. *Neurolology* **54**: S14–20.

Elan D. Louis, Blair Forsd, *et al.* (1998) How normal is normal? Mild tremor in a multiethnic normal cohort. *Arch Neurol* **55**: 222–7.

Elble RJ (2000). Diagnostic criteria for essential tremor and differential diagnosis. *Neurolology* **54**: S2–6.

Gorman WP, Cooper R, Pocock P, *et al.* (1984). A comparison of primidone, propranolol, and placebo in essential tremor, using quantitative analysis. *J Neurol Neurosurg Psychiatry* **49**: 64–8.

Louis ED, Ferreira JJ (2010). How common is the most common adult movement disorder? Update on the worldwide prevalence of essential tremor. *Mov Disord*, **25**:534–41.

Hemiballismus: medical management

Definition

Hemiballismus is a form of chorea characterized by involuntary violent flinging movements of the limbs on one side of the body. Less commonly, both sides (biballismus) and both legs (paraballismus) may be affected. In contrast to chorea, movements are persistent during the waking hours and the predominant involvement of the proximal muscles accounts for their flailing nature. However, the distinction is not clear-cut since proximal ballismic movements may coexist with distal choreic movements, symptoms may be intermittent in less severe cases, and in many patients a change from ballismus to chorea is seen spontaneously or in response to treatment. Other coexisting movement disorders include orofacial movements or prolonged dystonic posturing. Hemiballismus is often severely disabling and injury due to the movements is common.

Aetiology

The causes of hemiballismus include

- stroke (infarct or haemorrhage)
- traumatic brain injury
- tumour (primary or secondary)
- infection (e.g. tuberculoma, cerebral toxoplasmosis, HIV)
- other focal lesions (e.g. vascular malformation, abscess, granuloma, multiple sclerosis plaque, motor neuron disease)
- hyperglycaemia (non-ketotic hyperosmolar state)
- Drugs (phenytoin, dopamine agonists in Parkinson's disease)

Although an increasing number of exceptions are recognized, hemiballismus most often results from structural lesions affecting the subthalamic nucleus of the basal ganglia or the connections between this nucleus and the globus pallidum. Subthalamic nucleus activity usually acts via the medial pallidum to exert an inhibitory effect on the motor thalamus and cortex; loss of this inhibition leads to enhanced motor activity and abnormal involuntary movements.

Although hemiballismus is a rare complication of stroke, stroke remains the most common cause of the condition. In a series of 23 patients with hemiballismus and two with biballismus, stroke was considered the likely aetiology in 16. In most cases, the movement disorder was preceded by hemiparesis and only two patients had hemiballismus in the absence of other movement abnormalities. In this series, only six patients had a lesion in the subthalamic nucleus on neuroimaging. Hemiballismus due to stroke is predominantly a disease of older people.

The second most common reported cause of hemiballismus in some series is non-ketotic hyperglycaemia, often occurring in older people. Characteristically, hemiballistic movements reduce over several hours as glucose levels return to normal. A hyperintense putamen on neuroimaging, probably due to petechial haemorrhage, is sometimes found. Hemiballismus is a complication of HIV infection and is sometimes the presenting symptom. Although most cases result from secondary infection, especially cerebral toxoplasmosis, hypoglycaemia due to pentamidine use has also been reported as a cause.

Management

Spontaneous improvement in many people with hemiballismus makes it difficult to judge the efficacy of pharmacological interventions. As usual, the primary treatment is to deal with any remediable causes such as hyperglycaemia, neoplasms or infections. Other treatments that may be useful include

- antidopamine therapy (dopamine depletors or blockers)
- anticonvulsants (topiramate or sodium valproate)
- neurosurgical interventions.

Dopamine-blocking agents such as haloperidol or chlorpromazine remain mainstays of treatment and are effective in most cases despite uncertainty as to why they are effective. Dopamine depleting agents such as tetrabenazine (also used in other movement disorders such as Huntington's chorea) are a useful alternative because of a rapid onset of action and a reduced risk of long-term complications such as tardive dyskinesia. Case reports suggest that anticonvulsants may also be helpful. Functional neurosurgery with lesioning of the globus pallidus should be reserved for those with severe persistent hemiballismus resistant to other interventions.

Prognosis

Most patients go into spontaneous remission, with or without persistence of milder distal choreiform movements. Even in those with persistent hemiballismus, current medical management is generally successful in ameliorating symptoms.

Further reading

Chang MH, Chiang HT, Lai PH, et al. (1997). Putaminal petechial haemorrhage as the cause of chorea: a neuroimaging study. J Neurol Neurosurg Psychiatry 63: 300–3.

Dewey RB, Jankovic J (1989). Hemiballism-hemichorea: clinical and pharmacological findings in 21 patients. Arch Neurol 46: 862–67.

Postuma RB, Lang AE (2003). Hemiballism: revisiting a classic disorder. Lancet Neurol 2: 661–8.

Huntington's disease

Genetics and epidemiology

HD is an autosomal dominant condition; most patients have an affected parent but the rate of new mutations may be higher than previously thought. The HD mutation is an expansion of a CAG repeat within a gene located on chromosome 4. Paternal inheritance tends to produce larger CAG expansions and earlier onset. Estimates of UK prevalence have ranged from 2 to 10 per 100 000 but may be higher.

Clinical features

The four cardinal features of HD are disturbances in movement, mood, cognition, and behaviour. Athetoid and dystonic movements are sometimes more prominent than chorea. Chorea is an abrupt, fleeting twitch in skeletal muscle; dystonia produces a more sustained change in posture. Other motor features include tics, gait apraxia, and dysfluent and dysarthric speech. Mood is typically volatile, with depression frequent and suicide a significant risk. Frank psychosis may occur. Cognition and behaviour disorders can be linked to frontostriatal pathology. Memory and executive functions are impaired; there is reduced impulse control and also rigid, obsessional thinking.

Natural history and complications

Onset is typically in mid life but may be early (juvenile HD) or in late life; age of onset is inversely correlated with number of CAG repeats. Any of the four types of impairment can be presenting features although typically the first indication of HD is involuntary movements, with dementia and behavioural disturbance gradually asserting themselves in the later stages. Survival after symptoms are clearly established is around 15 years but is variable. The profile of involuntary movements evolves over time; they typically become much less obvious in the terminal phase.

When onset is in later life the presenting symptoms are often primarily motor. HD was sometimes misdiagnosed in the past as 'senile chorea'. In one retrospective study of those with onset aged 60–79, death was often related to diseases of old age. Falls were a major risk. The majority were the first in the family to be diagnosed.

The most common physical complication is malnutrition. The increased energy demand associated with involuntary movements may combine with the effects of dysphagia, motor feeding difficulties, apathy, memory impairment, depression, and possibly other neuroendocrine factors. Without nutritional support, the HD patient will typically become increasingly malnourished and may die from general inanition or aspiration pneumonia. Percutaneous endoscopic grastrostomy (PEG) feeding can greatly enhance quality of life in some patients. Other risks to consider include aspiration, falls and fire (many patients smoke).

Diagnosis and differential diagnosis

Clinical diagnosis is more reliable if all the above features are considered and less so when involuntary movements are taken as the key criterion. Diagnosis can be established by DNA testing but the process of diagnosis must be handled sensitively: family members as well as patients have a stake in the results and much distress is caused by omitting pre- and post-test counselling.

HD is too often confused with Parkinson's disease. Other, rarer degenerative conditions presenting with dementia or with a psychiatric syndrome may present more of a diagnostic challenge.

Management approach

A whole-family approach is essential in HD where many of the individual's problems rebound on the partner, family members and others. Patients and family have a range of needs at every stage of the condition and require support from clinicians experienced in HD. Counselling is important in pre-symptomatic patients undergoing DNAs but is also vital (although often neglected) when a heritable condition is identified in the course of diagnostic investigations.

Ethical issues sometimes arise when the patient appears to be less concerned than the family about symptoms and disability (however, there is an increased risk of suicide in HD). Later in the condition there may be ethical concerns about the use of interventions such as PEG feeding. As in other dementing illnesses, it is important not to make negative assumptions about quality of life in late-stage HD.

Drug treatment

Tetrabenazine is overprescribed for chorea. Most HD patients are not personally troubled by their involuntary movements, and those with dramatic movements will rarely respond to drug treatment usefully without experiencing side-effects such as depression, parkinsonism, and postural hypotension. With these provisos, tetrabenazine can be useful if prescribed judiciously in individuals who are specifically disabled by involuntary movements.

Drugs are useful for behavioural and mood disorders. An SSRI can be helpful in depression and potentially for obsessional traits. Patients liable to volatile mood with explosive outbursts will often benefit from an atypical antipsychotic. There is no evidence as to which is preferable. Classical antipsychotics such as haloperidol have higher potency as D1 dopamine receptor blockers and may have some efficacy in reducing involuntary movements but are thought to be less specific in their behavioural effects. At the opposite end of the spectrum, an atypical antipsychotic such as quetiapine has less potential to benefit movements but may be more likely to improve behaviour without sedation. Olanzapine is often useful and has the added benefit for many patients of promoting weight gain. With any antipsychotic, the advice in HD is to 'start low and go slow': effective doses are lower than in standard psychiatric practice. Postural hypotension is an important complication of drug treatment.

Referral pathways and useful resources

Clinical genetics support is essential at the time of diagnosis and DNA testing. In the UK, ongoing management of people with HD may fall to rehabilitation medicine physicians, neurologists, psychiatrists, or occasionally clinical geneticists. In all cases, input from a specialist nurse is invaluable. A network of regional specialists is currently funded by the Huntington's Disease Association

Physiotherapy has no known value in improving quality of movement or in reducing risk of falls. Speech and language therapists are helpful in managing dysphagia, together with dietitians. Environmental interventions through occupational therapy can be helpful although few patients can safely use a walking aid. Specialised armchair seating is often required in the non-ambulant stage. Imaginative social services support can make a large difference to quality of life.

Further reading

Almqvist EW, DS Elterman, PM MacLeod, et al. (2001). High incidence rate and absent family histories in one quarter of patients newly diagnosed with Huntington disease in British Columbia. *Clinical Genetics* **60**: 198–205.

Bates G, Harper PS, Jones L (2002). *Huntington's Disease*. Oxford University Press.

Lipe H, Bird T (2009). Late onset Huntington Disease: Clinical and genetic characteristics of 34 cases. *J Neurol Sci* **276**: 159-62.

Spinney L (2010). Uncovering the true prevalence of Huntington's disease. *Lancet Neurol* **9**: 760-1. Further information: Huntington's Disease Association: www.hda.org.uk

Neurological investigations

Investigations can help to determine the aetiology of various neurological illnesses, but are no substitute for a well taken history and appropriate clinical examination. The following categories will be discussed:

- structural imaging
- functional brain imaging
- neurophysiology
- cerebrospinal fluid analysis.

Structural imaging (Table 13.5)

Computed tomography (CT) of the brain

CT scans are fast and readily available. They are useful in the investigation of acute head injury, stroke, and suspected intracerebral and subarachnoid haemorrhage. They can also detect ventricular enlargement or displacement, calcified lesions, infection, and bone pathology. Contrast-enhanced CT demonstrates areas of increased blood supply and oedema more clearly. CT angiography is emerging as the preferred imaging modality for both arterial and venous pathology.

Magnetic resonance imaging (MRI) of the brain

MRI provides excellent visualization of parenchymal lesions, disorders of the meninges, brainstem, and cerebellum. It can detect inflammation, infection, tumours and blood products (Table 13.6). Different sequences are available to look for specific features. These include:

- T_1 weighted imaging (T_1WI). Water/cerebrospinal fluid (CSF) appears dark. Lesions containing fat appear bright (hyperintense). Subacute haemorrhage also appears bright, as does proteinaceous fluid such as abscesses.
- T_2 weighted imaging (T_2WI). CSF appears bright. Inflammatory lesions, acute and chronic infarcts, acute bleeds and some tumours appear bright compared with brain tissue signal.
- FLAIR (fluid attenuated-inversion recovery). The high signal intensity of CSF is cancelled out, but otherwise maintaining the characteristics of T_2WI. It is excellent for detecting lesions close to the ventricles (e.g. multiple sclerosis) and meningeal pathology.
- DWI (diffusion-weighted imaging) and ADC (apparent diffusion coefficient). These sequences detect areas of

Table 13.5 Use of MRI and CT in common clinical problems

Diagnosis suspected clinically	Radiological investigation of choice
Acute stroke	CT or DWI MRI if available
Subarachnoid or intracerebral haemorrhage	CT
Hydrocephalus	MRI
Bony injury	CT
Brainstem or cerebellar pathology	MRI
Encephalitis	MRI
Meningitis or meningeal pathology	MRI
Spinal cord compression	MRI

Table 13.6 Appearance of haemorrhage on T_1 and T_2 MRI images depending on age

Age of haemorrhage	Appearance on T_1WI	Appearance on T_2WI
Less than 24 h	Isointense	Hyperintense
24–72 h	Isointense to hypointense	Hypointense
3–7 days	Hyperintense	Hypointense
7–14 days	Hyperintense	Hyperintense
>14 days	Hypointense	Hypointense

cell damage, particularly ischaemia, which becomes apparent within 30 minutes of onset. When cells are damaged they swell, and this restricts diffusion of water molecules amongst them. Restricted diffusion appears bright on DWI and black on ADC images. Although DWI is highly sensitive for acute ischaemia, it is not 100% specific. Other causes of hyperintensity on DWI with hypointensity on ADC are pyogenic infection, HSV encephalitis, diffuse axonal injury and Creutzfeldt–Jacob disease (CJD). In addition, lesions that are bright on T_2WI, such as small vessel disease or inflammation, also appear bright on DWI because DWI are T_2-weighted scans; this is known as 'shine through'. Shine-through also appears bright on ADC, in contrast to ischaemia which appears black.

- Gradient echo. This detects blood products (haemosiderin), which appear black (hypointense). The distribution of blood products is helpful in determining the aetiology. Bleeds from cerebral amyloid angiopathy typically affect the cortex, particularly in the frontal and parietal lobes. Haemorrhages caused by traumatic brain injury usually occur at the junction of grey and white matter. Hypertensive bleeds affect basal ganglia, thalamus, brainstem and cerebellum. Lobar haemorrhages need further investigation to exclude an underlying cause such as vascular malformations and tumours.
- Post gadolinium T_1WI. Enhancement (hyperintensity) on T_1WI after intravenous injection with gadolinium containing contrast agents is a reflection of breakdown in the blood–brain barrier (BBB), and is seen in any condition that causes abnormalities in the BBB such as inflammation or infection.

MRI of the spine

MRI is the best modality for imaging the spinal cord and can identify many pathologies including spondylytic disease, ischaemia and infections such as discitis and osteomyelitis.

On T_1WI, the spinal cord is brighter than the CSF and the vertebral bodies are brighter than the intervertebral discs. T_1WI is useful for identifying osteophytes and other lesions obliterating exit foramina. On T_2WI, CSF is bright compared with the spinal cord and discs are brighter than vertebral bodies. T_2WI is useful to look at the cord itself and the nerve roots. Spinal cord inflammation, infarction and myelomalacia due to cord compression will all appear bright on T_2WI.

Functional brain imaging

The main functional brain imaging modalities are single photon emission computed tomography (SPECT) and positron emission tomography (PET). Both involve intravenous injection of a chemical ligand labelled with a radioisotope. The ligand has chemical properties that result in its accumulation in different regions of the brain. PET and SPECT scanners detect the radioactivity emitted by the attached radioisotope and the data is then used to create multicoloured images that reflect ligand concentration. PET and SPECT differ in the ligands and isotopes used and in the way they detect the radioisotope. PET has higher spatial resolution but SPECT is cheaper and more widely available.

The main uses for functional imaging are in the differential diagnosis of dementia and parkinsonism. PET is not routinely available in clinical practice and therefore only SPECT will be discussed. Functional MRI is also used as a research tool to assess brain function by determining localised changes in blood flow.

Functional imaging in parkinsonism

DaTSCAN is the trade name for a SPECT scan using a dopamine transporter protein. In healthy individuals, these ligands are taken up by dopamine active transporter (DaT) proteins on the presynaptic membrane of dopaminergic neurons in the corpus striatum (caudate and putamen). The main use of DaTSCAN is to differentiate essential tremor, drug induced parkinsonism and vascular parkinsonism, conditions in which DaT is normal, from idiopathic Parkinson's disease (IPD). In patients with IPD, there is loss of presynaptic dopaminergic terminals in the putamen, meaning that the isotope is only taken up by the caudate nuclei, giving rise to a 'full stop' appearance (see Figure 13.1) instead of the normal 'comma' appearance. This is usually asymmetrical, with the putamen contralateral to the most severely affected side of the body being most deficient in DaT. Presynaptic nigrostriatal degeneration also occurs in 'Parkinson plus' syndromes and dementia with Lewy bodies (DLB) and therefore DaT is unable to distinguish IPD from these conditions.

Functional imaging in dementia

The most commonly used SPECT scan in dementia is ^{99m}Tc-HMPAO-SPECT. This radioligand is taken up by brain tissue in a manner proportional to cerebral blood flow. Blood flow within the brain is tightly coupled to local brain metabolism and therefore this technique acts as a surrogate marker for brain metabolism. ^{99m}Tc-HMPAO-SPECT is most helpful in distinguishing Alzheimer's disease (AD), in which there is parietal and occipital hypoperfusion from vascular dementia (VD), in which there is patchy hypoperfusion, and frontotemporal dementia (FTD), in which there is hypoperfusion in the frontal and temporal lobes. It cannot be used to differentiate between AD and dementia with Lewy bodies (DLB), or between VD and FTD. DaT scans can be used to differentiate DLB from AD. This is the most frequent source of diagnostic confusion in clinical practice in older patients. In DLB, even in patients with no clinical parkinsonism, there is loss of dopamine from the striata, which can be picked up on DaT scan. In AD, a DaT scan is normal.

Neurophysiology

Nerve conduction studies (NCS)

NCS are helpful to confirm the presence of a neuropathy and its severity. They also provide information on whether the neuropathy involves motor or sensory nerves or both, and can determine whether the neuropathy is axonal or demyelinating, all of which are helpful in establishing the

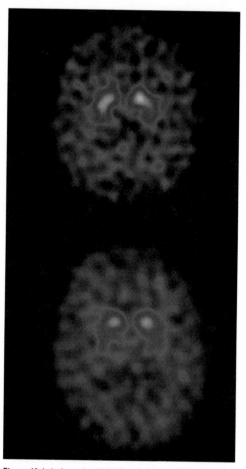

Figure 13.1 (colour plate 7) DAT scan in idiopathic Parkinson's disease.

underlying aetiology. They can also localise focal neuropathies such as carpal tunnel syndrome.

In NCS, both sensory and motor nerves are studied. The amplitude and latency of sensory nerve action potentials and compound muscle action potentials (CMAPs) are recorded along with conduction velocities (normal 50 meters/second). Electrical stimulation of the nerve results in a delayed muscle twitch due to the impulse travelling antidromically to the anterior horn cell, and returning back down the nerve. This is called the 'f-wave'.

Neuropathies can be broadly divided into axonal and demyelinating. Axonal neuropathies result in small or absent action potentials with relatively normal conduction velocities, whereas demyelinating neuropathies cause delayed, dispersed action potentials and slowed conduction velocities (<35 meters/second). Conduction block can also be seen where the CMAP amplitude is less on proximal stimulation when compared with distal stimulation. F waves are delayed in demyelinating neuropathies but are normal or absent in axonal disorders.

Repetitive stimulation of a muscle can demonstrate decrement in the amplitude of the CMAP in myasthenia gravis and the Lambert Eaton myasthenic syndrome.

Electromyography

This involves inserting a needle into a muscle and recording the electrical activity of the muscle (motor unit action potential (MUAP)). A motor unit consists of all the muscle fibres innervated by a single motor nerve. In diseased muscles, muscle fibres atrophy and die. On electromyography (EMG) this is seen as short duration low amplitude MUAPs. Healthy resting muscles are electrically silent. Diseased muscles produce electrical activity at rest. Acute denervation causes spontaneous fibrillation potentials and positive sharp waves. In chronic diseases of longer than 6 months, an additional type of spontaneous activity known as 'complex repetitive discharges' may be seen. In chronic partial denervation with reinervation, the motor units are larger due to axonal re-sprouting. This results in a reduced volitional interference pattern with giant MUAPs firing at high frequency. Single fibre EMG is used to identify neurophysiological abnormalities at the neuromuscular junction.

Electroencephalography

Electroencephalography (EEG) is a recording of cerebral electrical activity. EEG abnormalities reflect general pathological processes and are rarely specific for one particular diagnosis. A normal EEG does not exclude intracranial disorders. EEG is most helpful in states of altered consciousness and in epilepsy.

In patients with altered consciousness, the EEG is usually non-specifically abnormal, with slowing of background activity and loss of reactivity to eye opening and other stimuli. These abnormalities are seen whether the underlying cause is infective, toxic or metabolic. Occasionally features suggestive of a particular aetiology are seen:

- Bilateral temporal lobe abnormalities, particularly high amplitude complexes known as periodic lateralising epileptiform discharges (PLEDS) are highly suspicious of herpes simplex encephalitis
- Continuous epileptiform activity in non-convulsive status, a rare but important cause of fluctuating consciousness or cognition
- Excessive fast activity is seen in delirium tremens and benzodiazepine toxicity
- Triphasic waves and diffuse slowing suggest a metabolic encephalopathy, particularly hepatic encephalopathy

An EEG cannot diagnose or exclude epilepsy. An interictal EEG may be normal in patients with proven epilepsy (50%), and abnormal in subjects with no history of epilepsy (2%). Ictal recordings will differentiate epileptic seizures from non-epileptic attacks and can help classify seizure type.

Cerebrospinal fluid (CSF) analysis

Normal CSF is clear and colourless, contains less than 5 white blood cells per mm^3, less than 0.5 g/L protein and has a CSF to serum glucose ratio of >50%. The protein can be raised in diabetics. A traumatic tap can artefactually introduce blood into the CSF. This can be differentiated from subarachnoid haemorrhage by a fall in red cell count in serial samples and by the absence of xanthochromia on spectrophometric analysis. In a traumatic tap, it is necessary to correct the CSF white cell count and protein by subtracting one white blood cell and 0.01 g/L of protein for every 1000 red blood cells per mm^3.

The most important role of CSF analysis is in patients with suspected CNS infection. Lumbar puncture (LP) is essential unless there are contraindications such as platelet count <50 × 10^9/L, INR >1.2 or local infection. It is necessary to perform CT brain prior to LP in patients with reduced conscious level (GCS <13), focal neurological signs, new seizures, history of CNS disease or suspected immunosuppression.

Lumbar puncture should be performed in the left lateral position, so that the CSF opening pressure can be measured. Samples should be sent for microscopy and culture, protein, glucose, viral PCR to include HSV, VZV and enterovirus and meningococcal and pneumococcal PCR. It is essential to assay a paired serum glucose. When demyelination is considered, immunoglobulin electrophoresis should be performed on paired CSF and serum to demonstrate local synthesis within the CNS. If malignant meningitis is possible, a large quantity (5–10 mL) of fresh CSF should be sent for cytology.

The typical changes seen in CNS infection are shown in Table 13.7.

Other causes of a CSF pleocytosis include malignant meningitis, cerebral abscess, neurosyphilis, neuroborreliosis, sarcoidosis, and other CNS inflammatory conditions.

Table 13.7 Cerebrospinal fluid findings in central nervous system infection

	Normal	Bacterial meningitis	Viral meningitis	Tuberculous meningitis	Viral encephalitis
Opening pressure	5–25 cmH$_2$0	Often elevated	Usually normal	Elevated in 50%	Normal or elevated
Appearance	Clear, colourless	Turbid or purulent	Clear	Clear or turbid	Clear
White cell count	<5 mm^3	Up to several thousand cells per mm^3	Up to 1000 cells per mm^3	Up to 1000 cells per mm^3	Up to 1000 cells per mm^3
Type of WBC	Lymphocytes	Predominantly neutrophils (unless partially treated when lymphocytes can predominate)	Predominantly lymphocytes	Predominantly lymphocytes but neutrophils can predominate in early disease	Predominantly lymphocytes
Protein	Approx <0.5 g/L	Elevated up to several g/L	Normal or slightly elevated (up to 1 g/L)	Elevated up to several g/L	Normal or slightly elevated (up to 1 g/L)
Glucose	>50% serum glucose	<50% serum glucose; often very low	>50% serum glucose	<50% serum glucose	>50% serum glucose

Further reading

Binnie CD, Prior PF (1994). Electroencephalography. *J Neurol Neurosurg Psychiatry* **57**: 1308–19.

Hasburn R, Abrahams J, Jekel J, *et al.* (2001). Computed tomography of the head before lumbar puncture in adults with suspected meningitis. *New Engl J Med* **345**: 1729–33.

Hughes RA (1998). *Neurological Investigations*. Oxford, Blackwell Publishing.

Maizlin ZV, Shewchuk JR, Clement JJ (2009). Easy ways to remember the progression of MRI signal intensity of intracranial hemorrhage. *Can Assoc Radiol J* **60**: 88–90.

Piccini P, Whone A (2004). Functional brain imaging in the differential diagnosis of Parkinson's disease. *Lancet Neurol* **3**: 284–90.

Schaefer PW, Grant PE, Gonzalez RG (2000). Diffusion-weighted MR imaging of the brain. *Radiology* **217**: 331–45.

Smith SJM (2005). EEG in neurological conditions other than epilepsy: When does it help, what does it add? *J Neurol Neurosurg Psychiatry* **76**:ii8-ii12.

Talbot PR, Lloyd JJ, Snowden JS, *et al.* (1998). A clinical role for 99mTc-HMPAO SPECT in the investigation of dementia. *J Neurol Neurosurg Psychiatry* **64**: 306–13.

Chronic disease and disability

Faecal incontinence in older people

Background

Faecal incontinence (FI) in older people is a distressing symptom with a major impact on quality of life, health, and independence. Older individuals with faecal incontinence often do not seek help through embarrassment and a common perception that incontinence is 'part of getting old'. Healthcare providers should actively enquire about the symptom in frail older people and other high-risk patients (those with cognitive and/or mobility impairment), but such case finding is not usually routine. Faecal incontinence is therefore very much a 'hidden problem', leading to a decline toward dependency, poor health, informal carer fatigue, and long-term care placement. Even when healthcare professionals do identify FI in older people, assessment of underlying cause(s) is often less than rigorous with the condition being managed more passively than actively. The NICE guidelines (CG 49) provide an evidence base for management in adults, but the National Continence Care audit shows that practice across all healthcare settings is often poor.

Prevalence and incidence of FI in older people

Faecal incontinence affects one in five people aged over 65 years living in the community. Prevalence increases with age, particularly in the eighth decade, with men and women being equally affected. Rates are even higher in institutionalized settings, affecting a third of acutely hospitalized older people and half of those in care homes. Prevalence in UK residential care ranges widely from 17% to 95% between individual care homes with comparable case mix, which implies this variation is in part reflective of different standards of care. The annual incidence of new-onset FI in newly admitted care home residents was 20% in one study; of the 38% of these patients who had persistent (rather than transient) incontinence, 26% died within 10 months, compared with 6.7% of those who remained continent. FI has also been linked to increased mortality in older people living at home, independently of age, gender, and poor general health. FI is a burden on healthcare resources, being associated with high usage of community nurses and home healthcare, and costly consequences (if not well-managed), such as pressure sores.

Case-finding

Physicians and nurses across all settings (primary care, acute hospital, and long-term healthcare) have a low awareness of FI in older people. NICE CG49 recommends that healthcare professionals should ask about FI in frail older people, who are classified as a high-risk group, especially as they may be reluctant to volunteer the symptom. UK studies show that only half of older primary care patients with FI (or indeed their carers) discuss the problem with their GP. Other studies show that older people who do to talk to a healthcare professional about incontinence feel that they receive dismissive responses. Even in the acute hospital setting where patients can be closely observed, only one in six of patients reporting FI have the symptom actually documented by ward nursing staff. Organizations must make commitments to improving detection of FI by:

(a) educating healthcare workers to recognize the value of identifying FI, and have the knowledge and confidence that it can be treated

(b) develop case-finding protocols (who will ask, how to ask, when to ask, and who to ask)

(c) make information/education available to patients and carers to empower them to report the symptom.

> **Author's Tip**
>
> Healthcare providers should routinely and sensitively enquire about FI in:
>
> - frail older people
> - care home residents
> - hospital inpatients aged 65+
> - people aged 70+ living at home.
>
> Do not expect patients to volunteer this symptom which they may view as embarrassing and as 'part of getting old'.

> **Author's Tip**
>
> Bowel dysfunction leading to FI and constipation in older people is primarily related to risk factors associated with ageing (e.g. comorbidities, immobility, drugs) rather than ageing itself. It is not an inevitable consequence of ageing; it is important to communicate this to older people with FI to encourage help seeking and treatment expectations.

Anatomy and physiology in FI

In normal defecation, colonic activity propels stool into the rectum causing distension and reflex relaxation of the smooth muscle of the anal canal (also known as the internal anal sphincter). This prompts reflex contraction of the external anal sphincter and pelvic floor muscles (skeletal muscles innervated by the pudendal nerve). The brain registers the urge to defecate, voluntarily relaxing the external sphincter to allow evacuation of the rectum assisted by Valsalva contraction of the abdominal wall muscles.

Studies of total gut transit time, colonic motor activity, and postprandial gastrocolic reflex show no differences between healthy older and younger people. Older people with chronic constipation do tend to have a prolonged total gut transit time (4–9 days), especially if less mobile (6–14 days). Transit is particularly slowed through the sigmoid colon and rectum, predisposing frailer older people to overflow FI from impaction.

Both internal and external sphincters show age-related decline in tone, though not until the eighth decade. This predisposes older people to FI when having loose stools. Women who sustain subclinical damage to the anal sphincters during childbirth may present earlier with FI. Pudendal neuropathy is also an age-related phenomenon that predisposes to FI and is more evident in women.

People with recurrent stool impaction predisposing to overflow tend to have reduced rectal tone, increased compliance, and impaired sensation, so they may have a large rectal bolus without feeling the urge to void. One underlying cause for this type of rectal dysfunction is reduced parasympathetic outflow from the sacral plexus from ischaemia or spinal stenosis.

Rectal dysmotility can also develop through persistent disregard or suppression of the urge to defecate as a result of dementia, depression, immobility, or painful anorectal conditions. The Valsalva manoeuvre increases intra-abdominal and hence rectal pressure during defecation producing more effective rectal evacuation; however, older people often have weakened abdominal musculature limiting its use in compensating for rectal outlet delay.

Causes of faecal incontinence in older people

Faecal incontinence is a symptom that rarely has a single cause in older people. Comprehensive geriatric assessment (assessing medical, functional and psychosocial factors in addition to the bowel) is key to identifying and treating all contributing causes.

Overflow incontinence secondary to constipation and stool impaction

Constipation is the most important cause of FI in frail older people, as it is treatable, preventable, and frequently overlooked. Faecal loading was found to be present in 57% of older acute hospital inpatients, and 52–70% of care home residents with FI.

Risk factors for constipation in older people include:
- polypharmacy
- medications: anticholinergic drugs, opiates, iron supplements, calcium channel antagonists, non-steroidal anti-inflammatory drugs
- immobility
- institutionalization
- Parkinson's disease
- diabetes mellitus
- low fluid intake
- low dietary fibre
- dementia
- depression.

Loose stools

Loose stool is a primary risk factor for FI in epidemiological studies and is likely to be an undertreated condition in frail older people (44% of cases of FI in a care home study were related to diarrhoea). Important causes of persistent loose stool in older adults include:
- Colorectal cancer is more prevalent with increasing age, and must be considered in all older patients with persistent loose stool.
- Overuse of laxatives is common in older people as they may believe that anything less than a daily bowel movement is undesirable (more than three bowel movements per week is normal), plus laxatives are often prescribed for constipation when lifestyle measures may be sufficient. A third of people aged over 65 years living at home regularly use laxatives. Laxative use (in particular the stool softener docusate) has been linked to FI in care home residents.
- Drug side-effects: laxatives, proton-pump inhibitors, selective serotonin reuptake inhibitors, magnesium-containing antacids, cholinesterase inhibitors, iron supplements, metformin, colchicine.
- Antibiotic-related diarrhoea: age, female gender, and nursing home residency significantly increases the risk for Clostridium difficile-associated diarrhoea in hospitalized people who have had antibiotics. Diarrhoea takes longer to resolve following treatment of C. difficile in frail older patients. Faecal incontinence in context of C. difficile is in itself a risk factor for recurrent C. difficile diarrhoea in hospitalized patients.

- Lactose intolerance increases with age: lactose malabsorption rate increases from 15% in healthy women aged 40–59 years to 50% in those aged 60–79.
- Caffeinated drinks increase transit time and can cause faecal urgency (especially if carbonated).

Anorectal faecal incontinence

Age-related sphincter dysfunction is an important contributing factor to FI. In studies of FI, younger women are more likely to have an isolated anal sphincter defect relating to obstetric injury, while older women have multiple causes including haemorrhoidectomy, diabetes, rectal and vaginal prolapse, and pudendal neuropathy. Faecal incontinence in older women is also linked to childbearing via structural damage to the external anal sphincter that worsens with age. Uterovaginal prolapse, rectocele, and rectal prolapse are associated with FI in older women, emphasizing the importance of observation while asking people to 'bear down' during assessment for FI.

Comorbidity-related incontinence

FI affects 30–56% of individuals acutely after stroke, but may then persist, affecting 11–22% at 1 year. Major FI is over four times more likely in stroke survivors than a comparable population. Primary risk factors are not, however, stroke severity and/or location, but treatable causes such as functional difficulties in using the toilet and anticholinergic medications.

Diabetes is an important cause, especially in men. Diabetic neuropathy impairs gut function causing (a) overflow FI from prolonged transit, (b) nocturnal diarrhoea and FI from bacterial overgrowth in the small bowel, and (c) complex anorectal dysfunction (reduced internal and external sphincter tone, spontaneous relaxation of the internal anal sphincter, poor rectal compliance and abnormal rectal sensation). Hyperglycaemia may make anorectal FI worse.

Transit through the rectosigmoid is severely affected in lower spinal cord injury or disease and Parkinson's disease, and this may result in overflow FI.

Author's Tip

Older people with comorbidities are at greater risk of FI and should be asked proactively about symptoms (NICE CG49—'healthcare professionals should actively yet sensitively enquire about symptoms in high-risk groups.')

Dementia-related incontinence

Dementia is an independent risk factor for FI, with cognitively impaired patients lacking cortical control of the defecation process. These individuals are usually also incontinent of urine. NICE classifies people with cognitive impairment (of any degree) as an at risk group in whom FI should be enquired about, and likewise cognitive assessment should be part of the baseline evaluation of an older patient with FI.

Functional incontinence

Functional incontinence occurs in individuals whose access to the toilet is delayed by impairments in mobility, dexterity, or vision. Risk of functional FI is evidently increased by having loose stool or weak sphincter, but it can also occur in patients with normal lower gut function. Poor mobility is a strong risk factor for FI in older people (in multiply adjusted risk models). It is also a primary risk factor for constipation and therefore a contributor to overflow FI.

> **Author's Tip**
>
> Where a change in bowel habit is unexplained, imaging should be considered to rule out colorectal cancer.

Assessment and investigations of FI in older adults

When FI is identified in older people, further evaluation is often not pursued, and this has been noted in acute hospitals, primary care and care homes. Trained nurses working in UK care homes placed advanced age as the top cause of urinary and faecal incontinence, demonstrating the knowledge gap leading to underassessment and lack of active treatment (in one care home study only 4% of patients with FI had been referred to the GP for further evaluation).

Key aspects of assessing FI in older people are that it:
- is multicomponent
- identifies underlying causes
- includes patient-focused quality of life.

NICE states, 'For most patients with FI, a thorough basic assessment will provide enough information for the clinician to recommend an initial management strategy without recourse to more formal testing.'

> **Author's Tip**
>
> This basic assessment MUST include bowel history, documenting duration of symptoms, and pattern of incontinence.
>
> A stool diary or bowel chart is a simple tool for documenting stool frequency, pattern, and consistency and should be used in any patient being assessed for causes of FI.

Self-report of bowel symptoms is reliable and reproducible in older patients, including those living in long-term care. Stool consistency should be established using the Bristol stool chart (pictorial scale 1–7). Overflow results in constant passive leakage of loose stool, while anal sphincter dysfunction causes small amounts of leakage. Patients may report urgency with external anal sphincter weakness, but tend to be unaware of faecal leakage with internal sphincter dysfunction. The pattern in dementia-related FI is passage of complete bowel movements, usually after meals.

> **Author's Tip**
>
> Frequency of faecal incontinence:
> - is an essential measure of severity
> - should always be documented at baseline assessment and at every review
> - was the primary outcome of interest in NICE CG 49
> - is strongly associated with impact on quality of life.

Assessment of FI must include symptoms of constipation as per 'Rome II' criteria: usually two or fewer bowel movements per week over at least 3 months, hard stool, straining with more than 25% of evacuations, and a feeling of incomplete evacuation (tenesmus). Rectal outlet delay is characterized by feeling of anal blockage during evacuation, prolonged defecation (more than 10 minutes) and/or need for manual evacuation. It affects 21% of older people living at home and may lead to rectal impaction and FI.

> **Author's Tip**
>
> An objective assessment for constipation is important in frail older people who may:
> - be unable to give a bowel history due to communication or cognitive problems
> - have daily bowel movements despite rectal or colonic impaction
> - have impaired rectal sensation and so be unaware of rectal stool impaction
> - have non-specific presentation of faecal impaction (e.g. delirium, leucocytosis, anorexia, functional decline).

Digital examination is essential to rule out anorectal disease and impaction. Easy finger insertion with anal gaping on removal indicates poor internal sphincter tone, while weak pressure around the finger when asking the patient to squeeze indicates external sphincter weakness. While on the examination couch, the patient should also be asked to strain as this will show up rectal or urogenital prolapse. Skin integrity should be carefully looked at, FI being a primary independent risk factor for pressure sores.

> **Author's Tip**
>
> Pelvic floor exercises and anal sphincter strengthening exercises can effectively be taught during a digital rectal examination by asking the patient to 'squeeze and pull up' and giving them positive verbal feedback when a tight contraction of the external sphincter is felt around the finger.

Certain symptoms associated with FI (abdominal pain, rectal bleeding, recent change in bowel habit, weight loss, anaemia) should prompt investigation for underlying cancer. Chronic constipation alone is generally not considered an appropriate indication for lower gastrointestinal endoscopy.

> **Author's Tip**
>
> Urgency and persistent loose stool should prompt assessment for diarrhoeal disease: stool culture, medication review, sigmoidoscopy/colonoscopy, malabsorption tests.

Older patients with FI and without rectal stool retention digitally should ideally undergo a plain abdominal radiograph to establish or rule out the diagnosis of overflow. A radiograph will also demonstrate bowel obstruction secondary to impaction and any acute complications such as sigmoid volvulus and stercoral perforation.

Urinary incontinence affects 50–70% of people with FI and should be enquired about and fully evaluated and co-managed.

Patients should be asked about toilet access and be objectively assessed with measures of function (e.g. Barthel Index), mobility (e.g. 'timed get up and go'), visual acuity, upper limb dexterity (undoing buttons), and cognition. The healthcare provider should be aware of the layout of patients' homes in relation to the toilet (location, distance, width of doorway for accommodating frame, presence of grab rails or raised toilet seat).

Relevant comorbidities must be identified (e.g. dementia, diabetes, neurological disease) and medications reviewed for side-effects of causing loose stool or constipation (see above). History of obstetric-related tears or complications should be asked about.

Psychological impact

Bowel-specific quality of life scores have been used in clinical trials of FI management, though not so much in older people. They are now being increasingly used in clinical practice (e.g. ICIQ-B). Even if a standardized tool is not used, impact on quality of life (limitations in usual activities, attitude to FI - passive, distressed, positive, or apathetic) should be discussed so that the patient (and carer where relevant) have the opportunity to express how FI is affecting their lives. In a survey of patients with neuropathic FI, the negative impacts they rated as being most important were on activities and 'getting out of the house' rather than physical aspects such as soiling and hygiene.

> **Author's Tip**
>
> NICE CG49
> Regular FI is known to impact quality of life and this impact should always be assessed.
> Measuring impact on quality of life is important for guiding specialist care—one indication for surgical repair in people with external anal sphincter defect is FI symptoms restricting quality of life.
> Treatment of FI should aim towards enabling a person to live with dignity and to participate in whatever social, work, cultural activities they wish to.

Management of FI in older adults

There are very few published trials of treatment of FI in older people, and no trials on prevention of FI. NICE recommendations are that people with the following causes should have condition-specific interventions with aim of resolving FI:

- faecal loading
- potentially treatable causes of diarrhoea
- warning signs for lower GI cancer
- rectal prolapse
- third-degree haemorrhoids
- acute anal sphincter injury
- acute disc prolapse / cauda equine syndrome
- medication effects.

The most important aspects of treatment are that it:
- is multicomponent and addresses underlying causes
- informs patients of options allowing them to identify their own goals and preferences for treatment
- leads to a care plan that is shared with patients/carers and is regularly reviewed to achieve treatment goals.

Faecal impaction and overflow FI

Care home studies of bowel clearance for overflow FI used a regimen of daily lactulose, daily suppositories and weekly enemas found that treatment was only effective when long-lasting and complete rectal emptying was achieved. Polyethylene glycol (PEG, Movicol, Macrogol) has since been shown to be an effective oral laxative for disimpaction in older people, but it is important to start at a dose of 1–2 sachets a day (rather than eight sachets a day

as in the current British National Formulary) and titrate up if needed.

For complete resolution of FI due to overflow, bowel clearance must usually be continued for at least four weeks using a combination of osmotic laxatives, suppositories, and enemas.

Arachis oil retention enemas are useful in treating colonic impactions. The commonly used enemas (phosphate and sodium citrate) should be administered with an extension nozzle to be more effective in higher impactions. Phosphate enemas should be used with caution in renal impairment, as dangerous hyperphosphataemia has been reported in older people. Glycerine suppositories should be used regularly in rectal outlet delay, with an explanation to patients on how to insert them.

Once an older person has had overflow FI, they are at high risk of recurrence and require regular laxatives to prevent faecal impaction. There is a general lack of constipation trials in older people, but available levels of evidence for effectiveness of laxatives in treating chronic constipation in older adults (>55 years) are:

- increased bowel movement frequency were observed with a stimulant laxative (cascara – similar to senna) [3] and lactulose [2]
- psyllium (bulk laxative) [2] and lactulose [2] improved stool consistency and constipation symptoms in placebo-controlled trials.
- level [1] evidence supports use of polyethylene glycol (Movicol) in adults.

A stepped approach to treating chronic constipation in older people is recommended - senna or bulk laxative, add lactulose if persistent, plus suppositories for rectal outlet delay – and should be used in addition to lifestyle measures (exercise, fibre, fluids, toilet visits after meals). Polyethylene glycol is indicated for colonic disimpaction as above (shown to be more effective than lactulose and safe in nursing home residents causing no dehydration or haemodynamic side-effects), and for treating chronic constipation in high risk patients (immobile, neurological disease, taking opiates).

Anorectal FI in older adults

> **Author's Tip**
>
> A combined approach should be used to treat anorectal FI:
> [1] sphincter strengthening exercises (similar to pelvic floor exercises – 'pull up and squeeze' and hold for 10 seconds, at least 20 times a day)
> [2] increasing firmness of stools consistency—diet, caffeine avoidance, bulk laxatives
> [3] loperamide if needed (start 1–2 mg a day and titrate).

An randomized controlled trial in adults with FI showed that technological biofeedback provided no greater benefit than teaching sphincter-strengthening exercises. Pelvic floor exercises are effective in older women with urinary incontinence, and contrary to some misperceptions, frail older people adhere well to such interventions. Caffeine stimulates gut transit and reducing significant intake of tea, coffee, and carbonated drinks can reduce stool looseness and improve bowel control (with additional benefit of reducing any concomitant bladder overactivity).

Refined foods and those high in calcium (white rice, bread, dairy products) slow transit and can improve control in individuals with weak sphincters and looser stool. Likewise, bulk laxatives will create firmer stools and can reduce anorectal incontinence, but the effect can vary between individuals. If problems persist despite these measures, loperamide (taken after an episode of loose stool, starting at low doses and titrating up) can improve control and greatly restore self confidence (e.g. can be taken before going out). Constipation should be monitored with regular use in older people. Older people with very poor sphincter tone are likely to have significant sphincter damage (assuming neurological disease has been ruled out by appropriate examination) and they merit further assessment by endoanal ultrasound and colorectal surgical review.

Dementia-related FI

Studies from the USA showed that prompted or scheduled toileting (preferably after meals) in frail care home residents can reduce frequency of FI and increase the number of continent bowel movements (benefits constipation) in care home residents. Those patients whose FI is primarily due to dementia (having excluded treatable overflow, loose stool etc.) should have an explicit bowel care programme whether at home (where it should be discussed with informal carers) or in institutions (regular toileting is preferable to managing incontinence with pads).

Self-care

An RCT in frail older stroke survivors with constipation and/or FI evaluated a one-off assessment (by a non-specialist nurse and geriatrician) leading to targeted advice and patient/carer education with booklet. At 1-year follow-up the intervention group (compared with controls receiving usual care) were more likely to be altering their diet and fluid intake to control their bowels, and at 6 months had a higher proportion of 'normal' bowel movements. Self-care for FI is very important, as people often live with the symptom as they would with a debilitating chronic disease. A study in US home-dwelling older people with FI found that the most common self-care practices were dietary change, wearing pads, and limiting activity (the latter potentially negatively impacting quality of life). Provision of containment products should also be patient-centred:

- disposable body worn pads in a choice of styles
- disposable bedpads
- pads in sufficient quantity for the individual's continence needs
- anal plugs (if tolerated)
- skincare advice covering cleansing and barrier products (e.g. Cavilon spray)
- advice on odour control and laundry
- disposable gloves.

People with FI (and where relevant their carers) must be fully informed about their condition and have access (in formats and languages suited to their individual requirements) to appropriate sources of information and support groups. Written information is very helpful and can guide the interactive discussions between people and providers. People can be usefully directed to websites run by charities (e.g. Bladder and Bowel Foundation, Parkinson's UK, Stroke Association).

Author's Tip

Toileting advice should include encouraging people to:
- empty their bowel after a meal to utilize the gastrocolic reflex
- adopt a sitting or squatting position (to strengthen Valsalva effect).

Privacy and dignity

A UK study asked frail older patients with FI about privacy during defecation – adequate privacy was reported by only 23% of nursing home residents, and 50% of hospital inpatients. Lack of privacy, particularly in dependent older people in institutions, is a major care issue and can adversely affect bowel habits.

The following measures should be taken for less mobile patients:
- avoiding bedpans
- transferring bedside commodes into private toilet areas
- including toilet access in rehabilitation goals.

Geriatricians will often find themselves at the forefront of promoting good continence care and should endeavour to influence provision at an organizational level:
- Putting processes in place to screen for FI in older people (e.g. embedding case-finding questions into routine nursing and medical assessments)
- Heighten awareness and knowledge levels among healthcare providers through education and good practice.
- Standardize care and assessment in ways that are specific to each healthcare setting (e.g. RCN continence framework for care homes, continence link nurses in hospitals)
- Integrate continence care with community continence services, therapies, colorectal surgery, urology, and urogynaecology
- Cyclical audit (with provider accountability) to identify gaps between current bowel care practice and evidence (NICE CG49) in order to (a) drive continuous quality improvement and (b) build business case for additional resources e.g. for bladder and bowel clinic for older people, Continence Nurse Specialist).

Further reading

Barrett JA, Brocklehurst JC, Kiff ES, et al. (1990). Rectal motility studies in geriatric patients with faecal incontinence. *Age Ageing* **19**: 311–17.

Bharucha AE, Zinsmeister AR, Locke GR, et al. (2005). Prevalence and burden of fecal incontinence: a population-based study in women. *Gastroenterol* **129**: 42–9.

Chassagne P, Landrin I, Neveu C, et al. (1999). Fecal incontinence in the institutionalized elderly: incidence, risk factors, and prognosis. *Am J Med* **106**: 185–90.

Chassagne P, Jego A, Gloc P, et al. (2000). Does treatment of constipation improve faecal incontinence in institutionalized elderly patients? *Age Ageing* **29**: 159–64.

Cotterill N, Norton C, Avery K, et al. (2008). A patient-centred approach to developing a comprehensive symptom and quality of life assessment of anal incontinence. *Dis Colon Rectum* **51**: 82–7.

Department of Health (2000). *Good Practice in Continence Services*. Report No PL/CMO/2000/2. London, NHS Executive.

Gallagher PF, O'Mahoney D, Quigley EM (2008). Management of chronic constipation in the elderly. *Drugs Ageing* **25**: 807–21.

Harari D, Norton C, Lockwood L et al. (2004). Treatment of constipation and faecal incontinence in stroke patients: randomised controlled trial. *Stroke* **35**: 2549–55.

Nakanishi N, Tatara K, Shinsho F, *et al.* (1999). Mortality in relation to urinary and faecal incontinence in elderly people living at home. *Age Ageing* **28**: 301–6.

NICE (2007). *Faecal incontinence.* Clinical Guideline 49. London: NICE.

Norton C, Chelvanayagam S, Wilson-Barnett J, *et al.* (2003). Randomized controlled trial of biofeedback for fecal incontinence. *Gastroenterology* **125**: 1320–9.

Norton C, Whitehead WE, Bliss DZ, *et al.* (2009). Conservative and pharmacological management of faecal incontinence in adults. In (Abrams P, Cardozo L, Khoury S, Wein A, eds) *Incontinence.* Health Publications Ltd; 1321–87.

Ouslander JG, Simmons S, Schnelle J, *et al.* (1996). Effects of prompted voiding on fecal continence among nursing home residents. *J Am Geriatr Soc* **44**: 424–8.

Petticrew M, Watt I, Sheldon T (1997). Systematic review of the effectiveness of laxatives in the elderly. *Health Technol Assess* **1**: 1–52.

Potter J, Norton C, Cottenden A (2002). *Bowel Care in Older People.* London, Royal College of Physicians.

Potter J, Peel P, Mian S, *et al.* (2007). National audit of continence care for older people: management of faecal incontinence. *Age Ageing* **36**: 268–73.

Robson KM, Kiely DK, Lembo T (2000). Development of constipation in nursing home residents. *Dis Colon Rectum* **43**: 940–3.

Talley NJ, Fleming KC, Evans JM (1996). Constipation in an elderly community: A study of prevalence and potential risk factors. *Am J Gastroenterol* **91**: 19–25.

Urinary incontinence

Anatomy of urinary incontinence

The urinary bladder is a musculomembranous sac that is a reservoir for urine. It is made of an outer connective tissue, middle detrusor muscle and inner transitional cell epithelium. It lies in the anterior pelvic cavity behind the pubic bone between the two ureteric orifices and the urethral meatus. This region is sensitive to distension as a result of the large number of sensory nerve endings present here. In addition, there are other sensory receptors in the whole of the bladder wall which can sense the degree of bladder fullness. The stretch receptors are stimulated as the bladder fills and this is transmitted to the frontal lobe micturation centres via the thalamus in the brainstem. The sacral centre between S2 and S4 is the nerve relay centre for the neural pathways between the bladder, urethral sphincters (internal and external), pelvic floor, and brain. The bladder has somatic, sympathetic, and parasympathetic innervations. The pudendal nerve innervates the external urethral sphincter and stimulation results in contraction of the sphincter. The external sphincter can only stay contracted for brief periods during rises in intra-abdominal pressures that occur during laughing, coughing, and sneezing. The internal sphincter is innervated by the sympathetic system that arise from the lower thoracic and upper lumbar segments of the spinal cord. The detrusor muscle is innervated by the parasympathetic system that arises from between the second and fourth spinal sacral segment. When stimulated, usually by a desire to void, detrusor muscle contraction occurs with a subsequent rise in intravesical pressure (see Figures 14.1 and 14.2).

As urine fills the bladder, the stretch receptors get stimulated and transmit the degree of fullness to the brain. At about 300 mL of urine, the brain recognizes a sense of fullness. Up till this point, usually the sympathetic nervous system is stimulated resulting in contraction of the internal sphincter, while the parasympathetic system is inhibited causing detrusor muscle relaxation. Once the desire to void is there, the reverse occurs with intravesical pressure exceeding urethral resistance and voiding takes place. One can delay voiding temporarily at this point by voluntarily contracting the external sphincter.

For one to be continent of urine requires the capability of the bladder to store urine adequately by accommodating increasing volumes of urine under low pressure, a closed bladder outlet, appropriate sensation of bladder fullness, and absence of involuntary bladder contractions. It also requires the ability to empty the bladder adequately by contracting, absence of obstruction to the flow of urine and a balance between bladder contraction and reduction of outlet resistance. Other factors that are very important in older adults include being able to walk to a toilet and manage ones clothing. The ability to recognize toileting needs and find a toilet, motivation to be continent, and environmental issues such as accessible toilets are important to the maintenance of continence. In the older adult, it can therefore be appreciated that the understanding of urinary incontinence needs to take not only anatomical factors into consideration but functional, psychological, and environmental factors.

With ageing, the bladder size gets smaller and the capacity is therefore reduced, thus increasing the frequency of voiding. In older adults of both genders there is an increased amount of fluids excreted at night, increased residual urine, and uninhibited bladder contractions. In older females there is a reduction in the bladder outlet and urethral resistance pressures, while in older males there is increasing outflow obstruction due to the prostate gland getting bigger with age. All these factors are the reasons

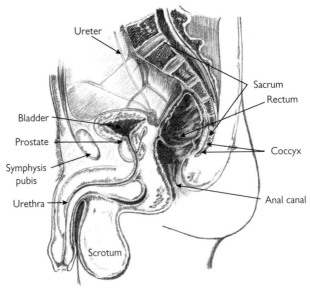

Figure 14.1 A cross-section of the male pelvis with the position of the bladder, prostate and urethra shown in relation to the pelvic organs. Figure kindly drawn by medical illustrator Mr Ken Jukes.

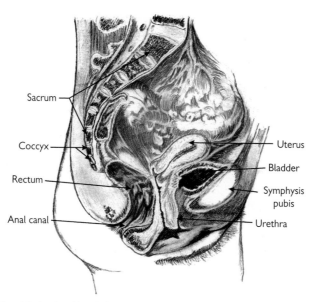

Figure 14.2 A cross-section of the female pelvis with the position of the bladder and urethra shown in relation to the pelvic organs. Figure kindly drawn by medical illustrator Mr Ken Jukes.

why an older adult is more prone to urinary incontinence when they either develop an acute illness or are given a new medication, as their threshold for maintaining continence is reduced (see Table 14.1).

Author's Tip

An understanding of not just anatomical but functional, psychological and environmental factors is critical to urinary continence especially in frail older adults.

Table 14.1 Summary of ageing changes that affect the continence status of older adults

Domain	Changes with ageing	Impact
Urinary tract	Decreased bladder contractions	Retention
	Decreased bladder capacity	Frequency
	Decreased urethral pressure	Stress incontinence
	Altered voiding pattern	Nocturia
	BPH	Obstruction
	Prolapse	Obstruction
	Atrophic vaginitis	Frequency/urgency
Cognition	Dementia	Disinhibition
	Depression	Self-neglect
Function	Impaired mobility	Urge incontinence
	Impaired dexterity	

BPH, benign prostatic hypertrophy.

Causes of urinary incontinence

In determining the root causes of urinary incontinence in older adults, factors to be considered are cognitive ability, functional ability, environmental issues, medications, and the lower urinary tract. Prevalence rates vary from 18% in community dwelling older adults to 60% in 24-hour care facilities, with 35% prevalence rates in older hospitalized adults. All these figures are most likely conservative as both healthcare professionals and those with incontinence share a reluctance to discuss this for a variety of reasons. This results in significant underreporting.

Cognitive impairment
Cognitive impairment of whatever origin, commonly delirium and dementia, can result in reduced awareness of bladder fullness or social disinhibition resulting in incontinence. Depression can result in a lack of self-care, including attention to remaining continent.

Functional ability
Functional ability refers to being able to walk to a toilet or its substitute, such as a commode, in time to undress and use the facilities. With neurological conditions and arthritis being commoner with age, as well as an increased prevalence of visual impairment, this action is affected and can contribute to urge incontinence.

Environmental factors
Environmental factors are important, with easy access for older adults to user-friendly toilets being the key.

Medications
Medications as illustrated in Table 14.2 can contribute to urinary incontinence via a variety of mechanisms.

Lower urinary tract
The state of the lower urinary tract is, of course, important and urinary incontinence can be classified based on pathophysiology and clinical features. Urge incontinence is the

Table 14.2 Drugs implicated in urinary incontinence

Drug	Mechanism
Anticholinergics	Urinary retention, loading and delirium
Antidepressants	Anticholinergic properties and sedation
Antipsychotics	Anticholinergic properties and sedation
Narcotics	Anticholinergic properties, sedation and delirium
Alpha-antagonists	Urethral relaxation
Alpha-agonist	Urinary retention
Beta-antagonists	Urinary retention
Diuretics	Excess urine output
Sedatives	Sedation and delirium
Anxiolytics	Sedation and delirium
Cholinesterase inhibitors	Pro-cholinergic effects
Antihistamines	Anticholinergic properties and sedation
Caffeine	Excess urine output
Alcohol	Delirium

involuntary loss of urine associated with a strong desire to micturate which is secondary to detrusor overactivity. This is responsible for between 50% and 70% of the urinary incontinence in older adults. There is frequent and repeated voiding with the person maintaining continence in between. Stress incontinence is the involuntary loss of urine when there is an increase in intrabdominal pressure such as in physical exertion, laughing, sneezing, and coughing. This is a consequence of underlying abnormalities of the urethral sphincters which can result from an idiopathic reason but more commonly in females as a result of the lax pelvic floor musculature. However, examination may also be normal and stress urinary incontinence is not always associated with uterine prolapse or a cystocele. Mixed incontinence can result from incomplete bladder emptying due to detrusor underactivity, bladder outlet obstruction, or a urethral diverticulum. Detrusor hyperactivity can also coexist with underactivity. Bladder outlet obstruction is much commoner in males than females and is secondary usually to benign prostatic hypertrophy including those who may have had surgery already. Detrusor underactivity due to neurological conditions is rare, as are urethral diverticula. A useful acronym to use in understanding causes of urinary incontinence is DIAPPERS:

D: Delirium
I: Infection of the urinary tract
A: Atrophic vaginitis and urethritis
P: Pharmacology
P: Psychological issues such as depression
E: Excess urine output, as in hyperglycaemia
R: Restricted functional ability/environment
S: Stools, as in constipation and faecal loading.

Clinical assessment

Acute urinary incontinence should be assessed systemically to look diligently for reversible factors using the DIAPPERS acronym and where it persists classifying it according to the various types of incontinence should be done in addition to identifying any contribution due to function or cognition.

> **Author's Tip**
>
> Cognition, functional capability, environment, medications, and the lower urinary tract are the components to be looked at when determining the causes of urinary incontinence in older adults.

Investigation of urinary incontinence

Older adults with urinary incontinence should have a urinalysis, urine culture, and selected blood tests. A bladder diary or frequency volume chart should then be requested, especially if the incontinence persists despite initial treatment of reversible causes. Additional investigations that may be necessary include a post-void residual urine volume and urodynamic testing.

Urinalysis

Normal, fresh urine is pale to dark yellow or amber in colour and clear. A red or red-brown colour could be from a food dye, eating fresh beets, a drug, or the presence of either haemoglobin or myoglobin. The actual test is done by immersing a strip in a urine sample. A strip may comprise up to 10 different chemical pads which react with the urine. The test should be read after one minute. The most common parameters to look for include:

pH
The glomerular filtrate of blood plasma is usually acidified by renal tubules and collecting ducts from a pH of 7.4 to about 6 in the final urine. Normal range is 5–7.

Ketone bodies
Normally negative. When the production of the ketones (acetone, aceotacetic acid, beta-hydroxybutyric acid) resulting from either diabetic ketoacidosis or some form of calorie deprivation (starvation) exceeds the ability of the body to metabolize these compounds, they accumulate in the blood and some are found in the urine.

Proteins
Normally negative. Proteins are very large molecules and are not normally present in measurable amounts in the urine. If this becomes positive by a urinary tract infection or it may be caused by other diseases that have secondarily affected the kidneys.

A small amount of filtered plasma proteins and protein secreted by the nephron (Tamm–Horsfall protein) can be found in normal urine. Dipsticks detect protein with an indicator dye, bromphenol blue, which is most sensitive to albumin but is poor at detecting globulins and Bence–Jones protein. Normal total protein excretion does not usually exceed 150 mg/24 hours or 10 mg/100 mL in any single specimen. Trace positive results are equivalent to 10 mg/100 mL or about 150 mg/24 hours (the upper limit of normal). For urine dipstick testing:

- 1+ corresponds to about 200–500 mg/24 hours
- 2+ to 0.5–1.5 gm/24 hours
- 3+ to 2–5 gm/24 hours
- 4+ represents 7 gm/24 hours or greater.

Nitrites
Normally negative. A positive nitrite test indicates that bacteria may be present in significant numbers in urine. Gram-negative rods such as *Escherichia coli* are more likely

to give a positive test. False positives can occur due to vaginal contamination and false negatives due to high urinary vitamin C.

Glucose
Normally negative. Less than 0.1% of glucose normally filtered by the glomerulus appears in urine (<130 mg/24 hours). The commonly used dipsticks for screening are specific for glucose but can miss galactose and fructose. False positives can occur in patients on L-dopa.

Red blood cells
Should be negative as none should be present. Positive if there are abnormal numbers of red cells in urine due to glomerular damage, tumours which erode the urinary tract anywhere along its length, kidney trauma, urinary tract stones, renal infarcts, acute tubular necrosis, urinary tract infections, nephrotoxins, and physical stress. Red cells may also contaminate the urine from the vagina in menstruating women or from trauma produced by bladder catheterization.

White blood cells
A positive test results from the presence of white blood cells either as whole cells or as lysed cells. Pyuria can be detected even if the urine sample contains damaged or lysed cells. A negative test means that an infection is unlikely.

Urine culture

This should be done if urinalysis indicates an infection or the history is suggestive. Chronic asymptomatic bacteriuria is not a cause of incontinence and treating it does not resolve the incontinence.

Blood tests

Urea and electrolytes to determine renal function and serum glucose and calcium especially when there is polyuria.

Post-void residual urine volume

This particular investigation is useful in determining whether there is reduced detrusor contractility or bladder outlet obstruction. A normal post-void residual volume should be less than 50 mL. The clinical significance of volumes between 100 and 200 mL is still unclear. However for now it is recommended that anything greater than 100 mL should result in further investigations which may include specialist investigations. With volumes greater than 300 mL, hydronephrosis and renal failure are likely to occur and the bladder should be drained while awaiting further investigations and treatment.

The gold standard for carrying out this investigation is by inserting a urinary catheter. The risks of infection by performing a sterile in and out catheterization are less than 2% and it allows for obtaining a clean mid-stream urine specimen from older adults with incontinence in whom it can be difficult to obtain this otherwise. The next best option if the clinician is not keen on inserting a catheter is to use a portable bladder scanner but one needs to be aware that it may not always detect significant residual volumes.

Frequency volume chart

A record kept by the person or their carer over a minimum of three days to record each episode of voiding including the incontinent episodes. The volume voided should be recorded using a measuring cup. The pattern of voiding and incontinent episodes can suggest the type of incontinence and the volume voided gives an idea of the functional capacity of the person's bladder.

Urodynamic testing

These include cystometry, urinary flow measurements, urethral pressure profiles, and some imaging studies.

Opinion is divided on the usefulness of these tests in the evaluation of lower urinary tract symptoms in older adults, especially those who are frail. The accuracy of the results is very dependent on not just the technical skill of the investigator, but the cooperation of the person being investigated. It becomes obvious that people with significant cognitive impairment or communication difficulties could have unreliable results. This can result in misdiagnosis and the wrong treatment. The tests themselves can cause discomfort, trauma and infection.

The best approach is to only proceed with these tests if surgery is being considered and medical therapy has failed.

> **Author's Tip**
>
> Most useful investigations are urinalysis, urine culture, serum urea, electrolytes, glucose and calcium, bladder diary, and where indicated post-void residual urine volume.

Management of urinary incontinence

Important factors to be considered in the management of urinary incontinence in older adults especially those who are frail, include choice and objective or goal of treatment, pharmacology of prescribed medicines and the involvement of care givers in these discussions where appropriate. The appreciation that, in addition to the lower urinary tract, cognitive ability, functional ability, environmental issues, and medications all contribute to urinary incontinence in the older adult is important to keep in mind when formulating a management plan.

The initial first step is to exclude any reversible causes of urinary incontinence which are discussed in detail in the section on causes. If the incontinence then persists, all the possible factors that could contribute to this should be listed. They tend to include moderate to severe cognitive impairment, reduced mobility and manual dexterity, medication, detrusor hyperactivity, lax pelvic floor musculature, and prolapse.

The next step is to agree with the person and their care giver where appropriate the preferences for care, goals of care and explain the expected benefits of intervention.

A careful consideration should be given to the contribution of any existing prescribed medication on the incontinence before prescribing any specific drugs for incontinence. Where a decision is then made to go ahead with drug therapy consider age related changes in pharmacokinetics when choosing a drug and the dose. Always aim to start with the lowest possible dose and where antimuscarinic agents are used monitor proactively for any effects on cognition.

Options for care

Lifestyle advice
Adequate oral hydration to increase voided volume in nursing home residents and for all older adults a reduction in caffeine intake and prevention of constipation should be attempted.

Prompted voiding
This should be offered to reduce daytime urinary incontinence in those with significant functional impairment such

as housebound, nursing home, and where applicable to hospitalized older adults. Care givers in these settings need to be educated, encouraged and motivated to comply with the agreed prompting schedule. For those with no cognitive impairment, they should be educated, encouraged and motivated to adhere to the agreed prompting schedule.

Supervised pelvic floor physiotherapy
This is appropriate for stress, urge, and mixed urinary incontinence as a lax pelvic floor musculature is very common in older females. The exercises should be initially supervised and should be done several times daily. This intervention would be inappropriate for those with significant frailty, severe cognitive impairment and those who are immobile.

Medications
This should only be considered where all contributing factors to the incontinence have been identified, lifestyle, and prompted voiding have failed and the person can physically toilet themselves or be assisted.

Antimuscarinic agents can be prescribed for urge or mixed incontinence.

The best antimuscarinics to use for older female adults, especially those with frailty, are tolterodine, solifenacin, and darifenacin. They are well tolerated and are very unlikely to cause cognitive impairment. They also reduce the number of incontinent episodes. Like all antimuscarinics, they can cause constipation and dry mouth. They should be reviewed after eight weeks and discontinued if they have not made any difference to the person's symptoms.

In males with symptomatic benign prostatic hypertrophy, alpha1-adrenoreceptor antagonists (e.g. tamsulosin, doxazosin) are used as first line. They act by causing relaxation of the smooth muscle in the bladder neck and prostate improving the flow of urine. The best one to use is tamsulosin, especially in frail older males, as postural hypotention is less likely to occur. Poor flow, hesitancy, and terminal dribbling will usually respond to treatment within four weeks, while urgency, nocturia, and increased frequency can take longer. 5-alpha-reductase inhibitors (finasteride or dutasteride) reduce the prostate size by blocking the formation of dihydrotestosterone from testosterone. They take about 6 months it to have the desired effect. They are especially useful where the prostate volume is greater than 40 mL and in combination with alpha-blockers better symptom relief is obtained.

Topical oestrogens (cream, tablet, ring) can be given for atrophic vaginitis.

All the medications mentioned above should be used long term if they relieve the symptoms that the person presented with.

Bladder relaxants in older frail males should only be prescribed where arrangements for monitoring post-void residual volume can be guaranteed.

Catheter
Condom catheters can be used to manage permanent urinary incontinence in males especially if the patient is dependent and has no urinary retention. Intermittent self catherization may be suitable for those with chronic urinary retention and care givers can be taught to do this if the person is unable to do it themselves. Indications for long-term indwelling catheters include urinary retention that has not resolved after medical or surgical treatment and where intermittent self catherization is not possible, skin wounds, or pressure sores are contaminated by urine, care of terminally ill, and those with severe cognitive impairment where bed and clothing changes will be disruptive and uncomfortable. It can also be considered in situations where either the person or their caregiver find toileting a significant burden and discomfort and they understand the risks associated with indwelling catheters.

Indications for insertion of urinary catheters include:
- assessment of urine output where clinically indicated
- as part of urodynamic studies
- surgery
- urinary retention
- bladder outlet obstruction
- atonic bladder
- pressure ulcers that could be contaminated by urine
- for comfort in terminally ill people.

Complications associated with urinary catheterization include:
- pain
- trauma
- infection
- obstruction
- bladder spasm
- calculi formation.

Surgery
In benign prostatic hyperplasia, this is usually indicated for recurrent urinary retention, bladder stones, haematuria, and failed medical therapy. The commonest procedure still performed is transurethral prostatectomy. Other procedures include laser prostatectomy, transurethral needle ablation, and microwave therapy.

In females, pelvic organ prolapse is commonly associated with urinary incontinence. It can result in cystocele, urethrocele, rectocele, enterocele, first- to third-degree descent of the cervix and vaginal vault prolapse. All of these can be managed initially with some pelvic floor exercises, insertion of vaginal ring or shelf pessary and in appropriately selected individual's surgery. Surgical techniques that can be carried out include vaginal wall repair, vaginal vault sacrospinous fixation.

For stress incontinence that has not responded to conservative measures in appropriately selected individuals, periurethral bulking agents and tension free vaginal tape are the most commonly carried out procedures. In urge incontinence where drug therapy and the other measures described have failed, procedures that are done include sacral nerve stimulation and injection of botulinum toxin A directly inside the bladder.

Author's Tip

Discuss management options.

Keep in mind that other factors other than the lower urinary tract play a major role.

Conservative treatment is first line.

Surgery only last option in appropriately selected individuals.

Further reading

Diokno AC, Brown MB, Brock BM, *et al.* (1988). Clinical and Cystometric characteristics of continent and incontinent nonistitutionalised elderly. *J Urol* **140**: 567–71.

Roe B, Akpan A (2009). Incontinence. In (M Gosney and T Harris, eds) *Managing Older People in Primary Care a Practical Guide.* Oxford, Oxford University Press.

Tan TL (2003). Urinary incontinence in older persons: A simple approach to a complex problem. *Ann Acad Med Singapore* **32**: 731–9.

Impaired vision: anatomy and physiology of vision (Figure 14.3)

Eyelids

Chief components
- Outer layer of skin
- Inner lining of conjunctiva that is continuous with the bulbar conjunctiva on the eyeball
- Orbicularis muscle
- Levator muscle in upper lid
- Tarsal plate containing meibomian glands
- Lid margin with eyelashes and orifices of meibomian glands

Key functions
- Protection: blink reflex and eyelid closure
- Secretion of tears by means of meibomian glands and conjunctiva

Main disorders
- Positional: ptosis, entropion, ectropion
- Blepharitis

Conjunctiva

Chief components
- The conjunctiva is a semi-transparent tissue. The bulbar conjunctiva on the eyeball and eyelid are continuous with each other through the superior and inferior fornices.

Key functions
- Secretion of tears
- Permits unrestricted movement of the eyeball

Main disorders
- Conjunctivitis: infective and non-infective
- Dry eye conditions

Cornea

Chief components
- Tear film
- Multilayered epithelium: binds the tear film
- Monolayer of endothelium: energy-dependent pump helps to maintain stromal dehydration
- Stroma: collagen lamellae and extracellular matrix, keratocytes, absence of blood vessels

Key functions
- Protection against micro-organisms
- Transmission of light: transparency is achieved by special arrangement of the collagen lamellae that minimise light scatter, a lack of blood vessels, and a low water content
- Refraction of light: through both higher-than-air refractive index and a convex anterior surface

Main disorders
- Infection (keratitis): chiefly bacterial (after disruption of the epithelial barrier) and viral (herpes simplex/zoster)
- Loss of clarity through overhydration due to insufficient number of endothelial cells (primary, Fuchs' endothelial dystrophy; secondary, usually after cataract surgery = pseudophakic bullous keratopathy).

Lens

Chief components
- Outer capsule (a basement membrane) that fully encloses the lens; attachments to the ciliary body via zonular fibres
- A central nucleus and an outer cortex
- Lens fibres that are elongated cells

Key functions
- Transparency: lens fibres contain specialized proteins to aid transparency
- Refraction: convex surface
- Accommodation: the convexity of the lens, and therefore its refractive power, can be varied by altering the tension of the zonules by contraction–relaxation of the ciliary body musculature

Main disorders
- Presbyopia: loss of accommodation. Starts at 45 years and progresses until complete at 65 years
- Cataract

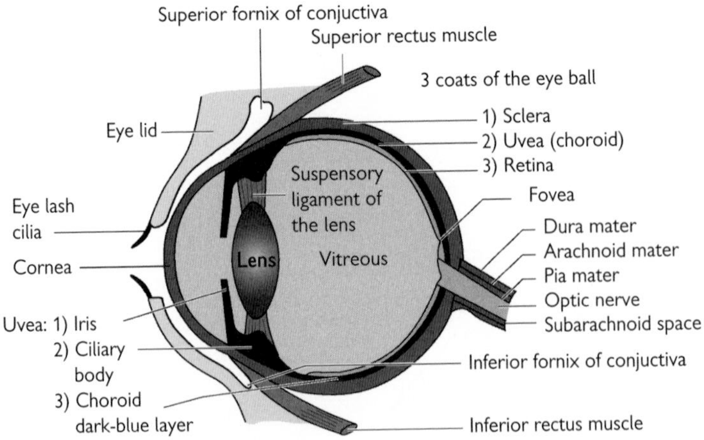

Superior fornix of conjuctiva
Superior rectus muscle
3 coats of the eye ball
Eye lid
1) Sclera
2) Uvea (choroid)
3) Retina
Suspensory ligament of the lens
Fovea
Eye lash cilia
Cornea
Lens
Vitreous
Dura mater
Arachnoid mater
Pia mater
Optic nerve
Subarachnoid space
Uvea: 1) Iris
2) Ciliary body
3) Choroid dark-blue layer
Inferior fornix of conjuctiva
Inferior rectus muscle

Figure 14.3 (colour plate 8) Anatomy and physiology of vision. Reproduced from Judith Collier, Murray Longmore, and Mark Brinsden, *Oxford Handbook of Clinical Specialities*, (7th edition), 2007, figure on p. 433, with permission from Oxford University Press.

Aqueous inflow/outflow system
Chief components
- Ciliary body makes aqueous humour by an active process
- Aqueous humour flows forwards through the pupil into the anterior chamber
- Aqueous leaves through the trabecular meshwork, which lies between the iris and the cornea, known as the anterior chamber angle

Key functions
- Aqueous humour secretion creates intraocular pressure (IOP)
- Aqueous humour contents maintain the health of the tissues bordering the anterior chamber (corneal endothelium, iris, lens, angle)

Main disorders
- Impairment of outflow, either through impaired function of the trabecular meshwork (as in primary open angle glaucoma, POAG) or proximity of the iris to the cornea (angle closure)

Retina
Chief components
- Neurosensory retina: light-sensitive photoreceptors connecting to ganglion cells via specialized modulating cells
- Ganglion cell axons pass across the retina and exit through the optic nerve at the optic disc
- Retinal pigment epithelium (RPE): monolayer of cells behind the neurosensory retina
- Choroid: highly vascular layer behind the RPE
- Retinal circulation: arterial and venous system on the retina; a capillary bed within the retina
- Photoreceptors subdivided into cones (confer acuity, colour) and rods (for low-light sensitivity, movement)

Key functions
- Photoreceptors change light energy into electrical energy
- RPE cells have a variety of functions, chiefly maintaining photoreceptor function
- Blood–retinal barriers (tight junctions between retinal vasculature endothelial cells and between RPE cells) limit movement of blood constituents into the retina to small molecules like glucose
- Cones: concentrated in the macula area (fovea) conferring high quality vision (acuity)
- Rods: peripheral retina is for field of vision

Main disorders
- Age-related macular degeneration (AMD, ARMD)
- Diabetic retinopathy
- Retinal vein/artery occlusion

Optic nerve
Chief Components
- Outer wall is extension of the dura mater
- Fibres are the axons of retinal ganglion cells that travel to the lateral geniculate nucleus by the thalamus
- Artery and vein are in the centre of the optic nerve; four subdivisions supply retinal quadrants
- An absence of photoreceptors creates the physiological blind spot

Key functions
- Transmission of ganglion cell axons from the globe to the occipital cortex

Main disorders
- Glaucomatous optic neuropathy (loss of axons)
- Ischaemic optic neuropathy (arteritic and non-arteritic)

Central pathways
Chief components
- Optic nerve, chiasm, optic tract; synapse in lateral geniculate body; optic radiation, visual cortex in occipital lobes.
- At chiasm, axons from nasal retina cross to contralateral tract.
- Primary visual cortex interlinks with visual association areas

Key functions
- Topographic localisation becomes more congruent the more posterior in the pathway

Main disorders
- Optic nerve disease: loss of acuity, central scotoma, red desaturation
- Compression of centre of chiasm: bitemporal hemianopia
- Left optic tract/radiation/cortex: right homonymous hemianopia (congruous)

Control of ocular position
Chief components
- Extraocular muscles: medial and lateral rectus for horizontal movement; inferior oblique and superior rectus for elevation; superior oblique and inferior rectus for depression; obliques also produce torsion (inferior, ex-superior, in-).
- Abducens (VI) to lateral rectus, trochlear (IV) to superior oblique; oculomotor (III) all the rest. (Oculomotor also constricts the pupil and stimulates upper lid levator.)
- Nuclei in brainstem. Complex system of controls with inputs and interconnections from a range of other nuclei and reflex centres ensures that the two eyes move in parallel.

Key functions
- Maintenance of single vision
- Three-dimensional vision

Main disorders
- Cranial neuropathies: usually due to a vascular disease
- Muscle disorders: dysthyroid eye disease and myasthenia gravis
- Progressive supranuclear palsy

Assessment of visual function
Acuity
- Snellen chart
- Logmar chart: Letters get smaller along the line

Fields
- Confrontational
- Computerized perimetry.

Colour
- Ishihara colour plates, designed to detect red-green disorders; also used for acquired disease.
- Red desaturation (loss of brightness of a red target) is sensitive for optic nerve disease

Pupils
- The swinging flashlight test is the most important test; can detect asymmetrical disease in the afferent limb of the light reflex along the optic nerve (RAPD, relative afferent pupil defect).

Investigation of sudden and chronic visual loss

Introduction

Patients who complain of symptoms relating to their eyes and visual pathway pose a challenge to non-ophthalmic trained physicians. A few inexpensive tools and a simple methodical approach can make life easy. We demonstrate in Figure 14.4 a simple approach to diagnosing and managing visual loss.

Assessment

Measurement of visual acuity is fundamental to the ophthalmic assessment and referral. Test distance vision with distance glasses/contact lenses using a 6 m or reduced size 3 m Snellen chart.

If the patient does not have glasses then the pin hole test is an acceptable alternative. Punch a hole through some paper using the nib of a ball point pen. Measure the distance vision without pinhole then with.

Each eye should be measured individually. Make sure the fellow eye is well occluded. Patients often peek through gaps in fingers – don't be tricked!

A simple exploration of the field of vision of each quadrant of each eye using a test object, even a finger, should be performed. A pen torch is used to look for the pattern of redness, to identify corneal clarity and to test the pupil reflexes.

Examination of the retina is hard but greatly helped by pupil dilation. Do not be afraid to dilate the pupils (see Table 14.3). The risk of precipitating angle closure glaucoma is in the region of 1/5000. It is better that it happen in the hospital setting than spontaneously elsewhere.

See other sections for age-related macular degeneration (ARMD); cataract; glaucoma.

Table 14.3 Drops for dilating pupils

Cylcopegic/ mydriatic agent (%)	Maximal effect (min)	Duration of action (h)
Tropicamide 0.5–1.0	20–30	3–6
Phenylepherine 2.5	20	3
Cyclopentolate 0.5, 1	20–45	24–36

Uveitis

Uveitis is inflammation of the uveal tract which comprises the iris, ciliary body, and choroid. Anterior uveitis can be considered to be synonymous with 'iritis', inflammation of the iris.

Presentation is usually of rapid onset (hours to days). Vision is often described as 'misty' or 'smoky'. Acuity can be reduced but usually no more than two to three lines less than the fellow eye. Photophobia and lacrimation are common.

The redness is circumcorneal, the cornea clear, the pupil small and may even be fixed.

Treatment should be by an ophthalmologist and patients should be seen within 24 hours of presentation. Management involves topical steroids and mydriatics.

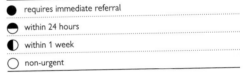

- requires immediate referral
- within 24 hours
- within 1 week
- non-urgent

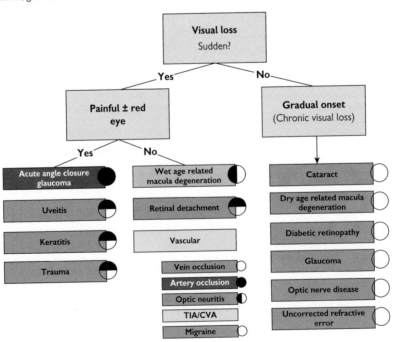

Figure 14.4 Visual loss decision tree.

Keratitis

Inflammation of the cornea identified by a collection of white cells seen as an opacity within the clear cornea. Keratitis may be bacterial, viral, fungal or autoimmune in origin and if untreated has the potential to lead to sight loss.

Presentation is with a painful, red eye with varying degrees of vision loss. Initially pain is described as a foreign body sensation noted primarily on blinking and can become felt through the side of the face. Photophobia and lacrimation frequently occur. A past history of 'ulcers', cold sores, or contact lens wear should increase the clinician's index of suspicion.

Use a pen torch to look at the pattern of injection around the cornea. The redness often 'points' to the lesion. A corneal opacity will prevent the visibility of iris detail through the cornea. A drop of fluorescein dye will illuminate bright green with a cobalt blue light indicating a breach of the corneal epithelium. Corneal abrasions and ulcers can be difficult to distinguish on history and bedside examination. The key difference is that there is no opacification with an abrasion which does not need specialist attention. However if the diagnosis is in doubt the patient should be seen the same day by an ophthalmologist.

Treatment involves biopsy of the ulcer and intensive topical antimicrobial treatment.

Retinal detachment

This is a separation of the neurosensory retina from the retinal pigment epithelium. It is often preceded by a degenerative detachment of the vitreous gel from its loose attachments to the retina (posterior vitreous detachment, PVD). Presentation can be thought of as the four 'Fs': Floaters, Flashes, Field defect, Fall in vision. PVD gives rise to symptoms of floaters, even a 'cobweb' or net-curtain-like visual disturbance, and flashing lights (photopsias) caused by vitreous traction on the retina.

A field defect perceived as a 'dark curtain' may be a late sign, not noticed if there is a complete field in the other eye. Occlude the fellow eye and perform a confrontational field test. A drop in acuity indicates detachment of the macula. Normal vision should not exclude urgent referral as macula 'on' detachment has a better post-operative outcome than macula 'off'. It is very hard to see the detachment with the ophthalmoscope unless fairly advanced.

Myopic patients and those with a history of previous retinal detachment in either eye are at greatest risk.

Sudden onset of symptoms of a PVD warrants referral within a few days; if there is loss of field of vision or drop in acuity, referral should be within 24 hours.

Vascular

There are multiple vascular pathologies that present with painless loss of vision. These include vein occlusions (branch, hemi or central), artery occlusions (branch or central), vascular pathologies in the visual pathway giving rise to transient ischaemic attacks, migraine and optic nerve related pathologies.

Vein occlusions are more common than artery occlusions and less devastating in their symptoms. Patients may describe a field defect or loss of central vision if the macula is involved. They are associated with age, hypertension, chronic glaucoma and, less frequently, blood disorders. Examination of the fundus will reveal large haemorrhages either distributed in one quadrant (opposite to the perceived field defect) in a branch occlusion or throughout the fundus in a central occlusion, engorged retinal veins and evidence of longstanding hypertensive changes. Patients should be seen on a non-urgent basis. Ophthalmic management will involve establishing a cause and minimising risk factors as well as regular follow up to ensure that the infrequent sequlae, particularly neovascular glaucoma, do not occur.

Artery occlusions are far more dramatic in presentation. There is painless, sudden, dense loss of vision, usually counting fingers acuity or worse, often noticed on waking but not reported till some time later. Signs can be subtle and need to be compared to the fellow eye. There should be a relative afferent pupil defect (RAPD). The fundus may look relatively pale due to oedema and a cherry red spot can be seen at the macula.

Referral should be made as an emergency as there are reports that if an embolus is dislodged within the first four hours of occlusion some sight can be restored, however the prognosis is very poor and the mainstay of management is prevention of disease in the fellow eye and reduction of risk factors.

Diabetic retinopathy

Diabetic retinopathy is a microangiopathy that results in vascular occlusion and leakage. Microvascular occlusion results in capillary non-perfusion and hypoxia of the retina. Angiogenic growth factors are released in a response to the retinal hypoxia leading to new blood vessel growth. New vessels are fragile and bleed leading to sight loss.

The mainstay of management is prevention of proliferative and sight threatening retinopathy through good systemic control of diabetes, hypertension and cholesterol and ophthalmic treatment with laser, intraocular steroids, or anti-vascular endothelial growth factors (anti-VEGF).

Patients with diabetes with poor control may report variable vision. This is due to changes within the lens related to fluctuating glycaemia. A report of a drop in central vision may indicate maculopathy and 'red blobs' or floaters may indicate a bleed from new vessels. These patients should be discussed with an ophthalmologist who will usually arrange to see the patient on a semi-urgent basis.

Further reading

Denniston A, Murray P (eds) (2009). Oxford Handbook of Ophthalmology, 2nd revised edn. Oxford, Oxford University Press; p. 976.

Kanski J (ed.) (2007). Clinical Ophthalmology: A Systematic Approach, 6th edn. Butterworth-Heinemann.

Cataract

Anatomy

The lens is a transparent, biconvex structure in the eye that provides about one-third of the focusing power of the eye (the rest is the cornea). The young lens, by changing its shape, changes the focal distance of the eye so that it can focus on objects at various distances. This adjustment of the lens is known as accommodation. The lens continues to grow throughout a person's lifetime. This steady growth results in gradual loss of accommodation until in middle age reading glasses are required. This is presbyopia.

The lens has three main parts: the lens capsule; the lens epithelium; and the lens fibres. The lens capsule is a smooth, transparent basement membrane that completely surrounds the lens. It is synthesized by the lens epithelium. The lens epithelium, located in the anterior portion of the lens between the lens capsule and the lens fibres, is a simple cuboidal epithelium.

It regulates most of the homeostatic functions of the lens and synthesises new lens fibres. These form the bulk of the lens. The bulk of the lens is a saturated solution of protein. If the lens epithelial cells die, the lens capsule is breeched, or the lens protein is chemically altered, then the protein comes out of solution and opacification occurs. To the ancient Greeks, this was similar to a river – clear when flowing smoothly, white and opaque when in the turbulence of a waterfall: hence the name 'cataract'.

Epidemiology

Cataract is a common and important cause of visual impairment world-wide. The prevalence of visually impairing cataract rises steadily with age (see Figure 14.5).

The treatment is always surgical, and delivery of surgical services represents a challenge to most healthcare systems. Cataract extraction accounts for a significant proportion of the surgical workload of most ophthalmologists in the UK and cataract surgery continues to be the commonest elective surgical procedure performed in the UK and the most likely operation that any patient will undergo.

The prevalence of cataract (after adjusting for age) was higher in women, the overall prevalence ratio (females: males) was 1.22 (95% confidence limits 1.07–1.40). Notably, the majority (88%) of people in the UK with treatable visual impairment from cataract were not in touch with eye

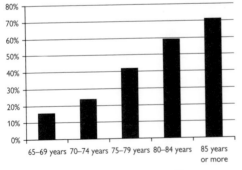

Figure 14.5 Prevalence of significant cataract with age. Data from: Reidy A, Minassian DC, Vafidis G, et al. (1998). Prevalence of serious eye disease and visual impairment in a north London population: population-based, cross sectional study. BMJ, **316**: 1643–46.

health services, representing the level of potentially unmet need for eye healthcare for cataract in the population. It is estimated that 2.4 million people aged 65 and older in England and Wales have visually impairing cataract in one or both eyes.

In addition, it is estimated that a further 225 000 new cases of visually impairing cataract are expected each year. The 5-year cumulative incidence is estimated at 1.1 million new cases among the population aged 65 years and older.

Risk factors

The causes for cataract are multifactorial. Apart from age, aetiological epidemiological studies have identified a number of risk factors for cataract:

- gender—commoner in females
- diabetes mellitus – glycosylation of the lens protein leads to opacity
- corticosteroids, especially topical to the eye
- nutrition
- low socio-economic status
- lifestyle: smoking and alcohol
- dehydration/diarrhoeal crises.

Exposure to ultraviolet light is commonly cited as a risk factor but generally now thought not to be.

Cataract surgery in this country is performed predominantly on older patients, with about 80% being over 70 years of age. Serious coexisting eye conditions such as glaucoma, age related macular degeneration, diabetic retinopathy or amblyopia, are present in 30% of patients having cataract surgery. With increasing life expectancy and the resulting expansion of the older population, both the prevalent cases of cataract and the demand for surgery will continue to rise.

Referral and assessment

Because cataracts build up slowly, many patients may not be aware of its development until quite advanced. Common complaints include loss of sharpness of vision, glare, and inability to read text on TV.

Cataracts are normally diagnosed by an optometrist but can be detected by any medical practitioner with a direct ophthalmoscope. Since the direct ophthalmoscope uses similar optics to the human eye, opacities seen as significant with this instrument will be so. One of the problems with severe cataracts is that it is not possible to see the retina, and the extent of coexistent eye disease that may preclude sight (such as advanced macular degeneration) is not recognized until after the patient has undergone the procedure.

Other indications for cataract surgery include facilitating treatment and/or monitoring posterior segment disease, e.g. diabetic retinopathy, correcting anisometropia or treating lens induced ocular disease. Contrary to common belief, surgery to the second eye is just as important to the patient's function as surgery to the first eye.

Following history taking and examination, the ideal refractive outcome should be considered. Because an intra-ocular lens implant can be obtained in many different dioptric powers, it is possible to correct significant refractive error as part of the cataract procedure, e.g. high myopia. Recently, toric intra-ocular lenses have been developed to enable the correction of astigmatism.

The vast majority of patients are suitable for day surgery under local anaesthesia.

Surgery

The aim of surgery is to remove the opacity and to replace the focusing power of the lens with an intra-ocular lens implant. Removal of the entire lens is termed intracapsular cataract extraction. This is rarely performed today. Instead the capsular bag is opened and the opaque nucleus and lens matter is removed either via a large incision (extracapsular cataract extraction or ECCE) or via a small incision (phakoemulsification). Phakoemulsification is the procedure of choice in the developed world.

Cataract surgery should include:

- Minimal trauma to ocular tissues: particularly the cornea, which has a limited ability to repair.
- Capsular fixation of the intraocular lens.
- Watertight incision closure with reduction of astigmatism where appropriate: often 10/0 nylon sutures are used to close the wound, but many small incisions are self-sealing and sutureless surgery is the norm.
- Prevention of infection: to date the only effective prophylactic measure in infection prevention has been Povidone iodine 5% aqueous solution irrigated into the conjunctival sac immediately preoperatively The use of intra-cameral or infusion fluid antibiotics remains controversial but a recent retrospective series has shown a reduced rate of postoperative endophthalmitis with intra-cameral cefuroxime.

Pre- and postoperative adverse affects

In the developed world 10% of patients undergoing cataract extraction are not improved by the procedure. This is because of coexisting macular degeneration that the cataract has prevented assessment, and the complications of surgery, particularly endophthalmitis (bacterial infection) and post-operative macular oedema due to uveitis usually associated with per-operative rupture of the capsular bag. The most common complication is reopacification of the residual posterior capsule behind the implanted intra-ocular lens. This complication is simply treated with a YAG laser capsulotomy (a non-invasive procedure). The risk of developing posterior capsule opacification is much greater in younger patients.

Further reading

AAO PPP American Academy of Ophthalmology. Preferred Practice Pattern (AAO 01) (http://one.aao.org/CE/PracticeGuidelines/PPP_Content.aspx?cid=6f2be59d-6481-4c64-9a3e-8d1dabec9ffa).

Ciulla TA, Starr MB, Masket S (2003). Bacterial endophthalmitis prophylaxis for cataract surgery: an evidence-based update. *Ophthalmology* **109**: 13–24.

Congdon NG, Taylor H (2003). Age related cataract. In Johnson GJ, Miassian DC, Weale R (eds) *The Epidemiology of Eye Disease.* London, Arnold Publishers, pp. 105–19.

Desai P (1999) UK NCS UK National Cataract Survey. RCO.

Desai P, Reidy A, Minassian DC (1999). Profile of patients presenting for cataract surgery: National data collection. *Br J Ophthalmol* **83**: 893–6.

Dolin P (1998). Epidemiology of cataract. In Johnson GJ, Miassian DC, Weale R (eds) *The Epidemiology of Eye Disease.* London, Chapman & Hall Medical, pp. 103–19.

Forrester J, Dick A, McMenamin P, Lee W (1996). *The Eye: Basic Sciences in Practice.* London, W.B. Saunders Company Ltd. p. 28 (http://www.doh.gov.uk/public/stats1.htm).

Minassian DC, Reidy A, Desai P, et al. (2000). The deficit in cataract surgery in England and Wales and the escalating problem of visual impairment : epidemiological modelling of the population dynamics of cataract. *Br J Ophthalmol* **84**: 4–8.

Montan Per G, Wejde G, Koranyi G, et al. (2002). Prophylactic intracameral cefuroxime – Efficacy in preventing endophthalmitis after cataract surgery. *J Cataract Refract Surg* **28**: 977–81.

Reidy A, Minassian DC, Vafidis G, et al (1998). Prevalence of serious eye disease and visual impairment in a north London population: population-based, cross sectional study. *Br Med J* **316**: 1643–6.

Royal College of Ophthalmologists (2007). *Cataract Surgery Guidelines.* London, RCO.

Glaucoma

Background

The term glaucoma refers to a group of conditions in which a progressive loss of retinal ganglion cells (RGC) results in a corresponding loss of visual field, usually in association with a characteristically cupped appearance of the optic nerve head (see Figure 14.6). Typically glaucoma is associated with elevated intraocular pressure (IOP), but in a proportion of cases progressive glaucomatous optic neuropathy occurs in the absence of demonstrable IOP elevation (normal pressure or normal tension glaucoma, NPG or NTG).

There are several types of glaucoma. The commonest in the UK is primary open angle glaucoma (POAG), which is typically a slowly progressive condition that affects around 2.5% of the population over 40 years of age. POAG has been nicknamed the 'sneak thief of sight' for its propensity to remain asymptomatic until the very late stages. NTG is not generally considered a separate entity but rather part of the POAG spectrum.

In contrast, the stereotypical presentation of primary angle closure glaucoma (PACG) is acute, with very high IOP, severe pain and vision loss. In reality, many patients with PACG also follow a chronic low-grade course and may be mistaken for POAG. There are also many types of secondary and developmental glaucomas.

Visual field loss is the hallmark of POAG, usually starting in the periphery and gradually eroding the visual field and affecting the central vision late in the course of the disease, leading eventually to varying degrees of visual disability and blindness in a small but significant proportion of patients. However in some, the central field is affected first, and these patients are at higher risk of losing central vision (see Figure 14.7).

Epidemiology

Glaucoma is the second commonest cause of blindness worldwide after cataract, and is the commonest cause of irreversible blindness. Quigley and Broman calculated that by 2010, there would be approximately 60 million sufferers worldwide increasing to 80 million by 2020, with those of West-African descent disproportionately affected.

The prevalence of undetected glaucoma is very high both in the industrialized and non-industrialized worlds.

More than 50% of people with glaucoma in the developed world are unaware of their condition. This figure has proven consistent and there has been no evidence of a reduction despite improvements in diagnostic techniques and therapy. The prevalence is higher still for underprivileged groups in developed countries (e.g. 62–75% of Hispanic residents in the southwestern USA) and greater than 90% in non-industrialized countries. In studies in southern India, only 1.5% in a rural population and 6% in an urban population were aware of their diagnosis. Delayed diagnosis, resulting in late presentation is an important cause of severe visual loss from this treatable condition in both the industrialized and non-industrialized world.

There are more than 500 000 estimated glaucoma sufferers in England and Wales and in the USA glaucoma affects approximately 5% of Medicare beneficiaries over the age of 65.

Classification

Glaucomas are usually classified as:
- Primary or secondary, according to whether there is an identifiable underlying ocular or systemic disorder causing the glaucoma (secondary) or not (primary)
- Open or closed angle, according to the mechanism of IOP elevation, i.e. whether there is a visible anatomical obstruction to aqueous outflow in the iridocorneal drainage angle (angle closure) or not (open-angle)
- Developmental (congenital).

Primary glaucomas are the most common, usually affecting both eyes asymmetrically. POAG is usually, but not always associated with IOP elevation whereas PACG, secondary and developmental glaucomas are always caused by IOP elevation. The latter groups have in common, obstruction of aqueous humour outflow either from primary obstruction of the iridocorneal angle with iris (PACG), another ocular or systemic disorder (secondary glaucoma), or a developmental anomaly of the angle (developmental glaucomas). IOP elevation in secondary glaucoma is often unilateral and may lead to much more rapid visual loss than POAG. IOP elevation is a late

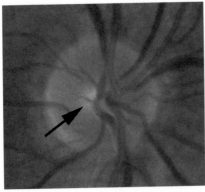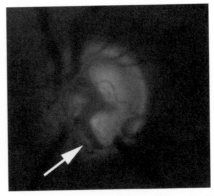

Figure 14.6 (colour plate 9) Normal optic disc (left). The black arrow points to the edge of the optic disc cup which occupies <30% of the disc area. Compare this with the glaucomatous optic disc (right) where the cup occupies around 80% of the disc area and the surrounding rim is pathologically thin. The white arrow points to a very thin area of optic disc rim (notch). Reproduced from Moorfields Eye Hospital with permission.

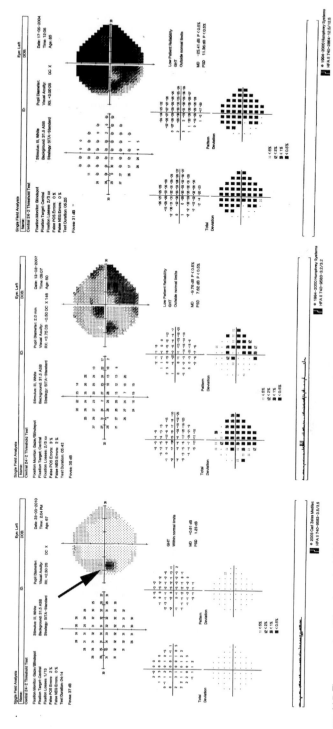

Figure 14.7 Three examples of Humphrey visual fields threshold test results in three left eyes. The plot at the top right of each of the 3 printouts represents the central 24° of each eye's visual field, except nasally where it extends to 30°. The first (left) is normal. The black arrow points to the physiological blind spot. The field in the middle has a paracentral defect, as well as the physiological blind spot, and additionally an inferonasal peripheral defect. This eye is at higher risk of central vision loss if the glaucoma is not well-controlled, because of the paracentral defect. The plot on the right is from an eye with advanced glaucoma which typically has only a small temporal island of vision less than 1° in diameter. First image: this image was created using Carl Zeiss Meditec software. Second and Third image: this image was created using Humphrey Systems software.

consequence of many serious ocular conditions and therefore there are many types of secondary glaucoma.

Primary open angle glaucoma is usually a diagnosis of exclusion, i.e. thorough examination reveals no evidence of angle closure, no secondary cause, and no evidence of a congenital or developmental cause.

Primary open angle glaucoma

Primary open-angle glaucoma (POAG) (formerly chronic simple or chronic open-angle glaucoma), is the most common type in Western Europe. The disease usually develops slowly, over years with gradual retinal ganglion cell and visual field loss. There is no cure and pre-existing damage cannot be reversed. The aim of treatment is to arrest progression.

Peripheral visual field loss often occurs first, with central vision usually affected relatively late in the course of the disease. In some patients paracentral visual field defects, close to central fixation develop before significant peripheral loss, and these patients consequently have a higher risk of loss of central vision (see Figure 14.7).

POAG may remain asymptomatic until extensive visual field loss has occurred. The reasons for this include the asymmetrical nature of the disease, in that advanced glaucoma in one eye may be missed if the fellow eye has good vision, and lack of awareness of peripheral visual field defects related to cortical plasticity which permits the brain to *fill in* missing gaps in the visual field so that they are not noticed.

Many patients present with significant sight loss at diagnosis. Because of the late development of symptoms, glaucoma is most likely to be diagnosed late in those who do not have regular eye tests. Reasons for this include poor economic circumstances, but also a lack of awareness in emmetropic individuals (no refractive error) who usually do not attend for routine eye examinations until their late 40s or early 50s when they become presbyopic and need reading glasses. Even then, routine eye tests may be avoided because of the trend to buy ready-made reading glasses from convenience stores and pharmacies.

There are a number of clinical presentations of POAG. These vary from patients with suspicious optic discs and normal IOP, through those with elevated IOP and normal optic discs, and to those with glaucomatous optic neuropathy (GON) with or without elevated IOP:

- POAG with elevated IOP
- POAG with normal IOP
- Ocular hypertension (OHT)
- POAG suspect.

This classification is somewhat arbitrary. Patients with OHT may never develop glaucoma, although they possess the most important modifiable risk factor.

POAG with elevated IOP

POAG, with or without elevated IOP, is characterized by a slow loss of retinal ganglion cells resulting in visual field loss, and a characteristic appearance of cupping of the optic disc (see Figure 14.6). While the rate of field loss is related to the degree of IOP elevation, individual patients vary greatly in the rate of progression. Men and women are affected equally.

IOP elevation is believed to result in mechanical damage to the retinal ganglion cell axons as they pass through the lamina cribrosa to exit the eye. The lamina cribrosa is a fine meshwork of pores in the scleral coat of the eye that permit retinal ganglion cell (optic nerve) axons to exit the eye on course to the lateral geniculate nucleus.

The structural integrity of the lamina cribrosa is believed to be important for the long-term health of these axons. Mechanical distortion of the lamina may impede axoplasmic flow. IOP elevation also reduces ocular perfusion which may adversely affect the health of the retinal ganglion cells and their axons. The role of ocular perfusion is less certain. Some patients with systemic hypertension that is aggressively treated are thought to be at risk of progression because of poor perfusion due to low systemic blood pressure. Classically nocturnal drops (*dipping*) in systemic blood pressure may negatively affect the health of a vulnerable optic nerve.

POAG with normal IOP (normal tension or normal pressure glaucoma, NTG)

Many glaucoma specialists dispute the existence of NTG as a separate entity. The relative risk of POAG increases with the degree of IOP elevation, but there is no evidence of a specific threshold IOP for the onset of the condition.

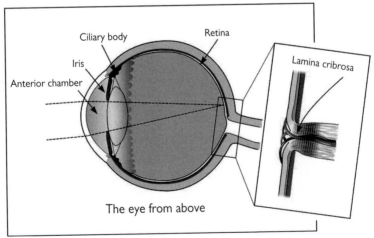

Ciliary body   Retina

Iris

Anterior chamber

Lamina cribrosa

The eye from above

Figure 14.8 (colour plate 10) Cross-sectional drawing of the eye showing the position of the *lamina cribrosa* and the optic nerve in relation to the other major structures. Reproduced from Moorfields Eye Hospital with permission. Figure kindly drawn by Alan Lacey.

There appears to be no difference in the appearance of the optic nerve between POAG and NTG.

Traditionally 21 mmHg (two standard deviations above the population mean) has been regarded as a cut-off point. There are many patients who develop glaucoma below this level, and some who remain healthy despite higher pressures. The term NTG has persisted because it is sometimes helpful when treating patients, to remember that a lower than usual treatment target IOP level may be required in those who have developed optic disc damage without a documented high IOP. Interestingly, most patients with NTG have documented IOP levels in the upper half of the normal range, and therapeutic lowering of the IOP does retard progression of the condition.

Some recent evidence suggests that an imbalance between IOP and intracranial pressure may be important in the pathogenesis.

As one might expect, in eyes with low IOP levels, disease progression tends to be slow. Despite this, the prognosis is not better than in those with elevated IOP because NTG patients tend to present later.

Ocular hypertension

By definition, patients with ocular hypertension have elevated IOP levels but without evidence of glaucomatous optic neuropathy. Not all patients with ocular hypertension require treatment but most specialists agree that high IOP levels, e.g. above 28–30 mmHg, do require treatment as conversion to glaucoma becomes inevitable.

POAG suspect

As examination techniques improve, increasing numbers of individuals present to the hospital eye service with abnormal optic discs or visual fields that are not glaucomatous. While a very small proportion of these have other forms of optic nerve disease, the majority have an optic disc appearance that cannot be distinguished easily from early glaucoma. Typically these eyes might be moderately to highly myopic with a stretched or *tilted* appearance to the optic disc in which the cup is not centred in the disc and one or more segments of the rim are thinner than usual. In others, the optic disc is congenitally larger than normal (>2.0 mm vertical diameter). Rims of large discs are thinner than normal, as they accommodate the same number

(1.2 million) of axons as smaller discs. The cups are therefore larger, creating a suspicious appearance.

The difficulty in differentiating the POAG suspect from definite POAG is the presence of an abnormal optic disc in the absence of other features of glaucoma. Usually, in such patients the retinal nerve fibre layer and visual field will both be normal and sequential examination over time will differentiate stationary anomalies from those with progressive glaucoma.

Primary angle closure glaucoma

Primary angle closure often occurs acutely in the elderly person with a dramatic IOP rise, associated with severe pain in a red, congested eye, with an oedematous cornea and vision loss, usually developing over the course of a few days. Acute primary angle closure is a medical emergency as the risk of severe permanent vision loss is high.

Angle closure occurs when the iridocorneal angle becomes obstructed with iris. Under normal circumstances, aqueous humour is actively secreted by the ciliary body behind the iris, flows through a narrow crevice between the posterior iris and anterior lens surface, through the pupil and leaves the eye passively through the trabecular meshwork in the iridocorneal angle, to rejoin the venous system (see Figure 14.9). The iridocorneal angle is the narrow recess occupying the angle between the anterior surface of the iris and the inner surface of the peripheral cornea.

In small eyes (hypermetropic or far sighted), the angle is normally narrower. Through life, the lens slowly enlarges and narrows the channel between the front of the lens and the back of the iris through which aqueous humour travels to reach the anterior chamber. This narrowing creates some resistance to aqueous flow and consequently a pressure difference between the anterior and posterior chambers. As a result, the iris bows forward, obstructing the angle and elevating the IOP precipitously (see Figure 14.10). This, the most common mechanism of angle closure, is known as *pupillary block*. Other, less common mechanisms include *plateau iris* which may develop in eyes that possess an anatomical variant of the ciliary body and iris root.

Angle closure is often seen with less dramatic presentation. In eyes where intermittent iridotrabecular contact

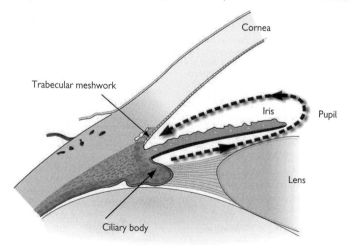

Figure 14.9 (colour plate 11) Cross-section of the anterior chamber periphery demonstrating the normal pathway of aqueous humour flow. Reproduced from Moorfields Eye Hospital with permission. Figure kindly drawn by Alan Lacey.

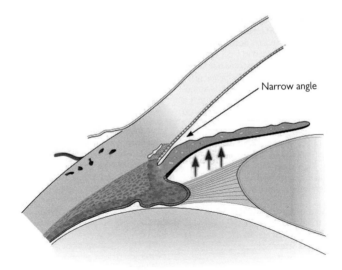

Narrow angle

Figure 14.10 (colour plate 12) Cross-section of the anterior chamber periphery showing the anatomical changes that occur in angle closure secondary to pupillary block. Reproduced from Moorfields Eye Hospital with permission. Figure kindly drawn by Alan Lacey.

occurs, adhesions may develop between the peripheral iris and trabecular meshwork, resulting in chronic primary angle closure glaucoma. This is more common and more visually destructive in Asian communities than either POAG or acute symptomatic PACG.

Secondary glaucomas

Secondary glaucomas develop as a result of other ocular conditions, trauma, intraocular surgery, systemic disease, or as a result of corticosteroid treatment. While some common ocular conditions such as exfoliation syndrome (*pseudo-exfoliation*) and pigment dispersion syndrome result in secondary open angle glaucoma, others such as neovascular glaucoma characteristically result in profound secondary angle closure, while uveitis typically may result in either or a mixture of the two.

Developmental glaucomas

Primary congenital glaucomas present from birth to 9 years of age and primary juvenile glaucomas from 10 to 35 years of age. Primary congenital glaucoma is rare in Europe (approximately 1:10 000 live births) but is relatively common in communities where consanguineous marriages are common. In primary congenital glaucoma, abnormal development of the angle impedes aqueous outflow, and the IOP elevates. In contrast to the adult eye, IOP elevation in the growing infant eye results in gross enlargement producing the characteristic *ox-eye* appearance (*buphthalmos*). The condition is usually bilateral but may be asymmetrical with a male preponderance. Severe visual disability is common, because of glaucoma, amblyopia and refractive error.

Primary juvenile glaucoma may be caused by mutations in the *myoc* gene which codes for the polypeptide Myocillin in trabecular meshwork. Mutations in this gene account for 2–4% of cases of POAG as a whole.

Diagnosis of primary open angle glaucoma

The diagnosis of POAG is based on a clinical pattern of a characteristic optic disc appearance (*cupping*), abnormal visual function (visual field defect) and usually IOP elevation.

There is no IOP level that provides a reasonable balance of sensitivity and specificity for detecting glaucoma, and the same applies to optic disc imaging and visual field testing. There are a number of methods of imaging optic disc surface topography and retinal nerve fibre layer thickness in fine detail, but there is no individual test that has sufficiently high sensitivity and specificity to detect early glaucoma. The diagnosis remains a clinical judgement based on the collective evidence of the parameters listed above.

Visual field testing

Visual field testing is performed using computerized automated perimetry in which light stimuli of variable intensity are presented to the eye under test, and the patient responds by pressing a button as soon as each stimulus is first seen. *Supra-threshold* testing is often performed in optometric practices, where a bright stimulus, above the normal visual threshold, is presented to the subject sequentially at different points in the visual field. Supra-threshold testing is used to confirm that the visual field is normal when no abnormality is suspected. This is inadequate for diagnosing and monitoring glaucoma, for which a *threshold* algorithm (e.g. the Humphrey Field Analyser using SITA or Swedish Interactive Threshold Algorithm) is required, whereby graded levels of stimuli are presented until the visual threshold has been identified.

Threshold testing gives detailed information about the visual threshold at individual points in the field, and also an indication of the patient's performance from test to test. The main advantage of threshold testing is the ability to look at subtle changes at individual points over time, providing a sensitive method of detecting disease progression

While the definitive diagnosis of POAG requires some visual field loss in addition to visible optic disc changes, it is accepted that significant changes in optic disc appearance may be manifest before any visual field loss can be detected. Glaucoma diagnosed prior to the development of a visual field defect is often called *pre-perimetric glaucoma*. A proportion of these patients will demonstrate visual field loss using other modalities such as short wavelength automated perimetry (SWAP), a modality that uses a blue stimulus on a yellow background, rather than the conventional 'white on white'. However, defects detected using SWAP are less specific for the diagnosis of glaucoma than those detected with 'white on white'.

Optic disc and retinal nerve fibre layer imaging
A number of devices are used to document optic disc and retinal nerve fibre layer structure. These include confocal scanning laser ophthalmoscopy (e.g. Heidelberg retinal tomograph, or HRT), optical coherence tomography (OCT), scanning laser polarimetry (e.g. GDx). As stated above, these devices give detailed documentation of a number of structural parameters but no individual device is sufficient to make the diagnosis. They are however of value in looking for subtle change over time.

IOP measurement
The intraocular pressure is usually measured by Goldman applanation tonometry (GAT), a technique whereby the IOP is measured from the force required to flatten a small area of anesthetized central cornea. The IOP end point is visualized using a cobalt blue light and fluorescein in the tear film. The accuracy of GAT is influenced by the thickness of the cornea and therefore corneal thickness is also measured, often using handheld ultrasound pachymetry. While there is no accurate IOP adjustment factor for corneal thickness, a thin cornea implies an under-reading of the IOP and a thick cornea the converse.

Non-contact methods of tonometry (eg. *air puff* devices) are widely used in optometric practices. These are useful methods of screening for IOP elevation but are not sufficient for the diagnosis and monitoring of glaucoma. Newer devices are available that appear to operate independently of corneal thickness and it is likely that one or more of these might replace GAT as the gold standard in the longer-term.

Gonioscopy
Gonioscopy is the examination of the iridocorneal angle. The main purpose of this is to exclude angle closure or an angle at risk of closure. Gonioscopy is performed on slit-lamp examination using a contact lens incorporating a prism.

Primary open angle glaucoma
Modifiable risk factors
In the past, the term glaucoma was often confined to patients with IOP elevation. This is no longer the case, and some optic nerves appear to withstand sustained IOP elevation for many years while others develop neuropathy when the IOP has never been elevated, IOP remains the single most important modifiable risk factor for POAG. Therapeutic lowering of the IOP is of benefit in preventing progression in eyes with NTG.

The only proven method of preventing progression of POAG is IOP reduction, whether by medical, laser or surgical means. In the majority, this reduces the likelihood of further damage and stabilizes the condition. It is uncertain, if there is a threshold below which further IOP reduction is ineffective, although there is some evidence that glaucoma progression is relatively rare when the IOP is consistently below 15 mmHg.

Other potentially modifiable risk factors
Though IOP elevation is the only modifiable risk factor, vascular risk factors, such as systemic hypertension may also play a role, although the exact nature of that role in the pathogenesis is uncertain. There is some evidence that low ocular perfusion pressure may increase the susceptibility of the optic nerve to damage. However, there is no evidence to support treatment of glaucoma by manipulating perfusion pressure.

Non-modifiable risk factors
Age
Increasing age is the most important single risk factor for glaucoma. The development and progression of glaucoma is highly age-dependent because of the cumulative loss of optic nerve fibres during a lifetime and the increase in risk factors with increased age.

In population-based studies, the prevalence increases consistently from around 1% in people of 43–54 years old to approximately 5% in those 75 years of age or older.

Ethnic origin
Individuals of African origin are more likely to have elevated IOP. In a US prevalence survey (Baltimore Eye Study), the prevalence of glaucoma was four to five times higher in black than white Americans. The prevalence was 11% in blacks aged 80 years or more. Glaucoma also appears to occur earlier in those of African origin than in white people.

Gender
There is a slight gender predilection for certain types of glaucoma. Pigmentary glaucoma is more common in men, and primary angle closure is slightly more common in women. Overall there appears to be no predilection for POAG to affect either gender.

Family history of glaucoma
First-degree relatives of glaucoma patients have a higher risk than other individuals. However, estimates of risk for first-degree relatives are highly variable and figures between 10% and 20% are commonly quoted. In the Baltimore Eye Study, the odds ratio of developing open-angle glaucoma was 3.69 for those with affected siblings and 2.17 for those with affected parents.

Myopia and hypermetropia
Low myopia does not appear to be a significant risk factor, whereas high myopia (>6 dioptres) is associated with an increased risk of POAG. Myopia is also a risk factor for pigmentary glaucoma.

Hyperopia carries an increased risk of both acute and chronic primary angle closure glaucoma.

Cerebrospinal fluid pressure
There is some evidence suggesting that the pressure gradient between the vitreous cavity and meninges may influence the development of glaucoma. It may be that reduced CSF pressure in relation to IOP, may have a similar effect to elevating the IOP.

Management
The management of secondary glaucomas and angle closure is often directed towards the cause. In primary angle closure, treatment is primarily directed at breaking the angle closure episode. Usually this consists of initial medial therapy followed by laser iridotomy or even lens extraction (cataract surgery) to relieve the pupillary block. Angle closure glaucoma is important to diagnose as it is the one form of glaucoma that may be curable with surgery.

Management of primary open angle glaucoma will depend on the degree of IOP elevation, the severity of the optic neuropathy at presentation, the age of the patient, the rate of progression and, to some extent, by the family history. Management of POAG usually begins with medical therapy. There are a choice of classes of IOP-lowering drugs available as eyedrops.

In general, prostaglandin agonists (latanoprost, travoprost, bimatoprost, tafluprost) lower the IOP by around 30–35% by enhancing aqueous outflow, as once daily topical treatment given at night. Beta-blockers (timolol, levobunolol), lower the IOP by around 30% by suppressing aqueous production. For maximal effect beta-blockers are used twice daily, although approximately 75% of their effect can be achieved with a once daily treatment. Alpha-agonists reduce IOP by around 25% (brimonidine) and topical carbonic anhydrase inhibitors (dorzolamide, brinzolamide) by about 15–20%. Additional pressure lowering can be achieved in emergency situations with the use of systemic carbonic anhydrase inhibitors (acetazolamide).

The topical prostaglandin analogues are the most popular first line treatment in the UK. They have relatively few systemic side-effects but may cause local intolerance, eyelash growth and, in those with green/hazel eyes, there may be some change in iris colour, but rarely to a noticeable degree. The side effects of topical beta-blockers are similar to their systemic counterparts. Alpha-agonists frequently cause allergy or chronic redness and this should be suspected in anyone using an alpha-agonist who develops a chronic sore itchy eye. They also cause dryness of the mouth and drowsiness in elderly patients. Topical carbonic anhydrase inhibitors may cause allergy, a bad taste in the mouth, and dorzolamide stings on instillation. Approximately half of POAG patients will be insufficiently well-controlled on one glaucoma mediation, and typically two or three drugs may be required. The addition of one or two additional medications usually results in additional pressure lowering. However, it is difficult to achieve more than 50% lowering in total with medical therapy and there is no evidence of a benefit in taking ≥3 IOP-lowering medications, while there is a significant increase in side-effects from polypharmacy.

It is also worth considering in patients with severe established visual loss whether multiple chronic topical glaucoma medications are worthwhile. Some patients with severe vision loss are reluctant to give up glaucoma medication, even though they are experiencing little benefit and sometimes adverse effects from its use. However, in many of these patients, the chronic use of topical medication is still justified as there may be a risk of loss of the little remaining visual field, though it may be worth considering if the intensity of the regimen could be lessened in patients using multiple medications.

Another common clinical problem is the use of systemic medications in older individuals which carry a warning that they should not be used in glaucoma. Most drugs that carry this warning are drugs that may precipitate angle closure in those who have narrow drainage angles. These include anti-histaminergic and anticholinergic drugs as well as alpha-adrenergic agonists. As angle closure is potentially devastating, it is important to try and identify those at highest risk. In general, most elderly patients with glaucoma have POAG and are not at risk, but a significant minority will be at risk. These are almost invariably patients who are hypermetropic (or hyperopic), i.e. their distance glasses contain plus or magnifying lenses and are similar to the glasses that emmetropic individuals wear for reading. Myopic patients (near or short-sighted) are rarely at risk of angle closure and neither are patients who have previously had cataract surgery, as cataract surgery widens the drainage angle.

Some antidepressants also increase the IOP in patients with POAG but this is rarely to a significant degree. Finally, topical and systemic corticosteroids do carry a significant risk of IOP elevation in predisposed individuals. However, with the exception of children, systemic corticosteroids usually require prolonged courses (one month or more) at significant levels (20 mg of prednisolone per day or more) to elevate the intraocular pressure. Topical ocular corticosteroids have a much higher propensity to elevate the IOP. Inhaled, nasal and topical skin preparations have an intermediate risk.

Laser treatment, either argon or selective laser trabeculoplasty are non-invasive techniques that may reduce the IOP by up to 30% and are useful techniques, especially in patient who cannot take topical medical therapy and in whom surgery is not indicated.

Surgical intervention is usually reserved for those with significant visual field loss that is progressing, those with high uncontrolled IOP levels and those with advanced glaucoma at presentation. While there has been a recent proliferation of new glaucoma surgical devices, the mainstay of surgical management, at the time of writing, remains trabeculectomy and aqueous shunt implantation, though some advocate non-penetrating procedures such as deep

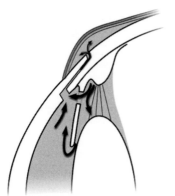
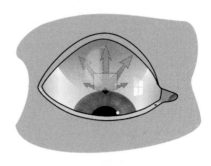

Figure 14.11 (colour plate 13) In a trabeculectomy operation, aqueous exits the anterior chamber through a guarded sclerostomy (a partial thickness flap in the sclera) to a drainage bleb at the superior conjunctival limbus, from whence it is reabsorbed via the venous system. Reproduced from Moorfields Eye Hospital with permission. Figure kindly drawn by Alan Lacey.

sclerectomy as an alternative to trabeculectomy. Trabeculectomy involves fashioning a partial thickness scleral flap over a partial thickness hole in the scleral wall. Aqueous humour drains through the hole. The scleral flap acts as a resistor, preventing excessive flow. Aqueous flowing through the trabeculectomy enters a low pressure conjunctival blister or bleb under the upper lid, from whence it is reabsorbed into the venous system. (see Figure 14.11)

Aqueous shunts (see Figure 14.12) are silicone tubes that function in the same way but route the draining aqueous further back to a plate that is behind the eyelid around the side of the eyeball.

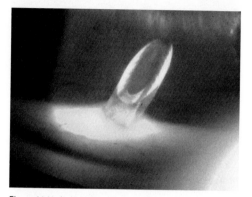

Figure 14.12 (colour plate 14) Aqueous shunts (commonly called *tubes* or *glaucoma drainage devices*) usually involve insertion of a small silicone tube of approximately 600 µm diameter into the anterior chamber (illustrated), which drains aqueous to a conjunctival bleb over an external plate. Reproduced from Moorfields Eye Hospital with permission.

Cyclodestruction (e.g. transscleral diode laser cyclophotocoagulation or *cyclodiode*) is a procedure whereby aqueous production is reduced by photocoagulating the ciliary body with an infrared laser. This is generally used in eyes in which the pressure cannot be controlled by other methods.

Further reading

American Academy of Ophthalmology (2011) *Basic Clinical and Science Course, 10 Glaucoma*. San Francisco, AAO.

European Glaucoma Society (2008). *Terminology and Guidelines for Glaucoma*, 3rd edn. Dogma, Savona.

Peter A Netland (ed.). 2008 *Glaucoma Medical Therapy, Principles and Management*, 2nd edn. New York, Oxford University Press.

Quigley HA, Broman AT (2006). The number of people with glaucoma worldwide in 2010 and 2020. *Br J Ophthalmol* **90**: 262–7.

Aqueous shunts: Information for Patients (www.keithbarton.co.uk/patient_aqsh_english.pdf).

Trabeculectomy: Information for Patients (www.keithbarton.co.uk/trab.pdf).

Age-related macular degeneration

Introduction

Age-related macular degeneration (AMD) is the term applied to ageing changes without any obvious cause that occur in the central area of the retina (macular), in people aged 50 years and above. AMD is the most common cause of severe visual loss in this age group with a prevalence of 10% in the 60–74 age group and 25% in over 74 years of age. AMD is divided in to dry (non-neovascular) and wet (neovascular) types.

Risk factors

- Increasing age is the main risk factor for AMD.
- Gender: many prevalence studies had shown a higher prevalence in women; however, this has been attributed to increased longevity in females.
- Immediate family members are at higher risk of developing AMD.
- Caucasians, blue iris colour and having AMD in the fellow eye are AMD risk factors.
- Tobacco smoking is the main modifiable risk factor. Current smokers have a two- to threefold increased risk of developing AMD, and there is a dose–response relationship with pack-years of smoking.
- Cardiovascular disease: raised blood pressure has been associated with AMD in some, but not all studies. There is no evidence that antihypertensive medication prevents the development or progression of disease. Lipid-lowering agents including statins do not appear to lower the risk of developing AMD.
- Alcohol intake has been shown to have weak or no association with AMD.
- Inflammatory: some studies have shown associations with inflammatory markers such as CRP, and in the gene coding for complement factor H in the inflammatory cascade.

Dry age-related macular degeneration

Dry AMD accounts for 90% of AMD.

Pathogenesis

Drusen (discreet lesions consisting of lipid and protein) deposit under the retinal pigment epithelium (RPE) and within Bruch's membrane. Hard drusen (less than 63 µm and well defined) do not appear to increase with age or predispose to advanced AMD. Soft drusen (larger than 63 µm and with ill-defined borders) often increase in size and number with increasing age. They are a hallmark of AMD are a significant risk factor for developing advanced AMD (see Figure 14.13).

Focal hyperpigmentation: focal areas of hyperpigmentation occur within the RPE, forming visible pigmented lumps.

Geographic atrophy: sharply demarcated areas of partial or complete depigmentation, reflecting atrophy of the RPE. Underlying choroidal vessels may be visible through atrophic RPE. Geographic atrophy indicates advanced dry AMD (see Figure 14.14).

Risk factors for progression of dry AMD include presence of large drusen (>125 µm), RPE abnormalities, and advanced AMD in one eye.

Clinical features

- Initially asymptomatic
- Patients generally have a gradual onset (over several years) of decreasing central vision and can have difficulty with reading and recognising faces.

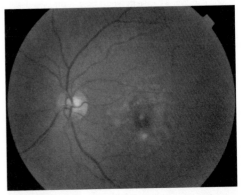

Figure 14.13 (colour plate 15) Colour fundus photo of left macular showing soft drusen. Reproduced from Venki Sundaram, Allon Barsam, Amar Alwitry, and Peng T. Khaw, *Training in Ophthalmology*, 2009, Figure 4.31, p. 170, with permission from Oxford University Press.

- Some patients with advanced AMD may experience visual hallucinations (Charles Bonnet syndrome) and alerting patients of this possibility can avoid further distress.

Management

- Cessation of smoking.
- Vitamin supplementation: the Age Related Eye Disease Study (AREDS) revealed a beneficial effect of very high doses of daily antioxidants in a small subset of patients. Vitamin supplements are indicated in patients with advanced AMD in one eye. Commercial products include ICaps and Ocuvite, although smokers are advised to take a lower dose of beta-carotene as there is a potential risk of lung cancer development.

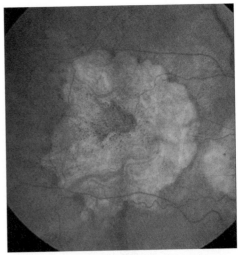

Figure 14.14 (colour plate 16) Colour fundus photo of right macular showing large area of geographic atrophy. Reproduced from Venki Sundaram, Allon Barsam, Amar Alwitry, and Peng T. Khaw, *Training in Ophthalmology*, 2009, Figure 4.32, p. 171, with permission from Oxford University Press.

- Amsler grid monitoring: the Amsler chart is a black grid pattern on a white background and evaluates the central 10° of visual field. Patients are asked to report any sudden changes in areas of the chart that are missing or distorted and is useful for monitoring worsening macular symptoms.
- Low visual assessment and aids.
- Supportive: counselling and linking to support groups/social services.
- Registration as sight impaired or severely sight impaired.
- Investigations are not usually necessary unless there is doubt about the presence of a choroidal neovascular membrane, where optical coherence tomography (OCT) or fundus fluorescein angiography (FFA) are indicated.

Future developments

Owing to the lack of current treatment options for dry AMD, considerable research is being conducted to develop viable therapeutic agents. These include ciliary neurotrophic factor, an injectable agent that may halt photoreceptor degeneration; complement C5aR, a slow-release injectable formula that may reduce progression to wet AMD; and OT-551 eye drops that have anti-inflammatory, anti-oxidant, and antiangiogenic properties.

Wet age-related macular degeneration

Although Wet AMD is less common, it accounts for 90% of cases of severe sight impairment due to AMD.

Pathogenesis

Choroidal neovascularization (CNV) is an ingrowth of permeable and fragile new vessels from the choroid into the RPE and subretinal space. These abnormal vessels can bleed causing disruption and damage to photoreceptors and eventually cause macular scarring (disciform scar). CNV are thought to arise and be stimulated by pathological secretion growth factors, one of which is vascular endothelial growth factor (VEGF).

Clinical features

Patients usually present with a sudden onset of reduced central vision and distortion of straight lines (metamorphopsia).

Clinical signs can include:
- grey-like subretinal membrane indicative of a CNV
- retinal, subretinal or sub-RPE haemorrhage (see Figure 14.15)

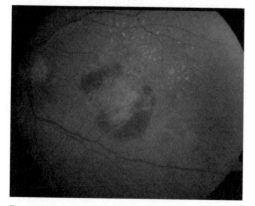

Figure 14.15 (colour plate 17) Colour fundus photo of macular haemorrhage due to choroidal neovascular membrane.

- subretinal fluid
- macular oedema
- retinal or subretinal exudates
- RPE detachment
- disciform scar
- associated features on dry AMD.

Investigations

- OCT gives high-resolution cross sectional images of the retina and can detect subretinal fluid, macular oedema and RPE detachment.
- FFA is the gold standard for diagnosing CNV and shows fluorescein leakage (hyperfluorescence) in the region of CNV.

Management

Previously, treatment of wet AMD was limited to laser photocoagulation, which was then superseded with photodynamic therapy (PDT) with intravenous verteporfin for targeting CNV, with both treatments aimed at reducing CNV activity.

In recent years, anti-VEGF agents such as Lucentis (Ranibizumab) and avastin (Bevacizumab) have become established treatments, and have been the first agents to show significant visual gain in wet AMD. Both agents bind to and block the effects of VEGF, however only Lucentis has been officially licensed for intravitreal use in AMD and became NICE approved in 2009.

NICE guidelines (which apply to either eye) for treating Wet AMD patients with Lucentis include:
- best corrected visual acuity is between 6/12 and 6/96
- no permanent structural damage to foveal centre
- evidence of recent disease progression (reduced visual acuity or blood vessel growth on FFA).

Treatment regimen: patients usually receive a loading dose of three intravitreal Lucentis injections at 1-month intervals. Patients are followed up at monthly intervals and further retreatment injections depend on CNV activity, which can be assessed with worsening visual acuity, recurrence or persistence of retinal fluid and new macular haemorrhage or CNV.

Complications of intravitreal injection are rare but include endophthalmitis, retinal detachment, and uveitis.

Prognosis

Left untreated, CNV lesions will result in severe visual loss in the majority of eyes. If CNV is present in one eye, there is a 50% of developing CNV in the fellow eye within 5 years.

The ANCHOR study showed that significantly fewer patients who were treated with Lucentis lost vision, compared with previous available treatment options. Also 40% of Lucentis treated patients gained vision, compared with only 6% of those treated with PDT.

Future developments

Future therapies for wet AMD may include longer acting Lucentis, other antiangiogenic agents such as Sirolimus, intra-ocular radiation application and combined treatment approaches.

Further reading

Brown DM, Michels M, Kaiser PK, et al. (2009). Ranibizumab versus verteporfin therapy for neovascular age-related macular degeneration: Two-year results of the ANCHOR study. Ophthalmology **116**: 57–65.e5.

www.rcophth.ac.uk/docs/publications/AMD_GUIDELINES_FINAL_VERSION_Feb_09

Registration of visual impairment

The registration of visual impairment was previously performed using a BD8 form, but since 2003 the process of registration has been modified with the introduction of a new Certificate of Visual Impairment (CVI), and was further updated in 2005. In conjunction, two additional forms, the Low Vision Leaflet and Referral of Vision Impaired Patient (RVI) were introduced to speed up the referral for social assessment and care.

In addition, the terminology of 'blind' or 'partially sighted' were replaced with the terms 'severely sight impaired' and 'sight impaired'.

Certificate of Visual Impairment (CVI)

This formally certifies someone as sight impaired (SI) or severely sight impaired (SSI) and is completed by a Consultant Ophthalmologist. Registration is voluntary but may entitle people to various benefits and concessions. The CVI acts as a referral to social care (if this has not already been done) and also acts as a method of recording diagnostic and other data that may be used for epidemiological analysis. The form comprises three parts:

• *Part 1* Patients consent to be registered, with Consultant counter-signature and confirmation for eligibility for SI or SSI registration.
• *Part 2* Documentation of visual acuity, visual field impairment and cause of visual impairment, according to ICD10 coding.
• *Part 3* Social situation, indication of urgency for social assessment, ethnic origin and preferred method of future correspondence (e.g. large print, on tape).

Low vision leaflet

This is a self-referral letter (obtained from opticians) that patients who encounter difficulties from sight loss can send to social services directly for further information and support.

Referral of vision impaired patient

Staff in the hospital eye service may issue an RVI to refer a patient (with their consent) for social care assessment. This should be done as soon as social needs become apparent, but when certification is not appropriate or cannot be carried out. The aim is to support people before their sight loss seriously affects their confidence and safety

Most ophthalmology departments will have an eye clinic liaison officer or sight care advisor, who provide a link between eye hospital services and community support.

Eligibility

Severely sight impaired

This has been legally defined by The National Assistance Act 1948 as a person 'so blind as to be unable to perform any work for which eye sight is essential'.

This is conventionally regarded as
• Snellen visual acuity of <3/60.
• Snellen visual acuity of 3/60 to 6/60 and with a very contracted field of vision.

• Snellen visual acuity of >6/60 with a contracted field of vision, especially if the contraction is in the lower part of the field.

Sight impaired

This has not been legally defined, but is conventionally regarded as:
• Snellen visual acuity 3/60 to 6/60 with full field
• Snellen visual acuity up to 6/24 with moderate contraction of field, opacities in media or aphakia
• Snellen visual acuity of 6/18 or better, with gross visual field defect.

Benefits

Potential benefits of visual impairment registration vary between authorities and might include:
• supporting an application for financial aid such as Attendance Allowance, Daily Living Allowance, Carers Allowance, Blind Person's Allowance and Council Tax benefits, Care home fees
• employment support
• home care, mobility training, and home modification
• low vision aids
• concessionary bus pass
• discounted rail travel
• taxi voucher scheme
• blue car badges to use disabled parking facilities
• TV licence reductions
• talking book service from the Royal National Institute for the Blind
• free BT telephone directory enquiries and aid with phone line installation
• postage concessions
• discounts on local leisure entertainment, e.g. cinema, theatre etc.
• free sight tests
• free NHS prescriptions: depends on age and income.

Low vision aids

There are a variety of commercially available low visual aids and these include hand magnifiers, stand magnifiers, illuminated magnifiers, electronic video CCTV magnifiers, TV magnifiers, magnifying mirrors and head-worn binoculars.

Further reading

www.rcophth.ac.uk/standards/cvi
www.rcophth.ac.uk/docs/profstands/ActionForSocialServices&
    Optometrists
www.rnib.org.uk

Psychosocial support for visual loss

The need for psychosocial support

Acquired visual impairment has been consistently associated with reduced psychosocial wellbeing. The event of receiving a diagnosis of irreversible vision loss has been described by patients as traumatic, which marks the transition in their lives from sighted to impaired and/or disabled status. The inevitable disruption to people's lives, including loss of independence in tasks of daily living and mobility, threatens valued activities such as driving and perhaps plans for retirement. All of these changes pose emotional challenges that not only effect mood, but identity, self-worth, personal relationships, and uncertainty for the future that may be blighted by fear of further vision loss. In addition, the presence of other health conditions can exacerbate a sense of loss of control and the functional impact of vision loss: A UK survey of 1000 people with visual impairment found that 73% aged 65+ had other chronic health problems or disabilities and 53% aged 75+ had difficulty with their hearing.

There is significant heterogeneity in how people respond to chronic disease, and it is expected that most adults will successfully adjust to vision loss. However, compared to their sighted peers, older people with visual impairment:
- are at an increased risk of clinical depression (odds ratio (OR) = 1.53, prevalence rate 20.57%)
- are twice as likely to report depressive symptoms (OR = 1.88, prevalence rate 23.4%)
- report lower mental health (mean difference (MD) = 20.17 out of 100)
- report lower social functioning (MD = 18.37/100).

In addition to the above, there are indications from qualitative studies and a small number of quantitative studies that older people with visual impairment are more at risk of reporting being socially isolated.

The role of rehabilitation

Much can be done to help patients cope with their visual impairment. Rehabilitation services help people come to terms with their new impairment and aid physical functioning by training patients to make use of their residual vision and perform tasks without sight. Healthcare staff would well serve their patients by directly referring them to rehabilitation services that assist with regaining lost skills, independence with activities of daily living, and mobility. In addition, many voluntary organizations assist people to learn new skills and engage in productive and meaningful activities. Enhancing independence and regaining skills will undoubtedly improve psychosocial wellbeing, as the two are intrinsically linked. However, a pattern that has emerged from the evidence is that rehabilitation in isolation appears insufficient to mitigate the negative psychosocial impact of visual impairment. It may be that there is currently an insufficient emphasis on the provision of psychosocial support in rehabilitation services, as rehabilitation only accounts for 7–12% of the variance in rates of mental health and depressive symptoms. In contrast, more direct approaches at promoting psychosocial well-being appear more effective.

> **Author's Tip**
>
> Although there may be no more that can be done to treat the patient's ocular disease, saying to patients with visual impairment that 'no more can be done' has been shown to inhibit psychosocial adaptation to acquired vision loss. Much can be done to help people adjust practically and emotionally to acquired visual impairment.

Provision of psychosocial support

As well as statutory support through social services, psychosocially supportive services are commonly provided by voluntary organisations both locally and nationally. Psychosocial support can be provided in a number of ways, as indicated by a number of pilot studies and reports from the grey literature:
- Group-based training in coping strategies/cognitive behavioural therapy
- Group-based health education facilitated by an occupational therapist
- Peer support groups facilitated by a trained peer with visual impairment
- Face-to-face counselling
- Telephone-based support in the form of counselling, peer support groups, buddy schemes, befriending, etc.
- Social activities/events organised by voluntary organizations for people with visual impairment
- Residential/weekly group-based seminars to educate those with newly acquired vision loss about the most frequent eye conditions, demonstrate the usefulness of low vision aids, and provide opportunity for peer support.

Although it is clear that there is a need to provide psychosocial support to those with visual impairment, and some demand for emotional support services among this client group, few studies have evaluated psychosocial support services/interventions.

From the published literature, two randomized controlled trials (RCTs) provide the strongest evidence for psychosocial interventions. One RCT provided information and advice through group-based self-management training that prevented clinical diagnoses of depression at the 6-month follow-up. Another RCT provided manual-driven problem-solving training to addresses negative cognitions that prevented clinical diagnoses of depression at the 2-month follow-up, but lost its efficacy at 6 months.

From the UK grey literature, the approach with the most reliable evidence is face-to-face counselling provided by a counsellor trained in integrative methods and in communicating with persons with visual impairment. A report showed that post-intervention, 36 out of 38 clients made a statistically and clinically significant improvement in emotional well-being including a reduction in the risk of suicide (from 26/38 to 1/38).

Signposting

Thus, emotional support, counselling, and peer support networks are to be made available to older people with visual impairment. From the current evidence base, it is unclear what the best content and delivery format is for providing psychosocial support to older people with visual impairment. Clearly some individuals require more psychosocial support than others, and severity of ocular disease does not reliably predict the level of support required.

Indeed, those with visual impairment below the threshold to be registered partially sighted or blind show signs of reduced emotional wellbeing. Although those with acquired visual impairment are more likely to require psychosocial support in initially adjusting to their new condition, others with deteriorating conditions may require support later when their vision reduces further, e.g. when they can no longer perceive faces or read standard print found in utility bills, newspapers, books.

As patients are unlikely to know where to obtain psychosocial support, and are likely to only receive a home visit by statutory support services weeks after their diagnosis of visual impairment, any information and advice healthcare staff can provide is valuable.

The social network

It must be remembered that the patient's social network (spouse, relatives, close friends, etc.) is affected by the life-changing diagnosis of visual impairment. Supportive others will be relied upon for instrumental and emotional support, and so the dynamic of some relationships may change. This has implications for the patient who may lose their esteemed social and occupational roles and statuses. As found in the wider literature with healthy populations, social support buffers against depressive symptoms in patients with visual impairment, and so patients are to be encouraged to accept help offered to them from their support network. Yet, the supportive social network may also require psychosocial support to adjust to the patients' vision loss. A pilot study has shown promise for group-based support for spouses of patients with vision loss, and voluntary organizations provide support for not just the patient but all those affected.

Special case: complex visual hallucinations

Community samples suggest that around 10% of older people with visual impairment experience complex visual hallucinations, otherwise known as Charles Bonnet Syndrome. It is believed that hallucinations occur in patients with ocular disease because the intact occipital cortex spontaneously generates activity due to under-stimulation; a theory supported by sensory deprivation experiments. Complex hallucinations are often the clear and detailed perception of an adult or child and experienced daily or weekly, while simple hallucinations would be seeing lights or unformed shapes. Complex visual hallucinations occur in cognitively intact individuals and are more common in those with poorer vision (e.g. severe contrast sensitivity). It appears that older people who experience complex visual hallucinations commonly fear the hallucinations signal the onset of insanity. Therefore, such patients would benefit from reassurance from healthcare staff that their hallucinations are believed and that such visions are benign. For those that find hallucinations distressing, medication could be prescribed such as anti-convulsants (e.g. carbamazepine, clonazepam, valproate, and gabapentin) or anti-psychotics (neuroleptics, e.g. thioridazine, haloperidol, risperidone, and melperone). However, caution should be exercised as the evidence is mixed with no universally effective drug.

> **Author's Tip**
>
> Provide patients and their significant others with information and the details of local and national organisations (statutory and voluntary) so they can seek psychosocial support services immediately.

Conclusion

Adaptation to visual impairment poses challenges both for physical functioning and emotional wellbeing. Holistic care for patients will involve psychosocial support services.

Further reading

Brody BL, Roch-Levecq A-C, Thomas RG, et al. (2005). Self-management of age-related macular degeneration at the 6-month follow up. *Arch Ophthalmol* **123**: 46–53.

Burmedi D, Becker S, Heyl V, et al. (2002). Behavioral consequences of age-related low vision. *Visual Impairment Res* **4**: 15–45.

Burmedi D, Becker S, Heyl V, et al. (2002). Emotional and social consequences of age-related low vision. *Visual Impairment Res* **4**: 47–71.

Casten RJ, Rovner BW (2007). Psychosocial interventions in age-related macular degeneration. *Expert Rev Ophthalmol* **2**: 191–6.

Dale S (2008). *RNIB Bristol counselling project report: Department of Health section 64 funded project October 2005-June 2008*. Bristol, RNIB.

Douglas G, Corcoran C, Pavey S (2006). *Network 1000: Opinions and circumstances of visually impaired people in Great Britain: Report Based on over 1000 Interviews*. Birmingham, Visual Impairment Centre for Teaching and Research, School of Education, University of Birmingham.

Horowitz A, Reinhardt JP (2000). Mental health issues in visual impairment: Research in depression, disability, and rehabilitation. In Silverstone B, Lang M, Rosenthal B, Faye E (eds) *The Lighthouse Handbooks on Vision Impairment and Vision Rehabilitation*. Oxford, Oxford University Press,. pp. 1089–109.

Menon GJ, Rahman I, Menon SJ, Dutton GN (2003). Complex visual hallucinations in the visually impaired: The Charles Bonnet syndrome. *Surv Ophthalmol* **48**: 58–72.

Nyman SR, Gosney MA, Victor CR (2010). The psychosocial impact of vision loss on older people. Generations Review. **20**. http://www.britishgerontology.org/DB/gr-editions-2/generations-review/the-psychosocial-impact-of-vision-loss-on-older-pe.html

Nyman SR, Gosney MA, Victor CR (2010). Emotional well-being in people with sight loss: Lessons from the grey literature. *Br J Visual Impairment* **28**: 175–203.

Nyman SR, Gosney MA, Victor CR (2010). Counselling for people with sight loss in the UK: The need for provision and the need for evidence. *Br J Ophthalmol* **94**: 385–6.

Nyman SR, Dibb B, Victor CR, Gosney MA (2011). Emotional well-being and adjustment to vision loss: A meta-synthesis of qualitative studies. *Disability and Rehabilitation*. http://informahealthcare.com/doi/abs/10.3109/09638288.2011.62

Rovner BW, Casten RJ (2008). Preventing late-life depression in age-related macular degeneration. *Am J Geriatric Psychiatry* **16**: 454–9.

Stanton AL, Revenson TA, Tennen H (2007). Health psychology: Psychological adjustment to chronic disease. *Annu Rev Psychol* **58**: 565–92.

Aids, appliances, and adaptations for visual loss

This chapter discusses the aids, appliances, and adaptations available to assist people with visual impairment.

There are three basic approaches:
- increase the visibility of the task
- use magnification (optical or electronic) to magnify the task
- use a non-sighted strategy to achieve the task's goal.

It should be noted that most people with visual impairment retain some residual vision and with appropriate help, will still be able to use vision to carry out tasks.

Clinicians often assume the problems faced by people with visual impairment relate primarily to seeing fine detail, such as reading text. However, for some, fine detail is not the issue. Rather, their main concerns are their ability to move around their local area, to shop, cook, socialize, and recognize people in the street.

The following five headings summarize the variety of aids, appliances and adaptations available.

Environmental adaptations

Most of the information people use to understand their location and identify possible routes and hazards is gathered visually. Inaccessible and hazardous streets, public buildings, shops, and homes create problems for people with visual impairments and good design of the built environment is particularly beneficial to them.

Good design practice includes adopting logical layouts and avoiding unexpected features and obstacles which project into circulation routes. Tactile paving and visual contrasts may be used to delineate steps, kerbs, and other hazards. Accessible signage such as audible signals and the rotating cones on pedestrian crossings indicate when it is safe to cross roads.

In the home, marking the edges of steps and introducing colour or tonal contrasts to highlight doorways, electrical switches, and furniture are all valuable adaptations.

Lighting

Good lighting for people with visual impairment should deliver uniform ambient light across a room or work space, so that a compromised visual system does not constantly have to adapt from one level of illumination to another. Good lighting design includes the control of glare, both from natural light through windows and from artificial light sources.

Sufficient local task lighting should be provided to enable reading and related activities to be carried out efficiently. The general rule is that a 70 year old needs around three times more light than a 20 year old for the same task. This multiplier is often increased for those with macular disease. Increased light is generally best provided by a dedicated reading lamp situated between the head and the task, rather than by ceiling or wall mounted light sources or natural light.

> **Author's Tip**
>
> If the magnifiers or spectacles aren't performing as well as they did in the clinic or consulting room, the problem is nearly always the lighting … or lack of it!

Aids to daily living

Commonly used aids to daily living include: talking or large print watches and clocks, writing frames and signature guides, bump-on markers for kitchen appliances and liquid level indicators to ensure the correct filling of cups. Talking books and newspapers are available, as are electronic readers. Everyday items such as medicines, foods, and correspondence may be effectively labelled with the PenFriend audio labeller available from RNIB.

Some people with visual impairment like to use a white support cane to indicate their disability. Others prefer not to highlight their disability: white 'symbol canes' are foldable and can be kept in a pocket until required. When appropriate, mobility techniques using a long (white) cane can be taught.

The simplest adaptations may be the most useful. These improve the visibility of tasks by maximizing size and contrast and include
- using a thicker blacker pen for writing
- using knives with handles which contrast with kitchen worktops
- chopping light-coloured foods on dark chopping boards and vice versa
- eating dark foods off light-coloured plates and vice versa
- replacing clear glass tumblers with coloured plastic alternatives
- using a mobile phone with more visible keys and display
- requesting large print bank statements and utility bills.

Optical aids

The foundational optical aid is a pair of spectacles. Spectacles may correct distance or reading vision. Specific spectacles may also be prescribed to correct for other working distances, such as for a computer or music stand. Bifocal or multifocal spectacles may combine corrections for different distances, although it has been suggested that elderly people have an increased risk of falls when these lenses are used for walking about.

Patients with loss of central vision, such as macular degeneration, often read best with separate reading spectacles. However, patients with cognitive impairment may find multiple pairs of spectacles confusing.

Low vision aids (LVAs) are optical devices designed to magnify objects making them easier to see. The most commonly prescribed low vision aids are simple hand magnifiers and stand magnifiers to assist reading text. Stand magnifiers are particularly useful in higher magnifications (6x or above) as they rest on the page and 'fix' the LVA in the correct position. Stand magnifiers are also useful for those who find it difficult to hold a hand magnifier still. Both hand and stand magnifiers may incorporate a light source. Less frequently, telescopic magnifiers may be mounted on a spectacle frame to give hands free magnification.

> **Author's Tip**
>
> Patients under ophthalmological care often go for many years without a review of spectacles or magnifiers. Always ask when these were last reviewed.

To improve the ability to spot distant objects and read distant text, such as bus numbers, hand held monoculars or binoculars may be prescribed. Spectacle mounted magnification may be used to help with television. However, the best strategy for improving television visibility is generally to use a larger screen or sit closer to it.

Author's Tip

Confused patients with dementia cannot easily use low vision aids. Their carers and families need advice on increasing size and contrast.

Glare control is needed by visually impaired people who find bright sunlight debilitating and for those who take time to adjust after coming in from outdoors. Glare may be effectively controlled with a tinted shield type appliance which cuts out light bouncing up from the ground and coming in from the peripheral visual field. Shields are removed on entering a shady area or a building. Photochromic lenses may also be used in normal spectacles. Although these do not control glare from the peripheral visual field, they do have the advantage of being more comfortable and less conspicuous than shields.

Electronic aids

A number of CCTV type devices are available for magnifying text. These incorporate a camera to capture an image electronically which is then magnified onto a screen. Manipulation of the image such as increasing its contrast may be possible. CCTVs may be desktop devices or handheld and pocket-sized. CCTV readers allow a 'mouse' type camera to be rolled across text while a magnified image is displayed on a TV screen. Electronic readers are available which scan printed text electronically and convert it to audible speech output.

People with visual impairment often struggle to see computer screens. In addition to in-built accessibility options, specialised software such as Guide, SuperNova and ZoomText make personal computers accessible and may be used alongside voice recognition software.

Conclusion

A wide variety of strategies are available to help older adults with visual impairment. Nearly always, something can be done to address particular concerns.

Those who are having difficulty may be directed to their optometrist, or to a low vision clinic if already under ophthalmological care. When issues of mobility or home safety are central, then a referral to a specialist sensory needs rehabilitation worker through social services is appropriate. Local voluntary organisations for the blind generally have resource centres where aids to daily living can be tried out.

Further reading

Jackson AJ, Wolffsohn JS (2007). *Low Vision Manual*. Butterworth Heinemann Elsevier.
www.rnib.org.uk

Impaired hearing: anatomy and physiology of hearing

The ears are a major part of our communication system. Hearing provides a defence mechanism and allows connection with the environment. The ears aid balance and this may be affected alongside hearing disorders.

Sound

Airborne sound travels at 340 m/s as a longitudinal pressure wave with sound packets vibrating around a fixed point. This is called sinusoidal oscillation and is subject to diffraction and interference effects.

Sound intensity is measured as a relative decibel (dB) logarithmic scale. A 20 dB increase corresponds to 100-fold increase in power. A 0 dB level depends on the scale. For the sound pressure level (dB SPL) scale 0 dB corresponds to 20 µPa. Frequency is expressed in hertz (Hz). The speech frequencies range from 250 Hz to 8 kHz.

The external ear

The external ear collects sound and helps with its localization. The pinna and lateral third of the canal are formed by elastic fibrocartilage. The bony medial two-thirds arches around the back of the temperomandibular joint, so to see the tympanic membrane (TM) with an auroscope, the pinna is pulled posterosuperiorly.

The ear canal is covered with skin which exhibits oblique maturation of the epidermis, such that surface layers effectively migrate towards the meatus at 0.1 mm/day.

The skin of the outer third has hairs, ceruminous (modified apocrine sweat glands), and sebaceous glands, which with desquamated cells form wax. This process does not change significantly with ageing. Wax found in the medial canal suggests patient instrumentation of the canal or on the TM may represent oxidized keratin obscuring underlying pathology such as cholesteatoma.

The middle ear cleft

Tympanic membrane (TM)

The TM is 10 mm in diameter and set at 55° to the long axis of the ear canal. Normally the appearance is of a slightly frosted window (see Figure 14.16). It comprises an outer layer of squamous epithelium, an inner mucosa with lamina propria between. The lamina presents differing fibrous architecture between the pars tensa and pars flaccida. The pars flaccida is least robust and is most likely to become retracted secondary to tympanic cavity pressure variations.

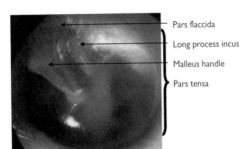

Pars flaccida

Long process incus

Malleus handle

Pars tensa

Figure 14.16 The normal tympanic membrane.

Tympanic cavity or middle ear

This air-filled space contains the ossicles (malleus, incus, and stapes), facial, and chorda tympani nerves. It is closely related to the middle and posterior cranial cavities. The roof of the middle ear (tegmen tympani) forms the floor of the middle cranial fossa and represents a route for transmission of suppuration.

The malleus inserts into the TM with each ossicle connected via a synovial joint. The footplate of the stapes sits in the oval window and allows sound vibrations to be transmitted to the cochlea. The round window niche sits just below the oval window.

The stapedius and tensor tympani muscles attach to the neck of stapes and top of manubrium of malleus respectively and are innervated with a reflex arc which protects the cochlear from loud noise damage. They also attenuate low-frequency sound increasing speech understanding at high intensity and reduce the mechanical resonances of the middle ear.

The middle ear functions as an impedance transformer accounting for the mismatch between the high-impedance cochlear fluids and low-impedance TM. This is achieved by the reduction in area between the TM and oval window (18.75×) and the lever advantage gained between the differing lengths of the malleus and incus (4.4×) giving a total transformer ratio of 82.5×. Around 50% of incident sound energy is transmitted to the cochlea.

TM defects and changes to the mobility/integrity of the ossicular chain can give rise to up to 60 dB predominantly low tone hearing loss.

The external and middle ear act as a broadly tuned band pass filter with peak transmission at the natural resonant frequency of 1 kHz.

The facial (VII cranial) nerve innervates the muscles of facial expression. From the fundus of the internal auditory meatus (IAM), it enters the middle ear near the malleus neck and traverses the medial wall in the (sometimes dehiscent) bony fallopian canal. It then descends to exit the skull base at the stylomastoid foramen medial to the mastoid tip.

The chorda tympani supplies taste to the ipsilateral anterior two-thirds of the tongue and traverses the tympanic cavity just medial to the tympanic membrane.

The Eustachian tube

The Eustachian tube (ET) is a dynamic channel connecting the anterior tympanic cavity to the nasopharynx. The lateral one-third is bony, the medial two-thirds cartilaginous. The tube opens on activation of the tensor palati, levator palati, and salpingopharyngeus muscles during swallowing, allowing equalization of pressure between the environment and middle ear cleft.

The mastoid

The mastoid probably functions to buffer pressure change in the middle ear cleft. The air cell system exhibits variable pneumatization, often poor in those with chronic ear disease.

The cochlea and its central connections

Cochlea (Figure 14.17)

The cochlea is situated in the inner ear and comprises a spiral tubular duct lined by membranes within the petrous temporal bone. It acts as a mechanoelectrical transducer. The basal turn presents the oval window containing the

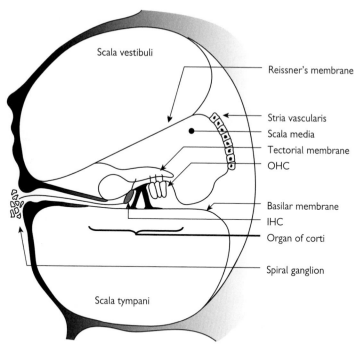

Scala vestibuli

Reissner's membrane

Stria vascularis

Scala media

Tectorial membrane

OHC

Basilar membrane

IHC

Organ of corti

Spiral ganglion

Scala tympani

Figure 14.17 Cochlea ultrastructure.

stapes footplate, and the round window, which releases pressure induced by sound stimulation at the oval window, to the middle ear. Pressure waves caused by sound enter the cochlea via the oval window and are analysed for frequency and amplitude by a complex and delicate sensory epithelium within the cochlear duct, the organ of Corti. This converts sound stimulus into electrical signals in the auditory nerve for transmission to higher centres for central processing.

Ultrastructure of the cochlea
The cochlear duct is divided into three by the longitudinally running Basilar and Reissner's membranes. The two outer channels (scala vestibuli and scala tympani) are contiguous via the helicotrema at the apex of the cochlea and contain perilymph at 0 mV potential (high sodium (Na+) concentration). The perilymph is continuous with cerebrospinal fluid via the cochlear aquaduct.

The scala media contains endolymph (high potassium (K+) and low Na+) with potential of +80 mV. This endolymphatic potential (EP) is maintained by the stria vascularis ('battery of the endolymph') situated at the lateral margin of the scala media. Animal models of presbyacusis suggest fibrocyte degeneration in the lateral wall leading to reduced EP and hair cell function.

Movement of the basilar membrane in response to cochlear fluid travelling wave motion causes mechanosensitive stereo cilia deflection and produces receptor potentials in the organ of Corti. The basilar membrane is highly sensitive and frequency selective (high frequencies at the base and low frequencies at the apex of the cochlea). Each point on the basilar membrane is passively and actively frequency tuned.

Organ of Corti
Inner hair cells
The single layer of inner hair cells (IHCs) subserve sensory transduction and processing in a passive manner. Mechanical movement of the reticular lamina in relation to the tectorial membrane causes radial shear deflection of the stiff, tip-linked stereocilia on each inner hair cell. Ion channels in the cell membrane open and K+ enters the cell via mechanotransducer channels. The cells are depolarised and neurotransmitter is released in synapses at the cell base giving an action potential in the auditory nerves.

Acoustic information is transmitted via both an oscillating AC response and DC depolarization. Stimulus and nerve depolarization frequency are linked. Nerve fibres themselves have different frequency selectivity (cochlear place coding). Auditory nerve firing rate increases with stimulus intensity.

The basilar membrane also generates non-linear response information such as frequency distortion products.

Outer hair cells
Three layers of outer hair cells (OHCs) respond to efferent higher control to allow active mechanical fine tuning and amplification of the travelling wave. The protein prestin is integral to the cellular shape change and mechanical tuning modulation of the basilar membrane. The OHC are the origin of otoacoustic emissions.

With age, the predominant cause for hearing loss relates to OHC function deteriorating, giving rise to increasing hearing thresholds, broad tuning and reduced frequency resolution (poor speech discrimination) with predominantly high-frequency loss.

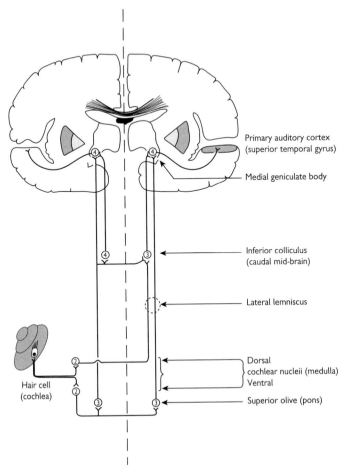

Primary auditory cortex
(superior temporal gyrus)

Medial geniculate body

Inferior colliculus
(caudal mid-brain)

Lateral lemniscus

Dorsal
cochlear nucleii (medulla)
Ventral

Superior olive (pons)

Hair cell
(cochlea)

The ascending auditory pathways - principal connections
(2 = neurone order)

Figure 14.18 Ascending auditory pathway principal connections. Numbers represent the neurone order. Drawn by Nicholas Mansell, reproduced with permission.

Central connections

Information from the cochlear is transmitted via the auditory component of the vestibulocochlear nerve to the ipsilateral cochlear nuclear complex in the brainstem. There is significant bilateral representation in the auditory cortex. Consequently unilateral cortical hearing loss is not commonly a presentation in the way that strokes can affect visual fields.

The cell bodies of the afferent fibres reside within the central spiral modiolus of the cochlea. The majority (95%) are related to IHC. A local circuit with multiple synaptic contacts exists within the functional hair cell unit.

Ascending pathway

The afferent auditory pathway (Figure 14.18) is complex and has many commissural and collateral connections. The ascending pathway takes auditory information toward the cortex. This data is modulated by various centres along the way via descending pathways (e.g. OHCs are acted upon by the descending neurons to affect basilar membrane activity and fine tune cochlea frequency reception.)

The most important sites between the cochlear nerve and auditory cortex are in ascending order:

- cochlear nuclear complex
- superior olivary complex
- inferior colliculus
- medial geniculate nucleus.

Within the cochlear nuclei the cochleotopic frequency map is maintained tonotopically. Neurones are influenced by interneurones and higher centres.

The pathway splits after the cochlear nuclei and rejoins at the superior olivary complex where binaural comparison occurs for the first time with sound localization ability. The inferior colliculus allows complex sound characteristic recognition and further localization. The auditory cortex corresponds to Brodmann's area 41 within the lateral fissure of the temporal lobe. This is arranged tonotopically with the high frequencies at the caudal end.

Descending pathway

Descending pathways exist from each named site down to the cochlear nuclei and from the superior olivary complex to the OHCs of the cochlea. The latter crossed olivocochlear feedback loop probably aids reduction in the masking effect of background noise. With age, this suppression is reduced and background noise becomes more intrusive.

Further reading

Kinsler LE, Frey AR, Coppens AB, Sanders JV (1999). *Fundamentals of Acoustics*. New York, Wiley.

Pickles JO (1988). An Introduction to the Physiology of Hearing, 2nd edn. London, Academic Press.

Robles L, Ruggero MA (2001). Mechanics of the mammalian cochlea. *Physiolog Rev* **81**: 1305–52.

Investigation of hearing loss

Investigations can confirm the presence of hearing loss suspected on clinical grounds. The degree and type of loss with assessment of functional compromise allows formulation of a management plan. The following categories of investigation will be considered:

- tuning fork (TF) tests
- psychoacoustic audiometry
  - pure tone audiometry (PTA)
  - speech audiometry
- evoked physiological testing
- imaging
- blood testing.

In the vast majority of patients with hearing loss a diagnosis and management plan can be made with the aid of PTA/tympanograms and magnetic resonance imaging (MRI).

Tuning fork testing

These can provide information on sensorineural asymmetry and conductive hearing loss.

Each frequency of TF will give information regarding the hearing at that frequency. The most commonly used is the 512 Hz, which is sufficiently high pitch not to stimulate by feel rather than sound, and sufficiently low pitch to maintain a tone without rapid decay.

The ear is designed to perceive airborne sound (i.e. via the ear canal) more efficiently than bone conducted sound. In a normal hearing ear a TF held (splines in line with the long axis of the ear canal) adjacent to the ear will therefore sound louder than when the base is placed firmly on the mastoid bone. This is described as Rinne positive. With significant conductive hearing loss (greater than about 25 dB) the test is reversed and bone conduction sound perception is greater (Rinne negative). In a dead/non-hearing ear there may be a false Rinne-negative result.

With normal hearing, a TF base held firmly on the central forehead will be heard in the centre of the head. If the sound lateralizes (it does so at about 5-10 dB asymmetry) there is either asymmetric sensorineural threshold (TF sound referred to the better ear) or a unilateral conductive loss (referred to the worse ear). The latter is known as Weber's test.

Psychoacoustic audiometry

Pure tone audiometry

The PTA is a subjective, behavioural measurement of hearing threshold enabling determination of degree, type, and configuration of any hearing loss. The test provides ear and frequency-specific data. It can provide both bone and air conduction thresholds. The test environment and equipment should be standardized and optimal with an experienced audiologist. The frequency range tested includes 250 Hz to 8 kHz. Threshold is recorded in decibels (dB). The threshold of the lower limit of normal is considered to be 20 dB. The scale is non-linear, such that 30 dB equates to the threshold of a whispered voice at 2 feet from the ear, 60 dB a conversational voice and 100 dB, a pneumatic drill in the street. Air conduction (AC) thresholds using headphones test the entire ear. In bone conduction (BC) testing, a stimulator is placed on the mastoid process and cochlear (sensorineural) thresholds are tested directly. If there is no difference between the two thresholds any

hearing loss will be sensorineural. A difference between the two will indicate a conductive hearing loss.

Some patients provide a significant challenge in testing. If testing the worse hearing ear, the better ear may need to be 'masked' during the audiogram (see Figure 14.19) with contralateral sound stimulation.

The PTA provides essential information when assessing and diagnosing hearing loss. However, it only provides data on pure tone stimulus and this may equate poorly to true functional loss.

Speech audiometry

The normal ear transfers acoustic speech signal into complex auditory nerve signal pattern. Sensorineural pathology may distort transformation and some data are lost. Frequency and temporal resolution is compromised and other extraneous sounds mask the desired speech signal. PTA does not assess the more complex transformation functions. Patients with identical pure tone audiograms may have significantly different functional deficits. Speech audiometry seeks to address this issue. Testing is more complex and assesses not only detection of stimuli but also identification and recognition of speech components, cognitive and linguistic function. Recorded speech (monosyllabic words up to full sentences) are presented monaurally through earphones or via sound field at different intensities. Various outcome measures are defined, the most commonly used is 'Speech Recognition Threshold level' which is defined as the lowest speech level at which the speech recognition score is equal to 50% for a given test subject, specified speech signal, and specified manner of signal presentation.

Testing can also give information regarding speech recognition in background noise. Speech testing is a very important tool in the assessment of patients using cochlear implants.

Evoked physiological assessment of auditory threshold

Otoacoustic emissions

Otoacoustic emissions (OAEs) are sounds generated by the active mechanical contraction of the outer hair cells (OHCs) of the cochlea. They can be spontaneous or evoked. Their main use is in screening very young children for genetic hearing loss. In adults they can provide information regarding the integrity of the OHCs and the differential diagnosis of cochlear and higher level hearing loss such as auditory neuropathy (= dyssynchrony). Objective testing correlates with audiometric threshold at 3–4 Hz within 5–10 dB.

Tympanograms

The tympanogram is a very simple, useful adjunct to the assessment of hearing loss, providing information on middle ear compliance. In the technique, middle ear impedance is measured continuously as air pressure in the sealed ear canal is varied. The result is a graph relating middle ear compliance and external auditory canal pressure. The results obtainable are:

- Type A: normal; peak compliance at 0 mmH$_2$O
- Type B: no peak of compliance/flat trace—fluid in middle ear cleft (e.g. otitis media with effusion)
- Type C: peak of compliance with negative middle ear pressure—Eustachian tube dysfunction

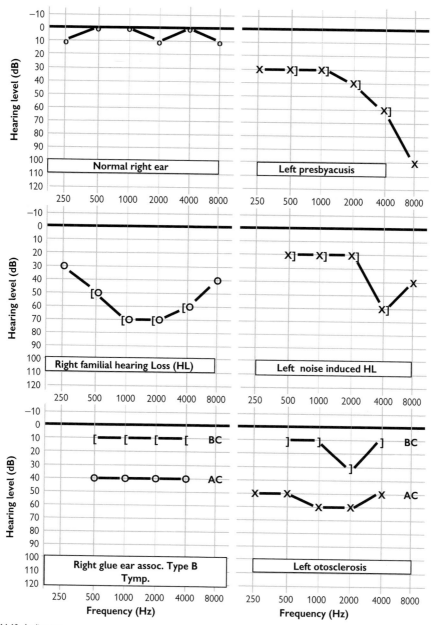

Figure 14.19 Audiogram.

- Low compliance peak—ossicular fixation
- High compliance peak—ossicular disruption/atelectatic TM
- High ear canal volume—TM perforation.

The tympanogram (see Figure 14.20) can also provide information regarding the acoustic–stapedial reflex arc and mobility of the stapes. Loud noise stimulates contraction of stapedius muscle to protect the inner ear. If the reflex is absent the stapes may be fixed or the neurological circuit may be compromised.

Neurogenic potentials

Electrical signals or evoked potentials generated by the auditory pathway from the cochlear to the cerebral cortex are a reliable, objective, and easily used method of assessing auditory function. Sound stimulation gives rise to potentials from the cochlear (cochlear microphonic, summating potential and compound action potential of the auditory nerve). A second potential occurs in the region of the entry of the auditory nerve into the brainstem. Subsequent potentials relate to levels on the auditory

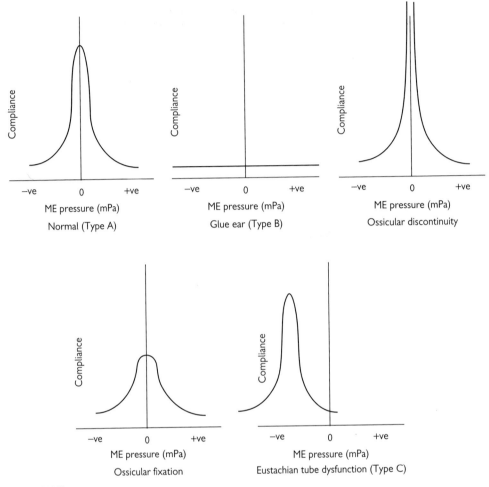

Figure 14.20 Tympanogram.

pathway, although their precise relationship to particular anatomical structures remains to be established. The potentials are recorded via scalp electrodes and complex electronics are used to clean and analyse the signals generated. The intact auditory pathway signal is symmetrical with similar peak latencies. Any asymmetry may suggest pathway pathology. The Auditory brainstem (or cortical) response can also be used to measure threshold; stimulus volume is slowly reduced until the waveform flattens and this gives an approximate objective level of hearing threshold.

Myogenic activity

The myogenic reflex arc, which protects the cochlear from loud noise and involves the stapedius muscle, may be used to assess the integrity of the neurological pathways and gives limited information regarding threshold. This information is readily available via the tympanogram.

Imaging

MRI: Asymmetric hearing loss or any indication of retrocochlear pathology, should be investigated by an MRI scan to rule out conditions such as a vestibular Schwannoma.

CT: This provides information on the bony anatomy of the temporal bone. Although a CT scan can define both congenital and acquired defects associated with hearing loss, they are most often ordered to assess the anatomy of the middle ear prior to surgery for Chronic Otitis Media. A CT may give helpful information for planning the management of patients with conductive hearing loss.

Angiography/magnetic resonance angiography
These are rarely used to further assess uncommon vascular lesions affecting the temporal bone (e.g. glomus tumours)

Blood tests

These rarely determine an underlying systemic cause for hearing loss and should therefore be targeted depending on presentation. Such tests include:
- full blood count: anaemia
- erythrocyte sedimentation rate: hyperviscosity syndrome
- blood sugar: diabetes
- thyroid function tests: hypothyroidism
- treponemal serology
- autoimmune profile
- genetic: Connexion 26.

Causes of hearing loss

Hearing loss can be conveniently divided into conductive problems (pathology related to mechanical transfer of sound vibration, e.g. ossicular defects) and sensorineural problems (the cochlea and its neural connections). Elucidation of the cause of any hearing loss involves establishing the history (presence of associated otalgia, otorrhoea, vertigo, tinnitus, past otological surgery, noise, ototoxic drugs, family history) and performing an examination to include otoscopy of both ears, tuning fork tests, and a neurological examination (cranial nerves, cerebellar testing, Romberg, Unterberger's tests). Full ear examination also includes assessment of the other ENT systems such as the nasal cavity, postnasal space, and palpation of the neck. Once it is established that the ear canals are clear of debris, a pure tone audiogram is the most useful investigation.

Prevalence of hearing loss

Hearing disorders constitute the most prevalent chronic impairment in the population (about 20% of people have 25 dB or greater loss in the better hearing ear over the four main speech frequencies), the major risk factor being age. With age, conductive hearing loss becomes a lesser proportion of aetiology and sensorineural loss becomes more dominant. Studies demonstrate that people with hearing disability and tinnitus have a significantly worse quality of life.

Presbyacusis results from reduction in cochlea cellular function with a parallel (but often less clinically evident) loss of labyrinthine (balance) function.

Conductive hearing loss (CHL)

External ear (pinna/external ear canal)

Wax

Wax can obstruct the ear canal if there are poor natural clearance mechanisms or the patient instruments the ear (e.g. cotton buds). The appearance is usually of hard dark brown material obstructing the ear canal and may give rise to a mild hearing loss. If there is functional compromise or doubt about the condition of the underlying tympanic membrane, initial treatment is with wax solvents such as sodium bicarbonate ear drops or olive oil. If this is ineffective referral to ENT may be necessary for outpatient microscope suction toilet.

Otitis externa/(OE) furuncle

Infection of the skin of the external ear canal is known as otitis externa. The common causative organisms are often multiple ear commensals which become pathogenic secondary to damp ear canal skin or an underlying exacerbation of eczema. The infection gives rise to skin swelling, erythema, discharge, discomfort, and mild hearing loss. A microbiology swab determines sensitivities to topical antibiotics and identifies fungal otitis externa, which requires a more protracted treatment of around 2 weeks. Treatment involves topical drops which often contain combined antibacterials, antifungals, and steroid. If cellulitis is present, oral antibiotics may be necessary. Poor response to treatment may necessitate an ENT referral.

Severe pain with localized swelling suggests a furuncle which should be treated with oral anti-staphylococcal drugs. Drainage is seldom required.

Immunocompromised patients (e.g. long-term steroid use, diabetes) with OE associated with severe pain may have 'malignant' OE, where the infection has progressed to

a skull base osteomyelitis. This requires expert specialist in-patient care. Mortality rate is now less than 10% with aggressive treatment, having previously been quoted as 50–60% in those with diabetes and a cranial nerve palsy at presentation.

> **Author's Tip**
>
> Persistent OE with poor response to treatment may be an external ear infection secondary to underlying middle ear pathology such as cholesteatoma.

Rare causes of ear canal obstruction giving rise to hearing loss include:

- external auditory canal (EAC) tumour (squamous cell carcinoma or adenocarcinoma)
- infective debris secondary to EAC cholesteatoma or radionecrosis of the temporal bone secondary to previous radiotherapy.

Middle ear

Acute otitis media (OM)

Bacterial or viral infection of the mucosal lining of the middle ear gives rise to suppurative effusion and a moderate hearing loss with a red bulging ear drum, fever, and otalgia. Purulent otorrhoea occurs after perforation of the tympanic membrane (TM).

The aetiology relates to the functional immunocompetence of the mucociliary clearance mechanisms of the middle ear mucosa and Eustachian tube.

The common responsible organisms are *Haemophilus influenza* and *Streptococcus pneumoniae*. In addition to the above history and otoscopic findings, testing will reveal a conductive hearing loss. Treatment includes analgesia and antibiotics are prescribed for the majority of cases although evidence for efficacy is weak. Complications include facial palsy and intracranial infection.

Otitis media with effusion

Chronic accumulation of mucus within the middle ear cleft gives rise to a mild to moderate hearing loss. Management aims at identifying and treating any simple causes, excluding serious underlying pathology and then treating the hearing loss.

Otitis media with effusion (OME) may follow an acute suppurative OM, rhinosinusitis, Eustachian tube dysfunction, or nasopharyngeal pathology (enlarged adenoids or nasopharyngeal carcinoma). Smoking and family history are predisposing factors.

Patients present with muffled hearing in the absence of pain or fever, though often preceded by a clear ENT precipitant. Autophony (the unusually loud perception of a person's own voice or breathing) and tinnitus may be present. Otoscopy reveals straw coloured fluid within the middle ear cleft and a CHL on tuning fork tests. Audiometry shows a mild hearing loss; tympanometry indicates poor middle ear compliance. Obvious underlying causes should be treated (e.g. with antibiotics, decongestants, antihistamines for rhinosinusitis). Persistent effusion necessitates a full ENT examination to exclude an underlying nasopharyngeal carcinoma. Where serious pathology is excluded and medical treatments have failed, management may include the insertion of a TM grommet under local anaesthetic, or in refractory cases the use of a hearing aid.

Chronic otitis media

Chronic otitis media (COM) is likely to be multifactorial in aetiology. The important factors are:

- previous acute OM or OME
- genetics and race (Innuit and Maoris)
- Eustachian tube dysfunction
- craniofacial abnormalities (cleft palate).

Chronic otitis media can be divided into five distinct categories:

Inactive (mucosal) chronic otitis media

This presents as a clean, dry permanent pars tensa tympanic membrane perforation with normal middle ear mucosa. This predisposes to middle ear infection with water exposure and hearing loss with larger defects. Surgery may be indicated in fit patients with lifestyle compromise or frequent infections. In experienced hands, surgery is highly successful.

Inactive (squamous) chronic otitis media

Imbalance of the middle ear environment (e.g. Eustachian tube dysfunction with negative middle ear pressures) may result in retraction of the TM. Such pockets can predispose to infection and may result in osteitic destruction of the ossicles with consequent hearing loss. Inactive stable cases require no action.

Active (mucosal) chronic otitis media

Chronic inflammation of the middle ear mucosa with permanent TM perforation results in chronic ear discharge and risk of suppurative complication. Resorptive osteitis of the ossicles is a feature. Such ears respond poorly to medical treatment and often require both closure of the TM defect (myringoplasty) and cortical mastoidectomy to clean the remaining middle ear cleft.

Active (squamous) chronic otitis media

Retracted TM squamous epithelial pockets may progress such that they become non-self-cleaning. Epithelial debris is retained within the pocket; infection and accelerated sac growth may result. Such pathology is known as cholesteatoma. Studies suggest a prevalence of around five per 100 000. Characteristically this presents as longstanding foul-smelling otorrhoea associated with hearing loss and occasionally complications. Because of the discharge, assessment of the TM and precise diagnosis may not be possible without special equipment (microsuction). Any patient with the above history should therefore receive a specialist opinion. The treatment is surgical, by the formation of a modified radical mastoidectomy to remove the sac of epithelium.

Complications of active chronic otitis media

Extracranial

- Sensorineural hearing loss
- Labyrinthine (dizziness)
- Facial nerve palsy

Intracranial

- Meningitis
- Intracranial abscess
- Venous sinus thrombosis
- Otitic hydrocephalus

Healed chronic otitis media

Some TM perforations heal spontaneously leaving an atelectatic area of the TM or hard white patches known as myringosclerosis which very rarely give rise to hearing loss.

Otosclerosis

This is a localized hereditary condition affecting endochondral bone of the otic capsule. In affected individuals, small regions of immature cartilaginous tissue become remodelled with fixation of the stapes footplate. Patients develop a slowly progressive unilateral conductive hearing loss from early middle age associated with a normal tympanic membrane, a normal tympanogram and a characteristic PTA.

In patients with functional compromise the first line treatment is a hearing aid. Some patients with cochlear otosclerosis and sensorineural loss may not find significant benefit.

If cochlear function is preserved and hearing aids fail, surgery may be considered. The complications of surgery include sensorineural deafness, vertigo and facial nerve palsy. These are rare but more likely to occur in an elderly person who has more sensitive labyrinthine function.

Trauma

Severe trauma to the ear may give rise to temporal bone fractures with cochlear, ossicular and possibly facial nerve damage. Hearing loss in such circumstances may not become apparent until long after the injury when the more serious life threatening consequences have been dealt with. Patients should be seen in ENT clinic at around two weeks post-injury for full hearing assessment. Lesser temporal bone trauma can result in dislocation of the incus and fracture of the incus long process. Complete ossicular discontinuity following trauma results in a 60-dB conductive hearing loss with high middle ear compliance. If cochlear thresholds are preserved, a hearing aid or surgery should be considered.

Sensorineural hearing loss (SNHL)

Cochlea

Age-related sensorineural hearing impairment

This term now replaces presbyacusis and describes high-frequency (HF) hearing loss in the elderly population. Six pathological types have been defined:

- sensory—hair cells lost at basal end of the organ of Corti; HF loss
- neural—most common, cochlear nerve. neuron degeneration with loss of ganglion cells; HF loss
- vascular/metabolic—flat threshold on audiogram; atrophy of stria vascularis (apical and middle turns)
- mechanical—increased stiffness of the basilar membrane
- intermediate—submicroscopic changes to the cochlear duct (endolymph composition and intracellular organelles)
- mixed.

Genetic factors are important and may determine thresholds; heritability appears to be around 30–50%. Proposed environmental factors include alcohol, smoking, systolic blood pressure, noise exposure, and blood hyperviscosity. Underlying potential systemic causes should be identified. Most patients present with a slow-onset hearing deficit with initial lack of clarity and speech discrimination in background noise. This progresses to frank communication problems. Tinnitus is often associated. Social isolation and depression may ensue. Diagnosis is based on age over 60, normal examination and a high tone symmetrical SNHL on audiometry. Any asymmetry (10 dB or more over the speech frequencies) warrants an MRI to exclude vestibular schwannoma. Management is matched to functional deficit and aimed at optimising the acoustic environment via advice from the hearing therapist and providing binaural hearing aids.

Noise-induced hearing loss

Exposure to significant noise exposure results in SNHL. Pathological changes within the cochlea include reduction in cochlear blood flow, stereocilia damage, outer hair cell necrosis and apoptosis. Genetic variance influences susceptibility as does smoking, diabetes, cardiovascular disease, drug use, and blue eye colour. Ototoxic drugs are synergistic. Typically there is a history of significant noise exposure, tinnitus, and hearing loss. Otological examination will be normal and the pure tone audiogram will indicate a ('boilermakers') notch at 4–6 kHz with recovery at 8 kHz. Asymmetric notch may suggest the use of rifles with the most damaged ear nearest the open barrel end.

Once the diagnosis is made, further noise exposure should be avoided. Management is matched to functional deficit and aimed at optimizing the acoustic environment via advice from the hearing therapist and providing binaural hearing aids. Psychological support may be necessary.

Genetic

Eight per cent of genetic HL is non-syndromic. Inherited hearing loss can be autosomal dominant (20% of non-syndromic genetic hearing loss) or autosomal recessive. Fifty such disorders have been identified. Genes coding for Connexion 26 account for 50% genetic hearing loss. Autosomal dominant deafness is usually apparent in childhood and progresses throughout life. Autosomal recessive forms tend to present later in life. Examination tends to be unremarkable and the PTA defect is consistent within families but varies with gene defect. A common pattern is U-shaped with relative preservation of high- and low-frequency thresholds.

Ototoxicity

This is a chemical injury to the labyrinth as a side effect of pharmacotherapy. The effect depends on drug and dose. The most commonly used agents causing such damage are the aminoglycosides and cisplatin. Salicylates, loop diuretics, quinine and erythromycin tend to cause a temporary loss at therapeutic dose.

Otoprotective agents used around the time of ototoxic drug administration have been shown to be effective in some animal studies. The challenge is to develop compounds which do not influence efficacy of the primary medication and lack side effects. Intratympanic administration may be most appropriate to protect the cochlea and avoid adverse systemic effects. Examples of such agents include Thiol compounds in cisplatinum therapy and aspirin to prevent aminoglycoside toxicity. Patients undergoing treatment should be monitored for high frequency loss with audiometry or with distortion product otoacoustic emissions (OAE). Early identification of toxicity is best management. Hearing loss should be treated with a hearing aid or if profound a cochlear implant with vestibular rehabilitation training for any balance deficit.

Idiopathic sensorineural hearing loss

The diagnosis and management of this condition is controversial. PTA findings are of a high frequency SN loss. Possible aetiologies include viral, vascular, immunological, or mechanical aetiologies. Initial investigations find a cause in less than 5% of individuals. Investigations include a full blood count, ESR, renal function and electrolytes, lipid screen, fasting blood sugar level, thyroid function tests, treponemal serology, autoantibodies, and a magnetic resonance imaging head scan. Spontaneous remission is common; 50% of patients recover with no treatment. There is no clearly effective evidence-based treatment, but common practice is to use a short course of oral steroids and antivirals.

Retrocochlear

Can be genetic or acquired congenitally or acquired postnatally.

Genetic

- Non-syndromal
- Syndromal (degenerative with peripheral neuropathy, e.g. neurofibromatosis type 2, Friedrich's ataxia, or degenerative without peripheral neuropathy, e.g. Usher's/Gaucher's

Congenital

- Cerebral palsy, asphyxia, respiratory distress syndrome, low birth weight, hyperbilirubinaemia.

Acquired

- Viral, e.g. cytomegalovirus, herpes zoster
- Bacterial, e.g. syphilis, meningitis
- Immune, e.g. Guillain–Barré syndrome, systemic lupus erythematosis, sarcoid
- Demyelination, e.g. multiple sclerosis
- Neoplastic, e.g. vestibular schwannoma, cerebellopontine angle lesion
- Metabolic, e.g. uraemia, cisplatinum
- Cerebrovascular, e.g. PICA syndrome

Author's Tip

Patients presenting with unilateral aural symptoms without an obvious benign cause should be referred for an ENT opinion e.g. unilateral deafness, tinnitus may be caused by a vestibular schwannoma.

Further reading

Gratton ME, Vasquez AE (2003). Age-related Hearing Loss: current research. *Curr Opin Otolaryngol Head Neck Surg* **11**: 367–71.

Gleeson M (ed.) *Scott-Brown's Otorhinolaryngology, Head and Neck Surgery*, 7th edn, vol **3**, 3311–593.

Hearing aids: helping your patient adapt to their use

Guidance is crucial in the hearing aid fitting process; a simple problem—as addressed in the next section—or difficulty with insertion or use of controls can all too easily lead to aid rejection.

Equally important is the counselling of patient expectation. For some, adapting to the new sound may take patience and perseverance. Hearing aids cannot 'magic back' perfect hearing but can offer to make the best use of remaining hearing.

Acclimatization

The brain needs to learn to listen to the new sound. Hearing aids rarely provide the gratifying 20/20 reaction found with glasses and the brain must be given time to 'acclimatize' or adapt. For those new to hearing aids, the most common complaints include:

'The sound is harsh, metallic and tinny!'
'My voice sounds funny!'
'I can hear the clock ticking loudly and the newspaper rustling—but I don't want to!'

What to say to your patient

Advise your patient that this is normal. The brain has been straining to hear these sounds for years and it will pay more attention to novel sounds. It can take 2–3 months to adapt to the sound from the hearing aid, but the more it is worn, the quicker the brain will adapt.

A strategy for adaptation: advising your patient

1 Start quiet: begin using the aids while sitting in a room with soft furnishings. Listen to everyday sounds, such as footsteps, turning the pages of a newspaper, etc.
2 Listen to people: start by listening to one person about 3–6 feet away. Then try talking to two or more people in a quiet room. It may be several days or even weeks before moving onto this situation.
3 Watch TV: to begin with, watch programmes where there is only one person talking at a time, such as the news. Gradually move on to programs with busier scenes. It may still be difficult with background music.
4 Get out and about: first try them in a familiar environment such as the garden. When comfortable here, try other places such as the shops or a park. Be wary of using the aids too soon in heavy traffic or busy shops, as these situations can be startling or unpredictable.

Hearing tactics

Busy situations with background noise may always be difficult. Remind your patient of the value of hearing tactics, for example:

• keep the speaker's face clearly visible and in the light
• cut down background noise where possible (e.g. turn down the TV/radio, shut the window, move away from a speaker in the pub)
• face the speaker, watch their lips
• in churches, theatres and similar, sit near the front or close to the loudspeaker
• use assisted listening devices.

Assisted listening devices

A range of equipment is available to help ease communication and listening in different situations. These 'assisted listening devices' aim to improve the signal-to-noise ratio.

Telecoil/loop systems

The hearing aid may be programmed with a telecoil, also known as a T-coil or loop system. Sound into a microphone is picked up by an inductive loop and sent direct to the hearing aid, so reducing background noise and helping the listener to hear more effectively.

The signal is picked up when sitting within the area of the loop and the hearing is switched to the 'T' or loop program. The loop system is installed in many public buildings, such as post offices, banks, supermarkets, cinemas, theatres, and places of worship. It is available wherever you see the loop sign (see Figure 14.21).

An induction loop can be installed as a cable that goes around the room. It will pick up the sound wherever the microphone is placed. Social Services should be able to provide advice on installing a loop in your patient's home.

Portable versions can also be purchased that loop round the neck or sit on the ear. The loop gets its signal from a direct connection with another sound source. This can be a sound system or TV set, or a microphone placed in front of the person speaking.

If the loop system appears not to be working, advise your patient to

• check the hearing aid is on and set to the loop program/'T' position
• ask staff in the building whether a loop system is available, and if so, whether it is switched on.

FM/infrared systems

An alternative to a loop system, here the signal is sent via infrared or FM instead of magnetically. The system comprises two parts – a transmitter placed near the source of sound (such as a TV set or stereo) and a receiver unit. As with the loop, the hearing aid must have a compatible program, but most modern hearing aids can switch automatically to the relevant program if set to do so at the fitting.

Direct audio input

Most behind-the-ear hearing aids have direct audio input, allowing the hearing aid to be directly coupled to a device (e.g. telephone, MP3 player) with special audio boots and cords. Wireless/blue tooth technology is now available.

Figure 14.21 Loop sign.

Environmental alerting

These devices use a visual or vibrotactile signal to alert the individual. Devices include alerts for the doorbell, telephone, alarm clocks, and smoke alarms.

Tinnitus relief

Tinnitus (hissing, buzzing, or other noises in the ears or head) can be extremely bothersome in some, resulting in disrupted sleep, anxiety, and depression. If your patient has tinnitus, it is likely to be reduced when using a hearing aid. This is because they are no longer straining to hear, and the perception of the tinnitus is decreased through 'sound enrichment'.

A sound generator may also help as part of a tinnitus management programme. These produce a soothing 'shhh' sound, known as 'white noise'. They may look like hearing aids and are usually provided by professionals. Alternatively, your patient can purchase a bedside sound generator that plays sounds, such as waves, fountains, birds, or rain.

Further details of the above devices can be found at the Action on Hearing Loss website or contact your local Social Services for further advice.

Referral to hearing therapy: why?

Most audiology departments have a hearing therapist.

Consider referral if your patient

• Struggles to fit their aid.
• Has usage and maintenance questions.
• Sometimes misses the doorbell/telephone/alarm clock/smoke alarm.
• Finds telephone conversation difficult.
• Wants the TV louder than those around them.

They can also provide advice on

• How to get the most out of their hearing aid.
• How to improve communication in the situations they find hardest.
• Equipment provision through Social Services.
• Hearing protection.
• Lip-reading classes and support networks.

Referral to other Audiology services: when?

• Drop-in repairs: easy access to fix basic problems.
• Volunteer service: for those patients unable to access the drop-in repairs service through immobility/transport issues, a home volunteer visit may be available. They may help with inserting the mould, operating the aid, re-tubing or just general support and advice.
• Tinnitus counselling and retraining therapy: to provide support, strategies and practical advice on tinnitus management.
• Adults with learning disabilities: to provide specialized assessment and rehabilitation services for this patient group.
• Balance assessment and rehabilitation: while balance problems in older people are most frequently multifactorial, they often involve some degree of labyrinthine dysfunction. Balance assessment and instruction in vestibular rehabilitation exercises can be helpful. General unsteadiness may benefit from assessment of dynamic gait and a tailored programme to improve standing balance and/or onward referral to physiotherapy, falls or social services.

Common questions asked by the patient

How long will it take to get used to my hearing aids?

It can take weeks or months. The more consistently they are worn, the quicker the adaptation process tends to be.

Will hearing aids make my hearing loss worse or make my ears lazy?

No. The opposite happens, as sounds are heard that would previously have been missed, attention, and discrimination improves. Aiding can prevent 'auditory deprivation', a condition where hearing is permanently impacted by the lack of neural stimulation.

Are two aids better than one?

Generally yes. When was the last time that an optician prescribed a monocle? Binaural aids could provide.

• better speech discrimination, especially in background noise, e.g. a noisy street or shop
• better ability to localize sounds
• a feeling of sound being balanced
• if one aid stops working, there is still another while the broken device is repaired
• *however*, consider dexterity/handling issues; two aids may prove difficult. Consider lifestyle issues; does the patient live alone in mostly quiet situations?

Why does the audiologist say my hearing has not changed yet I can't hear as well as I did?

Pure tone audiometry is referred to as a 'hearing test', when it is really a test of ability to detect sounds within a quiet environment at a number of discrete frequencies. 'Hearing' is the ability to understand complex speech in everyday, sometimes difficult, listening conditions.

There is a natural decline in our ability to process speech (or 'auditory processing') from the age of 40. In fact, cochlear and peripheral neural function as well as visual processing and cognitive skills all generally worsen with age. Level of cognitive function can influence the adaptation process, thus counselling your patient to understand their condition and to have realistic expectations is vital.

I refuse to wear it!

While encouragement and perseverance will see most patients benefiting from hearing aids, some may resolutely refuse. Or frustratingly, some are willing but unable. This may be influenced by dexterity issues or the level of cognitive function. Do not give up; other options may be available, such as a different type of aid, mould, or a personal listener. Help is available to reinstruct on aid use and insertion.

Summary

Physicians can play a central role in motivating and counselling a patient to comply and adapt to their hearing aids—not always a quick and easy task. While aids cannot give a patient perfect hearing, they can help them access quiet speech sounds and hear the everyday sounds they have been missing, such as the doorbell ringing or clock ticking. As a result, their confidence in conversation and social situations can improve with positive effects on their general well-being.

Further reading

Erber NP (2003). Use of hearing aids by older people: influence of non-auditory factors. *Int J Audiol* **42**: S21–25.

Lesner SA (2003). Candidacy and management of assisted listening devices: special needs of the elderly. *Int J Audiol* **42**: S68–76.

Pichora-Fuller MK (2003). Cognitive aging and auditory information processing. *Int J Audiol* **42**: S26–S32.

HearingLink. www.hearinglink.org

Hearing aids and their problems: a practical guide

Older people are major users of hearing aids which can be vital for effective communication, particularly in those with additional health problems or sensory deficits. This section deals with hearing aid basics and the management of common problems. Most problems are simple to fix and can be resolved at the point of care. With just a bit of know-how, you can prevent your patient being left without a hearing aid for longer than necessary.

Hearing aid basics

Hearing aids are used to increase audibility and make the most of an individual's residual hearing. Most are behind-the-ear (BTE) models, but some may be in-the-ear (ITE), or completely-in-the-canal (CIC). Increasingly, receiver-in-the-canal (RITC) or open-fit models are being fitted (for mild–moderate losses), which do not require the traditional mould but rather a flexible thin-tube and dome (see Figure 14.22).

The vast majority of aids are now digital models with automatic volume control. For those with good dexterity and cognition, manual program options are available through a button on the hearing aid. These typically include a directional program to aid speech in noise and a 'T setting' to access the loop (see following section).

For others, simplified operation with one basic program (traditionally called 'M') will be more appropriate, activated by simply closing the battery compartment. A few analogue units still persist; these may have a switch with M, T, and O settings ('mic', 'loop', and 'off' respectively).

Common problems and their solutions

Hearing aid appears 'dead'
- Hearing aid not switched on: turn hearing aid on (close battery compartment).
- Hearing aid is in 'T' mode: make sure the hearing aid is on the microphone 'M' setting. If the program order is unknown, try switching the unit on/off as the aid will automatically start in 'M' setting.

- Battery not inserted correctly: check the battery is inserted correctly, with '+' and '−' symbols the correct way round. Is it the correct size battery?
- Battery compartment not properly closed: ensure it is closed; is the battery upside down and preventing proper closure?
- Dead battery: replace battery. Batteries typically last 7–10 days if turned off at night, reducing to 3–5 days if left on; the battery compartment should be opened when not in use. Are the battery contacts clean? Clean gently with a cotton bud if dirty/damp/corroded if not.
- Blocked earmould tubing – wax or moisture (behind-the-ear and body-worn hearing aids only): clean earmould. Check sound outlet for wax. Moisture droplets in tube? Detach aid from tubing and blow through to clear (use a 'puffer' if available). Change tubing if blocked/more than 6 months old.
- Blocked sound bore (wax/ debris): clear blockage.
- Blocked filter on ITEs/RITCs and some BTEs: seek audiologist advice on how to change filter.
- Start-up delay: some aids are set with a delay (6–12 seconds) to provide the wearer with sufficient time to insert the aid before powering up.

Hearing aid makes a whistling sound (feedback)
- Earmould not inserted properly: ensure top part of the mould goes into the crease of ear (see Figure 14.23). An open fit dome should be inserted at sufficient depth into the ear canal
- Earmould does not fit properly: can occur after rapid weight loss or if an old mould. Remove the aid, put a finger over the earmould hole. If the whistling stops, the earmould was either not properly inserted or is not a good fit. Try it again in the ear; if the whistle continues, consult Audiology.
- Break in tubing: replace.

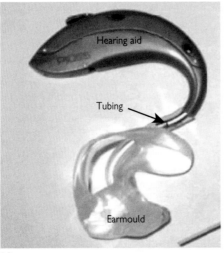
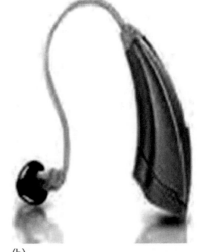

(a)   (b)

Figure 14.22 (a) Behind-the-ear aid with mould; (b) receiver-in-the-canal.

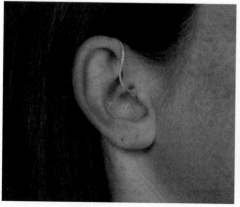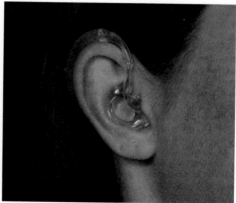

Figure 14.23 (colour plate 18) Inserting the earmould.

- Internal feedback: check by placing a finger securely over the sound outlet of the aid, which should stop the whistling. If not, a replacement aid is needed.
- Excess wax: sound is reflected back to the microphone, forcing a feedback loop. Dewaxing is required.
- Scarf/hat covering aid: again, reflected sound encourages feedback. Remove, loosen, or adjust the item.
- Volume set too high: turn down volume if volume control (VC) wheel activated; seek Audiology help if sound is then too quiet.
- Consult an audiologist if feedback persists; they may consider such options as use of a more occluding mould if insufficient gain before feedback or activation of a feedback cancellation program.

> **Author's Tip**
>
> As a stop-gap measure to reduce feedback, smear a water-based lubricant on the mould to create an acoustic seal, or try reducing the volume slightly.

Sound is intermittent
- Weak/dead battery: replace battery.
- Moisture: use a drying pot or leave in warm, dry place.
- Kink in tubing (open fit, RITC): replace.

Sound distorted
- Weak battery: replace.
- Volume set too high: reduce volume. Contact Audiology as a more powerful aid may be required.

Sound weaker than usual
- Weak battery: replace
- Sudden drain or batteries not lasting as long as expected: try a different batch of batteries first, then seek advice
- Hearing aid tubing damaged: replace if necessary.
- Earmould clogged with wax: clean with alcowipe. If blocked tubing, soak overnight in water soapy water. If still unable to remove, contact your hearing aid provider to have it cleaned/retubed.
- Moisture in tubing: see above.
- Drop in hearing: refer to Audiology for assessment. For sudden or asymmetrical changes, refer to ENT.

Moulds exacerbate ear infections
- Poor hygiene: stringent hygiene regime essential using alcowipes, frequent soaking in liquid disinfectant and use of a spare set of moulds to allow cleaning/alternation.
- Poor aeration: remove moulds regularly to let ear 'breathe'; use an open-fit/RITC if within fitting range; use bone conductor aid for conductive losses.

Moulds uncomfortable
- Not inserted properly: ensure mould inserted at helix.
- Poor fit: contact Audiology, may need new mould.
- Allergy: itching and otitis externa may be helped by use of a non-allergic mould material. Open fit/RITC aid?

'My voice sounds funny'
- Patient not acclimatized to sound: counsel patient and encourage consistent use.
- Good compliance but ongoing problems: refer Audiology; may need fine-tuning or mould adjustment.

Problem persists?
- Hearing aid may be defective: seek Audiology advice

> **Author's Tip**
>
> Most problems with hearing aids are due to a dead battery or blocked tubing. To quickly check, remove the tubing (simply pulls off). Does the aid whistle when cupped in your hands with a new battery?

Where can I get further help?
If despite your best efforts the problem resists fixing, consider these options:
- Service may also be available to help the patient Most Audiology centres have a drop-in repair service; if your patient is mobile, this is the quickest route to problem resolution.
- If your patient is immobile, send the aid to the drop-in repairs service; it may be possible to fix a simple problem without the patient present.
- If your patient is immobile or house-bound, contact the Audiology service for advice; a domiciliary or ward visit may be available. A volunteer manage the aid (e.g. practise mould insertion, use of controls, etc.).

- If the hearing aid cannot be fixed immediately (e.g. a patient is on the ward), other options may be available to prevent social isolation, such as the use of personal listeners (headphones and amplifier).
- If appropriate, arrange for a sign language interpreter.

What do I do in the meantime?

If your patient is without a hearing aid, simple hearing tactics will ease communication:
- Get your patient's attention before speaking to them.
- Face your patient directly so they can see your lips.
- Speak clearly and at a normal pace—do not shout. Shouting distorts words as well as your lips, making it harder to hear or lip read. Do not speak slower than usual. This, again, can distort your lips and make it harder to lip read.
- Lip-reading is 70% guesswork; many words look the same. Using whole sentences rather than one-word replies gives contextual clues
- Gestures and facial expressions can help to explain what you are saying.
- Be patient; when asked to repeat something, try slight changes to the sentence to make your point clearer.
- Don't give up! If still not understood, try writing it down.

Protection and storage of hearing aids

While reasonably robust, hearing aids should be treated as the mini-computers that they are.

Avoid
- Shock: dropping on hard surfaces
- Extremes of temperature
- Moisture: remove when bathing/washing hair, store in a drying pot overnight

Storage
- Use the case provided; avoid storing in tissues since these tend to end up in the bin
- Use a silica drying pot if the patient is prone to getting condensation in the tubing or conditions are humid

General tips
- Turn off the aid at night (open battery compartment) to save power (and to prevent whistling).
- The sound tubing becomes hard and brittle and will benefit from being replaced every 6 months. This is a simple job that anyone with reasonable dexterity can do. Tubing and instructions can be obtained from your local Audiology department.
- Remember all the 'Rs': if the hearing aid units become detached, convention denotes that a red marker relates to the right aid, a blue marker the left. Important if there is marked asymmetry in hearing levels.
- Use stetoclips (allows a normally hearing person to monitor the performance of a hearing aid) to perform a subjective sound check.
- If you send a patient to Audiology, ensure the ears are clear of wax. This will save your patient an extra journey back to the general practitioner and allow for prompt action

Further reading

Dillon H (2001). *Hearing Aids* (Northern J, ed.). Thieme.
Royal National Institute of the Deaf. www.rnid.org.uk
Royal Berkshire Foundation Trust. Audiology Fact Sheets. (http://www.royalberkshire.nhs.uk/wards__departments/a/audiology.aspx).

Rehabilitation

What is rehabilitation?

Defining rehabilitation

Rehabilitation has been described as the 'secret weapon' of geriatric medicine and, in tandem with comprehensive assessment, is among the most important interventions available to the discipline. Much of our working day is spent in the process of rehabilitation, but how well do we understand this process? Geriatricians and indeed most healthcare professionals would profess to an intuitive understand of rehabilitation as a concept. However, attempts to formally define rehabilitation reveal its inherent complexity.

There is no universally accepted definition of rehabilitation. In the broadest sense, 'rehab' encompasses concepts from addictions work to musculoskeletal interventions for injured athletes to functional rehabilitation of the older adult. These seemingly disparate areas highlight that the rehabilitation concept is applicable across a range of health and social science domains and within groups definitions evolve in tandem with scientific, social, and demographic change. Thus, definitions of rehabilitation will necessarily be context and client specific. Even within 'geriatric rehabilitation' there is no clear consensus.

Definitions of rehabilitation

Oxford Medical Dictionary

Treatment of an ill, injured or disabled patient with the aim of restoring normal health and function.

Rehabilitation of the Disabled (1956)

Rehabilitation must be a continuous process, beginning with onset of sickness or injury and continuing throughout treatment until final re-settlement in most suitable work and living conditions is achieved.

Kings Fund

A process aiming to restore personal autonomy to those aspects of daily life considered most relevant by patients or service users, and their family carers.

World Health Organization

To maximize function and minimise limitation of activity and restriction of participation resulting from an underlying impairment or disease.

The difficulty in defining rehabilitation is of more than academic interest. As we increasingly move towards evidence based practice, robust randomised controlled trials are required. The development of international multicentre collaborative working with generalizable study protocols to allow for meaningful comparative and meta-analysis, necessitates an understanding of what rehabilitation means. A common language is needed to describe the field and interventions contained within it.

Although specific content and taxonomies differ, shared constructs emerge from the various definitions of rehabilitation proposed. Rather than seek a precise definition, it is more useful for the clinician to tease out the themes that are common to these definitions and that are likely to contribute to successful rehabilitation. A description of key rehabilitation components, from a geriatric medicine perspective, is offered with the important concepts highlighted. In this sense, rehabilitation can be seen to differ from services supplied to the non-participating client (care) and from spontaneous/time-dependent improvement in function (recuperation).

Key concepts for a working definition of rehabilitation

Geriatric rehabilitation is not (usually) a single intervention, rather it is an active process with a holistic, individualized focus. It will often involve multiple professions, the patient, and other relevant parties such as carers, working as a team but with a final common goal of impacting on functioning; enabling patients and carers to live their lives to the fullest potential.

Rehabilitation in geriatric medicine

A review of the theory underpinning rehabilitation can be insightful and key references are provided for the interested reader. Practising geriatricians may find that ideas explored in some of these theoretical texts do not 'ring true' for their patients. Historically, rehabilitation has emerged from interventions involving injured soldiers where there is an expectation of recovery to 'normality'. It remains true that rehabilitation theory primarily relates to the younger disabled. Although much of this theory is also applicable to our patient group, in practice expectations, interventions and outcomes can be very different.

It is worth considering the ways in which geriatric rehabilitation differs from rehabilitation in other groups. Functional deterioration in the context of acute illness of any aetiology is commonplace in older adults. The 'medical' trigger to rehabilitation will rarely be a single insult, rather multiple acute and chronic pathologies are the norm and appropriate medical assessment and intervention is an important part of the rehabilitation process. Age itself is not a disease, but physical deconditioning is common in older adults, as are degenerative physical and cognitive disease processes. As a result the aim of rehabilitation in the older adult may be maintenance of function or slowing decline rather than achieving full recovery. Even in healthy old age, physiological reserve is reduced and therapy prescriptions have to be modified accordingly. Complications and concomitant illnesses are prevalent and may further impede progress. Ultimately, the rehabilitation process may take substantially longer and repeated interventions are often required. Finally, geriatric rehabilitation must take account of social and environmental issues. Support mechanisms for older adults will differ according to local culture and government. Care for the disabled, from family or friends, cannot be assumed and discharge planning is vital throughout the rehabilitation process. These differences are summarized in the British Geriatrics Society, Good Practice in rehabilitation document.

Good practice in rehabilitation

- Rehabilitation is a process that begins at admission and continues beyond discharge.
- Rehabilitation is necessary to restore daily living skills and mobility in older people recovering from illness and (planned or emergency) surgery.
- Rehabilitation requires medical contribution to ensure treatable illness is not missed; multidisciplinary input and robust evidence base.

Models of disease relating to rehabilitation

Central to many theories of rehabilitation are models of illness. For example, the World Health Organization describes a classification of disease where effects can be considered at levels of pathology (the disease itself)

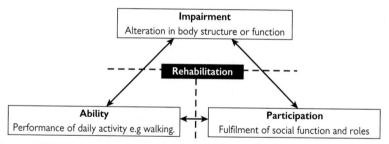

Figure 15.1 Illustrating WHO classification of disease and the role of rehabilitation. Data from WHO Expert Committee on Disability Prevention and Rehabilitation (1981). World Health Organization Technology Reports Series, **668**: 1–39.

impairment; activity (formerly disability), and societal participation (formerly handicap). Using this model, interventions aimed at pathology can be thought of as purely 'medical', while interventions at other levels may represent rehabilitation (see Figure 15.1).

The non-linear relationship between categories is worth exploring as it is not in keeping with a classical medical model. For example, in a person who falls and fractures their neck of femur (pathology), it cannot be assumed that repairing the broken bone alone (impairment) will return pre-fracture mobility (activity) or allow the patient to return to previous hobbies and activities (participation). An optimal rehabilitation intervention will target each of these levels simultaneously, although the primary focus may change as the patient progresses. Such an approach is efficient and prevents the formation of 'feedback loops' where problems at one level of the classification impact on others, for example fear of falling, leading to reduced mobility and physical deconditioning.

Classification of overall satisfaction or quality of life is out with the scope of the WHO system, although this is likely to be the most important to the patient. To impact on quality of life may require an even broader perspective, incorporating physical, psychological, social, and spiritual dimensions.

Down with rehabilitation culture

A criticism of many of the rehabilitation definitions described, is the implicit assumption that the person can and wants to return to a previous level of 'normal' function. We must be careful that we do not paternalistically assume the goals of rehabilitation for the patient. For example, we may assume that the recent amputee will desire independent mobility with a prosthesis and target physiotherapy interventions accordingly, when the patient may be happy to be wheelchair independent.

Disability is not an illness and vocal groups of rehabilitation service users have criticised rehabilitation that focuses on improving function to meet societal norms. As example, some patients with mobility problems argue that the goal should not be to improve walking to allow access to buildings but rather society should adapt to prevalent disability by improving availability of ramps or level access. While the applicability of these arguments to the client group seen in geriatric medicine is questionable, few would argue that central and local government have an important role in successful rehabilitation of the older adult (for example, through benefits, day centres, disability legislation).

Further reading

Blaxter M (1976). *The Meaning of Disability*. London, Heinemann.

British Geriatrics Society (2005). *Position Paper. Rehabilitation in the NHS and Social Care*. London, British Geriatrics Society.

Expert Group on Healthcare of Older People (2002). *Adding Life to Years*. Edinburgh: Scottish Executive.

Lazar RB (ed.)(1998). *Principles of Neurological Rehabilitation*. New York: McGraw Hill.

Nocan A, Baldwin S (1998). *Trends in Rehabilitation Policy*. London, Audit Commission.

Post MW, de Witte LP, Schrijvers AJ (1999). Quality of life and the ICIDH: towards an integrated conceptual model for rehabilitation outcomes research. *Clin Rehab* **13**: 5–15.

Wade DT (1998). A framework for considering rehabilitation interventions. *Clin Rehab* **12**: 363–8.

Wade DT, de Jong BA (2000). Recent advances in rehabilitation. *Br Med J* **320**: 1385–8.

WHO Expert Committee on Disability Prevention and Rehabilitation (1981). *World Health Organization Technology Reports Series* 668: 1–39.

Young J, Robinson J, Dickson E (1998). *Rehabilitation for Older People*. *Br Med J* **316**: 1108–9.

Who should receive rehabilitation?

Selecting patients for rehabilitation

In any service there will be a finite capacity to offer intervention, a reality that is especially pertinent for complex health treatments such as rehabilitation. Robust evidence describes the benefits of specialist assessment and rehabilitation for certain patient groups, for example following acute stroke, and these patients should be universally considered for such services. For the more 'general geriatric medicine' patient cohort, the evidence base to guide patient selection for rehabilitation is less robust.

Traditionally choice of patients for rehabilitation has been more of an 'art' than a 'science' based on clinicians intuition and past experience. Ideally services should be directed to those patients most likely to benefit, however often the best way to explore potential efficacy of rehabilitation is to offer the patient a time limited 'trial' period of rehabilitation. Should we then adopt an inclusive policy, accepting all referrals for inpatient rehabilitation? The practical answer is no, and arguments against this approach are included in the text box. To achieve a balance between sensitivity (selecting those patients likely to benefit) and specificity (not accepting patients unsuitable for rehabilitation) some form of 'triage' is usually necessary.

Why not accept all older patients for rehabilitation?

- Direct unselected referral from community or hospital wards could quickly overburden even a large service.
- Referral for 'rehabilitation' is often a sign that the referring team are struggling to cope, or more cynically want to transfer a challenging patient. Those referred are often complex older patients who need comprehensive assessment but they do not always need dedicated rehabilitation.
- A universal acceptance policy will raise false expectation and may result in inappropriate intervention in those who will not benefit from rehabilitation.
- Non-discriminate rehabilitation may divert the team's time and attention from those who would benefit most from the service.

Selecting patients for rehabilitation

Accepting that some form of assessment for rehabilitation is required, how should this be facilitated? Some units may operate explicit admission policies for inpatient rehabilitation beds, for example age over 65 or previously community dwelling. Although these criteria are useful to prevent inappropriate use of a limited resource, a degree of pragmatism is optimal. For example, it is difficult to argue that a 64 year old, disabled, stroke survivor should be denied access to specialist rehabilitation as they are 1 year 'too young'.

Even with simple admission criteria, 'demand' is likely to be greater than availability and further triage is necessary. When faced with rationing, we may ask the question – will this patient benefit from rehabilitation? In reality most patients will benefit from some form of rehabilitation, it is the extent of benefit and the input required to facilitate benefit that is important and difficult to predict.

More useful questions to inform decisions regarding rehabilitation are considered below.

Does the patient require any rehabilitation?

It is worth considering, what will happen if the patient is not accepted for rehabilitation. Many older adults will recover well from even serious systemic illness with little functional impairment. Admission to a specific rehabilitation service is not warranted if the patient only needs a few more inpatient days to finish treatment and allow spontaneous recovery.

Is the patient ready for rehabilitation?

Patient and therapist safety must always be considered and a period of medical or psychiatric stabilization is often preferred before commencing active rehabilitation. For example, a patient with recent myocardial infarction and ventricular arrhythmia may not be appropriate for transfer to an 'off-site' rehabilitation facility with limited capacity for monitoring or resuscitation. These decisions are time-sensitive and after a short period of medical stabilization, the same patient may be entirely appropriate for rehabilitation.

Predicting outcome from rehabilitation

A number of potential predictors of good and poor outcome in rehabilitation have been suggested and these will be considered in turn. However, it is often difficult to translate from observational studies to the individual and the extent that these variables actually contribute to outcome is probably modest at best. In addition, although certain groups may have poorer outcomes following rehabilitation this does not equate to lack of effectiveness. Often in geriatric rehabilitation the aim is maintenance of function or delaying decline.

Age

Older age is seen by many non-geriatricians as the *raison d'etre* of rehabilitation. It is recognized that the older patient is particularly vulnerable to the problems associated with immobility (venous thromboembolism, decubitus ulcer, hypostatic pneumonia). Although all older patients will benefit from good medical and nursing care with early mobilization if possible, not all require dedicated rehabilitation. It is debatable whether age itself is a predictor of outcome from rehabilitation. The 'oldest old' have longer lengths of stay and fewer will return home; however, differences in outcome are less evident when analyses are corrected for comorbidity.

Cognitive impairment

The efficacy of rehabilitation services for those with advanced cognitive impairment has been debated. It is recognised that this group often have poor functional outcomes. However, a direct association between standard measures of cognitive function and change in functional status during rehabilitation has not been consistently demonstrated. It can be frustrating to work with a patient group with limited capacity to learn. However, beneficial effects such as strength and balance training are possible; education and training of family/carers can be useful and many therapists have reported that repeated interventions do translate into meaningful improvement. For this particular patient group, an adaptive, rather than restorative approach, may often be beneficial; for example, through the provision of assistive technology.

Pre-morbid ability

Functional ability at time of admission and 'pre-morbid' ability are powerful predictors of functional gain. It is self-evident that the greater the disability, the greater the potential benefit from intervention. It is less apparent if there is a minimum level of functioning required for successful rehabilitation. Patients with complex needs and dependency are unlikely to improve in general medical wards. Case series of rehabilitation interventions in severely impaired older adults suggests relative improvement but at the cost of substantial input from the team. Rehabilitation should not be denied simply because it will be 'a lot of work'. For example, the older, incontinent, sensory impaired woman sustaining a fractured neck of femur has a poor prognosis. However, with focused intervention meaningful gain can be made and even modest improvements in functional ability may allow a supported return home rather than long-term care.

Care home domicile

A return home is often the ultimate goal of rehabilitation in the older adult. Extrapolating from this, it may be argued that rehabilitation is not justified for those patients already in a care home environment, particularly those already in higher level 'nursing care'. We should be wary of assuming universally poor outcomes for nursing home residents that experience functional deterioration. Rehabilitation interventions delivered in care homes may prevent unscheduled hospital admission and some functional gain can be safely achieved through inpatient rehabilitation of care home residents.

Other factors such as race, gender, educational level, financial resources, and living arrangements have been described as impacting on rehabilitation outcomes.

It is difficult to disentangle whether these direct causative effects simply reflect the complex socio-cultural context in which rehabilitation takes place. Certainly, few would advocate withholding rehabilitation based on cultural or demographic factors.

Even factoring all this information, we may still select patients who ultimately do not benefit from rehabilitation. This is not a failure of selection, often the best assessment of rehabilitation success is a trial of rehabilitation itself. For services to operate efficiently, early appropriate placement for those patients unable to return home and not requiring further inpatient rehabilitation would be optimal but remains uncommon in many healthcare settings.

Further reading

Diamond PT, Felsenthal G, Macciocchi SN, *et al.* (1996). Effect of cognitive impairment on rehabilitation outcomes. *Am J Phys Med Rehabil* **75**: 40–3.

Foster A, Lambley R, Hardy J, *et al.* (2009). Rehabilitation for older people in long-term care. *Cochrane Database Syst Rev* (1):CD004294

Patrick L, Knoefel F, Gaskowski P, Rexroth D (2001). Medical comorbidity and rehabilitation efficiency in geriatric inpatients. *J Am Geri Soc* **49**: 1471–7.

Stroke Unit Trialists' Collaboration (2007). Organised inpatient (stroke unit) care for stroke. *Cochrane Database Syst Rev* (4):CD000197.

Wade DT (2003). Selection criteria for rehabilitation services. *Clin Rehabil* **17**: 115–18.

Models of rehabilitation

Just as there is no agreement on a formal definition of rehabilitation, so there is no consensus on the best model to facilitate rehabilitation. Services have to adapt to changing demographics and healthcare infrastructures. Although geriatric rehabilitation is a relatively new discipline, its delivery has taken many permutations. Although flexibility in the service is welcome, national audits have recognized substantial variation and inequity in practice and delivery of rehabilitation services for older people.

The 'original' geriatric rehabilitation model

To better understand successful models of geriatric rehabilitation, it is useful to consider the work of Marjory Warren – 'The Mother of Geriatrics'. In the chronic sick beds of West Middlesex County Hospital, Warren developed a system of single centre, individualized assessment and multidisciplinary intervention. The success of this novel intervention was evidenced by the fact that most of Warren's 'incurable' patients returned home.

> "treatment should be undertaken by a team whose central theme is optimism and hope. It is wise to get elderly up as soon as their physical condition warrants. It is of great value to get them dressed in their own clothing..." (Warren 1943)

Conversely, a successful rehabilitation model can also be appreciated by considering the models of care that Warren argued against and that unfortunately may still be seen in contemporary practice.

How NOT to rehabilitate

A previously independent older adult with complex comorbidity is admitted as an emergency with deterioration in mobility related to intercurrent illness. The presenting illness is treated promptly. However, nurses' concerns over mobility result in a protracted period of bed rest. With declining functional ability, ward staff take on more tasks 'for the benefit' of the patient, with gradual institutionalization. After a period of time, ward staff take the decision that the patient is not 'safe' to return home and the patient is transferred to a care home.

Rehabilitation: where, what, by whom?

A plethora of differing approaches to rehabilitation have been described (for example, in neurological rehabilitation, therapy approaches include: 'Bobath'; 'motor relearning'; 'neuromuscular facilitation'). All have vocal proponents; however, there is little robust evidence to distinguish them. Guidelines now recommend that teams to do not limit practice to one particular model or style, rather that interventions should be selected according to the needs of the patient.

At a more pragmatic level, key questions relating to models of care are: Where should rehabilitation take place? How should interventions be delivered? Who should deliver them? These will be considered in turn.

Rehabilitation environment

Many will be familiar with the traditional rehabilitation hospital. However, rehabilitation can be delivered in a number of settings. An emergent literature suggests that efficacy of rehabilitation is sensitive to organizational structure with a central rehabilitation unit, often the optimal model.

This area has been best explored in the field of stroke rehabilitation, although certain concepts may apply to more 'general' rehabilitation.

Models of rehabilitation delivery with reference to stroke

Inpatient care

Dedicated stroke unit
Proven superior, in terms of mortality, functioning to:
- general medical ward
- general ward with peripatetic stroke team
- general ward with integrated care pathway
- hospital at home services.

Dedicated stroke unit with early supported discharge
Proven superior to all for mild–moderate stroke.

Post-discharge

Outpatient hospital-based services (e.g. day hospital)
    Proven equivalent to:
- domiciliary interventions.

Ideally, the traditional geriatric rehabilitation hospital is characterized by greater space around beds for equipment and storage of the patients own clothes; day room for social activity; gym for physiotherapy interventions and kitchen/bathroom area for activity of daily living assessment. The strengths of a dedicated rehabilitation unit probably relate to more than physical structure and environmental modifications. The components that seem to account for superiority of stroke unit care include: a geographically distinct ward; a dedicated specialist team; multidisciplinary working and a focus on education and training. It seems probable that these elements will be equally important in non-stroke rehabilitation. In particular, a single unit should allow for easier communication, audit and research, with improved team dynamics and 'knock-on' effects on morale.

With increasing pressure on acute hospital beds, alternatives to acute hospital admission have been explored. Options include therapy in the patient's own home or delivered in various community locations that are often referred to collectively using the rubric 'intermediate care'. Interventions delivered in local communities are intuitively attractive but evidence base is lacking. A Cochrane review comparing, care-home, own home and hospital delivered rehabilitation for older adults described several relevant studies. All had methodological weaknesses and, using stringent exclusion criteria, no study was felt to be sufficiently robust to inform decision making.

Frail adults are prone to unexpected deteriorations in health and early accessible intervention for those requiring inpatient services should not be lost in the drive towards community delivered care. One possible solution would involve community 'out-reach' and hospital 'in-reach' teams, all operating from a central rehabilitation unit 'hub'.

The amount of therapy is equally important, as increasing intensity of therapy has beneficial effects on functional outcomes. The reported gain from increasing therapy is variable and the relationship may be non-linear, particularly at extremes. 'Overdose' of rehabilitation is a possibility, although with current models it would seem unlikely that patients will reach this theoretical treatment ceiling.

Delivering more frequent rehabilitation may necessitate changes in working practice or infrastructures. Reports of impressive functional outcomes in centres offering seven-day-a-week therapy are thought provoking but without robust randomized control trial evidence are not enough to warrant an overhaul of traditional working patterns.

In interpreting these data, we must not equate rehabilitation solely with active 'therapy' time. Interactions with nurses and carers who promote independence are an essential, albeit difficult to measure, part of any rehabilitation model. Achieving this therapeutic environment may represent a radical change in philosophy for ward staff used to providing direct supportive care. The temptation may be to wash and dress an older patient, rather than hold back and supervise while the patient attempts such activities independently.

The rehabilitation team

Central to the success of rehabilitation is a number of individuals or agencies working together towards a shared goal. The effect of this team approach should be greater than the sum of its component disciplines. Traditionally, the geriatric rehabilitation team has consisted of representatives with backgrounds in medicine, nursing and therapy (occupational, speech, physiotherapy). As the scope of rehabilitation has expanded, so have the potential members of the team.

The make up of any rehabilitation service will be dependent on local services, expertise and client group. A common approach is to have a core membership with ad-hoc input from a more extended group. It is out with the scope of this piece to describe the evidence base behind all the possible disciplines potentially involved. In practice, if a team dynamic underpins therapy, there is often considerable overlap.

Dynamics within rehabilitation teams have changed and it is no longer assumed that the 'doctor' will lead the team. For the older adult, presenting complaint(s), co-morbidity and propensity to develop complications justify substantial initial medical input and leadership. With time the need for direct medical input may decrease and others may better lead rehabilitation with access to medical advice as required.

Prehabilitation

All the above models describe rehabilitation as a reactive process, triggered by functional change or disease. The medical truism of prevention being better than cure remains apparent in rehabilitation. The ageing phenotype is highly variable. Functional decline is not inevitable and 'disuse atrophy' can be prevented and reversed with exercise programmes. Perhaps the future of rehabilitation research and practice should focus on pro-active exercise schemes instituted before functional decline is evident—'prehabilitation'.

Further reading

Diserens K, Michel P, Bogousslavsky J (2006). Early mobilisation after stroke. *Cerebrovasc Dis* **22**: 183–90.

Kwakkel G, van Peppen R, Wagenaar RC, et al.(2004). Effects of augmented exercise therapy time after stroke. *Stroke* **35**: 2529–39.

Kwan J, Sandercock P (2005). In hospital care pathways for stroke. *Cochrane Database Syst Rev* (4): CD002924.

Langhorne P, Holmqvist LW, Early Supported Discharge Trialists (2007). Early supported discharge after stroke. *J Rehabil Med* **39**: 103–8.

Langhorne P, Pollock A, Stroke Unit Trialists' Collaboration (2002). What are the components of effective stroke unit care. *Age Ageing* **31**: 365–71.

Scottish Executive (2007). *Coordinated, Integrated and Fit for Purpose. A Delivery Framework for Adult Rehabilitation in Scotland.* Edinburgh, Scottish Government.

Shepherd S, Doll H, Broad J, et al. (2009). Early discharge hospital at home. *Cochrane Database Syst Rev* (1): CD000356.

Stroke Unit Trialists' Collaboration (2007). Organised inpatient (stroke unit) care for stroke. *Cochrane Database Syst Rev* (4): CD000197.

Ward D, Drahota A, Gal D, et al. (2008). Care-home versus hospital and own home environments for rehabilitation of older people. *Cochrane Database Syst Rev* (4): CD003164.

Warren MW (1943). Care of the chronic sick. *Br Med J* **2**: 822–3.

Evidence base and cost-effectiveness of rehabilitation

Demographic and fiscal pressures impact on both health and delivery of healthcare. The population is ageing in most Western countries where care of older adults accounts for a substantial and growing proportion of total healthcare spending. Government and service funders will increasingly demand clinical and cost efficacy data for interventions in this population group. Complex interventions such as rehabilitation, with its multiple component parts and potential large initial economic cost, will come under particular scrutiny.

We recognize the compelling evidence base for disease specific rehabilitation resources, for example cardiac rehabilitation. Selected older patients can benefit from such intervention. However, these services are rarely delivered or coordinated by Geriatric Medicine specialists and will not be considered further in this chapter.

Evidence base for rehabilitation

Geriatricians will be used to comments from colleagues in other disciplines that rehabilitation represents 'soft' science with little supporting evidence. In fact, a robust and growing body of work describing efficacy of rehabilitation is available. Good-quality trials supporting multidisciplinary team based, rehabilitation in multiple sclerosis, chronic pain and head injury have been available for many years. The exponential increase in stroke rehabilitation work has shown that rehabilitation of the older adult is also amenable to good quality scientific research. Progress made is evidenced by recent guidelines. The European Stroke Organisation guidelines on rehabilitation contained seven recommendations based on class 1 evidence (meta-analysis or robust large-scale randomized control trial), whereas the more recent Scottish Intercollegiate Guideline Network (SIGN) clinical guideline on stroke rehabilitation is a 100 page document with 17 grade 'A' or 'B' recommendations and 300 supporting references, hardly 'soft' science.

Evidence base in other areas pertinent to geriatric medicine is less extensive but the available data supports belief in the efficacy of a rehabilitation approach. For older adults with fractured neck of femur, previous systematic reviews have suggested improved outcomes with coordinated inpatient rehabilitation but heterogeneity and small numbers precluded robust summary data. Trials of 'orthogeriatric' rehabilitation continue to inform the debate and the recent meta-analysis reports significant improvements in mortality, functioning and care home avoidance. Away from the traditional hospital setting, review of rehabilitation interventions for care home residents describes functional improvement with few adverse effects.

Studies relating to 'general' geriatric rehabilitation are also available. Recent meta-analysis of multidisciplinary rehabilitation (physiotherapy, occupational therapy) in patients aged over 65 years, included summary data from eight trials (n = 2927 patients). Rehabilitation was associated with greater return home and improved outcomes at discharge; longer term benefits were less apparent (see Table 15.1). This may not represent rehabilitation failure; rather, it reflects propensity for future functional deterioration in older frail cohort.

In summary, there are robust data supporting effectiveness of multidisciplinary rehabilitation as a complex package of care for the older adult. There remain many unanswered questions, however in the words of Wade

Table 15.1 Efficacy of multidisciplinary inpatient rehabilitation

Meta-analysis of published trials	
Improved functioning at discharge:	1.34 (1.12–1.60)
(3 trials, n = 1918)	
Improved functioning follow-up:*	1.02 (0.86–1.21)
(6 trials, n = 2712)	
Admission to care-home at discharge:	0.53 (0.33–0.86)
(4 trials, n = 572)	
Admission to care-home at follow-up*: 0.90 (0.71–1.13)	
(7 trials, n = 2877)	
All cause mortality at discharge:	0.76 (0.54–1.06)
(3 trials, n = 867)	
All cause mortality at follow-up*:	0.88 (0.75–1.94)
(7 trials, n = 2877)	

Data from Bachman (2010).

Data are odds ratio and 95% confidence interval.

*Follow-up at between 3 and 12 months.

'it is no longer tenable to depict rehabilitation as an expensive placebo service'.

The challenge of rehabilitation research

We have evidence that rehabilitation in certain situations is beneficial but finer details are less clearly defined. There is a pressing need for more research, making for an exciting time in the field. It could be asked why the evidence base is not more advanced and why it has taken so long to get where we are. There are many historical, political and economic reasons why rehabilitation research does not appear as advanced as some single organ specialities. An important factor is the inherent difficulty in design, implementation and analyses of a rehabilitation intervention.

Population

Trials in a frail older adult cohort are prone to attrition bias (loss of participants). Without large scale studies, impact of an intervention may be lost in the 'noise' related to health states associated with ageing (polypharmacy, comorbidity, cognitive decline and mortality).

Standardization

Traditionally, the rehabilitation process has been customized to the patient. However, to translate outcomes to routine practice, a consistent approach with standard protocols is required. Some therapists argue that it is individualisation of treatment that accounts for success.

Intervention

If trial data do suggest efficacy, it may be difficult to tease out the important components from the many interrelated processes comprising the intervention. For this reason, rehabilitation is often referred to as a 'black box'. We know it works as a concept but we are not sure how. Examining individual components separately risks 'type III' error, i.e. finding non-efficacy of individual components of a system and concluding that the whole system has a neutral effect.

Comparator

Most studies to date have been comparisons against 'usual' care. These studies have been instrumental in proving that rehabilitation 'works' and have progressed the rehabilitation agenda. We now need comparative studies of one rehabilitation intervention or model against another – doubling the complexity and decreasing statistical power. Blinding patients and trialists to rehabilitation input also poses methodological challenges.

Outcomes

Measuring efficacy of rehabilitation is difficult. For example, how should a trialist measure increased societal participation? Even measuring less abstract concepts is not straightforward. Multiple tools exist for clinical and trial use, however there is little consensus on the optimal instrument to use and all outcome measures have clinometric weaknesses. A common taxonomy and uniform methods of measuring rehabilitation effect are necessary. To this end, professional societies have suggested standard tools e.g. Barthel Index for activities of daily living.

Numbers

Many studies in rehabilitation have been statistically underpowered to provide definitive data. Two complimentary solutions are meta-analysis and multi-centre recruitment. Meta-analysis is only as good as the input data and in the rehabilitation literature, heterogeneity and methodological weaknesses limit the validity of many individual trials. Multicentre trials require substantial economic investment and as there is usually no investigational medical product, pharmaceutical funding is not an option. Furthermore, international multi-centre trials still face the challenge of potential heterogeneity between centres.

Cost-effective rehabilitation

Compared with other disciplines, there are few direct economic analyses in rehabilitation. All of the systematic reviews described in the 'further reading' section cite a lack of economic data as a potential weakness in rehabilitation research. Where data are available, conclusions can be contradictory, highlighting the difficulties inherent in performing economic analyses of complex interventions. For example, in a review of day hospital provision, studies claiming increased, decreased and cost neutral expenditure were described (albeit only one study found cost benefit). Unequivocal cost benefit is demonstrated for certain specific services or patient groups, for example, early supported discharge for mild–moderately disabled stroke survivors, but the economic case for general rehabilitation of the older adult remains to be proven.

The initial expenditure of setting up a rehabilitation service may be substantial. This investment is made in the anticipation that overall health is improved and future health care resource use is less. Standard inpatient stays are expensive and interventions that reduce length of stay or reduce future unscheduled admission make economic sense. The wider financial implications of disability, both direct (care homes) and indirect (lost productivity through family members adopting a carer role) make a rehabilitation approach intuitively attractive. However, we should be wary of assuming economic efficacy without appropriate analyses. The move away from central hospital care, to a greater emphasis on community delivered services was advocated with the anticipation of substantial cost savings. United Kingdom analyses comparing cost of traditional hospital care with novel community services have reported cost-equivalence.

Although clearly important to attract continued funding, demonstration of cost benefit of rehabilitation packages in an older, frail population poses its own challenges. A rehabilitation 'success' may involve allowing for a heavily supported return home with ongoing, unpredictable hospital use rather than admission to a care home. Although clearly desirable to the patient, this may be seen as less of a success to the health economist. To take this fiscal argument to an extreme, reducing mortality in a 'costly consumer' cohort may not be economically desirable. In addition to concrete measures such as mortality or length of stay, we need to add measures of satisfaction and quality of life. A valid methodology for describing these outcomes in an older cohort is not yet agreed – another opportunity for the budding rehabilitation researcher.

Further reading

Bachmann S, Finger C, Anke H, et al. (2010). Inpatient rehabilitation specifically designed for geriatric patients: systematic review and meta-analysis of randomised controlled trials. *BMJ* **340**: 1718.

Foster A, Lambley R, Hardy J, et al. (2009). Rehabilitation for older people in long-term care. *Cochrane Database Syst Rev* (1):CD004294.

Handoll HG, Cameron ID, Mak JC, Finnegan TP (2009). Multidisciplinary rehabilitation for older people with hip fractures. *Cochrane Database Syst Rev* (4): CD007125, 2009.

Langhorne P, Holmqvist LW, Early Supported Discharge Trialists (2007). Early supported discharge after stroke. *J Rehabil Med* **39**: 103–8.

O'Reilly J, Lowson K, Green J, et al. (2008). Post-acute care for older people in the community – a cost effectiveness analysis within a multi-centre randomised controlled trial. *Age Ageing* **37**: 513–20.

Quinn TJ, Paolucci S, Sivenius J, et al. (2009). European Stroke Organisation Executive Committee. European Stroke Organisation Writing Committee. Evidence-based stroke rehabilitation: an expanded guidance document from the European stroke organisation (ESO). *J Rehabil Med* **41**: 99-111.

Scottish Intercollegiate Guidelines Network (2010). *Clinical Guideline 118. Management of Patient with Stroke: Rehabilitation, Prevention and Management of Complications and Discharge Planning.* Edinburgh, SIGN.

Rehabilitation goals

The multiple disciplines involved in a patient's rehabilitation need to work together effectively. Therefore, a shared understanding of what the team are trying to achieve is needed. Goal setting is the preferred term for this process of focusing and coordinating the team's efforts around the progress of the individual patient. Historically, therapists assessed patients individually assigning relevant unidisciplinary goals. These may have been presented at multidisciplinary meetings but were rarely collaborative. A move towards truly collaborative, team-based goal setting is now recommended with emphasis on early, active engagement with the patient.

For the purposes of this discussion we will use the following definitions:

- Goal: a future state that is desired, with the implication that some form of intervention or change is necessary to achieve this state.
- Goal setting: process of agreeing on goals, usually between patient and all other interested parties.

Why set goals

Most human behaviour is goal directed. Doctors often set goals (sometimes subconsciously) for themselves and their patients. However, for these goals to be realized they need to be made explicit and agreed on by all the relevant parties. Potential benefits of team-based goal setting include

- improved efficiency through cooperation and avoiding duplication of effort
- comprehensive planning, ensure all relevant goals at levels of impairment, activity and participation are considered
- the goal provides both a target for the patient and the team, and is a yardstick to measure success of interventions
- the process may be therapeutic in itself, motivating and educating the patient, their family and the team.

Goal setting: the evidence

For a process that is perceived to be fundamental to rehabilitation practice, there are surprisingly few trials evaluating goal setting. The theory and initial 'evidence base' for goal setting derives from the field of business management and it is not difficult to see how strategies used to build effective teams, maintain motivation and work towards deadlines in complex business projects could translate to the rehabilitation setting.

Some evidence relating to efficacy of goal planning in chronic disease is emerging. For example, a study of care-home residents described reduced dependency through a combined goal planning and behaviour modification approach. General themes that emerge from the goal setting literature describe:

(a) The importance of patient involvement for effective goal setting.
(b) The use of supported goal setting to effect behavioural change.
(c) The superiority of setting short, medium and longer terms goals compared to long term goals alone.

The area continues to evolve and more research is needed. In particular, there is little published evidence to guide the process of goal setting. (For the interested reader, contemporary models for goal setting include: Goal Attainment

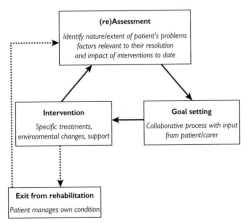

Figure 15.2 The rehabilitation cycle.

Scaling; Contractually Organized Goal Setting; Canadian Occupational Performance Measure). Furthermore, goal setting requires time and effort on the part of the team. This 'cost' may be substantial, particularly if there is disagreement within the team. As yet, there are no studies describing cost effectiveness of a goal setting strategy.

Despite the many theoretical advantages and emergent literature, use of goal planning strategies is not universal across rehabilitation teams and when employed, there is heterogeneity in application. A postal survey of British Society of Rehabilitation Medicine members found that a problem based approach was prevalent but standardized goal setting and active patient involvement was less common.

Goal setting in action

The conventional approach to rehabilitation is a cyclical process of assessment, goal setting, intervention and reassessment. It should have an end point where patients exit the process, but there should be opportunity to re-enter the cycle as required (see Figure 15.2).

An essential first step in setting goals is assessment: defining the underlying problems and issues. A problem list approach is useful and increasingly common in geriatric practice. A common challenge in assessment is having suitable tools to allow definition (and where appropriate, quantification) of problems and to allow a common understanding across all team members. The patient is central to the assessment process and their specific problems and aspirations must be established as the framework for future goal setting. The problem list may also be informed by collateral information from family, carers, general practitioner, etc.

Having described the underlying problems, a common next step is to separate out proposed short, medium and long-term intent. (Some textbooks use the terminology of long term *aims*, and short term *targets*.) This can assist with the goal setting process and prevents the patient and team from becoming overwhelmed at an early stage. The targets may be linked and progressive. Thus, while the ultimate aim for a patient with stroke related hemiparesis may be a return home, shorter term interventions may focus on sitting balance and transfers.

Focused goal setting

Generic goals of rehabilitation have been defined and include: maximizing participation of the patient in their chosen social setting; minimizing patient's symptoms and distress; and minimizing stress on carers. While useful as a template, these abstract goals may have little direct meaning to patients and therapists.

To focus goal setting, many teams use the SMART acronym. The origins of the acronym are unclear and various words and phrases have been associated with each included letter. A common description is of Specific (to that patient), Measurable (it is clear when goal is achieved), Achievable, Relevant (to the overall rehabilitation process) and Time limited goals. Examples of two goals proposed for a recent bilateral amputee are given in Figure 15.3.

Collaborative goal setting and assessment

Communication is vital for the team to progress towards goals. In a rehabilitation unit, regular informal exchange of information is common. However, regular formal multidisciplinary meetings should also be held. These discussions should include all those agencies actively working with a patient and can cover a variety of areas. Core points to be covered in a multidisciplinary meeting include progress and complications, discharge planning, current and new or revised goals. Patients are not usually present at all multidisciplinary meetings, however ongoing patient and carer involvement is recommended. In some instances a formal rehabilitation contract may be drafted with explicit goals and proposed timelines. In other situations intermittent progress meetings can serve a similar purpose.

Patient-led goal setting

For rehabilitation to be effective, all members of the team, family/carers and most importantly the patient must agree with proposed goals. Patients and carers can be unrealistic about what can be achieved with rehabilitation. This may

be no bad thing, as patients with greatest aspiration often progress better than those who set less ambitious goals. The team should try to ensure that goals are broadly achievable for the individual, mindful of their pre-morbid functioning, presumed prognosis and socio-cultural context. However, a challenging but achievable rehabilitation goal should usually be attempted. Patients should be pushed to work towards their limits of physical, functional and mental ability. To successfully achieve rehabilitation goals requires flexibility and creativity on the part of both patient and team. Unfortunately in goal setting, we cannot divorce rehabilitation from the reality of limited resources. In theory, patients with any level of dependency could remain at home; however, the resources required to facilitate this discharge may not be available or practical.

Discharge home as a primary goal

For most patients the primary aim will be a return home and to maintain motivation it is often prudent to allow for early discharge, continuing rehabilitation as required in the community. Although desired by most patients, transfer from the relative safety of the rehabilitation unit to their own home can be daunting. A supervised assessment within the home environment, 'home visit', can be useful to identify actual and likely problems. This should be performed well before proposed discharge to allow organisation of necessary modifications and equipment. Return home does not signal an end to the rehabilitation process, rather it is a change in location. Ongoing input, either in the patient's own home or as an outpatient, may be required to achieve maximal potential or maintain current level of functioning.

Further reading

Bovend'Eerdt TJH, Botell RE, Wade DT (2009). Writing SMART rehabilitation goals and achieving goal attainment scaling: a practical guide. *Clin Rehab* **23**: 352–61.

Guthrie S, Harvey A (1994). Motivation and its influence on outcome in rehabilitation. *Rev Clin Gerontol* **4**: 235–43.

Holliday RC, Antoun M, Playford ED (2005). A survey of goal setting methods used in rehabilitation. *Neurorehab Neural Repair* **19**: 227–31.

Kirusek TJ, Smith A, Cardillo JE (1994). Goal attainment scaling applications theory and measurement. Hillsdale, NJ.

Playford ED, Dawson L, Limbert V, et al. (2000). Goal setting in rehabilitation, report of a workshop to explore professionals' perceptions of goal setting. *Clinical Rehab* **14**: 491–6.

Ronan WW, Latham GP, Kinne SB (1973). The effects of goal setting and supervision on worker behaviour in an industrial situation. *J Applied Psychol* **58**: 302–7.

Schut HA, Stam HJ (1994). Goals in rehabilitation teamwork. *Disabil and Rehabil* **16**: 223–6.

Goal	Improve walking and get home	Independent wheelchair transfer in two weeks
Specific	x	✓
Measurable	x/?	✓
Achievable	x	✓
Relevant	x	✓
Time limited	x	✓

Figure 15.3 SMART goal setting. Data from Bovend'Eerdt TJH, Botell RE, Wade DT. Writing SMART rehabilitation goals and achieving goal attainment scaling: a practical guide. *Clinical Rehabilitation*. 2009; **23**: 352–61.

Physiotherapy

Role of the physiotherapist

Physiotherapists are an integral part of the multidisciplinary team (MDT). In order to be able to work as an effective MDT, it is important to understand the subset of skills that each profession brings to the team.

Since the National Service Framework for Older People (2001), there has been an emphasis on the development of intermediate care, stroke, falls, and mental health services, splitting many aspects of rehabilitation for older people into specialist areas. This has enabled the development of a specialist workforce and pathways, but is not always helpful to the older client who may fulfil the referral criteria to all. Thus, physiotherapists involved in the rehabilitation of older people should retain a level of generic skill to be able to assess and treat or effectively triage to other services, while also specializing in their chosen field, e.g. neurology.

To this end, physiotherapists assess and treat compromise in the neuromuscular, musculoskeletal, cardiovascular, and respiratory systems when this compromise either risks or has caused mobility impairment. Physiotherapists also consider the psychosocial aspects of presentation (in line with the WHO International Classification on Function), including an overview assessment of environment, social support, and cognition behaviour/mood in their initial screening.

Treatment is indicated for a wide range of conditions, ranging from simple exercise intolerance caused by deconditioning, to a stroke patient with an associated aspiration pneumonia and dense hemiparesis.

Physiotherapists aim to reduce the functional consequences of impairments such as

- muscle weakness
- pain
- hemiparesis
- spasticity
- sensory loss
- loss of joint range
- respiratory compromise such as poor basal expansion and retention of secretions
- amputation.

This list is by no means exhaustive. Acknowledging that functional compromise can cause secondary impairments, physiotherapists also have a role in secondary prevention. For example, teaching self-pressure-relieving techniques to a wheelchair-bound patient in order to prevent sacral sores, and identifying suitable physical activities for mobility-compromised patients so that cardiovascular and respiratory health is not compromised further. Thus, rehabilitation comprises assessment, treatment, and secondary prevention roles.

Assessment and treatment planning

It is beyond the scope of this text to describe physiotherapy assessment and treatment interventions in depth. The key principles of assessment and problem solving in rehabilitation will be outlined.

A problem solving approach is taken, with emphasis on initial identification of functional compromise. In the past, physiotherapists have been thought of as a profession that prescribes exercises with little context or meaning for the patient and their activities of daily living.

However, a problem-solving approach encourages starting from a point of functional compromise and drilling down to causative factors, be they impairments or environmental or social factors. Subsequent treatment may be aimed at directly addressing the impairment, such as in the use of targeted training at weak hip extensors/abductors for patients with Trendelenberg's gait. Alternatively, compensatory strategies may be used, such as walking aids to reduce the weight-bearing load on an arthritic hip. A skilled practitioner should be able to identify those impairments that can be treated and those that cannot, and require adaptations. This is particularly challenging when dealing with older people, as it is likely that they will present with a complex mix of longstanding, fixed impairments and newly acquired impairments. Accurate identification of the treatable impairments can save many hours of ineffective therapy time.

Underpinning this process are objective measures designed to quantify at either impairment, activity or participation level (for definitions see the WHO, ICF). In order to adequately monitor effectiveness of interventions, it is recommended that measures at all three levels are used. The following examples illustrate why.

A patient presents with a history of persistent falls. On assessment, weak dorsiflexion is identified ('drop-foot'), caused by a previous mild stroke. Poor foot clearance during the swing phase of gait and poor ability to use the ankle strategy in standing result in both a tripping hazard and increased postural sway respectively. By issuing an ankle foot orthosis, the tripping hazard and subsequent falls risk can be reduced, and function (activity and participation) improved. However, presentation of initial impairment, weak dorsiflexion, will remain and show no change on objective measurement. Conversely, changes at impairment level may be effected with little to no functional change. For example, administering botulinum toxin to the wrist and finger flexors to reduce spasticity in the forearm flexors and to increase joint range at the wrist and fingers. This may enable a carer to gain access to the palm for maintenance of the patient's skin integrity and reduce pain, but will not necessarily change the patient's functional use of their hand. If all levels of measure are not used, proof of efficacy of input would be compromised.

A whole range of activity and participation level measures exist. Decision-making regarding which assessments are used is dependent upon validity and reliability studies and personal preference on the part of the therapist. Examples include the functional independence measure (FIM), Barthel index, Rivermead Mobility Index and Hauser ambulation index to name but a few. Objective impairment level measures used include assessments such as peak flow, dynamometry and goniometry, used to assess respiratory function, muscle strength and joint range respectively. Ordinal scales for motor strength and control and sensation have also been devised. For example the Nottingham Sensory Assessment, the Ashworth scale to assess spasticity and the Motricity Index to assess motor control.

In many of these tests, performance of a task is observed and scored using an ordinal scale against standardized descriptors. For example, on the Hauser ambulation scale, zero is scored if the patient has normal gait and the score of four is attributed to a patient walking with a unilateral aid. Although this type of measure provides a simple measurement tool, there is a level of subjectivity, which compromises inter-rater reliability, limiting their value across a pathway when several treating therapists have been involved. This can be overcome, to some extent, in specialist pathways if internal consistency checking is performed, and agreement reached across the pathway regarding interpretation of the descriptors. Unless this is done, objective measurement data transferred across a pathway should be treated with caution, particularly if using it to assess recovery, response to therapy and prognosis.

For the cognitively intact patient, the advent of greater emphasis on patient reported outcome measures may serve to overcome across pathway issues of measurement.

For the cognitively impaired patient, 'service user' reported outcomes have been devised which canvas the carers/relatives, rather than the patient, in order to gain insight into the patient's functional performance. Some questionnaires modified for dysphasic patients, by using pictographs and underscoring of key words, have had some success in gaining patient reported outcomes with this client group. However, accurate assessment and measurement of movement can be particularly challenging in patients with cognitive impairment. Poverty of movement and function may be directly attributable to cognitive impairments rather than true motor impairments. For example, patients with dyspraxia are unable to plan and sequence and may be unable to complete simple motor tasks such as standing up from a seated position, washing and dressing or feeding themselves. This may be despite having otherwise intact musculoskeletal systems.

Author's Tip

It is essential that assessment of the cognitively compromised patient include psychology, speech and language and occupational therapy input.

Treatment

Physiotherapists have a variety of treatment modalities available. For example, simple exercise prescription, provision of aids, electrotherapy, complex handling techniques to manage neurologically impaired patients, soft tissue techniques such as massage, specific mobilization and manipulation of joints, gait retraining, and chest vibrations or shaking to aid sputum expectoration along with the active cycle of breathing technique. Many of these will be employed in rehabilitation.

Generally patients with cognitive compromise have a poorer rehabilitation outcome. This should not preclude them from rehabilitation, for example if procedural memory is relatively intact approaches such as task specific, step by step, training may enable relearning of motor tasks, use of pictographs, gesture and demonstration may assist motor rehabilitation of patients with coexisting communication deficits and use of augmented feedback may aid in rehabilitation of patients with insight and safety awareness deficits.

Substantial work is underway to unpack the 'black box' of conventional therapy in order to aid research and identify efficacy of treatments. Several Cochrane reviews are available. Unfortunately, unequivocal research evidence for the efficacy of these interventions is, at present, limited.

Goal setting

Goal setting is an essential feature of physiotherapy treatment planning, and should be done in conjunction with the multidisciplinary team; placing the patient at the centre of the process. Goals should be specific, measurable, achievable, realistic, resourced, and timed (SMARRT). Most importantly, they should be functionally meaningful and expressed in a patient friendly language.

Physiotherapists use goal setting as an opportunity for the patient to express their expectations and priorities and for the patient to start taking a lead role in their own care planning. It is used as an educational platform, allowing the therapist to raise the patient's insight, as it provides a structure for the patient to self-monitor. It is also used by physiotherapists to motivate patients, by placing small hard-earned achievements into a functional context.

More generally, goal setting provides an opportunity to coordinate the actions of the team, by attributing shorter term goals and actions to individual team members, but at the same time keeping a focus on the longer term goal. As such, it is an invaluable tool for effective multi-disciplinary working and can facilitate interdisciplinary working.

Summary

Physiotherapists bring a broad scope of knowledge and skill to the multidisciplinary team. They are specialists in assessing mobility and physical compromise, but are mindful of the psychosocial presentation. They use a problem solving approach, starting from the point of functional compromise, and use these functional indicators, in conjunction with the patient, to inform goal setting.

Further reading

Ashworth B (1964). Preliminary trial of Carisoprodol in multiple sclerosis. *Practitioner*,**192**: 540–2.

Collen FM, Wade DT, Bradshaw CM (1990). Mobility after stroke: reliability of measures of impairment and disability. *Int Disabil Stud* **12**: 6–9.

Collin C, Wade DT, Davies S, et al. (1988). The Barthel ADL index: a reliability study. *Int Disabil Stud* **10**: 61–3.

Department of Health (2001). *National Service Framework for Older People*. Crown Copyright, UK.

Hastings M, Squires A (2002). *Rehabilitation of the Older Person. A Handbook for the Interdisciplinary Team*, 3rd edn.

Lincoln NB, Crow JL, Jackson JM, et al. (1991). The Unreliability of Sensory Assessments. *Clin Rehabil* **5**: 273–82.

Smith P, Hamilton BB, Granger CV, (1990). *The Fone FIM*. Buffalo, NY, Research Foundation of the State University of New York.

Wade DT (1992). *Measurement in Neurological Rehabilitation*. Oxford, Oxford University Press.

World Health Organization (2001). *International Classification of Functioning, Disability and Health* (ICF). Geneva, Switzerland, WHO.

Occupational therapy

Background

Occupational therapy aims to increase participation through improving body function and structure and reducing activity imitations in activities of daily living for people of all ages with physical, cognitive, and psychological limitations. Occupational therapy is mostly undertaken by occupational therapists (www.cot.co.uk) who are part of the Allied Health Professions (AHP) in the UK working in a multidisciplinary team. Occupational therapy for older people is delivered in hospital wards and the Emergency Departments, outpatients, day hospitals, health centres, community centres, and increasingly in the patient's home. Occupational therapists are mostly employed by the NHS or Social Services in the UK, but are gradually being employed by other organisations such as Job Centres, charities, GP practices, housing associations, residential and nursing homes, and private health organizations.

Occupational therapy interventions for the older person

Occupational therapy follows the rehabilitation process and is a recognizable series of sequential actions by the therapist that hopefully lead to actions by the participant. Creek has described 11 different actions that an occupational therapist might use: referral, assessment, goal setting, action, and others through to discharge. Occupational therapy interventions for an older person can be wide ranging, such as dressing practice, getting back to work, looking after grand children, cooking, shopping, hobbies, and using the computer. Goals are broken down by the therapist and patient into achievable tasks which are documented in the notes and updated weekly.

There is a growing research literature which indicates that occupational therapy can be very effective at helping older patients regain independence after an acute medical incident and in living with a long-term condition. The most effective interventions are targeted to a particular limitation such as mobility, occur over a few months, and have been most successful in the community. For stroke patients, the use of occupational therapy can lead to an increase in activities of daily living such as dressing oneself, increased outdoor mobility, and leisure activities. This is mostly achieved by patients getting the chance to practice activities over many sessions in a graded way but may be achieved through the timely prescription and supply of assistive technology, such as a raised toilet seat or second star rail. Pre-discharge home visits organized by occupational therapists are a routine part of rehabilitation, but care needs to be taken when they are organized as although they have been found to alleviate carers concerns, they can make patients more anxious. However, a feasibility study in Australia suggested that home visits had a positive effect on independence in activities of daily living 12 weeks after discharge. Occupational therapy as part of a team approach for falls prevention has been proven to reduce the rate of falls in high-risk patients.

Duration of occupational therapy

An occupational therapy session is routinely 45–60 minutes. However, the total number of sessions required is very variable. The provision and teaching use of equipment may take only two sessions while enabling a stroke patient to live at home independently may take many months. Occupational therapy can be sometimes delivered in group sessions where patients are encouraged to share their experiences. Occupational therapists will include family, carers and employers in the treatment sessions if needed.

Referral to an occupational therapist

All occupational therapists should be registered with the HPC (www.hpc-uk.org) but may be listed as part of a team such as the Falls Prevention team or Early Supported Discharge Team. The referral process depends on who funds the rehabilitation service. Most NHS and Social Service Occupational Therapy services in the UK will accept referrals from the patient or carer plus other health professionals, police, ambulance service, fire service as long as the patient is aware of the referral.

> **Author's Tip**
>
> There is evidence that occupational therapy for older people is more effective in their own home. If possible refer to community-based services.

Conclusion

Occupational therapy is an essential part of an older person's rehabilitation package as it has been shown effective at improving quality of life indicators such as personal activities of daily living, outdoor mobility, and leisure activities.

Further reading

Atwal A, McIntyre A, Craik C, Hunt J (2008). Older adults and carers' perceptions of pre-discharge occupational therapy home visits in acute care. *Age Ageing* **37**: 72–6.

Creek J (2002). *Occupational Therapy Defined as a Complex Intervention*. London, College of Occupational Therapists.

Department of Health (2001). National Service Framework for Older People. London: Department of Health.

Drummond AE, Walker MF (1995). A randomised controlled trial of leisure rehabilitation after stroke. *Clin Rehabil* **9**: 283–90.

Lannin N, Clemson L, McCluskey A, et al (2007). Feasibility and results of a randomised pilot-study of pre-discharge occupational therapy home visits. *BMC Health Serv Res* **7**: 42.

Logan P, Ahern J, Gladman J, Lincoln N (1997). A randomised controlled trial of enhanced Social Service occupational therapy for stroke patients. *Clin Rehabil* **11**: 107–13.

Logan P, Gladman J, Avery A, et al. (2004). Randomised controlled trial of an occupational therapy intervention to increase outdoor mobility after stroke. *BMJ* **329**: 1372–5.

Logan PA, Coupland C, Gladman JRF, et al. (2010). Community falls prevention for people who call an emergency ambulance after a fall: randomised controlled trial. *BMJ* **340**:c2102.

Wade DT, A de Jong B (2000). Recent advances in rehabilitation. *BMJ* **320**: 1385–8.

Walker MF, Drummond AER, Lincoln NB (1996). Evaluation of dressing practice for stroke patients after discharge from hospital: a crossover design study. *Clin Rehabil* **10**: 23–31.

Aids and appliances

Aids and appliances, otherwise referred to as 'community equipment', or 'assistive technology', cover a range of devices and technologies designed to help older and disabled people with daily living in their usual environments. Some products are related to particular health needs, whereas others are designed to help in carrying out particular activities. However, the provision of aids has the potential to transform the lives of people with a variety of different impairments, enhancing their functional activity, and contributing to their independence.

Different types of aids and appliances

Equipment relating to particular health needs is usually available through local health services. Examples of this type of product include pressure relieving cushions and mattresses to avoid the development of pressure ulcers, garments and pads to contain incontinence, elastic stockings which provide compression to relieve aching symptomatic varicose veins, or prevent post-thrombotic syndrome, and products for ileostomies and colostomies such as bags and belts.

Another specific type of equipment comprises those items which provide or assist mobility. Wheelchairs are perhaps the most obvious, but other products include walking sticks or canes, three-wheel rollators, quad sticks, walking frames, and ramps, which can help when crossing door thresholds or enable wheelchair users to avoid the need to climb steps when accessing buildings. Fixed hoists, ceiling tracking, and slings also fall into this category, as do transfer aids such as boards and slides.

The largest group of aids are those which are designed to help performance in activities of daily living, such as eating, food preparation, and personal hygiene. This wide range of products includes those with padded or elongated handles to help with reach and grip. Such products range from the very simple, such as slip-resistant mats and jar openers, to larger powered items, such as motor powered bath lifts (see Figure 15.4), which enable users to get into and out of the bath, either independently, or with support from a carer.

A more specialized group of products are those designed for people with sensory impairment, such as hearing or sight loss. Websites run by voluntary organizations are often a good source of information, and many products can be purchased directly from such sites. An example in the UK is the RNIB (Royal National Institute for the Blind), whose pages include information about their Talking Books service and their online shop, stocking items such as braillers, electronic key locators, magnifiers, and light bulbs.

Another closely related group are communications aids, designed to help people to communicate more effectively with those around them. These include books or charts, symbols or systems (such as Makaton), and aids which 'speak', using either pre-recorded or computer-generated language.

The final group of aids and appliances considered here are prosthetic limbs and surgical appliances such as artificial breasts (used following mastectomy), wigs, and bespoke footwear.

Functional challenges which aids and appliances can address

Long-term conditions and sudden illness episodes can result in a wide variety of problems in carrying out

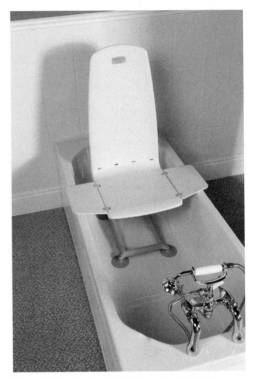

Figure 15.4 Archimedes Bath Lift. Reproduced with kind permission of Mangar International Ltd.

activities of daily living. Although some equipment has been designed to address very specific requirements, other products can be of use to older people with a wide range of impairments. This section considers the impairments and resulting disabilities which aids and community equipment can help address.

Products with wide application are those designed to assist function where there is restricted or painful movement, often caused by arthritis. These include raised toilet seats, toilet frames, and chair raisers, of help to those with painful or immobile hips caused by osteoarthritis, for example, and a range of homeware and personal care items with enlarged and elongated handles which can assist those with rheumatoid conditions, resulting in problems particularly in the small joints of the hands. Many mobility aids will also be of use to people with arthritic conditions, with walking sticks, rollators, and walking frames frequently used by those who experience pain and difficulty walking.

Similarly, items which can help relieve fatigue and conserve energy have wide application, for example for those with neurological conditions (such as Parkinson's disease or multiple sclerosis), and within palliative care. Products in this category include stair lifts, shower stools, and devices which can help the user guide food to their mouth, enabling them to eat independently.

Specific conditions for which equipment has been designed include stroke, hearing and visual impairment and communication difficulties. A range of devices designed to facilitate everyday activities for those with use of one hand is available. These include the 'spork' (an item of cutlery incorporating spoon, knife, and fork), footwear with Velcro fastenings (rather than shoelaces), and can openers and cheese graters which can be operated with one hand.

Equipment provided for health reasons, such as pressure relieving equipment and incontinence aids, are used in a variety of scenarios, but can substantially contribute to the care and dignity of very frail and confused older people.

One of the most important considerations in working with older people is the high likelihood of multiple impairments and challenges. Although there may be an obvious presenting functional problem, there will often be additional issues which need to be considered in the provision of equipment. An individual whose primary problem appears to be loss of function due to a dense hemiplegia might, for example, also be experiencing confusion or impairment which could preclude the use of some of the one handed kitchen items (see Case study).

Perhaps some of the most exciting recent developments in the field of assistive technology have been those designed to help people with cognitive problems, such as memory loss and perceptual difficulties. These are considered more fully in the section entitled Recent developments in assistive technology.

Considerations in supplying aids and appliances

In reviewing the prerequisites for successful supply and use of assistive technology, the Assist UK's Trusted Assessor Competence Framework initiative identifies a number of considerations in the provision of aids and equipment:

- the service user
- the task or activity for which a solution is required
- the environment within which the activity is carried out
- the equipment (or alternative solution).

Recommendations are also influenced by the reasoning skills of the practitioner, the professional regulations governing their practice, and the supply process.

This section will review each of these issues in turn, and provide examples to demonstrate their influence, and the interplay between them.

Service user

Some of the elements in relation to the service user (i.e. the potential impact of function impairments on an individual's lifestyle and daily activity) have been briefly considered within the previous section.

However, it is critical to reinforce the inclusion of the service user as an active partner in the centre of considerations about appropriate equipment provision, rather than assume a level of need in relation to their impairment. Effective and empathetic communication is essential in order to understand the individual's priorities and preferences for daily living activities. This could be more challenging in some circumstances, for example, if the individual has dysphasia or dysarthria following a stroke, or is confused. In such scenarios, reference to family members or carer will also be important.

The provision of most aids and appliances should be accompanied by education and advice about how the products should be used. Ideally, this will be provided *in situ*, with demonstration and practice. However, this is not always possible, and in such circumstances, the information provided will be of particular importance. In addition to visual demonstration supported with verbal explanation,

the supply of written information (including further contact details in case of problems) to which the service user can refer is helpful.

Case study

Mr T, a 72-year-old man living at home with his wife, experienced a stroke resulting in left hemiplegia, left-sided neglect, and some cognitive difficulties.

He was admitted to hospital, and at 2 months is ready to commence more active rehabilitation with the full support of his wife and two sons. Jane, the occupational therapist, carries out a full assessment, in conjunction with the multidisciplinary team on the ward, and establishes that while initial cognitive difficulties with planning, memory, and left-sided visual neglect seem to be improving, Mr T still has left-sided weakness and oedema. Practically, this means that Mr T still has difficulties with washing, dressing, eating, and mobilizing (walking and transfers). In discussion with Mrs T, Jane establishes that Mr and Mrs T do not have a shower at home.

Jane, Susan, the physiotherapist and Dave, the allied health professions assistant, begin working daily with Mr T, focusing on personal care and eating, transferring on and off the bed, toilet and in and out of the chair, and independent walking.

Mr T is taught to use a tripod to help with walking, strategies to dress himself and begins to practise using a bath board and bath seat in order that he can get into and out of the bath more easily. The chairs on the ward are all of sufficient height for Mr T to be able to rise relatively easily, and several of the toilets in the ward area have toilet frames and raised toilet seats, which Mr T also finds useful. At mealtimes, he practices using a plate surround as he has difficulty holding a knife in his left hand. As his rehabilitation progresses, Mrs T regularly visits to encourage, support, and learn with her husband in preparation for his return home.

Mr T makes good progress, and the team plan for his discharge. Jane carries out a home visit with Mr and Mrs T, to enable the couple to determine what difficulties he might experience once home. She arranges the loan and delivery of bath aids, toilet aids and Mr T purchases a plate surround from the small aids store at the hospital. He is able to take the walking aid home, also on long-term loan. Jane discusses the possibility of fitting some bed risers under each leg of the bed to elevate it in order to assist with rising. However, Mr and Mrs T decide to purchase a new bed, which is both higher and has a firmer mattress. Mr T's existing armchair is upright and has arms, and he is able to sit and stand independently.

Six months following discharge, Mr T has continued to make a good recovery, and he has regained more use of his left hand. He has bought a large handled knife, and no longer needs his plate surround. He is now using a walking stick rather than a tripod to walk.

Task or activity

The professional or carer assisting the older person to make a choice about potential options should be able to consider the component parts in carrying out the relevant tasks. Another factor sometimes overlooked is the ease with which a carer can use or operate the assistive device. In such scenarios, it may be equally important to focus on the learning of the carer.

Another consideration is the activity for which the individual is requiring help, and the meaning that this has for them. In a powerful example in Seymour (1998), a young mother with a spinal cord injury, Francis, tells how her rehabilitation focused on managing stairs and getting to and from the bathroom, but never within the context of her role as a mother, and considering how her mobility solutions impacted on this and on her baby. Older people potentially have a number of important social roles such as spouse, mother/father and grandparent, and in addition, may themselves be carers. It will therefore be important to accommodate the equipment within the context of the person's daily routines, which may involve other people.

Environment

In considering environmental factors in the provision of aids and equipment, the emphasis is usually on the physical barriers present which present challenges to the service user. Steps or high door thresholds for those with mobility problems, for example, can present problems with access. In such a scenario, there is a range of potential solutions, including the use of ramps, levelling of door thresholds, and the installation of a stairlift. A focus on physical barriers to function is undoubtedly important. The environment, however, can also be interpreted more widely to additionally include geography (for example, urban or rural location), attitudes, and culture. An understanding of the impact of geography or location on activity might suggest alternative solutions. In preference to enhanced mobility in order to carry out grocery shopping, for example an older person with limited mobility living in a more remote region might prefer to consider use of the internet to order shopping, or to arrange for a carer to do a regular shop.

Louise-Bender Pape et al highlighted how attitudinal or culture environments can impact on the acceptability of assistive technology. In their exploration of personal meanings, they highlight how the use of equipment within some cultures could signify 'dishonour, disgrace and embarrassment'. This reinforces the importance of exploring the possible provision of aids with sensitivity and with the full involvement of the service user, and where appropriate, their carer and/or family.

Equipment

New solutions to functional challenges are continuously being developed and marketed. In considering options for assistive devices, it is often useful to access individuals or resources with specialist knowledge about different ranges of equipment, such as occupational therapists (considered further below). The different types of aids have been outlined initially, but further considerations in supply include sources, cost, and the potential for customizing. In fitting the equipment, an appreciation of technical factors such as fitting or stabilising is important (for example, some types of assistive devices used in bathing are not recommended for plastic baths). The installation of major adaptations such as fixed hoists, walk in showers and stair lifts requires the input of specialists such as a surveyor or builder.

Other important considerations with respect to the equipment include maintenance and cost, and in the case of large adaptations, such as stairlifts, cover for breakdown or malfunction.

Other considerations

Further suggestions impacting on equipment provision include the importance of a comprehensive risk assessment, an appreciation of the legislative and professional practice frameworks surrounding equipment provision, and knowledge about local policies and procedures for equipment supply.

Mechanisms for supply

Internet searching will confirm the large number of manufacturers and retailers in the field of assistive technology from whom products can be purchased directly. Some simple items may not require any additional advice or information to support their use. However, with larger or more complex items, it is important to consider if the retailer has the prerequisite knowledge, skills, and experience to make suitable recommendations.

Independent advice can be sought from some of the organizations identified in the Further reading section at the end of this chapter. Additionally, demonstration centres resourced by statutory or voluntary organizations can provide an opportunity to view equipment. In the UK, for example, Assist UK leads a national network of over 60 Disabled Living Centres (alternatively known as Independent Living or Assistive Technology Centres). It is possible to try a range of different types of equipment at such centres, and also to receive impartial advice from experienced staff, many of whom are qualified occupational therapists.

Also in the UK, social service departments (England and Wales), social work departments (Scotland) or health or social services boards/trusts (Northern Ireland) can also provide some products such as beds, chairs, bathing, and personal care equipment, hoists, and products to help with activities of daily living. The range of equipment and funding available will vary, but an assessment usually by an occupational therapist or other professional is generally required.

Local authorities can also fund major home adaptations, such as fixed hoists, walk in showers and stairlifts. Again, an assessment by an occupational therapist will be required.

Equipment to assist with mobility and communication is in general supplied through the NHS in the UK, through referral to physiotherapy and speech and language therapy departments. Similarly, aids to help with health needs such as incontinence products will be supplied by community or district nurses, accessed through referral by a general practitioner.

Grants and equipment may also be available through both local and national charities and welfare associations.

Addressing problems with provision

Research into the provision of assistive technology suggests there are high rates of non-use. This represents a waste of resource and continuing levels of unmet need. Factors influencing use include a perception of equipment as heavy or cumbersome, concerns about safety, and negative views about the appearance of the product.

Following in-depth interviews with 67 older people, all of whom had received some form of assistive technology, a model to explain the acceptability or otherwise of assistive technology to older people was developed. The first component of the model influencing acceptability was described as the 'felt need for assistance', itself dependent on service user characteristics (individual preferences, disability, living arrangements and carer needs), and the housing type and design. The second component related to the assistive technology, in that users wanted products or solutions which worked 'properly, reliably and safely'.

The third element influencing acceptability of assistive devices for older people focuses on access to such products. This may be dependent on knowledge that support is available, the systems or processes used by organizations to determine need, or the financial resources of the older service user themselves.

Consideration of all the elements outlined previously in relation to aids and equipment should help to ensure a match between the different elements of McCreadie and Tinker's model, resulting in the successful provision of assistive technology which meets need and is perceived as useful.

Recent developments in assistive technology

Innovations in computer programming and software have had a significant impact on the design and applications of assistive technology in recent years. This section provides information about two developments reflecting these changes: telecare and smart housing. The topic is covered in more detail in Chapter 26, Gerotechnology.

Telecare is generally understood to mean remote systems and devices which automatically alert help if there is a lack of response from a service user. This technology can be applied in a variety of different ways to help support older people to continue to live independently, although risk has been acknowledged. Automatic sensors can modify the environment if, for example, gas or water is left turned on, and temperature can also be monitored remotely. Discreet devices can also monitor a change in activity, for example if an older person does not get into bed at their usual time, or if they don't appear to have moved for a considerable period, perhaps because of a fall or loss of consciousness. Telecare systems can be installed to remind people with memory loss about their daily routines, such as the time to take their medication, and the need to remain indoors at night. Telehealth devices can also monitor body systems such as circulation and breathing, and alert services if there are sudden and unexpected changes.

Smart houses are designed so that key appliances and services can be operated simply, using technology such as a mobile phone, or can ensure that some functions occur automatically. Examples of the application of technology in such houses include automatic temperature setting for water and heating; lights which operate automatically at night; settings which simulate occupancy of the home when the owner is out; programming of the television to record remotely; fridges that alert owners to food past its sell-by date; electrical appliances which trigger a service call when a component fails.

The application of computer technology in products used in everyday living such as talking labels, keyless locks, and height-adjustable surfaces is increasingly featured in everyone's lives and it has perhaps the potential to make most difference to a group of older people for whom assistive devices have had limited use, those with dementia. Many of the systems described here can enable people with dementia to continue to live independently and safely at home for longer.

Conclusion

Aids and equipment have the potential to significantly improve the lives of older and disabled people. The design, manufacture and retail of such products is increasing exponentially as the population ages. In addition, health and social care and voluntary organizations have invested significant resources in assistive technology, understanding that it is cost-effective and can support older peoples' aspirations to continue living independently.

However, it is easy to view assistive technology as a panacea, and McCreadie and Tinker identify several notes of caution which should be heeded in the supply of aids and equipment.

- First, that there may be a difference in perception of need for equipment between the professional and the service user, and that in order for aids to be optimally useful, older people should be fully involved in their provision
- Second, that older people value their homes as expressions of their identity and enjoy their comfort and familiarity. Potential alterations to the character of a home through the provision of equipment may be unwelcome, and affect the product's acceptability
- Finally, that although there may be cost benefits associated with assistive technology, it should not replace human contact, care, and support.

Further reading

Louise-Bender PT, Kim J, Weiner B (2002). The shaping of individual meanings assigned to assistive technology: a review of personal factors. *Disabil Rehabil* **24**: 5–20.

McCreadie C, Tinker A (2005). The acceptability of assistive technology to older people. *Ageing Soc* **25**: 91–110.

Ricability (2007) What's new? Newer devices and gadgets for older and disabled people (http://www.ricability.org.uk/consumer_reports/at_home/whats_new).

Seymour W (1998). *Remaking the Body: Rehabilitation and Change.* London, Taylor and Francis.

Winchcombe M, Ballinger C (2005). *A Competence Framework for Trusted Assessors.* London, Assist UK (http://www.cot.co.uk/Mainwebsite/Resources/Document/Competence_framework.pdf).

Disabled Living Foundation Website (http://www.dlf.org.uk).

Foundation for Assistive Technology Website (http://www.fastuk.org/home.php)

Assist UK Website (http://www.assist-uk.org)

Royal National Institute for the Blind Website (http://www.rnib.org.uk/Pages/Home.aspx).

Speech and language therapy

Speech and language therapists (SLTs) have a role in the assessment and management of older people with acquired speech, language, and swallowing difficulties within acute and community settings. Accurate identification of breakdown in both communication and swallowing is essential for effective rehabilitation and for the differential diagnosis of types of communication/swallowing disorders.

Common causes of language and communication disruption in older people include degenerative diseases such as Parkinson's disease, cerebrovascular disease, head injury, and dementia. These may result in dysphasia and/or motor speech disorders such as dyspraxia or dysarthria and dysphagia.

Aphasia

Ageing does not result in speech and communication disorders but some changes occur with age such as naming difficulties, reduced syntactic complexity, increased verbosity and tendency to not maintain the reference of discourse.

The most common cause of aphasia is cerebrovascular disease. Aphasia is a multimodal disorder potentially affecting all aspects of language including

- speaking
- listening
- reading (acquired dyslexia)
- writing (acquired dysgraphia).

Twenty per cent to 30% of stroke survivors experience aphasia; 15% have ongoing problems up to 6 months post stroke. Early assessment and diagnosis is essential. Historically, labels for types of aphasia reflected their presumed neuroanatomical origin in the left hemisphere, such as Broca's or Wernicke's aphasia. Currently linguistic symptoms are identified in the consideration of assessment and treatment. The terms below are not exhaustive but characterise types of aphasia.

Fluent aphasia
- Reduced comprehension of language
- Long often incoherent utterances with intact intonation
- Jargon: words are linked to make meaningless utterances
- Neologisms (creation of new words) e.g. an 'ommah' for a watch
- Difficulty monitoring and correcting their own output
- Perseveration
- Lexical retrieval problems (word finding difficulties)

Non-fluent aphasia
- Relatively preserved comprehension
- Awareness and frustration with language production difficulties.
- Short utterances with reduced sentence structure
- Loss of function words and verbs results in telegrammatic speech e.g. instead of 'I will go for a walk' says 'I walk'
- Semantic paraphasias, e.g. chair for table

Assessment

Linguistic assessment of language breakdown is essential. Language screens may be used, such as the Frenchay Aphasia Screening Test (FAST) and more in depth language batteries such as the Boston Diagnostic Aphasia Examination (BDAE). It is not clear, however, whether linguistic performance on assessment gives a true picture of someone's communicative abilities at conversational level, thus it is essential to investigate how a person's language is affected in everyday situations.

Aphasia rehabilitation

Paramount is the establishment of a method of communication prior to any impairment work. Realistic communication goals will be set with the patient and family.

Rehabilitation will include one or more:

- Individual work on specific language impairments. May involve a number of modalities per time such as writing and comprehension. May address specific areas of language such as syntax or semantics.
- Consideration of alternative/augmentative communication (AAC).
- Explanation of language breakdown and how to support communication, with all communication partners (including MDT).
- Training of conversational partners. This has been shown to be effective.
- Use of total communication via all modalities such as writing, drawing and gesture.
- Consideration of group rehabilitation: studies demonstrated psychosocial benefits.

> **Author's Tip**
>
> Ensure opportunities for communication on a daily basis. Consider the environment, is it conducive to communication?

Consideration of the psychosocial impact of aphasia is needed to ensure that lack of confidence and anxiety does not reduce the desire to communicate or result in social isolation. Quality of life measures, such as the stroke and aphasia quality of life scale (SAQOL) by Hilari and colleagues can be used throughout the rehabilitation period to monitor this.

Motor speech disorders

Dysarthria – disruption in the force, range and coordination of movements required for breathing, phonation, resonance, and articulation. Results in unclear or unintelligible speech, ranging from mild articulatory difficulties to severe unintelligibility. Differential diagnosis of type of dysarthria is essential for treatment planning via assessments such as the Frenchay Dysarthria Test.

Dyspraxia—a disorder in the motor programming for speech. Speech may be effortful with obvious groping movements of the oral articulators to find the correct articulatory position. Awareness of difficulties and frustration are common.

Management
- Establishment of optimal method of communication.
- Specific techniques to improve intelligibility using motor programming principles.
- Consideration of AAC, such as alphabet charts or electronic communication aids.
- Work with communication partners to support strategies.

Comorbidities common in older people may impact on rehabilitation, such as cognitive impairment, cerebrovascular disease, chronic obstructive pulmonary disease, fatigue, poor vision and hearing. This may restrict frequency of practice, selection of, for example AAC, or intensity/ choice of intervention for speech and communication.

Dysphagia

There is evidence of some prolonged oropharyngeal transit times with ageing. The impact of poor dentition, possible weakening of oral and pharyngeal musculature and psychosocial issues such as depression must be considered in differential diagnosis in the older people and not mistaken for dysphagia.

Dysphagia may result in malnutrition, dehydration, aspiration, and pneumonia with a marked impact on quality of life. The SLT role is to assess and manage the dysphagia with the MDT to maintain nutrition, reduce risk and optimize enjoyment of eating and drinking. Over 40% of conscious individuals have dysphagia following stroke. Up to 30% of older people are admitted to hospital with dysphagia.

Breakdown of swallow

Impaired lingual, labial or buccal musculature results in reduced manipulation, control and formation of a food / liquid bolus ready for swallowing. There may be overspill and aspiration prior to the swallow. Breakdown at the reflex pharyngeal stage of swallowing may result in delayed swallowing, poor clearance of food/liquids, reduced laryngeal protection and thus potential for aspiration.

Author's Tip

Risk factors for aspiration pneumonia include lack of self-feeding, poor oral hygiene and dentition.

Assessment

- Bedside assessment—screening for dysphagia and aspiration risk, but variable reliability.
- Instrumental and radiological techniques such as videofluoroscopy and fibreoptic endoscopic evaluation of swallowing (FEES) when appropriate.
- Quality of life measures such as the swallowing quality of life tool by McHorney et al. SWAL-QOL.
- Liaison with the MDT – dietician, nurses physiotherapists, occupational therapists.

Management

There are three main approaches in management strategies used in dysphagia:

- Dietary modification of texture, bolus size and temperature.

Soft food if difficulty chewing or thickened fluids for delayed pharyngeal swallow/poor oral control. Reduced compliance with modification of diet and liquids has been demonstrated. An increased adherence to advice on swallowing was shown after brief training sessions to relevant professionals.

- Compensatory strategies (chin tuck on swallowing, small mouthfuls with a double swallow).
- Direct intervention techniques (such as effortful swallow).

Consideration of non-oral feeding with the MDT will take place if a patient appears unsafe to continue with oral intake, in order to maintain hydration and nutrition. However, it should be noted that non-oral feeding routes, such as percutaneous gastrostomy do not abolish the risk of aspiration completely.

Conclusion

SLT are involved in the rehabilitation of communication and swallowing disorders in older people in close liaison with the rest of the MDT.

Further reading

Carnaby G, Hankey G J, Pizzi J. (2006) Behavioural intervention for dysphagia in acute stroke: a randomised controlled trial. *Lancet Neurol* **5**: 31–7.

Cummings L (2008). *Clinical Linguistics.* EUP, Edinburgh

Cunningham R, Ward D (2003). Evaluation of a training programme to facilitate conversation between people with aphasia and their partners. *Aphasiology* **17**: 687–707.

Enderby P, Wood V, Wade D (2006). *Frenchay Aphasia Screening Test.* Chichester, Wiley.

Goodglass H, Kaplan E, Barresi B (2001). *Boston Diagnostic Aphasia Examination*, 3rd edn. Baltimore MD, Lippincott Williams & Wilkins.

Hilari K, Byng S (2009). Health–related quality of life in people with RCSLT (2006). *Communicating Quality 3*. London, RCSLT.

Hilari K, Byng S (2009).Severe aphasia. *Int J Lang Commun Disord*, **44**: 193–205.

Kendall K, Leonard R, McKenzie S (2004). Common medical conditions in the elderly: impact on pharyngeal bolus transit. *Dysphagia* **19**: 71–7.

McHorney C, Bricker D, Lomax K, et al. (2002). The SWAL-QOL and SWAL-CARE outcomes tool for oropharyngeal dysphagia in adults III: Documentation of reliability and validity. *Dysphagia* **17**: 97–114.

Rosenvinge SK, Starke D (2005). Improving care for patients with dysphagia. *Age Ageing* **34**: 587–93.

Ross A, Winslow I, Marchant P, Brumfitt S (2006). Evaluation of communication, life participation and psychological well-being in chronic aphasia: the influence of group intervention. *Aphasiology* **20**: 427–8.

Systems of care in older people

Systems of care for older people in hospital

Not all cases of acute illness can be managed in the community. Some, such as hip fracture, stroke, or severe acute medical illness requiring intensive supportive care, require admission to hospital for specific diagnosis and management.

Only 50 years ago, the debate was not about how to meet the needs of sick and frail older people, but how to secure access to hospital inpatient facilities. It is often forgotten these days, but previous generations of sick older people were often denied access to diagnosis, treatment, and rehabilitation, instead being confined to long-stay facilities which were a legacy of the Victorian workhouse infirmaries. Even after access to hospital inpatient care had been secured for older people, it was not uncommon for them to have only partial access to the range of available inpatient technologies (such as, for example, coronary or intensive care units).

The battle of access has been largely won, and today the majority of hospital inpatients are older people, with up to two-thirds of acute hospital admissions for General Medicine in the UK being over the age of 60 years. The debate has moved on and it is now important to try and ensure that the inpatient assessment process and care environment are optimized for the best outcomes for older people.

In the absence of comorbidity and/or factors indicating a degree of frailty (such as, for example, loss of physical or cognitive functioning, incontinence, or falls), older inpatients can probably be managed most effectively using the usual inpatient care processes for their presenting complaint. However, patients presenting with geriatric clinical syndromes need a need a more broad-based diagnostic/ therapeutic approach.

Comprehensive geriatric assessment (CGA) provides such a broad-based approach. The use of CGA with hospital inpatients is supported by evidence from multiple sources, including systematic literature reviews and meta-analysis of randomized controlled trials. However, there is still some debate about the best ways of organizing and delivering hospital inpatient care to meet the needs of those inpatients who are most likely to benefit from CGA.

Assessment of frail older inpatients are structured and multifactorial. They include paying due attention not just to the diagnosis of immediate health problems but also cognitive and psychosocial functioning and the use of standard approaches to improve self-care, continence, nutrition, mobility, sleep, skin care, mood, and transition.

Dedicated inpatient units in various forms have been shown to be effective ways to deliver CGA and are associated with health benefits. Examples include condition-specific units for stroke and hip fracture management, inpatient evaluation and management units, including specific Acute Care Environments (or ACE units) for general acute inpatient care. These units include the provision of safe flooring and orientation cues (such as large clocks and calendars). Ideally aids to mobility and self-care (such as handrails and raised toilet seats) should be integral to the care environment.

Delirium is a specific problem which is common in acute care of frail older people. Appropriate management of frail older people in acute hospital care includes measures to minimise the incidence and impact of delirium and multi-component interventions which meet this aim have been described. These include care processes that emphasize non-pharmacological approaches to difficult or challenging behavioural symptoms, and the avoidance of physical restraint and catheterisation.

The delivery of CGA in other ways for hospital inpatients, for example by providing CGA as a consultation service, have a less profound effect on outcomes.

Finally, best practice in inpatient care for frail older people values the process of care transfer after the acute episode and so planning for discharge begins as soon as the admission has occurred. Discharge arrangements are most effectively organized across the hospital/community interface, involving cooperation between hospital and community services which are focused on the patient's best interest and can make a significant contribution to minimizing unplanned hospital readmission after discharge.

Further reading

Baztán JJ, Suárez-Garc´a FM, López-Arrieta J, et al. (2009). Effectiveness of acute geriatric units on functional decline, living at home, and case fatality among older patients admitted to hospital for acute medical disorders: meta-analysis. Br Med J 338: b50.

Parker G, Bhakta P, Katbamna S, et al. (2000). Best place of care for older people after acute and during sub-acute illness: a systematic review. J Health Serv Res Policy 5: 176–89.

Case management

The origins of care or case management lie in the need for coordination of a range of support, provided from a range of sources to achieve a common goal of effective care and support. A definition of intensive care/case management can be found in the presence of several features as shown in the box. Intensive care/case management is designed for the community care of vulnerable people with complex and fluctuating needs. These patients often require a multi-service response rather than those with less complex needs which are often met by a single service response provided by one agency.

Features of intensive care/case management

- **Core tasks**: case finding and screening; assessment; care planning; monitoring and review
- **Functions:** coordination and linkage of care services
- **Goals**: providing continuity and integrated care; increased opportunity for home-based care; make better use of resources; promote well-being of older person
- **Small caseloads**: to permit attention to fluctuating need and risk; titrating resources to needs
- **Target population**: long-term care needs; multiple service requirements; risk of institutional placement
- **Differentiating features of long-term care**: intensity of involvement; breadth of services spanned; lengthy duration of involvement with older person
- **Multi-level response**: dual function of Intensive Case Management in coordinating care at user level and generating information to help inform service commissioning to develop more appropriate support

Source: Challis 2003

Rationale

The development of case management has been the focus of many policy discussions in both the health and social care sectors internationally over a considerable period of time. Both the terms *care* management and *case* management have been regularly used to describe this practice.

A key component of the community care reforms in the 1990s was the introduction of care management arrangements. These had the underlying aims of cost containment and promoting choice. The aim was to shift the delivery and accountability of social care away from institution based services towards care at home. Some of the earliest studies of care management in the UK were the Kent, Gateshead, Darlington, and Lewisham Schemes undertaken by PSSRU based in social care, primary care, geriatric services, and old age psychiatry. This model of care management was designed to ensure that improved performance of the core tasks of care management could contribute towards more effective and efficient long-term care for highly vulnerable people. Devolution of control of resources, within an overall cost framework, to individual care managers was designed to permit more flexible responses to needs and integration of fragmented services into a planned pattern of care to provide a realistic alternative to institutional care for highly vulnerable older people. Overall, the findings of these intensive care management studies suggest an increased efficiency in the provision of social care with improved outcomes at similar or slightly lower costs. Subsequently, it has become important to distinguish between a 'care management approach' to care coordination for the majority of cases and 'intensive care management' for those cases where needs are more complex and risk greater.

Similarly, the later introduction of the NHS and social care model in England for long-term conditions attempts to offer a move away from a reliance on high-cost acute services towards treating more patients with enduring long-term health problems in community settings. Long-term conditions case management is intended to focus on patients with multiple complex needs. It is targeted predominantly towards older people. The role of community matrons, case managers with clinical nursing skills, was created to undertake the case management function, including medicine management and the provision of self-care skills training as appropriate. Personal care plans have been identified as a means of achieving coordinated care for people with long-term conditions. It has been suggested that case management within the long-term conditions service in England is differentiated from other programmes for frail elders by the inclusion of psycho-social support. However, there is some evidence that within the nurse/patient relationship one of the barriers to self-management is the dependent role accorded to the latter. Furthermore, the efficacy of self-care must be seen in the context of the patient's expectations, their history of health service use and the wider system of healthcare provision.

In both health and social care approaches, the emphasis is on providing a coordinated link between the range of agencies and organizations delivering care and those receiving it, in order to minimize the fragmentation of service provision for those with multiple health and social needs.

Settings

In the UK, there are three settings where case/care management is particularly evident. First, within local authority social care services, taking one of two forms: either a generic care coordination or care management approach or, for a much smaller group with complex health and social care needs, intensive care management is sometimes provided. Second, the latter approach can sometimes be seen in old age mental health services, where it is particularly used to support older people with dementia in the community. Third, more recently a form of intensive case management in primary care in conjunction with self-care support services is intended for those with long-term conditions as an alternative to unplanned hospital admissions. Case management for long-term conditions, therefore, has the broad aim of identifying 'very high-intensity users' of unplanned secondary care and actively managing their care to enable them to remain at home longer and require less unplanned reactive care from specialist services. However, currently the evidence for the presence of intensive case management in this service model is limited.

Effective case management

Studies indicate that intensive care/case management allied to social care is an approach which has a use in social care, primary care, geriatric medicine services, and old age mental health. It is sometimes, though not exclusively, delivered through a multidisciplinary team. With regard to intensive case management for long-term conditions, there is less UK evidence for effectiveness, with this being a relatively new development. It would appear that although patient and carer satisfaction may improve, the evidence that case management for patients with complex long-term conditions contributes to outcomes such as reducing hospital admission, length of stay and improving patient well being is equivocal.

Most studies of intensive care/case management have focussed upon populations with a high probability of admission or readmission to hospital or long-term care settings. The issue of programme fidelity, ensuring that the intervention continues to deliver the key elements through time, remains very important. It is possible to infer some common operational, organizational and financial success factors as shown in the box below. A recent review of case management for patients with long-term conditions confirmed this, identifying three key issues for developing a coherent and sustainable implementation of case management. These were fidelity to the core elements of case management; caseload size; and case management practice, incorporating matters relating to continuity of care, intensity, and breadth of involvement and control over resources.

Factors associated with positive outcomes

- **Integrated programme funding**—to reduce perverse incentives that can arise from narrow budgetary confines permitting effective integrated teams
- **Logical linkages between model of care, objectives of programme and practice level incentives**—so that the day to day world and pressures of practice remain congruent with the overall objectives (e.g. capacity to permit flexible response)
- **Clear service objectives with clearly articulated values**—offering a basis to manage and monitor programmes in terms of needs of recipients, service process such as costs and outcomes such as hospitalization, community tenure or quality of life
- **Precision and clarity of target population**—so that case management is directed upon those for whom it is most appropriate
- **Continuity of involvement**—with staff staying responsible for assessing, monitoring and reviewing cases and gaining feedback from effective and ineffective strategies, both at the individual level and more generally
- **Adequate service networks**—in the absence of a local service network intensive support at homes and choice are difficult to achieve
- **Flexible resources and responsive services; care/case manager influence upon services**—these may be devolved finance; care/case manager held personal budgets to permit creation of personalized responses

---

- **A single point of access**—offering uniform assessment and case management (organizational rather than geographic) and clarity about eligibility
- **Integrated programme funding**—to reduce perverse incentives that can arise from narrow budgetary confines permitting effective integrated teams

Source: Challis 2003.

Conclusion

As the British Geriatrics Society has stated: geriatricians provide high quality clinical care for older people as part of a multidisciplinary team during acute illness, chronic illness, rehabilitation and at the end of life, in both hospital and community settings. These are settings where case management for older people could flourish by providing care at home for patients who might otherwise be admitted to hospital or a care home. However implementation of effective case management will require coherent and logical models of intervention employing the key components listed above.

Further reading

Béland F, Bergman H, Lebel P (2006). A system of integrated care for older persons with disabilities in Canada: results from a randomized control trial. *J Gerontol A Biol Sci Med Sci* **61**: 367–73.

Challis D (2003). Achieving co-ordinated and integrated care among long term care services: the role of care management, in Brodsky J, Habib J and Hirschfeld M. (eds) *Key Policy Issues in Long Term Car.* Geneva, World Health Organization.

Challis D, Davies B (1986). *Case-Management in Community Care.* Aldershot, Gower.

Challis D, Darton R, Johnson L, et al. (1991). An evaluation of an alternative to long stay hospital care for frail elderly Patients: I. The model of care. *Age Ageing* **20**: 236–44.

Challis D, Darton R, Johnson L, et al. (1991). An evaluation of an alternative to long stay hospital care for frail elderly patients: II. Costs and effectiveness. *Age Ageing* **20**: 245–54.

Challis D, Darton R, Johnson L, et al. (1995). *Care Management and Health Care of Older People: The Darlington Community Care Project*, Ashgate, Aldershot.

Challis D, Chesterman J, Luckett R, et al. (2002). *Case Management in Social and Primary Health Care: The Gateshead Community Care Scheme*, Aldershot (Ashgate).

Challis D, von Abendorff R, Brown P, et al. (2002). Care management, dementia care and specialist mental health services: an evaluation. *Int J Ger Psychiatry* **17**: 315–25.

Challis D, Hughes J, Sutcliffe C, et al. (2009). *Supporting People with Dementia at Home.* Aldershot, Ashgate.

Challis D, Hughes J, Reilly S, et al. (2010). *Self Care and Case Management in Long Term Conditions: the Effective Management of Critical Interfaces* (http://www.sdo.nihr.ac.uk/projdetails. php?ref=08–1715–201).

Gravelle H, Dusheiko M, Sheaff R, et al. (2006). Impact of case management (Evercare) on outcomes for frail elderly patients: controlled before and after analysis of quantitative outcome data. *Br Med J* **334**: 31–4.

Reilly S, Hughes J, Challis D (2010). Case management for long-term conditions: implementation and processes. *Ageing Soc* **30**: 125–55.

Primary care perspective

Background

Current estimates predict that the proportion of people over 65 years will increase from 20% in 2000 to 35% in 2050; those aged 85 and over, the oldest old, are now the fastest growing sector of the population. Our ageing populations will lead to an increase in age-related illnesses, such as dementia and osteoarthritis. This may present considerable challenges for healthcare in the UK but particularly for primary care as current policy stipulates that care for older people, and for those with long-term conditions, should be delivered as close to their homes as possible.

The role of the general practitioner

In the UK, general practitioners (GPs), and their primary care teams, are an integral part of the NHS. The role of the GP has been defined as a doctor who gives personal, primary, and continuing care to individuals, families, and a practice population, irrespective of age, gender, and illness. His or her aim is to

- make early diagnoses;
- include and integrate physical, psychological, and social factors in considerations about health and illness
- undertake the continuing management of patients with chronic, recurrent, or terminal illnesses
- know how and when to intervene, through treatment, prevention, and education.

This concept of care gives GPs a unique involvement with the full range of health problems of older people, which are usually interwoven with personal and social problems. Good primary care also involves the rational use of hospital based resources which is achieved through the GP's 'gate-keeping' role.

The GP and the primary care team

Team working in primary care is essential to manage the complex demands of caring for an increasingly ageing population with long-term, multiple health problems. Within primary care, the trend is towards large multiple-partner practices; single-handed GPs account for only a fifth of all practices. The primary healthcare team may include a range of other professionals including

- practice-based nurses and community nurses
- nurse practitioners
- health visitors
- practice managers and administrative staff
- counsellors and community psychiatric nurses.

The last decade has seen an expansion in the role of nurses within primary care. Nurse practitioners are nurses with advanced clinical skills who can prescribe from a limited formulary; they increasingly deal with the acute, self-limiting illnesses presenting in primary care such as infections and musculoskeletal problems. Practice nurses can also become specialists in specific chronic illness management.

Primary care teams may also have access to physiotherapists, a social worker and other allied professionals depending on local service provision.

Organization of primary care services

In 2004, a new General Practice Contract was introduced into the NHS which classified GP services into essential core services and optional enhanced services that are additionally remunerated.

Within this contract, the implementation of a Quality and Outcomes Framework (QOF) linked achievements in both clinical care, and the organization of GP services, to financial rewards. In addition to receiving healthcare via registration with a local GP, older people may access a range of innovative primary care services such as:

- Walk-in centres: These are located in public places such as railway stations and supermarkets, although older people are less frequent consulters in these settings
- NHS Direct: A nationwide direct access telephone service. These centres are staffed with 24-hour availability by nurses who use computer based decision pathways to advise on self-care and initial management of illnesses.

Since 2004, statutory responsibility for ensuring the provision of out-of-hours care has been transferred from GPs to local Primary Care Trusts. GPs can choose to provide practice based 24-hour care 7 days a week, often within a 'cooperative' with other GP practices to share the workload or, through opting out of out-of-hours care and transferring responsibility to the Primary Care Trust who coordinate out-of-hours care either through GP deputizing services or via cooperatives based in emergency centres. For patients aged over 65, about half of all out-of-hours calls result in a home visit, and, of these, those aged over 75 had a hospital admission rate which was seven times that of infants.

Primary care, or practice-based, commissioning

The restructuring of the NHS has brought about a shift of resources from hospital to community. The greater emphasis on preventative care, the transfer of clinical responsibility for some chronic diseases from secondary to primary care, and the shift in service provision in order to deliver care closer to patients' homes has contributed to these demands.

In England, a new White Paper published in 2010, *Equity and Excellence: Liberating the NHS,* announced innovative changes for the commissioning and delivery of healthcare services. This recommended that local groups of general practices be in charge of commissioning services to meet the needs of their local populations through the formation of GP consortia which work together to develop innovative ways of contracting clinical patient services. The GP consortia will work closely with secondary care, mental health services and community partners with a focus on integrated, join-up services for all patients; this will be especially important for older people. This process is being fast-tracked through the GP Consortia Pathfinder Programme, in which early adopters of the consortia system will create new commissioning networks and test new ways of working

Innovative community services for older people

Locality commissioning of specialist services by Primary Care Trusts, or practice based commissioning, influences the development of healthcare strategies for local populations.

Through primary care-based commissioning initiatives, specialist community-based services for older people have been created to facilitate home-based care. These can include

- older people's assessment and management teams
- older people's mental health teams
- outpatient or 'outreach' clinics, which may be in the GP surgery
- domiciliary visiting by secondary care specialist, e.g. old age psychiatrists/geriatricians.

Intermediate care services

The development of rehabilitation and care schemes which are intermediate between acute hospital care and long-term institutional care has led to a range of alternative provision termed intermediate care. Such services are designed to maximize independence and prevent unnecessary hospital admissions. Most schemes offer short-term interventions (1–6 weeks) and involve cooperative working with other agencies including local authority social services, and the voluntary and private sectors. Examples of intermediate care services include:

- 'Hospital at home' or 'supported discharge' schemes: these involve early patient discharge from hospital with support from intensive home nursing.
- 'Rapid response' community nursing teams: maintain acutely ill patients at home via 24-hour care.

Another care option for frail older people, when insufficient home care or community support makes home care impossible and when hospital admission is declined, is admission to a community hospitals or nursing home; GPs and their multidisciplinary teams also provide first-line care in these situations with support from specialist colleagues.

Epidemiology of primary care of older people

The average list size for a general practice in the UK is between 6000 and 8000 for an average partnership, and corresponds to an average workload for each doctor of approximately 1700 patients. A full-time GP with an average list size can expect to care for approximately 140 patients aged 65–74 (8.1%), 95 patients aged over 75 (5.6%), and about 30 (1.8%) aged over 85 years.

Information from the General Practice Research Database showed that the mean age-standardized consultation rate for patients of all ages was 3.85 (3.01 for males and 4.71 for females). In 2004, the General Household Survey reported an average annual consultation rate for persons aged over 65 years of six for men and seven for women, in addition to an annual average of 3–4 consultations with a practice nurse. For older people, there tends to be fewer patient-initiated GP practice visits and more professional-led follow-up of established chronic illness care by either the GP or practice nurse.

Most GP practices offer appointments that are between 7 and 10 minutes in length; however, the average consultation time for patients of all ages is 13.3 minutes, with older patients tending to consult for longer than younger age groups.

General practitioner contact rates are 17% higher for older people living in communal establishments and 8% higher in older people living alone than those living in standard accommodation; to compensate for this additional workload, GPs receive weighted capitation fees for patients aged over 65 years.

Monitoring chronic disease care in older people

The Quality and Outcomes Framework system encourages the delivery of optimum care, derived from evidence-based practice, in key clinical domains. The QOF framework has an emphasis on chronic disease management with targets for

- diabetes
- epilepsy
- hypertension
- atrial fibrillation
- coronary heart disease and heart failure
- asthma and chronic obstructive pulmonary disease
- hypothyroidism
- chronic renal failure
- stroke
- mental illness
- dementia
- cancer and palliative care.

Because the incidence of most of these long-term conditions increases with age, care tends to be focused on older patients and can be delegated to practice nurses or nurse practitioners. The QOF system requires practices to produce patient disease registers to demonstrate the percentage of registered patients diagnosed with these specified long-term conditions.

Challenges of caring for older people in primary care

Key challenges for primary care services in providing care for our increasingly older populations include

- multimorbidity
- polypharmacy
- cognitive impairment
- assessment of capacity and best interests' decision-making
- legal and ethical issues
- carer support
- palliative and end-of-life care.

Multimorbidity and older people

Multimorbidity is defined as the presence of two or more chronic illnesses in patients; multimorbidity increases with age. The management of older people with multiple long-term illnesses is the norm, rather than the exception, in primary care consultations. This leads to an increasingly complex case mix for GPs to manage within a short consultation time. Consequently, the Royal College of General Practitioners has recently recommended extending the length of a routine GP appointment to 15 minutes in recognition of the increasing complexity of care required by our ageing population.

Polypharmacy

The monitoring of prescribing in general practice has been improved by the use of computerized prescribing systems and electronic patient records which facilitate medication review. The Quality and Outcomes Framework stipulates that patients who are prescribed four or more medicines should have an annual medicines review; this may be undertaken by a GP or by the patient's pharmacist.

Author's Tip

For older people taking multiple medications and for whom adherence is becoming a problem, taking their drugs can be simplified via a 'dosette' box, with daily dosage compartments dispensed on a weekly basis by a pharmacist.

Assessing cognitive function in primary care

Tests are available for use in the community to make an initial assessment of a person's cognitive function. The most commonly used tool is the Mini-Mental State Examination (MMSE) which is scored out of 30; a score of <24 is suggestive of dementia. It is important to note, however, that in dementia, a person's functional ability may not be reflected by the MMSE, as MMSE scores have been influenced by social status and education.

In practice, the MMSE can take up to 20 minutes to complete and so an Abbreviated MMSE or other brief cognitive tests, like the General Practitioner Assessment of Cognition (GPCOG), which takes around 7 minutes to complete (4 minutes: patient; 3 minutes: carer) can be used. Both the MMSE and GPCOG are recommended for use in primary care in the National Institute of Clinical Excellence guidance on dementia care.

Assessment of capacity: Mental Capacity Act

A significant number of the oldest old, especially those in nursing homes, will have cognitive impairment, even if a formal diagnosis of dementia has not been made. In the UK, the Mental Capacity Act (Adults with Incapacity Act in Scotland), stipulates that people must be assumed to have capacity regardless of their age, appearance, or behaviour. However, if capacity has been lost, specific guidance must be sought and an appropriate consultee, usually the next of kin or immediate carer, identified who will be then responsible for issues of consent.

If the older person does not have any immediate family or close networks to help in making a best interests decision, a referral to the Independent Mental Capacity Advocate (IMCA) may be made.

Assessment of capacity in practice is a complex and difficult area for GPs and advice may be needed from colleagues in old age psychiatry. Protocols, or clinical pathways, which assess the key areas that define capacity may be helpful. These comprise

- the ability to understand information specific to the decision to be made
- the ability to retain information relevant information
- the ability to use the information to make a decision
- their ability to communicate that decision.

Legal and ethical issues: advance care planning

The GP is well placed to provide sensitive and timely discussion of legal and financial matters, including information or advice about seeking lasting power of attorney (LPA). Advance Care Planning (ACP) is a process of discussion between a patient and professional carer, and sometimes family carers. Potential outcomes include

- 'advance statement': patient preferences for future care
- advance decision' or living will: informed consent to refuse certain treatment in specific circumstances, if loss of mental capacity ensues
- Lasting Power of Attorney: where a person names another to act on their behalf, should they loose capacity to consent, in areas of both their health and/or financial welfare.
- The last two are legally binding documents. Guidance on how to approach ACP exists for both patients and professionals, but there still appears to be a knowledge transfer gap into practice as the number of written ACP documents in practice is very small.

Caring for the carers: the role of the general practitioner

The provision of informal care to older people living at home will often be via families and friends, who may themselves be older and have long-term health problems. Usually the carer and the carer's family are registered with the same practice as the patient. The current General Practitioner Contract has encouraged a more pro-active approach in supporting informal carers, with practices rewarded for implementing a management system that includes the creation of a carer register. Carers can be referred for an individual assessment by social services in accordance with the Carers Act 2004.

The primary care team should have access to a regularly updated directory of local services covering NHS, local authority and voluntary and private sector provision, to ensure carer access to self-help and support groups; services should be adapted to the individual circumstances of the carer and the patient. The GP's role should include offering advice to carers on their personal health and the problems they experience, acknowledging the carer's crucial role in the care of the older patient and giving emotional support by counselling the carer on their attitudes and expectations.

Nursing and residential care

Patients in care homes register with a local GP and have access to general medical care in the same way as the general population; this has led to care home staff having to deal with multiple GPs for all their clients. Recently local initiatives have led to a one GP–one care home approach, whereby one general practice takes responsibility for the medical care of all the home residents in order to provide greater continuity of care.

In terms of the decision as to whether an older person is no longer able to live independently at home, the GP has a key role together with social services. Patients and their relatives considering admission to a home may wish to discuss the situation with the patient's GP and community nurses caring for the patient. The decision to transfer a patient into residential care is difficult and should only be taken after all possible community support services in the home have been explored with the patient's relatives and other involved community staff.

Palliative and end-of-life care

An individual GP can expect six or seven deaths annually of older patients suffering from dementia, frailty, and multimorbidity. Predicting how long an older person with problems like multimorbidity and dementia may live is extremely difficult in practice; however, GPs need to recognize when treatment or intervention is unnecessary in older people with multiple problems and when extra care or support is needed. The GP should advise patients with a palliative illness about the special attendance allowance (DS1500).

Through the QOF framework, the palliative care indicator requires a GP practice to have a register of patients considered to be in need of palliative or supportive care, if their death in the next 12 months can be reasonably predicted. The palliative care register should

- include people with both cancer and non-cancer illnesses
- facilitate regular review of patients, and their carers, by the multidisciplinary primary care team

- encourage early referral to specialist palliative care services to ensure more pro-active and supportive care.

Author's Tip

In order to identify people who may be in need of palliative care, remember to ask the 'surprise question': Would you, as a health professional, be surprised if this patient died within the next year?'

The National Institute for Clinical Excellence has recommended the use of care pathways to improve the quality of care at the end of life. These care pathways contain detailed guidance on how to transfer the principles of specialist palliative care as given in hospices, to other settings in which patients are cared for during their last few days of life and enable the GP, nursing and care staff in the community to deliver a high standard of end-of-life care. ACP has an important role in influencing the care received by older people in nursing homes and, although there is evidence that unnecessary hospital admissions can be reduced, a better understanding of how to translate theory into practice in this area is urgently needed.

Conclusion

In caring for older people in the community, the case below outlines a typical scenario of for the GP and their associated team. The case demonstrates the roles of the GP and other primary care team members and how co-ordinated teamwork can enable older people to remain in their own homes, for as long as possible, and die there should they choose to do so.

Coordinated care in the community: a typical case for the GP and primary care team

Mrs W is a 76-year-old lady with osteoarthritis of the hip, type II diabetes, and angina. She has been the main carer for her husband, who has advanced Parkinson's disease, for many years. Following an emergency admission for abdominal pain, she underwent surgery for bowel cancer. She is fully informed of the diagnosis and offered post-surgery chemotherapy, which will only be palliative. On her return home, the community nurse attends to provide wound care; she also organizes a social services referral to discuss temporary home care support for both Mrs W and her husband and an occupational therapy assessment.

During a visit from Mrs W's GP, the diagnosis and prognosis of the illness are rediscussed and the pros and cons of undergoing chemotherapy reviewed. Mrs W decides to forego this, as she feels it will not greatly alter her prognosis and may affect her ability to continue to care for her husband. She wishes to remain at home for as long as possible but acknowledges that they may not be able to cope when her health deteriorates.

The GP refers Mrs W to the Palliative Care Team for support and to the local hospice, as both Mrs W and her husband wish to attend for day care and complementary therapies. This will also allow Mrs W to visit the hospice and become comfortable with this environment, as she may wish to consider this an option for future care. The GP also advises Mrs W about the special attendance allowance (DS1500). The GP adds Mrs W's name to the practice cancer and palliative care registers.

In the above example, the GP would traditionally discuss the diagnosis and prognosis of the disease, act as gatekeeper to secondary and community care services, provide information on practical, emotional and financial assistance, and anticipate care requirements. Meanwhile, the community nurse would provide general hands on nursing care, organize aids and equipment, provide emotional support and coordinate and access other services.

Both would liaise closely with palliative care services, especially specialist palliative care nurses (often termed Macmillan nurses in recognition of the charity that supports their role), in order to access specialist advice and hospice-based services, such as day care and respite care. In some areas, a 24-hour community nursing service is available; a night sitting service may also be accessed, sometimes provided by Marie Curie nurses. It would be part of the GP's role to discuss where Mrs W would choose as her preferred place of care and provide care options.

Further reading

Brodaty H, Pond D, Kemp NM, et al. (2002). The GPCOG: a new screening test for dementia diagnosed for general practice. *J Am Geriatr Soc* **50**: 530–4.

Department of Health (2005). The Mental Capacity Act 2005. (http://www.opsi.gov.uk/acts/acts2005/ukpga_20050009_en_1)

Department of Health (2008). *End of Life Care Strategy: Promoting High Quality Care for All Adults at the End of Life*. London, Department of Health.

Folstein MF, Folstein SE, McHugh PR (1975). Mini-mental state: a practical method for grading the cognitive state of patients for the clinician. *J Psychiatr Res* **12**: 189–98.

Help the Aged (2006). *Planning for Choice in End-of-life Care*. Educational Guide.

National Health Service (2009). *Advance Care Planning: A Guide for Health and Social Care Staff*.

NICE/SCIE. (2006) *Dementia: Supporting People with Dementia and their Carers in Health and Social Care*. London, National Institute for Clinical Excellence and Social Care Institute for Excellence (NICE/SCIE).

Discharge planning

Background

Admission and discharge from an acute hospital setting is a stressful time for older people, their carers, and families. It is a process rather than an isolated event and if the process is not communicated well to all involved it can cause conflict, lack of trust, complaints, readmission and increased length of stay (LOS). Long LOS is associated with hospital-acquired infections and harm from iatrogenic causes, as well as functional decline to such an extent that patients never regain independence to allow return home.

Older people are frequently admitted to acute hospital care. In the UK, the majority of admissions are of patients over the age of 65 years. For many, admission to an acute hospital is associated with a decline in physical and mental functioning which may not have recovered fully by the time discharge is considered. How we support patients back in their own homes is often a source of frustration, with lack of communication and collaboration between agencies and cross-border partners. After longer stays, formal and informal support may be so disrupted as to make returning to their usual place of residence very difficult. The longer the stay in hospital, the more iatrogenic functional deterioration occurs. Older people make up a disproportionate number of those waiting for services to support discharge and these are often delayed.

This chapter will give an overview of the pathways that enhance safe but effective discharge in a timely fashion ensuring older patients are not exposed to unnecessary harm in hospital and unnecessary delay in returning to their own environment. It adopts a UK perspective, but many of the issues will apply in other settings.

Barriers to discharge

Many complaints stem from what patients and more often carers perceive as poor discharge arrangements. They feel that they are not involved, and that either the discharge occurred too soon or was overly delayed.

Reasons for poor/delayed discharge
- Lack of involvement of patient and carers
- Limited choice options
- Timings of ward rounds
- Diagnostic delays
- Delays in functional/social assessments
- Delays in pharmacy for take home medications
- Delays in transport
- Poor quality documentation
- Delays in writing discharge letter
- Poor use of third sector
- Limited rehabilitation beds
- Few private agency carers
- Limited planning beds, especially for people with dementia
- Multiple assessments repeat processes
- Lack of information sharing between secondary and primary care
- Electronic systems that do not communicate
- Mental capacity issues
- Continuing care assessments

Elective admissions

Discharge planning should start before admission in those older patients coming into an acute care setting for elective procedures. There are well established pre-assessment clinics in most acute hospitals that have occupational therapy input and some with an integral geriatrician. Here comprehensive geriatric assessments (CGA) are carried out to ensure that the equipment and care is in place once patients are deemed medically stable post surgery thus ensuring discharge is not delayed.

Benefits of pre-assessment clinics
- Information can be gathered in a detailed way
- Functional ability assessed
- Community agencies can be contacted in advance and interventions planned for discharge
- Communication of concerns regarding admission
- Reassurance for the individual and their families that there will be adequate support on discharge.

Unplanned admissions

Although it is desirable that a discharge strategy has been considered before unplanned admissions as well as elective admission, it is not always possible for those taken suddenly ill.

Health services are trying to reduce the number of unplanned admissions to secondary care. This may involve diverting resources into identifying and case managing frail older people with long-term conditions in the primary setting. These initiatives include
- allocation of case managers
- identifying those frail older people who might benefit from early intervention
- emergency care plans for long-term conditions
- 'step up' beds in community hospitals
- 'step up' beds in local nursing homes
- telemedicine to monitor vital signs within step up facilities
- telemedicine in patient's own homes.
- third sector involvement with patient advisors for financial assessment.

Whether these measures actually reduce the number of older people coming to hospital is debatable. These services, however, do appear to be what older people would prefer; that is to be treated closer to home and in familiar surroundings with known carers and their own support networks.

Older people with cognitive impairment are particularly likely to suffer harm from secondary care and the need to support them in their own environment is vital. There is also real emphasis on increased information sharing across the primary and secondary divide.

Education of first response paramedical staff to make them aware of alternative pathways for older people who may have fallen but not injured themselves may be helpful. Such pathways should offer clear guidance on the assessment of patients who fall and who may need admission on the one hand and those that can be cared for in their own home. Alternatives to emergency admission and access to community and secondary care falls services may reduce the use of secondary care services. However, the safety of such schemes remains to be robustly evaluated.

Once older patients reach the emergency department or medical assessment units, it is important that the pathway for discharge begins, although not at the expense of managing urgent conditions. Alongside acute treatments, the receiving doctor should ensure that all information needed to inform discharge planning is gathered and is correct.

Essential information
- How they usually walk: stick/frame/independently
- Can they wash and dress themselves
- Do they cook for themselves
- Do they go out
- Do they drive
- Do they have carers
- How often do they have carers
- Do they have family support
- Whether care home is residential or nursing (front door staff need to know the difference)
- Type of housing, flat, bungalow
- How do they manage stairs
- Do they live in Housing with Care

Even if the patient is unable to give this information, they may be accompanied by relatives or other informants. Care homes can be contacted, relatives at home telephoned and general practitioners (GPs) asked for more information.

Geriatricians might consider attending emergency care settings to better understand the pressure the staff there are under. They might also give assistance with difficult discharge decisions and train the front door staff that functional assessment can be a quick but vital piece of their work. The identification of reduced functional independence and the provision of appropriate support on discharge may avoid readmissions.

Earlier assessment by a geriatric multidisciplinary team (MDT) may allow an earlier assessment of the likely trajectory of the patient, and better discharge planning.

Multidisciplinary early intervention teams located in the emergency department can assess patients quickly and issue equipment to aid mobility, access community beds for rehabilitation and contact primary care agencies that can rapidly support discharge. Referral to such teams may come from a variety of sources. The role of social care workers is a critical part of multi-agency working. The holistic emergency assessment needs to be clearly and rapidly communicated in order to be effective. Carers should also be listened to and supported. Support services in primary care need to be able to react quickly at extended hours of the day.

Discharge planning from inpatient beds
Practicalities allowing flow through ward
- Daily board rounds so staff on ward know where in the discharge planning process patients are.
- Clear discharge goal setting.
- Clear documentation of management plan.
- Clear documentation when patient becomes medically stable.
- Clear documentation of communication with patients and with families.
- Regular reviews by experienced medical staff.
- Clear MDT documentation.
- MDT meetings twice a week but do not wait for MDT for decisions to be made.
- Criteria lead discharge.

- Ward OT, physiotherapist and ward allocated social worker who attends MDT.
- Effective use of intermediate care beds.
- Efficient inter disciplinary referral systems (electronic).
- Discharge planning 7 days a week.
- Named coordinator for each patient to enhance communication and ensure patient-focused care.
- Integrated care pathways for specific chronic conditions.
- Rapid assessment of baseline function both physical and social.
- Assessment of discharge destination.
- Organized transport provision.
- Effective pharmacy provision.
- Transcribing pharmacists.
- Timely equipment provision.

This whole process has to have 'buy-in' from all disciplines to allow this to operate efficiently: a shared common vision for how the service should operate.

In the UK, the discharge planning process is increasingly 'performance managed', in order to drive up standards. Explicit targets and LOS information might be displayed on each ward. Variation from established targets can be openly challenged. Patient satisfaction surveys might be used to ensure that quality is not sacrificed in the drive for efficiency.

All of the factors listed above for planning discharge of complex older patients should be in place for all wards, whether surgical or medical in the hospital However, it is often the case that discharge planning for a complex frail older person is much harder on wards where the multidisciplinary team do not have 'ownership' of the patient. Length of stay may be longer on outlying wards and there is an increased likelihood of harm occurring to the patient. Staff may not have 'focus' on the needs of the older person especially those with dementia. Staff may not have the training to deal with challenging behaviour. The MDT may not be in place. Targets for surgical wards are different and the focus is usually on getting relatively fit and uncomplicated patients attending for elective procedures through the system efficiently. Liaison services might offer some support to these settings, though the evidence to date for such services has been somewhat disappointing.

Early supported discharge
This has been proven to be clinically and cost-effective for patients with stroke and fractured neck of femur, at least in urban settings. However, it is possible that these intensive enablement teams could be used for all manner of long term conditions seen in older and younger individuals giving patients the chance of rehabilitation in their own environments.

Mental capacity
It is always good practice to ensure every patient is assessed for rehabilitation potential before permanent decisions on future long-term care are made. This is the case whether the individual has cognitive impairment or not. Mental capacity assessments can be seen as difficult and time-consuming. They can also be wrongly seen as the remit of the old age psychiatrist. Any clinician or social worker can undertake a mental capacity assessment. In relation to discharge, the clinician must take time to gather as much information as possible about the individual's ability to judge the risks involved in discharging back to their own home. There is a need to make certain that they are

basing their assessments of their ability to cope at home on recent events and not past abilities. Functional assessments in hospital are often flawed and do not genuinely reflect the person's abilities. All this must be taken into account, as well as carers insights in to behavioural difficulties. Give some thought to whether the patient has completed an advance directive and/or power of attorney. This should then be marked on the notes.

Continuing care assessments

Continuing care assessments are a peculiarity of the UK National Health Service, and relate to the split in funding for long term care between health and social care. These are required if the person is deemed to require nursing home care and then pre-check screening is required to assess whether their health needs fall into the category that will meet the need for NHS funding. Funding needs to be confirmed by the authorities and this can result in delays.

Good practice relies on the commissioners of health and social care working closely together to provide services that meet the needs of the local population in a collaborative and positive way. Physicians should be influential in planning the services required. Managers of health and social care within acute settings need to work closely together in the best interests of the patient. Front line staff need the training and the experience to feel confident that they are doing all they can to ensure a safe, efficient and appropriate discharge.

Conclusion

Discharge planning is a complex process that has many pathways and many agencies involved in it. To make sure the process is as smooth and timely as possible, communication between disciplines, agencies, primary and secondary care has to be excellent and coordinated. Patients and carers should be at the centre of this decision making process and their views heard at all stages.

Further reading

Cunliffe AL, Gladman JRF, Husbands SL, et al. (2004). Sooner and healthier: a randomised controlled trail and interview study of an early discharge rehabilitation service for older people. *Age Ageing* **33**: 246–52.

Department of Health (2003). *Discharge from Hospital: Pathway, Process and Practice*. (http://www.dh.gov.uk/en/Publicationsandstatistics/Publications/PublicationsPolicyAndGuidance/DH_4003252).

Gilbert R, Todd C, May M, et al. (2010). Socio-demographic factors predict the likelihood of not returning home after hospital admission following a fall. *J Public Health* **32**: 117–24.

Gladman J, Forster A, Young J (1994). Hospital-and home-based rehabilitation after discharge from hospital for stroke patients: Analysis of two trails. *Age Ageing* **24**: 49–53.

Huby G, Stewart J, Tierney A, et al. (2004). Planning older people's discharge from acute hospital care: linking risk management and patient participation in decision-making. *Health Risk and Society* **6**: 115–32.

Jones D, Lester C (1993). Hospital care and Discharge: Patients' and Carers' Opinions. *Age Ageing* **23**: 91–6.

Katikireddi SV, Cloud GC (2008). Planning a patient's discharge from hospital. *BMJ* **337**: a2694.

Rowland K, Maitra AK, Richardson DA, et al. (1990). The discharge of elderly patients from an accident and emergency department: Functional changes and risk of readmission. *Age Ageing* **19**: 415–18.

Stewart R, Bartlett P, Harwood HR (2005). Mental capacity assessments and discharge decisions. *Age Ageing* **34**: 549–50.

Intermediate care

The term intermediate care (IC) was first coined in the British medical literature in 1985, describing a GP-led 20-bed facility in London doing a mix of activities including what we now call step-up care, plus respite. The first domiciliary based hospital discharge support services emerged soon after. The description IC seemed to fit, as these services were positioned between primary and secondary care, and for the patient, intermediate between clinical instability and stability, for example between acute illness and recovery

Why did intermediate care get started?
Hospitals are changing
Hospitals and what we use them for have changed dramatically in recent decades. Developments in medical technology and clinical knowledge, societal and individual attitudes and government policy have all played a part. Emergency hospital admission rates have risen, 11.8% in the NHS over the five-year period to 2008/09, with demographic change accounting for less than half of this. Meanwhile, the long term trend for reducing average lengths of stay in hospitals continues, with averages having fallen several fold in recent decades.

What are the consequences?
The majority of older people leave hospital with poorer functional capacity than they had in the immediate period before the acute illness, injury or surgery that resulted in the hospital admission.

However, among health policy-makers in the UK and increasingly elsewhere, the predominant view is that staying longer in hospital to regain optimum recovery is not the solution, for several reasons:
- hospitals are ineffective at promoting recuperation or rehabilitation,
- hospitals discourage expression of individual autonomy,
- hospitals are unsafe, as the risk of adverse events is associated with longer spells in hospital, and both the public and policy makers are more aware of healthcare acquired infections etc,
- hospitals are expensive, whereas community care is cheap.

Some of these assertions may be true. Anticipating this development, over 10 years ago the Audit Commission in England pointed out many older people remained in hospital 'inappropriately'. Evaluation of this idea of 'appropriateness' has been formalised in US and Europe but is not in common use in the UK. However, the Audit Commission also pointed out that there were insufficient opportunities after hospital discharge to fully recover lost functionality and health. A vicious cycle of poor recovery, loss of functional reserve and subsequent readmission was the result. Hence the need for a new approach, an alternative to hospital, but something which was not yet present in traditional primary or community based healthcare: intermediate care.

What services are we talking about?
The early Department of Health (DH) guidance and reviews set out the criteria characterizing services which could be bracketed under IC:
- Targeted at people who would otherwise face unnecessarily prolonged hospital stays or inappropriate admission to acute inpatient care, long-term residential care or continuing NHS in-patient care.
- Provided on the basis of a comprehensive assessment, resulting in a structured individual care plan that involves active therapy, treatment or opportunity for recovery.
- Having a planned outcome of maximizing independence and typically enabling patients and service users to resume living at home.
- Time-limited, normally no longer than 6 weeks, and frequently one to 2 weeks or less.

Service models
- Rapid response: designed to prevent avoidable acute hospital admission.
- Hospital at home: intensive support in the patient's own home, including investigations and treatment which are above the level that would normally be provided in primary care.
- Residential rehabilitation: a short-term programme of therapy and enablement in a residential setting (such as a community hospital, rehabilitation centre, nursing home, or residential care home) for people who are medically stable but need a short period of rehabilitation for 1–6 weeks. Residential rehabilitation may be 'step down', i.e. following a stay in an acute hospital; or it may be 'step up'.
- Supported discharge: a short-term period of nursing and/or therapeutic support in a patient's home, typically with a contributory package of home care support.
- Day rehabilitation: a short-term programme of therapeutic support, e.g. at a day hospital.

Methods of working
The expectation in the English DH guidance was that all these would involve inter-professional working within an agreed framework for multidimensional assessments, shared protocols, and unified records. The work would typically involve nurses working with unqualified healthcare assistants, allied health professionals (e.g. physiotherapists, occupational therapists, speech/language therapists, psychologists, dieticians), and care managers with medical input from general practitioners; support from other specialists such as geriatricians was ill-defined. In practice, the pattern of services has undergone considerable change since the first policy targets were set out, as shown by the evaluation commissioned by the DH. Hospitals and mainstream community services are constantly evolving, so inevitably intermediate care services must adapt. Indeed, this suggests indeed a new connotation of the term 'intermediate', a service which is developmentally transitional.

Does intermediate care work?
From the discussion above, it is obvious that asking the question "Is Intermediate Care safe, effective and efficient?" is not helpful. Rather we need to look at what any particular type of IC is trying to achieve, for whom, and how. So, what is the evidence for particular types of services for particular clinical challenges?

Evidence for types of IC
Admission avoidance: Hospital at Home (H@H)
As the heading implies, this type of service is not intermediate in content, but is included as it represents an attempt

to provide in the patient's home inputs which would and elsewhere still do require an acute hospital admission. Of the ten studies included in the most recent 2008 Cochrane Review, seven were limited to one condition only: cellulitis (New Zealand), chronic obstructive pulmonary disease (COPD) (UK and Australia), stroke (UK and Italy), community-acquired pneumonia (NZ), and severe dementia (Italy); three with mixed casemix, mostly older people (Australia, NZ and UK). The summative conclusions were drawn from meta-analyses of individual patient data where available (five of 10 studies, 850 of total 1333 patients).

Main conclusions

- A non-significant reduction in mortality at 3 months for the admission avoidance H@H (adjusted HR 0.77, 95% CI 0.54–1.09; p = 0.15).
- A significant reduction in mortality at 6-month follow-up (adjusted HR 0.62, 95% CI 0.45–0.87; p = 0.005).
- A non-significant increase in admissions was observed for patients allocated to H@H (adjusted HR 1.49, 95% CI 0.96–2.33; p = 0.08).
- No notable or significant differences in functional ability, quality of life, or cognition.
- Patients reported increased satisfaction with H@H.

Interpretation

These data indicate the possibility of safely substituting hospital care by high-intensity home-based care. All the services included nurses, doctors (sometimes with hospital specialists being prominent or sole medical providers) and a range of allied health professionals. Nursing intensity varied up to 24 hours a day. Both stroke studies predated thrombolysis, which for suitable patients changes entirely the desirability of emphasizing admission avoidance rather than a short admission followed by early supported discharge.

The UK evidence

The sole UK study finished recruitment in May 1997, since when much has changed. A further caveat with that study is that of the 97 of 199 patients randomized to hospital, 23 were not admitted for various reasons, suggesting that a H@H service offered to these would not have in fact been an alternative to hospital. Nevertheless, the acuity of patients generally was high and over a quarter had died within 3 months. Excluding the costs of informal care, H@H was less expensive than admission to an acute hospital ward.

The proportion of the total acute medical admission cohort suitable for this type of service is unclear. Likewise, it is not clear that the opportunity costs of management and clinical leadership effort justifies this sort of initiative in an urban setting where access to an acute hospital is quick. Although there are several such initiatives currently operating in the NHS, there is no published data from them to assess their utility. Perhaps it is an option for well defined conditions with reasonably predictable clinical course. For example, a review of such schemes for COPD patients with exacerbations included two each in England and Scotland, and concluded that hospital readmission and mortality were similar in hospital and H@H (relative risk 0.89, 95% CI 0.72–1.12, and 0.61, 95% CI 0.36–1.05, respectively), but that H@H was associated with substantial cost savings as well as freeing up hospital inpatient beds.

Admission avoidance, rapid response services

Assessing these schemes is challenging as there is an ambiguity at its heart. Most have been set up to meet the needs of users who do not need the type or intensity of care which would justify an acute medical admission, i.e. they may provide a semblance of this but the reasoning behind them is that people end up being admitted through lack of locally available acutely accessible personal and nursing care. Usually a key ingredient is support from care assistants to meet functional care needs. Without them, hospital admission probably would have occurred, but it would have been inappropriate from the viewpoint of what hospitals are 'really' for. It is unlikely that any of the services included in the Cochrane Review analyses described above had many of these patients. Therefore, we have to rely on alternative sources of evidence, some distinctly grey.

The Partnerships for Older People Projects in England, 2006–2009 (POPP) were a wide variety of English DH funded but locally designed and managed projects in 29 local authorities. Some of these services had objectives which included reducing acute hospital admissions. Users targeted by these initiatives included attendees at Emergency departments, people with multiple hospital admissions or those predicted to be at high risk for future admissions. Services included elements of intermediate care, along with case management and enhanced community support from non-health professionals. The national evaluation concluded that these services could be very cost-effective, as they resulted in reduced attendances and admissions to hospitals, with cost savings which exceeded the running costs of the projects. None of these evaluations were randomised trials. Most depended upon historical comparative data, extrapolations of trends or subjective views of users and providers. Local effects are clearly highly contingent on context, which makes generalisable conclusions problematic, perhaps impossible.

Early and/or supported hospital discharge services

These are services that provide active treatment by health care professionals in the patient's home for a condition which would otherwise require longer acute hospital inpatient care. The updated Cochrane Review in 2009 presented the results of meta-analyses done on an intention-to-treat basis, and using individual patient level data where available, (received from the trialists for 13 of the 21 eligible trials). The findings were analysed according to two casemix groups – stroke or older patients with a mix of conditions. The main conclusions were:

- No evidence of a difference in mortality between groups for patients recovering from a stroke (adjusted HR 0.79, 95% CI 0.32–1.91; n = 494) or older patients with a mix of conditions, (adjusted HR 1.06, 95% CI 0.69–1.61; n = 978).
- Short-term readmission rates were higher in the early discharge group for older patients with a mix of conditions (adjusted HR 1.57; 95% CI 1.10–2.24; n = 705).
- For both conditions, the chance of being in residential care at follow up were lower (RR 0.63; 95% CI 0.40–0.98; n = 4 trials, stroke; RR 0.69, 95% CI 0.48–0.99; n = 3 trials, older people).
- Satisfaction was higher with earlier discharge.
- Evidence about costs was inconclusive due to limited data and different cost counting approaches.

Interpretation

These conclusions are tempered by the significant heterogeneity in casemix, even though the review included only patients being discharged from surgical or medical wards. This was reflected by heterogeneity of outcomes, so applicability is problematic. Perhaps more can be gleaned from well conducted individual trials, as long as their context is understood as an explanatory factor in local effectiveness.

The UK evidence

For example, one of these studies has reported the service outcomes, the success factors and the cost-effectiveness evaluation. Its focus was early discharge coupled with a home-based rehabilitation and care programme for up to 4 weeks. The description showed that this encompassed aspects which others call recuperation or, more recently, re-enablement as conducted now by social service departments in England. Main findings were:

- The early discharge group spent fewer days in hospital at 3 months (mean difference 9, median difference 4 days, 95% CI of median difference 2–8).
- The early discharge group were functionally more able at 3 months in personal care (mean difference in Barthel scores 1.2, 95% CI 0.4–1.9, and instrumental ADL).
- The early discharge group had better General Health Questionnaire scores at 3 months (mean difference 2.0, 95% CI 0.1–3.8).

Supported by their linked studies which showed that the service addressed physical, psychological, social and environmental issues, the authors concluded that 'some older people can be discharged from hospital sooner, with better health outcomes using a well-staffed and organized patient-centred early discharge service providing rehabilitation' and was likely to be more cost-effective than usual care.

Related evidence about hospital discharge

The process of hospital discharge support IC variably includes enhanced discharge planning, rehabilitation input at home, enhanced home care and follow-up with an element of short term case management. It is difficult to unpick these components in the reported studies and to attribute effects to them. These broader aspects are by no means novel aspects confined to IC services. A recent review of 15 systematic reviews addressing this broader scope concluded that there is some evidence that some may have a positive impact, particularly those with educational components and those that combine pre-discharge and post-discharge interventions. However, overall there was limited collective evidence that discharge planning and discharge support interventions have a positive impact on patient functioning after discharge, on health care use after discharge, or on costs.

Community hospitals and care homes

Despite there being hundreds of community hospitals in the UK and internationally, there is a paucity of experimental data on effectiveness. There is little commonality of meaning of the term community hospital. In US research literature, hospitals identified are more akin to small district generals in UK. In the context of IC, community hospitals may be either step up or step down. Step up is for admissions usually from home direct or via brief attendance at an urgent care facility, with less severe acute problems, with medical care being the responsibility of primary care, often the patients' own general practitioner. This was a traditional pattern of service inherited by the NHS in 1948. The research literature contains no randomized controlled trials comparing outcomes or costs. History may help here. During the 1970s and 1980s, hundreds were closed in favour of centralizing care in district generals and the reasons usually given were safety, improved outcomes and greater efficiency.

Step-up services

More recently, step up has been promoted as part of more explicit care pathways into traditional community hospitals or new build primary care bedded units or care homes supported with additional NHS funded staff, usually allied health professionals. In the IC era, no randomized controlled trials or even quasi-experimental studies of this approach have been published, though it is likely that many local evaluations of varying degrees of methodological rigour have been conducted. Since the outcomes and costs are likely dependent upon details of patient selection, transfer of information and knowledge and specifics of care received in the alternative venue, it is questionable whether these or indeed a randomized controlled trial in one setting will help planners and or clinicians in another.

Step-down services to care homes

In contrast, step-down or post acute care in alternative settings, have been studied. The Cochrane review included 56 studies and five reviews which were assessed. However, comparability between intervention and control groups was poor:

- description and specification of the environment was unclear, or
- the components of rehabilitation in either setting were not adequately specified or
- if specified, other methodological weaknesses or lack of detail precluded meaningful comparison.

Step-down to NHS community hospitals

There is one multisite randomized controlled trial of using community hospitals in the NHS for post-acute care and rehabilitation. The community hospitals were mostly recently opened, rather than the longer established traditional model. At a median of 6 days after acute admission, 490 patients who were then clinically stable but not recovered, were randomized to remain in their acute hospital or transfer to their local community hospitals in the north of England. Participants would be familiar to UK geriatricians: mostly female, in their mid-80s, living alone, nearly 30% with cognitive impairment, and half with preadmission limitations in activities of daily living (ADLs). The main findings were:

- At 6 months, greater improvements in instrumental ADL in the community hospital group (mean adjusted Nottingham ADL score group difference 5.30; 95% confidence interval 0.64–9.96).
- Length of hospital stay, mood, mortality, discharge destination and patient service satisfaction were similar for each group.
- Costs for the community hospital group were slightly higher (mean £8946 versus £8226)
- A small non-significant lower difference in quality-adjusted life-year values for the community hospital group, translating into an incremental cost-effectiveness ratio estimate of £16 324 per quality-adjusted life year.

Thus, overall the impact of secondary care district hospital and the community hospital approaches to post-acute care are comparable; the additional benefits in extended ADLs would not appear to command reconfiguration of services without other considerations favouring it. Capital costs to create new community hospitals would not appear justified on these findings.

Nurse-led inpatient units (NLU)

There is no consistent model of care for these units, which have sometimes been established pragmatically on hospital sites losing 24-hour medical cover. The theoretical justification is that an alternative, nursing model of care may be more holistic, patient centred and therefore effective for optimizing post-acute recovery and preparation for independent living. The Cochrane review analysed results from ten random or quasi-random controlled trials reported on a total of 1896 patients.

- Patients leaving NLU were better prepared for discharge but it is unclear if this is simply a product of an increased length of inpatient stay.
- No statistically significant adverse effects were noted but there was a trend towards increased early mortality and a real difference could not be discounted.
- Costs of care on the NLU were higher for UK studies but lower for US-based studies, which are probably quite different contexts.

The momentum behind the early enthusiasm for stand alone NLUs is now waning and evidence would suggest that promoting truly multidisciplinary care incorporating the benefits of nurse leadership is the way forward.

How does intermediate care work best?

Arguably, until IC services have established how to do what it is that theoretical or policy propositions deem necessary, then randomised trials of effectiveness and cost benefit may be premature. Much of the grey literature which informs national policy is drawn from observational studies which seek to explore what characteristics might make IC more effective and sustainable. Such a study was conducted by researchers at the University of Leeds for the Department of Health. The fieldwork in 2002–2004 was in a purposive sample of five areas, with varied levels of IC development. Quantitative data was obtained for 7452 service users, plus more detail from 153 tracked over 6 months. Qualitative interview data was from 64 service users and 247 staff working in or potentially affected by the local IC service. There was considerable variety in stated purpose, structure and staffing, and delivery content of the services studied.

The researchers concluded from triangulating data from service users, providers, and the wider localities that three elements of good user-centred intermediate care were

- an enabling ethos built around activities and goals of value to individual users
- recognition of and partnership with informal support networks to maintain and sustain progress
- links into on-going practical, clinical and social support from services where necessary.

Similar conclusions were drawn from other studies, such as the POPP evaluation described above.

For services which sustain quality and performance, partnership working has to encompass clinical governance and this is poorly implemented so far, according to the English DH's recent updated guidance, which recommended stronger primary–secondary care partnerships.

Overall, has intermediate care delivered on promise?

The DH commissioned evaluation of the National Service Framework identified uneven development of intermediate care, with some services having poorly defined objectives, though in general local problems with 'delayed discharges' seemed the main impetus to set up services. Users' comments were generally positive and consistent with the notion of enhanced support for recovery: 'it set me up', 'got me on my feet—literally', 'gave me a boost over the worst part' etc. The DH commissioned study described above, however, found no evidence from high level indicators to prove or not whether the presence of IC rendered the local health and social care economies in the study areas either more effective or more efficient.

The only peer-reviewed study to address this question concerned a fairly well resourced IC service in Leeds, England, consisting of short-term home or care home-based rehabilitative and support services available for patients in the post acute phase of a hospital stay for a mix of geriatric syndromes. Two cohorts were compared, before and after introduction of the IC service. This was supplemented by a more detailed study of matched samples from each cohort. Clinical outcomes, including functional ability, mood and mortality were similar between the groups. Uptake of IC was lower than anticipated at 29%. The detailed study demonstrated increased hospital bed days used over 12 months (mean 8 days; 95% CI 3.1–13.0). Thus, their objectives of reducing long-term care and hospital use were not achieved.

Conclusions

- 'Intermediate care' only has meaning as a general description related to the policy intentions of reducing hospital use while attempting to promote clinical recovery and independence.
- Several distinct service models exist and specific service models may be needed to suit the casemix in question.
- Overall, there is some evidence that early and/or supported hospital discharge services and step down to community hospitals provide care which is as safe and effective as prolonged stays for recovery in hospital, but they are not cheaper.
- Acute care hospital at home may work well for selected conditions.
- There is no consensus IC model to deliver rapid response, hospital admission avoidance; this outcome may be achievable by a variety of community healthcare developments.

The essential first step in developing IC in any locality is to define what the problem is that needs solving and design the service accordingly, and then to make sure there is sufficient performance data and clinical governance to keep it on track.

Further reading

Askham J (2008). *Health Care Service and Older People: putting national service framework principles to work.* A review report of research to support the NSF for older people, OPUS project final report. London, Kings College.

Blunt I, Bardsley M, Dixon J (2010). Trends in emergency admissions in England 2004–2009: is greater efficiency breeding inefficiency? London, The Nuffield Trust (www.nuffieldtrust.org.uk/publications).

Cunliffe AL, Gladman JR, Husbands SL et al. (2004). Sooner and healthier: a randomised controlled trial and interview study of an early discharge rehabilitation service for older people. *Age Ageing* **33**: 246–52.

Department of Health (2001). *Intermediate Care:* HSC. 2001/01. London, DH.

Department of Health (2001). *National Service Framework for Older People*. London, DH.

Department of Health (2009). Intermediate Care-Halfway Home. Updated guidance for the NHS and Local Auithorities (http://www.dh.gov.uk/en/Publicationsandstatistics/Publications/PublicationsPolicyAndGuidance/DH_103146).

Griffiths PD, Edwards ME, Forbes A, *et al.* (2007). Effectiveness of intermediate care in nursing-led in-patient units. *Cochrane Database Syst Rev* (2): CD002214.

Higgs R (1985). Example of intermediate care: the new Lambeth Community Care Centre. *Br Med J (Clin Res Ed)* **291**: 1395–7.

Institute of Health Sciences and Public Health Research, University of Leeds (2005). *An Evaluation of Intermediate Care for Older People - Final Report*. Leeds.

Lorenzo S, Lang T, Pastor R, *et al.* (1999). Reliability study of the European appropriateness evaluation protocol. *Int J Qual Health Care* **11**: 419–24.

Miller P, Gladman JR, Cunliffe AL, *et al.* (2005). Economic analysis of an early discharge rehabilitation service for older people. *Age Ageing* **34**: 274–80.

Mistiaen P, Francke AL, Poot E (2007). Interventions aimed at reducing problems in adult patients discharged from hospital to home: a systematic meta-review. *BMC Health Serv Res* **7**: 47.

O'Reilly J, Lowson K, Green J *et al.* (2008). Post-acute care for older people in community hospitals—a cost-effectiveness analysis within a multi-centre randomised controlled trial. *Age Ageing* **37**: 513–20.

PSSRU (2009). National Evaluation of Partnerships for Older People Projects. Final Report. University of Kent. (http://www.dh.gov.uk/en/Publicationsandstatistics/Publications/PublicationsPolicyAndGuidance/DH_111240).

Ram FS, Wedzicha JA, Wright J, *et al.* (2004). Hospital at home for patients with acute exacerbations of chronic obstructive pulmonary disease: systematic review of evidence, *Br Med J* **329**: 315.

Shepperd S, Doll H, Angus RM, *et al.* (2008). Admission avoidance hospital at home. *Cochrane Database Syst Rev* (4): CD007491.

Shepperd S, Doll H, Broad J, *et al.* (2009). Early discharge hospital at home. *Cochrane Database Syst Rev*, (1): CD000356.

Shepperd S, Harwood D, Gray A, *et al.* (1998). Randomised controlled trial comparing hospital at home care with inpatient hospital care. II: cost minimisation analysis. *Br Med J* **316**: 1791–6.

University of Leicester. *A National Evaluation of the Costs and Outcomes of Intermediate Care for Older People: Executive Summary*. Leicester Nuffield Research Unit (http://www.hs.le.ac.uk/nccsu/indexa.html).

Ward D, Drahota A, Gal D, *et al.* (2008). Care home versus hospital and own home environments for rehabilitation of older people. *Cochrane Database Syst Rev* (4): CD003164.

Wilson A, Parker H, Wynn A, *et al.* (1999). Randomised controlled trial of effectiveness of Leicester hospital at home scheme compared with hospital care. *Br Med J* **319**: 1542–6.

Young J, Green J, Forster A *et al.* (2007). Postacute Care for Older People in Community Hospitals: A Multicenter Randomized, Controlled Trial. *J Am Geriatr Soc* **55**: 1995–2002.

Young JB, Robinson M, Chell S, *et al.* (2005). A whole system study of intermediate care services for older people. *Age Ageing* **34**: 577–83.

Community geriatrics

History

Old age was not uncommon in ancient times, yet 'geratology'—the study of old age—was born by an American IL Nascher in 1909, and clinical geriatrics was pioneered by a Londoner, Dr Marjory Warren, in 1936. She worked in workhouses – long-stay hospitals now equivalent to our nursing homes. In 1948, workhouses became part of the new NHS and geriatricians were appointed with responsibility for these homes, but were excluded from main hospitals and private practice. Thus the first geriatricians worked exclusively 'in the community'. In the 1970s, geriatricians were increasingly given responsibility for acute care of ill older people, rather than purely taking those patients no-one else wanted. 'Integrated' models of care emerged, where geriatricians worked alongside other consultants on a joint ward. The 1990s saw widespread closure of long-stay NHS wards, as this was transferred to privately owned nursing homes, where medical care was the responsibility of the general practitioner. Thus geriatricians, who had started with duties solely in the community had gained access to the acute hospitals, and now worked solely in the acute setting.

In the USA, geriatrics was initially restricted to nursing home practice, and the specialty continues to provide predominantly subacute care in most European countries.

Re-emergence of community geriatrics

The National Service Framework for Older People (NSF-OP) set out a plan for the optimal health and social care for the start of the twenty-first century and, although introduced for the NHS in England, it includes many central elements that are held to be true in any country and at any time. This NSF was written in a period during which health policy in England was moving towards a model where care is delivered in community settings as opposed to hospitals, on the basis that this might be more cost-effective or preferable to users. With this, the NSF-OP stimulated the growth of intermediate care services and subsequent policy initiatives have continued this process by introducing community matrons for certain frail older people in the community.

There are a range of settings where the interface between the geriatrician and primary care has moved outside of the district hospital and beyond the traditional outpatient clinic. Those settings are principally the community hospital, intermediate care services, care homes, domiciliary visits, and community matrons. The strength of these interfaces varies greatly across the country. There are policy directives and cost pressures to attempt to deliver specialist care for older people without admission to the district hospital. The arguments for and against delivering this specialist care in the community may be summarized.

Benefits of community-based care
- Care closer to home
- Reduction of risks associated with hospital admission
- Greater continuity of home support systems with less disruption of care
- Easier to deliver integrated care across services
- Financial savings from reduced hospital admissions

Disadvantages and risks
- Ageism—older people managed differently
- Inadequate medical assessment and diagnosis
- Inefficient use of specialist staff time in travelling
- Weak clinical governance structures.

A critical question for each of the service models is whether there is evidence of better or worse patient outcomes. For some service models, there is evidence and this is discussed in related chapters. However, it is always difficult to determine whether a particular service evaluation is generalizable to another setting because of crucial dependence on the quality and quantity of staff, as well as other factors, in each model. Expediency in the local health economy is often more likely to drive service design changes rather than evidence from controlled trials.

Developing an effective service model

Where geriatricians find themselves working at least in part within a community geriatrics service, it is important to identify factors critical for success. These have been split into challenges faced; critical elements for success; and qualities required in the geriatrician.

Challenges faced

Community-based services for frail older people will often adopt a pragmatic problem-based approach to care, usually centred around loss of functions. This can appear person-centred and acceptable to patients. However, it may fail to recognise that a treatable medical condition underlies this loss of function. It also may fail to think ahead in terms of secondary prevention to try and reduce future events.

There are potential tensions around professionalism or clashes of individuals regarding who should take lead responsibility. This can easily occur between the general practitioner and a consultant in community hospitals or care homes. This is where new models of shared care challenge more traditional separation. This can lead to ambiguity regarding who indeed is carrying professional responsibility.

Communication failure may be a common source of poor care or heightened tensions. Consultants will be familiar with communication problems so often at the root of user complaints.

Critical elements for success

Teamwork

Teamworking is crucial for success in managing a crisis in a frail older person. The team must meet regularly, knowing each other and their respective competencies. This enables the team to respond quickly and act decisively. Comprehensive assessment and accurate diagnosis are critical, alongside clear delegation for who is responsible for each task. Many community services for older people, especially outside community hospitals, are trying to deliver this without full membership of the team and/or with fragmentation and boundaries. This results in a loose grouping of disparate individuals.

The boundary of social and healthcare is one example. There is a need to drop the old languages of 'social model' and 'medical model' and adopt an 'integrated model,' where all staff understand the importance and valuable contribution of each other. Some successful teams are based around a neighbourhood or a large Primary Care centre, while others may identify with a locality with a population of around 40 000. A locality network might combine neighbourhood teams with specialist staff covering a larger area. Community Matrons and 'virtual ward' models of care need to find their optimal size for their situation. Health and social care must agree on a structure for their locality. Once structures are agreed, relationships can develop and strengthen. Where team or network members know each other and have agreed 'rules of engagement', emails, and mobile phones can enhance integration and information sharing perhaps less painfully than establishing a shared IT system!

Time

As well as acting quickly, assessment of older people in a crisis needs sufficient time to reach a correct answer. History taking may be difficult and interviews required with several people. Information needs to be gathered from several sources as the clinical picture is pieced together and the process may be spread out over several assessments. All of this is time-consuming, which requires appropriate allocation of resources. Risks from insufficient time may be most pertinent where the patient remains at home.

Accessing specialist expertise

In the district hospital, specialist advice is generally at hand. There are many specialists with community responsibilities and others who are accessible for telephone advice even if they do not work in the community. Establishing and maintaining this network is important. Training programmes can improve expertise and teams should be regularly reviewing their training needs.

Accepting responsibility

General practitioners meeting a crisis in an older person at home or other settings need a service that can be trusted to take over responsibility for the patient for the next part of their journey. Where this trust is not established, general practitioners will opt for the more familiar emergency referral to hospital, perceived as the safer option. There can be ambiguous understanding of responsibility in settings outside hospital and so clear and precise communication is vital.

Qualities required in the geriatrician

Experience

Working outside the comfort zone of the district hospital is not easy: it is not for the faint-hearted! Making a diagnosis in geriatric medicine is often difficult and relies upon investigation results, which may not be immediately available.

Nevertheless, experience and training provide the geriatrician with valuable skills which should not be under-rated. Often a judgement can be made regarding the most probable diagnosis or the chances of the patient benefiting from investigation and treatment. This can be enormously valuable in discussions with patient and family and decisions regarding place of treatment.

Friendly manner

Teamworking and communication have been stressed above and require of the doctor an easy manner to foster strong trusting relationships with colleagues and patients.

Leadership

The risk of fragmentation of the team is high when working in community settings, though may be less of a problem in care homes or community hospitals. Nevertheless, confident leadership engenders commitment and quality of care which is so important when services are delivered away from the constant supervision of seniors. The geriatrician must know when it is right to point out failings in management or treatment by the service.

Going the extra mile

It is difficult to manage every situation that presents within the proscribed timetable. Often, it may require being available on the mobile phone, seeing a relative or going back to the house. Flexible interfacing with general practitioners and others is needed. Geriatricians will recognise this as part of the job. The gratitude of staff, patients and relatives easily repays the extra effort.

Conclusion

In our ageing society there are a growing number of people living at home with multiple long-term conditions. Although geriatricians have a key contribution to episodes of care necessitating hospital admission, there is a strong desire to minimize the frequency and duration of hospital admissions without sacrificing the person's access to specialist care. Consultant geriatricians have a unique contribution within the complex environment of community care and will be welcomed warmly if they adopt the principles described here. It must be hoped that new models of commissioning bring down some of the financial and organizational boundaries that currently inhibit flexible working across the hospital/community interface.

The domiciliary consultation

The domiciliary consultation involves an assessment of a patient in their own home by a hospital specialist at the request of a general practitioner. Home visiting by specialists varies considerably across the world being, for example, uncommon in the USA but more frequent in Australia.

Historically, it involved a joint review of the patient by both the general practitioner and the hospital consultant. The necessity for domiciliary consultation varies considerably between specialities. Due to this variation in workload it was recommended (in the UK) that such visits should incur a fee. The majority of domiciliary visits are requested for geriatric medicine (25%) or psychiatric (23%) consults.

Over recent years, the joint review has become less common. The majority of domiciliary visits are now undertaken by a hospital specialist who will then inform the general practitioner of his or her opinion. The visit cannot be for the purpose of reviewing the urgency of a proposed admission or to continue to supervise treatment already initiated in hospital or clinic. In the UK, the frequency of such consultations has declined since their introduction and the involvement of a fee has led to some criticism within the medical press.

Indications to request a domiciliary review
The reasons for a domiciliary visit are varied. The traditional criterion for a visit is that the patient should be, on medical grounds, unable to attend the hospital. Referrals of older patients are commonly for psychiatric symptoms (disorientation, depression, and disturbed behaviour) and non-specific physical symptoms (especially immobility and repeated falls).

Indications include:
- General practitioners requiring a patient to be seen urgently as an outpatient.
- Patients needing geriatric or psychiatric input where a home consultation is thought more appropriate as the patient can be assessed in their own environment.
- Practitioners wanting confirmation that a terminally ill patient is beyond curative intervention and a palliative approach is appropriate.
- Where reassurance with a second opinion is required for a patient or family.
- Advice on management is required but attendance to an outpatient department would be an uncomfortable or distressing experience for the patient.
- When faced with an acutely unwell patient whom the general practitioner feels does not require inpatient admission but would value assistance with diagnosis and/ or management.

Note that the domiciliary visit is not a prerequisite for admission to secondary care.

Advantages of the home assessment for the geriatrician
- Developing a closer association with primary care services.
- Appropriate use of multidisciplinary resources available.
- Improved understanding of the demographics and health needs within the region.
- Most appropriate treatment decided early, reduction in unnecessary investigations and length of inpatient admission.
- Prioritizing admissions.

For the general practitioner
- Advice obtained for patients with challenging diagnoses or complex health problems.
- Reassurance of a second opinion.
- Sharing responsibility of care with a specialist.
- Help with managing patients who are reluctant to be admitted or unable to attend clinic.
- Developing a closer association with local secondary care.

For the patient
- Developing a relationship and building trust with their consultant.
- An opportunity to discuss treatment options prior to admission, investigation or further review.
- Avoiding unnecessary admissions or investigations.

Getting the most from a domiciliary visit
Assessing a patient in a non-clinical environment can be challenging, with a lack of both an ideal setting for an examination and available equipment. However the domiciliary visit can also provide the clinician with vital information including:
1 Detailed history from relatives and neighbours.
2 Mental state examination may be more favourable in a familiar setting.
3 Signs of self neglect may be more apparent.
4 Medications not taken, alcohol abuse, lack of fresh food, poor social conditions, or an unused bed may be evident.
5 The environment can be assessed. Are the stairs too steep, grab rails required, chair too low, bathroom accessories required, etc.?

Author's Tip

Agree with the general practitioner how to discuss the outcome

Telephone ahead. Being expected will ensure your journey is not wasted and your patient will not be distressed by the arrival of a stranger

Arrange to meet a relative, neighbour, or district nurse (especially when removing dressings is required)

Come equipped. Do not forget the referral letter, notebook, disposable gloves, phlebotomy equipment, examination kit, including low reading thermometer and possibly ECG machine

Wear a stout pair of shoes and have warm clothing!

Further reading
National Health Service Act 1946. 9&10. London: HMSO, 1946.
Donaldson LJ, Hill PM (1991). The domiciliary consultation service: time to take stock. Br Med J 302: 449–51.
Interdepartmental Committee on the Remuneration of Consultants and Specialists. Report. London, HMSO, 1948.
Littlejohns PC (1986). Domiciliary Consultation – who benefits? J R Coll Gen Pract 36: 313–15.
Wattis JP (1980). Home assessment: a study of different needs. Geriatric Med 10: 91–5.

Long-term care

The medicine of care homes and specialist housing

Care homes and specialist housing form part of a spectrum of care provision for older people with physical and mental disability. One of the key changes of the last three decades has been that institutional residential care, once primarily concerned with caring for the poor and homeless, has increasing focused around disability in later life. Dementia and its associated dependencies account for much of the workload. The spectrum of housing solutions available, in order of increasing volume and complexity of care, comprises:

Specialist housing

'Sheltered Accommodation', 'Assisted Living', or 'Warden aided' facilities. These will have some supervision by wardens, who largely provide reassurance by their presence on site. Traditionally wardens would have been resident and available 24 hours per day but this practice has become increasingly uncommon since the inception of the European Working Time Directive, which limits their availability to routine working hours. Outside of these, most residents will be reliant on visiting services and alarms linked to call centres for support and surveillance. Unless specifically arranged, residents will receive no personal care or assistance with activities of daily living.

Extracare housing

This has developed over the last decade, supported by funding from central government, to promote independent living in later life and reduce the need for residential care. It typically comprises 'flatlet' or suite style accommodation provided by a housing agency, usually a charity or housing association, together with domiciliary care to help with activities of daily living. Care is provided by a separate organization from the housing element or by a specialist provider arm of the housing agency. The premise is that care and support can be provided more efficiently to a campus of housing than by staff travelling to individual homes. Extracare probably works best for people with good cognitive function and fixed disabilities such as those related to a stroke. It is less appropriate for those with major cognitive impairment and/or rapidly progressive conditions, as it is likely that such residents would require admission to a more definitive care setting a short time after moving to Extracare.

Care homes without nursing, or residential care homes

These predominantly provide care for people with dementia and/or modest physical disability whose care needs cannot be met in the community. Transition to care in this setting will be driven by a combination of frailty, disability, comorbidity, and more holistic concerns of quality of life and the practicality of care delivery. Many residential homes specialize in the care of people with dementia, although the prior classification of homes as elderly mental infirm (EMI) no longer exists. The manager and staff of a residential care home will often not have professional qualifications. They do, however, in many cases possess both a strong sense of vocation and a considerable body of expertise, for example in the non-pharmacological management of behavioural and psychiatric symptoms of dementia. This expertise is not in the delivery of nursing or healthcare but rather in the day-to-day practicalities of caring. Residents of these homes are therefore reliant upon NHS staff for healthcare expertise.

Care homes with nursing, or nursing homes

These provide 24-hour nursing support for residents with more severe and complex mental and physical disability. As in a hospital ward, nurses provide both technical expertise—for example in pressure care and wound dressings—and a supervisory presence, with care workers conducting many of the more routine care activities. Nursing homes now perform a range of differentiated activities—such as rehabilitation, convalescence, support of long-term conditions, and end-of-life care—that map very closely to the work undertaken in NHS community hospitals. There has been a trend towards NHS providers commissioning increasingly complex services from nursing homes—for example as the provider of intermediate care services—and, were this to continue, these facilities might become much more aligned with the health than social care sector.

Place, person, and capability

The proportion of older people with activity limitation is falling. However, the absolute number of older people is rising to the extent that the functional dependency ratio (physically dependent: independent people within a population) will rise across all developed market economies for the foreseeable future. Older people constitute the main users of institutional care services and their impairments and disabilities are driven by long-term neurological diseases, and their problems are often more cognitive and social than physical.

The move to specialist housing and Extracare requires forethought and planning and will usually take place electively in the context of gradual, predictable decline in functional status. An acute deterioration in physical function driven by illness more commonly precipitates admission to a care home.

The placement of an older person in a care home may mean that a residential home is able to support increasing dependency and medical complexity in a well known and established resident supported by the primary care team, much in the way that many people are supported by their families in the community. Such arrangements are dependent on the good-will of all involved and should not be taken to imply that a residential facility has the capacity to manage repeated referrals of similar dependency, as the reserve of care capability may quickly become exhausted, overstretching staff and risking the health and wellbeing of all the residents.

An alternative way to understand the spectrum of care is to recognize the variation in length of stay and admission route. For residential care homes the average length of stay is currently 22 months, compared with 10 months for care homes with nursing. This includes a significant minority of short-stay residents who receive respite, intermediate, or end-of-life care, and a smaller group of very long-term residents, some of whom have been resident in the home for years and represent a more physically robust cohort who may not have been admitted under current criteria.

Intrinsic to most descriptions of frailty is the understanding that a person may not regain their pre-morbid functional status following an acute illness. A consequence is that those living in sheltered or Extracare housing, or residential care homes, may have deteriorated beyond the level of support which they can reasonably be expected to receive in their current setting following such an episode. At a more practical level, a fall, episode of infection or other acute illness may be a marker that the infrastructure of support in a given setting is no longer adequate. A particularly common circumstance is the reality of the person with advancing dementia in specialist housing who becomes unable to manage with intermittent care and support and must move to a residential care home as a consequence.

The organization of care homes varies considerably, at one extreme there are large corporate providers with portfolios of hundreds of homes and on the other an owner-managed single home. In England, the large corporate providers account for 54% of provision, small companies with one or two homes for 37%, and local councils for 6%. The local authority share of the market is rapidly shrinking, as authorities seek to rationalize their spending in the light of recent economic pressures. There remain, for historical reasons, small pockets of NHS provision (0.003% of the market) but the health service is rapidly divesting itself of these. Single home businesses, sometimes referred to as 'mom and pop' homes, are often run as family businesses, with the owner also managing the home and playing a role in hands-on care delivery. This model allows smaller homes (there are still single resident homes in parts of the UK) to remain financially viable and is more applicable in the residential than nursing sectors, where the cost of employing professional nurses precludes such small-scale operation.

Care homes are principally funded for the provision of board, lodging, and personal care, which will include, in nursing homes, nursing support. In both cases, medical support comes from general practitioners and their allied professionals. The division of responsibilities between nurses employed by nursing homes and NHS community nurses is blurred and requires to be negotiated on a home-by-home basis, depending on the specific skill-base of the nurses employed by the home and the needs of their residents.

Care homes do not enjoy a hugely supportive public profile. They are, however, a vital part of care and support of older people. It is salutary to recognize that for every NHS bed (of all types), there are three care beds. This spares the NHS the responsibility of long-term care for frail older people and almost certainly also protects the health service from recurrent inappropriate admissions, simply by providing a more supported living arrangement for those who require it. Recent trends in commissioning also show a trend towards medicalization of the care home sector—with rehabilitation, intermediate and end-of-life care all being provided through contracts with the NHS. Whether such medical provision can be easily nested within a highly socialized model of care without making the environment more hospital-like is unclear. It may be that the sector diverges to allow the emergence of more medicalized long-term care facilities alongside the more homely social care settings to which we have become accustomed.

Funding and care

Specialist and Extracare housing are funded by residents from their own incomes and no formal mechanism for state funding exists. Residents are, however, frequently in receipt of state benefits such as disabled living and attendance allowances and it could therefore be argued that, through these indirect mechanisms, some state subsidy is provided.

State funding is provided for some care home residents but the system is complex, even for the initiated. Potential residents and their families face a considerable learning curve when tackling it for the first time and it is reasonable to expect that they may not fully have grasped all of the nuances of the system by the time they move to a home. It is important for physicians involved in discharge planning to understand this and both to signpost families to social workers for advice and allow families sufficient time to come to terms with the system.

One reason for the considerable complexity within the system is the distinction drawn between health and social care funding—present since the inception of the NHS in the 1940s. Thus healthcare is controlled and funded from central government and free at the point of delivery, whereas social care is controlled and funded at a local authority level and means-tested.

The assessment for admission to a care home will involve assessment by a local authority-employed social services assessor to assess the social care contribution and, if necessary, an NHS-employed nursing assessor to assess the need for, and amount of, any NHS continuing care funding. Following this, residents will find themselves in one of four broad categories:

1 Fully funded continuing care by the NHS, with eligibility determined on the basis of complexity of needs, dependency and/or end of life determination by primary care trust (PCT) nursing assessor.

2 Combined social and healthcare funding, with means-tested social care determined by a local authority assessor and a non-means tested registered nursing care contribution (RNCC) payment for professional nursing determined on the basis of need by a PCT nursing assessor.

3 Means-tested residential care without nursing, determined by local authority assessor.

4 Fully privately funded if savings too great for local authority assistance.

The decision to fund, or not to fund, a resident under NHS continuing care depends upon a, somewhat arbitrary, distinction between what is health and what is social care. A consequence is that the decision not to classify residents as NHS continuing care has been subjected, successfully, to legal challenge. The NHS response has been to tighten up and standardize assessment frameworks considerably, thus minimizing but not negating the possibility of such a challenge.

The means-testing framework for social care depends upon assessing a resident's assets against upper and lower payment thresholds. At the time of writing, any person with assets above £23 000 would be required to fully fund their own care, whereas those with assets less than £14,000 would have their care fully funded by the state. Assets include any property owned by the resident which, with an average UK house price of £168 202, means that anyone who owns a property will pay their own way. Currently 42% of residents fund some or all of their care, 52% are fully state funded, and 7% are funded by the NHS continuing care.

A few issues cloud the picture further. A preferred home's fees may exceed the rate which a local authority is prepared to pay for care. A consequence of this is that 25% of residents in receipt of government-funded care currently have a top-up payment made by families or friends to meet their fees despite, ostensibly, being regarded by the state as too poor to pay. Though very uncommon, some people will have a long-term insurance policy that may have relevant benefits. There are, in addition, benefits such as the attendance allowance and pension and other benefits that may be either amended, or counted towards the cost of care after admission to a care home. The crucial message is that this is a complicated system that is widely considered to be in need of radical reform.

The issue of top-up fees highlights that care homes, even those run by charities and not for profit organizations, have to be commercially successful to survive. The margins of error between success and failure are relatively slim for what in commercial terms is a utility service with considerable risk in terms of liability to clients. Successful operation is a product of good levels of occupancy, satisfactory fee levels, and well-managed costs (of which staffing is the single most important). These parameters are very much shaped by supply, demand, reputation, and affordability.

The shape of social care is driven as much by politics as by common sense or the needs of the population. It has not, thus far, been shaped to any great extent, by evidence-based social policy, as health services research has been slow to identify the care sector as key to broader provision. At the time of writing, in spring 2010, a new coalition government has pledged to ring-fence NHS-funding against cuts, without similar pledges for social care funding, despite the demonstrated interdependency of the two sectors and without any clear idea of how cuts in one will affect the other.

Over the last decade, dementia has emerged as a major health problem. In the UK in 2008, 700 000 people had dementia, with this number predicted to be as high as 1.4 million by 2038. Dementia now competes with cancer, cardiovascular, and cerebrovascular disease as a major healthcare challenge. Unlike these other conditions, however, much of the day-to-day care for dementia is non-pharmacological, non-medical, and provided in a care home setting. It is thus provided by social (means-tested) care rather than health (free at the point of delivery); this is not without controversy.

Presently, dementia is the most common reason for admission to a care home and, based upon the above projections for prevalence, the care home provision within the UK will be inadequate to meet the needs of dementia over the next 25 years. There is no evidence, at present that drug treatments, increased community care, or telecare innovations will substantially reduce the demand for care home placement among people with dementia.

What is clear to seasoned geriatricians is that the line between healthcare and social care has shifted, with much illness-driven disability now being classified as personal care. At the time of writing, the variety of assessment procedures for eligibility testing to satisfy national and local criteria reflect more on a broken system than a personalized approach to care.

Going forward, the funding for long-term care will centre on how our nations decide to manage dementia between health and social care budgets. Is it a social disease, or a medical one, or both? Equality of access to healthcare may have influence, in that a just society should treat the care and support of dementia in the same way as learning difficulties or brain injury. The debate is likely to continue for some time yet.

The medical role in long-term care

The principal medical responsibility to older people, as indeed it is to all ages, is to diagnose and formulate an opinion regarding diagnosis, the nature, and potential reversibility of a patient's functional impairment and their likely trajectory both in terms of longevity and personal functional capacity. This responsibility remains the same in a care home setting. The dynamics of healthcare delivery in a care home setting are, however, influenced by the fact that a third stakeholder, the 'care home', may considerably be affected by the output of a consultation.

The current mantra of healthcare provision to care home residents in the UK is based around the assertion that, as they live in 'homes', they should receive the same medical care as anybody else. Thus general practitioners are responsible for day-to-day care, without any additional time or resources allocated for the increased demands of this cohort. There are some problems with this approach. Because of their frailty and cognitive impairment, care home residents are frequently unable to get to, or use, a phone and unable to attend their doctor, relying instead on home visits. To contact the doctor they often must first convince a care home staff member that their request for a visit is legitimate—an additional gatekeeping measure not faced by community dwellers. Thus the system is more unequal than the rhetoric would suggest. There are also logistical issues, with the mean number of general practitioners per home being seven (range 1–50), making it difficult to standardize care between residents.

Many primary care trusts have now recognized this inequality and a number of innovations have emerged in response. In some regions, enhanced contracts for GPs have been developed to encourage increased focus on supporting care home residents. These payments are, however, small and it is not clear that they make any difference to the quality or quantity of care developed. More novel strategies have looked at systematizing the interaction between healthcare staff and care homes by developing care home practices—where all nursing home residents within a geographical radius, usually a city, are listed with a single group of GPs, sometimes with integrated geriatrician support—or appointing community matrons with specific responsibility for care homes. Again, there is very little evidence surrounding the effectiveness of such services and further evaluative work is required.

History-taking and clinical examination in care homes

Care homes are not clinical settings and can pose a challenge to detailed medical assessment. An attending doctor must carry with them all of all of the equipment required—equipment for neurological examination, fundoscopy, otoscopy, and rectal examination may all be routinely required during a care home assessment and will not be available from the home. Another key issue is to remember that, however institutional some homes might feel, you are visiting a resident in their home, and a room should only be entered and a chair taken at the invitation of the resident. The day room, although providing a useful arena in which to examine the residents' interactions, transfers, and mobility, is an inappropriate place to take a history or conduct an examination and help should be sought from the staff to get the resident to their own bedroom.

Care home staff, although often not healthcare qualified, work with residents with a frequency, intensity, and duration not encountered in any other setting. This can provide a considerable asset in terms of establishing a detailed collateral history and can provide insight into aspects of the history—for example nocturnal behaviour—which might be harder to establish in other settings. In a nursing home, staff should be expected to be able to assist with intimate examinations—it should not be taken for granted that this will be the situation in a residential home.

Homes have a number of tools which aid in diagnosis. Weight charts should be available for all ambulatory residents—although not always for bed- or chair-bound ones. Although variable, many care homes will also keep charts detailing behaviour, nutritional intake, bowel habit, continence, and checks on pressure areas. Nursing homes may also keep regular blood pressure records. Most homes will keep a record of current drug prescriptions and administration in a Medication Administration Record (MAR) book—which is often kept centrally in a nursing station or office.

Because care home staff are often not healthcare professionals, they may describe presentations in terms focused around non-specific functional decline. The onus, therefore, is on the physician to make sense of it all. An important consideration is to reflect upon what might have caused a decline sufficiently insidious to prompt a review *in situ* rather than an emergency transfer to an acute hospital. Iatrogenesis is common in care homes and adverse drug events particularly so. It is also regrettably true that fractures and pressure sores are missed. If a resident has had a fall and has suddenly become unable to weight bear, a radiograph is indicated even in the absence of classical signs of a femoral fracture. If there is a smell suggesting infection, make sure the pressure areas are examined.

The high prevalence of dementia in a care home setting and the short time that a visiting physician will spend with a resident make the diagnosis of delirium particularly challenging. Here, again, the staff can be an asset and assertions that a resident is behaving unusually should not be dismissed out of hand.

For the most part, despite being delivered on a small budget, menus in care homes are carefully designed to be appealing and nutritious to residents. Formal meal times in a dining room setting, as is the norm in care homes, have been shown to improve nutritional intake. Some homes also have provision for families to bring in food and more ambulant (and affluent) residents may choose to dine out. Despite this array of possibilities, the high prevalence of physical and cognitive impairment means that residents are significantly at risk of malnutrition. As well as protein–energy malnutrition, consider that thiamine, pyridoxine, and vitamin C deficiency—and their corresponding syndromes—may be present.

Finally, any new skin condition especially one with irritation, should lead one to consider scabies.

Treatment

Medicines management and prescribing reviews

Care home residents are prescribed on average seven or eight medicines. This figure incorporates a wide variation in practice between residents and homes. Although more independent residents can choose to look after their own medications, care homes will commonly deal with this on their behalf. This will include liaising with general practitioners and community pharmacies to ensure prescriptions are dispensed on time and may involve collecting medications from the pharmacy—although these are now more commonly delivered.

The recent trend has been away from individual packet prescribing to monitored dosing systems—either blister pack or cassette based—where drugs are placed into dispensing trays marked by time and day by pharmacy staff. This takes some of the onus away from care home staff and allows for less qualified staff to aid in administration.

The regulation of medicines management in care homes is stricter than within the NHS, with even minor documented omissions or errors constituting unacceptable breaches. A 100-bed care home with an average of seven prescriptions per resident and an average administration rate of twice daily will conduct 1400 medication administrations per day. It is therefore, perhaps, unsurprising that medication errors occur. These errors happen throughout the drug administration chain with a recent study reporting prescribing errors in 39%, dispensing errors in 32%, administration errors in 37%, and medication monitoring errors in 18% of residents. Fortunately, most of these represented minor errors, resulting in little clinical harm, but the potential for mistakes when working with drugs on such an industrial scale are large.

These findings are based on the presumption that prescriptions are appropriate in the first place. However, up to 70% of residents are reported to be prescribed one or more inappropriate drugs. Good practice is to conduct a critical review of a resident's medication after initial settlement in a new setting with attention to cessation, dose reduction, and frequency reduction where possible and introduction of new medications only where absolutely necessary. Medication reviews should be undertaken at 6-monthly intervals thereafter—or more frequently if the patient is in the last days of life. The practice of conducting medication reviews remotely from the patient, using care staff as a proxy for face-to-face meetings, is to be discouraged. Unexplained symptoms should always be thought of as being iatrogenic in origin and the maxim 'last in first out' is often useful when a new potential adverse drug reaction occurs.

A key issue is to understand that prescribing errors will be minimized if changes to medications are conducted by the patient's usual prescriber. Although the evils of polypharmacy cannot, for the most part, be overstated, drug cessation is rarely so pressing an issue that it cannot be conducted in discussion with—or preferably by—the patient's general practitioner.

It is also likely that patients will become more concordant with their prescriptions when they enter a home—this will be particularly the case for those on many medications. A consequence is that patients may become hypotensive, dehydrated, confused, constipated, incontinent, or over-anticoagulated a short while after moving to care as a consequence of being given the drugs they were always erroneously believed to be taking.

Certain classes of drugs are particularly common in care settings and deserve particular mention.

Antipsychotic medications

These are often commenced in acute hospitals where people with severe cognitive impairment may become agitated, disturbed, and a danger to themselves and those around them. Sedation and behavioural control with antipsychotics may be a poor response but is often the only practicable solution. A big problem is that often the short-term therapeutic objective is lost and such prescriptions become embedded into routine. Although these medications may have a role in the transition to the new surroundings of a care home, it should be normal practice for them to be critically reviewed after a week or two with a clear intent to reduce and withdraw them. Clearly these drugs are used outside their usual licences in dementia and are often used in inappropriately high doses. Although no clear advice is given in the British National Formulary, a pragmatic approach to withdrawal is to half doses weekly until a medication can be withdrawn or symptoms suggest a continued need. A good home, particularly one with specialist dementia registration, should not require routine use of these drugs. What is clearly important is for the prescribing doctor to be clear on what symptom or behaviour the treatment is attempting to resolve and that critical follow-up is made. The dubious clinical benefit is compounded by the high risk of stroke among patients on atypical antipsychotics. These drugs are therefore now so contentious that the prescription and rationale should be clearly communicated with care home staff and families and a risk–benefit assessment made using a shared decision-making framework.

Diuretics

These are often prescribed in acute heart failure and the doses are then not critically reviewed as the patient stabilizes. Patients often moderate their fluid intake on moving to a care home and dehydration may follow. Beware that many non-specialists use these medications for orthostatic oedema, where they rarely work and increase the risk of incontinence, orthostatic hypotension, and falls such that the risk–benefit ratio is almost never in their favour. In this circumstance, they should be stopped.

Statins

Although the role of statins in controlling cardiovascular risk from hypercholesterolaemia is well established in younger patients, there are no specific trials or data justify their continuation in care home residents who may be at risk of malnutrition and who are likely to suffer more from muscle pain that may well contribute to immobility. Their use in advanced old age is often justified by plaque regression data from large multicentre studies in coronary artery and cerebrovascular disease. In practice, the doses required to obtain such effects are rarely achievable in frail older patients.

Antihypertensive medication

Reviewing the need for antihypertensive medication is often rewarding. In all nursing homes and many residential care homes, blood pressure readings can be taken for attending doctors. Lying and standing blood pressures should be a routine part of the care home examination in all but the most functionally impaired patients.

Antibiotics

There is evidence that the commensal organisms colonizing care home residents are different from the wider population but no evidence that modifying antibiotics from standard recommended community regimens has any role in the UK setting. In older care home residents, the widely used CURB-65 criteria for establishing severity of community-acquired pneumonia have a low specificity and positive predictive value and there is no evidence that moving residents to hospital improves outcomes. There is therefore a strong incentive for treating care home residents with pneumonia *in situ* using oral antibiotics, except where there is a clear indication for either oxygen therapy or intravenous fluids. The difficulty of diagnosing urinary tract infections in older patients should be acknowledged and antibiotics reserved for patients who are symptomatic. Fastidiousness in antibiotic prescribing is essential, as this group are particularly vulnerable to antibiotic-associated infections.

It is very difficult to effectively care for a patient with *Clostridium difficile* diarrhoea in care home setting because of the fabric of the building (carpets and soft furnishings), unenforced freedom of movement for residents around their home and the lower staffing ratios in care homes, which are tested to the limit if a resident suddenly becomes faecally incontinent several times per day.

Analgesics

Assessing pain in patients with dementia is notoriously difficult. Two conflicting issues are that patients should not be denied pain relief simply because they cannot express their pain in abstract terms and that both opioid and non-steroidal analagesics have considerable side-effect profiles in this cohort. Non-verbal cues are important and close attentiveness of care home staff to these can help to identify when analgesics are indicated.

Communication

Communication between agencies is particularly important for care home residents because they will be dependent on others—care home staff, primary care staff and general practitioners—for care. These agencies can only provide care effectively if informed of the key healthcare issues.

On discharge from hospital

It is commonplace for older people to change general practitioner on taking up residence in a care home and effective decision making and clinical management in this context will rest heavily on the adequacy of available information. Over 50% of care home admissions are transfers from acute hospitals. These residents are also potentially more medically unstable than those moving from their own home, further emphasizing the need for clarity of communication. Medical discharge transfer documentation should have the following;

1 biographic data
2 reason for hospital admission
3 current status and predicted prognosis, the reason for transfer to care and expectation of care (is the transfer for convalescence, long-term care or end of life care)
4 full diagnostic synopsis and indication of whether each diagnosis is active in the condition of the patient
5 simple justification for each prescribed medication whether it is a planned long term treatment or newly introduced treatment (to facilitate identification of adverse drug reactions)
6 resuscitation status. If 'Do not resuscitate' decisions have been taken or legitimate advance care plans or decisions have been agreed they should be clearly communicated

Armed with the above information and assisted by clear observations from home staff, attending doctors in emergency situations will be much better informed and able to make decisions in the best interest of patients in the event of sudden change. They may also have the confidence to manage people in situ when it is clear that the burden of illness will make a further hospitalization more of a risk than opportunity.

Urgent referral to hospital

A general practitioner called to see an older person in a supported housing setting or a residential care home may not have access to sufficient background medical information and may have to make a default decision to refer the patient to hospital. Although it is undeniably true that there is much unwarranted variation in decision-making, the standards of communication should enable the receiving hospital doctor to understand the basis of referral from the doctor. In the present operation of primary care, many such referrals will not come from the general practitioner with whom the patient is registered but an out of hours service. If a doctor is unfamiliar with the resident and is only able to rely on the evidence of a temporary care worker or nurse clearly their threshold for referral will be lower.

1 Biographic data including the name of any key worker, manager and their contact number.

2 Reason for referral which should provide clear information as to the patient's status whether they are for active treatment, palliation or whether this is unknown.

3 Full summary of active and managed diagnoses. diagnostic synopsis and indication of whether each diagnosis is active in the condition of the patient.

4 Medication record whether it is a planned long-term treatment or newly introduced treatment (to facilitate identification of adverse drug reactions)

5 Resuscitation status, if known.

Keeping staff in the loop

A common dilemma in communications about care home residents is how much information, if any, to disclose to care home staff who—for the most part—are employed in a social rather than healthcare role. Although these staff have no right of access to patients' medical records, it is certainly the case that their job is made easier by a comprehensive understanding of their residents' healthcare problems. Such enlightenment can, for example, allow them to look for changes in behaviour or functional status that may indicate a change in residents' health status. It may also allow them to identify a problem, for example recurrent pain, is now fully understood and therefore not a reason for repeated calls to a general practitioner. Finally, the care home records are available to out-of-hours general practitioners, whereas notes from the residents' own doctors are not. A copy of recent correspondence, along with a list of up-to-date diagnoses, can significantly aid decision making in this context.

Gold standard practice is probably to seek a resident's consent to copy correspondence to the care home manager and then to ensure that you do so, addressing correspondence directly to the manager. Where a resident does not have capacity to provide such consent, an assessment of best interests will have to be made but it is difficult to envisage a scenario where it will not be in a resident's interests for the agency providing most of their care to understand their current health status.

Regulation of care

The level of regulatory scrutiny of care homes exceeds that experienced by the NHS and public services and many practitioners joining the care sector are surprised by the importance placed on risk assessment and governance frameworks. The care sector has historically been regulated separately to health services but now regulation has merged into the responsibility of the Care Quality Commission (CQC).

At the time of writing, the regulations governing CQC inspections are in a state of flux, with both the frequency and triggers for inspection due to change in the near future in response to the Health and Social Care Act of 2008. However, consistent features between new and old systems are that inspections are more frequent and less likely to be announced for care homes categorized as 'average' or 'poor' than for those thought to be 'excellent' or 'good'.

Inspection is conducted according to Key Lines of Regulatory Assessment (KLORAs), which provide detailed descriptors of what constitutes an 'excellent', 'good', 'fair', or 'poor' home against 38 national minimum standards across seven domains comprising: choice of home, health, and personal care, daily life and social activities, complaints and protection, environment, staffing, and management and administration. Although healthcare features among the minimum standards, it is not at the centre to the inspection process. This is perhaps reasonable, given the remit of care homes as social rather than healthcare providers.

Copies of all care home inspection reports produced by the CQC can now be found online and can be a considerable asset to potential residents, or their families, in trying to choose a home. In some respects the detailed descriptions in the reports are more useful than the overall ratings, since homes frequently move between ratings and the KLORAs are sufficiently subjective to allow for inconsistency between inspections. One of the truisms of regulation is that what can be counted, or easily described, is likely to be regulated more intensively/obsessively than less tangible aspects of care. Thus the ethos and 'feel' of a care home cannot easily be included in assessments. It is therefore essential that residents, or at the very least their families, visit the home and speak to the staff and manager before arriving at a decision to move there.

An additional level of inspection is imposed by local authorities on all providers from whom they commission social care and the NHS on all providers whom they pay for NHS continuing care. These inspection processes are less standardised and vary from area to area, although attempts are currently under way to make them more uniform.

Further reading

Barber ND, Alldred DP, Raynor DK, et al. (2009). Care homes' use of medicines study: prevalence, causes and potential harm of medication errors in care homes for older people. *Qual Saf Health Care* **18**: 341–6.

Bowman C, Whistler J, Ellerby M (2004). A national census of care home residents. *Age Ageing* **33**: 561–6.

Donald IP, Gladmam J, Conroy S, et al. (2008). Care home medicine in the UK- in from the cold. *Age Ageing* **37**: 618–20.

Gordon A, Ewan V (2010). Pneumonia and influenza? specific considerations in care homes. *Rev Clin Gerontol* **20**: 69–80.

Mitchell A (ed.) (2009). *Care of the Elderly People UK Market Survey 2009*. London, Laing and Buisson.

Owen T (2006). *National Care Homes Research and Development Forum. My Home Life: Quality of Life in Care Homes*. London, Help the Aged

Geriatricians and continuing care

Individuals may need services to meet long-term health and social care needs which have arisen from acute illness or the progression of chronic disease. Health care from the NHS is provided free whereas personal and social care is arranged by local authorities (LAs) and means-tested.

For some individuals, health needs are sufficiently severe to make them eligible to have both their continuing health and personal care needs met by the NHS. In other words, some people who are deemed eligible for free continuing NHS healthcare (NHS CHC) have all their care home costs met by the NHS for as long as they remain eligible at each review.

Decisions about eligibility for NHS CHC are made in line with the National Framework for NHS Continuing Healthcare the latest version of which, at the time of writing, was released in July 2009. The process as it applies to an individual is overseen by the primary care trust to which the patient's general practitioner belongs and depends on information about health needs. Geriatricians have an important role supplying this for their patients.

Terminology

The National Framework sets out the current definitions of continuing healthcare. The general term continuing care means 'care provided over an extended period of time, to a person aged 18 or over, to meet physical or mental health needs that have arisen as a result of disability, accident or illness'. Very often individuals receive means-tested services from LAs and free healthcare from the NHS as a joint care package.

NHS continuing healthcare means a package of care that is arranged and funded solely by the NHS for those with a 'primary health need' and can be provided in a person's own home or a care home in which case the accommodation costs are also met.

Primary health need

It is important to understand that a primary health need refers to the situation where the ongoing health needs are the main reason for the provision of services. If the main need is for personal care arising from a medical condition, then those services are arranged by the LA on a means-tested basis or by those individuals funding their own care labelled as 'self-funders'.

For example, a person with a stroke that leads to the need for personal care without any health interventions would receive means-tested services. If that person were to have ongoing health needs, such as management of convulsions, broken skin, behavioural, cognitive or communication problems, diabetes needing alterations in treatment, then the health needs would mount up. The purpose is to decide if the totality of health need amounts to a primary health need rather than being ancillary or incidental to the need for accommodation.

> **Author's Tip**
>
> A primary health need confers eligibility for NHS CHC and refers to the ongoing healthcare needs as being the main reason for care and *not* to the primary diagnosis or medical event that led to the need for personal care.

General procedures

The process for deciding eligibility is still evolving. Until recently the primary care trust (PCT) would assemble information about a person's care needs and convene a continuing care professional review panel to decide eligibility. The information would include contributions from a nurse, a doctor, a social worker, and where necessary a therapist, dietician, or community psychiatric nurse.

In line with Department of Health guidance, recommendations for eligibility of hospital inpatients are now made by the multidisciplinary team (MDT) providing care, assisted by the PCT. Similarly, arrangements are evolving for MDTs in the community to make recommendations for eligibility for people at home or in care homes. The PCT checks the soundness of the MDT decision before ratifying it. A PCT panel will also review cases from another panel when the patient or family appeal a 'no' decision. If dispute continues the next steps are the Strategic Health Authority and then the Ombudsman.

The foregoing describes the NHS system as it operates in England. Differences in process and documentation apply in the devolved countries of the UK.

> **Author's Tip**
>
> Sound decisions on eligibility for free NHS continuing healthcare depend on good clinical information about the ongoing healthcare needs caused by disease. A list of diagnoses is insufficient.

The geriatrician's role

Geriatricians should be aware that it is a legal obligation for hospitals to 'take reasonable steps to ensure that an assessment for NHS continuing healthcare is carried out in all cases where it appears … the patient may have a need for such care' before giving notice of an individual's case to the LA in accordance with the Community Care Delayed Discharges Act 2003. This means that whenever hospitals are planning to discharge a person who needs ongoing care (and is not, of course, already receiving NHS continuing healthcare), they should use a checklist to consider whether a full continuing care assessment should take place.

Geriatricians and the MDT provide information about health needs and ongoing treatment to support the full assessment. The documentation varies using a single assessment process or separate contributions.

A fast track system is available for those with a limited life expectancy.

Decision-makers will consider the case in line with the Decision Support Tool (DST) in the National Framework. Geriatricians should therefore be aware of the contents of the DST so that important clinical factors are not omitted.

The decision support tool

The DST is used to decide whether a person's needs constitute a 'primary health need' and has two main sections. The first is a list of health domains covering behaviour, cognition, psychological needs, communication, mobility, nutrition, continence, skin, breathing, medication, altered states of consciousness, and a section for other situations not covered by the list. The features of an individual case are weighted from 'no needs' through 'low', 'moderate', and 'high' according to the DST wording with 'severe' and 'priority' for some of the domains.

The second considers the health needs under the general headings of nature (who can provide the care), intensity (quantity), complexity (quality, interactions), and unpredictability. In general, one 'priority' or two 'severe' weightings are strong indicators of eligibility, which can also arise from a combination of lesser weightings.

The decision on eligibility therefore rests on full consideration of the person's health needs under the domains with their nature, intensity, complexity, or unpredictability.

Medical information

Geriatricians providing medical information will appreciate that a list of diagnoses should be accompanied by brief comment relevant to the DST. For example, diabetes mellitus might be stable and subject to planned review, or unstable necessitating vigilance and action by care home staff to deal with unpredictable hypoglycaemia, more so if the person is cognitively impaired or unable for whatever reason to signal their symptoms.

Geriatric medicine is synonymous with unique combinations and interactions of clinical disorders for individuals. Geriatricians with their expertise have an important role to ensure all factors are available so the assessment is fair and complete and to ensure their junior colleagues become familiar with the system for awarding NHS continuing healthcare.

Acknowledgement
I am grateful to Sue Cooper, independent advisor on continuing care, for help with this chapter

Further reading
Department of Health (2009). *The National Framework for NHS Continuing Healthcare and NHS-funded Nursing Care July 2009 (revised)*. Gateway reference 11509. London, Central Office of Information.

Falls and fall prevention

Prevalence of falls and injuries

Prevalence

Falls are common among older people and are a major public health concern in terms of morbidity, quality of life, mortality, and cost to health and social services. It is estimated that 28–35% of community-dwelling older people aged 65 years and above fall each year. This figure rises to 42% in people aged 75 years and over. In institutionalized older people, there is an even higher prevalence. In surveys conducted of nursing home populations, the percentage of patients falling each year ranged from 16% to 75% with a mean of 43%. This may be due to the frailer nature of the nursing home population, together with more stringent reporting by staff. About half of those who fall do so repeatedly.

Location of falls

Of those who fall:

- Approximately 65% of women and 44% of men fall inside their usual residence and garden.
- In the home, most falls occur in the most frequently used rooms—bedroom, kitchen, and dining room.
- Falls in the hallway or bathroom tend to be associated with urinary incontinence.
- People aged <75 years are more likely to fall outdoors than those aged 75 years and over.
- Indoor falls are associated with frailty, whereas outdoor falls are associated with compromised health status in more active people.
- Most falls in the community occur during the day with only 20% occurring during the night.

Mortality

Accidents are the fifth leading cause of death of older people, behind cardiovascular disease, cancer, stroke, and pulmonary disease. Falls account for two-thirds of these accidental deaths. Fall-related mortality increases dramatically with advancing age, particularly over 70 years of age with men having a higher mortality rate than women. Nursing home residents account for one-fifth of all fatal falls.

Morbidity

Falls related injuries are more common in the older population due to a higher prevalence of underlying disease, e.g. osteoporosis, than younger counterparts. There are also age-related physiological changes with limited functional reserve. This can lead to a precarious physiological and physical balance with the potential to fall and injury from seemingly minor intrinsic and extrinsic risk factors:

- 40–60% of falls lead to injuries
- 30–50% of injury results in minor trauma
- 10–15% of injury leads to serious injuries
- 5–10% of serious injury results in fracture, 1–2% of these being hip fractures
- the proportion of falls leading to serious injury is the same in community dwelling and institutionalized older people.

Many older fallers are unable to get up again without assistance and are at risk of a 'long lie'. This can lead to hypothermia, dehydration, bronchopneumonia, pressure sores, rhabdomyolysis, and death.

> **Important impact of falls**
> - Significant morbidity
> - Mortality
> - Functional decline
> - Social Isolation
> - Depression
> - Loss of confidence
> - Hospitalization
> - Institutionalization
> - Expenditure to health and social care services

Hip fractures

Hip fractures can have a devastating effect on physical and social wellbeing. So much so that 80% of older women would prefer death than experience the loss of independence and quality of life that results from a bad hip fracture resulting in nursing home admission. Seventy-five per cent of hip fractures occur in women. There is significant associated mortality:

- 10% die within 1 month
- 20% die within 6 months
- 33% die within 1 year.

Morbidity is mainly associated with immobilization and includes venous thromboembolism, bronchopneumonia, and muscular deconditioning.

Fifty per cent will no longer be able to live independently in the community, and 10–20% of people will need to move from their own home into residential or nursing care.

Approximately half of hip fractures occur in people whose bone mineral density is above the osteoporotic range. Several studies have shown that there is an association between risk of hip fracture and falls risk factors. In a large epidemiological study the risk of hip fracture increased by 30% per fall from zero to five or more falls.

> **Falls risk factors which have shown to predict hip fractures**
> - History of falls
> - Fall to the side
> - Self reported health
> - Self reported physical activity
> - Impaired cognition
> - Slower walking speed
> - Type 2 diabetes mellitus
> - Parkinson's disease
> - Poor vision and depth perception
> - Lack of exercise in the last year
> - Frailty
> - Muscle composition

Fear of falling

Fear of falling is well recognized in older people with a history of falls and in itself can lead to an increased risk of falls. One-third of fallers will develop this after an incidental fall. This can lead to self-imposed restrictions on activities of daily living. This, in turn, can lead to depression, social isolation, loss of confidence, and functional decline.

Social morbidity

Repeated falls is a common cause of institutionalization in older people who were previously living independently. If a serious injury occurs, the risk of institutionalization is three times higher than after a non-injurious fall.

Financial implications

Falls also represent a significant cost to health and social care. In 1999, an analysis of the cost of unintentional falls was undertaken. It estimated that falls cost the UK government £1 billion per year with 59% of the cost being borne by the NHS and the remainder by social services. Falls in people aged 75 or above accounted for 66% of the overall cost. The highest overall cost component was inpatient admission followed by long-term care provision. The cost of A&E admissions and GP follow up was comparatively small. A more recent study from 2008 comprising an international comparison of the cost of falls in older people living in the community estimates an annual cost of US$1.6 billion to the UK government.

Further reading

Austin N, Devine A, Dick I, *et al.* (2007). Fear of falling in older women: a longitudinal study of incidence, persistence and predictors. *J Am Geriatr Soc* **55**: 1598.

Bath PA, Morgan K (1999). Differential risk factor profiles for indoor and outdoor falls in older people living at home in Nottingham, UK. *Eur J Epidemiol* **15**: 65–73.

Cummings SR, Nevitt MC, Browner WS, *et al.* (1995). Risk Factors for hip fracture in white women. Study of Osteoporotic Fractures Research Group. *N Engl J Med* **332**: 767–73.

Davis JC, Robertson MC, Ashe T, *et al.* (2010). International comparison of cost of falls in older adults living in the community: a systematic review. *Osteoporos Int* **21**: 1295–306.

Guesens P, Van Geel T, Van Den Bery J (2010). Can hip fracture prediction in women be estimated beyond bone mineral density measurement alone? *Ther Adv Musculoskelet Dis* **2**: 63–7.

Masud T, Morris RO (2001). Epidemiology of falls. *Age Ageing* **30**(4): 3–7.

Rubenstein LZ, Josephson, KR (2002). The epidemiology of falls and syncope. *Clin Ger Med* **18**: 141–58.

Salkeld G, Cameron ID, Cumming RG, *et al.* (2000). Quality of life related to fear of falling and hip fracture in older women: A time trade off study. *Br Med J* **320**: 341–6.

Scuffham P, Chaplin S, Legwood R (2003). Incidence and cost of unintentional falls in older people in the United Kingdom. *J Epidemiol Community Health* **57**: 740–4.

Aetiology of falls

Definition of falls and fallers

Numerous definitions for a fall have been employed in the research literature. The prevention of Falls Network Europe (ProFaNE) organization has standardized the definition to 'an unexpected event in which the participant comes to rest on the ground, floor or lower level'.

A faller can be defined as someone who has fallen at least once over a defined period of time, normally 6 months or 1 year. Fallers can be further subdivided according to the frequency of their falls. The category into which they fall can reflect their underlying physiology as well as predict the types of injuries likely to be sustained. A recurrent faller is usually defined as someone with more than one fall (often two or more falls, or sometimes three or more falls) over a period of time, usually 1 year. The term 'once-only faller' is also sometimes used—someone who has fallen only once during a defined period of time.

Physiological parameters such as visual contrast sensitivity, reaction time, body sway, quadriceps strength, and vibration sense are similar between non-fallers and once-only fallers. In recurrent fallers, these parameters are significantly worse.

Classification of falls

Falls can be classified in several ways.

- Intrinsic, where some event or condition affects postural control, or extrinsic, where an environmental factor is the main contributing factor.
- Explained (e.g. simple trip, arrhythmia) versus unexplained (cause or causes not entirely clear).
- Injurious or non-injurious.
- Accidental versus non-accidental falls; this can be misleading. The implication is that accidental falls are purely random events whereas other causal factors, intrinsic or extrinsic, may also be involved.
- Syncopal versus non-syncopal.

Risk factors for falls

There have been over 400 potential risk factors for falling identified in the literature and they can be classified in several ways. One classification categorizes risk factors according to whether they are intrinsic (inherent to the individual) or extrinsic (environmental).

Important intrinsic and extrinsic risk factors contributing to falls

Intrinsic Factors

Central Processing
- Cognitive impairment
- Depression

Neuromotor
- Parkinson's disease
- Parkinson's related syndromes (e.g. PSP, MSA, LBD*)
- Gait and balance disorder
- Stroke
- Decreased muscle strength
- Neuropathy

Musculoskeletal
- Chronic musculoskeletal pain
- Arthritis

Vision
- Decreased visual acuity
- Decreased depth perception
- Decreased contrast sensitivity

Cardiovascular
- Dizziness
- Orthostatic hypotension
- Carotid sinus hypersensitivity
- Neurocardiogenic syncope
- Arrhythmias
- Valvular heart disease

Other
- Low body mass index/nutritional deficiency
- History of Falls
- Age ≥80
- Female Sex

Extrinsic factors
- Medication
- Alcohol
- Environmental obstacles
- Poor lighting
- Inappropriate clothing and/or footwear

LBD, Lewy body dementia; MSA, multisystem atrophy; PSP, progressive supranuclear palsy

---

The causes of falls are often multifactorial with a number of risk factors involved. Often the faller has many chronic, predisposing factors making them prone to falls. Any superimposed acute precipitating factors can then trigger the fall (e.g. infection, myocardial infarction, dehydration, new medication). A previous history of falls is also a significant risk factor for further falls. Several studies have shown that the risk of falling increases dramatically as the number of risk factors increases. One study reported the percentage of people falling increased from 27% for those with no or one risk factor, to 78% for those with four or more.

Vision

Poor vision increases the risk of falling. It has been shown that improving vision, such as through early cataract surgery, can lead to a significant reduction in falls. However, it has also been shown that by improving vision quickly through new prescription lenses the rate of falls can actually increase. This is particularly true if the change in prescription is large and it is likely a period of adjustment is needed. Regular eye assessments are recommended to avoid sudden dramatic changes in lens prescription. Bifocal and varifocal lenses are not recommended in those at high risk of falls, as they can further increase risk of falls due to altered depth perception.

Cognitive impairment

There is a 70–85% annual incidence of falls in people with cognitive impairment and dementia. This is double the falls risk of the cognitively intact older population. Cognitive impairment can impair judgement, visuospatial perception and cause an inability to orientate oneself to the surroundings. Once a fall has occurred, the prognosis tends to be poorer with less likelihood of good recovery from a significant injury. For example, one year mortality after a neck of femur fracture is 71% in the cognitively impaired versus 19% in the cognitively normal. Patients with vascular dementia and Lewy body dementia tend to fall more often than those with Alzheimer's dementia. This is thought to be due to the more marked gait abnormalities seen in the first two syndromes.

Gait disturbance, muscle weakness, and physical activity

These can arise from specific medical conditions, e.g. stroke, Parkinson's disease, arthritis, or through deconditioning through inactivity. Up to two-thirds of people experiencing a fall will have some form of gait disturbance. The prevalence of grossly detectable muscle weakness ranges from 48% in community-dwelling older people to 57% in intermediate care facilities to over 80% among nursing home residents. Levels of physical fitness also play a part. People with low levels of cardiorespiratory fitness and low levels of activity are more likely to fall while walking than those with high levels of fitness.

Fear of falling

This is not only a consequence of falling, it is a psychological risk factor for further falls. This occurs in around a third of older people after an incidental fall.

Urinary incontinence

Urge incontinence is an independent risk factor for falls, whereas stress incontinence is not. Urinary frequency, nocturia, and rushing to the toilet all contribute.

Syncope

There is a significant overlap between syncope and falls. The majority of patients with syncope will suffer a fall. Twenty per cent of unexplained falls will be due to syncope from a neurally mediated cardiovascular disorder or hypotensive syndrome. 'Pre-syncope' can also lead to falls. Causes of syncope and pre-syncope commonly include arrhythmias (brady- and tachy-), orthostatic hypotension, neurocardiogenic (vasovagal) syndrome, carotid sinus syndrome, and valvular heart disease (e.g. aortic stenosis).

Medication

Medication is commonly implicated as a contributing factor in falls in older people. This can either be due to the direct effect of the drug, e.g. clouding of consciousness with psychotropic medication, or due to the combined effects of polypharmacy. It has been shown that being on four or more medicines increases the risk of falls. Poor medication compliance can also increase risk of falls by up to 50%. This is one of the reasons why medication review is an essential part of comprehensive geriatric assessment.

Medications implicated in increased risk of falls in elderly people

- Benzodiazepines
- Neuroleptics
- Antihypertensives
- Antidepressants
- Anticholinergics
- Class IA antiarrhythmic medications

Environmental factors

Twenty-five per cent to 45% of falls are attributed to 'accidents' due to environmental hazards. There is often an interplay between the hazard and the faller's intrinsic factors making them more susceptible to the fall. Common hazards found within the home include clutter, loose carpets and rugs, poor lighting, slippery surfaces and lack of hand rails. Stair-related falls account for 10% of all fall related deaths. Seventy-five per cent occur during descent. Characteristics that make falls more likely include the stair design, step height and depth, stair maintenance and lighting.

Further reading

Cummings RG, Ivers R, Clemson, L, et al. (2007). Improving vision to prevent falls in frail older people. A randomised trial. *J Am Geriatr Soc* **55**: 175–81.

Harwood RH, Foss AJ, Osborn F, et al. (2005). Falls and health status in elderly women following first eye cataract surgery: a randomised control trial. *Br J Ophthalmol* **89**: 53–9.

Lamb SE, Jorstad-Stein EC, Hauer K, et al. (2005). Prevention of Falls Network Europe and Outcomes Consensus Group. Development of a common outcome data set for fall injury prevention trials. The Prevention of Falls Network Europe consensus. *JAGS* **53**: 1618–22.

Masud T, Morris RO (2001). Epidemiology of Falls. *Age Ageing* **30**: 3–7.

Mertz K, Lee D, Sui X, et al. (2010). Falls among adults. the association of cardiorespiratory fitness and physical activity with walking-related falls. *Am J Prev Med* **39**: 15–24.

Rubenstein LZ, Josephson, KR (2002). The epidemiology of falls and syncope. *Clin Ger Med* **18**: 141–58.

Shaw FE (2002). Falls in cognitive impairment and dementia. *Clin Ger Med* **18**: 159–73.

Tinetti ME, Speechley M, Ginter SF (1988). Risk factors for falling among elderly people living in the community. *N Engl J Med* **319**: 1701–7.

Investigation of falls

Screening

All older people should be asked whether they have fallen in the past year. Falls are under-reported, so should be specifically asked about. If a person reports a fall, a full history of the frequency and circumstance(s) of falls should be taken. Further assessment depends on the level of future falls risk for that individual.

The American Geriatrics Society/British Geriatrics Society (AGS/BGS) Guideline recommends three questions should be asked of all older people (aged 65 and over) who report any falls in the last 12 months:

1 Have you had two or more falls in the last 12 months?
2 Have you presented acutely with a fall?
3 Do you have problems with walking or balance (not necessarily restricting activity)?

If a person gives a positive answer to any of these questions, they should be considered at **high-risk** of further falls and assessed as such. Those who have had a single, non-injurious fall are categorized as **low-risk**.

Assessment of low-risk fallers

Carelessness is not the sole preserve of the young. Older people can, of course, have accidental falls with no underlying physical impairment. However, a single fall could be the first sign of difficulties with walking and/or balance, which may not yet be apparent to the patient, and provides an opportunity for early intervention. The majority of older people who fall have an underlying musculoskeletal reason for falling. Therefore, all older people reporting a single fall should undergo a simple assessment of gait and balance.

There are many tools for assessing gait and balance, none of which are sufficiently sensitive or specific to allow recommendation as the 'best' test for predicting falls risk. One simple tool in widespread use is the Timed Up and Go Test, subjects begin seated and are instructed to stand from the chair, using their arms if necessary, to walk to a line 3 metres in front of the chair; to turn round, return to the chair and sit down again. The time for the subject to complete this task is predictive of their risk of falling. Different thresholds have varying degrees of sensitivity and specificity, but the commonly used cut-off is 13.5 seconds. Fallers taking more than 13.5 seconds to complete the timed up and go test are at high-risk of further falls and require further assessment. In addition, some people will manage the task within 13.5 seconds but appear unsafe in doing so. These patients should also be assessed further as high-risk.

Alternative tools for predicting falls risk include the Berg Balance Scale, which assesses balance but not gait, and the Performance-Oriented Mobility Assessment (POMA) Score, which assesses gait and balance in detail but takes 10–15 minutes to complete.

In subjects with cognitive impairment, falls are more often due to a failure of multitasking. One simple way to assess this is the see if the person can walk and talk at the same time. If they need to stop walking in order to engage in conversation, or if their walking speed is significantly slower if asked to perform simple mental arithmetic while walking, this is strongly predictive of future falls.

An older person who has had a single non-injurious fall and who has normal gait and balance (normal Timed Up and Go Test) does not require further assessment or intervention. They should be rescreened a year later, or sooner in the event of a further fall.

Assessment of high-risk fallers

'There is always a reason why someone falls', but many older people possess several risk factors for falling and there may not be a single treatable cause. Consequently, high-risk fallers should receive a multifactorial assessment for falls risk factors, with intervention tailored to modify the identified risks (see section Management of falls). Assessment should be performed by one or more clinicians with the necessary skills and training. Many falls services benefit from a multi-disciplinary team approach to falls risk factor assessment, including a geriatrician, physiotherapist, nurse specialist, occupational therapist and pharmacist. Assessment must allow the identification of the minority of fallers that have a 'medical' reason for falling, including syncope, as well as those who will benefit from further investigation or intervention.

Investigation of falls begins with the clinical assessment to determine underlying falls risk factors. The history should begin with a detailed description of the most recent fall including any preceding or concurrent symptoms and any injuries or other consequences (including fear of further falls). Where possible, this should be accompanied by a collateral history from a witness. Specific consideration should be given to the possibility of loss of consciousness, bearing in mind that there may be amnesia for syncope. Therefore, treat with caution the patient who says they 'must have' slipped, but cannot remember doing so.

The history should also include a review of medication and other medical problems. A detailed medication review, including non-prescribed medication, is required, with particular regard to medications that have sedative or hypotensive effects. The history should also include any relevant acute or chronic medical problems, such as osteoporosis, osteoarthritis, incontinence, alcohol misuse, cardiovascular disease, or neurological disorders.

Clinical examination should include the following aspects.

- Detailed assessment of gait, balance, mobility, and the joints and muscles of the lower limbs.
- Cognitive assessment using a validated tool.
- Neurological assessment including tests of cortical, extrapyramidal, cerebellar, and vestibular systems, peripheral sensation and proprioception.
- Romberg test, which is positive in both proprioceptive and vestibular disorders.
- Pulse rate and rhythm, postural (lying and standing) blood pressure, heart sounds.
- Visual acuity (Snellen chart) with usual glasses or other visual aids.
- Feet and footwear.

These examinations can be performed by any appropriately trained member of the multiprofessional team, although a geriatrician should be trained in all of the above assessments.

All patients should have an assessment of function, including activities of daily living and any perceived impairment in relation to falls or the fear of falling. An assessment of the home environment will also be appropriate in most cases.

Unless the history clearly excludes syncope as a potential cause for falls, most patients should have a 12-lead ECG to look for abnormalities of rhythm or conduction. Other investigations, including blood tests, imaging, Holter monitoring, and tilt testing, will depend on the clinical findings.

The multifactorial risk assessment should be recorded and an intervention plan devised to address any modifiable risk factors that have been identified.

Some important conditions

Only a minority of older people fall due to a single medical cause, but it is important that such diagnoses are made. Details on these conditions can be found in other chapters.

Neurological disorders

These may present for the first time as a fall or falls. Clinical assessment should include consideration of a neurological cause for falls:

- Cervical myelopathy: patients present with impaired balance sometimes, but not necessarily with altered peripheral sensation. Gait is classically high-stepping, stamping and slightly wide based due to sensory ataxia. Proprioception is impaired and Romberg test will be positive. The absence of neck pain and deformity does not exclude the diagnosis. If suspected, an MRI of the cervical spine is indicated. Surgical decompression should prevent progression and may produce improvement.
- Peripheral neuropathy: patients usually describe altered peripheral sensation as well as impairment of balance. Gait is wide based due to sensory ataxia and there will be reduction of sensory modalities in a stocking (and glove) distribution. Ankle jerks will be absent. The diagnosis may be confirmed with nerve conduction studies and further tests for underlying important or treatable causes should be performed, particularly glucose and vitamin B12 levels. The value of syphilis serology is uncertain.
- Lumbar stenosis: most patients will primarily report pain and/or paraesthesia in the legs on walking or prolonged standing (neurogenic claudication) in association with low back pain. Falls occur due to impairment of balance or mild lower limb weakness. Neurological examination may be normal, but gait is often wide-based and Romberg test is usually positive. MRI of the lumbar spine is indicated if the patient has typical symptoms along with an abnormal gait or Romberg test.
- Cerebellar ataxia: the gait is wide based, lurching, and unsteady. There will be associated cerebellar signs of nystagmus, finger-nose and heel-shin ataxia, dysdiadochokinesis, dysmetria, intention tremor, and slurred or staccato speech. There are many causes of cerebellar dysfunction. In practice, ataxic falls clinic attendees are much more likely to have sensory ataxia than cerebellar ataxia.
- Parkinson's disease: falls can be an early symptom of Parkinson's disease, as well as related parkinsonian syndromes. A shuffling, small-paced gait and the presence of tremor, rigidity and bradykinesia should lead to further assessment and referral, as appropriate. Vascular parkinsonism should be considered in patients with a classical parkinsonian gait but minimal features in the upper limbs, which typically does not respond well to dopaminergic therapy.
- Dementia: the falls clinic may be the first occasion for dementia to be identified as some dementia sufferers experience problems with falls early in the disease due to impairment of executive function or risk awareness. Vascular dementia and Lewy body disease are more commonly associated with early gait disturbance, with this being a later feature in Alzheimer's disease. A standard screen of cognitive function, such as the Abbreviated Mental Test Score or Mini-Mental State Examination, should be performed, leading to further assessment if the screen is positive. Patients with dementia often have a higher level gait abnormality due to frontal lobe dysfunction. This leads to difficulties in initiation of gait (so-called gait ignition dyspraxia) and walking is often hesitant or lacks a clear stepping rhythm. Although classically described as part of the triad of symptoms in normal pressure hydrocephalus (NPH), along with dementia and urinary incontinence, similar gait abnormalities are often found in vascular dementia and in Alzheimer's disease. A CT scan of the head should be performed, in particular looking for ventriculomegaly as a sign of NPH. It is worth remembering that NPH is a rare cause of dementia, falls, and incontinence, all of which are common syndromes in older people and often coexist. Treatment for NPH rarely leads to significant sustained clinical improvement.

Cardiovascular disorders

These can cause falls with or without a history of loss of consciousness. Vasovagal syndrome, orthostatic hypotension and carotid sinus hypersensitivity syndrome may all present as falls. The history will usually reveal symptoms suggestive of syncope or pre-syncope. However, amnesia for loss of consciousness is common, particularly in the presence of cognitive impairment.

Vestibular disease

This can lead to vertigo, imbalance and/or falls. Many patients with vestibular disease do not describe the typical rotational illusion of vertigo due to the presence of other falls risk factors or causes of imbalance. However, a history of falling to one side, or falls related to turning of head or body, is suggestive of ipsilateral vestibular disease. Romberg test will be positive with the patient falling in the direction of the lesion. The gait will be unsteady and the patient will often veer to the side of the lesion, particularly if they attempt to walk with eyes closed (supervised, of course).

Patients with bilateral vestibular impairment do not report vertigo, which requires the combination of a normal vestibule with an abnormal one. Instead, patients report 'oscillopsia', the sensation that objects do not appear to be fixed in position and oscillate from side to side. This is due to the failure of the vestibular-ocular reflex in maintaining visual fixation.

There is also a phenomenon of cervical vertigo, often in older people with neck deformity due to osteoarthritis. These patients report unsteadiness or falls on head turning but without loss of consciousness (and with negative testing for carotid sinus hypersensitivity) and without vestibular symptoms or signs. This is probably due to impairment of cervicovestibular neurological connections or disrupted central proprioception. There is some doubt as to whether vertebrobasilar insufficiency really exists as a condition, or whether most falls due to head-turning are due to vestibular, cervical or carotid disease.

Summary

Falls are a common problem for older people, often resulting in injury and disability. Falls are not an inevitable part of ageing and are often due to underlying disease or dysfunction that may be amenable to treatment or modification. It is essential that falls are investigated and that all clinicians working with older people receive training in the assessment and management of falls risk.

Further reading

AGS/BGS (2010). *Clinical Practice Guideline: Prevention of Falls in Older Persons* (http://www.medcats.com/FALLS/frameset.htm).

Lord SR, Sherrington C, Menz H, Close J (2007). *Falls in Older People: Risk Factors and Strategies for Prevention*. Cambridge, Cambridge University Press.

Podsiadlo D. Richardson S (1991). The timed 'Up & Go': a test of basic functional mobility for frail elderly persons. *J Am Geriatr Soc* **39**: 142–8.

Prevention of Falls Network Europe (ProFaNE) (www.profane. eu.org).

Shumway-Cook A, Brauer S, Woollacott M (2000). Predicting the probability for falls in community-dwelling older adults using the Timed Up and Go Test. *Phys Ther* **80**: 896–903.

Management of falls

Most older adults who fall possess more than one risk factor for falling. The principle of falls prevention is to reduce their risk of future falls and injuries through risk factor modification. In the unusual situation that a single treatable cause for falling is identified, this should be the main focus for treatment. For most other fallers, intervention is likely to consist of a combination of some or all of the following:

- strength and balance training
- home environment modification (where appropriate)
- footwear and foot care
- vision optimization (usually by referral)
- medication optimization, particularly psychotropics
- management of postural hypotension
- fracture risk assessment, osteoporosis treatment and vitamin D
- patient education and information.

Multicomponent risk factor modification

These interventions may be tailored to the individual, which is the most effective approach in community-dwelling older adults, or offered as a package to all individuals in a group setting, such as a long-term care facility. Tailored multifactorial interventions have been studied in a number of trials and meta-analysed by the Cochrane collaboration. Trials have been heterogeneous, but most contain the key components above. Fall rate reductions vary from trial to trial, but pooled data suggest a modest reduction in the order of 10%. To date there is no robust evidence for cost effectiveness.

Interventions can be delivered in a variety of settings, including acute and community hospitals, day hospitals and other intermediate care sites, and people's homes.

Strength and balance training

The strongest evidence of falls risk reduction is for exercise, in the form of strength and balance training. All older adults who have fallen, or who are at risk of falling, should be offered this intervention unless there are clear contraindications. Exercise is also the most effective single intervention for falls reduction and may be offered separately from multifactorial interventions in low-risk fallers (see section Investigation of falls) if other falls risk factors have not been shown to be present.

Falls exercise programmes must be tailored to the individual, progressive (becoming more challenging as the programme goes on) and comprise both muscle strengthening and balance retraining components. Exercise is typically undertaken at least three times a week and programmes last for a minimum of 12 weeks, although some trials continued intervention for 36 weeks.

Examples of evidence-based falls exercise programmes include

- Otago exercise programme
- FaME: Falls Management Exercise
- some forms of tai chi

Exercise should be led by an appropriately trained individual, typically a physiotherapist, exercise instructor, or nurse. The exercise may be individualized, in a clinic or a person's home, or performed as a group in a hospital or community setting.

Intervention will often include assessment for, and provision of, a suitable walking aid.

Home environment modification

Minimization of home hazards and provision of assistive aids and adaptations can reduce the risk of falls at home. Most successful trials of multifactorial falls risk management included home hazard assessment and intervention, usually led by an occupational therapist.

Footwear and foot care

Foot problems, such as bunions, ulcers, and deformities of toes or nails, are common in older age and are associated with impaired balance. Footwear that is inappropriate or in disrepair is also a risk factor for falls. Foot abnormalities should be identified and treated and advice should be given regarding appropriate footwear (well-fitted with a low heel and maximal area of ground contact). Although popular with the public and managers, there is no evidence that 'sloppy slipper' exchanges are effective as a single intervention.

Vision optimization

Visual problems are common in older age and contribute to balance impairment. Low visual acuity is most recognized as a risk factor for falls. Visual field defects, reduced contrast sensitivity and diplopia can also increase falls risk. Patients reporting, or found to have, visual disorders will normally be referred on to the appropriate service, rather than managed by the falls service.

One trial demonstrated that expedited cataract surgery in older women with cataracts resulted in a reduced falls risk. Falls clinic may be the first or best opportunity for cataracts to be identified in some individuals.

Bifocal or multifocal glasses are associated with an increased risk of falls due to the effect on distance perception created by looking at the ground through a lens designed for near sight. Advice should be given not to wear such glasses when walking, particularly on stairs.

Medication optimization

Medication, prescribed and non-prescribed, can increase falls risk. Prescription of multiple (four or more) medications is an independent risk factor for falls, as is use of psychoactive medication (sedatives, anxiolytics, antidepressants, and antipsychotics). Most successful trials of multifactorial intervention for falls prevention have included medication management.

Medication optimization requires the active review of all medication to ensure that all prescribing is rational (not rationed) and risks and benefits of each drug are considered, particularly in light of falls risk.

In particular, psychoactive medication should be stopped or reduced whenever clinically appropriate. In a clinical trial of psychoactive medication withdrawal as a single intervention for falls prevention, falls were reduced, even though only a minority of subjects successfully stopped the medication. It is important to remember that some sedative medication, such as antihistamines, may be prescribed for other indications. Some drugs are also inappropriately prescribed with the intention of using sedative effects to manage challenging behaviour, such as wandering, even though this increases the risk of harm.

Management of postural hypotension

Both falls and postural hypotension are common. In older adults who fall and who have postural hypotension, it can be difficult to determine if the two are causally linked. Where there is a clear history of pre-syncopal symptoms prior to falling, this would be strongly suggestive of causation, but this is uncommon. Some successful trials of multifactorial intervention included identification and management of postural hypotension. Therefore, postural hypotension should be sought routinely as part of falls assessment and treatment offered, if required. Similarly, if history or ECG indicates that cardiac dysrhythmia may be present, this should be investigated further and treated as necessary.

Fracture risk assessment, osteoporosis treatment and vitamin D

Older adults who fall, or who are at risk of falling, should also be assessed for their risk of fracture. If they have already sustained a fragility fracture, then osteoporosis should be diagnosed and treated.

In addition, many older adults, particularly older women who are housebound or in long-term care, are deficient in vitamin D. As well as affecting bone density and structure, vitamin D deficiency leads to proximal muscle weakness and increases the risk of falling. Vitamin D supplementation has had mixed fortunes in trials. The current consensus is that vitamin D supplementation (at least 800 IU per day) should be offered to all older adults who have confirmed deficiency and also considered for those with suspected deficiency (based on diet and sun exposure) and at risk of falls.

Vestibular disease

Although vestibular problems are increasingly recognized as causing balance impairment and falls, there is no evidence that treatment of vestibular disease reduces the risk of falls. Nevertheless, if pathology is identified, it should be treated. In particular, treatment of benign positional vertigo with a successful Epley manoeuvre will result in a better balanced and grateful patient.

Older people with cognitive impairment

Trials of interventions to reduce falls in older people with cognitive impairment have not shown benefits. Furthermore, treatment of dementia symptoms (e.g. with acetylcholinesterase inhibitors) does not reduce fall rates. It is unknown whether this lack of evidence is due to the inability of people with dementia to comply with, or follow through, interventions such as exercise recommendations or reflects the challenges of performing trials in this population.

It is hypothesized that people with dementia fall for different reasons to those without cognitive impairment. For instance, executive dysfunction affects multitasking and increases falls risk during complex activities such as toileting. Some people with dementia lack risk awareness. Postural instability and gait dyspraxias are common.

Despite the evidential gap, it is still advisable to manage modifiable falls risk factors in this population, but with lower expectations of falls reduction. It is likely that there will be benefits at an individual level, for instance with the identification and treatment of syncope and withdrawal of psychotropic medication.

Older people in long-term care and hospital

Falls are more common in residents of long-term care facilities than in community-dwelling older people. Approximately 50% of residents will fall per year and all falls risk factors are more common in this population. In hospital, there is approximately 1 fall per 100 bed days, although fall rates vary widely. Falls, and their consequences, are the most common reason for older adults to be admitted to hospital and this population occupy more bed-days than any other diagnostic group.

Whole-system multicomponent interventions are likely to afford more benefit than individual multi-factorial risk management. The key components are strength and balance training (in long-term care and long-stay wards), medication optimization (particularly reduction in psychotropic drugs), environmental adaptation and training of staff in falls prevention. Dementia is common in older residents and inpatients, so falls interventions may be ineffective.

Falls management should concentrate on reducing harm from falls, as well as falls themselves. Osteoporosis and vitamin D deficiency should be treated. Assistive, rather than restrictive, technology can be useful in some residents. The resident or inpatient, or their carer, should be involved in decisions regarding falls management and prevention.

Summary

Falls prevention requires the systematic identification and modification of falls risk factors. In low-risk fallers, exercise training for strength and balance may be offered as a single intervention. Falls in long-term care and hospital settings require a different approach, though there are common elements in all settings.

Further reading

AGS/BGS (2010). *Clinical Practice Guideline: Prevention of Falls in Older Persons*(http://www.americangeriatrics.org/health_care_professionals/clinical_practice/clinical_guidelines_recommendations/2010)

Bischoff-Ferrari HA, Dawson-Hughes B, Willet WC, et al. (2004). Effect of vitamin D on falls: a meta-analysis. *JAMA* **291**: 1999–2006.

Campbell AJ, Robertson MC, Gardner MM, et al. (1999). Psychotropic medication withdrawal and a home-based exercise program to prevent falls: A randomized controlled trial. *J Am Geriatr Soc* **39**: 142–8.

Gates S, Fisher JD, Cooke MW, et al. (2008). Multifactorial assessment and targeted intervention for preventing falls and injuries among older people in community and emergency care settings: systematic review and meta-analysis. *Br Med J* **336**: 130–3.

Gillespie LD, Gillespie WJ, Robertson MC, et al. (2003). Interventions for preventing falls in elderly people. *Cochrane Database Syst Rev* **4**: CD000340.

Harwood RH, Foss AJ, Osborn F, et al. (2005). Falls and health status in elderly women following first eye cataract surgery: a randomised controlled trial. *Br J Ophthalmol* **89**: 53–9.

Li F, Harmer P, Fisher KJ, et al. (2005). Tai Chi and fall reductions in older adults: a randomized controlled trial. *J Gerontol A Biol Sci Med Sci* **60**: 187–94.

Lord SR, Sherrington C, Menz H, Close J (2007). *Falls in Older People: Risk Factors and Strategies for Prevention*. Cambridge, Cambridge University Press.

Prevention of Falls Network Europe (ProFaNE) (www.profane.eu.org).

Robertson MC, Campbell AJ, Gardner MM, et al. (2002). Preventing injuries in elderly people by preventing falls: a meta-analysis of individual level data. *J Am Geriatr Soc* **50**: 905–11.

Skelton DA, Dinan SM, Campbell MC, et al. (2005). Tailored group exercise (Falls Management Exercise - FaME) reduces falls in community-dwelling older frequent fallers (an RCT). *Age Ageing* **34**: 636–9.

Wolf SL, Barnhart HX, Kutner NG, et al. (1996). Reducing frailty and falls in older persons: an investigation of Tai Chi and computerized balance training. Atlanta FICSIT Group. Frailty and Injuries: Cooperative Studies of Intervention Techniques. *J Am Geriatr Soc* **44**: 489–97.

Falls in the cognitively impaired

Cognitive impairment is a well recognized independent risk factor for falls. The differential diagnosis is extensive and includes acute potentially reversible conditions such as delirium as well as more chronic conditions such as dementia. The annual incidence of falls may be as much as three times that in the normal elderly population. The consequences are also significantly more serious. Older people with confusion are three times more likely to sustain a fracture, five times more likely to be institutionalized, and have a mortality of 71% within 1 year after a fracture neck of femur.

Why do cognitively impaired patients fall?

For a fall to occur during any activity, at any age, postural control must be impaired relative to the amount by which it is stressed. Continuous muscle corrections maintaining the upright posture are made on the basis of proprioceptive and other sensory information about body position. Vision is probably the most important, supplemented by the vestibular apparatus and various propioceptors in muscle spindles, joints, skin surface, and importantly the joints of the neck. Information is referred for central processing within the cerebrum, cerebellum, basal ganglia, and brainstem, and efferent fibres subsequently control muscular contraction. Gait dyspraxia and falls occur early in the natural history of cerebrovascular disease.

Age-related changes, as well as disease and medication, adversely affect the ageing adult's ability to maintain the upright position, resulting in abnormalities of gait and balance. Indeed, gait abnormalities are often identified as the single most independent risk factor for falls in dementia patients, increasing the risk further if associated with risk taking behaviour or agitation.

The main causes of falls in cognitively impaired patients are summarized in the box.

Factors often leading to falls in cognitively impaired subjects

- Abnormal gait
- Dyspraxia
- Drugs (sedatives, neuroleptics, antidepressants)
- Wandering/exhaustion in agitated patients
- Undiagnosed comorbid pathologies
- Decreased ability to verbalize
- Inability to observe environmental hazards
- Deconditioning
- Malnutrition/vitamin deficiency
- Dysautonomia
- Alterations in sleep wake cycle
- Associated incontinence
- Inability to use appropriate walking aids
- Impaired vision
- Fear of falling
- Neurocardiovascular disorders
- Environmental hazards
- Perception that patients are inappropriate for rehabilitation

---

Structural and neurochemical degeneration associated with dementia leads to abnormalities in gait and balance. Although falls present early in progressive supranuclear palsy, there is often an evolution of falls risk as diseases causing cognitive impairment progress. Early stage Alzheimer's patients have cognitive problems, depression and anxiety. With disease progression, patients develop intellectual deterioration and psychiatric or behavioural complications increasing falls risk. Late stage Alzheimer's patients will have severe intellectual loss and forget how to perform basic bodily functions such as eating and walking. Muscular strength is maintained through the early and middle phase of the illness but by late stage patients lose weight and manifest muscular wasting further increasing falls risk.

Sedating medications, like benzodiazepines, phenothiazines, and antidepressants, have been implicated as independent risk factor for falls in patients with dementia by causing sedation, muscle weakness, orthostatic hypotension, and extrapyramidal side-effects. Prescription of these classes of drugs doubles the risk of falls in the cognitively impaired. Patients with Lewy body dementia are particularly sensitive to phenothiazines, with 50–60% of patients experiencing severe neuroleptic sensitivity associated with increased mortality.

Cardiovascular disorders are common in cognitively impaired patients. Orthostatic hypotension may be a prominent presenting feature in Lewy body dementia due to failure of the autonomic nervous system. Carotid sinus hypersensitivity is more common in cognitively impaired patients with a fractured neck of femur, suggesting a possible association between dementia, carotid sinus hypersensitivity, and falls. Patients with dementia are less likely to recall a history of syncope, often resulting in the diagnosis being missed and remaining untreated.

The environment and how the cognitively impaired patient interacts with it is an important risk factor for falls in this group. Patients, particularly if wandering and agitated, do not appreciate the risks of mobilization and do not take precautions to prevent falls

Is it possible to prevent falls in patients with dementia?

Evidence for reducing falls in cognitively impaired patients is limited and often contradictory. Many studies on fall prevention measures were community based and excluded patients with cognitive impairment. A study of cognitively impaired patients admitted to an accident and emergency department after a fall has shown that multidisciplinary intervention was ineffective at reducing falls. On the other hand, a very small study of focused supervision of high risk patients in a dementia unit suggested that such a strategy might lead to less falls. The role of medication manipulation is also unclear. Although it is accepted that tranquilizer use increases the risk of falls, one study suggested that using risperidone reduced falls in a group of patients with dementia. Judicious use of sedation to control agitation may thus have a role in prevent falls and clinical decisions need to be taken on an individual basis.

Systematic reviews of studies that included cognitively impaired patients based in care home and hospital looked at single and multifaceted interventions Single interventions such as bed alarms or identification bracelets were ineffective. One meta analysis of multifaceted intervention trials showed a modest reduction (18%) on fall rate ratios in hospital, but no clear effect on relative risk of falling or fracture rates. This positive finding however is not universal and a subsequent Cochrane Review was inconclusive. Multidisciplinary interventions were varied and included setting up falls prevention teams, medication reviews, identifying risk factors like orthostatic hypotension, tailored exercise programmes, and environmental assessments in variable combinations. There is debate that differences in components of multifaceted interventions and how they are applied may account for differences in results between studies.

In view of the multifactorial nature of falls in patients with dementia, a successful intervention strategy to reduce falls would need to be multidisciplinary, tailored to the patient and address the risk factors and specific causes of falls identified as being important. Further general interventions are covered in The management of falls section.

Restraint

As the evidence base for effective ways to prevent falls is limited, the subject of restraint as a falls prevention measure is often considered in the cognitively impaired. The Mental Capacity Act 2005 provides a precise legal definition of restraint. It is the use or threat of force to help do an act which the patient resists, or the restriction of the patient's liberty of movement, whether or not they resist. In its broadest context, restraint is any physical method of limiting a patient's freedom of movement, physical activity or normal access to his or her body. For most purposes a restraint may take the form of a physical device (ranging from physical binding to bed rails and motion alarms) or a drug. It may also include seclusion, which is the involuntary confinement of a patient in a room or an area where the patient is physically prevented from leaving. Psychopharmacological restraint refers to the use of drugs to control behaviour when not a standard treatment for the patient's medical or psychiatric condition.

The primary consideration in deciding whether to restrain a patient or not should be what is the best interests of the patient, and those persons in the immediate vicinity. Patients have the right to be free from the use of restraints or seclusion unless there is an emergency, i.e. the patient's behaviour presents an immediate and serious danger to the safety of self or others. There is no evidence from experimental studies that shows restraint is effective at reducing falls and injury. It has the potential to produce serious adverse consequences such as physical or psychological harm, loss of dignity, violation of a patient's rights, and even death. Because of the associated risks and consequences, methods must be sought to decrease restraint use through effective use of alternatives. When used the restraint should be the least restrictive possible. This is best done as a component of an approved protocol stating what is acceptable and unacceptable practice. Under no circumstances should restraining methods be used as a substitute for clinical supervision. A key principal in assessing a patient for restraint is proportionality. The means of restraint should be proportional to the level of risk to the patient or others on the ward (patients, staff, or visitors) at risk of harm. This involves an assessment of the likely harm to the patient and/or others if restraint is not used and the potential harm (physical, psychological and social) to the patient of using the particular method of restraint.

Conclusion

Falls are a cause of substantial morbidity and mortality in patients with cognitive impairment. Abnormal gait and balance, medication, cardiovascular pathology, and the environment can all contribute to falls in this patient group. Multidisciplinary intervention to modify these risk factors for falls is feasible in patients with dementia, although data on effectiveness is lacking. As the population ages, the prevention of falls in patients with dementia is becoming increasingly important as a wider health service issue.

Further reading

Mental Capacity Act 2005

Alzheimer Europe. Position Paper Guidelines on the use of various measures designed to restrict liberty of movement. Guidelines on the use of various measures designed to restrict liberty of movement 2001.

Gillespie LD, Gillespie WJ, Robertson MC, et al (2003). Interventions for preventing falls in elderly people. Cochrane Database Syst Rev **1**: 17.

Oliver D, Connelly JB, Victor CR, et al (2007). Strategies to prevent falls and fractures in hospitals and care homes and effect of cognitive impairment: systematic review and meta-analyses. Br Med J **334**: 82–5.

The third report from the Patient Safety Observatory. Slips, trips and falls in hospital. NHS National Patient Safety Agency 2007.

Falls in the care home population

Background

Given the ageing processes and comorbidities that result in care home admission, care home populations are likely have very high levels of risk factors for falls, including impaired mobility, cognitive impairment, incontinence, polypharmacy, and depression. These risk factors result in around a threefold higher incidence of falls for care home residents than for older people living in the community, with reported rates of around 1.5 falls per resident year and around 0.04 hip fractures per resident year in the UK. For a care home with 100 beds, this would represent around four hip fractures per year and around three resident falls each week, each of which may cause significant distress and further impairment for residents whose functional reserve and capacity for rehabilitation may already be very limited.

The aetiology of falls and appropriate investigation and intervention are described elsewhere, but there are special considerations for care home residents and some evidence specific to the care home community.

> **Author's Tip**
>
> In care home populations, falls and injury prevention should include:
> - vitamin D supplementation
> - medication review
> - multifactorial interventions with multidisciplinary input
> - identification and treatment of osteoporosis.
> - There is currently no convincing evidence of effectiveness of hip protectors, exercise, and unidisciplinary interventions in the care home population.

Multifactorial interventions

Multifactorial interventions involving only nursing or therapy staff do not appear successful in care home settings, but where multidisciplinary teams are involved in applying multifactorial interventions, a reduced rate of falls and risk of being a faller is found. The importance of medical involvement in the multifactorial intervention is plausible given the high level of medical and medication risk factors for falls seen in the care home population. Key components in the multidisciplinary trials included review by a geriatrician, referral to optometry and podiatry, continence care, environmental hazard assessment including improvements to lighting, staff and resident education, walking aid review and repair, and alert signs.

Vitamin D

Pooled trials in care home populations indicate that vitamin D supplementation appears to reduce the rate of falls. It is likely that vitamin D supplementation is only effective in residents who are vitamin D deficient, but the majority of care home residents, who may be relatively less exposed to sunshine, are likely to be vitamin D deficient.

Medication review

There is strong association between the following medication types and falls:
- benzodiazepine sedative/hypnotics
- other sedatives/hypnotics
- antidepressants
- antipsychotics
- diuretics.

These medication types are in common use in the care home population, with serious concerns that antipsychotics are prescribed inappropriately to residents with dementia, leading to increased mortality in addition to increased falls risk. Studies of medication reviews in care home residents have demonstrated that it is possible to reduce and discontinue a wide range of medications where the risks had come to outweigh the benefits, and that this significantly reduced the number of falls. Risk of falls for these medications is in most cases dose dependent, so the lowest dose for the lowest duration should be the default. In addition to specific 'culprit' drugs, polypharmacy *per se* increases risk of falls, so review should encompass all medication. Residents need to be engaged in this review where possible; in community settings many chose to continue taking psychoactive medication even when aware of the increased risk of falling.

> **Author's Tip**
>
> Do not discontinue benzodiazepines abruptly in habituated patients as this can precipitate a distressing agitated confusion in older people.

Osteoporosis

The age and comorbidities of care home residents result in a high prevalence of osteoporosis; in addition to the standard assessment and intervention, in care home settings educating staff on correct administration of bone-strengthening medication is important, and care homes should seek to provide calcium-rich diets in addition to any prescribed calcium supplementation.

Bedrails

Systematic review suggests that both routine bedrail use and evangelical elimination of bedrails can increase falls and injury; care homes should undertake individual assessment rather have a blanket policy on bedrail use or non-use. This assessment should avoid bedrails for those residents who do not want them, who could be independently mobile without them, or who are mobile enough and confused enough to be at risk of climbing over their bedrails. However, for patients unable to mobilize without help from carers, who have alternating pressure mattresses, poor postural stability, restlessness, spasms, or epilepsy, bedrails may reduce the risk of falls and injury. Used in these circumstances, bedrails would be unlikely to fit the definition of restraint (see below). If bedrails are used, it is vital the combination of mattress, bed and bedrail is assessed to ensure there are no gaps that could trap the residents head, neck or chest; outdated equipment or 'hybrid assembly' (where bedrails, bed and mattress have been obtained from different manufacturers without consideration of compatible measurements) is particularly likely to create entrapment risks.

Restraint

The controversial issue of restraint is best approached using an ethical definition of 'stopping them from doing something they appear to want to do'. Restraint can be physical (holding a resident still), mechanical (using a belt or straps to keep the resident in their chair), chemical (using medication with the intent of controlling behaviour, not disease), or psychological (creating a situation where they are afraid to move without permission). Although any use of restraint in many debates has been equated to an unacceptable infringement of personal liberty or to abuse, the reality is not so black and white. In certain circumstances (e.g. a delirious resident attempting to leave a care home during a snowstorm), failing to use restraint would be dereliction of the duty of care. Additionally, in practice, intent and effect are often blurred—heavy automatically closing doors may have been installed for fire protection purposes, but also to stop patients vulnerable to falls from walking far. Resources exist to support care home staff to recognize when their actions could constitute restraint and how to choose the least restrictive method of managing risk (see further reading), whilst issues of abuse are covered in more detail elsewhere.

Exercise

The effect on falling of exercise programmes in care homes remains uncertain, with the majority of trials showing no significant effect. Although exercise may have other benefits in terms of physical health and mental wellbeing, it may not be beneficial in terms of falls prevention, and some trials suggest the risk of falls may be increased if frail residents are encouraged to exercise outside a multifactorial intervention where underlying risk factors for falls are also addressed.

Hip protectors

Although the updated Cochrane review suggests a possible benefit from the use of hip protectors in care home populations, this may only be an artefact of the earlier and less methodologically sound cluster randomized trials taking place in care homes. This interpretation is supported by a large-scale care home trial of hip protectors in the UK setting that showed no effect on fracture rates. Until there is more convincing evidence for any benefit from hip protectors, environmental changes to reduce the impact of falls may be more appropriate; observational studies suggest that carpeted flooring with underlay may reduce the likelihood of fracture.

New technology

Although movement alarms (infrared or pressure sensitive devices), and ultralow beds are in increasingly common use in care home settings, there is relatively little evidence of their effect on preventing falls or injury. Careful patient selection and the capacity of care home staff to respond promptly to the alarms is likely to be crucial, and the potential for these devices to be used inappropriately to restrain rather than support patients needs consideration.

Addressing other risk factors

The care home population has high levels of dementia, depression, visual deficit, malnutrition, chronic pain, and foot problems. Routine screening for these problems in the care home setting followed up by appropriate referrals and treatment cannot be proven to reduce falls, but will improve quality of life.

Further reading

Cameron I, Murray GR, Gillespie LD, et al. (2010). Interventions for preventing falls in older people in residential care facilities and hospitals. *Cochrane Database Syst Rev* **1**: CD005465.

Hartikainen S, Lonnroos E, Lohivouri K (2007). Medication as a risk factor for falls: Critical systematic review. *J Gerontol A—Biolog Sci Med Sci* **62**: 1172–81.

Healey F, Oliver D, Milne A, et al. (2008). The effect of bedrails on falls and injury: a systematic review of clinical studies. *Age Ageing* **37**: 368–76.

Medicine and Healthcare products Regulatory Agency (2006) *Device Bulletin 2006(06) the safe use of bedrails*. London, MHRA.

National Institute for Health and Clinical Excellence (2004). *The assessment and prevention of falls in older people*. London, NICE.

Oliver D, Connelly J, Victor C, et al. (2007). Strategies to prevent falls and fractures in hospitals and care homes and effect of cognitive impairment. Systematic review and meta-analyses. *Br Med J* **334**: 82–7.

Royal College of Nursing (2008) *Let's Talk about Restraint: Rights, Risks and Responsibilities*. London, RCN.

Fear of falling

Background

It is perhaps understandable that people are aware of their risk of falling, especially older people in whom falls are more prevalent and are more likely to result in injury. It can be argued that some insight is a normal adaptive response to challenged equilibrium. However, if people become overly concerned about falling, this may result in a persistent and dysfunctional disruption of attention and behaviour. Fear of falling may then have a detrimental effect upon several domains of life, including restricting activities of daily living and enjoyable pastimes, which may, then, lead to physical inactivity and social isolation (see Table 18.1).

Conceptualizations

- *Fear of falling*: continuous concern regarding falls which may limit activities of daily living
- *Falls efficacy*: perceived ability to confidently undertake activities of daily living without falling

Prevalence

- 29–92% in those who have suffered previous falls.
- 12–65% in those who have not suffered previous falls.
- Women are more commonly affected than men.
- Prevalence increases with age.

Examples of fear of falling assessments are listed in Table 18.1.

Associated factors

Fear of falling may reflect a realistic appraisal of reduced functional abilities and consequent increased risk of suffering a fall and fall injuries. Such a fear may result from

- first-hand experience, e.g. a near fall or a recent fall that resulted in pain, embarrassment or injury
- actual falls risk, as is reflected in the high correlation between objective measures of physiological factors and fear of falling (see Figure 18.1).

Fear of falling can also be irrational, excessive, or phobic and needlessly restrict participation in physical and social activities with a consequent negative impact on quality of life.

Table 18.1 Fear of falling assessment

	Concept	Indoor	Outdoor	Social	Items
Single item					
Are you afraid of falling	fear	NA	NA	NA	1
Multiple item					
FES	Efficacy	Yes	No	No	10
MFES	Efficacy	Yes	Yes	No	14
FES-I	Concern	Yes	Yes	Yes	16
ABC	Confidence	Yes	Yes	No	16
SAFFE	Fear/activity avoidance	Yes	Yes	No	14

All assessments are brief self-completed questionnaires. FES, Falls Efficacy Scale; MFES, Modified Falls Efficacy Scale; ABC, Activities-Specific Balance Confidence Scale; SAFE, Survey of Activities and Fear of Falling in the Elderly.

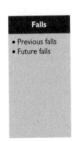

Figure 18.1 Associated factors with fear of falling based on prospective and retrospective cohort studies.

Few studies on fear of falling have been able to unravel the 'chicken and egg' question regarding interrelationships among associated factors as shown in Figure 18.2. Recent developments have suggested that fear of falling itself can induce falls in older people.

- By manipulating the environment in a way that exacerbates the potential consequences of a fall, it is possible to investigate whether fear of falling induces gait adaptations. Several experimental studies have suggested that fear of falling decreases walking speed and step length, and increases double support time (where both feet are on the ground simultaneously). This so-called 'cautious' gait, however, decreases walking stability and could increase falls risk, rather than protect against it.
- A prospective cohort study has investigated the effect that a disparity between perceived and actual fall risk can have on falls and related factors. In people with similar actual balance abilities:
  - high levels of fear of falling were related to future falls, mainly through psychological pathways such as depression
  - low levels of fear of falling were protective for falling through a positive outlook on life, and maintained physical activity and community participation.

Fear of falling interventions

Cognitive behavioural therapy has been shown to reduce fear of falling and recurrent falls, especially in combination with exercise.

- Cognitive behavioural therapy: with a focus to improve self-efficacy and sense of control over falling, reduce symptoms of depression and promote active and healthy lifestyle
- Exercise programmes: with a focus on high intensity balance training

Some fall prevention programmes that were successful at reducing falls, also showed a reduction in fear of falling.

Further reading

Delbaere K, Close JCT, Brodaty H, et al. (2010). Fall risk and fear of falling in older people: the vigorous, the anxious, the stoic and the aware. *Br Med J* **341**: c4165.

Jorstad EC, Hauer K, Becker C, et al. (2005). Measuring the psychological outcomes of falling: a systematic review. *J Am Geriatr Soc* **53**: 501–10.

Legters K. Fear of falling (2002). *Phys Ther* **82**: 264–72.

Zijlstra GA, van Haastregt JC, Ambergen T, et al. (2009). Effects of a multicomponent cognitive behavioral group intervention on fear of falling and activity avoidance in community-dwelling older adults: Results of a randomized controlled trial. *J Am Geriatr Soc* **57**: 2020–8.

Palliative care

Recognizing dying

'In order to care for the dying patients it is essential to 'diagnose' dying'. This is possible in up to half of all UK deaths and allows time, appropriate planning, important communication, withdrawal of futile treatments, and aids provision of spiritual support and enhancement of the patient's autonomy. It also anticipates the need for care after death and bereavement support for families, relatives and carers.

The imbalance between preferred place of death (in the patient's own home in the majority of cases) and the actual place of death (acute hospitals in the majority of cases) has led to the development of systems of care designed to facilitate discussions between doctors (especially general practitioners) and patients and their families. Systems such as the 'Gold Standard Framework', initially used for cancer patients, have been used more widely and their use expanded to include patients dying from other disease processes. Once discussions have taken place and the patient's wishes identified, communication with emergency services, palliative care, district nursing services and other relevant groups can occur to ensure the patient's wishes are respected. For the majority of patients who die of long-term conditions, such advance planning is possible and desirable. Symptoms may be controlled and the need for a hospital admission at the end of life avoided.

In other cases, it may be more difficult to anticipate that a further exacerbation marks the last phase of the patient's illness and hospital admission may be felt to be appropriate. Scores and scales which guide assessment of the severity conditions (such as the 'CURB-65' score in pneumonia) and generic measures of illness severity may be helpful in identifying those patients who are acutely severely ill or deteriorating, so that an assessment of the appropriate balance between active treatment and palliation may be considered.

Recognizing the key signs and symptoms is an important clinical skill in diagnosing dying. Some are condition specific, but there are many predictable generic changes occurring at reasonably well-defined points that can also be recognized by the untrained eye of informal carers and relatives.

The physical changes that become apparent in the last few months and weeks prior to death are often dependent on the underlying disease process. These can include, for example, loss of ambulatory function and impaired speech in advanced dementia, reduction in muscle mass and development of cor pulmonale in end-stage chronic obstructive pulmonary disease, and systolic hypotension and arrhythmia development in chronic heart failure. As disease progresses to the terminal stages, the physical changes follow a common pathway in spite of individual variations. They do not apply to patients who have a rapid decline following, for example, massive haemorrhage or large pulmonary embolism. There is a further category of patients who tip rapidly into respiratory failure, leading to sudden decline and death, when trivial illness occurs in the context of severe lung disease and poor respiratory reserve. The more generic signs and symptoms associated with death from any terminal condition can be broadly divided into time periods approaching death.

Signs of approaching death in next few days

- Profound global weakness (bed-bound, assistance with all care)
- Gaunt physical appearance
- Drowsy or reduced cognition (disorientated, extreme difficulty concentrating, scarcely able to cooperate with care)
- Diminished intake of food/fluid
- Difficulty swallowing

The final few hours

- Decreased urine output
- Minimal or no oral intake
- Decreased interaction
- Clouding of consciousness
- Death rattle
- Cyanotic extremities/mottling
- Pulselessness on radial artery (often in final 6 hours but earlier if there is lung disease)
- Change in respiratory pattern—fast shallow breaths then irregular breathing pattern
- Cooling of extremities

Clouding of consciousness accelerates as death approaches. As patients drift in and out of consciousness, there may be attempts at communication—it is recognized the patient may frequently try to convey messages. This can either be describing what they are experiencing in real or metaphoric terms, or asking for something they need in order to die peacefully. This can sometimes be confused with terminal agitation.

The moment of death

Breathing stops, following moments to minutes later by the heart stopping. This can occasionally be associated with a reflex respiration. Pupils become fixed and dilated and the eyes may remain open. Sphincters can relax, sometimes releasing urine or stool.

Frequently occurring symptoms

The death rattle

As death approaches, the tongue and the tissues of the soft palate sag. The gag reflex and cough reflex decline and secretions pool in the oropharynx and bronchi. It is the sound of air passing through these secretions that creates the loud gurgle descriptively named 'the death rattle'. Death rattle occurs in up to 92% of dying patients and often precedes other terminal signs.

Breathing pattern

Changes in breathing pattern are indicative of significant neurological deterioration rather than a primary respiratory dysfunction. Initially, breaths become shallow and frequent with a diminishing tidal volume. The lack of physiological response to the rising carbon dioxide results in the breathing pattern becoming irregular, where periods of shallow breathing alternate with periods of apnoea, lasting 5–30 seconds. This is also called 'Cheyne–Stokes' respiration.

Mottling

Blood volume decreases and as hypoxia develops, both heart rate and blood pressure decrease. This leads to a decrease in peripheral circulation and perfusion which in turn causes a change in appearance from uniformly pale to mottled. It usually occurs on the soles of the feet and over bony prominences such as the knees. As the perfusion decreases further, blood pools in the sacrum and lower back causing these areas to darken.

Reduction in temperature

This is due to slowing of the basal metabolic rate. It is also due to a reduction in cardiac output, in combination with a reduced circulating blood volume.

Importance of recognizing the dying phase

There are a number of both patient- and physician-centred barriers to recognizing and accepting the dying phase.

- Hope that the patient will recover
- No definitive diagnosis
- Unrealistic expectations
- Pursuance of futile interventions
- Disagreement about the patient's condition
- Failure to recognize key symptoms and signs
- Lack of knowledge about how to manage the dying phase—in particular the prescription of appropriate drug therapies
- Poor communication
- Concerns about withdrawing or withholding treatment
- Fear of foreshortening life
- Concerns about resuscitation
- Cultural and spiritual beliefs
- Medicolegal issues

Accurately predicting prognosis, especially in non-malignant conditions, is fraught with difficulty and can be a barrier to effective anticipation of the dying phase. According to the disease trajectory of chronic progressive life-limiting illness, where a patient can come close to death numerous times, it is difficult to be precise about the timings of the final terminal decline. Doctors tend to be inaccurate and overoptimistic in their estimations of prognosis in non-malignant conditions.

If the terminal phase is not recognized, unnecessary treatments may be continued, via inappropriate routes. There is likely to be a lack of realistic goal setting and the patient and carers may hold unrealistic expectations regarding the future, and their own personal chance of survival. It is unlikely that the patient's religious and spiritual needs are attended to. The patient may not have swift access to medications primarily aimed at relieving symptoms, increasing the risk of dying with uncontrolled pain, breathlessness, or other symptoms such as agitation or anxiety. Inappropriate cardiopulmonary resuscitation may also be instituted. Integrated Care Pathways for patients imminently approaching death are now in widespread use and act as a framework to prompt recognition and advance planning of patient needs, ensuring these issues are attended to (for example, the Liverpool Care Pathway).

Other detrimental effects on the family of not recognizing the dying phase are

- patient and family unaware that death is imminent
- loss of trust in medical professionals
- dissatisfaction

- distress
- complex grief reaction
- formal complaints
- family unable to be present as moment of death not anticipated
- missed opportunity to take patient home if this is their wish.

Conclusion

There are a number of recognized physiological and psychological changes that occur as death approaches, and if these are recognised in a timely fashion by experienced clinicians, a number of preparatory steps can occur to afford the patient a comfortable and dignified death. It is also extremely important and helpful for families and carers to be involved in this process. Planning and open, sensitive communication is key to achieving a 'good death', both for the patient and those entering their bereavement process.

Further reading

Al-Qurainy R, Collis E, Feuer D (2009). Dying in an acute hospital setting. The challenges and solutions. *Int J Clin Pract* **63**: 508–15.

Callanan M, Kelley P (1992). *Final Gifts: Understanding the Special Awareness, Needs and Communications of the Dying*. New York, Bantam Books, pp. 76–84.

Coventry PA, Grande GE, Richards DA, et al. (2005). Prediction of appropriate timing of palliative care for older adults with non-malignant life threatening disease: A systematic review. *Age Ageing* **34**: 218–27.

Ellershaw J (2003). Care of the dying patient: the last hours or days of life. *Br Med J* **326**: 30–4.

Emanuel L, et al. (2010). The last hours of living: practical advice for clinicians. Medscape Nurses. (http://www.medscape.com/viewarticle/716463).

Morita T, Ichiki T, Tsunoda J, et al. (1998). A prospective study on the dying process in terminally ill cancer patients. *Am J Hosp Palliat Care* **15**: 217–22.

Murray SA, Kendall M, Boyd K, Sheikh A (2005). Illness trajectories and palliative care. *Br Med J* **330**: 1007–11.

National Council for Hospice and Specialist Palliative Care Services (2006). *Changing Gear - Guidelines for Managing the Last Days of Life in Adults*. London, National Council for Hospice and Specialist Palliative Care Services, London.

Pitorak E (2003). Care at the Time of Death: How nurses can make the last hours of life a richer, more comfortable experience. *Am J Nurs* **103**: 42–52.

The Marie Curie Palliative Care Institute Liverpool (2009). Liverpool Care Pathway for the Dying Patient. (Available from http://www.mcpcil.org.uk/liverpool-care-pathway/).

Wee B, Hillier R. (2008). Interventions for noisy breathing in patients near to death. *Cochrane Database Syst Rev* **23**(1).

Care after death

Preparation

The preparation and support of families both when death is imminent and when it has occurred can reduce anxiety and distress. Families may want to contribute to the caring process by highlighting the patient's religious, spiritual, cultural or personal requirements, e.g. desire to donate tissue.

Cultural and religious requirements

It is impossible to understand the laws and prohibitions about handling human bodies after death without having some idea of what that particular person's religion or philosophy has to say about the nature of human life and its value. As the UK today is a multicultural and multifaith society, this offers a great challenge to nurses who need to be aware of the different religious and cultural rituals that may accompany the death of a patient. There are considerable cultural variations within and between people of different faiths, ethnic backgrounds, and national origins and their approach to death and dying. There are a multitude of websites that offer religion specific guidance and each acute hospital trust will have information available. There may be a request for burial within 24 hours. If this is the case, the medical certificate of cause of death will need to be completed promptly. The death will also need to be registered prior to the funeral. It may be appropriate to transfer a patient home to die so that the religious and cultural rituals may be followed without interruption by hospital and mortuary procedures.

Verification and certification of death

Ensure that the death has been verified (this can be done by a medical practitioner or nurse dependent on local policy) and must be documented in accordance with the code of practice for the Diagnosis and Confirmation of Death (Academy of Royal Colleges 2008). A registered medical practitioner who has attended the deceased person during their last illness is required to give a medical certificate of the cause of death (MCCD). The certificate requires the doctor to state on which date he/she last saw the deceased alive and whether or not he/she has seen the body after death (the doctor must have attended the patient within the previous 2 weeks to avoid the need for referral to the coroner). Prior to completion of the MCCD, the following questions should be considered: do the circumstances leading to this death indicate the need for referral to the coroner? Do you have the appropriate registration? Were you in attendance during the last illness? Did you see the body after death? Do you have sufficient data about the patient and the circumstances of death to make a confident diagnosis of the cause of death? Can you describe the cause of death in the format required by the MCCD? Are you confident that the registrar of births and deaths will receive the MCCD?

Deaths in the community

Families should be prepared in advance for an expected death at home. Such preparation includes families having the number of the medical practitioner (in hours) or the out of hours service to notify them of the death. They should be aware to state this was "an expected death" to prevent the unnecessary calling of an ambulance or police. Although funeral directors require notification, the deceased can be kept at home to allow time for family to visit and religious, cultural or social rituals to be followed.

Death in hospital

If the family are not present at the time of death, then this significant news should be given by a senior member of staff, preferably known to the relative/carers. When the relatives/carers arrive on the ward, every effort should be made to ensure information is given in a suitably private and appropriate environment. When necessary, a decision to tell the relatives over the telephone can be made, considering the circumstances for that particular patient and their family/carers. Considerations include whether the next of kin lives alone, has a medical condition that could be affected by the news and has ready access to support from family/friends. The patient's death should be communicated across all appropriate healthcare teams, including to the general practitioner.

Infection control and identification of hazards

The healthcare professional should ascertain if the deceased had any notifiable infection, has had any radiological procedures, has an implantable cardiac defibrillator, or any other potential hazards.

- Implantable cardioverter-defibrillators (ICDs) can still generate high voltage shocks to the body after death. Accordingly, they must be deactivated and the mortuary/funeral directors should be made aware that one is *in situ*.
- Certain extra precautions are required when handling a patient who has died with an infectious disease. However, the deceased will pose no greater threat of an infection risk than when they were alive. It is assumed that staff will have practised universal precautions when caring for all patients, and this practice must be continued.
- If the patient has undergone any procedure involving radioactive material, advice should be sought from the local physics department regarding removal of any radiological devices and/or precautions in handling the body.

Last offices

The care of the immediately deceased and their family is an activity that in healthcare is almost unique to nursing and is the final part of the pathway of care of the dying patient, as documented in the End of Life Strategy.

Last offices, sometimes referred to as 'laying out', is the term for the nursing care given to a deceased patient which demonstrates continued respect for the patient as an individual and, in contemporary society, it is focused on attending to health, safety, and legal requirements, making the body safe to handle and pleasant for others to see, while also respecting religious beliefs and cultural norms. When someone dies at home, the funeral directors will undertake any preparation of the body required. For deaths within hospital, each Trust will have its own protocol to follow.

Rigor mortis can occur relatively soon after death and last offices should be carried out promptly and at least within 2–3 hours of death.

Some families and carers may wish to assist with last offices and within certain cultures it may be unacceptable for anyone except a family member or religious leader to wash the patient. Families and carers should be supported and encouraged to participate if possible and desired as this may help to facilitate the grieving process.

Lay the patient in alignment and close their mouth. Remove any mechanical aids such as syringe drivers. Dependent on local policy, catheters and lines can be left *in situ*. Clamp drains with an umbilical cord clamp, then pad around the exit site with gauze and occlude with an occlusive dressing. A record should be made in the medical notes of all lines and drains left *in situ*. When a death is being referred to the coroner or for post-mortem, all lines, devices, and tubes should be left in place until instructed otherwise by the coroner's office.

Close the patient's eyes by applying light pressure to theeyelids for 30 seconds. This will provide protection in case of corneal tissue donation. Drain the bladder by applying firm pressure over the lower abdomen. Apply pad and pants because the body can continue to excrete fluids after death.

Leakages from the oral cavity can be contained by the use of suctioning. Patients who do continue to have leakages from their orifices after death should be placed in a body bag following last offices. The packing of orifices can cause damage to the body and should only be done by professionals, such as mortuary technicians, who have received specialist training.

Exuding wounds or unhealed surgical scars should be covered with a clean absorbent dressing and secured with an occlusive dressing. Stitches and clips should be left intact. Stomas should be covered with a clean bag.

Wash the patient, unless requested not to do so for religious/cultural reasons or carer's preference. Clean the patient's mouth using a foam stick to remove debris and secretions. Clean dentures and replace them in the mouth if possible.

Remove all jewellery unless requested by the patient's family to do otherwise. Religious jewellery should be left *in situ* (e.g. Sikh bangle). Jewellery remaining on the patient should be documented.

Dress the patient in a shroud or personal clothing depending on relatives' wishes. Ensure a correct hospital identification band is attached to the patient's wrist and attach a further identification band to one ankle. Wrap the body in a sheet, ensuring that the face and feet are covered and that all limbs are held securely in position with arms placed at the patient's side.

Tissue donation

Specific considerations may need to be made during last offices if the patient is donating organs or tissues. It is important to liaise with the NHSBT tissue services on 0800 432 0559 to ascertain if there are specific preparations required.

Referral to the coroner

The Coroner will need to be informed when the person has died in the following ways:
- cause of death is unknown
- trauma, homicide, assaults
- road traffic collisions
- fractures, falls
- industrial accidents/disease
- suicide
- suspicious death
- death in police custody, prison, detention centre, or psychiatric unit (particularly if detained under a section of The Mental health Act)

- neglect of any kind by any person
- death during an operation or before recovery from an anaesthetic
- death within 24 hours of hospital admission or within 24 hours of an operation
- where a member of the healthcare staff may be the subject of criticism in connection with the death
- suspicion of poisoning (occupational, accidental, suicidal, or homicidal)
- any matter, which may be of concern to the public.

In these cases the deceased patient must not be washed and must be prepared for the mortuary by leaving all intravenous attachments, cannulae, endotracheal tubes, drains, catheters as they were when the person died. Additionally, in suspicious deaths, where a police investigation is necessary, the deceased patient should not be touched by relatives or anointed by anyone of their faith unless express permission has been given by the police.

This is the current situation at time of writing. When the Coroners and Justice Act (2009) become law in 2012, there will be a statutory duty on doctors to refer certain deaths to the coroner and the MCCD issued by the doctor will be scrutinized by a medical examiner.

Care of the family after death

After death, the family should have written guidance regarding
- where/when to collect the death certificate
- how to register the death
- what happens when the coroner is involved
- what will happen to the deceased person until they reach the undertaker
- the 'What to do after death' DWP1027 can be offered
- it is useful to provide simple guidance that identifies features of loss and grieving and contact telephone numbers for local bereavement support agencies.

Further reading

Dougherty L, Lister S (2008) *The Royal Marsden Hospital Manual of Clinical Nursing Procedures*, 7th edn Chichester, Wiley-Blackwell.

Frost PJ, Leadbeatter S, Wise MP. (2010) Managing sudden death in hospital. *Br Med J* **340**: 1024–8.

Green, J. Green, M. (2006) *Dealing with Death: A Handbook of Practices, Procedures and Law*, 2nd edn. London, Jessica Kingsley Publishers.

MRC (2008) *A code of practice for the diagnosis and confirmation of death*. Academy of Medical Royal Colleges

Neuberger J (1999) Cultural issues in palliative care. In (Doyle D, Hanks G, MacDonald N, eds) *Oxford Textbook of Palliative Medicine*. Oxford, Oxford University Press.

NMC (2008) *The Code: Standards of Conduct, Performance and Ethics for Nurses and Midwives*. London, Nursing and Midwifery Council,.

RCN (1996) *Verification of Death by Registered Nurses*. Issues in Nursing and Health, 38. London, Royal College of Nursing.

The Shap working group—Shap world religions in education

Religion or Belief—a practical guide for the NHS Jan 09

www.mapofmedicine.co.uk

www.mfghc.com/resources/resources_faithindex

www.religionandcultures.co.uk

Recommended reading

Guidance for staff responsible for care after death (last offices). National End of Life Care Programme 2011

Managing death and dying

Background

Around half a million people die in England each year of whom almost two-thirds are over the age of 75. The majority of these follow a period of chronic illness such as heart disease, stroke, chronic respiratory disease, or dementia. Most deaths (58%) occur in NHS hospitals, with around 18% at home, 17% in care homes, 4% in hospices, and 3% elsewhere.

How we care for the dying is an indicator of how we care for all sick and vulnerable people. Care of the dying is urgent care, with only one opportunity to get it right to create a potential lasting memory for relatives and carers.

Recognition of the dying phase (the last hours or days of life)

In order to achieve a good death, one of the key challenges is recognition of the dying phase. The type of care required in the last days of life can be quite different from the palliative measures used earlier in a patient's illness. Identification of this transition phase can be difficult and is not an exact science. It is also often harder when caring for somebody with a long-term chronic illness.

Signs and symptoms of death approaching

As the patient approaches death they may show some of the following signs:

- profound tiredness and weakness
- reduced interest in getting out of bed
- less interested in things happening around them
- diminished intake of food or fluids
- drowsiness or reduced cognition
- difficulty swallowing medicine.

It is likely that few of these features are new ones, but what can suggest that a patient is entering the dying phase is when most of these become evident at the same time.

It can also be difficult to decide whether the patient is entering the dying phase or possibly having an exacerbation of a chronic condition, from which there might be a recovery as has happened in the past. An example of this could be a severe acute exacerbation of chronic obstructive pulmonary disease. It is therefore important where clinically appropriate to exclude any potentially reversible causes.

Possible reversible causes to be considered include

- infection
- hypercalcaemia
- renal failure
- medication changes
- opioid toxicity
- raised intracranial pressure.

On such occasions where there is uncertainty as to whether the patient is entering the dying phase, the situation needs to be fully explained to the patient, and, when appropriate, to the relatives. They need to be aware why investigations are being done, what is hoped to be achieved with any treatment and be reassured that this 'active' treatment will be withdrawn should it prove futile. It is important not to promote false hope with patients and relatives by ordering unnecessary investigations or futile treatment.

A multidisciplinary decision

It is important that considering whether or not a patient is entering the dying phase is a multidisciplinary decision. Although individuals can possess the skills to recognize and diagnose dying, input from other members of the multiprofessional team is vital. Providing good-quality care at the end of life requires a team approach. No single member of the palliative care team, no matter how committed, can meet all the palliative care needs of a patient and his/her family.

If there is doubt as to whether a patient is dying, you can always seek a second opinion and specialist palliative care support as needed.

The Liverpool Care Pathway for the Dying Patient

The Liverpool Care Pathway for the Dying Patient (LCP) is a multiprofessional document that incorporates evidence based practice and appropriate guidelines related to care of the dying. It is unrealistic to expect specialist palliative care teams to be involved with every dying patient. Therefore, a key feature of the LCP is that it empowers generic health care workers in the hospital and the community to ensure that dying patients and their relatives and carers receive a high standard of care in the last hours and days of their life.

It is well recognized that hospices are synonymous with high-quality care of the dying and the LCP allows the transfer of this model of best practice to other settings such as hospitals and the community.

Key themes

- To improve knowledge related to the process of dying
- To improve the quality of care in the last hours or days of life

Key Sections

- Initial assessment and care
- Ongoing assessment
- Care of the relatives after death

Initial assessment and care

This should be a joint assessment by the doctor and nurse and identifies that active care of the dying patient should include

- assessment of baseline symptoms
- communication with the patient and family
- assessment of insight
- religious and spiritual needs are assessed with patient/carer
- reviewing medication and discontinuing non-essentials
- anticipatory prescribing of prn (as required) medications for pain, agitation, respiratory tract secretions, nausea and vomiting and dyspnoea.
- reviewing the need for interventions such as blood tests and antibiotics
- reviewing the need for clinically assisted nutrition by the MDT
- reviewing the need for clinically assisted hydration by the MDT
- informing the patients primary healthcare team/GP practice.

The LCP does not preclude the use of clinically assisted nutrition or hydration or antibiotics. All clinical decisions should be made with the primary aim of symptom relief. When the patient lacks capacity to guide treatment themselves, a best interests approach is mandatory.

Ongoing assessment

The LCP emphasizes the need for regular reassessment with at least 4-hourly observations of symptom control and the need to take appropriate action if there is a problem.

If a goal is not achieved, this should be coded as a variance. It is important to stress that this is not a negative process reflecting bad care, but rather that it is demonstrating the individual nature of the patient's journey and is highlighting areas that need to be addressed in order to optimize the care and symptom control of that patient.

It is recommended that in addition to the regular assessments, a formal full MDT review is undertaken every three days. There are situations when a patient who is thought to be dying lives longer than expected or vice versa. There are also occasions, highlighting the complexity of diagnosing dying, when patients (approximately 3%) will actually improve and the LCP will be discontinued for that particular patient at that point in time.

Care of the relatives after death

Here the LCP focuses on care and support for family and carers immediately after death. It includes catering for the information needs of the family and any special requests regarding the care of the body. Obviously, if there were specific requests, perhaps of a religious nature then these should ideally have been identified earlier in the initial assessment in order to minimize any further distress to the family at this stage.

Author's Tip

As with all clinical guidelines and pathways the LCP aims to support but does not replace clinical judgement

The LCP is only as good as the people using it and a robust continuous learning and teaching programme must underpin the use of the LCP

Symptom relief in the dying patient

The main symptoms in the terminal phase are pain, nausea and vomiting, agitation/restlessness, retained respiratory secretions, and breathlessness. Other problems may include constipation, urinary problems, and less commonly bleeding and seizures.

Managing these symptoms can be a continuation of what has already being done. However, previously well managed symptoms can recur and new symptoms develop.

An important factor in achieving good symptom control is being proactive rather than reactive. This involves anticipating what symptoms may develop and prescribing appropriate medications for use as required. Anticipatory prescribing in this manner will ensure that there is no delay in responding to a symptom if it occurs.

Pain

In general, pain will often not be troublesome at the end of life if it has previously been well controlled. However, careful evaluation is still vital and new pains can develop. If a new pain appears to have developed, then consideration should be given to

- whether pain control has been lost when changing drugs or routes of administration

- urinary retention or constipation has developed
- painful pressure sores have developed.

Most patients in the dying phase will have difficulty swallowing oral medication. If a patient is on a regular strong opioid then this needs to be given via an alternative route such as a continuous subcutaneous infusion (CSCI). Abrupt discontinuation of an opioid runs the risk of a return of pain and possible withdrawal symptoms.

Restlessness/Agitation

Similarly, when evaluating pain, it is important to consider reversible causes of agitation. For example

- pain
- urinary retention
- constipation
- nausea
- cerebral irritability
- anxiety and fear
- medication side-effects

Once any reversible cause of the agitation has been excluded or treated, it is important to inform the family of ongoing management options, emphasizing clearly the goals of treatment which in this case are alleviating suffering and maintaining comfort.

Commonly used drugs to manage restlessness and agitation at the end of life include benzodiazepines, such as midazolam, and if symptoms remain uncontrolled despite this, second line agents such as levomepromazine may be considered.

Respiratory tract secretions

Weakness in the last few days of life can result in an inability to clear respiratory secretions, leading to noisy rattling breathing. This is due to fluid pooling in the hypopharynx and can occur in up to 50% of dying patients.

General measures include reassurance for the family, for whom it is often more distressing than for the patient, and repositioning the patient. Specific treatments should be started as early as possible and commonly used drugs include glycopyrronium and hyoscine hydrobromide. Hyoscine hydrobromide can be sedating and cause confusion.

Nausea and vomiting

Nausea and vomiting can be a very unpleasant symptom and prompt action to control it is essential. The use of antiemetics in palliative care is guided by the probable cause of the nausea and vomiting in relation to the mechanism of action of the drug. However, establishing the precise cause in the dying phase can be difficult. If a cause cannot be identified, then the use of a broad spectrum anti-emetic is suggested. Cyclizine is usually prescribed in this situation and, if cyclizine does not work, levomepromazine should be considered.

Dyspnoea

The commonest causes of breathlessness in the dying phase include

- chest infection
- anxiety or panic
- pulmonary oedema
- extensive lung metastases or lymphangitis.

Non-pharmacological treatments include simple advice about opening windows, the use of a fan, or relaxation techniques.

Drug treatment usually comprises the administration of an opioid such as morphine, which may be given via a continuous subcutaneous infusion. If anxiety appears to be contributing significantly to the breathlessness, then consideration of a sedative/anxiolytic, such as midazolam, in addition to the opioid may be appropriate.

Further information on recommended doses of medications to help treat these symptoms can be obtained from the Palliative Care Formulary.

Ethical issues

Clinically assisted (artificial) hydration

The provision of clinically assisted nutrition and hydration is regarded as a medical treatment and not part of basic care. Therefore a clinician should only offer it if he/she feels it is likely to lead to symptomatic benefit. Loss of interest and a reduced need for food and drink are part of the normal dying process

There is insufficient evidence to draw firm conclusions about either the beneficial or harmful effects of fluid administration to the dying patient. Such conflicting data emphasizes the need for individual evaluation on a case-by-case basis. A blanket policy of clinically assisted hydration, or of no clinically assisted hydration, is ethically indefensible and, in the case of adults lacking capacity, prohibited under the Mental Capacity Act (2005). When a decision is made that clinically assisted hydration is not of overall benefit to the patient, you must monitor the situation and be prepared to reassess the benefits, burdens and risks of providing clinically assisted hydration in light of changes in their condition.

The LCP does not preclude the use of clinically assisted hydration. When there is uncertainty about the potential benefits, a time limited trial with specific goals could be undertaken. For example, giving 1 L of fluid over 24 hours and assessing the response.

Cardiopulmonary resuscitation

Decisions about CPR are complex and should be undertaken by experienced clinicians and documented carefully.

Decisions need to be tailored to the patient's individual circumstances and decided following an assessment of benefits versus burdens.

The decision not to resuscitate is usually based on the ineffectiveness of CPR in the presence of overwhelming disease(s). To inform patients of a decision not to resuscitate in these circumstances can cause unnecessary distress. In such circumstances, it is not a requirement to inform the patient of this decision. If it is decided not to inform the patient, the reason for this should be documented in the medical records. However, some patients express a wish to discuss CPR and it is important to ascertain early how much information the patient wants. Often the decision not to resuscitate will fall out naturally from a more general discussion with the patient about their condition and prognosis.

Truth telling at the end of life

Healthcare professionals may censor their information giving to patients in an attempt to protect them from potentially hurtful or bad news. This can also sometimes be at the request of relatives.

Although the motivation behind economy with the truth is often well meant, a conspiracy of silence usually results in a heightened state of fear, anxiety, and confusion rather than one of calm and equanimity.

Prognosticating is more difficult in non-malignant disease than in cancer patients but some of the conclusions from studies with cancer patients can still be applied. Evidence suggests that there are potentially negative consequences for an individual who lacks insight into their disease stage. These can include unsatisfactory management of the advanced stage of the illness, such as unnecessary and unwanted hospital admissions, a higher proportion of hospital deaths, and lack of or late referral to palliative care, poorer symptom control, less end of life advance care planning and consequently reduced patient choice. There is also documented mistrust and feelings of abandonment in patients who have information withheld from them. It would therefore seem that open communication and awareness are desirable objectives in caring for patients with advanced disease.

However, not all patients want this information and it is therefore important that disclosure is not an active procedure undertaken by the professional with the patient a passive recipient. Instead, it requires a skilled approach to provide the appropriate level of prognostic information that they need as individuals to meet their own goals and priorities in the final phase of their lives.

Further reading

Department of Health (2008) *End of Life Care Strategy. Promoting High Quality Care for all Adults at the End of Life* (http://www.dh.gov.uk).Department of Health (2009) *End of Life Care Strategy. Quality Markers and Measures for End of Life Care.* (http://www.dh.gov.uk).

Fallowfield LJ, Jenkins VA, Beveridge HA (2002). Truth may hurt but deceit hurts more: communication in palliative care. *Palliat Med* **16**: 297–303.

Fürst CJ, Doyle D (2005). The terminal phase. In (Doyle D, Hanks G, Cherny, et al. eds) *Oxford Textbook of Palliative Medicine*. Oxford, Oxford University Press, pp. 1119–33.

General Medical Council (2010) Treatment and care towards the end of life: good practice in decision making (www.gmc-uk.org).

Glare P, Dickman A, Goodman M (2003) Symptom control in the care of the dying. In Ellershaw J, Wilkinson S (eds) *Care of the Dying. A Pathway to Excellence.* Oxford, Oxford University Press, pp. 42–61.

Innes S, Payne S (2009). Advanced cancer patients' prognostic information preferences: a review. *Palliat Med* **23**: 29–39.

Kinder C, Ellershaw J. (2003) How to use the Liverpool Care Pathway for the Dying Patient? In (Ellershaw J, Wilkinson S, eds) *Care of the Dying. A Pathway to Excellence*, Oxford, Oxford University Press, pp. 11–41.

Marie Curie Palliative Care Institute Liverpool (2009) *What is the LCP? Information For Healthcare Professionals.* (www.mcpcil.org.uk).

NCPC (2006) *Changing Gear—Guidelines for Managing the Last Days of Life in Adults (revised edition).* London, National Council for Palliative Care.

NCPC (2007) *Artificial Nutrition and Hydration- Guidance in End of Life Care for Adults.* London, National Council for Palliative Care.

Resuscitation Council UK (2007) Decisions relating to cardiopulmonary resuscitation. (www.resus.org.uk).

Twycross R, Wilcock A (eds) (2011) *Palliative Care Formulary*, 4th edn. Nottingham, Palliativedrugs.com Ltd.

Twycross R, Wilcock A, Stark Toller C (eds) (2009). *Symptom Management in Advanced Cancer*, 4th edn. Nottingham, Palliative Drugs Comp Ltd, Chapter 13.

Watson M, Hoy A, Beck A, et al. (eds) (2009) *Oxford Handbook of Palliative Medicine*, 2nd edn. Oxford, Oxford University Press, Chapter 16.

Advance care planning

Definitions

Advance Care Planning (ACP) is a process enabling individuals to discuss and prepare for their care in the event of future decisional incapacity. A written output is not obligatory, but any of the following, in isolation or combination, may be recorded (replacing previous terms of 'Advance Directives' and 'Living Wills') and come into force in the event of decisional incapacity.

- Advance Statements (AS) indicate preferences for care following loss of decisional capacity; they are not legally binding.
- Advance Decisions on Refusal of Treatment (ADRT) are legal records of informed consent for refusal of specific treatments in certain scenarios and must be in writing, signed and witnessed.
- A healthcare proxy may be appointed (Lasting Power of Attorney (LPA), England and Wales): applications through Office of the Public Guardian.

Rationale

The intention of ACP is to increase an individual's control over their future (and particularly end-of-life) care.

- By guiding health professionals once a patient has lost decisional capacity, it attempts to reduce the gap between a patient's prior preferences and physician behaviour.
- It may allow patients to reflect on and communicate their aspirations and goals, thereby better preparing them for the 'end-of-life' period.

Other benefits may also arise:

- It can alleviate anxiety and depression in caregivers, exacerbated by the decision-making burden that is often incumbent upon them in end-of-life situations.
- It affords an opportunity to improve all round communication between patients, caregivers, and medical professionals.

Initiating and undertaking ACP

ACP often involves multiple conversations between patients and care providers and is subject to wide variations between cultural groups and individuals.

- Healthcare providers should be the initiators of ACP, although patients should not be pressurized to partake in these discussions.
- Timing of discussions can be prompted by clinical indicators of advanced disease and physician-intuition regarding prognosis (Gold Standards Framework).
- ACP has been initiated in both in- and outpatient settings, but should not happen too close to an acute illness or new diagnosis, when patients are unwell or coming to terms with a condition.
- Inadequate mental capacity and depression should be excluded before embarking on discussions.
- Generic requirements for ACP are good communication skills, sensitivity, time, and ensuring any sensory impairments have been optimized and the patient made as comfortable as possible.
- Discussions may progress through stages of considering, discussing, and planning end-of-life care.
- It is important to recognize an individual's stage in the process and understand barriers to progression.

Postponing or ceasing discussions may be an entirely appropriate action.

- Undue focus should not be given to completion of formal documents per se, which are not necessarily associated with improvements in patient-physician communication.
- It is preferable that any recorded documents are reviewed periodically, typically following a change of patient circumstances, to allow for potential changes in preferences.

> **Author's Tip**
>
> Advance Care Plans need to be accessible to relevant care professionals. Distributions lists may include GPs, out-of-hours services, care homes, and local hospitals.

Advance care plan content

A number of downloadable tools exist to facilitate and document ACP discussions. Examples include: 'Thinking Ahead', 'Preferred Priorities of Care', 'Let Me Decide', 'Expression of Healthcare Preferences', 'The Medical Directive'.

ACPs tend to record patient preferences predominantly with one of the following approaches.

- A documentation of the patient's values.
  - e.g. 'If you were dying, how important would it be for you to avoid pain and suffering, even if it means that you might not live as long?'
- A consideration of specific treatments in a range of different clinical scenarios.
  - e.g. 'If I am aware but have brain damage that makes me unable to recognize people, speak meaningfully, or live independently, and I do not have a terminal illness: then I would/would not want artificial ventilation.'

More specific medical care plans may give patients a feeling of greater control over future care, albeit with concerns that they provide less guidance on routine decisions compared to critical treatments and cannot inform on situations outside of their specific remit.

> **Author's Tip**
>
> A suggested strategy is an individually tailored plan, elaborating a strong expression of positive values and preferences (included in an AS). This can be combined with preferences for refusal of specific treatments (life-sustaining measures such as artificial ventilation, nasogastric/PEG feeding and CPR). Legal assistance can be sought for formulation of such ADRTs where there is uncertainty.

ACP practitioners

- ACP discussions may be carried out by physicians and other care professionals such as specialist nurses and social workers, given prior training.
- Ideally, an ACP facilitator should possess knowledge relating to condition(s) pertinent to that patient, so that questions regarding natural history of the illness and prognosis can be discussed.

- In practice, the whole process may involve discussions with a range of professionals to benefit from the knowledge offered by each group.

Cognitive impairment and incapacity

Future 'care planning' may still have a role for patients lacking capacity to inform ACP discussions, though such a process cannot legally support an ADRT or appointment of an LPA. Discussions may be instigated by caregivers or physicians if there is a perceived risk of future care not being in the patient's best interests.

Such a process of 'care planning' requires

- identifying relevant participants who can inform discussions (family, informal carers, professionals)
- eliciting values and preferences of the patient based on information from invited participants.

Further discussion may include:

- Ensuring a shared understanding of diagnoses and trajectories of illnesses with participants.
- Discussing prognosis, anticipating future clinical events, and considering the effects of potential lines of management.
- Physician-led advocacy for the patient, establishing 'best interests' in a range of situations. This may be recorded as a statement of values and preferences (e.g. preferred place of death, preferences to avoid certain treatments).
- Where consensus between physicians and caregiving participants is not attained, discussions may be postponed, with care being managed expectantly.

Does ACP improve patient care?

There is a paucity of data relating to the effectiveness of ACP in the UK. With some exceptions, experience from the North American continent and Australia, demonstrates little improvement in medical or end-of-life care following ACP and variability in both interpretation and adherence to the plans. Any benefit is mainly from improved communication, giving patients a sense of empowerment over their care and preparing them for death. General 'care planning' and ACP may, however, have an impact in care homes, resulting in fewer (potentially unnecessary) hospitalizations without increase in overall mortality.

'Is ACP acceptable to patients?'

ACP discussions can promote increased satisfaction with care, including in older people. There is increasing public acknowledgement of its potential benefits, but this has yet to translate into significant completion of Advance Care Plans (only 8% of people in England and Wales have some documented Advance Care Plan).

'Could ACP deny treatments to older people?'

There is a concern that Advance Care Plans, particularly ADRTs, may limit appropriate active treatment before an individual reaches the state of illness and/or incapacity to which the ADRT pertains. Safeguarding against this requires more detailed care plans and education to improve interpretation of these documents by healthcare professionals. ADRTs can also express treatments in a graduated fashion, with licence to withdraw once a more accurate prognosis is known.

'How can ACP discussions be facilitated?'

The following methods have been shown to improve rates of ACP discussion and documentation:

- Video decision support tools have been utilised in planning end-of-life care for cancer and dementia.
- Structured questionnaires have been evaluated within an inpatient setting, where an accessible clinician–patient relationship and an environmental context of death and illness, may promote end-of-life discussions.

'Can ADRTs be overruled once capacity is lost?'

- If an LPA is appointed with powers to make decisions covered in the ADRT, then the decisions of the LPA take precedence.
- The following may raise questions concerning the validity of an ADRT.
  - An individual acting in a manner suggestive of a change of view on the ADRT.
  - Concerns about capacity at the time the ADRT was devised.
  - Changes in circumstances which may not have been anticipated by the person and might have affected their decision (e.g. a recent therapy that radically changes the outlook for their particular condition).

Where such doubt exists, ADRTs could be overruled according to the principle of 'beneficence'.

Further reading

Caplan GA, Meller A, Squires B, et al. (2006). Advance care planning and hospital in the nursing home. *Age Ageing* **35**: 581–5.

Conroy S, Fade P, Fraser A, et al. (2009). Advance Care Planning: concise evidence-based guidelines. In (Turner-Stokes L, ed.) *Concise Guidance to Good Practice Series*. London, RCP.

Molloy D, Guyatt GH, Russo R, et al. (2000). Systematic implementation of an advance directive program in nursing homes. A randomized controlled trial. *JAMA* **283**: 1437–44.

Schiff R, Shaw R, Raja N, et al. (2009). Advance end-of-life healthcare planning in an acute NHS hospital setting; development and evaluation of the Expression of Healthcare Preferences (EHP) document. *Age Ageing* **38**: 81–5.

Teno J, Lynn J, Wenger N, et al. (1997). Advance directives for seriously ill hospitalized patients: effectiveness with the patient self-determination act and the SUPPORT intervention. SUPPORT Investigators. Study to Understand Prognoses and Preferences for Outcomes and Risks of Treatment. *J Am Geriatr Soc* **45**: 500–7.

Thomas K. (2010). The GSF Prognostic Indicator Guidance. *End of Life Care Journal* **4**: 62–4.

Volandes AE, Paasche-Orlow MK, Barry MJ, et al. (2009). Video decision support tool for advance care planning in dementia: randomised controlled trial. *Br Med J* **28**: b2159.

Euthanasia

Introduction

Euthanasia is illegal in most countries except for Belgium (2002), the Netherlands (2002), and Luxembourg (2009). In Belgium, the law on euthanasia came into force together with laws on patient's rights and on palliative care. These three laws have emerged from the growing support for respect of patient autonomy. In Belgium, euthanasia is considered to be an extension of good palliative care (Federation of Palliative Care, Flanders).

The countries in which euthanasia is legal all use a specific definition of euthanasia:

'the administration of lethal drugs, with explicit intention of ending the patient's life at the patient's explicit request'

Incidence of euthanasia in Belgium

The Federal Control and Evaluation Committee publishes data concerning *reported* euthanasia cases in Belgium. (The numbers presented here are data from 2007.)

- 495 cases of euthanasia were reported, representing 0.44% of all deaths
- 85/495 (17%) of registered cases were 80 years and older
- It mostly concerned requests from competent patients (98%) with terminal malignant illness (82%)
- There was usually a combination of physical and mental suffering.

Previous studies showed that euthanasia is rare in patients older than 80 years (1% of all deaths) compared with other end-of-life decisions, such as withdrawing or withholding life-sustaining therapies (23%) or symptom relief (20%). Additionally, there is relatively less symptom relief and more non-treatment decisions in older patients than younger patients.

Belgian Act on euthanasia

- No physician can be compelled to perform euthanasia
- The law allows euthanasia *only under strict conditions* (see Box on p. 452).

Legal criteria for euthanasia in Belgium

Actual request for euthanasia

Terminally ill patient

- Patient is a major and is competent at the time of the request.
- Request is voluntary, well considered, and repeated, and does not result from any external pressure.
- Patient has an incurable condition with constant and unbearable physical or mental suffering that cannot be alleviated.
- Physician must discuss the possible therapeutic and palliative courses of action and their consequences.
- Second physician (expert) must confirm the incurable nature of the disease and the fact of unbearable suffering.
- Physician must discuss the request with the nursing team and with the relatives of the patient (after patient's consent).
- The request for euthanasia must be written down and signed by the patient.

Not terminally ill patient

- Third physician (expert or psychiatrist) must confirm that there is unbearable suffering and that the request is voluntary, well considered, and repeated.
- A period of at least 1 month must pass between the time of the written request and the act of euthanasia.

Advance directive concerning euthanasia

- Only applicable when the patient is in an irreversible coma.
- Second physician (expert) must confirm the irreversibility of the coma.
- The directive must be discussed with the nursing team.
- The directive must be discussed with the surrogate decision-maker.
- Directive must be renewed every 5 years.

The physician who has performed euthanasia is required to send a registration form to the Federal Control and Evaluation Committee.

What to consider when confronted with a request for euthanasia?

- Physicians and other healthcare providers need to be sensitive to signals indicating a desire to talk about end-of-life issues.
- The exploration of end-of-life preferences should be the priority in these discussions in order to provide insight into patient's thoughts and feelings.
- Practical stepwise recommendations are given in Figure 19.1.

Nurses and euthanasia

Nurses often are with the patient and his/her relatives 24 hours a day. As a consequence, they are more often confronted with patient's anxieties and questions regarding prognosis or end-of-life issues than physicians. Nurses are sometimes the first to detect the patient's wish to die. Moreover, nurses (can) have a meaningful contribution in further exploring the patient's request.

Nurses (can) provide assistance in administering lethal medication by supporting the patient and family members, also after the patient has died.

Controversies concerning euthanasia in the older patient

Dementia

Only in the early stages of dementia (in which the patient can still be considered as being competent) can an actual request for euthanasia be made. However, it remains difficult to assess competence in the patient with dementia.

In the later stages of dementia, an actual request is no longer possible given the lack of competence of the patient. In Belgium, advance directives concerning euthanasia are not applicable for the patient with advanced dementia (only in the case of irreversible coma). Although advance directives are also applicable for advanced dementia in the Netherlands, there has not been a case registered before 2010.

Existential suffering in old age

In order to have a legal request, there should be 'an incurable condition' present. The discussion remains if frailty and old age may be considered as such.

1. Exploration of the request

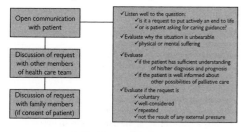

Open communication with patient	✓ Listen well to the question: 　✓ is it a request to put actively an end to life 　✓ or is patient asking for caring guidance? ✓ Evaluate why the situation is unbearable 　✓ physical or mental suffering
Discussion of request with other members of health care team	✓ Evaluate 　✓ if the patient has sufficient understanding 　　of his/her diagnosis and prognosis 　✓ if the patient is well informed about 　　other possibilities of palliative care
Discussion of request with family members (if consent of patient)	✓ Evaluate if the request is 　✓ voluntary 　✓ well-considered 　✓ repeated 　✓ not the result of any external pressure

2. Decision-making

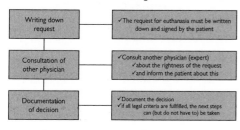

Writing down request	✓ The request for euthanasia must be written down and signed by the patient
Consultation of other physician	✓ Consult another physician (expert) 　✓ about the rightness of the request 　✓ and inform the patient about this
Documentation of decision	✓ Document the decision 　✓ if all legal criteria are fulfilled, the next steps can (but do not have to) be taken

3. Accomplishment

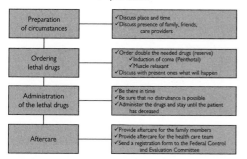

Preparation of circumstances	✓ Discuss place and time ✓ Discuss presence of family, friends, care providers
Ordering lethal drugs	✓ Order double the needed drugs (reserve) 　✓ Induction of coma (Penthotal) 　✓ Muscle relaxant ✓ Discuss with present ones what will happen
Administration of the lethal drugs	✓ Be there in time ✓ Be sure that no distrubance is possible ✓ Administer the drugs and stay until the patient has deceased
Aftercare	✓ Provide aftercare for the family members ✓ Provide aftercare for the health care team ✓ Send a registration form to the Federal Control and Evaluation Committee

Figure 19.1 A practical approach to requests for euthanasia in Belgium. Reproduced from Grame Rocker, Kathleen A. Puntillo, Élie Azoulay, Judith E. Nelson, *End of Life Care in the ICU*, 2010, Figure 7.1, p. 219, with permission from Oxford University Press.

Additionally, a constant and unbearable physical or mental suffering that cannot be alleviated, should be present. However, physicians and other team members do not always feel confident in assessing and alleviating existential suffering and spiritual needs.

Key points

- Euthanasia is rare compared with other end-of-life decisions.
- Euthanasia is illegal in most countries except for Belgium, the Netherlands and Luxembourg. In these countries:
- a specific definition of euthanasia is used, namely:
  - the administration of lethal drugs with the explicit intention of ending the patient's life at patient's explicit request.
  - euthanasia is considered to be an extension of good palliative care.
  - euthanasia can only be performed after the clarification of the patient's request through good communication.
  - euthanasia should be the result of interdisciplinary communication and decision-making.
  - euthanasia in patients with dementia and/or existential suffering is controversial.

Further reading

Bernheim J, Deschepper R, Distelmans W, *et al.* (2008). Development of palliative care and legislation of euthanasia: antagonism or synergy? *Br Med J* **336**: 864–7.

Van der Heide A, Deliens L, Faisst K, *et al.* (2003). End-of-life decision-making in six European countries. *Lancet* **362**: 345–50.

Orthogeriatrics

Principles of orthogeriatrics

Introduction

Fractures in older people, often related to falls, are common, with approximately 300 000 fragility fractures each year in the UK. Many of these patients are frail with multiple medical comorbidities and complex rehabilitation and discharge needs. Traditionally, their post-surgical care was left to orthopaedic junior doctors who lacked the skills and support to care for this vulnerable group. The principles of geriatric medicine can be applied in orthopaedics and have the potential to improve the quality of care. The 'core business' of an orthogeriatrician is the care of hip fracture patients, the number of whom are expected to double by 2050.

Definition

The concept of orthogeriatrics can be interpreted in a number of ways and service models vary. However, an orthogeriatric service should provide certain key components. The aim is to see patients preoperatively to optimize existing medical problems and review them perioperatively, so that any decompensation of these conditions can be resolved, as can any new problems that develop (such as sepsis, atrial fibrillation, perioperative myocardial infarctions, etc.). Barriers to rehabilitation are identified and dealt with and discharge planned in a multidisciplinary setting. The drive for this service is to reduce perioperative complications, decrease morbidity and mortality, increase the number of patients returning to independent living, and reduce length of stay. Patients with long lengths of stay in orthopaedics are usually due to medical and social issues rather than surgical ones.

History

Orthogeriatrics is not a new concept. Before the Second World War, patients with hip fractures were treated non-operatively and remained bed bound. The death rate was high due to complications of immobility such as venous thromboembolic events, bronchopneumonia, and sepsis from pressure sores. In the 1940s, a surgeon, Lionel Cosins, started working with his physiotherapist to provide rehabilitation for patients, with the result that many started to mobilize and returned home. The first orthopaedic and geriatric collaboration was in Hastings in 1957, when Professor Michael Devas (an orthopaedic surgeon) and Dr Bobby Irvine (a physician) did combined ward rounds. Michael described himself as a humble carpenter requiring a physician to inform him what was wrong with his patients. They advocated early surgery for even the frailest old followed by early mobilization. After these beginnings, the subspecialty has continued to increase in popularity.

National guidelines

There are national guidelines indicating what a good orthogeriatric service should provide. The Royal College of Physicians (RCP) Hip Fracture Report recommends that the assessment and treatment of medical problems should not be left to orthopaedic doctors alone and that we should strive for early surgery. The National Service Framework states that every hospital should have a ward for orthogeriatrics but accepts that the type of service can be decided locally. The Scottish Intercollegiate Guidelines Network (SIGN) produced evidence-based guidelines in 1997, which have been revised twice. The 'bible' of orthogeriatrics is 'the Blue Book', a collaboration between the British Geriatrics Society (BGS) and the British Orthopaedic Association which sets out six standards for Orthogeriatric Care.

1 All patients with hip fracture should be admitted to an acute orthopaedic ward within 4 hours of presentation.
2 All patients with hip fracture who are medically fit should have surgery within 48 hours of admission, and during normal working hours.
3 All patients with hip fracture should be assessed and cared for with a view to minimising their risk of developing a pressure ulcer.
4 All patients presenting with a fragility facture should be managed on an orthopaedic ward with routine access to orthogeriatric medical support from the time of admission.
5 All patients presenting with fragility fracture should be assessed for antiresorptive therapy to prevent future osteoporotic fractures.
6 All patients presenting with a fragility fracture following a fall should be offered multidisciplinary assessment and intervention to prevent future falls.

Models of orthogeriatric services

There are various models of care in practice and it is this diversity that makes it difficult to evaluate the usefulness of orthogeriatrics. Large meta-analyses have failed to demonstrate much improvement in outcomes such as length of stay, mortality and return to functional independence. However, there are many individual case studies that would suggest otherwise.

Traditional orthopaedic care

Patients are admitted by and cared for by orthopaedic surgeons. Patients requiring medical input can be referred to a physician. This is not an orthogeriatric model of care but is included as a reference point.

Orthogeriatric units

These are units separately located from acute orthopaedic wards. Patients are transferred a few days postoperatively. Identification of individuals may be by nurses, doctors, or therapists. The unit is under the care of an orthogeriatrician with discharge planning proceeding as it would in geriatric medicine.

Orthogeriatric liaison service

Patients are admitted by and cared for by orthopaedic surgeons. Geriatric input is provided on a timetabled basis, often in the form of a ward round. Patients can be referred to the service by the orthopaedic doctors or may be identified by a liaison nurse. An additional benefit is the opportunity to provide support and education to the orthopaedic junior staff.

Combined orthogeriatric care

Patients are admitted under the joint care of the orthopaedic surgeons and geriatricians. There is preoperative assessment by the geriatricians and this regular review continues throughout the patients stay. Rehabilitation may occur on the same or a different unit.

Early supported discharge schemes

Community rehabilitation schemes are being introduced in many branches of medicine and orthogeriatrics is no exception. These can be new services or may make use of existing schemes. There is evidence to suggest that these reduce length of stay (although this is offset somewhat by a non-significant trend towards readmissions) and an increased return to independent living.

Components of care

Preoperative assessment

Although often recorded as a 'mechanical fall', this is rarely the case in older people. Medical conditions predispose to falls and a small but significant number of patients will fall as a result of an acute medical condition such as acute delirium, cardiac events, or stroke. Although patients may be unfit for surgery on admission, often minimal medical input can rectify this. Electrolytes can be corrected, fast atrial fibrillation controlled, and infection managed. The geriatrician may intervene directly or through the production of guidelines managing common preoperative issues, such as warfarin reversal.

The importance of early surgery cannot be overstated and there is evidence to suggest that for every 8-hour delay to surgery there is a 24-hour increase in length of stay. This requires collaboration not just with the surgeons but also the anaesthetists. Any delay to surgery must be with a clear intent to medical optimisation. The blue book states a time from admission to theatre of 48 hours and the Best Practice Tariff (additional payment for best practice) requires 36 hours.

One source of controversy is the management of systolic murmurs which are found not uncommonly and echocardiography is often requested. The consensus from leading experts is that these should not be done if they result in surgical delay. Individuals should instead be treated as high risk with anaesthetic type and monitoring chosen to reflect this.

It should also be remembered that surgery is the best pain relief for a hip fracture, so should be considered even if life expectancy is very short with or without surgery. Surgery undertaken in such high risk patients should be in full discussion with the patient and/or relatives and the geriatrician can have a key role in this.

Perioperative care

Most of the postoperative problems encountered by older patients are medical rather than orthopaedic. Issues such as fluid management with hypovalaemia and hyponatraemia are common. Early mobilization is key to reducing complications such as constipation, pressure ulcers, bronchopneumonia, and venous thrombotic events. This requires good pain relief and therapists and nurses skilled in the care of older people. Nutrition is important, with 20% of patients with hip fracture malnourished on admission, and inpatients consuming only half the recommended daily amount of calories. Intervention with nutritional supplements may improve outcomes, although trials to date have not been encouraging. Thromboprophylaxis should be instigated as clinically significant DVT occurs in 3% of hip fractures and PE in 1%. The recent NICE guidance reviews the evidence for mechanical and chemical methods and suggests leg compression devices and low molecular weight heparin as best, although local policies may vary.

A frequent complication after surgery is delirium, which occurs in 35–65% of patients and is associated with poor functional recovery. It is generally multifactorial and may be due to pain, disorientation due to an unfamiliar environment, medication, constipation, hypoxia, intercurrent

infection etc. There is evidence to suggest that proactive geriatric intervention can reduce the incidence with subsequent improvement in outcome.

A condition referred to as postoperative cognition dysfunction is increasingly recognized; its cause is unclear. It is thought to occur in as many as 25.8% of patients at 1 week post surgery, 9.9% at 3 months and has been recognized as persisting for as long as a year and may even be permanent. Whether this is a prolonged postoperative delirium or an unmasking of dementia or independent of both is unclear. Postoperative confusion of any kind is distressing to patients and relatives and requires good communication from staff to reduce anxiety.

Falls and osteoporosis assessments can also be completed in the perioperative period.

Rehabilitation and discharge planning

Services available locally will dictate the model used but involvement of the multidisciplinary team is central. Although the aim is for patients to return home, often with community rehabilitation, some will require a period of inpatient rehabilitation which may be provided in community hospitals or off site rehabilitation units. Ten to twenty per cent of patients will need transfer to care homes. The geriatrician can assist in selection of appropriate patients for rehabilitation schemes. Barriers to rehabilitation can be identified and managed, such as inadequate pain relief, intercurrent illness, and depression. Loss of independence and lack of confidence can be considerable following a fall and may impact on the rehabilitation process.

Palliative care

Ten per cent of patients with hip fracture die in the first month following the fracture and for most this will occur in hospital. The role of the geriatrician is in recognizing these individuals and changing the focus of care to one of symptomatic relief. Unfortunately 20–30% will die within a year of the fracture reflecting the frailty of this patient group.

Further reading

British Orthopaedic Association (2007). *The Care of Patients with Fragility Fracture ('The blue book')*. East Sussex, Chandlers Printers Ltd,.

Cameron I, Crotty M, Currie C, et al. (2000). Geriatric rehabilitation following fractures in older people: a systematic review: *Health Technology Assessment* **4**: 1–121.

Currie C (2009). Orthogeriatric Care. In Rai GS and Muller GP (eds) *Elderly Medicine: A Training Guide*, 2nd edn,. London, Churchill Livingstone, pp. 124–34.

Gupta A (2005). Orthogeriatric service: models of care. *Geriatric Medicine* **35**: 43–9.

Handoll HH, Cameron ID, Mak JC, et al. (2009). Multidisciplinary rehabilitation for older people with hip fractures. *Cochrane Database Syst Rev* **4**: 1–80.

Marcantonio ER, Flacker JM, Wright RJ, et al. (2001). Reducing delirium after hip fracture: A randomised controlled trial. *JAGS* **49**: 516–22.

National Institute for Clinical Excellence (2010). Venous thromboembolism: reducing the risk. NICE clinical guideline, 92. London, NICE.

Royal College of Physicians (1989). *Fracture Neck of Femur. Prevention and Management*. London, RCP.

Seymour DG (2008). Pre-operative assessment of the older surgical patient. *CME Journal Geriatric Medicine* **10**: 85–93.

Scottish Intercollegiate Guideline Network (SIGN) (2009). Management of hip fracture in older people: a national clinical guidance. *SIGN* **111**: 1–56.

Osteoporosis

Introduction

Osteoporosis is the commonest bone disease in adults and is characterized by a reduction in bone density, a disruption of bone architecture and a subsequent increased risk of fracture after low impact trauma. The lifetime risk of a fragility fracture is one in two for women over 50. Osteoporosis results in significant morbidity and mortality; for example, following a hip fracture, 20% of people will die within the first year and 30% will have significant disability. Falls and fractures account for more hospital bed days than stroke and cardiovascular disease, yet less medical attention is given to osteoporosis. Studies show that only 30% of those with fractures have any osteoporosis assessment done. This is despite a previous fracture resulting in a two- to fivefold increased risk of subsequent fracture (see Table 20.1).

Clinical features

Osteoporosis can be asymptomatic but usually presents with fractures. Certain fracture types are commonly associated with osteoporosis and these are referred to as fragility fractures. The definition of these can vary. The National Falls and Bone Health Audit in Older People (FBHOP) includes fractures of the hip, vertebrae, radius/ulna, humerus, and pelvis. The NICE definition is more useful in practical terms and states 'fragility fractures are those associated with low trauma; that is, a fracture sustained as the result of a force equivalent to the force of a fall from a height equal to or less than of an ordinary chair'.

In practice, the commonest types of fractures associated with osteoporosis are those of the proximal femur, distal radius/ulna, and vertebrae. Proximal femur and wrist fractures rarely go unnoticed, presenting with pain and deformity following a fall. However vertebral fractures are often silent, with only 25% resulting in pain. They are therefore found as incidental findings or as a progressive kyphosis known as a dowager's hump. Even silent fractures are associated with significant morbidity and mortality, as the resultant posture predisposes to loss of balance, falls, respiratory compromise and pneumonia.

Diagnosis

The diagnosis should be considered in patients presenting with a fragility fracture, progressive kyphosis, or acute-onset back pain with no or minimal trauma. Plain radiographs used to diagnosis the incident fracture can give an indication of bone density. The diagnosis of vertebral fractures on spine radiographs can be difficult requiring expert opinion.

The gold standard investigation for osteoporosis is the dual X-ray absorptiometry (DEXA) scan. This measures BMD usually at the hip and the spine and compares it to that of a young healthy woman. The standard deviation (SD) from the young adult mean is the T score. The World Health Organization (WHO) has diagnostic categories for osteoporosis based on T scores:

- normal bone density: T score above −1 SD
- osteopenia: T score −1 to −2.5 SD
- osteoporosis: T score −2.5 or less SD
- severe osteoporosis: T score −2.5 or less and fragility fracture.

Less commonly, Z scores are used which compare BMD to age/gender/weight-matched controls. Management of osteoporosis in the older population is often independent of BMD, so these scans are most useful in the younger old.

Biochemical investigations are used mainly to exclude secondary causes which are commoner in men. Basic bone biochemistry should be normal apart from alkaline phosphatase, which rises immediately post fracture. Investigations to exclude secondary causes:

- full blood count and erythrocyte sedimentation rate—multiple myeloma, malabsorption
- serum electrophoresis and urine for Bence–Jones protein if suspicious of multiple myeloma
- bone profile—primary hyperparathyroidism, osteomalacia
- renal function—chronic renal impairment and renal osteodystrophy
- liver function—chronic liver disease
- parathyroid hormone/vitamin D—osteomalacia, secondary hyperparathyroidism
- testosterone in men—hypogonadism
- additional tests, e.g. coeliac autoantibodies, 24-hour urinary calcium measurements, overnight dexamethasone suppression test.

Treatment

Various guidelines have been established to aid management, but these are not without controversy. The revised NICE technology appraisal guidelines (TAG 161) for secondary prevention were first published in 2008 but were contested by the National Osteoporosis Society (NOS). In a statement published in January 2011, Nice confirmed the original guidance following a review of further evidence. The main controversies were the lack of guidance on osteoporosis in men and for those on corticosteroids and the reliance on DEXA scanning. There was also concern that if patients failed to tolerate first-line treatment, there was difficulty in them 'qualifying' for alternative treatments within the guidelines. NICE does, however, recommend treatment for women over the age of 75 with fragility fractures without the need for a DEXA scan.

Table 20.1 Risk factors for osteoporosis and fractures

Age	Perhaps the best predictor of fracture risk
Gender	Commoner in females, bone loss is accelerated after the menopause
Parental history of fracture	Both paternal and maternal, this appears to be independent of BMD
Previous fracture	A powerful indicator, following initial fracture there is a two- to fivefold increase risk of a subsequent fracture
Low body mass index (BMI)	Especially with BMI <20 kg/m². In premenopausal women amenorrhoea resulting from a low BMI exacerbates bone loss
Low bone mineral density (BMD)	Fracture risk increases by 1.5–3 for each Standard deviation (SD) decrease in BMD.
Smoking Alcohol	This is dose dependent. Alcohol >3 units a day
Drugs	Steroids, anticonvulsants, heparin, cyclosporin, aromatase inhibitors, hormone treatment for prostate cancer

The National Osteoporosis Guidelines Group (NOGG) produced guidance incorporating the WHO approved FRAX tool, which is independent of DEXA results. This assessment can be easily carried out using the online tool found at www.shef.ac.uk/FRAX. It calculates the 10 year probability of a fracture and stratifies patients into three groups: treatment, further investigation with DEXA scan, or lifestyle advice. Critics of NOGG claim that the non-BMD-related risk factors used in the assessment may not respond to treatment and that older people require a higher fracture risk before treatment. A practical approach is to use NICE guidance for those over 75 and NOGG for those under 75.

Once a decision to treat has been made the next step is to decide on which of the many therapies is most appropriate.

HRT

Since the Women's Health Initiative (WHI) data were published, the use of HRT in post-menopausal osteoporosis has decreased. HRT reduces the risk of fractures by 30%. However, the increased risks of breast cancer, stroke, and cardiovascular disease outweigh the benefits. HRT is no longer recommended for treatment of osteoporosis in postmenopausal women.

Raloxifene

Raloxifene is a selective oestrogen receptor modulator (SERM) with a mixture of anti-oestrogen (in breast) and oestrogen-like (in bone) effects. There is no evidence that it reduces hip fracture in postmenopausal women but it does decrease the risk of vertebral fractures by 40%. It is occasionally useful in younger post menopausal women who have a significant risk of both vertebral fractures and breast cancer.

Calcium and vitamin D supplementation

There is evidence to suggest that many older people are deficient in vitamin D. This may be due to lack of sunlight exposure and chronic renal impairment. The Chapuy study provides evidence for calcium and vitamin D supplementation as monotherapy in frail institutionalized older people. This showed that 1.2 g of calcium and 800 IU of vitamin D resulted in a 43% reduction in hip fractures. There is also a suggestion that vitamin D may have effects on fracture reduction outside effects on BMD, by reducing body sway and thereby reducing the risk of falls. A recent study has suggested the converse is true: high doses of vitamin D may upset balance.

Calcium and vitamin D should also be coadministered with the antiresorptive agents described below. The trials of these agents were conducted against a control group taking supplements and there is a suggestion that the increase in BMD seen with bisphosphonates is blunted in vitamin D deficiency.

Bisphosphonates

Bisphosphonates inhibit osteoclast activity and are therefore antiresorptive agents. The first bisphosphonate was cyclical etidronate and it was a weak antifracture agent. There is no evidence it prevents hip fractures and it has been superseded.

Generic alendronate is the cheapest and is therefore recommended first line. It reduces hip and vertebral fractures by approximately 50%. The main disadvantage of the bisphosphonates is their gastrointestinal intolerability. They should be avoided in patients with oesophageal ulceration, erosion, stricture or significant dyspepsia. In order to reduce the incidence of gastrointestinal side-effects, bisphosphonates should be taken on an empty stomach, 30 minutes before food with the patient remaining upright for 30 minutes after treatment. It is these side-effects and complex dosing regimen that result in poor compliance with treatment.

There is a suggestion that risedronate has fewer gastro-intestinal side-effects and NICE guidance recommends this as an alternative for those who are unable to tolerate alendronate.

Patients with osteoporosis, like those with other chronic diseases, are poorly concordant with therapy, with only 50% taking their bisphosphonate after 12 months. The introduction of weekly and monthly therapies has improved concordance. Intravenous bisphosphonates can also be used to improve this and are given 3 monthly (Ibandronate) or 12 monthly (zolendronate).

The timing of commencement of therapy can cause concern. However, there is no evidence that starting the drug during the acute phase will delay fracture healing. In practice, if therapy is not started immediately the opportunity may be lost.

Bisphosphonate therapy is required for many years, although the exact duration of treatment is not clear, 5–10 years is recommended.

There have been reported cases of osteonecrosis of the jaw with oral bisphosphonate therapy. However, it is rare and patients taking high doses of intravenous bisphosphonates for malignancy are most at risk.

More recently bisphosphonate related atypical subtrochanteric features have been reported in some patients with prolonged exposure to treatment. These present with a prodrome of uni- or bilateral thigh pain following by a 'snap' indicating fracture. Although rare, advice is that patients on bisphosphonates presenting with such symptoms should be imaged with plain X-rays followed by MRI to look for characteristic radiographic features.

Strontium

Strontium has two main actions; as an antiresorptive drug and promoters of bone growth. It has particularly good data in the oldest old and has been shown to reduce non-vertebral fractures by 41% and vertebral fractures by 59%. The advantage of strontium is that it has no increased risk of upper gastrointestinal side-effects. It is also considerably easier to take than bisphosphonates. It should be taken 2 hours after and before food, which is typically easiest to achieve by taking it at bedtime. Its main side-effect is diarrhoea, which tends to be self-limiting. Other side-effects include the development of a rash and a slight increase in venous thromboembolic risk.

Denosumab

Denosumab is a monoclonal antibody to the receptor activator of RANKL that blocks it binding to RANK inhibiting the development and activity of osteoclasts, decreasing bone resorption and increasing bone density. It is administered as a subcutaneous injection every 6 months and can therefore be given in primary care. Patients must be calcium and Vitamin D replete prior to administration. Relative risk reduction of fractures reported in trials are 68% in vertebral fractures and 40% in hip fractures.

Adverse effects are urinary and respiratory infections, rashes, eczema and skin infections. The main advantages of denosumab are its contribution to improved compliance and its apparent safety in renal impairment patients.

Teraparatide

Teraparatide is an anabolic drug derived from human parathyroid hormone. It is NICE approved for those with very high fracture risk. For secondary prevention, it requires intolerance to other therapies, treatment failure and a very low T score. Practically speaking, many primary care trusts have strict constraints on whom they will fund it for, making its usage very limited.

Practical dilemmas

Renal impairment

Many older people have chronic renal impairment and this can prove problematic in selecting treatment for osteoporosis. The bisphosphonates are only licensed for those with an estimated glomerular filtration rate >30 mL/min/1.73 m^2 (risedronate eGFR ≥20 mL/min/1.73 m^2), likewise with strontium. Some clinicians recommend a dose reduction with fortnightly administration, though this is off-licence. There is suggestion that bisphosphonates are safe down to an eGFR of 15 mL/min/1.73 m^2 with fracture reduction still occurring and no detrimental effect on renal function. However, further studies are required.

1-Alpha-calcidol is not licensed in the UK for osteoporosis, only osteomalacia. There is also a high risk of hypercalcaemia, so additional calcium is not given. Denosumab is showing promise in the treatment of osteoporosis in renal failure patients.

Treatment failure

Another area of controversy is what to do in those who fracture while on bisphosphonate therapy. The first thing to do is to look for poor compliance, as this is the commonest cause. Poor compliance may be due to gastrointestinal intolerance and the complex dosing regimen. In these patients, Strontium, intravenous bisphosphonates or denosumab can be used instead. In older patients, poor compliance can be due to cognitive impairment and dosette boxes and NOMAD systems may be helpful. Intravenous bisphosphonates also have a place in poor compliance due to dementia.

If fractures have occurred while taking bisphosphonates, further options are limited. Teraparatide may be considered, but local restrictions often make this unfeasible. In practice, a change to strontium or denosumab is useful although the evidence base for this is limited.

Further reading

Campbell G (2009). Current thoughts on osteoporosis. *CME Geriatric Medicine* **11**: 54–72.

Chapuy MC, Arlot ME, Duboeuf F, et al. (1992). Vitamin D3 and calcium to prevent hip fractures in the older women. *New Engl J Med* **327**: 1637–42.

Chapuy MC, Arlot ME, Delmans PD, et al. (1994). Effect of calcium and cholecalciferol treatment for three years on hip fractures in older women. *Br Med J* **308**: 1081–2.

Cummings SR, San Martin J, McClung MR, et al. (2009). Denosumab for prevention of fractures in postmenopausal women with osteoporosis. *NEJM* **361**: 750–65.

Johnell O, Kanis JA (2006). An estimate of the worldwide prevalence and disability associated with osteoporotic fractures. *Osteoporos Int* **17**: 1726–33.

Kanis JA, Johnell O, Oden A, et al. (2008). FRAX and the assessment of fracture probability in men and women from the UK. *Osteoporos Int* **19**: 385–97.

Keene GS, Parker MJ, Pryor GA (1993). Mortality and morbidity after hip fracture. *Br Med J* **307**: 1248–50.

Meunier PJ, Roux C, Seeman E, et al. (2004). The effects of strontium ranelate on the risk of vertebral fracture in women with postmenopausal osteoporosis. *New Engl J Med* **350**: 459–68.

Miller P (2005). Treatment of osteoporosis in chronic kidney disease and end stage renal disease. *Curr Osteoporos Rep* **3**: 5–12.

National Institute for Health and Clinical Excellence (2011). Alendronate, etidronate, risedronate, raloxifene, strontium ranelate and teriparatide for the secondary prevention of osteoporotic fragility fractures in postmenopausal women. NICE Technology Appraisal Guideline 161.

National Osteoporosis Guideline Group (2008). Guideline for the diagnosis and management of osteoporosis in postmenopausal women and men from age of 50 years in the UK.

Reginster JY, Seeman E, De Vernejoul MC, et al. (2005). Strontium ranelate reduces the risk of nonvertebral fractures in postmenopausal women with osteoporosis: treatment of peripheral osteoporosis (TROPOS) study. *J Clin Endocrinol Metab* **90**: 2816–22.

Thompson P, Cooper C, Carr A (2005). Factors influencing adherence to bisphosphonates for osteoporosis. *J Bone Miner Res* **20**: S394.

Fractured neck of femur

Introduction

Hip fracture is the most common serious injury of older people. In the UK approximately 70 000 hip fractures occur per year, with current projections predicting that the number of hip fractures could double by 2050. The increase in hip fractures reflects the ageing population, but in addition there is also an increase in age specific incidence. The average age of people sustaining a hip fracture is 80 years and 80% of fractures occur in those over 75 years of age. Approximately 80% of hip fractures occur in women. People living in residential and nursing homes are at nine times greater risk than the general population of sustaining a hip fracture.

Hip fractures cost the NHS about £1.4 billion per year; if social care is also considered then the financial burden of hip fractures doubles. As well as the economic burden, hip fractures cause significant problems to the individual sustaining the fracture and their family/carers. Following hip fracture there is up to 37% mortality at 1 year, with about 30% of these deaths directly attributed to the fracture. Of those who survive, there will be significant decline in the individual's ability to perform daily activity, with only half returning to their previous level of independence. Up to 20% will require a change to a more dependent residential status.

Aetiology

Hip fracture aetiology is multifactorial and reflects general frailty and falls risk as much as bone fragility. Most hip fractures in older people will be sustained after minimal trauma, for example, falling from standing height or less to the ground.

Classification of hip fractures

A hip fracture refers to any fracture of the femur from the hip joint articular cartilage to a point 5 cm below the distal part of the lesser trochanter. Hip fractures can be classified anatomically according to their relationship to the capsular attachments of the hip joint, into intracapsular and extracapsular fractures (see Figure 20.1). This subdivision of fractures is important when considering management options and potential fracture complications. Intracapsular fractures occur proximal to the point at which the hip joint capsule attaches to the femur, and can be further divided into displaced and undisplaced fractures. Displaced intracapsular fractures may be associated with avascular necrosis

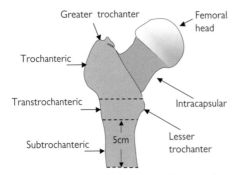

Figure 20.1 Key landmarks for classification of femoral neck fractures.

through disruption of the blood supply to the head of the femur. Extracapsular fractures occur distal to the hip joint capsule and are subdivided into trochanteric and subtrochanteric. Subtrochanteric fractures are those in which the fracture is predominantly in the 5cm of bone immediately distal to the lesser trochanter. Trochanteric fractures are those that are extracapsular, but proximal to the lesser trochanter.

Clinical features

Hip fractures usually present after a fall, resulting in pain in the hip and an inability to walk. Some people can still mobilize after fracturing the hip, so an index of suspicion should be maintained if a person has fallen and complaining of significant hip pain, even if they are still managing to mobilize. Following the fracture the affected limb is often shortened and externally rotated; however, this can also be observed in people who have undergone hip replacements. In addition, 15% of individuals have undisplaced fractures and this will not cause shortening and rotation of the limb. Most people who have fractured their hip will be unable to straight leg raise and rotation of the hip will cause pain. Whilst assessing for hip fracture, a full falls history should be elicited as well as an osteoporosis history.

Pathological fractures

Pathological fractures need to be considered in cases where there is minimal trauma, in younger people, especially men, and if the individual already has a known cancer. Sometimes the fracture can precede the fall and this should make one particularly suspicious that a pathological process occurred. If suspicion of pathological fracture has arisen then the individual should be investigated accordingly, in particular bone reamings taken during surgery should be sent for histology.

Investigation

Plain radiographs of the hip are the first-line investigation, two views should be obtained, anteroposterior (AP) and lateral. Fractures can be difficult to identify, especially impacted/undisplaced fractures, so it is always worth getting the orthopaedic team or radiologist to review them. In 1% of individuals with a hip fracture the initial radiograph will appear completely normal. If a fracture is not apparent on plain films, but clinical suspicion of a fracture remains high, then the next line investigation would be computed tomography or magnetic resonance imaging of the hip (subject to local policy).

If a fracture has been identified then as a minimum all patients should have the following tests:

- full blood count: it is not uncommon to lose several units of blood following fracture
- group and save
- INR – will need correcting if raised and the patient is going to theatre
- urea and electrolytes/liver function tests/glucose
- other 'osteoporosis' bloods, as outlined in the section Osteoporosis
- chest radiograph
- ECG
- urine dip/mid-stream urine.

These tests are in part to investigate the individual from a falls and osteoporosis viewpoint, but also to allow any problems that might impair surgery to be quickly identified and thus remedied.

Management

There are a number of guidelines published on hip fracture management. Comprehensive guidelines have been published in Scotland (SIGN 2002) and also the Blue Book, a joint collaboration between the British Geriatrics Society and the British Orthopaedic Association. The National Institute for Health and Clinical Excellence (NICE) published guidelines on the management of hip fracture in June 2011. All of these guidelines stress the importance of multi-disciplinary working, including orthopaedic surgeons, physicians, anaesthetists, and allied health professionals. Broad principles for the management of hip fractures include high-quality fracture care, high-quality secondary prevention through falls assessment and bone protection and rigorous information collecting through audit and feedback to ensure standards are met and care continuously improved. For the remains of this section we will concentrate on fracture care, as falls assessment and bone protection are covered elsewhere in this textbook.

Preoperative care

Preoperative care involves prompt diagnosis and investigation of the individual as outlined above. Other areas that need to be addressed include good pressure area care – all hip fracture patients are at risk of developing pressure sores, so should be nursed on a pressure relieving surface. All patients should receive analgesia and fluid resuscitation and should be moved to a specialist trauma ward as quickly as possible. The Blue Book has outlined that all patients should be on a dedicated trauma ward within four hours of admission as one of the standards of care. All patients should also receive comprehensive assessment by an anaesthetist and orthogeriatrician to allow optimization of the individual and facilitate prompt surgery. There is evidence from cohort studies that early surgery (within 48 hours of admission) is associated with reduced lengths of stay and also with reduced pain and reduced dependency. Consequently both SIGN and the Blue Book advocate early surgery.

Fracture management

The management of the fracture can be divided into operative and non-operative (conservative). Historically, fractures were managed conservatively; however, this approach is rarely used now, as conservative management tends to result in ongoing pain, inability to weight bear, and continuing dependency. Non-operative management is also associated with a high rate of non-union of the fracture and higher mortality rate.

Occasionally, hip fractures are still managed conservatively, in the following circumstances:

1 The individual has a short life expectancy and the risks of surgery outweigh the benefits (although operative management would still provide good pain relief and facilitate easier nursing care).

2 Late presentation of the fracture with evidence of healing.

3 Totally immobile patient (though again, operative management provides good pain control and enables easier nursing).

Intracapsular undisplaced fractures

Internal fixation is recommended, the most common methods utilized are parallel screws or a sliding hip screw. Individuals tend to recover from this procedure rapidly,

facilitating early mobilization. Arthroplasty is not appropriate because of the increased surgical risk and postoperative complications. The most common surgical complication after this surgery is failure of the fracture to heal, which will manifest as displacement of the fracture and non-union. Avascular necrosis is a potential complication that occurs 1–2 years after the fracture; this has to be managed by replacement arthroplasty. Occasionally the screws used to fix the fracture can cause local irritation; replacing the screw with shorter ones or removing the screw if the fracture has healed can remedy this.

Intracapsular displaced fractures

There are two surgical options for these fractures: internal fixation or arthroplasty. Internal fixation is a smaller operation, thus conferring lower operative morbidity and mortality, including less chance of infection and wound haematoma. These advantages are offset by the increased risk of non-union and avascular necrosis and thus much higher reoperative rates (20–36%). If arthroplasty is employed then there are lower re-operative rates (6–18%). However, there are increased risks of haematoma, infection, peri-prosthetic fracture, implant loosening, and acetabular wear. The decision over which way to manage these fractures is influenced primarily by the risk of non-union, which in turn is determined by the presence of delayed time to theatre, presence of pathological lesions of the bone and rheumatoid arthritis. In the younger patient (generally considered less than 70 years old) then internal fixation is the preferred method of management, as the life expectancy in these individuals is expected to be longer than the life of the implant used in an arthroplasty.

Trochanteric fractures

These fractures are managed by utilizing implants. The commonest implant to be used is the sliding hip screw. Short intramedullary nails are also utilized, although these have higher complication rates, including increased reoperative rate and increased risk of fracture-healing complications. With respect to the sliding hip screw, the most common complication is for the implant to cut out (1–5% cases), resulting in it protruding into local tissues or cutting into the acetabulum. This will result in pain and impaired mobility. Management options for this include revision of the sliding hip screw, hemi-arthroplasty or removal of the sliding hip screw.

Subtrochanteric fractures

These fractures are difficult to treat as the high mechanical forces in this area of bone increases the risk of fixation failure. For the more distal fractures, an intramedullary nail is often the surgical management of choice. For the more proximal fractures, sliding hip screws tend to be the management of choice, though these are technically difficult to perform, requiring considerable surgical skill.

Postoperative care

Postoperative care requires ongoing excellent collaboration between the surgeons, anaesthetists, physicians with an interest in orthopaedics, and other allied health professionals. The aim of postoperative care is to rehabilitate the individual, but also to prevent and manage potential complications.

Wound complications

Complications related to the wound include wound haematoma and infection. Wound haematoma will occur in up to 10% of individuals after hip surgery. Smaller haematomas can be managed conservatively, while larger haematomas will need to be drained surgically. Wound infection can be divided into superficial infections, which are limited to the subcutaneous tissue, and deep infections, which are those penetrating the deep fascia and often involving the implant used. SIGN recommend that all patients undergoing hip surgery should receive antibiotic prophylaxis to reduce the risk of both deep and superficial infection. Superficial infections can be adequately managed with antibiotics, but need to be monitored carefully to ensure they are not progressing to deep infection. Deep infection occurs in up to 5% of hip fractures and is commoner in arthroplasty, and it can lead to chronic infection of the hip joint. It carries a mortality rate of up to 50%.

Treatment is surgical, with debridement of the infected tissue and sometimes removal of the implant. After removal of the implant, new implants are often not employed until it is clear that all infection has been adequately treated. This can result in a patient being left with a Girdlestone hip (a hip without the femoral head). Weight bearing on Girdlestone is possible; though many older people will find this particularly difficult and may never regain mobility.

Analgesia

Nearly all patients will experience pain after surgery. Poor management of pain will result in impairment in rehabilitation and the resultant increased risk of complications associated with immobility, for example pressure sores and infection. Most hospitals have an acute pain team and their help can be utilized if necessary. All patients should be prescribed paracetamol and a weak opioid such as codeine. Stronger opioids should be made available if required. Non-steroidal anti-inflammatory drugs should be avoided in older people as they come with a heavy burden of side effects and complications in the older age group.

Pressure care

Up to one-third of hip fracture patients will develop a pressure ulcer. As soon as an individual has fallen and sustained a fracture, they are at increased risk of pressure ulcers. All patients should be assessed for their risk of pressure ulcer development and then managed appropriately with pressure relieving mattresses, regular repositioning and early mobilization. Other mainstays of pressure ulcer prevention are good nutrition, adequate analgesia (to allow mobility), and maintaining a dry environment (use of barrier creams/pads in incontinent individuals). If an individual develops a pressure ulcer, then involvement of the tissue viability team can improve care and outcome.

Thromboprophylaxis

All patients who are immobile and who have undergone surgery are at risk of developing both deep vein thrombosis (DVT) and pulmonary embolus (PE). The clinical incidence of symptomatic DVT after hip surgery is 3%, and for PE is 1%. PE is responsible for 0.5% of deaths after hip surgery.

A number of methods have been investigated with regard to preventing DVT and PE. These include wearing pressure stockings, cyclic leg compression devices and foot pumps, and chemical prophylaxis. Pressure stockings can be painful to put on in patients who have had hip surgery and also can cause skin damage; at present there is no good evidence that these prevent DVT in post-operative hip fracture patients. Cyclic leg compression is difficult to use and expensive. However, there is evidence that it does reduce DVT incidence. Chemical prophylaxis with aspirin or heparin has been shown to be effective in reducing the number of DVTs and PEs. However they are both associated with side effects, including increased bleeding rates and increased wound complications, e.g. haematoma.

After reviewing the potential benefits and side-effects, NICE and SIGN advise using chemical prophylaxis in the form of heparin (unfractionated or low molecular weight) or fondaparinux for four weeks after surgery, as long as there are no major contraindications. They both also recommend mechanical prophylaxis while the patient has significantly reduced mobility. There are two new drugs which have currently been approved by NICE for thromboprophylaxis in elective hip and knee surgery, dabigatran (direct inhibitor of the enzyme thrombin) and rivaroxaban (inhibits activated factor X). In the future these might also be recommended in emergency hip surgery. The complexity of thromboprophylaxis management should not distract from the need for early surgery, prompt mobilization and not over-transfusing individuals to help prevent thrombotic complications.

Nutrition/fluid and electrolytes

The frailty of hip fracture patients means that many of them will present with poor nutritional reserves and with electrolyte imbalance. In the perioperative period, electrolytes need to be monitored carefully and replacement instituted as necessary. Particular care has to be taken when reviewing drug charts, for example, diuretics that were used by the patient when at home might no longer be appropriate and could contribute to electrolyte disturbance. Caution also has to be exercised when prescribing intravenous fluids as these can often contribute to electrolyte disturbance. An additional risk in the postoperative period is the syndrome of inappropriate antidiuretic hormone release (SIADH).

With regard to nutrition, only 50% of hip fracture patients achieve their daily energy, protein and nutritional requirements. The evidence base for providing nutritional supplements is lacking and generally the tolerability of these by the individual is poor. A pragmatic approach to managing the nutritional needs of hip fracture patients is making all staff aware of the importance of good nutrition, for patients' intake to be monitored and for supplements to be given if they are tolerated. Those struggling to eat due to physical difficulty should be provided with help as required and those who would benefit from dietician review should be referred promptly.

Infection

All postoperative patients are at risk of infection and the underlying frailty of hip fracture patients places them at increased risk. The patients need to be monitored carefully for evidence of infection and treatment started promptly if an infection is identified. Common sites to find infection are the urinary tract, the surgical wound and the chest.

Avascular necrosis

Avascular necrosis is a complication observed after intracapsular fracture. It normally occurs 1–2 years after the fracture and is due to disruption of the blood supply to the femoral head. In avascular necrosis, the weight-bearing part of the femoral head collapses. The management of the condition is either replacement arthroplasty, or in younger patients, sometimes the femoral head can be salvaged by osteotomy or revascularization.

Dislocation

A potential risk after hemiarthroplasty is dislocation of the hip. However, with modern surgical techniques, in particular an anterolateral approach during surgery, this risk is minimized. Traditionally after hemiarthroplasty individuals were required to restrict hip flexion in-order to reduce the risk of dislocation, however this is no longer necessary. There is a risk of dislocation in total hip replacement and these individuals still require limitation of hip flexion.

Rehabilitation

Rehabilitation should start the day after surgery. With current surgical techniques and operative options there are very few situations in which weight bearing is not possible. Consequently the patient should be transferred out of bed and start to stand the day after surgery. Rehabilitation should be multidisciplinary, as outlined in the section Principles of orthogeriatrics.

National Hip Fracture Database (NHFD)

The National Hip Fracture Database (NHFD) is a web-based audit tool for hip fracture care that was set up in 2007 by the British Geriatrics Society and British Orthopaedic Association. It allows hospitals in England, Wales, Northern Ireland, and the Channel Islands to input data about hip fracture management and bench mark their management against national management in order to optimize the care they provide. The database collects information on key areas in hip fracture care as outlined in the standards in the Blue Book. In 2010, the NHFD report showed that 97% of hospitals are now signed up to the database and 87% of hospitals regularly input data.

Author's Tips

Hip fracture is the commonest serious injury of older people.

Mortality is up to 10% in the month after the fracture and 30% in the year after.

Most patients should be treated surgically.

Hip fracture care involves multi-disciplinary working.

Further reading

Bergeron E, Lavoie A, Moore L, et al. (2006). Is the delay to surgery for isolated hip fracture predictive of outcome in efficient systems? *J Trauma* **60**: 753–7.

BOA (2007). *The Blue Book*. British Orthopaedic Association (http://www.nhfd.co.uk/).

Brennan nee Saunders J, Johansen A, Butler J, et al. (2003). Place of residence and risk of fracture in older people: a population based study of over 65 year olds in Cardiff. *Osteoporos Int* **14**: 515–19.

Burge RT, Worley D, Johansen A, et al. (2001). The Cost of Osteoporotic Fractures in the UK: Projections for 2000–2020. *J Med Econ* **4**: 51–62.

Cummings SR, Melton LJI (2002). Epidemiology and outcomes of osteoporotic fractures. *Lancet* **359**: 1761–7.

Department of Health. Hospital Episode Statistics (England) 2006. Available from: http://www.hesonline.org.uk/Ease/servlet/ContentServer?siteID=1937&categoryID=192

Duncan D, Murison J, Martin R, et al. (2001). Adequacy of oral feeding among older patients with hip fracture. *Age Ageing* **30**: S2–22.

Grimes JP, Gregory PM, Noveck H, et al. (2002). The effects of time-to-surgery on mortality and morbidity in patients following hip fracture. *Am J Med* **112**: 702–9.

Handoll HH, Farrar MJ, McBirnie J, et al. (2002). Heparin, low molecular weight heparin and physical methods for preventing deep vein thrombosis and pulmonary embolism following surgery for hip fractures. *Cochrane Database Syst Rev* **4**: CD000305.

Lyons AR (1997). Clinical outcomes and treatment of hip fractures. *Am J Med* **103**: 51S–64S.

Moran CG, Wenn RT, Sikand M, et al. (2005). Early mortality after hip fracture: is delay before surgery important? *J Bone Joint Surg Am* **87**: 483–9.

National Hip Fracture Database Annual Report (2010). Available at: www.ccad.org.uk/nhfd.nsf/NHFD_National_Report_2010.pdf

Orosz GM, Magaziner J, Hannan EL, et al. (2004). Association of timing of surgery for hip fracture and patient outcomes. *JAMA* **291**: 1738–43.

Parker MJ (2002). Trochanteric and subtrochanteric fractures. In (Bulstrode C, Buckwalter J, Carr A, et al, eds) *Oxford Textbook of Orthopaedics and Trauma*. Oxford: Oxford University Press, pp. 2228–39.

Parker MJ, Anand JK (1991). What is the true mortality of hip fractures? *Public Health* **105**: 443–6.

Parker M, Johansen A (2006). Hip fracture. *BMJ* **333**: 27–30.

Rosell PAE, Parker MJ (2003). Functional outcome after hip fracture: a 1-year prospective outcome study of 275 patients. *Injury* **34**: 529–32.

Scottish Intercollegiate Guidelines Network. Prevention and Management of Hip Fractures in Older People. A National Guideline. SIGN 56. January 2002. Available from http://www.sign.ac.uk/guidelines/fulltext/56/

Siegmeth AW, Gurusamy K, Parker MJ (2005). Delay to surgery prolongs hospital stay in patients with fractures of the proximal femur. *J Bone Joint Surg Br* **87**: 1123–6.

The PEP Trial Collaborative Group (2000). Prevention of pulmonary embolus and deep vein thrombosis with low dose aspirin: Pulmonary Embolism Prevention Trial. *Lancet* **355**: 1295–302.

Thorngren K-G (2002). Femoral neck fractures. In: Bulstrode C, Buckwalter J, Carr A, et al, Eds. *Oxford Textbook of Orthopaedics and Trauma*. Oxford: Oxford University Press, 2216–27.

Venous Thromboembolism – reducing the risk. NICE Guidance 2010

Versluysen M (1985). Pressure sores in elderly patients. The epidemiology related to hip operations. *J Bone Joint Surg Br*, **67**:1:10–13

Other common fractures

Epidemiology

Records taken from the General Practice Research Database in England and Wales for the incidence of fractures during the period of 1988 and 1998 found that, after the age of 60 years, the incidence of all fragility fractures steadily rises. Different fracture sites showed a different distribution with age. Fractures of the radius and ulna tend to start to increase from an earlier age with women in their sixth decade, although no increase in forearm fracture incidence was seen in men of any age. Fractures of the vertebrae and pelvis began to increase in patients of both genders in their seventh decade and fractures of the proximal femur were seen to increase more when patients reach their eighth decade.

It is well known that the standardized mortality rate is elevated in patients who have had a hip fracture, but it has also been shown to be raised in the first five years following other major fragility fractures, such as vertebrae, pelvis, proximal tibia, and proximal humerus.

This section will discuss the management of wrist, proximal humerus, pelvis, tibial plateau, ankle, and vertebral fractures, which along with hip fractures are grouped as fragility fractures and are related to osteoporosis and low impact trauma. There is a need to be aware that there is a heightened risk of fractures at all sites in those with low bone density and adults who fracture at one site are at a substantially greater risk of sustaining another fracture at a different site.

Wrist fractures

These are usually sustained by falling onto an outstretched hand, which then forces the wrist backwards. The fracture site is usually seen 2cm from the wrist joint where the radius starts to narrow and the relatively soft cancellous bone meets the harder cortical bone of the shaft of the radius. The fracture may extend into the wrist joint itself. The result is shortening of the radius in comparison to the ulna with angulation. The deformity seen in 97% of cases is the 'dinner fork' deformity of the Colles fracture

Management

The main aims of treatment are to reduce the fracture into the correct position and stabilize it while healing takes place. The most common way of doing this is by manipulating the wrist while the patient has a local anaesthetic block and the arm is put in plaster. Initially this may be a backslab until any early swelling has settled and this can then be converted into a full cast. The fracture takes an average of six weeks to heal. If the fracture is particularly unstable there are various options for fixation such as K wires, external fixator, internal plates and screws, and intermedullary devices. The choice will depend on the comminution and angulation of the fracture.

Radial fractures appear to be a good indicator for risk of future hip fracture and therefore it is important to target these patients for treatment for osteoporosis. Patients who have sustained a radial fracture have twice the relative risk of a future hip fracture. They can be thought of as an early marker for fragility.

Common problems

- Malunion of the fracture. The radius may heal in the wrong position causing deformity and pain where the ulna catches on the carpal bones. This may require rebreaking of the radius.

- Nerve injury. The median nerve may be compressed by swelling in the carpal tunnel.
- Ligamentous damage. Strain of the ligaments surrounding the wrist can lead to pain and weakness in the joint even after the fracture has healed.

Proximal humeral fractures

The most common fracture site is due to falling on an outstretched hand, which leads to a fracture of the proximal surgical neck of the humerous. The tuberosities may also be fractured and the head split. The vast majority are closed fractures. Owing to impaction of the bone, they can be extremely painful.

Management

Conservative management is felt appropriate if the fracture is an undisplaced two-part fracture, which is most common. An arm sling was found to be more comfortable than a body bandage in one study but this does not appear to influence union or functional end result. An issue in many older people is one of compliance with having an arm in a sling particularly if they have poor cognition. Having an arm in a sling also interferes with using a standard zimmer frame. An alternative frame may be required. The fracture usually unites within 6 weeks.

Operative management with either a hemiarthroplasty or tension band wiring may be considered for fixation of more severe injuries that are comminuted and displaced. However studies looking at functional outcome of operative versus conservative management did not show a significant improvement. Osteopaenia in older patients provides poor fixation for plates and screws and open reduction may further disrupt the blood supply to the humeral head leading to avascular necrosis.

Common problems

Joint stiffness is a common problem post-fracture. Exercise as early as possible can help minimize this.

Pelvic fractures

The pelvis is made up of an anatomical ring of bones consisting of the ilium, ischium, pubis and sacrum. Disruption of this ring requires a lot of force. Those pelvic fractures seen in older people due to falls and osteoporosis are most likely to involve the pubic ramus. Studies that have performed magnetic resonance imaging (MRI) scans on patients with fractured pubic rami showed that they nearly always involve sacral injury. The fracture is caused by lateral compression of the pelvis. As the pubic ring is still intact in these fractures they are considered to be stable and there should not be any damage to the intrapelvic structures. The patient will generally complain of pain in the hip/groin region.

Management

Management is to mobilize as pain allows. Most will be able to walk moderately comfortably in 1–2 months.

Tibial fractures

In tibial fractures, one or more of the condyles may be split and displaced. They result from axial and bending forces across the knee. Central depression fractures of the lateral tibial plateau typically occur in older osteopenic patients. The joint is swollen and has the doughy feel of a haemarthrosis. CT scan may be needed to show the full extent of the fracture.

Management

These fractures all involve the articular surface. The aim is to restore the congruity of the surface. The depressed articular fragment is raised with impacted bone graft and can be fixed by a subchondral lag screw. Obsessional surgery to restore a shattered surface can produce a good radiographic appearance but can cause poor function due to a stiff knee.

Undisplaced fractures of the lateral condyle may be treated conservatively with aspiration of the haemarthrosis and a compression bandage. Once the swelling has subsided, a hinged brace can be fitted. However the patient is not allowed to weight-bear for a number of weeks. Mobilizing non- or even partial weight bearing in the older person can be extremely difficult, particularly for those whose poor balance led to the initial fall which caused the fracture. The alternative is bed rest whilst the fracture heals, which is usually 8–9 weeks, but is fraught with complication risks such as pressure sores, and can lead to an irreparable amount of deconditioning, which means that the patient is not able to mobilize even after the fracture has healed. Internal fixation with a lag screw may be more appropriate.

Complications

- Joint stiffness. This is reduced by starting movements early. If the patient is unable to regain full knee bend this can lead to major issues with mobility.
- Deformity. Some residual valgus or varus deformity is quite common but it is still possible to have good function. Constant overloading of one compartment can predispose to osteoarthritis.
- Osteoarthritis. If, at the end of treatment, there is marked depression of the plateau, deformity of the knee or ligamentous instability the patient can develop osteoarthritis.

Ankle fractures

Fractures and fracture-dislocation are common and usually result from the ankle being twisted, causing the talus to tilt or rotate. This leads to a low-energy fracture of one or both malleoli. Patients will describe a history of a twisting injury and that they are then unable to put any weight through the leg. The ankle will appear swollen and deformity may be obvious.

Care has to be taken to consider whether there has been associated injuries of the ligaments and displacement of the talus. The most obvious change seen on radiograph is a fracture of one or both malleoli; however, the less visible part of the injury involving rupture of the collateral and/or distal tibiofibular ligaments needs to be considered. Collateral ligament damage is suggested by displacement or tilting of the talus.

Management

Swelling is usually rapid and severe. If the injury is not treated within a few hours, definitive treatment may have to be deferred for several days while the leg is elevated so that the swelling can subside.

As with all fractures involving a joint, the anatomy must be accurately restored and held until the healing is complete. Residual displacement or incongruity of the joint will lead to osteoarthritis. The level of the fibular fracture gives an idea as to the congruity and stability of the joint. Undisplaced fractures below the level of the tibiofibular joint can be treated with plaster immobilization for 4–6 weeks. Fractures above the tibiofibular joint, displaced fractures and fracture-dislocations require accurate reduction and internal fixation.

Postoperatively the ankle and the foot will be immobilized in a below-knee cast. The patient is allowed to walk about, partial weight-bearing with the aid of crutches. As already discussed this may prove very difficult for an older person even with a lightweight cast. For stable, low-level fractures, the cast can usually be discarded after four weeks. For unstable and operatively treated fractures, the cast is required for 6–8 weeks.

Complications

- Joint stiffness. Swelling and stiffness of the ankle are usually the result of neglect in treatment of the soft tissues. This can be a particular problem if the patient does not walk correctly in the plaster. Physiotherapy is helpful.
- Complex regional pain syndrome. Recurrent swelling and regional osteoporosis are fairly common after ankle fractures.
- Osteoarthritis. Malunion and/or incomplete reduction will eventually lead to secondary osteoarthritis of the ankle.

Vertebral fractures

Vertebral fractures are the most common fragility fracture. They can occur after low intensity activity, such as bending forward, standing from a seated position, coughing, or sneezing. Many patients may be asymptomatic or have very minimal pain. They may report loss of height otherwise it may be diagnosed as an incidental finding on radiological examination. However, there are a significant number in which pain can lead to significantly reduced quality of life and disability.

Vertebral fractures are usually mechanically stable, but can lead to progressive kyphosis. The thoracolumbar spine is particularly susceptible to fracture. This is where the relatively fixed thoracic spine meets the more mobile lumbar spine.

Plain radiographs are used to diagnose the fracture and to look at the degree of kyphosis. Fractures most commonly appear wedge shaped, on lateral radiograph of the spine, because the anterior portion of the vertebral body collapses and the posterior portion remains relatively intact. Care needs to be taken to ensure that a pathological fracture is not missed. If there is any doubt then computed tomography or MRI of the spine should be organized. If there is any neurological compromise an MRI must be performed. Further imaging can be particularly useful when looking at the upper thoracic spine as the scapula and shoulders can obscure the view on a plain radiograph.

Management

Management previously was conservative by limiting activity, physiotherapy, analgesia and possibly a back brace. Most patients will become symptom free using these measures. The challenge is to try and limit the amount of time spent in bed rest. To prevent deconditioning, thromboembolus, pneumonia, and pressure ulcers, pain needs to be controlled so that activity can be resumed. Bisphosphonates have been shown to reduce the number of days that a patient needs bed rest due to severe pain. They have the added benefit of protecting the patient from other fragility fractures. Diazepam can help to reduce muscle spasm, but must be used continuously in the very frail elderly individual. The use of bracing has become controversial because of concerns that it may put increased stress on the posterior elements of the spine. Immobilization of the spine can aggravate bone loss and muscle wasting around the spine.

If there is significant pain or wedging of the vertebrae, kyphoplasty and vertebroplasty may be considered.

These are minimally invasive procedures involving the injection of a bone filler to restore height and strength to the vertebrae. (see Vertebral augmentation section).

If patients are unable to have vertebral augmentation but still have severe pain they should be admitted for daily calcitonin injections for 10–14 days. Calcitonin is a potent antiresorptive agent, which effects osteoclast function. This has been shown to relieve acute pain within 1–2 days and result in increased rate of mobilization over the next two weeks. There is also an intranasal spray preparation if a patient is unable to attend hospital.

Surgery with spinal fusion is usually a last resort due to the difficulty in securing fixation to weakened osteoporotic bone. Surgery would be considered if there is neurological impairment or there is evidence of an unstable fracture, which might lead to compromise of the spinal canal.

Most patients who develop significant back pain from a vertebral fracture have resolution of pain without intervention in 6–8 weeks. For patients who have persistent disabling pain, kyphoplasty and vertebroplasty have shown excellent results, substantially relieving pain and improving functional levels.

Complications

- Kyphosis – once there has been one vertebral fracture, additional stress can be put on other vertebrae causing malalignment, particularly those vertebrae that are adjacent to the original fracture. In turn, this can cause progressive kyphosis and further pain. This can also lead to a reduction in vital capacity of the lungs, which can be a particular problem in those with chronic lung disease.
- Neurological injury – symptoms of bowel or bladder changes and neurological deficits are not characteristic of vertebral fractures and should prompt further investigation with MRI scanning.

Further reading

Center JR, Nguyen TV, Schneider D, et al. (1999). Mortality after all major types of osteoporotic fracture in men and women: An observational study. Lancet 353: 878–82.

Van Staa TP, Dennison EM, Leufkens HG, et al. (2001). Epidemiology of fractures in England and Wales. Bone 29: 517–22.

Vertebral augmentation

Background

Vertebral compression fractures (VCFs) occur in 20% of people over 70 years old and 16% of postmenopausal women. One large population based study identified that VCFs were due to osteoporosis in 83%, trauma in 14% and cancer in 3% of cases. Both asymptomatic and symptomatic vertebral insufficiency fractures have been associated with increased morbidity and mortality.

The 5-year survival for patients with symptomatic vertebral insufficiency fractures is 61% compared with 76% for age-matched peers. Following a vertebral insufficiency fracture there is a three- to five-fold increased risk of developing adjacent vertebral collapse over the ensuing three years. One study showed a one in five risk of subsequent fracture in the following 12 months in post-menopausal women. Altered vertebral biomechanics are thought to increase the risk of further adjacent fractures.

Percutaneous vertebroplasty (PVP) and percutaneous kyphoplasty (PKP) are techniques that aim to maintain or improve residual vertebral height, and restore strength and therefore function following a compression fracture. Percutaneous vertebroplasty involves the percutaneous injection of bone-filler directly into the vertebral body, typically polymethylmethacrylate (PMMA) via an introducer and under fluoroscopic guidance. Galibert and Deramond et al. pioneered PVP in 1984. Percutaneous kyphoplasty, introduced by Reiley in 1998, involves the additional step of the insertion of an inflatable bone tamp (balloon) that compacts the cancellous bone, not performed in PVP, and aimed at elevating the end plates, restoring the vertebral height, and reducing cement leakage pathways prior to the injection of bone-filler.

PVP and PKP both aim to

- Relieve pain in the acute setting
- Avoid the development of chronic pain
- Prevent progressive vertebral collapse with resultant loss of height
- Prevent fractures at adjacent levels due to altered spinal kinematics
- Prevent progressive kyphosis, thus helping maintain balance
- Avoid reduced pulmonary function from kyphosis
- Improve overall mobility
- Avoid the complications of conservative management
- PKP has the additional potential for restoring previous vertebral height

Mechanism for vertebral augmentation

Vertebral augmentation is thought to anatomically restore and stiffen the affected vertebral body thereby reducing pain and potential neural damage. In an ex vivo study of osteoporotic VCFs, the injection of 2mL of polymethylmethacrylate restored vertebral strength (the ability of the vertebral body to bear load). However, between 4 and 8 mL of cement was required to restore stiffness to the vertebra (the ability to resist deformation).

The exact mechanism of action for vertebral augmentation has yet to be scientifically proven, but several mechanisms of action have been hypothesized, including: halting micro-motion; prevention of further collapse and deformity; thermal damage of the pain fibres and tumour tissue by the exothermic reaction of the cement; toxic effects of PMMA cement; and the placebo effect.

Indications

PVP is a minimally invasive technique currently indicated in the treatment of:

- osteoporotic vertebral compression fractures
- spinal metastases.
- vertebral haemangiomas.
- avascular necrosis.

Patient selection

Typically patients are referred after six weeks of failed conservative management and anywhere up to a year after fracture. Clinically, patients should have localisable intense focal pain corresponding to the level of fracture. It should be a midline, non-radiating axial pain which is worse on weight bearing. There is no absolute degree of vertebral compression that precludes treatment.

The amount of pain may vary widely between patients. If a precise source of pain is difficult to localize, then magnetic resonance imaging (MRI) or isotope bone scan may help identify the affected level. MRI investigations are also helpful in identifying the affected vertebra when multiple fractures are seen on the radiographs.

Contraindications

Absolute

- Locally active infection
- Coagulopathy
- Neurological signs of cord compression
- Cardiopulmonary compromise preventing the patient lying prone

Relative

- Lack of definable vertebral collapse
- Collapse <20% of the vertebral height
- Unstable fracture patterns preventing safe access
- Deficient posterior cortices that may lead to the extrusion of cement
- Allergy to cement constituents
- Intraoperative difficulty viewing the fracture

Preoperative planning

To include:

- Physician confirms that the back-pain correlates with the VCF.
- A thorough neurological examination is necessary to rule out any neurological compromise (note pain radiating around the trunk in a dermatomal manner often accompanies VCFs).
- Clotting screen.
- Anteroposterior and lateral preoperative radiographs of the affected vertebra.
- Further imaging (MRI or CT) is not necessary for routine VCFs.
- CT imaging can be useful for preoperative planning as it helps determine pedicular size, involvement and whether there is posterior vertebral wall involvement and canal compromise.
- MRI imaging is useful for distinguishing between acute and chronic VCFs, in addition to determining whether the fracture aetiology is osteoporotic, malignant or infective.
- Pulmonary function testing may be required in patients with advanced kyphosis, as they are potentially a higher

anaesthetic risk through difficulties in achieving adequate ventilation when prone.

- Fractures above T7 are more likely to represent tumour, so further investigation is recommended.
- Consent.
- NICE recommend that vertebral augmentation should not be performed in centres with without access to a spinal surgical service.

Techniques

For both techniques, the patient is positioned prone on the operating table, usually with bolsters supporting their shoulders and pelvis. Patient positioning may help improve the fracture position and reduce any acute kyphosis. Both techniques are routinely performed under either local anaesthesia with conscious sedation (e.g. with midazolam) or general anaesthesia. Biplanar fluoroscopic guidance is required throughout the procedure.

A transpedicular approach is typically used for access to the lumbar vertebra while an extrapedicular approach, due to the reduced pedicle diameter, is typical in the thoracic vertebra. For vertebroplasty, the trocar is advanced to the junction of the anterior and middle thirds of the vertebral body, then between 2 and 5 mL of cement (PMMA) is injected under fluoroscopic control.

Cement may be introduced either unilaterally or bilaterally. Unilateral (asymmetrical) filling may lead to single sided load transfer and an effect known as toggle. The clinical significance of toggle is unknown. Most physicians therefore favour a unilateral approach as it theoretically halves the chance of a procedure specific complication, reduces operative time and radiation exposure.

Outcomes

The results of vertebral augmentation vary depending on the indication, patient selection, operator skills and complication rates. The majority of published results are based on retrospective case series and there have been very few prospective controlled trials.

In general, augmentation for osteoporotic fractures successfully relieves pain in 57-97% of patients, with around 10% having recurrent painful episodes. The analgesic effects typically occur at 6–48 hours after the procedure. Improved functional levels and a reduced requirement for analgesia are seen in 60–100% of patients who have undergone augmentation for VCFs. PVP and PKP have the similar analgesic effects. Mobility has been shown to improve by 60–100% in patients with osteoporosis who undergo vertebral augmentation. Seventy-four per cent and 50% of patients had improved quality of life and reported improvement in sleep respectively.

PKP tends to be more effective when performed early on after fracture and can improve kyphosis by less than 50% if performed within 3 months. PKP has been shown to improve spinal kinematics more towards normal than PVP. In a cadaveric study, PKP restored 97% of vertebral height compared to 30% in PVP. The restoration of height helps reduce kyphus and correct sagittal balance that is important in preventing falls in the older population.

Complications

Complications are either anaesthetic or procedure specific. The complication rate is 1–5%. The majority of complications occur due to instrument malplacement or cement leakage. Extravertebral cement leakage occurs in up to 65% of cases and may reside in the epidural space, paravertebral soft tissues, adjacent disc spaces, or intraforaminally. Despite the substantial prevalence of cement leakage during vertebral augmentation, the risk of a clinically significant complication has been reported to be low.

In general, vertebral augmentation is a day-case procedure, with patients discharged home when comfortable, with a vertebral augmentation advice sheet. Both immediate and late complications rely upon an amicable agreement between the hospital radiological and spinal surgical services where hospital admission and further management is necessary. Otherwise, the ongoing management is predominantly the responsibility of the referring clinician. Management of the underlying disease (osteoporosis) with appropriate pharmacotherapy is paramount in preventing disease progression and further fracture.

The cost of a single level vertebroplasty is around £700 with kyphoplasty costing around four times as much. Multiple level augmentation does not increase the cost of the procedure in a linear fashion. NICE recommend that the current evidence on the safety and efficacy of percutaneous vertebroplasty appears adequate to support the use of the procedure. The true cost/benefit analysis of vertebral augmentation has yet to be determined.

General

- Hypotension
- Allergic reaction to cement
- Drug reaction

Procedure specific

- Cement leakage (extravasation out of the vertebral body)
- Nerve damage
- Radiculopathy – secondary to the exothermic reaction of cement curing
- Infection
- Dural puncture
- Cerebral cement embolism
- Pulmonary cement embolism
- Epidural haematoma
- Acute paraplegia

Further reading

Evans AJ, Jensen ME, Kip KE, et al. (2003). Vertebral compression fractures: pain reduction and improvement in functional mobility after percutaneous polymethylmethacrylate vertebroplasty – retrospective report of 245 cases. Radiology 226: 366–72.

Lieberman IH, Dudeney S, Reinhardt MK, et al. (2001). Initial outcome and efficacy of kyphoplasty in the treatment of painful osteoporotic vertebral compression fractures. Spine 26: 1631–8.

Masala S, Ciarrapico AM, Konda D, et al. (2008). Cost-effectiveness of percutaneous vertebroplasty in osteoporotic vertebral fractures. Eur Spine J 17: 1242–50.

Truumees E, Hilibrand A, Vaccaro, AR (2004). Percutaneous vertebral augmentation. Spine J 4: 218–29.

Stroke and transient ischaemic attack

Definition of stroke and transient ischaemic attack

Stroke is defined by the World Health Organization (WHO) as 'a clinical syndrome characterized by rapidly developing clinical symptoms and/or signs of focal, and at times global (applied to patients in deep coma and those with subarachnoid haemorrhage), loss of cerebral function, with symptoms lasting more than 24 hours or leading to death, with no apparent cause other than that of vascular origin'. The classical definition of a transient ischaemic attack (TIA) is of 'a sudden, focal neurological deficit lasting for less than 24 hours, of presumed vascular origin, and confined to an area of the brain or eye perfused by a specific artery'.

The majority of patients with TIA do not come to medical attention before their symptoms have resolved and the diagnosis is therefore usually made by history alone. The 24-hour criterion that divides TIA from ischaemic stroke is arbitrary. Recently there have been proposals to replace this definition with a new one. A diagnosis of TIA would then exclude symptoms lasting for more than one hour and would require the absence of evidence of infarction on imaging of the brain. This new definition has the advantage that it distinguishes clearly between symptoms with and without obvious evidence of tissue injury and stresses the fact that truly transient symptoms without demonstrable tissue injury rarely last longer than one hour. In many patients whose symptoms resolve within 24 hours, diffusion-weighted magnetic resonance imaging (MRI) can show evidence of tissue damage. Also, in the era of thrombolysis when patients present early for treatment, it avoids some confusion whether or not to diagnose a stroke or TIA.

Nevertheless, there are disadvantages.

- This definition can only be applied to patients who have had brain imaging.
- It does not take into account the differences in sensitivity of different scanning methods; standard computed tomography (CT) will not show many of the lesions revealed by diffusion-weighted MRI and there is considerable interobserver variability in interpreting ischaemic lesions on CT.
- Evidence of tissue injury critically depends on the timing of the examination. Relatively minor tissue injury takes many hours before it becomes apparent on CT, whereas restricted diffusion on DWI, although usually signifying irreversible tissue injury is transient.

Moreover, abandoning the current definition would severely hamper comparability of studies with different access to imaging or patient behaviour and would make comparisons with older studies impossible. There is therefore no need to replace the standard definition, as long as it is not taken as an excuse for therapeutic nihilism.

Classification of stroke

There are three main types of stroke: ischaemic stroke, primary intracerebral haemorrhage, and venous infarction. Occasionally subarachnoid haemorrhage is counted as a stroke, although it usually does not cause focal symptoms.

Ischaemic stroke

Ischaemic stroke can be further subdivided. Some of the most popular classifications, such as the one used in the Trial of Org 10172 (TOAST), are based on the likely pathophysiological mechanism leading to stroke:

- large artery disease caused by atherosclerosis of the large extra and intracranial arteries supplying the brain and subsequent thromboembolism
- small vessel disease caused by lipohyelinosis of the small perforating arteries of the brain
- cardioembolic strokes
- other determined rare causes (e.g. arterial dissection, infarction in water-shed territories secondary to hypotension, cerebral vasculitis, genetic stroke syndromes such as MELAS or CADASIL)
- unknown causes with no apparent source despite exhaustive investigations.

Not uncommonly patients have several competing potential causes for their stroke. The classification requires comprehensive investigations including brain imaging with CT or MRI, vascular imaging, particularly of the carotid bifurcation, and cardiac investigations, especially ECG. Aetiological classifications aid in tailoring secondary prophylaxis.

The Oxfordshire Community Stroke Project definition in contrast classifies strokes by clinical syndrome only and can be used without prior brain imaging. It is particularly useful for prognosis and assessing and planning rehabilitation potential but also suggests likely aetiologies (see Table 21.1).

Common types of infarct

Total anterior circulation infarct

Patients with complete hemiplegia or severe hemiparesis, hemianopia, and higher cortical dysfunction (e.g. aphasia, visuospatial disturbance) attributable to a brain lesion contralateral to the hemiplegia at the time of maximum deficit are classified as having a total anterior circulation infarct (TACI). Often this is accompanied by at least some impairment of consciousness. This syndrome is caused by occlusion of the proximal main-stem of the middle cerebral artery usually by artery-to-artery or cardiac embolism, although it can be mimicked by extensive intraparenchymal bleeds.

Not surprisingly given the extent of damage, it carries a poor prognosis. Recurrent major strokes are relatively rare. This reflects the usually permanent occlusion of the affected cerebral arteries, which prevents further embolic ischaemia, and the extent of brains damage to the territory dependent on these, which renders any further insult functionally and clinically irrelevant.

PACI (Partial Anterior Circulation Infarct)

Any of the following deficits are classified as partial anterior circulation infarct if they reflect damage in the same cerebral hemisphere at the time of maximum deficit:

- Motor/sensory deficit + hemianopia
- Motor/sensory deficit + new higher cerebral dysfunction (eg aphasia, visuospatial disturbance)
- New higher cerebral dysfunction + hemianopia
- Pure motor/sensory deficit less extensive than for lacunar syndromes (e.g. monoparesis)
- Isolated new higher cerebral dysfunction (e.g. aphasia).

Table 21.1 Oxford stroke classification with cause and prognosis

Classification	TACS	PACS	LACS	POCS

Typical presentation	- Higher cortical dysfunction
	- Hemiparesis
	- Hemianopia
		Two of
		  - Motor or sensory deficit
		  - Higher cortical dysfunction;
		  - Hemianopia
			Hemiparesis or Hemisensory loss	- Brainstem or cerebellar symptoms
				- Isolated hemianopia

CT scan	Extensive hemispheric infarct	Limited hemispheric infarct	Small subcortical infarct	Brainstem/cerebellar/occipital infarct
Cause	Thrombo-embolism (heart, carotid artery)	Thrombo-embolism (heart, carotid artery)	Occlusion of deep perforating arteries (Lipohyalinosis)	Thrombo-embolism (heart, vertebro-basilar arteries)
Problems	Motor/sensory loss, dysphasia, neglect, dysphagia, hemianopia	Motor/sensory loss, dysphasia, neglect, dysphagia, hemianopia	Motor/sensory loss, ataxia	Ataxia, motor/sensory loss, dysarthria, dysphagia, double vision, vertigo, hemianopia
Prognosis at 1 year				
Survival	60%	85%	90%	80%
Recurrence	5%	20%	10%	20%
Independence	5%	60%	70%	70%
Mobility	40%	70%	80%	80%

This usually reflects (partial) occlusions of branches of the middle cerebral artery but again can be mimicked by intracerebral haemorrhage.

Although the majority of patients are alive after 1 year, a significant proportion will still be dependent. The risk of further major strokes is high and potential sources of emboli, particularly at the carotid bifurcation or the heart, should be looked for and treated.

LACI (lacunar infarct)

Lacunar infarcts are characterized by the absence of any new deficits of higher cerebral function attributable to cortical lesions (e.g. visual field defects, aphasia, neglect). The classical lacunar syndromes are

- pure motor stroke causing hemiparesis (usually affecting face, arm, and leg)
- pure sensory stroke (affecting face, arm, and leg)
- ataxic hemiparesis
- dysarthria, clumsy hand syndrome
- homolateral ataxia and crural (leg) paresis syndrome

These are most often caused by non-embolic occlusions of small perforating arteries but can be mimicked by small embolic strokes or haemorrhages. It is generally difficult in these cases to differentiate clinically between lesions affecting the anterior or posterior circulation.

Patients with lacunar strokes have the best short term prognosis and more than 90% will be alive at one year and around 70% independent. Furthermore, the recurrence risk is relatively low, although still higher than for TACI. Nevertheless, long-term morbidity, in particular cognitive dysfunction, is high and risk factors, in particular hypertension, should be looked for and treated vigorously.

POCI (posterior circulation infarct)

Posterior circulation infarcts can result in a great variety of deficits:

- ipsilateral cranial nerve palsy (III–XII), in various combinations with contralateral hemiparesis and/or sensory deficit
- bilateral motor or sensory deficit
- disorders of conjugate eye movement
- cerebellar dysfunction
- isolated hemianopia or cortical blindness.

These are mainly caused by thromboembolic occlusion of the vertebral, basilar, and posterior cerebral arteries or their branches but can be mimicked by intracerebral haemorrhages. It is also worth bearing in mind that the posterior cerebral artery can infrequently arise as a branch of the internal carotid rather than the basilar artery.

The prognosis for mortality, independence and recurrence risk is similar to PACI, reflecting similar aetiology.

Primary intracerebral haemorrhage

Primary intracerebral haemorrhage refers to non-traumatic spontaneous bleeding into the brain parenchyma. It should be differentiated from secondary haemorrhagic transformation of a primary ischaemic stroke, as treatments differ. However, this is often very difficult in practise and (neuro-) radiologists commonly disagree in their assessment whether a bleed is primary or secondary. Most patients who have had a cerebral bleed will require a follow up scan after 4–6 weeks to exclude any underlying pathology.

The most common sites affected are the basal ganglia, lobar regions, thalamus, pons, and cerebellum. Occasionally the bleed can extend into the intraventricular or subarrhachnoid space. The most common risk factors are hypertension and a bleeding diathesis, but there are multiple possible aetiologies including vascular malformations, tumours, angiopathies such as cerebral amyloid angiopathy, moya moya, aneurysmata, or vasculitis. Cerebral amyloid angiopathy should be suspected in older patients with (recurrent) lobar bleeds, and in patients who have multiple (asymptomatic) lobar microhaemorrhages, visible on gradient ECHO MRI sequences. Young patients can occasionally be affected, particularly if there is a family history.

Venous infarction

Thrombosis of the venous sinuses that drain the brain or less commonly thrombosis of cerebral deep veins can cause brain infarction, often with haemorrhagic transformation.

Classification of transient ischaemic attack

Most transient ischaemic attacks are of presumed embolic aetiology. It is useful to differentiate between purely monocular symptoms (amaurosis fugax) and hemispheric TIA, with or without additional monocular symptoms as the former have a lower risk of subsequent stroke. Anterior circulation hemispheric TIAs result in cortical symptoms (with the exception of isolated hemianopia), unilateral hemisensory or motor symptoms in the absence of additional brainstem symptoms, whereas posterior circulation TIA can cause isolated hemianopia, vertigo, double vision, ataxia, and crossed sensory or motor signs. Various combinations of these symptoms are possible. The risk of subsequent stroke differs little between these.

Low-flow haemodynamic TIA are a rarity, including in the posterior circulation. These are usually precipitated by postural changes or low blood pressure, for instance, recent introduction or increase in anti-hypertensive medication, not by neck movements (as the concept of vertebro-basilar insufficiency proposed). Patients with true low flow TIA are at a very high risk of subsequent stroke.

The so-called capsular warning syndrome is characterised by recurrent stereotyped transient lacunar symptoms (hemiparesis or hemisensory loss without symptoms attributable to cortical dysfunction). The aetiology is not fully understood. Patients with capsular warning symptomatology have a very high risk of an early subsequent infarct.

Further reading

Adams HP, Bendixen BH, Kappelle LJ, et al. (1993). Classification of subtype of acute ischemic stroke. Definitions for use in a multicenter clinical trial. TOAST. Trial of Org 10172 in Acute Stroke Treatment. *Stroke* **24**: 35–41.

Albers GW, Caplan LR, Easton JD, et al. (2002). Transient ischemic attack – proposal for a new definition. *N Engl J Med* **347**: 1713–16.

Bamford J, Sandercock P, Dennis M, et al. (1991). Classification and natural history of clinically identifiable subtypes of cerebral infarction. *Lancet* **337**: 1521–6.

Warlow C, Sudlow C, Dennis M, et al. (2003). Stroke. *Lancet* **362**: 1211–24.

Warlow CP, van Gijn J, Dennis MS, et al. (2008). *Stroke: Practical Management*, 3rd edn. Oxford, Blackwell Science.

Aetiology of stroke

Stroke refers to any acute vascular injury of the central nervous system. There are, however, a number of distinct aetiological mechanisms that can cause stroke. Most share common risk factors for vascular disease, such as high blood pressure, diabetes mellitus or smoking, and several aetiologies can coexist in an individual patient. Nevertheless, there are important differences, in particular regarding prognosis and treatment, that are essential to consider when evaluating and treating patients who have had a stroke.

The most basic distinction is between ischaemic and haemorrhagic stroke; the latter must not be confused with haemorrhagic transformation of an ischaemic stroke. Most stroke in Western Europe, Australia, and North America is ischaemic (c. 80%), whereas in East Asia and the Indian subcontinent haemorrhagic stroke is as common as ischaemic stroke.

Burden of stroke

According to the WHO in 1990, stroke was the second most common cause of death worldwide and the third leading cause of death in rich countries after ischaemic heart disease and all cancers combined. In 1999, there were 5.54 million deaths caused by stroke worldwide. However, only a minority of strokes are fatal and stroke has many other detrimental consequences for affected individuals, their families, and society at large. For instance, stroke is the leading cause of long-term disability and is a major cause of dementia, depression, epilepsy, etc. This leads to enormous costs in addition to the personal suffering. This burden is likely to rise as populations age, and contrary to common belief low- and medium-income countries will be affected most severely. Despite the enormous burden of stroke, funding of stroke-related research has been considerably less than for comparably prevalent conditions such as ischaemic heart disease and cancer. Indeed, therapeutic nihilism has been pervasive up until recently.

Incidence and mortality

Most reliable studies of stroke incidence were conducted in rich countries and there are no reliable data from Africa, most of South America, with the exception of Bolivia and the French West Indies, and most of Asia, with the exception of Japan, Russian Siberia, and Taiwan. In these studies, the incidence ranged from 1.3 to 4.1 per 1000 person years.

Management of stroke differs considerably between countries, with 41% of stroke patients being admitted to hospital in Japan versus 94.6% in Germany. The mean age of onset also varied considerably from 60.8 years for men in Uzhgorod, Ukraine, to 75.3 years in Innherred, Norway, and 66.6 years for women in Uzhgorod to 78.0 years in Perth, Australia. Around a quarter of all strokes were fatal (death within one month after stroke onset).

Most studies that investigated time trends showed a decline in stroke incidence through to the late 1970s and early 1980s but this decline reached a plateau or even reversed in the late 1980s and early 1990s, with exceptions in Oxford, UK, Perth, Australia, and Oyabe, Japan.

Stroke mortality rates have declined steeply in western Europe, North America, Australasia, and Japan but have increased in eastern Europe and Russia.

Ischaemic stroke

The most widely used aetiological classification of ischaemic stroke is the TOAST classification (more memorable than Trial of Org 10172 in Acute Stroke). It differentiates (1) large artery atherosclerosis, (2) cardioembolism, (3) small vessel occlusion, (4) stroke of other determined aetiology, and (5) stroke of undetermined aetiology.

The relative importance of vascular risk factors differs between the pathophysiological subtypes of ischaemic stroke; large vessel stroke is particularly associated with smoking, male sex, and raised cholesterol. Hospital-based studies had previously suggested that there was a particularly strong link between small vessel stroke and hypertension and diabetes. However, this observation could not be confirmed in the population-based studies that were free of referral bias and included the whole spectrum of disease severity.

Large-artery atherosclerosis

Atherosclerosis of the large intra- and extracranial brain-supplying vessels (aortic arch, common and internal carotid artery, vertebral arteries, basilar artery, circle of Willis and its branches) accounts for up to a fifth of ischaemic strokes. Stroke can be caused by several mechanisms, mainly artery-to-artery embolism and in situ thrombosis. Furthermore, atherosclerotic plaques can obliterate origins of perforating vessels, causing lacunar infarction. Artery-to-artery embolism is the most common of these mechanisms. Sites predilected for atherosclerosis are the branching points of large vessels. These act as the most common donor sites for emboli, which cause stroke if they lodge in downstream functional end-arteries. Complex genetic and environmental factors can influence the actual site of atherosclerosis; the carotid bifurcation is the single most important site in patients of European descent, intracranial vessels are commonly affected in patients with diabetes mellitus, and in many non-European ethnic groups, e.g. in the Far East, Indian subcontinent, and patients of African descent. Atherosclerosis is typically a systemic process; patients with large vessel strokes frequently have significant disease in other vascular territories (e.g. ischaemic heart disease).

Any atherosclerotic plaque can give rise to emboli if ruptured; the risk however increases significantly if there is haemodynamically significant stenosis (i.e. >50%).

Cardioembolic stroke

Systemic sources of emboli, most commonly cardiac sources account for about a third of ischaemic strokes. Numerous pathological processes can cause formation of emboli inside the heart, e.g. atrial fibrillation, recent (within 3 months) myocardial infarction, left ventricular aneurysms, severe heart failure, endocarditis, prosthetic mitral or aortic valves, rheumatic mitral stenosis, and atrial myxoma. Furthermore, right-to-left shunts (e.g. patent foramen ovale) allow embolic material from the systemic venous circulation to embolise to the brain. Atrial fibrillation, even if only intermittent, is by far the most important of these. The actual composition of the embolic material varies depending on different pathophysiological mechanisms, e.g. platelet aggregates, thrombi, cholesterol crystals, calcium, septic emboli, neoplastic emboli.

Small vessel disease

The perforating vessels that supply the deep white matter of the cerebral hemisphere and brainstem can be harmed by a number of mechanisms and insults (e.g. genetic factors, hypertension, diabetes mellitus) resulting in endothelial damage and lipohyalinosis that leads to dysfunction of the blood–brain barrier, thickening of vessel walls, and subsequent reduction of lumen, and hardening of vessels. This can in turn lead to chronic ischaemic damage. Cerebral small vessel disease commonly coexists with microhaemorrhages visible on gradient ECHO MRI sequences. This might be a factor explaining the higher risk of symptomatic haemorrhages in patients with small vessel disease.

Perforating vessels are physiological end vessels, and sudden occlusion of these results in lacunar strokes. This accounts for between a fifth to a quarter of ischaemic strokes. This mostly affects vessels afflicted by lipohyalinosis. Therefore, chronic small vessel ischaemic damage and lacunar strokes frequently coexist. Nevertheless, other pathological processes, namely embolism (either of large vessel or cardiac origin) or atherosclerotic plaques in the larger parent vessel occluding the orifice of a perforating artery can also lead to lacunar strokes.

Stroke of other determined aetiology

This category contains any stroke that is caused by a defined cause other than large vessel atherosclerotic, small vessel or cardioembolic. There are numerous different aetiologies, most of which are rare. Some conditions require specific treatments, such as immunosupression for vasculitis. It is therefore important to consider them in the differential diagnosis of ischaemic stroke, particularly when the patient has no conventional risk factors, is young, has a strong family history of stroke or related disorders, or has other features of a specific syndrome. Important examples to consider are outlined below.

Arterial dissection

Arterial dissection is an important cause of stroke, particularly in young patients. Two main mechanisms are implicated: first, an intimal tear or, second, a bleed into the medial layer that can lead to secondary intimal tear or formation of a pseudoaneurysm if expanding towards the intima or adventitia. The extracranial internal carotid and vertebral arteries are most commonly affected; dissection of intracranial arteries can result in subarachnoid haemorrhage. In many cases a history of trauma, often trivial such as violent coughing, or recent systemic infections can be elicited. Most patients have no obvious underlying condition, although certain genetic conditions such as type IV Ehlers–Danlos syndrome predispose to arterial dissection. Strokes are usually caused by a combination of embolization of thrombi that form when the endothelial layer is breeched and haemodynamic factors through narrowing of the true lumen. Most strokes occur within hours to days of the dissection; strokes beyond 1 month are very rare.

Genetic stroke syndromes (CADASIL, MELAS)

There are also a number of single gene disorders that can cause ischaemic stroke and examples of single gene disorders have been described for each of the major pathophysiological subtypes of ischaemic stroke.

The most common, known classic Mendelian stroke syndrome, is cerebral autosomal dominant arteriopathy with subcortical infarcts and leukoencephalopathy (CADASIL). It is transmitted in an autosomal dominant fashion and leads to disease of mainly the small vessels of the brain and is characterised by recurrent strokes and dementia with pseudobulbar palsy.

The syndrome of mitochondrial encephalomyopathy, lactic acidosis, and stroke-like episodes (MELAS) is a progressive neurodegenerative multisystem disorder. Most patients present before the age of 20. Symptoms are generalized tonic–clonic seizures, recurrent headaches, anorexia, vomiting, and proximal muscle weakness. Seizures are often associated with stroke-like episodes with altered consciousness. There is a gradual impairment of motor abilities, vision, hearing, and intellectual function.

Venous infarction

Thrombosis of cerebral veins or venous sinuses can lead to infarction of the drained cerebral tissue, frequently accompanied by haemorrhage. Predisposing factors include:

- thrombophilia
- oestrogen-containing contraception
- pregnancy and puerperium
- infectious mastoiditis
- sinusitis
- meningitis
- nephrotic syndrome
- trauma
- mechanical obstruction of veins
- chronic inflammatory condition, (e.g. Behçet's disease, colitis)
- haemoglobinopathies, (e.g. polycythaemia vera, paroxysmal nocturnal haemoglobinuria).

Stroke symptoms are frequently accompanied by headaches and seizures.

Vasculitis

Vasculitis can lead to often multiple cerebral infarctions, but can also result in parenchymal or subarachnoid haemorrhage. The vasculitic process can be confined to the cerebral vessels as in primary cerebral angiitis, be part of a systemic vasculitis (e.g. giant cell arteritis, Wegeners), or is associated with a connective tissue disease (e.g. systemic lupus erythematosus, rheumatoid arthritis). Secondary vasculitis is caused by infections (e.g. herpes zoster), drugs (e.g. amphetamines, cocaine) or malignancy.

Vasoconstriction

The reversible cerebral vasoconstriction syndrome is a newly recognised entity characterized by a monophasic course with an acute severe headache with or without seizures, segmental vasoconstriction of cerebral arteries on angiography and complete normalization on repeat angiography. It can be associated with localized cortical subarachnoid haemorrhage, and parenchymal ischaemic or haemorrhagic strokes. Many cases are secondary, mainly postpartum or after ingestion of vasoactive substances (e.g. cannabis, cocaine).

Haemodynamic infarction

Transient hypotension, especially if there is pre-existing vessel obstruction due to atherosclerosis or other factors, can lead to infarction in watershed territories. Watershed areas, however, are also sites predilected for emboli.

Moya moya disease

Moya moya disease is a rare non-atherosclerotic, non-inflammatory disorder of hyperplasia of smooth muscle cells resulting in progressive stenosis and luminal thrombosis of the intracranial carotid arteries and their proximal branches leading to the development of compensatory collaterals. It typically affects both carotid and spares the vertebrobasilar arteries.

Stroke of undetermined aetiology

The number of strokes classified to this category depends on the amount, quality and thoroughness of investigations. For instance, paroxysmal atrial fibrillation is more often detected the longer the ECG is monitored. Nevertheless, the aetiology of around a third of ischaemic strokes remains undetermined despite exhaustive investigations. It has been suggested that strokes of undetermined aetiology are mainly due to unrecognized large vessel disease. However, the relative importance of risk factors differs in the systematic review between large vessel strokes and strokes of undetermined aetiology.

Haemorrhagic stroke

There are numerous causes of intracerebral haemorrhage, these are particularly common in patients with bleeding diathesis, e.g. patients on anticoagulation, haematological malignancies. The most basic distinction is between subarachnoid and parenchymal haemorrhage.

Subarachnoid haemorrhage

Subarachnoid haemorrhage is most commonly caused by rupture of intracranial aneurysmata that typically form at branching points of intra-cranial vessels, especially the circle of Willis. Other causes include so-called perimesencephalic subarachnoid haemorrhage of presumed venous origin, vascular malformations, reversible vasoconstriction and vasculitis.

Intraparenchymal haemorrhage

Deep intraparenchymal haemorrhages affecting the basal ganglia, internal capsule, brainstem or cerebellum are most commonly caused by hypertensive damage to the deep perforating arteries.

Lobar haemorrhages are frequently caused by amyloid angiopathy, particularly in older patients. Other common causes are underlying vascular malformations or tumours. Venous sinus thrombosis can lead to haemorrhagic infarctions.

Further reading

Warlow C, Sudlow C, Dennis M, et al. (2003). Stroke. Lancet **362**: 1211–24.
Warlow CP, van Gijn J, Dennis MS, et al. (2008). Stroke: Practical Management, 3rd edn. Oxford, Blackwell Science.

Investigation of suspected transient ischaemic attack

A transient ischaemic attack (TIA) is a clinical diagnosis based on a careful detailed history from the patient or a witness; only rarely will a clinician directly observe a TIA.

TIA is defined as a sudden focal neurological deficit affecting brain, retina, or spinal cord of presumed vascular origin that is fully reversible within 24 hours. TIA and stroke are fundamentally caused by the same pathophysiological mechanisms and any distinction is therefore likely to be arbitrary to some degree. This is particularly true for the time limit of 24 hours and restricted diffusion on diffusion-weighted magnetic resonance imaging (MRI) suggestive of permanent tissue injury (i.e. infarction) can be seen in nearly half of patients whose symptoms have clinically reversed within 24 hours of tissue injury can be seen.

A new definition of TIA has therefore recently been proposed that requires there is no evidence of infarction on brain imaging. This new definition stresses that any benign connotation that symptoms lasting for less then 24 hours might have are misplaced. It relies on patients presenting promptly and the rapid imaging with diffusion-weighted MRI as pathological diffusion restriction is often reversible within a few days. However, this would make the diagnosis dependent on the local availability of modern imaging facilities and the time delay between symptom onset and evaluation. Amongst other disadvantages this would seriously compromise epidemiological studies of incidence in different settings and would make the study of time trends and other historical comparisons impossible. Furthermore, contrary to its intentions it might foster complacency in patients who do not have areas of restricted diffusion on diffusion-weighted MRI.

Anterior circulation TIA may cause unilateral weakness, clumsiness or sensory symptoms involving face, arm, hand and/or leg, speech disturbance (dysphasia or dysarthria), visual symptoms, amaurosis fugax or any combination of these. Posterior circulation TIA may cause a combination of weakness or sensory symptoms (unilateral or crossed with facial symptoms on the opposite site of limb symptoms), ataxia, vertigo, double vision, dysarthria, isolated hemianopia but occasionally any of these can occur in isolation. It is therefore clinically difficult to distinguish the vascular territory of symptoms with certainty. Furthermore, isolated posterior circulation symptoms such as vertigo or double vision are difficult to distinguish from similar symptoms of non-vascular aetiology. Transient loss of consciousness without focal neurological symptoms or isolated transient memory loss are not typical features of TIA. The differential diagnosis of apparent transient focal neurological symptoms is wide and examples of the diagnoses people receive who are initially referred with suspected TIA include:

- Partial epileptic seizures: typically repeated episodes with stereotypical features (responsive to antiepileptic medication).
- Transient global amnesia (TGA): characterized by loss of short term memory with some anxiety and repetitive questioning for a few hours, and no other neurological deficit. Only recurs rarely, and so diagnosis should be reviewed if recurrent episodes.
- Migrainous aura: suspect if symptoms evolve over a few minutes rather than occurring suddenly, particularly if the patient has a history of migraines. New onset migrainous auras can be difficult to differentiate from TIA; if in doubt investigate and treat as if TIA.

- Hypoglycaemia: often causes focal symptoms.
- Brain tumours: do not always present with gradual onset of symptoms, e.g. focal seizures or haemorrhage into the tumour.
- Subdural haemorrhage: suspect if symptoms vague and onset not clear, particularly in patients prone to falls.
- Bell's palsy.
- Central nervous system demyelination: tends to affect younger patients, but not exclusively.
- Peripheral neuropathy: e.g. mononeuritis multiplex can present as sudden deficit usually affecting motor and sensory fibres in a typical nerve territory. Compressive neuropathies (e.g. radial nerve palsy) often become apparent after sleep, coma or anaesthesia. Radiculopathies can present with neck or lower back pain and deficit of motor and sensory function in a typical territory.
- Myasthenia gravis: transient double vision or dysphagia/dysarthria are symptoms that can be confused with TIA. Initially, predominantly dysphagic symptoms rather than ophthalmoplegic ones are not uncommon in older patients.
- Motor neuron disease: patients referred to the TIA clinic are usually in the early stages and might present with dysarthria/dysphagia. The more typical features of progressive mixed upper and lower motor neurone signs might not be apparent until later.

The diagnosis of TIA is often made indiscriminately in any patients with vague transient neurological symptoms. This often leads to unnecessary and inappropriate investigations and long-term pharmacological therapy with its inherent risks and cost. It is thus essential that competent clinicians, preferably in a specialist TIA clinic, assess patients.

TIA and minor stroke should be regarded as medical emergencies as both carry a similarly high risk of subsequent major strokes, mainly within hours or days. Thus patients should be referred to specialist TIA clinics without delay and should be assessed, fully investigated and appropriate treatment commenced as soon as possible, ideally within 24 hours of the event.

Risk stratification/prognosis

Risk stratification helps to focus limited resources at patients most at risk of subsequent stroke. The most commonly used way of risk stratification is the ABCD^2 score, which uses easily available patient data, namely **A**ge, first available **B**lood pressure reading after the TIA, **C**linical features such as weakness or speech disturbance, **D**uration of symptoms, and pre-existing diagnosis of **D**iabetes mellitus.

A (age); 1 point for age >60 years,

B (blood pressure ≥140/90 mmHg); 1 point for hypertension at the acute evaluation,

C (clinical features); 2 points for unilateral weakness, 1 for speech disturbance without weakness, and

D (symptom duration); 1 point for 10–59 minutes, 2 points for ≥60 minutes.

D (diabetes); 1 point

Patients with a score ≥4 should be seen and investigated within 24 hours. The ABCD^2 score works less well for posterior circulation TIA, which compromise approximately

20% of TIA. Nevertheless, they have a similar if not some-what higher risk of stroke compared to anterior circulation TIA.

The predictive value of the $ABCD^2$ score can be further improved if the results of brain imaging (either CT or DWI/MRI) are incorporated. Evidence of brain infarction (either new or old) is an independent risk factor for further strokes.

Investigations

The main aim of investigations is to establish the aetiology of the TIA and identify sources of emboli so that the subsequent risk of stroke can be diminished with appropriate treatment. Moreover, investigations might reveal an alternative explanation for the patient's symptoms such as brain tumours, seizures, subdural haemorrhages, or central nervous system demyelination.

Investigations need to be tailored to the individual patient and take account of local resources. Most patients will be investigated as outpatients. One-stop clinics offering an assessment by a neurologist or stroke physician, brain and vascular imaging, blood tests, electrocardiogram (ECG) on the same day should be established in order to avoid delay in treating patients. It might be justified to admit selected patients at high risk to an acute hospital, in particular patients with symptomatic haemodynamically (>50%) significant large vessel disease, in particular at the carotid bifurcation. This would facilitate carotid surgery or endovascular treatment, expedite investigations and would also afford the chance to thrombolyse patients rapidly in case of a subsequent stroke.

Brain imaging

All patients with hemispheric TIA should have brain imaging to look for signs of new or old ischaemia and rule out TIA mimics. Diffusion-weighted MRI is the most useful modality although CT is still widely used as a first-line investigation.

Diffusion weighted imaging (DWI)

Areas of restricted diffusion closely match with regions of recently infarcted tissue. Areas of restricted diffusion can be demonstrated in up to 30–50% of patients in the first couple of days after a TIA, and can persist for a few weeks. This confirms the diagnosis in the appropriate clinical context and effectively rules out non-vascular causes.

Beyond establishing the diagnosis DWI lesions inform about prognosis and can give useful clues about the likely aetiology of the TIA. The presence of infarction on DWI is a strong predictor of subsequent stroke. Multiple areas of restricted diffusion (see Figure 21.1) in more than one vascular territory suggests a cardiac embolic source (a), multiple areas of restricted diffusion in a single vascular territory suggest an upstream embolic source in a single vessel (b), restricted diffusion in the territory of a deep perforator suggests impaired blood-flow rather than embolism in patients with recurrent TIA with lacunar symptomatology (capsular warning).

MRI is also superior to CT in demonstrating potential old vascular lesions, leukoaraiosis, and diagnosing non-vascular disorders that might mimic TIA.

Computed tomography

CT will only rarely identify an area of infarction that corresponds to the TIA symptoms. It is therefore increasingly replaced by MRI but still has value if MRI is contra-indicated

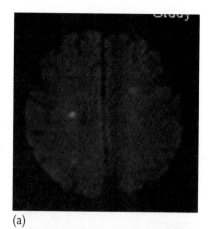

(a)

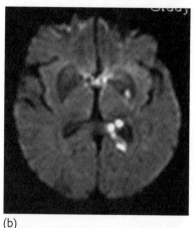

(b)

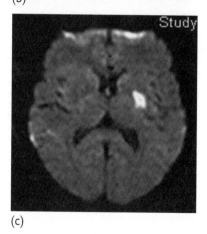

(c)

Figure 21.1 MRI images showing ischaemic changes.

or unavailable. The main utility of the CT is to investigate for alternative diagnosis and to demonstrate leukoaraiosis or old strokes.

Vascular imaging

The most important role of vascular imaging is identifying patients with critical stenosis (i.e. ≥50%) at the origin of the internal carotid artery. Symptomatic patients with critical stenosis are at high risk of further ischaemic events including major strokes. Carotid endarterectomy without delay is the single most effective intervention to prevent major strokes in this context.

Imaging of the large brain-supplying arteries from the aortic arch to the intracranial vessels often provides useful clues about the aetiology of the TIA, e.g. critical stenosis in a blood vessel that supplies the brain territory affected by ischaemia, arterial malformations, aneurysmata. Imaging of the intracranial circulation should be considered in otherwise unexplained TIA (no obvious cardiac or extracranial arterial disease), patients with diabetes mellitus and patients from certain ethnic groups with a high prevalence of intracranial disease (black people, oriental people, Indians, Hispanics).

However, reliable data about the effectiveness of intervention in the vertebral and intracranial arteries is not yet available. In the absence of definitive data from randomized trials, angioplasty, or stenting can be considered in selected patients with critical stenosis, particularly if there is insufficient collateral blood supply resulting in recurrent TIA because of poor flow. These interventions should only be performed in experienced centres, if possible patients should be enrolled in trials or at least be entered in registries.

Imaging can often help to identify the underlying pathology of vascular disease, i.e. hint whether identified lesions are atherosclerotic or suggest rarer aetiologies such as arterial dissection, dolichoectasia, vasculitis and moya moya (a non-inflammatory vasculopathy leading to progressive occlusion of the circle of Willis.).

Widely available modes of vascular imaging are ultrasound, magnetic resonance angiography (MRA), computed tomography angiography (CTA), and conventional digital subtraction angiography.

Ultrasound

Modern vascular ultrasound usually combines Doppler ultrasound with colour Duplex methods. It is relatively cheap, non-invasive, not associated with ionizing radiation, contrast is only rarely employed, the equipment is portable, and ultrasound examinations can therefore be repeatedly carried out in an individual patient if necessary. Furthermore, it is the only non-invasive technique that allows haemodynamic investigations. Ultrasound is therefore in many centres the method of choice to screen for stenosis of the internal carotid artery. Nevertheless, it requires considerable technical expertise and should only be used routinely where this is available.

In expert hands it is a reliable method to visualize the extracranial carotid artery and estimate the degree of stenosis. Heavily calcified plaques however, can occasionally make accurate estimations difficult. The vertebral and intra-cranial arteries are more difficult to visualise. Nevertheless, Doppler studies can provide reliable indications of downstream stenosis even if direct visualization is not possible. Intracranial ultrasound relies on adequate bone windows, which mainly depend on age, sex, and race. The quality of images can be substantially improved by use of intravenous contrast. The detection of micro-emboli in the middle cerebral artery with semi-automated methods is a promising technique that is likely to be valuable in refining stratification of risk for stroke. It is however, not yet widely available.

MR angiography (MRA)

MR angiography allows imaging of all brain supplying large arteries. It can be combined with MRI/DWI of the brain offering a comprehensive assessment of vessels and for tissue injury. MRI is, however, relatively expensive, time consuming, and some patients have contraindications such as cardiac pacemakers, cannot lie still long enough, or are claustrophobic.

Several different techniques are available for imaging blood vessels with MRI; time of flight MRA, phase-contrast MRA and contrast-enhanced MRA. Phase contrast MRA is time-consuming and rarely used in the evaluation of patients with TIA. Time of flight MRA does not require contrast injection. However, it takes approximately 15 minutes to image from the aortic arch to the base of skull, which makes it susceptible to movement and breathing artefacts. Furthermore, this technique frequently overestimates degrees of stenosis. It is more suitable for imaging the circle of Willis, which requires less time. Contrast-enhanced MRA is the fastest and most accurate MR imaging modality but requires injection of contrast and appropriate timing of image acquisition.

CT angiography (CTA)

CTA with a spiral CT offers a fast and reliable way of imaging the brain-supplying arteries. It requires contrast injection and is associated with considerable radiation exposure.

Conventional digital subtraction angiography

Conventional digital subtraction angiography is still the gold standard of vascular imaging and, apart from ultrasound, the only technique that provides haemodynamic information. Its spatial resolution is superior to non-invasive techniques and is currently the only routinely available mode to image smaller intracranial vessels. However, it is invasive, associated with potentially significant complications, time-consuming and is therefore rarely used first-line in the routine evaluation of patients with TIA.

Which imaging modality?

The choice of imaging modality depends on local availability, experience and individual patient characteristics.

Anterior circulation TIA

Carotid Doppler ultrasound offers a cheap, fast and in experienced hands accurate method of evaluation the extracranial carotid artery and is therefore the method of choice in most centres for assessing patients with anterior circulation TIA. Additional investigations with MR or CTA are only necessary if an accurate estimation of stenosis is not possible or if intracranial disease is suspected.

Two common methods are used to describe the angiographic degree of stenosis of the internal carotid artery named after the studies where they were employed, the NASCET (North American Symptomatic Carotid Endarterectomy TRIAL) and the ECST (European Carotid Stenosis Trial) methods; a combination of angiographic and haemodynamic measurements are usually employed in sonography. These measurements are not equivalent, and it is important to clarify which method is used locally.

There is an on-line "Carotid Stenosis Risk Prediction Tool" to predict 1 and 5 year risk of stroke after a TIA or minor stroke, taking into account degree of stenosis, age, sex, co-morbidities, and time from event (http://www.stroke.ox.ac.uk/.) This helps to decide whom to refer for endarterectomy.

Posterior circulation

Contrast-enhanced MRA and CTA are the preferred non-invasive equally reliable modalities for investigating the posterior circulation. Although ultrasound Doppler investigations can also provide valuable information about haemodynamically relevant stenosis in the intra- and extracranial posterior circulation, it requires considerable technical expertise. Carotid Doppler ultrasound or alternative imaging of the carotid bifurcation should be considered in patients presenting with ischaemia attributable to the posterior cerebral artery (isolated hemianopia or cortical blindness) as in a substantial minority the posterior cerebral artery is a branch of the internal carotid artery rather than the basilar artery (the so called fetal origin).

Intracranial circulation
CTA, MRA (either time of flight or contrast enhanced), and intracranial Doppler are the available non-invasive methods. There are no studies so far, that have compared the reliability of different imaging modalities in the intracranial circulation.

Blood tests

Blood tests help to identify risk factors for vascular disease such as diabetes mellitus, hypercholesterolaemia, renal impairment, polycythaemia, conditions associated with raised C-reactive protein. The following blood tests are recommended:

- full blood count
- urea and electrolytes
- fasting serum glucose
- fasting cholesterol
- inflammatory markers (erythrocyte sedimentation rate, C-reactive protein).

Consider:

- a lipid profile including high-density lipoprotein and low-density lipoprotein cholesterol, triglycerides)
- prothrombin and partial thromboplastin time
- thyroid function tests
- autoimmune antibodies (e.g. antinuclear antibodies, ANCA)
- syphilis serology, HIV test
- drug screen (younger patients. e.g. cocaine, amphetamines).

Cardiac investigations

Cardiac emboli are an important cause of cerebral ischaemia. Furthermore, cardiac disease is closely linked with cerebrovascular disease and shares similar risk factors. The identification of a potential cardioembolic source potentially alters treatment as anticoagulation with coumarin derivatives or direct thrombin inhibitors is superior in these patients to usual prophylactic treatment with platelet inhibitors. Cardiac investigations are therefore an essential part of the evaluation of TIA patients.

An ECG recording is an essential part of investigating patients with a TIA. This may show evidence of atrial fibrillation or other emboligenic dysrhythmias, (silent) cardiac ischaemia or hypertension.

Further investigations should be considered, especially if no other cause for the TIA is apparent or in patients with a high likelihood of cardiac disease. The appropriateness of investigations depends on individual factors. Paroxysmal atrial fibrillation is an important risk factor for stroke, especially in the presence of other risk factors including age.

Holter ECG recordings or continuing telemetry recording may reveal paroxysmal atrial fibrillation in patients with sinus rhythm on a standard ECG. Prolonged recordings

(e.g. 72-hour recordings) have a higher rate of detection than standard 24-hour recordings. These should be considered particularly if prior investigations have not shown any obvious other cause of the TIA.

An echocardiogram should be considered, especially in young patients without vascular risk factors who might have structural heart conditions that predispose to cerebral ischaemia and in patients with possible endocarditis. Its main use is to look for structural cardiac disease that predisposes to emboli, such as right-to-left shunts, valvular disease, and left ventricular aneurysm. It may also show evidence of longstanding hypertension (left ventricular hypertrophy), previous myocardial infarctions or show enlarged atrial appendages, which increase the risk of atrial fibrillation.

A bubble transthoracic echocardiogram using agitated saline is a useful first line test and will detect most clinically relevant right-to-left shunts.

Transoesophageal echocardiography is more sensitive for most conditions important in patients with cerebral ischaemia then transthoracic studies but is more invasive and might not be easily available everywhere. It is particularly useful in visualising the left atrial appendage, the most common site of cardiac emboli, in demonstrating endocarditic vegetations and showing abnormalities of the intra-atrial septum (septal defects, patent foramen ovale, interatrial septal aneurysm). Furthermore, it is the best method to demonstrate aortic atherosclerosis and spontaneous ECHO contrast within the left atrium, which is associated with thrombi. It should be considered if finding a cardiac source of emboli would alter management.

Further tests to consider

A number of further investigations might be appropriate in selected patients, in particular if alternative diagnoses need to be ruled out.

- An electroencephalogram (EEG) may reveal an epileptogenic focus, which should be considered if a patient has recurrent stereotyped focal symptomatology. A normal EEG however, does not rule this possibility out.
- Nerve conduction studies or MRI of the cervical spine might be appropriate if a peripheral neuropathy (carpal tunnel syndrome, ulnar or radial neuropathy) or radiculopathy are possible differential diagnosis.
- A lumbar puncture and examination of the cerebrospinal fluid is appropriate to investigate for possible inflammatory conditions such as multiple sclerosis or vasculitis of the central nervous system.

Further reading

Giles MF, Rothwell PM (2006). Prognosis and management in the first few days after a transient ischemic attack or minor ischaemic stroke. *Int J Stroke* **1**: 65–73.

Johnston SC, Rothwell PM, Nguyen-Huynh MN, et al. (2007). Validation and refinement of scores to predict very early stroke risk after transient ischaemic attack. *Lancet* **369**: 283–92.

Merwick A, Albers GW, Amarenco P, et al. (2010). Addition of brain and carotid imaging to the ABCD[2] score to identify patients at early risk of stroke after transient ischaemic attack: a multicentre observational study. *Lancet Neurol* **9**: 1060–9.

Rothwell PM, Giles MF, Flossmann E, et al. (2005). A simple score (ABCD) to identify individuals at high early risk of stroke after transient ischaemic attack. *Lancet* **366**: 29–36.

Rothwell PM, Warlow CP (2005). Timing of TIAs preceding stroke: time window for prevention is very short. *Neurology* **64**: 817–20.

Transient ischaemic attack

A transient ischaemic attack (TIA) is defined as stroke symptoms and signs that resolve within 24 hours, although more typically within a few minutes or hours. Approximately 70 000 TIAs are diagnosed per annum in the UK, with up to 20% of stroke patients having sustained a preceding TIA. This provides a significant opportunity for stroke prevention, and this section will focus on aspects of symptom recognition, early prognosis following TIA including risk factors for early recurrence, optimum investigation, and its timing, and strategies for early therapeutic intervention and their effectiveness.

Symptom recognition

A review assessing factors explaining delays in seeking medical attention showed that patients with TIA compared with stroke are less likely to receive emergency and/or timely specialist assessment, and often never seek medical attention. This reflects a lack of patient recognition of symptoms, no event witness to promote medical contact, general practitioner (GP) rather than emergency medical services (EMS) contact, and the event occurring outside GP surgery hours, including weekends. Specific tools are increasingly used to promote symptom recognition. The most common pre-hospital scale used is the Face Arm Speech Test (FAST) with 89% (range 84–94%) positive predictive value for subsequent vascular neurological diagnosis, and by EMS the Recognition Of Stroke In the Emergency Room (ROSIER) with a positive predictive value of 90% (85–95%).

Risk assessment

Early symptom recognition is important because the risk of disabling stroke is front-loaded following TIA and minor stroke. A large systematic review of stroke risk reported a 3.1% (95% CI 2.0–4.1) stroke risk within two days of TIA and a 5.2% (3.9–6.5) 7-day risk. Recent work has therefore focussed on identifying a population at highest risk; the $ABCD^2$ score has been well validated and is the most commonly used (see Table 21.2).

In a validation study of the $ABCD^2$ score, patients were classified as high (score 6–7), moderate (4–5), or low risk (0–3) with 2-day stroke risks of 8.1%, 4.1%, and 1.0%, respectively (see Figure 21.2). Subsequent specialist assessment should be prioritized on the basis of risk; those at highest risk ($ABCD^2 \geq 4$) being assessed within 24 hours. However, posterior circulation TIA is associated with

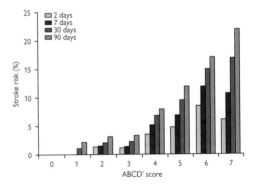

Figure 21.2 Short-term risk of stroke by $ABCD^2$ score. Reprinted from *The Lancet*, **369**, S Claiborne Johnston, Peter M Rothwell, Mai N Nguyen-Huynh, Matthew F Giles, Jacob S Elkins, Allan L Bernstein, Stephen Sidney, pp. 283–92, Copyright 2007, with permission from Elsevier.

increased risk but these are poorly recognized by the $ABCD^2$ score. One meta-analysis quoted an odds ratio of 1.47 (95% CI 1.1–2.0) for risk of recurrent stroke in patients presenting acutely with a vertebrobasilar compared with a carotid event; another reported an odds ratio of 1.70 (95% CI 1.3–2.2) for recurrent vertebrobasilar TIAs. Furthermore, crescendo TIA, defined as multiple TIAs of increasing duration, severity and/or frequency over a several day period, requires urgent assessment.

Assessment

Sufficient capacity should be available to ensure timely specialist assessment. This is considered in more detail in the Investigation of suspected TIA section, but the key principles are:

- careful history and examination, including exclusion of stroke mimics
- identify the vascular territory
- identify the likely cause: cardioembolic, carotid atheroma, *in situ* thrombus, other (e.g. vasculitic, septic embolus)
- investigation to confirm diagnosis and exclude differentials: CT/MRI head. Diffusion-weighted MRI (MR-DWI) is the preferred technique but should not delay secondary prevention. One study of patients assessed within 48 hours finding that a positive MR-DWI and an ABCD2 score ≥4 was associated with a significantly increased 7-day (5.4%) and 90-day (9.7%) stroke risk
- investigations to guide secondary prevention: includes urgent carotid imaging to identify significant stenosis in patients suitable for endarterectomy.

Early secondary preventative therapeutic intervention initiated in an open-access clinic compared with recommendations to GPs prior to hospital appointment was assessed in the early use of Existing PREventive Strategies for Stroke (EXPRESS) study, and resulted in a highly significant reduction in 90-day stroke recurrence (adjusted hazard ratio 0.20, 95% CI 0.08–0.49; p = 0.0001). As well as a reduced delay in specialist assessment, there was an increased uptake of antiplatelet, statin and BP-lowering therapies.

Table 21.2 The $ABCD^2$ score

Risk factor		Points
Age	≥60 years	1
Blood pressure	Systolic >140 mmHg and/or diastolic ≥90 mmHg	1
Clinical features	Unilateral motor weakness	2
	Speech disturbance	1
	Other	0
Duration of symptoms	≥60 minutes	2
	10–59 minutes	1
	<10 minutes	0
Diabetes mellitus	Present	1

Secondary prevention

A detailed critique of secondary prevention strategies is provided in the Secondary prevention of stroke section, but recommendations specific to TIA include:

Antiplatelet/anticoagulant therapy

The FAST Assessment of Stroke and TIA to prevent Early Recurrence (FASTER) and EXPRESS trials have assessed the addition of clopidogrel to aspirin; the former showing no significant benefit, and the latter reporting benefit of an urgent treatment strategy rather than antiplatelet therapy per se. The immediate (<24 hours) compared with delayed (>7 days) introduction of modified-release dipyridamole to aspirin was investigated in the EARLY trial, and was not associated with a significant improvement in 90-day Modified Rankin score. A strategy of aspirin and modified-release dipyridamole with or without clopidogrel, and aspirin with or without clopidogrel immediately for short-term use in high risk patients are being assessed in the ongoing Triple Antiplatelets for Reducing Dependency after Ischaemic Stroke (TARDIS) and Platelet-orientated Inhibition in New TIA (PILOT) trials, respectively. Therefore, current UK guidance is for the immediate introduction of aspirin at 300 mg, continued until 2 weeks, at which time long-term treatment should be initiated. This comprises aspirin 75 mg in combination with modified-release dipyridamole (if tolerated). Long-term treatment can be started earlier in those discharged before 2 weeks.

Cholesterol/lipids

In the Stroke Prevention by Aggressive Reduction in Cholesterol Levels (SPARCL) trial, patients were randomised between one and six months following TIA and non-disabling stroke, and a significant reduction in recurrent ischaemic stroke reported with a low-density lipoprotein (LDL) decrease of 1.4 mmol/L. In the FASTER trial, early statin use was associated with an absolute non-significant increased risk of 90-day stroke of 3.3% (−2.3 to 8.9), although this trial was stopped early as increased use of statin therapy meant that patients were not recruited at the pre-specified minimum enrolment rate. Early specialist assessment in the EXPRESS study was associated with an increased use of statin therapy, at 84% compared with 65%.

Blood pressure

This also included blood pressure-lowering therapy, a combination of angiotensin-converting enzyme inhibition and thiazide diuretic, if systolic blood pressure was ≥130 mmHg. Therefore, current UK guidance recommends the continuation of pre-existing statin therapy or its de novo introduction following stroke, and acknowledges the lack of evidence to inform blood pressure-lowering recommendations in acute stroke. No specific guidance is issued in respect of TIA, though early risk factor modification with statin and blood pressure-lowering therapy appears sensible.

Carotid artery stenosis

Evidence shows that for significant (≥50%) symptomatic carotid artery stenosis the greatest benefit of carotid endarterectomy is in those treated within 2 weeks, when the number needed to treat (NNT) is five, compared with 125 if surgery is delayed by over 3 months.

Atrial fibrillation

Atrial fibrillation patients, who have survived an acute stroke or TIA, are at highest risk of recurrent stroke at 12%

Table 21.3 Risk factor modification strategies

Strategy	Target population	Strokes avoided per year	Inferred NNT for target population
Carotid surgery	300	9	33
Aspirin	9240	60	167
Aspirin + DP-MR	7800	51	125
Clopidogrel	7800	51	125
Anticoagulation	960	70	13
BP lowering*	10800	184	59
LDL lowering†	9600	58	167
Stop smoking	2400	58	42

Adapted from GJ Hankey, J R Coll Physicians Edin b 2010. DP-MR, modified-release dipyridamole; BP: blood pressure; LDL, low density lipoprotein; *by 10 mmHg systolic BP; †by 1 mmol/L LDL.

per annum. In the context of TIA, current UK guidance recommends the immediate introduction of anticoagulation following TIA, though intracranial haemorrhage should be excluded and hypertension controlled first. (See also Chapter 5, and Stroke rehabilitation section.)

Lifestyle

Healthy lifestyle aspects of secondary prevention, include smoking cessation, alcohol consumption, exercise, healthy diet, etc. The educational opportunity in terms of TIA and stroke symptom recognition and the need for urgent action should be undertaken, and the patient appraised of relevant Driving and Vehicle Licensing Agency regulations.

The following table provides an indication of size of the group suitable for individual risk factor modification (see Table 21.3) and the number of strokes prevented per annum, applied to 10 000 prevalent and 2000 incident strokes and TIAs per million population.

Summary

TIA is an important risk factor for future stroke; this risk is front-loaded and validated scoring systems are available to identify those at highest risk. Patients should undergo timely specialist assessment and investigation, and risk factor modification therapy should be introduced urgently. In addition, ongoing public and healthcare professional education remains an important component of reducing the burden of disabling stroke by the initial inadequate management of TIA.

Further reading

Calvet D, Touze E, Oppenheim C, et al. (2009). DWI lesions and TIA etiology improve the prediction of stroke after TIA. *Stroke* **40**: 187–92.

Flossmann E, Rothwell PM. (2003). Prognosis of vertebro-basilar transient ischaemic attack and minor stroke. *Brain* **126**: 1940–54.

Giles MF, Rothwell PM (2010). Systematic review and pooled analysis of published and unpublished validations of the ABCD and ABCD2 transient ischemic attack risk scores. *Stroke* **41**: 667–73.

Giles MF, Rothwell PM (2007). Risk of stroke early after transient ischaemic attack: a systematic review and meta-analysis. *Lancet Neurol* **6**: 1063–72.

Hankey GJ (2010). Ischaemic stroke – prevention is better than cure. *J R Coll Physicians Edinb* **40**: 56–63.

National Collaborating Centre for Chronic Conditions (2008). Stroke: national clinical guideline for diagnosis and initial management of acute stroke and transient ischaemic attack (TIA). London, United Kingdom: Royal College of Physicians.

Rothwell PM, Eliasizw M, Gutnikov SA, *et al.* (2004). Endarterectomy for symptomatic carotid stenosis in relation to clinical subgroups and timing of surgery. *Lancet* **363**: 915–24.

Sprigg N, Machili C, Otter ME, *et al.* (2009). A systematic review of delays in seeking medical attention after transient ischaemic attack. *J Neurol Neurosurg Psychiatry* **80**: 871–5.

Acute stroke management

Access

Acute stroke management is a specialist endeavour. Almost all patients with stroke should be admitted to hospital, unless,

- symptoms are transient, with minimal disability (which can be difficult to tell without a full multidisciplinary assessment), and the patient can be assessed in a TIA clinic within a day or so
- the patient has severe prior disability, and a decision is taken that they are approaching the end of life.

Time spent in emergency departments and acute medical units is lost time. Admission should be directly to an acute stroke unit. The Face, Arm, and Speech Test (FAST) performed by paramedics will identify 80% of strokes and is sufficiently accurate to guide this decision. Many interventions are likely to have greater impact when delivered immediately, and complications can arise very early.

The first assessor should establish time of onset, and ask if thrombolysis might be possible (see section Thrombolysis).

Diagnosis

The initial task is to make, confirm or refute the diagnosis. 10–20% of patients referred to hospital with suspected stroke will have something else. These include hypoglycaemia, tumours, subdural haematomas, venous sinus thrombosis, cerebral abscess, seizures, and many non-specific symptoms with only a remote likelihood of being caused by stroke.

Diagnosis is primarily clinical ('sudden onset of focal neurological symptoms of presumed vascular origin and lasting more than 24 hours'). This requires careful history taking and perceptive neurological examination. Classification according to the Oxfordshire Community Stroke Project classification (see Table 21.4) gives information on

- anatomical localization
- likely pathology and possible aetiology (e.g. stroke likely to be embolic may be due to carotid disease, atrial fibrillation (AF) or endocarditis);
- prognosis.

Efforts should be made to explain the mechanism of the stroke, but in at least 30% of cases no convincing cause can be found despite comprehensive workup.

Investigation includes:

- *CT scanning* to diagnose haemorrhage and exclude mimics, rather than to diagnose infarcts. Bleeds cannot be reliably distinguished from infarcts clinically, but can be seen immediately on CT scans. Early features of infarction can appear within a few hours of onset, but CT is not sensitive.
- *MRI scanning* with diffusion-weighted imaging (DWI) is the best way to diagnose (and exclude) infarction, and can be extended to give carotid and intracranial angiography as well. The characteristic changes on DWI scans are apparent from 30 minutes after onset until about 10 days after the stroke.
- *ECG* will identify cardiac rhythm and ischaemia. Echocardiography is only needed in selected cases, where cardiac embolism is suspected, or no other cause has been found. Younger patients with unexplained stroke should have bubble contrast echo or transoesophogeal echocardiogram to exclude a patent foramen

Table 21.4 Oxfordshire Community Stroke Project Stroke Classification

Type	Features
Posterior circulation infarct (POCI)	Cranial nerve deficit with contralateral hemiparesis or sensory deficit, or bilateral stroke, or disorders of conjugate eye movement, or isolated cerebellar stroke, or isolated homonymous hemianopia
Lacunar infarcts (LACI)	Pure motor or pure sensory deficit affecting two out of three of face, arm and leg, or sensori-motor stroke (basal ganglia and internal capsule), or ataxic hemiparesis (cerebellar-type ataxia with ipsilateral pyramidal signs—internal capsule or pons); or dysarthria plus clumsy hand, or acute onset movement disorders (hemichorea, hemiballismus—basal ganglia)
Total anterior circulation infarct (TACI)	1. New higher cerebral function dysfunction: dysphasia/dyscalculia/apraxia/neglect/visuospatial problems plus 2. Homonymous visual field defect plus 3. Hemi-motor and/or sensory deficit of at least two areas of face, arm and leg motor and sensory deficit. In the presence of impaired consciousness, higher cerebral function and visual fields deficits are assumed
Partial anterior circulation infarct (PACI)	Two of the three components of TACI, or isolated dysphasia or other cortical dysfunction, or motor/sensory loss more limited than for a LACI

Reproduced from Harwood RH, Huwez F, Good D (2010). *Stroke Care: a practical manual* 2nd edn. Oxford University Press, Oxford.
See also: http://www.nle.nottingham.ac.uk/websites/stroke/

ovale. 24-hour ECG will pick up a few cases of paroxysmal AF that would otherwise be undetected, but is not required as a routine.

- *Early vascular imaging* (duplex ultrasound, MR or CT angiography) to identify carotid stenosis, occlusion or dissection. Imaging can also identify aneurysms, arteriovenous malformations, venous sinus thrombosis or tumours underlying bleeds, and may need repeating once a haematoma has resolved.
- *Blood tests* for inflammation (causal, complicating or co-morbid infection or vasculitis), thrombophilia, or other comorbidities.
- *In younger patients* think especially about the possibility of arterial dissection, drug abuse, HIV, and cardiogenic causes.

Management

Seven key elements are:

- accurate diagnosis
- reperfusion (thrombolysis), if <4.5 hours from onset
- physiological normalization
- prevention, detection, and aggressive treatment of complications
- early rehabilitation
- early institution of secondary prevention
- information and education, emotional support.

In very severe cases a decision to pursue end-of-life care may be appropriate. But predicting death early after stroke is unreliable; keep an open mind, and review plans if unexpected improvements are made.

Acute nursing care

The patient may be very ill, drowsy, immobile without sitting balance, and unable to communicate or swallow. Immediate plans should be made for physiological and neurological monitoring, pressure area care, manual handling, therapeutic positioning, and swallow should be assessed using a water swallow test. This assessment may require (very) early collaboration with a physiotherapist.

Patients less severely affected should sit out of bed, and attempts made to transfer or walk as soon as possible.

Plans should be made for nutrition, continence, venous thromboprohylaxis, explanation and giving of information to the patient and family.

The prevention of complications appears to be one of the most important elements of stroke unit care, including chest and urinary infections, falls, pressure sores, shoulder pain, and early development of abnormal muscle tone. Urinary catheters should be avoided, but can be difficult to argue against for a very 'heavy' drowsy patient with no sitting balance, especially if pressure areas are vulnerable.

Prevention of deep vein thrombosis (DVT) is contentious: early mobilization and good hydration are sensible; aspirin and low molecular weight heparin reduce DVT but have no impact on survival or function; elasticated compression stockings are of no benefit and can cause skin or vascular complications.

Half of stroke patients admitted to hospital have neurogenic dysphagia (unsafe swallow), and will tend to aspirate orally administered food and fluid (and saliva). This can result in aspiration pneumonia. A doctor or nurse should assess by observing swallowing of small volumes of tap water, usually following a set protocol. A 'safety-first' philosophy is adopted: if swallow is unsafe, the patient is made 'nil by mouth', and parenteral fluids given. Swallowing is retested daily. An assessment by a speech and language therapist may be required.

Acute management of intracerebral bleeds

- Haematomas expand within the first few hours. If the patient is anticoagulated, reverse it immediately with prothombin complex concentrate and vitamin K, even in cases where there is a metallic prosthetic heart valve. Risk of thrombosis or valve failure is about 0.2% per day when not anticoagulated (for both mitral and aortic valve positions.) Anticoagulation should be withheld for 2–4 weeks.
- Liaise with neurosurgeons. Following the negative STICH trial, many are reluctant to intervene, but this nihilism may be overdone, especially in relatively young patients, with moderate depression of conscious level (GCS 9–13) and relatively superficial haematomas. The STICH trial could have been falsely negative: it was underpowered, it excluded patients whom surgeons thought likely to benefit from operation, and had a moderate crossover rate in medically treated patients.
- Otherwise treat as for infarcts.
- Some international guidelines call for the reduction of systolic BP to 160 mmHg. This is probably safe, if not done too quickly or too much (no more than 25% reduction in mean blood pressure in 24 hours). However, there is a risk of cerebral under-perfusion, and as yet, no evidence of clinical benefit. In the UK, standard current management is not to lower blood pressure unless there

is another indication (such as encephalopathy) or blood pressure is very high (>220/120).

Most bleeds should have further imaging 4–6 weeks after the event to rule out abnormal underlying vascular pathology.

Physiological monitoring and normalization

The effectiveness of individual components of physiological normalization are uncertain, but a combination of interventions appears to be beneficial:

- Blood pressure: the greater danger is probably low blood pressure rather than high, and optimal blood pressure appears to be 140–180 mmHg systolic. Correct tachyarrhythmias (usually AF), keep well-hydrated (intravenous fluids if unable to swallow or for all but the mildest cases), and stop prior anti-hypertensive drugs if need be. Very high blood pressure may promote oedema formation and increases (by a small amount) the risk of vessel rupture and haemorrhagic transformation. Some guidelines suggest cautiously reducing very high blood pressure (e.g. >220/120).
- Hemicraniectomy: patients under 60 years within 48 hours of a very large middle cerebral artery infarct, with prominent oedema, and progressive drowsiness, may benefit from hemicraniectomy (forming a large bone flap) to release intracranial pressure. Fewer die, and some recover with no more than moderate disability, although the chances of survival with severe disability are increased.
- Glucose: observational studies suggest that high initial blood glucose is associated with poorer outcomes. Trial evidence on reducing glucose is inconclusive, but it seems sensible to reduce it to 5–10 mmol/L.
- Temperature: observational studies suggest that increases in initial blood glucose are also associated with poorer outcomes. Search for infection in those with pyrexia, and then administer paracetamol and a fan to try to reduce raised temperature. More aggressive attempts to reduce body temperature are not yet justified.
- Oxygen: monitor pulse oximetry and keep oxygen saturation above 95% using careful positioning and supplementary oxygen if needed.
- Early anticoagulation (initially with low molecular weight heparin) is rarely indicated, even in AF or other cardioembolism, but may be considered in cases of arterial dissection, venous sinus thrombosis (including where there is intracerebral bleeding), or if there is an underanticoagulated patient with a metallic heart valve. Typically warfarin is started 2 weeks after the acute stroke, often with relatively low doses owing to the initial potential for a prothrombotic state to develop. Some guidelines suggest omitting warfarin for 2 weeks after an infarct in a patient anti-coagulated for AF in order to reduce the risk of haemorrhagic transformation. If someone has an infarct whilst on anti-coagulants there is no clear indication for adding other agents (e.g. antithrombotics), nor for increasing target INR. Both of these increase the rate of subsequent intracranial haemorrhage.

Feeding and hydration

About half of patients admitted to hospital following a stroke cannot swallow safely. Feeding problems continue through both acute and sub-acute phases. Of those with problems initially:

- half are dead by 6 weeks
- 30% can feed orally within 2 weeks

- most of the rest recover safe swallowing over the next month
- long-term survival without safe swallowing is relatively uncommon.

There are good theoretical reasons for ensuring adequate hydration and nutrition:
- 10–30% of stroke patients are undernourished at onset, their outcomes are worse, and may improve with food supplements.
- venous thrombosis and pressure sores are more likely in dehydrated patients.
- inadequate cardiac filling pressure may result in decreased blood pressure, which may be harmful to brain perfusion.
- muscle is catabolized under conditions of subnutrition, causing atrophy and weakness.
- death results after 1–2 weeks with no fluid intake.

Some guidelines assist safe oral feeding:
- Thickened liquids and cold, soft, single consistency foods are easier to swallow.
- Ensure patient is sufficiently alert before attempting feeding.
- Sit the patient up (which can be difficult if there is poor trunk control).
- Risk of aspiration can be reduced by flexing the neck ('a chin tuck') before swallowing (which closes the airway and opens the gullet).
- Feed slowly, allowing time for each mouthful to be cleared before giving another.

If, despite these measures, swallowing is unsafe by day 2, consider nasogastric feeding. Mouth care and monitoring for recovery of swallowing should continue. A standardised tube-feeding regimen can be used initially. Refer to a dietician for assessment of individualized nutrition requirements and an appropriate feed prescription.

Nasogastric feeding has problems:
- Tubes are uncomfortable, both when inserted and when in place, and are often pulled out.
- Occasionally they can be misplaced into the trachea, and ensuring that this has not occurred causes much testing, delays, and missed feed or medication. If an acid pH (<5.5) can be detected on indicator paper after aspiration of stomach contents from the tube, then the tube is in the stomach. If not, a chest radiograph is needed. Auscultating over the stomach while blowing air down the tube with a syringe is unreliable.
- A loop or bridle passed behind the nasal septum can effectively secure a nasogastric tube, reducing the need for reinsertion and increasing feed volume delivered.

As an alternative, percutaneous endoscopic (PEG) or radiologically guided gastrostomy (RIG) can be used.
- They cause little discomfort, are difficult to dislodge, and can be managed outside acute hospitals.
- They may cause fewer problem with oesophageal reflux than nasogastric tubes.
- In the longer term they require some maintenance to prevent embedding in the gastric mucosa. The tube should be loosened, and rotated every 3–4 weeks.

Early gastrostomy placement brings no overall improvement in long term outcomes, and so can be deferred until there is a clear need:

- If a nasogastric tube cannot be tolerated.
- If long-term gastrostomy feeding is required (judged 4 to 6 weeks after onset).
- If transfer to a rehabilitation facility that cannot manage a nasogastric tube is planned.

Periprocedure mortality is about 1%, and local complications seen in up to 10%. RIG may be possible even if the patient is not fit for endoscopy. The procedure requires formal consent or a best interests assessment if the patient lacks capacity. If someone is clearly dying, inserting a feeding tube may not represent appropriate care, but keep an open mind as circumstances can change. Close liaison with family members and carers is required.

Beware the possibility of re-feeding syndrome if starvation has been prolonged: electrolyte derangement, rhabdomyolysis, heart and respiratory failure, hypotension, arrhythmias, seizures, and coma. To minimize the risks, give thiamine, start feed slowly, monitor serum phosphate, potassium, magnesium, and calcium daily for first 4 days, and correct if necessary. If phosphate is less than 0.5 mmol/L, give iv phosphate 50 mmol over 24 hours and repeat if necessary.

Speech and language therapists will assess more persistent cases. They will advise on the timing of reintroducing oral food and fluid, usually of modified consistency initially (appropriately trained nurses may also do this in some places).

Videopharyngography ('videofluoroscopy', a radiographic test of swallowing) may be required where 'silent aspiration' is suspected, usually on the advice of a speech and language therapist.

Early rehabilitation assessment

- In cases of severe disability, physiotherapists advise on positioning (to promote normal muscle tone, and avoid spasticity developing, and maximize lung ventilation), transfers, sitting and may even try early supported standing.
- In less severely affected cases, a physiotherapist should assess mobility and identify rehabilitation needs.
- Speech and language therapists mostly work assessing and treating with neurogenic dysphagia, but early plans should also be made for communication, especially in those with aphasia and relatively mild other disabilities (who may be discharged quickly). In these cases, there are almost always subtle visuospatial problems or apraxia, so an occupational therapy assessment is needed as well.
- Occupational therapy assessment may enable early discharge, identify cognitive or visuospatial abnormalities, or permit some rehabilitation in severely aphasic patients through engagement in familiar functional tasks.

Early complications

The prevention, detection and aggressive management of compilations is a key part of how stroke units work. 'Complications' is often used loosely to include neurological features such as neglect, or dysphagia, comorbidities such as arthritis or dementia, or recurrent vascular events (such as early recurrence of stroke or heart attack). True complications are new conditions arising as a result of the stroke, including:
- spasticity development
- aspiration pneumonia

- shoulder subluxation or shoulder pain
- delirium
- deep venous thrombosis and pulmonary embolism
- pressure sores
- catheter associated urinary infections
- psychological adjustment reaction
- malnutrition.

Acute stroke care is 'medically active' and at least one medical complication can be expected in half of hospitalised stroke patients. Stroke physicians therefore need a good grounding in acute general medicine.

Deep vein thrombosis and pulmonary embolism (PE) warrant some comment. PE is a common cause of death in the subacute phase after stroke (2–8 weeks). If they occur after an infarct standard anticoagulation is used (the benefit outweighs any theoretical increased risk of haemorrhagic transformation of the infarct). After an intracerebral bleed, anti-coagulation is usually unwise, but an inferior vena cava filter may be inserted instead.

Information

Tell patients and their relatives what a stroke is, the prospects for recovery, anticipated length of stay, and what is likely to happen next. Keep them updated with progress. They may be needed to help inform early decision-making. Driving regulations must be explained. Do not include too much too soon, however.

Multidisciplinary working

Teams work better than individuals in isolation. Nurses are key (being with the patient 24 hours per day). Allied health professionals have considerable expertise and should not be ignored or dominated by doctors. A neurological examination done by a neurophysiotherapist is at least as detailed as that done by a doctor (but subtly different: it is directed towards function rather than diagnosis). Occupational therapy is founded on sophisticated neuropsychology. Speech and language therapists are both expert in communication, but also act as advocates for people with communication disorders, especially where difficult decisions are to be made. Doctors should know what their particular expertise and responsibilities are, namely diagnosis and medical therapy. In the early stages, review and team communication should be daily.

Further reading

Harwood RH, Huwez F, Good D (2010). *Stroke Care; A Practical Manual*, 2nd edn. Oxford, Oxford University Press.

National Collaborating Centre for Chronic Diseases. National clinical guideline for diagnosis and initial management of acute stroke and transient ischaemic attack (TIA). Royal College of Physicians/NICE, 2008. (www.nice.org.uk).

Warlow CP, van Gijn J, Dennis MS, et al. (2008). *Stroke: Practical Management*, 3rd edn. Oxford, Blackwell.

Thrombolysis

Rationale

Stroke is a common and devastating condition. In the Western world, the lifetime risk of having a stroke after 55 years is one in five for women and one in six for men. One in four strokes occur in adults below 65 years old. After a stroke, one in three patients will die and half of all survivors will remain disabled at 1 year.

Ischaemic stroke, which accounts for 85% of all strokes, is usually caused by an acute occlusion of one or more intracerebral arteries with thrombus originating either from a proximal arterial atherothrombotic lesion or from a cardiac source.

Thrombolysis aims to restore vessel patency, which may in turn lead to an improvement in, or reversal of, the acute neurological syndrome.

Ischaemic core and penumbra

After arterial occlusion, there are two major zones of brain injury:

- The ischaemic core (central core of severely ischaemic or infarcted brain tissue).
- The ischaemic penumbra (a rim of mild-moderately ischaemic brain tissue surrounding the ischaemic core).

The ischaemic penumbra is at risk of neuronal death, but it is also potentially salvageable if timely recanalization of the occluded vessel restores perfusion (e.g. by thrombolysis).

Evidence to support the use of thrombolysis

Intravenous recombinant tissue plasminogen activator (rt-PA) is licensed for the treatment of acute ischaemic stroke if administered within 3 hours of stroke onset in selected patients.

In one meta-analysis, intravenous rt-PA given within 3 hours of onset reduces the odds of death or dependency compared to placebo (OR 0.64, 95% CI 0.5–0.83).

One recent randomized controlled trial (ECASS-3) found that intravenous rt-PA may also be effective when given between 3–4.5 hours after stroke onset.

The balance of benefit and risk for intravenous rt-PA given within 3 hours of stroke onset can be summarized as follows:

- For every 100 stroke patients thrombolysed using intravenous rt-PA, 32 will benefit and three will be harmed (due to intracranial haemorrhage).
- Intravenous rt-PA is 10 times more likely to help than to harm eligible stroke patients.

Time saved is brain saved

Approximately 2 million neurons die during every minute after an acute ischaemic stroke. Reperfusion should therefore be attempted as quickly as possible.

The earlier the thrombolysis is performed after stroke onset, the higher the likelihood of a favourable outcome at 3 months after stroke (i.e. the lower the number needed to treat, NNT) (see Table 21.5).

Methods of improving speed of thrombolysis include:

- better public awareness of stroke symptoms and how to respond in the event of an acute stroke (call for an ambulance)
- faster recognition of stroke symptoms by the paramedics (e.g. using the Face, Arm, and Speech Test, FAST) and immediate transfer to the hospital with the appropriate expertise

Table 21.5 Timing of thrombolysis can determine outcome at 3 months

Time of thrombolysis after stroke onset (min)	NNT for good outcome at 3 months after stroke
60	2
90	4
180	8
270	14

- faster access to neuroimaging
- more efficient emergency stroke pathway within the hospital including a protocol for thrombolysis
- use of telemedicine to enable remote decision-making by stroke specialists without delay.

Pre-thrombolysis medical assessment

- Acute stroke can be a difficult diagnosis to make. One in three emergency admissions with suspected stroke may be a mimic, especially those who present with cognitive impairment and abnormal physical signs in systems other than the neurological system.
- An efficient but careful clinical assessment should distinguish stroke from mimics such as migraine, epilepsy (Todd's paresis) and hypoglycaemia.
- Simple assessment tools such as the Recognition of Stroke in the Emergency Room (ROSIER) can improve the accuracy of diagnosis (positive predictive value 90%, negative predictive value 88%).
- Brain scan (usually CT, sometimes MRI) should be performed immediately (see below).
- Stroke severity should be assessed using the National Institute of Health Stroke Scale (NIHSS, www.nih-strokescale.org).
- Patient should be screened according to the inclusion and exclusion criteria below:

Inclusion criteria
- Definitive diagnosis of acute stroke
- Clear time of onset (or last known feeling normal)
- Age 18–80 years old

Exclusion criteria
- Brain scan showing intracranial haemorrhage, any suspicious lesion (e.g. tumour) or a very large area of ischaemia (>1/3 middle cerebral artery territory)
- Rapidly improving or very minor stroke symptoms
- NIHSS score >25 (i.e. very severe stroke)
- BP >185/110 mmHg (can lower with iv glyceryl trinitrate or labetolol before administering bolus)
- On heparin or warfarin (with INR >1.7)
- Blood glucose <2.7 or >22 mmol/L
- Previous stroke or serious head injury <3 months
- Any history of intracranial haemorrhage, aneurysm, tumour, arteriovenous malformation, spinal or cranial surgery, haemorrhagic retinopathy
- Symptoms suggestive of subarachnoid haemorrhage (even if brain scan is normal)
- Major surgery, external cardiac massage, or obstetric delivery <14 days

- Gastrointestinal or urinary tract haemorrhage <21 days
- Known clotting disorder or platelets <100/mm^3
- Epileptic seizure as the initial symptom
- Bacterial endocarditis, pericarditis, acute pancreatitis, oesophageal varices, peptic ulceration <3 months, aortic aneurysm, active hepatitis, cirrhosis
- Prior history of stroke and concomitant diabetes
- Puncture of non-compressible blood vessel <14 days
- Comorbidities e.g. renal failure, liver failure, or malignancy are not contraindications *per se*, hence no need to wait for laboratory results before treatment

Administration of rt-PA

Decision on the use of intravenous rt-PA should only be made by senior physicians who have received appropriate experience and training in acute stroke management and thrombolysis.

The balance of benefit and risk should be clearly explained to the patient (and family/carer if available)

Intravenous rt-PA is administered at a dose of 0.9 mg/kg body weight (maximum dose of 90 mg):

- 10% of the total dose is given as a bolus injection over 2 minutes
- 90% of the total dose is infused over 1 hour.

Post-thrombolysis care (first 24 hours)

- Patient should be managed in the Acute Stroke Unit with high-dependency nursing care.
- Patient requires continuous monitoring of cardiac rhythm, blood pressure, oxygen saturation and Glasgow Coma Score (GCS).
- Patient should be kept nil by mouth if water swallow test has shown that swallowing is unsafe.
- No urinary catheter, nasogastric tube, central venous line, or arterial line.
- NIHSS score should be repeated at two hours and 24 hours post-thrombolysis to exclude neurological deterioration.
- Brain scan should be repeated at 24 hours to exclude haemorrhage. No aspirin, heparin or warfarin should be given until after the repeat scan.

Post-thrombolysis complications

High blood pressure
- Patients with blood pressure over 185/110 mmHg after thrombolysis are at a significantly higher risk of developing intracranial haemorrhage.
- Blood pressure over 185/110 mmHg must be rapidly controlled using iv glyceryl trinitratrate infusion or labetolol (as bolus injection or infusion).

Neurological deterioration
- Intracranial haemorrhage should be suspected and a repeat CT brain scan should be performed immediately.
- Any haemorrhage (intracranial or systemic) should be treated according to local protocol, including obtaining an urgent senior haematology opinion.

Anaphylactic reaction (or angioedema)
This rare complication should be treated as usual by stopping the infusion and the administration of hydrocortisone and antihistamine intravenously and adrenaline 1mg subcutaneously.

Ongoing clinical trials

There are a number of ongoing clinical trials in stroke thrombolysis. For example, combining standard rt-PA thrombolysis with antiplatelet therapy (ARTIS trial), using a new thrombolytic agent such as Desmoteplase (DIAS-4), and extending the window of treatment up to 6 hours (IST-3).

Importantly, more data are needed on the effects of rt-PA in the following subgroups of patients:
- older patients (>80 years)
- patients with very mild or severe stroke
- patients with prior history of stroke and diabetes
- patients with different findings on neuroimaging (e.g. presence of visible infarct, cerebral atrophy and white matter ischaemia)
- prior use of medications e.g. antiplatelet agents.

Clinical governance

It is important to monitor the outcome and performance of stroke patients who have received thrombolysis, (e.g. through Safe Implementation of Treatments in Stroke Registry, SITS, https://sitsinternational.org).

Further reading

Demaerschalk BM (2007). Thrombolytic therapy for acute ischemic stroke: the likelihood of being helped versus harmed. *Stroke* **38**: 2215–16.

Hacke W, Kaste M, Bluhmki E, et al. (2008). Thrombolysis with alteplase 3 to 4.5 hours after acute ischemic stroke. *N Engl J Med* **359**: 1317–29.

Hand P, Kwan J, Lindley RI, et al. (2006). Distinguishing between stroke and mimic at the bedside: the Brain Attack Study. *Stroke* **37**: 769–75.

Kwan J, Hand P, Sandercock P (2004). A systematic review of barriers to delivery of thrombolysis for acute stroke. *Age Ageing* **33**: 116–21.

Lees KR, Bluhmki E, von KummerR, et al. (2010). Time to treatment with intravenous alteplase and outcome in stroke: an updated pooled analysis of ECASS, ATLANTIS, NINDS, and EPITHET trials. *Lancet* **375**: 1695–703.

Wardlaw JM, Murray V, Berge E, et al. (2009). Thrombolysis for acute ischaemic stroke. *Cochrane Database Syst Rev* **7**(4): CD000213.

Stroke rehabilitation

Stroke can be a devastating condition. Stroke disease accounts for 4% of the NHS budget and is the leading cause of adult disability. Recovery after stroke is of two types, intrinsic and adaptive. Intrinsic recovery is as a result of either the ischaemic penumbra regaining function or cerebral plasticity whereby other areas of the brain adapt and compensate for the damaged areas to maintain a particular function. Adaptive recovery involves an individual or those involved with his/her care adopting strategies to overcome disability.

The aims of rehabilitation are twofold. The first aim is to optimize function, through minimizing any deficits and optimizing residual function. The second is to help the patient come to terms with any residual deficits and adapt to life at a different functional level. Aspects of rehabilitation such as goal setting are covered in Chapter 15, Rehabilitation.

This chapter will also discuss some of the longer term consequences of stroke, many of which become apparent during the rehabilitation period.

Stroke units

These are dedicated wards specializing in caring for patients after a stroke. Their success reflects the benefits of multi-disciplinary team working and importance of specialist knowledge of stroke disease and its complications. Management of these complications includes early addressing of issues such as dysphagia, nutrition and oral care, continence, early management of pressure care, through to vigilance over the development of aspiration pneumonia. They also provide early mobilization and rehabilitation, alongside appropriate information and psychological support for the patient and their families.

Stroke rehabilitation should start from the day of admission, with ascertaining the patient's pre-morbid function and knowledge of their background and personal interests, which in turn can guide goal setting.

Driven by the National Sentinel Audit for Stroke and Stroke Improvement Programme, the majority of patients in the UK are now cared for on dedicated stroke units. When compared with non-specialist care, the benefits of these include

- 3% absolute reduction in mortality (odds ratio 0.86; 95% CI 19–67)
- 5% absolute reduction in death institutional care (odds ratio 0.81; 95% CI 15–40)
- 6% absolute reduction in death/dependency (odds ratio 0.79; 95% CI 0.71–0.88).

An alternative way of presenting this is that for patients treated on an organized stroke unit:

- for every 29 patients there will be one extra survivor
- for every 20 patients treated there will be one extra patient discharged home
- for every 18 patients treated there will be one extra independent survivor.

These benefits are seen regardless of age, gender, stroke type, and stroke severity, and have been shown to persist up to 10 years after the original admission.

The team on the stroke unit should include specialists from medicine, nursing, physiotherapy, occupational therapy (OT), speech and language therapy (SALT), and dietitians, as well as support, from psychology and counselling services and social work.

Patients should be treated on a stroke unit throughout their inpatient stay.

Assessment of function

Functional scales for the objective assessment of patients are described in Chapter 2. The scale most commonly used for stroke patients is the Oxford Handicap Scale (see Table 21.6), a modification of the Rankin scale. At a very simplistic level, patients scoring 2 or less are deemed to have had a good outcome, while those scoring higher a poor outcome.

Deficits following stroke

It is important that all patients are screened for common problems, e.g. swallowing, hemianopia, depression.

Mobility

The main presenting feature with most strokes is unilateral weakness. Most patients cite a return of independent mobility as one of their key aims from the rehabilitation process. Early mobilization is a key feature of stroke unit care. Nurses and physiotherapists work closely together to optimize mobility with active involvement of carers where possible.

There are differing approaches to physical rehabilitation, with the two main types being neurophysiological and motor learning. Biofeedback and training with a moving platform are promising interventions to improve balance. Repetitive practice of functional tasks, high intensity therapy and fitness training appear to be effective ways of improving mobility. The current stroke quality standard as outlined in the National Clinical Guideline for Stroke is that 'patients should be offered a minimum of 45 minutes for a minimum of 5 days per week at a level that enables the patient to meet their rehabilitation goals for as long as they are continuing to benefit from therapy and are able to tolerate it'.

Trunk control is essential for sitting balance, and in turn standing balance and walking. Prior to this returning, patients can sit out in appropriate chairs, such as a tilt and space chair, which through leaning the patient back to varying degrees according to their needs, enables them to get used to a sitting posture. Mirrors can also aid the patients in seeing their own posture and learning to correct this for themselves.

Table 21.6 Oxford Handicap Scale

0	No symptoms.
1	Minor symptoms which do not interfere with lifestyle
2	Minor handicap. Symptoms which lead to some restriction in lifestyle but do not interfere with the patients' ability to look after themselves.
3	Moderate handicap. Symptoms which significantly restrict lifestyle and prevent totally independent existence.
4	Moderately severe handicap. Symptoms which clearly prevent independent existence although not needing constant care and attention.
5	Severe handicap. Totally dependent, requiring constant attention day and night.

Bamford JM, Sandercock PAG, et al. (1989). Interobserver agreement for the assessment of handicap in stroke patients. Stroke **20**: 828.

Other options for helping motor recovery include orthoses: e.g. an ankle–foot orthoses (AFO) for foot drop, to prevent the foot tripping the patient over. Functional electrical stimulation (FES involves stimulation of the nerve (or occasionally muscles) directly. It can be considered in patients where an AFO is not effective in improving foot drop sufficiently

Upper limb rehabilitation

Between 50% and 70% of stroke patients have persistent arm functional limitations in the longer term. Repetitive functional task practice appears to be beneficial in improving upper limb function.

Constraint-induced movement therapy (CIMT) is a valuable intervention for carefully selected patients. This involves restraining the unaffected limb, thus ensuring that the affected limb is used as much as possible. It should only be considered for patients more than 2 weeks after their stroke, who can walk independently and are able to consent to the treatment. Patients should have at least 10° of voluntary finger extension. Other interventions which look promising but which require further evaluation include mental practice, EMG biofeedback, and robotics.

Spasticity

This is common and develops in the weeks following a stroke with the imbalance of flexors and extensors, resulting in the typical flexed position of arms and legs of a pyramidal weakness. Discriminating between how much of a patient's deficit relates to spasticity *per se* or their other deficits (e.g. motor) can be difficult. Early intervention from the therapists with passive stretching and/or splinting is essential, as is controlling any pain which may be contributing to the problem. The evidence base for the management of spasticity post-stroke is weak, though options include:

- Medication e.g. baclofen, tizanidine or gabapentin. (NB these may all cause sedation, increased falls, and delirium).
- Local injection of botulinum toxin where there is focal spasticity affecting one or two joints. This treatment is an adjunct to ongoing physiotherapy and injections may need to be repeated every few months.
- Intrathecal baclofen infusion.
- Phenol nerve block: this is irreversible and is only for patients with severe spasticity which precludes comfortable positioning (e.g. the patient is unable to sit out in a wheelchair).

The last two of these options should only be administered in the context of a specialist service or clinical trial. The Modified Ashworth Scale can be used to objectively assess improvements with spasticity.

Neglect

Neglect is the lack of awareness of one side of the body despite the presence of sensory input on this side. It can result, for example, in patients not eating a full meal or bumping into things on the affected side. With therapy, the aim is to improve aspects such as tracking across to the affected side and stimulation on this side (for example, patients should not be in beds adjacent to a wall on the affected side.) Other approaches include securing the unaffected limb (with patient consent; see above), such that the patient must use the affected limb, with faster improvements on this side.

Visual loss

The visual loss associated with stroke is usually a hemianopia. Sudden visual loss can be devastating for patients. While the stroke will usually result in a specific field defect rather than bilateral visual loss, many older patients may well have other pathology which reduces vision, such as glaucoma, or macular degeneration. Helping patients adjust to this deficit, including with help from sensory deprivation teams, can help improve function.

Hearing loss

The exact nature of stroke-related hearing loss is unclear, though hearing does not tend to be affected in the same way as vision by stroke disease because there is bilateral cerebral representation. However, it may be an issue which limits rehabilitation, either through further deficits from the stroke or the communication problems associated with hearing loss. Basic interventions such as ensuring the ears are clear from wax and the hearing aid is working should not be overlooked (see Chapter 14).

Cognitive impairment

A significant number of patients will have some cognitive impairment prior to having a stroke, and with others, underlying cognitive impairment becomes apparent follow a stroke which is not entirely explained through the region of brain affected by the acute event. All patients should be screened for cognitive impairment. Many patients have varying degrees of leukoaraiosis evident on imaging, although the image appearances do not always correlate with the degree of functional deficit.

Rehabilitation for patients with cognitive deficits can be difficult, with little or no carry over between therapy sessions. Many patients with cognitive impairment need support, such as repeated prompts. Other problems associated with this include increased impulsivity (e.g. patients getting up from their chairs despite a high falls risk) or poor attention span.

Approaches in rehabilitation are the same as for general advice here, including: not jumping from topic to topic; early establishment of a routine; optimizing sensory input through ensuring that spectacles are clean and worn, possibly avoiding bifocals (can increase falls risk with downward vision making the floor out of focus) and optimizing hearing; and placing calendars with days crossed out and clocks to help orientation. Further help can be through including pictures of the key members of staff caring from them, including the doctors, nurses and therapists.

Dysphasia

This can limit progress even when the patient has made a good physical recovery. It often occurs alongside severe perceptual problems, such as the inability to recognise common objects. Sometimes it is not initially recognised and patients may be labelled as being confused.

The speech and language therapists are essential with assessment and treatment here, and often do joint sessions with the other members of the multidisciplinary team and family. Communication can be enhanced through

- keeping to one topic of conversation at a time so things are in context
- maximizing use of non-verbal communication, such as gestures for drinking when asking if thirsty
- mixing written and verbal communication: patients may be able to understand better with sensory input from both
- communication books with pictures illustrating what you are trying to say e.g. pictures of a toilet, or illustrating symptoms such as pain.

Dysphagia and feeding

All stroke patients should remain nil by mouth and be rapidly assessed for their ability to swallow on arrival to hospital, whether through specialist SALT input or through appropriately trained nursing staff doing an initial screen.

Patients who are unable to swallow should receive intravenous or subcutaneous fluids until supplementary feeding is established. Maintaining good mouth care is also very important. Early initiation of supplemental feeding should be instigated where the patient is unable to meet their nutritional requirements, typically with a nasogastric tube of the first instance, and then subsequently via percutaneous endoscopic gastrostomy (PEG) tube or equivalent. Patients who are unable to swallow should be reassessed regularly to see if the swallow has improved and they may then be offered a modified or normal diet. More formal assessments of swallowing can be done through videofluoroscopy. Caution should be exercised as swallowing can vary with time, such as with fatiguing through the course of a meal or being worse when the patient is tired.

Typical problems seen with swallowing following a stroke include:

- delayed swallow initiation
- incomplete clearance of a food bolus, often with the need for prompts for a second swallow to clear it
- poor cough reflex; when the cough reflex is absent, can cause false reassurance that the bolus has been cleared unless voice is subsequently assessed and found to be 'wet'
- the presence or absence of a gag reflex is not helpful in assessing whether or not a patient can swallow safely.

Often the voice is dysarthric, which should prompt suspicions that the swallow is weak. Basic measures to optimise swallowing include ensuring the patient is awake and alert, giving patients enough time to eat without rushing them and positioning them as upright as possible prior to feeding (ideally sitting out). Some patients will improve with smaller meals or snacks given frequently, rather than being reliant on one or two main meals through the day. Patients should be monitored carefully for development of aspiration pneumonia.

For patients with minor dysphagia, achieving a reasonable oral intake with a palatable diet is not usually a major problem. Difficulties come with more severe levels of dysphagia requiring very thickened drinks, which many find unpalatable and so stop drinking. Thickened drinks are reported to taste like wallpaper paste. The Frazier free water protocol allows dysphagic patients free access to water, assuming it does not cause distress through gagging. They argue that the risks from aspiration (which can occur anyway) are outweighed by the benefits of improved fluid intake.

In order to try improving quality of life for patients with severe dysphagia, tasters can still be given, whereby the patient enjoys the gustatory sensations from food though without necessarily swallowing them.

Some patients have problems with pooling of secretions in the valleculae. This can be eased in some with atropine 1% one or two drops given sublingually up to three times per day (the same drops as are used in glaucoma; unlicensed for this indication) or ipratropium spray to the mouth. These methods avoid the systemic side effects, such as confusion, seen with measures such as hyoscine patches.

Where patients are to be discharged home with feeding tubes, either they or their family/carers will need training on day to day care of them and the possible complications associated with them.

Continence

Loss of continence is a common consequence of severe stroke and its presence/absence at 1 week is a helpful guide for independence at 1 year. Continence problems are a major source of distress to the patient and significantly increase the risk of pressure sores. The extra burden for carers from incontinence can preclude a patient's discharge home.

The evidence base for managing post-stroke incontinence, both urinary and faecal, is unfortunately limited, with the mainstays of treatment being the same as for non-stroke patients. This includes the exclusion of urinary tract infections; optimizing fluid intake; and avoidance of medication that may affect continence (e.g. diuretics, alcohol, caffeine, cholinesterase inhibitors). Pelvic floor exercises and regular toileting can reduce the number of episodes of incontinence and can be used to gradually retrain the bladder, albeit with varying degrees of success. Indwelling urinary catheters should only be used once other measures have failed or where there are specific concerns such as pressure area damage.

Faecal continence can be improved with ensuring an optimal stool consistency through dietary modification and adequate fluid intake, often with extra stool softeners combined with establishing a regular pattern. For other patients, regular enemas or suppositories may be required, which can ensure there is some control over when the bowels are opened and distress minimized.

Psychological effects of stroke

Strokes give patients no time to adjust to their sudden change of circumstances. For minor strokes, adjustment is usually fairly straightforward. However, for more major strokes the impact can be devastating both to the patient and their family. An adjustment period is common in these early phases, following along similar stages to those seen following bereavement, and the stroke team's role is to support the patient and their families through this with information and encouragement.

Depression and/or anxiety are very common following a stroke. Precise figures for their incidence and prevalence are variable, though they probably affect around 30% of patients. National stroke guidelines recommend all stroke units should screen patients for depression using validated tools. Depression is treatable in around 80% of patients and causes suffering both to the patient and their family, and so it is essential that it is not missed. However, prior to starting medication for this, it should be noted that the depressive symptoms in many patients improve in parallel with motor and functional improvements.

Presentation of depression may be atypical, which in turn accounts for why it is difficult to detect. Sometimes, it will present with the patient not engaging with therapy sessions. All patients should be screened for this regularly (e.g. with the General Health Questionnaire (GHQ-12) or Patient Health Questionnaire (PHQ-9)). Support from a clinical psychologist can be invaluable. Treatment is with support from the team and family, though finding the balance between being encouraging and positive without giving false hope and raising unrealistic expectations is sometimes difficult. Antidepressant medication, such as with SSRIs, and counselling services are also key to helping. Where anxiety is sufficient to require medication, either a short-term course of benzodiazepines can be tried, or anti-depressants with significant anxiolytic properties, such as mirtazapine, can be used.

Emotionalism, or emotional lability, may be seen following a stroke. With this, the patient flips from being happy to sad and then back again, often without major attached emotion. This often improves with time, although sometimes depression can develop which will need treatment as outlined above. Reassurance and explanation about what is happening is often sufficient, though in other patients it can be quite severe, and mood stabilizing agents, such as sodium valproate, have been tried with varying degrees of success.

The psychiatric sequelae from a stroke can be very difficult for the family as well as the patient, and so they will also need support and clear explanations of why they have occurred, the treatment plan and the prognosis. For patients in the community, it can also add to the sense of burden and carer strain.

Other complications
Stroke patients may develop a number of complications during the rehabilitation period. For in-patient rehabilitation patients, Langhorne et al found post-stroke complications occurred in 85% of patients, including recurrent stroke (9%), epileptic seizure (3%), urinary tract infection (24%), chest infection (22%), other infections (19%), falls (25%), and those with serious injury (5%), pressure sores (21%), thromboembolism (3%); shoulder pain (9%) and other pain (34%), and confusion (56%).

With regard to falls, there is a paradox, whereby as patients go from being immobile to mobile following a stroke, their falls risk increases. Osteoporosis is a common condition, and its prevalence is even higher in patients unable to get outside. Osteoporosis is increased specifically in the paretic limb. Treatment with high-dose vitamin D and calcium is required, often combined with a bisphosphonate (caution with dysphagic patients; consider intravenous zoledronate) or strontium (although will increase risk of venous thromboembolic disease).

Patients may develop pain following a stroke. Sometimes this relates to a pre-existing problem, such as osteoarthritis. On other occasions, it reflects the tonic imbalance following the stroke, such as with shoulder pain, which can also be associated with subluxation. Analgesia, physiotherapy, and botulinum toxin may be helpful. Central neuropathic pain should be suspected where there is hyperaesthesia and no obvious other focus for the pain. It can be difficult to treat, and medications such as amitriptyline, gabapentin, and sodium valproate can all be tried. Where mood is also a problem, medication such as duloxetine can improve both.

Barriers to rehabilitation and failure to progress
The factors affecting rehabilitation potential are discussed in Chapter 15. Specific issues related to stroke are predominantly associated with the severity of the stroke, though younger patients tend to have better potential to overcome even quite severe disability.

The natural history of strokes involves patients getting to their worst functional level at onset. From there, patients usually improve. Where patients deteriorate further, the most common reasons are concomitant infection or other medical illness, medication, or a further stroke. Failure to engage in rehabilitation or failure to

progress despite expectations should prompt a review of the patient's mood to ensure there is no underlying depression. Some patients deteriorate significantly on the wards, most commonly associated with problems such as aspiration pneumonia. For some of these patients, rather than active management, such as with antibiotics, a palliative approach may be more appropriate. Strokes can have a huge impact on quality of life, and this can be at a level the patients would not have wanted.

Discharge planning
Discharge planning should be an ongoing process and the patient and their family should be actively involved in decision-making.

The timing of discharge is dependent on functional level and cognitive ability, availability of local community rehabilitation schemes, and family support. Some patients may be impulsive as a result of cognitive deficit or pre-morbid personality, thus exposing themselves to increased risks such as falls. Ideally all patients with ongoing rehabilitation or social care needs and their families should have discharge planning meeting with all the therapists, nurses and doctors involved being present. Frequently the discussions are around acknowledging the risks, making conscious plans and decisions around these, and jointly assessing the acceptability of these risks and discussing expectations and available services. There are often compromises that have to be made, such as with the patient remaining downstairs, or not being able to get outdoors.

Early supported discharge
Most patients are keen to return home as soon as possible and benefit from continuing rehabilitation in familiar surroundings. Early supported discharge services, which provide levels of specialist services equivalent to stroke unit care, can reduce long term dependency and admission to institutional care as well as reducing the length of hospital stay for carefully selected patients. 44% of stroke services in the UK currently provide early supported discharge. Targeted rehabilitation to address mobility, leisure, and transport may be effective in reducing the longer term consequences of stroke.

Approaches to rehabilitation
Formal rehabilitation sessions are typically done as one-to-one sessions with the patients and their therapist. This enables assessment and feedback which in turn helps focus on specific issues for the rehabilitation.

Sometimes it can help for family members to be present during the session, with benefits including the sense of inclusion for the families. A family's presence aids communication and understanding of the impact of stroke, such that they can see for themselves how the patient is progressing, rather than hearing about it second hand. It also helps the family see how to conduct transfers and care for the patient safely (both for them and the patient). From this, it can also aid discharge planning, as the families have a direct feel for how much support is required after discharge. From the patient's perspective, it helps them to feel supported by their family and gives more time together with them. Group sessions can also be helpful, and increase interaction between patients and thus increasing their social interactions as well as the specific issue being addressed. These include:

- Cooking sessions: rather than individual kitchen assessments, patients together can make, for example, cakes.

These can also help with patients with poor appetites, as they encourage snacking between meals and so increase calorie intake.

- Balance classes: for patients at risk of falls, it can help to see that they are not alone and to share the sessions with others, analogous to going to the gym by oneself or playing in a team. Sessions can include exercises such as passing a ball to each other.
- Gardening sessions: many patients love gardening and this has the advantage of getting them outside during periods of good weather, and facilitating hobbies and interests after discharge.
- Thinking groups/newspaper groups: these can be tailored to the cognition of the class. It encourages social interaction while stimulating the patient mentally.

Much of rehabilitation is with what happens between the formal sessions. With the aim of developing maximal independence, through doing the day-to-day activities, patients will improve. Typically this is with the nurses and care assistants on the wards or just through being at home, where the transfers and independent washing and dressing are done throughout the week and weekends. Often this aspect of rehabilitation is unappreciated, with all the focus being on the specific sessions.

Other issues arising following stroke

Legal and financial
The nature by which strokes come out of the blue often leaves people unprepared. Patients may be intestate or have nobody who can take care of their finances. If they are dysphasic or have become very cognitively impaired, it can be very difficult and time consuming to address this. Also, difficult decisions regarding ceiling of care or placement, if they are unable to express their own wishes, can also complicate matters. Issues regarding capacity are discussed in Chapter 12.

In order to optimize communication, the Speech and Language Therapists (SALT) are invaluable. Communication can be enhanced with visual aids, such as photographs, with patients being able to choose whom to give Power of Attorney to. While there is a presumption of capacity, clearly extreme caution needs to be used in these decisions, and the patient asked the questions on a number of different occasions and by different members of the team (e.g. SALT, consultant, social worker). A number of patients can be shown to give reliable 'yes/no' answers, and thus demonstrate capacity to enable them to make the decision. Where the patient is unable to demonstrate capacity and/or is inconsistent with their answers, then the Court of Protection must be involved. In England and Wales, for patients without anyone close to them who is able to represent their interests, support from an Independent Mental Capacity Advocate (IMCA) should be sought (or equivalent.) This help will also be needed where long-term placement may be required.

Driving
In the UK, patients are not allowed to drive following a stroke until at least 4 weeks after and on the advice of a doctor. Factors that affect the resumption of driving include: functional deficit and the ability to use the controls (or have a car adapted sufficiently); cognitive impairment; visual field defects; and sensory inattention. Specialist assessments are available in many areas for patients with residual neurological deficits who wish to return to driving.

Prognosis following strokes
Predicting the extent of improvement is difficult as patients all progress differently, although through the Oxford Community Stoke Project classification, some objective information can be given (see section Definition of stroke and transient ischaemic attack). Another simple means of predicting the likelihood of being independent in activities of daily living at 1 year is through maintaining or losing continence at 1 week following the stroke.

Patients tend to improve quite quickly early on, and then their rate of progress slows and plateaus. Typically the majority of the improvements will be in the first 6 months following the stroke, although smaller improvements can be seen even years afterwards. Recognizing the stage where patient's improvements slow down is important, as it marks the stage at which time one should concentrate on working with the patient to accept the level of recovery where they have plateaued. Clearly, other medical issues such as new infection or depression should be considered.

Prognosis following cerebral haemorrhage is harder to predict than for ischaemic strokes. While the mortality is higher in the acute phase, after this, often patients seem to do 'disproportionately' well for the extent of their initial deficit. Patients with a cerebral bleed should have further imaging after 6 weeks to exclude any underlying conditions such as a space-occupying lesion or vascular abnormality, which in turn may affect prognosis.

Secondary prevention
For patients who are relatively independent and have a good prognosis, decisions on secondary prevention are generally straightforward and follow contemporary evidence based guidelines. However, for many of the frailer older patients with an uncertain prognosis, things can be more complex. On the one hand, one does not want to deny them appropriate medical care or have further strokes; on the other, one wants to keep the medication burden and side effects down to a minimum. Typically these patients would not have been included in the clinical trials, and the same level of benefit cannot be assumed. These patients may well be cognitively impaired or dysphasic, thus making conversations regarding their wishes harder. It is sometimes appropriate to concentrate just on giving medicines that will directly improve quality of life, such as antidepressants, rather than those to improve longevity, such as statins and antiplatelet agents.

Conclusions
Stroke rehabilitation requires careful assessment and input from a multidisciplinary team. Active involvement of patients and carers where possible, aids the rehabilitation process. Stroke units and ongoing rehabilitation with an early supported discharge team have been shown to improve patient outcomes and are the cornerstones of high-quality stroke care.

Further reading
Bamford JM, Sandercock PAG, et al. (1989). Interobserver agreement for the assessment of handicap in stroke patients. Stroke 20: 828.

Intercollegiate Stroke Working Party (2008). National Clinical Guideline for Stroke, 3rd edn. London, Royal College of Physicians.

Johansson BB (2000). Brain Plasticity and stroke rehabilitation: the Willis lecture. Stroke 31: 223–30.

Harwood RH, Huwez F, Good D (2010). *Stroke Care: A Practical Manual*, 2nd edn. Oxford Care Manuals. Oxford, OUP.

Kalra L, Wolfe C, Rudd A (2010). *A Practical Guide to Comprehensive Stroke Care*. World Scientific Press.

Langhorne P, Coupar F, Pollock A (2009). Motor recovery after stroke: a systematic review. *Lancet Neurol* **8**: 741–54.

Langhorne P, Stott DJ, Robertson L, *et al.* (2000). Medical complications after stroke: a multicenter study. *Stroke* **31**: 1223–9.

Panther K (2005). The Frazier Free Water Protocol. Perspectives on Swallowing and Swallowing Disorders. *Dysphagia* **14**: 4–9.

Stroke Association: www.stroke.org.uk

Warlow CP, van Gijn J, Sandercock P, *et al.* (2008). *Stroke: Practical Management*, 3rd edn. Oxford, UK: Blackwell Science.

Secondary prevention of stroke

Background

Acute treatment of ischaemic stroke has limited applicability (thrombolysis) or only marginal benefit (early aspirin). Thus a comprehensive approach, incorporating co-ordinated multidisciplinary rehabilitation in a designated stroke unit and preventive interventions is essential to tackle the 'stroke epidemic'.

There is convincing evidence to support the efficacy of interventions for prevention of stroke. Although the relative benefits from primary prevention (of first stroke) are small and the target population is difficult to define, secondary preventive intervention (in those with cerebrovascular disease including previous transient ischaemic attack (TIA) or previous ischaemic stroke) can be focused on a well-defined subset of the population who are at considerably higher risk. Effective secondary prevention has the potential to reduce the annual 53 700 recurrent strokes in England and Wales by a half to two-thirds.

Preventive interventions

Secondary preventive interventions can be classified into three main categories: lifestyle changes; medical therapies; and surgical intervention for carotid disease.

Lifestyle changes

Most evidence in this category is in relation to primary prevention. Tobacco use increases the incidence of stroke by 50%, the risk falling to similar levels as non-smokers after about 5 years of cessation. A combination of professional support and pharmacological therapy can double rates of cessation. Dietary measures which may reduce stroke risk include reduced sodium intake in hypertension, increased consumption of fish/fish oils, and fruit and vegetables. Exercise can halve the relative risk of stroke (RR 0.41), and more strenuous activity is associated with greater benefits. Since each unit increase in body mass index (BMI) is associated with a 6% relative increase in stroke risk, maintaining an optimal weight is important (BMI 20–25 kg/m^2).

Medical

Antithrombotic

In a meta-analysis of trials studying antithrombotic therapy, people with a history of TIA/stroke had a 21.4% risk of further vascular events (over a mean of 29 months), with antiplatelet therapy reducing the absolute risk by 3.6% (number needed to treat (NNT) 28). Adding dipyridamole MR to aspirin is associated with an 18% reduction in vascular events. Clopidogrel monotherapy is equivalent to the aspirin–dipyridamole combination.

Although the SIGN guidelines accept both as initial therapy, the NICE/RCP guidance suggests clopidogrel only when there is genuine intolerance to aspirin. The CAPRIE study suggested that clopidogrel is slightly more effective than aspirin in reducing vascular events in a population at high risk, though the relative risk reduction of 7.3% in those with previous stroke/TIA was not significant. A recent NICE appraisal (TA210) advocates generic clopidogrel as the most cost-effective antiplatelet for secondary prevention following a stroke (Note: clopidogrel is not licensed for prevention following a TIA).

The combination of aspirin and clopidogrel is used rarely by specialists in the short term, where there is a high risk of cerebrovascular events from documented significant carotid disease, based on a significant reduction in a surrogate endpoint (microembolic burden). Prolonged use is associated with a reduction in ischaemic stroke, however this is balanced by an increase in major bleeding.

Blood pressure reduction

Elevated blood pressure (BP) is the most prevalent risk factor for stroke. There is a linear association between BP's and stroke risk across the ranges commonly encountered in clinical practice. Consistent with this, BP reduction has been shown to be beneficial across a range of BP from normotensive to hypertensive values. To achieve target BP values, combination therapy will be needed in 75% of people, and should be considered at initiation.

Angiotensin-converting enzyme inhibitors/angiotensin-2 receptor blockers, thiazide diuretics and dihydropyridine calcium channel blockers have direct evidence from trials in patients with cerebrovascular disease. Beta-blockers have fallen into disrepute following an observed increased incidence of diabetes and are generally reserved as fourth line agents, followed by alpha-blockers, spironolactone, and centrally acting agents. Other compelling indications for a particular drug class may influence this hierarchy e.g. beta-blockers for arrhythmia or coronary artery disease.

Lipid modification

Elevated total cholesterol (TC) and low-density lipoprotein (LDL) cholesterol (LDLC) levels are well recognized risk factors for coronary artery disease. However, the observational evidence for stroke is less clear, perhaps because epidemiological studies have failed to make the distinction between ischaemic and haemorrhagic stroke, and to divide ischaemic strokes into their pathophysiological subtypes, cholesterol levels being more relevant to particular subtypes e.g. large vessel atherosclerosis. Nonetheless, as for BP, TC and LDLC reduction is known to be beneficial across the ranges commonly encountered in clinical practice. Also, low high-density lipoprotein cholesterol is now recognized as an independent risk factor for ischaemic stroke.

Statin therapy significantly reduces recurrent stroke, with a 21.1% relative reduction of stroke risk for every 1 mmol/L reduction in LDLC. Atorvastatin is the only agent with direct evidence of benefit in secondary prevention, while generic simvastatin is recommended by guidelines as a cheaper alternative, with evidence in primary prevention of stroke. Other statins have not been shown to reduce clinical endpoints. Hydrophilic statins (e.g. rosuvastatin, lovastatin, fluvastatin) should be considered if the above choices are not tolerated.

Although there is no direct evidence that HDL elevation is beneficial in secondary prevention, gemfibrozil use in people with coronary heart disease was associated with a significant 31% relative reduction in stroke risk and fibrates may be considered where BP and LDLC levels have been controlled to target.

Atrial fibrillation

Atrial fibrillation is the commonest aetiology of cardioembolic stroke, which has a worse prognosis than other stroke subtypes. In this group, there is clear evidence that dose-adjusted warfarin is highly efficacious at reducing recurrent stroke (OR 0.55) with a small increase in major extracranial bleeds. Where warfarin is clearly unsuitable due to high risk of bleeding complications, practical difficulties with monitoring or informed patient choice, aspirin or aspirin plus clopidogrel may be considered as less effective alternatives. In rough terms, aspirin reduces stroke risk by a third and warfarin by two-thirds. Other novel agents are being investigated as alternatives to warfarin, e.g. dabigatran.

Glycaemia
Observational evidence indicates that post stroke hyperglycaemia is common and associated with higher in hospital mortality, worse prognosis, longer hospitalization and associated costs. Unfortunately there is no clear evidence to guide early management of dysglycaemia. Poorly controlled diabetes is also associated with increased risk of microvascular and macrovascular complications. The NICE guidelines for diabetes mellitus type 2 (CG 66) advise a target glycosylated haemoglobin (HbA1c) of <6.5% generally. However as one climbs up the treatment ladder and reaches insulin, this may be relaxed to <7.0%. More aggressive targets are not advised, due to an association with increased mortality, presumed to be due to increased risk of hypoglycaemia.

Surgical intervention
An early carotid scan should be carried out to identify significant underlying carotid artery stenosis in those without significant dependency prior to or as a result of their stroke/TIA, where carotid endarterectomy (CEA) may be beneficial. Early liaison with a vascular surgeon is vital since expedited intervention is significantly more effective than delayed intervention e.g. one stroke is prevented for every five operations within 2 weeks of symptoms, and for every 125 operations beyond 3 months. While the NICE guidelines advocate CEA in appropriate patients within 2 weeks of symptoms, only 20% undergo the procedure within that timeframe in current UK clinical practice.

Early versus late secondary prevention
For minor ischaemic stroke and TIA, early initiation of secondary prevention is essential, and has the potential to reduce stroke risk by 80%. Direct evidence of early initiation of individual therapies though, is lacking. In fact, early statin therapy in the FASTER study was associated with a trend towards worse outcome.

For major stroke, aspirin should be given as soon as possible after haemorrhage is ruled out by brain imaging for major stroke, except in the context of thrombolysis where a delay of about 24 hours is advised. There is no clear evidence to suggest that routine early initiation of dipyridamole MR (modified release), BP or lipid intervention is beneficial or harmful in this situation.

Pragmatic application of evidence in subgroups
There is a clear discrepancy between trial and real-life populations. Antiplatelet therapy is associated with similar reductions in vascular event risk irrespective of age, gender, diagnosis of hypertension or diabetes. The safety and efficacy of warfarin has been demonstrated clearly in the over 75 age group. Most of the participants in secondary prevention studies looking at BP reduction were under 75 years of age. While the Heart Protection Study included people up to the age of 80 years, most participants in SPARCL were under 65 years. Thus, one should be guided by chronological age and estimated survival when applying these interventions.

Post-stroke secondary prevention studies have generally excluded dependent people with significant residual deficit following a stroke, favouring those with minor strokes, e.g. lacunar or partial anterior strokes (at a higher risk of recurrent stroke ~20%, compared with the lower risk of 4% per year with total anterior circulation strokes). The absolute benefit for the more dependent group is therefore likely to be significantly less, and the risks possibly greater. Thus more research is required to create an evidence base that will guide appropriate secondary prevention in this group.

As with all medical interventions, an experienced physician must estimate life expectancy and weigh the balance of risk and benefit before initiating interventions with potential side-effects.

Intracranial haemorrhage
Haemorrhagic transformation of infarct
Minor asymptomatic bleeds into cerebral infarcts do not have a significant impact on the outcome and management is unchanged. Larger/symptomatic bleeds suggest the need to delay initiation of antithrombotic therapy, though there is no clear guidance to help define the duration of delay. Since the underlying problem is the structural damage, all interventions to reduce recurrent ischaemic vascular events remain relevant.

Primary intracerebral haemorrhage
The key interventions for prevention of recurrence of primary intracerebral haemorrhage (PICH) are treatment of hypertension as for ischaemic stroke, and avoidance of antithrombotic medication. Statins are generally avoided due to an observational association between low cholesterol and increased PICH rates.

In the longer term, if the risk of ischaemic events is felt to be high, then antithrombotic and/or statin therapy may be reconsidered after a frank discussion of the potential higher risk of recurrent PICH.

Current Practice
Guidelines
The Third National Clinical Guidelines for Stroke UK 2008 outlined the appropriate management strategy for secondary prevention of stroke, with clearly specified threshold and target values for BP and cholesterol (see Table 21.7).

Current application
It is clear that the current application of secondary prevention is poor. In the British Regional Heart Study, only the minority received an appropriate combination of antiplatelet, antihypertensive and statin. With increasing recognition of stroke as a major preventable and treatable illness in the last decade, it is hoped that implementation of secondary prevention will improve.

Risk factors are inadequately controlled after a stroke or TIA, even in the hands of specialists. The proposed reasons for this include: lack of information and advice about secondary prevention; system failure in terms of organised follow up; poor medication adherence; drug side effects;

Table 21.7 Risk factor thresholds and targets

Risk factor	Threshold	Target
BP	130/90 mmHg	<130/80 mmHg
TC	3.5 mmol/L	<4.0 mmol/L & >25% fall
LDLC		<2.0 mmol/L & >30% fall
HbA1c	-	<6.5% early, <7.0% late

Data from the *RCP National Guidelines for Stroke*, 3rd edn, 2008 and the NICE *Guidelines for Diabetes*.

lack of patient involvement in the long-term, and difficulty in comprehending the balance of real side-effects of drugs with the perceived benefit in terms of reduced stroke risk.

Novel methods of service delivery

Research into novel methods of service delivery to enhance application of secondary prevention is still in infancy. A combined approach including evidence-based recommendations, audit and feedback, interactive educational sessions, patient prompts, and outreach visits led to increased detection of atrial fibrillation and improved compliance with guidelines for management of TIA and was cost effective. Nursing intervention and brief behaviour modification was not associated with improved risk factor control. Monthly pharmacist intervention and use of electronic medical records and regular performance reports has the potential to improve adherence to guidelines.

In summary, a multifaceted organized approach with patient involvement is suggested. As in other fields, it remains a challenging task to establish benefits and cost-effectiveness of changes to service delivery.

Conclusion

A preventive strategy is ideal for stroke owing to the high prevalence, high disability and societal cost, well-known modifiable risk factors, and availability of effective evidence-based preventive measures. Comprehensive application of preventive interventions has the potential to reduce recurrent stroke by up to two-thirds.

An individualised strategy to address lifestyle and medical risk factors should be generated in partnership with the patient. Annual review of vascular risk factors in conjunction with a pre-defined target, with emphasis on long-term compliance is recommended.

Long-term compliance remains a significant challenge, with further research needed to establish the underlying reasons and potential solutions.

Direct evidence in older people and those with significant post-stroke dependency is not always available and an experienced physician must implement evidence-based therapies in a pragmatic fashion.

Further reading

Amarenco P, Labreuche J (2009). Lipid management in the prevention of stroke: review and updated meta-analysis of statins for stroke prevention. *Lancet Neurol* **8**: 453–63.

Mant J, Hobbs FD, Fletcher K, et al. (2007). Warfarin versus aspirin for stroke prevention in an elderly community population with atrial fibrillation (the Birmingham Atrial Fibrillation Treatment of the Aged Study, BAFTA): a randomised controlled trial. *Lancet* **370**: 493–503.

NICE Clinical Guideline 68 - Stroke: diagnosis and initial management of acute stroke and transient ischaemic attack (TIA) – nationally relevant guidelines.

NICE Primary Care Concise Guideline for Stroke 2008 - Abbreviated guidance on primary care roles in management of TIA and stroke.

PROGRESS Collaborative Group (2001). Randomised trial of a perindopril-based blood-pressure-lowering regimen among 6,105 individuals with previous stroke or transient ischaemic attack. *Lancet* **358**: 1033–41.

Ramsay SE, Whincup PH, Wannamethee SG, et al. (2007). Missed opportunities for secondary prevention of cerebrovascular disease in elderly British men from 1999 to 2005: a population-based study. *J Public Health* **29**: 251–7.

Rothwell PM, Eliasziw M, Gutnikov SA, et al. (2004). Endarterectomy for symptomatic carotid stenosis in relation to clinical subgroups and timing of surgery. *Lancet* **363**: 915–24.

Rothwell PM, Giles MF, Chandratheva A, et al. (2007). Effect of urgent treatment of transient ischaemic attack and minor stroke on early recurrent stroke (EXPRESS study): a prospective population-based sequential comparison. *Lancet* **370**: 1432–42.

Saxena R, Koudstaal PJ (2004). Anticoagulants for preventing stroke in patients with nonrheumatic atrial fibrillation and a history of stroke or transient ischaemic attack. *Cochrane Database Syst Rev* **1**: CD000185.

Schrader J, Luders S, Kulschewski A, et al. (2005). Morbidity and mortality after stroke, eprosartan compared with nitrendipine for secondary prevention: principal results of a prospective randomized controlled study (MOSES). *Stroke* **36**: 1218–26.

Scottish Intercollegiate Guidelines Network. Management of patients with stroke or TIA: assessment, investigation, immediate management and secondary prevention 2008 – relevant guidelines for Scotland.

Wright J, Bibby J, Eastham J, et al. (2007). Multifaceted implementation of stroke prevention guidelines in primary care: cluster-randomised evaluation of clinical and cost effectiveness. *Qual Saf Health Care* **16**: 51–9.

Skin problems: acute and chronic

Scabies

Scabies is a contagious disease due to the ectoparasitic mite *Sarcoptes scabieii*. It is endemic in many care homes and is transmitted by skin to skin contact. Carers and 'kissing contacts' may be infected asymptomatically. The incubation period before itching begins is up to 3 weeks but shorter in recurrent infestations. The female mite burrows into skin to lay eggs. Itch and eczematous rash are due to an immunological reaction to the mites or their products. Scratching contributes to the typical appearance of excoriated papules. Creases, genitals, and breasts are often affected, with the head and neck being spared. Burrows can be seen on close inspection in good light and the mite extracted and identified on light microscopy. There may be very few burrows in spite of widespread rash.

Management
Only topical agents are licensed for this condition. Permethrin cream appears to be the most effective. Application must be to the whole skin, including creases and genitals and should remain on the skin overnight before washing off. Reapplication to some areas may be needed, e.g. after using the toilet. All contacts and all care home staff and residents should be treated. Treatment should be repeated 7–14 days later but should not be used continuously.

Ivermectin is an effective systemic treatment, given as a single oral dose (100–200 µg/kg). This is not, however, licensed in the UK for scabies. It tends to be reserved for cases of crusted scabies (see below) and where topical therapy is impossible. Side-effects include headache and hypotension but are rare in practice; increased mortality in older people has been reported, but this has not been confirmed.

Itching may persist for several weeks after treatment. Topical steroids, emollients and short-term systemic antihistamines may be helpful.

It is a wise precaution to wash bedding and clothing after treatment.

Treatment failure
Treatment failure may be due to inadequate primary treatment, compliance being difficult in patients with

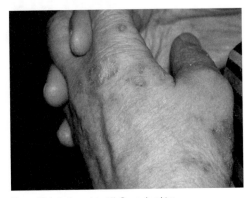

Figure 22.1 (colour plate 19) Crusted scabies.

physical disability, cognitive failure, and flexion contractures. Ivermectin may be needed. Failure to treat contacts may result in reinfestation. Resistance to topical antiscabetics is rare but has been reported.

Crusted scabies
Crusted or Norwegian scabies (see Figure 22.1) is the situation where there is a very heavy infestation with the scabies mite. This occurs in those who are unable to scratch or in whom treatment has been delayed. There is a build-up of scaly skin which can be at any site, including the face and scalp. Microscopy of the scale reveals multiple mites. This requires systemic ivermectin unless contraindicated.

Further reading
Barkwell R, Shields S (1997). Deaths associated with ivermectin treatment of scabies. *Lancet* **349**: 1144–5.

Strong M, Johnstone P (2007). Interventions for treating scabies. *Cochrane Database Syst Rev* **3** :CD000320.

Pruritus

Pruritus or itching is a distressing symptom which can have a devastating effect on quality of life in older people. It is important to establish if there is a skin disease or an underlying significant systemic disorder. 'Senile pruritus' or 'Willan's itch' remains a diagnosis of exclusion. The cause is not known but may be xerosis (dry skin) or a disorder of cutaneous sensation. Management is aimed at symptom relief

Epidemiology

Studies are unfortunately lacking. Itching was reported in 29% of non-institutionalized older adults with an average duration of 21 months. In cohort studies, mainly of care home residents, itch was complained of in up to two-thirds, more commonly in women and increasing in prevalence with advanced age.

Causes

Itchy skin diseases and systemic illness which should be excluded are shown in Table 22.1. Although drugs may cause an itchy rash, itch alone accounts for 5% of drug reactions. This may be due to hepatic causes, especially cholestatisis, neurological in origin (as in opiates) or of unknown mechanism.

A search for a systemic cause for itching should be made. In addition to clinical history and examination, it can be fruitful to do baseline blood tests including full blood count, renal and hepatic function, inflammatory markers, thyroid function, and ferritin levels. The evidence for iron deficiency is conflicting but in practice, supplementation with oral iron can be helpful. Further investigations should be dependent on clinical suspicion and continued vigilance is recommended since itching can precede clinical features of malignancy.

Management

Having excluded a correctable cause, management is aimed at combating xerosis, controlling the itch and distress. Xerosis is present in the majority of older adults. Treating dryness should prevent development of asteatotic eczema. Standard advice is the introduction of a moisturising agent in place of soap or detergents together with regular application of a moisturiser, preferable containing urea or an anti-pururitic agent such as calamine. It is not always possible for those living alone to thoroughly apply topical agents to the whole skin. Use of a commercially available applicator, long-handled sponge roller or similar home-made gadgets can help.

Table 22.1 Causes of pruritus

Common itchy skin problems	Systematic causes of itching
Dry skin	Malignancies (notably haematological including lymphoma)
Photoaged skin	
Multiple seborrhoeic warts	
Scabies	Haematological problems (including iron deficiency in absence of anaemia)
Eczemas	
Psoriasis	Renal failure
Bullous disorders	Hepatic disease (cholestatic)
Drug rashes	HIV disease

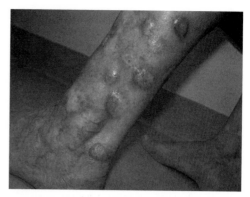

Figure 22.2 (colour plate 20) Multiple lesions of nodular prurigo on lower legs.

Comparative trials of soap substitutes and moisturisers are lacking; therefore, it can be necessary to try a number of agents to find the one which is best tolerated. Aqueous cream BP is very inexpensive. However some brands contain sodium lauryl sulphate which may irritate. There is a small risk of contact dermatitis due to the preservative. There is no evidence that laundry detergents cause a problem and it is usually fruitless to change brands. It is however unwise to use detergents for washing by hand without wearing waterproof gloves.

Systemic antihistaminic drugs can be useful. In the absence of comparative trials, it is wise to use those of low sedative potential. Consideration should be given to addition of a sedative antihistamine at night. Topical steroids of low potency may be a useful short-term adjunct. Topical doxepin and crotamiton may help some cases. Pruritus may precede appearance of malignancies so follow-up is wise.

Nodular prurigo

Nodular prurigo (see Figure 22.2) is mysterious, driving the sufferer to scratch and rub the skin uncontrollably, resulting in the appearance of multiple excoriated nodules of varying size and age which may be painful. Itch may be denied. A clue to diagnosis is the absence of lesions on areas which the patient cannot reach. Bandaging affected parts allows temporary rapid improvement. Biopsy should be considered to exclude the rare nodular form of bullous pemphigoid. Management strategies include emollients and potent topical steroids, sometimes under short-term occlusion together with systemic antihistamines. UV phototherapy and systemic immune suppressants may be necessary. Thalidomide has been shown to be effective in intractable cases.

Further reading

Beauregard S, Gilchrest BA (1987). A survey of skin problems and skin care regimes in the elderly. *Arch Dermatol* **123**: 1638–43.

Ward JR, Bernhard JD (2005). Willan's itch. *Int J Dermatol* **44**: 267–73.

Weisshaar E and Greaves M (2008). In *Evidence Based Dermatology*, 2nd ed. Williams H (ed). Blackwell, London

Leg ulcers and pressure ulceration

Leg ulcers

Overview

Ulceration of the lower leg is an archetypal disease of the older person and represents a significant burden in the UK for patients, families, and to the healthcare system. Leg ulcers are often present for many months, and are painful and disabling; they result in greatly reduced quality of life and occasionally social isolation. Yet, with appropriate diagnosis and treatment, much of this burden can be reduced.

Epidemiology

Conservative estimates are that leg ulceration affects between one and three per 1000 people in the UK; thus, there are between 70 000 and 190 000 individuals with lower leg ulceration at any one time in the UK. The number of individuals affected increases with age, so that the disease affects 1% of adults, 3.6% of those over 65 years of age and upwards of 4% for those greater than 80 years.

Over 80% of leg ulcers are cared for in the community by the primary healthcare teams and in particular community nurses, more recently under the guidance of regional tissue viability teams. The resources consumed by leg ulcer care are estimated to cost the National Health Service upwards of £500 million per annum.

Pathophysiology

Tissue repair is characterized by an overlapping sequence of processes divided into three discernable functional phases: (1) haemostasis and inflammation, (2) tissue proliferation and migration, and (3) tissue remodelling (see Figure 23.1). The temporal relationship of these cellular processes are coordinated by a host of extracellular proteins that are released by cells and interact with cell surface receptors to provide signals for recruitment (chemotaxis), activation, and proliferation (growth factors). Under normal circumstances, these biological processes work in harmony so that there is clinically apparent reduction in wound size within 6 weeks. However, certain pathologies can intervene and hinder healing, resulting in a chronic ulcer. Diseases commonly associated with chronic lower leg ulcers include chronic venous insufficiency, peripheral arterial disease, diabetes mellitus, and rheumatoid arthritis. With appropriate management of these diseases responsible for chronic lower limb ulcers, in the majority of cases (~70%) it is possible to restore the healing potential of the wound. The pathophysiological basis of the common causes of chronic lower leg ulcers is described in Figures 23.2–23.4.

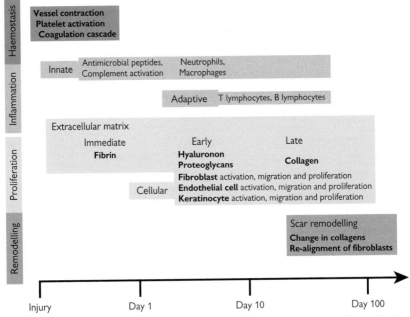

Figure 23.1 The Biology of Wound Healing. Wound healing biology can be subdivided into three sequential but overlapping phases: (1) haemostasis and inflammation, (2) tissue proliferation and migration, (3) tissue remodelling. Soon after injury, vessel contraction prevents excessive blood loss, which is followed soon after by thrombus formation from the combined effects of platelet and coagulation cascade activation. The formation of a thrombus (clot) in addition prevents bacteria from entering the circulation and also acts as a provisional extracellular matrix. The local wound environment simultaneously reacts to forestall tissue infection by first activating the innate and then later the adaptive immune system. Cells of the immune system release cytokines that further refine the immune reaction and together with local cells provide extracellular signals for tissue migration and proliferation. Even when the wound defect is eventually closed, cells and the extracellular matrix continue to undergo changes so that the scar tensile strength and pliability is maximal, albeit not to the standard of unaffected skin.

Aetiology

There is a long list of causes that result in lower leg wounds (see Table 23.1), but most result in an acute wound that will heal with conventional wound care in a timely manner once the precipitating disease is managed. Of the causes of chronic lower leg ulcers, the most common by far is venous leg ulceration (~70%). Figure 23.5 highlights the typical location of these common chronic wounds; for example, 87% of all venous ulcers arise in the 'gaiter' area. In addition, both a squamous cell carcinoma (called a Marjolin's ulcer when it arises within a venous leg ulcer) and a basal cell carcinoma can masquerade as chronic wounds.

The new patient

Each leg ulcer patient is different, in terms of the effect the wound has on their quality of life, the impact of coexistent diseases, the concomitant medications they are taking, their acceptance of treatments, and the rate at which the wound will heal. History, examination, and investigations are necessary to determine the wound aetiology first and foremost, elucidate coexistent diseases that may further impair healing, and the presence of wound infection or osteomyelitis if present.

History

All wounds initially begin as acute wounds; it is the lack of response to conventional treatments or continued enlargement over a period of 6 weeks that is used to define whether it is a chronic wound. In some cases, there may be a simple explanation for why a wound has persisted during this time, such as the presence of an underlying stitch abscess. For the classical causes of

Table 23.1 Causes of lower leg wounds

Vascular	Arterial	Atherosclerosis, thromboangiitis obliterans, arteriovenous malformation, cholesterol embolus
	Venous	Chronic venous insufficiency, acroangiodermatitis
	Vasculitis	Small vessel: idiopathic or hypersensitivity vasculitis secondary to drugs, connective tissue disease, malignancy; Wegner's granulomatosis, Churg–Strauss syndrome, microscopic polyangitis, Henoch–Schonlein purpura, essential cryoglobulinaemia
		Medium vessel: polyarteritis nodosum, Kawasaki disease
		Large vessel: Takayasu's arteritis, giant cell arteritis
	Lymphatics	Lymphoedema
Neuropathic	Diabetes, tabes dorsalis, syringomyelia	
Metabolic	Diabetes, gout, prolidase deficiency, Gaucher's disease	
Haematological	Red blood cell	Sickle cell anaemia, spherocytosis, thalassaemia, polycythaemia rubra vera
	White blood cells	Leukaemia, chronic granulomatous disease
	Dysproteinaemia	Cryoglobulinaemia, cold agglutinins disease, macroglobulinaemia
Trauma	Pressure, cold, radiation, burns, facticial	
Neoplasia	Epithelial	Squamous and basal cell carcinoma
	Sarcoma	
	Lymphoproliferative	Systemic or cutaneous lymphoma
	Metastases	
Infection	Bacterial	Furuncle, ecthyma, ecthyma gangrenosum, septic emboli, Gram-negative septicaemia, anaerobic infections, mycobacterial infection (including atypical mycobacteria), spirochetes
	Viral	Epstein–Barr virus, Herpes simplex, cytomegalovirus, human papilloma virus
	Fungal	Majocchi's granuloma, deep fungal infection
	Protozoa	Leishmania
	Infestations and bites	
Panniculitis	Weber–Christian disease, pancreatic fat necrosis, alpha-1-antitrypsin deficiency, necrobiosis lipoidica	
Neutrophilic dermatoses	Pyoderma gangrenosum, Bechet's	
Marotell's ulcer		

chronic lower leg wounds, the history should elucidate the characteristics of the disease, such as a history of chronic venous insufficiency in patients with venous leg ulcers (see Table 23.2).

Important historical features:
- Precipitating event e.g. trauma, insect bite, cellulitis
- Duration
- Whether the wound is healing or deteriorating and the rate of change
- Previous ulceration
- Pain (including claudication and rest pain)
- Mobility e.g. claudication, fixed joints
- Coexistent diseases, such as diabetes, rheumatoid arthritis, systemic sclerosis, hypertension
- Family history
- Concomitant medication

Pain is a common feature in a number of different causes of lower leg ulceration. In patients with venous disease, approximately 45% complain of discomfort/pain within the wound, and typically this is relieved by resting the leg in an elevated position. In contrast, arterial disease, which may coexist with venous or diabetic ulceration, patients complain of claudication or, in more severe disease, rest pain which is relieved by lowering the affected leg. Also, pain can be a feature of localised wound bed infection or spreading cellulitis. The absence of pain should raise the possibility of peripheral neuropathy, as is often the case in patients with diabetic foot ulceration.

Examination

A general examination of the patient is often necessary to elucidate the cause of the lower leg ulcer. For example, in rheumatoid arthritis, it is necessary to define the extent and severity of the disease including both articular and extra-articular involvement. Often in connective tissue diseases, lower leg ulceration develops at a time of increased systemic disease activity. The typical examination findings for the common chronic wounds are described in Table 23.2.

Examination of the wound itself should include an assessment of
- site
- size
- surrounding skin
- ulcer edge
- wound bed granulation tissue
- exudate.

The ulcer margin in venous leg ulcers is shallow, in contrast to the punched out appearance observed in arterial ulcers.

The appearance of a white margin is not specific to venous leg ulceration, but instead is a sign of maceration from either uncontrolled oedema or local wound infection. Occasionally, this may also be the appearance of adherent topical therapies in patients who do not regularly wash their legs, often due to the misconception that washing their leg will make the ulcer worse.

Inflammatory diseases, such as pyoderma gangrenosum often present with painful lower leg ulceration with margins that are typically violaceous and overhung.

Heaped up granulation tissue at the ulcer edge, which is common, together with an enlarging wound are characteristic features of squamous cell carcinoma (Marjolin's ulcer).

Ankle brachial pressure index

The measurement of an ankle brachial pressure index is both sensitive and specific for detecting significant peripheral arterial disease that may impact on wound healing. If the ankle brachial pressure index is 0.7 or less, then further arterial studies are required (arterial duplex scan or arteriogram) to assess the suitability for surgical intervention.

Peripheral arterial disease is most commonly due to atherosclerosis, which in turn may be associated with the following reversible factors: smoking, hypercholesterolaemia, raised C-reactive protein and hypertension.

Table 23.2 Common causes of chronic lower limb ulceration

	Venous leg ulcer	Arterial leg ulcer	Diabetic foot ulcer	Rheumatoid arthritis ulcer
History	A history of lower limb trauma, personal and family history of varicose veins, previous deep vein thrombosis, pain relieved by leg elevation, and/or previous venous surgery	A history of smoking, claudication, rest pain, smoking history, hypertension, ischaemic heart disease, cerebrovascular disease, and/or arterial surgical intervention	Duration of diabetes, claudication, rest pain, smoking history, hypertension, ischaemic heart disease, cerebrovascular disease, loss of lower limb sensation, and/or arterial or orthopaedic surgical intervention. Family history	Duration of rheumatoid arthritis, severity of disease, medication (in particular steroids and methotrexate), associated vasculitis, joint surgery
Examination	Lower limb oedema, haemosiderin deposition, atrophie blanche, lipodermatosclerosis, varicosities, venous flares	Loss of lower leg hair, thin shiny skin, absent or diminished peripheral pulses. Blood pressure	Loss of lower limb sensation, loss of lower leg hair, thin shiny skin, absent or diminished peripheral pulse.	Rheumatoid joint disease, rheumatoid nodules, vasculitis
Investigations	Venous duplex (not always necessary)	Lipids, ABPI, arterial duplex, angiography	ABPI, arterial duplex, angiography, investigations for osteomyelitis	Inflammatory markers (erythrocyte sedimentation rate or C-reactive protein level), rheumatoid factor level

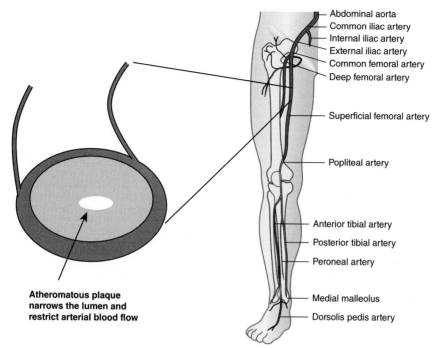

Abdominal aorta
Common iliac artery
Internal iliac artery
External iliac artery
Common femoral artery
Deep femoral artery

Superficial femoral artery

Popliteal artery

Anterior tibial artery
Posterior tibial artery
Peroneal artery

Medial malleolus
Dorsolis pedis artery

Atheromatous plaque narrows the lumen and restrict arterial blood flow

Figure 23.2 (colour plate 21) Pathogenesis of arterial ulcers. Is associated most commonly with atheroma formation from atherosclerosis. The large artery walls accumulate lipid that induces local inflammation and intimal proliferation; progressively leading to narrowing of the lumen. The distal blood supply gradually reduces and as the lumen narrows, beyond the watershed tissues undergo atrophy. Occasionally, the atheromatous plaque will rupture and either embolize or thrombose, whereupon the affected distal tissues suddenly become necrotic. The distribution of tissue atrophy and necrosis follows the distribution of the arterial branches that are involved. Arterial flow duplex scan can be used to determine the size, location and blood flow; thus provide useful information regarding the need for surgical intervention.

Examination reveals a cool limb, with absent hair, reduced capillary refill, and diminished peripheral pulses. However, these signs are not sufficient to rule out mild peripheral arterial disease that may be exacerbated by compression therapy for coexisting venous disease, hence the need for an ankle brachial pressure index measurement.

Initial investigations

Investigations are used to further characterize and confirm the underlying diseases (see Table 23.2). In addition, investigations are used to elucidate factors that may further hinder healing, such as wound infection (see below) and nutritional status.

Wound healing is a catabolic process, which requires adequate nutrition. All patients with large or longstanding wounds, require assessment of their nutritional status, and each patient should have documented (1) a history of daily food intake, (2) serum albumin, and (3) serum transferrin.

Microbiology

Local wound infections are an extremely common complication in the management of chronic wounds. Local wound infection typically presents with increased wound pain, tenderness, pungent discharge, a 'beefy' red wound bed, overgranulation, and contact bleeding. Infection of the surrounding tissues, cellulitis, may cause erythema, tenderness, and increased warmth of the surrounding skin.

Empirical antibiotic regimens are often effective while awaiting tests to confirm the organism responsible and sensitivity profiles are important. The chronic wound bed often contains multiple different bacteria. However, during wound infection, there is often overgrowth of the pathogenic organism. Microbiology swabs taken from the wound bed surface, not just from one part of the wound, after cleansing with saline and in a zig-zag fashion, can help identify the organism. However, the most sensitive test is a wound bed biopsy for microbiological culture, also undertaken after cleansing the wound bed surface. Blood cultures are only useful when there is bacteraemia or septicaemia.

As mentioned earlier, chronic wounds are usually colonised by multiple bacterial organisms, thus taking a microbiological swab of a chronic wound bed that does not exhibit signs of local wound infection will also yield bacterial colonies. Antibiotics for bacterial colonisation with no sign of local wound infection does not improve wound healing, but instead will lead to the development of antibiotic resistant strains. In contrast during wound infection, the overall number of bacteria within the wound increases, due to overgrowth of the infecting bacteria.

The most common organisms responsible for chronic wound infection are *Staphylococcus aureus*, enterococci, group B beta haemolytic streptococci, and *Pseudomonas aureginosa*. In patients with deep wounds, such as those in diabetic foot ulceration, anaerobes may also be present.

Therefore pencillins, or macrolides for those who are penicillin allergic, together with a quinalone offer good coverage. In addition, metronidazole may be added to the regimen if anaerobes are suspected. Often local wound infections respond to oral antibiotics, as tissue penetration is adequate. However, intravenous antibiotics should be used when treating rapidly progressive cellulitis, such as those caused by group B beta haemolytic streptococci.

The use of compression during the treatment of local wound infection remains controversial, although most patients will not be able to tolerate compression due to pain. Some compression is, however, beneficial as this will increase antibiotic tissue penetration into the wound bed by reducing tissue oedema. It is important to also remember that dressings need to be changed frequently, as bacteria will often reside on dressings only to reinfect the wound again. Thus the choice of compression system needs to be modified to facilitate daily or alternate day antimicrobial dressing changes.

Primary dressing

Although wound dressings represent an important aspect of ulcer care, in isolation they will not necessarily achieve healing. The ideal dressing should be (1) easy to apply and remove, (2) have low allergenic potential, (3) be sterile and impermeable to micro-organisms, (4) provide a moist wound environment but remove excess wound exudates, (5) reduce wound pain, and (6) not add to the wound debris.

For superficial ulcers a simple contact dressing (paraffin gauze, knitted viscose, silicone-coated net, gel-impregnated viscose net, or hydrocolloid) or foam dressing should be used. For the deeper ulcers, an interactive dressing should be used to pack the wound, such as hydrocolloids, hydrogels, hydrofibres, or alginates. These dressings are kept in place with a superficial absorbent and adherent dressing such as foam.

Where there is maceration of the surrounding skin, topical barrier preparations (e.g. zinc oxide, titanium dioxide, dimeticone, benzalkonium, or white soft paraffin) can be employed to prevent further moisture associated tissue damage.

Secondary dressing

These hold in place the primary dressing; they can be as simple as a tubifast retention bandage. Alternatively, it may have an additional functional role such as surgical pads or adhesive foam dressing to absorb moisture.

Definitive treatment

Arterial leg ulcers: restoration of blood flow

Arterial ulceration is typically caused by progressive arterial narrowing from atherosclerosis of large and medium sized vessels. The subsequent reduction in blood flow, results in tissue hypoxia, inability to repair and eventually skin breakdown. The risk of arterial ulceration is dependent upon the rate of arterial narrowing, but gradual arterial narrowing is associated with the formation of collateral blood flow that can circumvent the occlusion and restore lower limb perfusion. The ankle brachial pressure index is often used as a screening tool to determine the level of lower limb perfusion, but when this is reduced (<0.7) additional investigation are required to define the site of occlusion; such as an arterial duplex scan or arteriogram. Restoration of blood flow is essential to ensure healing

and this can be achieved either by angioplasty or reconstructive vascular surgery.

Venous leg ulcers: compression bandaging

In simple terms compression squeezes the limb, thereby reducing tissue oedema and aiding venous return to the heart.

Normal venous return from the lower limb is aided by the calf muscle pump, which during walking forces blood up the lower limb with the help of venous valves that prevent retrograde blood flow, so that venous pressures at the ankle remain between 10 and 20 mmHg (see Figure 23.3). In chronic venous insufficiency, the calf muscle contraction results in retrograde blood flow and so adds to the already elevated ankle venous pressures from damaged or absent venous valves. Ambulatory venous pressures at the ankle in a patient with venous diseases can be as high as 100 mmHg, which in turn forces fluid out of the capillaries into the tissue to cause oedema.

Graduated compression, with 40–50 mmHg at the ankle reducing to ~10 mmHg at the calf, provides extra tissue pressure that counteracts oedema formation. However, such compression is only applicable if there is normal arterial systolic flow to maintain blood flow into the limb, hence why all patients receiving compression require an ankle brachial pressure index measurement. There are a number of different compression systems available, elastic bandages are the most commonly used in the UK (see Table 23.3).

Diabetic foot ulcers

The management of diabetic foot ulcers due to its more complex aetiology involves multiple components: debridement, nail care, re-distribution of pressure, regular vascular assessment, and the aggressive management of wound infection (see Figure 23.4)

Debridement of callus is a critical component in the management of all diabetic patients, and is an essential component in managing diabetics with peripheral neuropathy. As discussed earlier, patients with diabetes have dry skin (due to autonomic neuropathy) that easily fissures/cracks and also develops callus formation (corns) from repeated rubbing over bony prominences. As the callus hardens, it can act as a sharp inward-facing mass that can cause breakdown of the underlying skin. Thus in all patients with diabetes, routine foot care must involve sharp debridement of callus.

All patients with diabetes, in addition to attending the diabetic foot clinic, should have regular visits with the podiatrist for both callus debridement as well as nail care. Such patients often find it difficult to cut their toenails for a number of reasons, including neuropathy, obesity, poor vision, and poor flexibility. For these reasons, toenail cutting can easily result in skin trauma and as such is a preventable cause of ulceration. Routine podiatry also provides a focus for foot care to detect, manage, and prevent ulcer formation.

Patients with diabetic peripheral neuropathy lose proprioception and pain sensation as well as small muscle tone in their feet. The combined effect of diabetic peripheral neuropathy results in abnormal pressure loads that predispose to pressure ulceration on the sole of feet. The use of felt pads, specialized shoe insoles, and deep orthopaedic shoes are used to redistribute foot pressure and thus prevent ulceration. The most efficient way to redistribute plantar pressure is to use prefabricated Aircast or

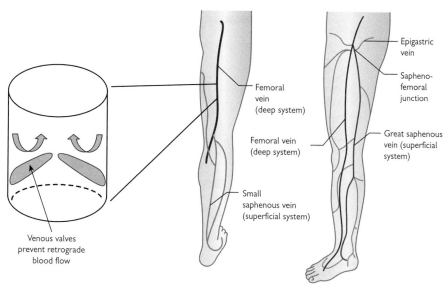

Figure 23.3 (colour plate 22) Anatomy of venous valves. Venous valves maintain blood flow back to the heart. When these valves are absent or destroyed by thrombosis, there is increased venous pressure. In such cases, contraction of the calf muscle pump results in retrograde flow, which is normally prevented by the presence of the venous valve, thus further increasing venous pressures at the ankle. This in turn leads to varicosities and local tissue oedema, a prelude to venous ulceration.

Scotchcast boots, which have a rocker sole that uniformly distributes pressure over the foot. They are often used when treating patients with plantar foot ulceration.

One in five patients with diabetes will develop foot ulceration in their lifetime as a consequence of ischaemia and/or peripheral neuropathy. Thus, all patients who present with foot ulceration should be assessed to evaluate the relative contribution of these two determinants. Assessment of the lower limb perfusion can be performed by measuring the ankle brachial pressure index or arterial toe pressure. Where there is reduced arterial perfusion,

further assessment is necessary to determine the type of vascular intervention necessary to restore blood supply, as for arterial ulcers discussed earlier. In the case of digital gangrene, these tissues can either be debrided surgically or alternatively left to autoamputate.

Diabetic foot ulcers are more prone to local wound infection, resulting in a static or an enlarging wound with abnormal wound bed that is 'beefy' red, friable, demonstrates contact bleeding and is malodorous. While waiting for microbiological confirmation of the pathogenic organism and antibiotic sensitivities, it is essential that early empirical antibiotic treatment is initiated. As the most common bacterial species are staphylococci, streptococci, pseudomonas and anaerobes, a commonly used empirical regimen is co-amoxiclav, ciprofloxacin, and metronidazole. However, it must be remembered that antibiotic therapy will not penetrate necrotic tissue, and therefore wound debridement remains an essential component of management. This is particularly true in wet gangrene where the infection causes septic vasculitis that further compounds tissue necrosis. In cases where the wound connects directly to the underlying bone, there is likely to be concomitant osteomyelitis, for which additional investigation and parenteral antibiotics with or without recourse to orthopaedic surgery may be necessary. The presence of osteomyelitis necessitates specialist care by a diabetic foot clinic or orthopaedic/vascular surgical team.

In summary, the management of diabetic foot ulceration remains a complex clinical entity, which may vary in its presentation with dramatic consequence for the patient. Careful monitoring of such patients together with appropriate early intervention, as outlined above, can achieve wound healing and also prevent lower limb amputation.

Table 23.3 Types of compression

Type of compression	Examples	Features
Elastic compression	Tensopress, Setopress, Surepress	Achieve sustained compression between 30 and 40 mmHg at the ankle. These are typically left on for up to 1 week
Multilayered bandaging	'Charing Cross' four-layer bandage, consisting of orthopaedic padding, crepe, Elset elastic bandage and Coban self-adhesive bandage.	Achieve sustained compression of up to 40 mmHg at the ankle. Typically left on for one week
Compression stockings	Class 2	Typically used to prevent venous ulcers in patients with chronic venous insufficiency

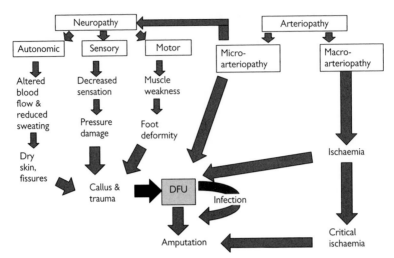

Figure 23.4 Causes of foot ulceration in diabetes mellitus. Diabetic foot ulceration can arise from neuropathy, arteriopathy, or a combination of the two diseases. Peripheral neuropathy through a combination of autonomic, sensory and motor loss results in pressure points that increase callus formation, which in turn act as a focus for wounds. In addition to macro-vessel disease, diabetics also develop microangiopathy that further reduces tissue perfusion and together they both predispose to lower limb ulceration. Patients with diabetes also demonstrate an increased propensity to develop local wound infection, occasionally in the absence of clinical signs that further hinder healing and risk osteomyelitis. If left untreated, diabetic foot ulceration is a major risk factor for lower limb amputation and today there are still 1200 amputations for this reason carried out in the UK each year.

Prevention

Venous leg ulcer

Approximately one-third of venous lower leg ulcer recurrences can be prevented by compression therapy after the ulcer has healed, this can be effectively achieved by the prescription of class 2 compression stocking. Class 1 compression stockings, a weaker level of compression, can be substituted for those unable to tolerate the higher compression hosiery. It is important to remember that these stocking lose their elasticity and so need to be replaced every 3–6 months.

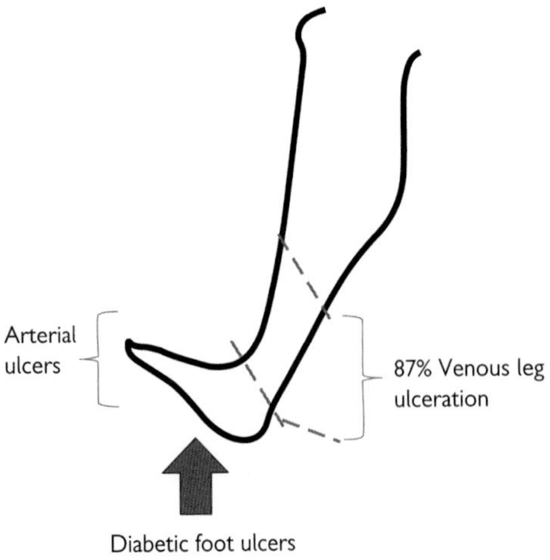

Arterial ulcers

Prevention of arterial leg ulcers is dependent upon reduction of potential risk factors for the underlying disease. For example in the case of atherosclerosis, the commonest cause this would involve optimisation of blood pressure, lipids and cessation of smoking. Continued exercise will increase collateral blood flow and so should be encouraged.

Diabetic foot ulcers

Patients who have lost their peripheral sensation require advice on how to care for their feet. Patients should be instructed to examine their feet daily for breaks in the skin. After washing their feet, care must be taken to ensure that they are completely dry and then moisturized. Emphasis should be made on conveying the importance of appropriate footwear and new shoes need to be 'broken in' gradually to avoid undue pressure. All patients should to be aware of the signs of infection (reddening of the skin, swelling, and warmth) as well as the importance of reporting breaks in the skin early.

Further reading

Boulton AJM, Connor H and Cavanagh PR (eds) (2000). *The Foot in Diabetes*, 3rd edn. Chichester, John Wiley & Sons.

Bowker JH, Pfeifer MA (eds) (2001). Levin & O'Neal's *The Diabetic Foot*, 6th edn. St. Louis, Mosby Year Book.

Edmonds M, Foster AVM, Sanders L (2004). *A Practical Manual of Diabetic Foot Care*. Oxford, Blackwell Science.

Grey J, Harding KG (eds) (2006). ABC of wound healing. *Br J Med* **332**: 347–50.

Arterial ulcers

87% Venous leg ulceration

Diabetic foot ulcers

Figure 23.5. Common sites of lower limb ulceration. Lower leg ulcers can be defined by the site of predilection, for example 87% of venous leg ulcers arise in the "gaiter" area. Whereas arterial ulcers are more common on the distal digits, diabetic pressure ulcers from neuropathy frequently occur on the plantar aspect of the foot.

Harding KG, Morris HL, Patel GK (2002). Healing chronic wounds. *Br Med J* **324**: 160–3.

International Working Group on the Diabetic Foot (1999 and 2003). International Consensus on the Diabetic Foot (http://www.iwgdf.org/).

NICE (2004). *Prevention and Management of Foot Problems: Clinical Guidelines for Type 2 Diabetes.* London, National Institute of Clinical Excellence

Pressure ulceration

Disconcertingly, despite increased vigilance, pressure ulcers remain an all too common problem. Annually more than 400 000 people develop a pressure ulcer in the UK. Prevalence in the acute setting ranges from 3% to 14%. In the surgical specialties, the rate varies from 2% (general surgery) to 10% (orthopaedics) reflecting, in part, the patient characteristics. Data for the community is not reliable but it is thought that the prevalence of pressure ulceration in nursing homes and the acute hospital setting is similar. The incidence in the acute setting is between 1% and 5%, rising to almost 8% in patients who are bed or chair bound for over a week. Approximately 20% of pressure ulcers develop at home and a further 20% in nursing homes.

Pressure ulcers are responsible for a significant degree of morbidity, both physical and psychological. Moreover, the mortality of an older person with a pressure ulcer is increased fivefold, with hospital mortality rates of between a quarter and a third. In addition, the financial burden is enormous, both to the State and the individual: £2 billion is a conservative estimate of the amount thought to be spent on pressure ulcer care annually, equivalent to 4% of the total NHS expenditure. The current figures for pressure ulcer epidemiology and costs may be underestimated given their reliance on data from hospital-based surveys, with Vowden and Vowden demonstrating that only 11% of patient with pressure ulcers were located in hospital.

The development of a new pressure ulcer imposes further financial burdens, as it is associated with a fivefold increase in length of hospital stay. There is a 10-fold increase in the cost of healing a grade IV pressure ulcer compared with healing a grade I pressure ulcer. Complications, including infections such as osteomyelitis, are associated with lengthy inpatient stays and increased financial cost. Most pressure ulcers are avoidable. Significant potential cost savings (to the patient and the healthcare system) can be made by preventing a pressure ulcer. Potential litigation also impacts on the financial cost of a pressure ulcer. The development of a pressure ulcer in a setting where a person is receiving care, for example, a care home or hospital, may be regarded as evidence of clinical negligence and may trigger a safeguarding investigation.

Pathogenesis

Extrinsic factors

A pressure ulcer may be defined as an area of localized damage to the skin and underlying tissue caused by the extrinsic factors of pressure (the load perpendicular to the tissue surface), shear (the load parallel to the tissue surface), friction (the load acting tangentially to the tissue surface) or a combination of these (adapted from European Pressure Ulcer Advisory Panel). Moisture (due, for example, to urinary or faecal incontinence, perspiration, or excessive wound drainage) exacerbates the deleterious effects of pressure, shear and friction.

Pressure ulceration may occur rapidly in the presence of sustained high pressures and more slowly at lower pressures sustained for longer periods. Intermittent pressure relief by, for example, regular turning or the use of pressure relieving devices (mattresses, cushions) helps to reduce the risk of pressure ulceration. However, the time/pressure threshold for skin damage to occur in an individual is also dependent on the presence of other intrinsic risk factors:

- acute illness
- extremes of age

- level of consciousness
- malnutrition/dehydration
- limited mobility/immobility
- history of pressure damage
- sensory impairment
- severe chronic or terminal disease
- vascular disease.

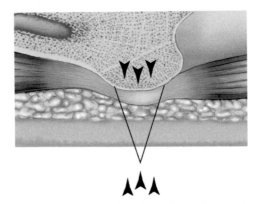

Figure 23.6 (colour plate 23) Distribution of external pressure at the bone/muscle interface

Shear forces occur as a result of sliding and relative displacement over a bony prominence of adjacent skin structures, which are restrained from moving due to frictional forces. The skin of older individuals contains less elastin than the skin of younger people, thus reducing its tensile strength and increasing the effects of shear. Pressure damage is greatly enhanced by the effects of shear forces. The effect of shear may be reduced through the use of vapour permeable mattress covers, which reduce the amount of moisture.

Frictional forces oppose the movement of one surface against another. Clinically, friction leads to damage of the epidermis, initiating pressure ulcer formation and is common

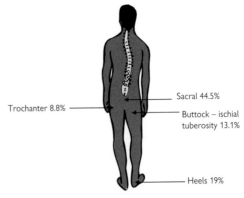

Figure 23.7 (colour plate 24) Common sites of pressure ulceration. Reproduced from Dealey, C., The size of the pressure-sore problem in a teaching hospital, *Journal of Advanced Nursing*, **16**, 6, pp. 663–70, Copyright Wiley 1991, with permission.

where the papillary layer is thin. Such forces occur, for example, when a patient is dragged across a bed sheet, pulling the sheet under the patient, sliding transfer from bed to chair, as a result of ill-fitting prosthetic devices or footwear, or uncontrollable spasms. Friction enhances the damage caused by pressure. Excess moisture (for example, as a result of incontinence; excess sweating in acute illness) leads to skin maceration and tissue breakdown and increases the effect of friction by up to five times.

The bone/muscle interface over bony prominences experiences the highest pressures. An external pressure may rise fourfold at a bony prominence (see Figure 23.6), resulting in deep tissue destruction, which may not be evident on the surface of the skin. Sustained high pressures may decrease transcutaneous oxygen tensions to almost zero. Pressures of 70–100 mmHg have been recorded over bony prominences of individuals nursed on standard NHS mattresses. Pressure reducing mattresses reduce this

pressure to between 30 and 40 mmHg. Regular relief from high pressures in the at-risk patient is, therefore, essential to prevent pressure ulceration.

The majority of pressure ulcers develop on the lower half of the body; Two-thirds of these occur around the pelvis and one-third on the lower limbs (see Figure 23.7).

However, pressure ulcers may arise wherever there is compression between a bony prominence and an external surface (see Figure 23.8).

Assessment of pressure ulceration risk

The effect of the extrinsic factors of pressure, shear, friction and moisture compounded by intrinsic factors predispose an individual to the development of pressure ulceration. Assessment of risk should involve the use of an established risk calculator suited to the individual patient. This ensures systematic evaluation of individual risk factors. Any scale should be used as an adjunct to clinical

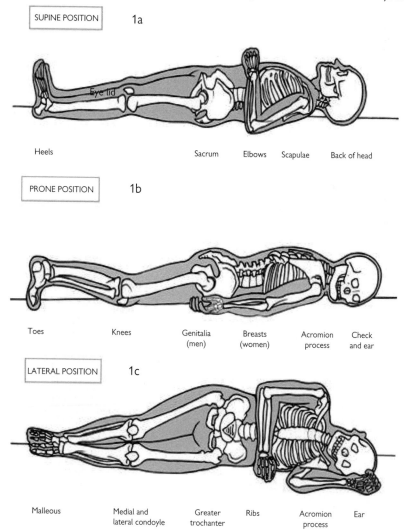

Figure 23.8 Areas prone to pressure ulceration.

judgement and not replace it. Several risk assessment scales have been developed. These scales include, among others, Waterlow (see Table 23.4) commonly used in the UK, Braden, Norton, Gosnell, and Anderson. Although some are more comprehensive than others, there are components common to all the scales:

- age
- mobility
- activity
- level of consciousness
- nutrition
- continence
- skin status
- illness severity.

There is little evidence that any one scale is superior to another nor that their use has led to a reduction in pressure ulcer incidence. They are all subject to interobserver error. They are designed for use in individuals who are bed or chair bound or who have limited ability to reposition themselves. All at-risk patients should be assessed at regular intervals. It should be self-evident that risk assessment scales are only of use if the at risk patient identified receives appropriate intervention.

A variety of guidelines and protocols on pressure ulcer prevention and treatment have been developed by international bodies. For example, The National Institute for Health and Clinical Excellence (NICE) and the Tissue Viability Society in the UK: the National Pressure Ulcer Advisory Panel (NPUAP) in the USA and the European Pressure Ulcer Advisory Panel (EPUAP). NICE has identified various risk factors associated with the development of pressure ulceration (see Table 23.5).

Intrinsic factors

Age

Physiologically, age-related susceptibility to skin breakdown may occur due to loss of dermal vessels, thinned epidermis, flattening of the dermoepidermal junction, decreased elastin content and increased skin permeability. However, despite the fact that more than two-thirds of pressure ulcers are found in those over 70 years of age, age alone is not an independent risk factor for pressure ulcer development. Rather, it is the comorbidities associated with ageing that predispose to increased pressure ulcer risk and impaired healing. Appropriate management of acute and chronic conditions is integral to pressure ulcer prevention and treatment.

Mobility

Poor mobility and immobility, secondary to a variety of factors, are associated with advancing age. Fractured neck of femur, more common in older people, is a risk factor for the development of a pressure ulcer. Up to 60% of such patients develop a pressure ulcer within 2 weeks of admission to hospital.

Immobility (the inability to reposition without assistance) or limited mobility are common sequelae of neurological problems such as stroke and spinal cord injury. Decreased muscle bulk and reduction of subcutaneous tissue consequent on paralysis further predisposes to pressure ulceration. Pain as well as joint deformity and lack of strength due, for example, to arthritis and orthopaedic problems may also lead to the inability to change position frequently.

A reduction in the number of nocturnal movements has been correlated with development of pressure ulcers. Factors leading to reduced nocturnal mobility include

Table 23.4 Waterlow pressure sore prevention/treatment policy. (Printed with the permission of Judy Waterlow MBE SRN RCNT http://www.judy-waterlow.co.uk" www.judy-waterlow.co.uk).

RING SCORES IN TABLE, ADD TOTAL. SEVERAL SCORES PER CATEGORY CAN BE USED

BUILD/WEIGHT FOR HEIGHT	★	SKIN TYPE VISUAL RISK AREAS	★	SEX AGE	★	SPECIAL RISKS	★
AVERAGE	0	HEALTHY	0	MALE	1	**TISSUE MALNUTRITION**	★
ABOVE AVERAGE	1	TISSUE PAPER	1	FEMALE	2		
OBESE	2	DRY	1	14–49	1	e.g.: TERMINAL CACHEXIA	8
BELOW AVERAGE	3	OEDEMATOUS	1	50–64	2	CARDIAC FAILURE	5
		CLAMMY (TEMP↑)	1	65–74	3	PERIPHERAL VASCULAR DISEASE	5
CONTINENCE	★	DISCOLOURED	2	75–80	4	ANAEMIA	2
		BROKEN/SPOT	3	81+	5	SMOKING	1
COMPLETE/ CATHETERISED	0						
OCCASION INCONT	1	MOBILITY	★	APPETITE	★	**NEUROLOGICAL DEFICIT**	★
CATH/INCONTINENT							
OF FAECES	2	FULLY	0	AVERAGE	0	e.g.: DIABETES, M.S, CVA, MOTOR/SENSORY PARAPLEGIA	4–6
DOUBLY INCONT	3	RESTLESS/FIDGETY	1	POOR	1		
		APATHETIC	2	N.G. TUBE/			
		RESTRICTED	3	FLUIDS ONLY	2	**MAJOR SURGERY/TRAUMA**	★
		INERT/TRACTION	4	NBM/ANOREXIC	3		
		CHAIRBOUND	5			ORTHOPAEDIC- BELOW WAIST, SPINAL	5
						ON TABLE > 2 HOURS	5

SCORE	10+ AT RISK	15+ HIGH RISK	20+ VERY HIGH RISK

MEDICATION	★
CYTOTOXICS, HIGH DOSE STEROIDS ANTI-INFLAMMATORY	4

© J Waterlow 1991 Revised March 1992

OBTAINABLE FROM: NEWTONS, CURLAND, TAUNTON, TA3 5SG

Table 23.5 Risk factors for pressure ulceration (Based on NICE guidelines for pressure ulcer prevention, 2005)

Acute Illness

Increased metabolic rate and demand for oxygen compromising tissues

Age

Chronic disease
Stroke
Impaired nutririon
Bed/chair bound
Faecal incontinence
Fractured neck of femur
Confusion

Level of Consciousness

Acute/chronic illness
Medication
    - sedatives
    - analgesics
    - anaesthetics

Limited Mobility/Immobility

Stroke
Spinal cord injury   - hemiparesis
                   - paraparesis
                   - quadriplegia
Spasticity
Arthritis
Orthopaedic problems, especially fractured neck of femur
Bed- or chair-bound individuals

Sensory Impairment

Neuropathies, e.g., diabetes
Decreased conscious levels
Medication
Spinal cord injury

Severe Chronic or Terminal Disease

Diabetes
COPD
Chronic cardiovascular disease
Terminal illness

Vascular Disease

Smoking
Diabetes
Peripheral vascular disease
Anaemia
Anti-hypertensives

Malnutrition/Dehydration

Weight loss
Lymphopenia
Low albumin, prealbumin, transferrin

History of Pressure Damage

paralysis, a high pressure ulcer risk score and iatrogenic factors such as the use of sedative medication. Analgesics and anaesthetics may also lead to altered conscious levels and reduced mobility. Appropriate pressure relieving surfaces as well as regular repositioning should be provided for those who are bed or chair bound. Pressure ulceration is more common in immobile patients who develop pyrexia. This leads to an increased metabolic rate and increased demand for oxygen by the compromised tissues making pressure ulceration more likely.

Other risk factors, which have been found to increase the incidence of pressure ulceration in the immobile patient, include dry skin, a pre-existing category of pressure ulcer (non-blanchable erythema of intact skin), and faecal incontinence. Obesity may lead to reduced mobility. Drugs, such as antihypertensives, may cause alteration in blood flow and predispose to pressure ulceration in the immobile individual.

A reduction in the ability to reposition is seen in those with sensory deficits as a result of an altered ability to perceive the pain and discomfort associated with persistent local pressure. Individuals at risk include those with neurological problems such as neuropathies (e.g. diabetes), which especially predisposes to heel ulceration. Decreased mobility may result from medical or psychological conditions which lead to altered conscious levels. Iatrogenic causes of altered conscious levels due to prescription medication are relatively common, for example due to sedatives. The effects of sensory loss in patients with stroke or spinal cord injury may be compounded by motor deficits or increased tone (spasticity), which limit mobility and the ability to reposition.

Intercurrent illness

Acute, severe chronic and terminal illness may predispose to pressure ulceration. For example, acute illness may lead to a general metabolic disturbance culminating in reduced tolerance of pressure and impaired healing. This may be exacerbated by poor nutrition and drug therapy. At least 4% of all people admitted to hospital develop pressure ulcers. It should be recognised that energy and protein requirements are increased in chronic diseases and should be addressed accordingly. All patients should be assessed for their risk factors, nutritional support provided and frequently repositioned.

Chronic and terminal illnesses are more common with advancing age. Diabetes may be associated with pressure ulcer formation, commonly in the form of diabetic foot ulceration, as a result of vascular disease, sensory, autonomic, and motor neuropathy. Poor tissue oxygenation as a consequence of chronic conditions, such as chronic obstructive pulmonary disease (COPD), chronic cardiovascular disease and peripheral oedema, or peripheral vascular disease, make individuals more prone to pressure ulceration. For the same reason anaemia should be addressed. Reduced blood perfusion as a result of peripheral vascular disease, often as a result of smoking and diabetes, leads to an increased risk of pressure ulceration particularly of the heels, feet and toes (see Figure 23.9 and 23.10).

The prevalence of pressure ulceration in terminally ill individuals has been estimated to be as high as 50%, reflecting the severity of the underlying disease and multisystem failure. Although the aim is generally to prevent and treat pressure ulceration, symptom control, dignity, and comfort should be paramount for the dying person who has pressure ulceration.

Nutrition

Adequate nutrition is pivotal both to the prevention and treatment of pressure ulceration. Protein–energy malnutrition, impaired oral intake, and the development of pressure ulceration are intimately related. The relative risk of pressure ulcer development in high-risk malnourished patients is more than double that of patients with normal nutritional status. Moreover, malnutrition retards the healing of pressure ulcers and there is a correlation between the degree of malnutrition and the extent and severity of pressure ulceration.

Studies on the prevention of pressure ulceration through nutritional intervention alone are inconclusive. However, there is general consensus that there is a need

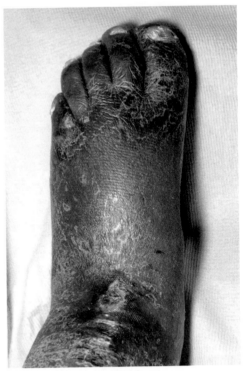

Figure 23.9 (colour plate 25) Feet and toe pressure ulcers.

for optimized protein, energy, and fluid intake with the addition of the recommended daily allowance of vitamins and trace elements. In individuals with established pressure ulceration nutritional demands may be greater.

Dietetic involvement for individuals at high risk and those with established pressure ulceration is essential. Temporary dietary supplementation, either assisted or enteral (via a nasogastric or percutaneous endoscopic gastrostomy tube), may be necessary to provide adequate nutrition. However, there may be a degree of morbidity associated with such interventions. These include diarrhoea and incontinence for individuals rendered immobile as a result of enteral feeding, in themselves risk factors for pressure ulcer formation. Supplementation with high protein dietary supplements for 15 days to critically ill older

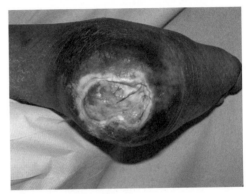

Figure 23.10 (colour plate 26) Heel pressure ulcer.

patients has shown a reduction in pressure ulcer development. Practically, however, this may prove difficult to maintain in many unwell patients. Adequate hydration is essential for prevention and treatment of pressure ulceration.

Measures of nutritional status predictive of pressure ulcer formation include decreased body weight, decreased triceps skin-fold thickness and lymphocytopenia. Serum albumin level is a commonly used surrogate marker, though its relatively long half-life does not provide an accurate reflection of nutritional status. More sensitive, though not routinely available, markers include serum pre-albumin and transferrin.

Pressure relieving strategies

Minimizing the effects of extrinsic factors (pressure, shear, friction and moisture) through pressure relief or redistribution is the main focus of prevention strategies. It is a *sine qua non* that control of intrinsic factors is also necessary for preventative strategies to be optimal. Patient and carer education will lead to early recognition of at risk individuals and timely preventative interventions.

Abolition of friction and shear forces is neither possible nor desirable, otherwise the patient would slip off the bed or chair! The individual should be repositioned by lifting (safely) to minimize these forces. Keeping the head of the bed at 30° or less minimizes shear damage and helps protects the sacrum, ischial tuberosities, and heels from pressure damage. The support surface should be kept clean and free of any debris (for example, food), which may exacerbate any pressure damage.

Individuals with established pressure ulcers, as well as those at risk, should be nursed on an appropriate pressure-relieving surface. These surfaces include mattresses, mattress overlays, and cushions. Risk assessment scales are used to identify at-risk individuals. They should be used as part of a holistic assessment of the individual and not be a substitute for clinical judgement.

Pressure-relieving surfaces fall broadly into two categories: the continuous low pressure (static) system designed to redistribute pressure; and the alternating (dynamic) pressure system which relieves the pressure under different parts of the body in a sequential and cyclical manner. The surface should not be able to 'bottom out', i.e. the mattress (or overlay) or any part of it providing less than 2.5 cm of support.

NICE recommends that individuals with category 1 or 2 pressure ulcers should be managed on a high specification foam mattress, although if there is any deterioration this should be changed to a high specification continuous low pressure or alternating pressure system. Individuals with category 3 or 4 ulceration should be managed on an alternating pressure system. Adherence to local pressure ulcer prevention protocols and liaison with local wound healing specialist or tissue viability nurses may help define the appropriate surface.

Appropriate seating is a further important adjunct to prevent pressure damage and to maintain a balanced, symmetrical seating posture. When choosing an armchair, attention should be paid to the seat base, cushion, backrest (with or without recline) and armrests. The main points of contact between the pelvis and seat are the ischial tuberosities, the tissue over which, not surprisingly, is particularly prone to pressure ulceration. Frail, immobile, and ill older patients are particularly at risk due to reduced muscle bulk around the pelvis and reduced skin elasticity.

Pressure relieving cushions may be classified as either static or dynamic (Figure 23.11). Static cushions are used mainly for pressure ulcer prevention, whilst dynamic cushions are used for individuals at elevated risk of

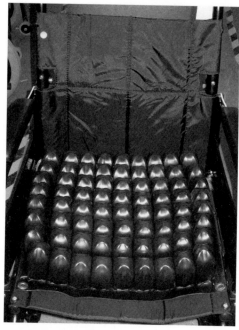

Figure 23.11 (colour plate 27) ROHO cushion.

pressure ulceration and those with established pressure ulceration. Cushions should be compatible with the chair or wheelchair. Ring, or 'Doughnut', cushions must not be used as they may cause rather than prevent pressure ulceration. Foam wedges or pillows may be used to avoid direct contact of bony prominences such as ankles or knees.

Management of pressure ulceration
Classification of Pressure Ulcers

A variety of systems have been devised to classify pressure ulcerations, none of which is perfect. The European Pressure Ulcer Advisory Panel (EPUAP) and the American National Pressure Ulcer Advisory Panel (NPUAP) have developed a four category system (see Figures 23.12–23.15) of level of injury. The term category has been adopted as a neutral term to replace the terms stage and grade, though the latter terms remain in common use. 'Category' has been adopted as a non-hierarchical term, attempting to dispel the idea of an ulcer 'progressing from I to IV' and 'healing from IV to I'. In one European study, the majority of the pressure ulcers identified were categories I and II. Full thickness, categories III and IV, pressure ulcers were less common.

Drawbacks to the system include the fact that in the USA, the NPUAP has added two further categories; unclassified/unstageable and deep tissue injury (see Box 23.1). In Europe these are generally graded as category IV. This may lead to some confusion when comparing international data. Difficulties also arise when, for example, trying to distinguish category 1 ulceration in people with darkly pigmented skin and accurately categorizing a pressure ulcer covered with Eschar (generally graded as category 4 due to the uncertainties as to what lies beneath). Undermining and sinuses commonly occur and may affect categorization as well as healing.

Tools, which are not widely used, have been developed in an attempt to assess the healing of pressure ulcers.

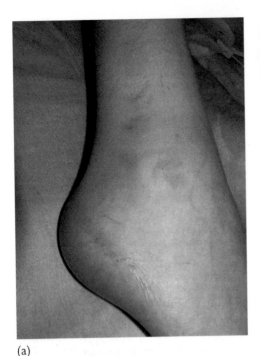

(a)

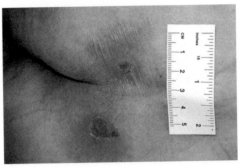

(a)

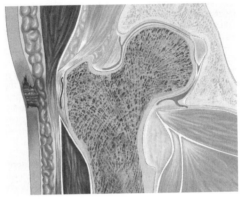

(b)

Figure 23.13a and b (colour plate 29a and b) *Category/stage II: partial thickness skin loss or blister.* Partial thickness loss of dermis presenting as a shallow open ulcer with a red/pink wound bed, without slough. May also present as an intact or open/ruptured serumfilled or sero-sanginous filled blister. Further description: presents as a shiny or dry shallow ulcer without slough or bruising. This category/stage should not be used to describe skin tears, tape burns, incontinence associated dermatitis, maceration or excoriation.

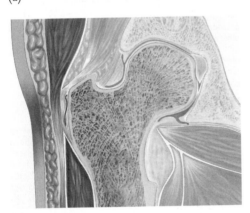

(b)

Figure 23.12a and b (colour plate 28a and b) *Category/stage I: non-blanchable redness of intact skin.* Intact skin with non-blanchable erythema of a localized area usually over a bony prominence. Discoloration of the skin, warmth, oedema, hardness or pain may also be present. Darkly pigmented skin may not have visible blanching. Further description: the area may be painful, firm, soft, warmer, or cooler than adjacent tissue. Category/Stage it may be difficult to detect in individuals with dark skin tones. May indicate 'at risk' persons.

These include the 'pressure sore status tool' (PSST) and the 'pressure ulcer scale for healing' (PUSH) tool.

Initial wound management

Effective management of pressure ulceration includes a detailed history, thorough examination, comprehensive evaluation of the wound characteristics (for example, site, size, depth, undermining, stage, drainage, wound infection, sinuses, underlying osteomyelitis) and the surrounding skin, and an assessment of the contributory intrinsic and extrinsic factors that have contributed to the formation of the ulcer. As part of the documentation the ulcer should be photographed. Management of any contributory underlying disease process should be optimised.

Initial cleansing of the wound may be undertaken with water (that is of potable quality) rather than more expensive sterile saline solutions. Showering with large amounts of water (directed above the wound so the water irrigates without too much force) helps cleanse the wound and reduce the bacterial burden on the wound surface and also provides psychological benefits to the patient.

Antiseptics should not be used in the cleansing process. Although they are intended to kill bacteria within a wound, they are also toxic to non-bacterial cells, such as fibroblasts and macrophages, found in the wound and necessary for effective repair.

Removal of necrotic tissue, eschar, and debris is essential both to facilitate wound healing and accurately to stage a pressure ulcer. High bacterial levels in wound tissues delays healing. Debridement helps reduce the bacterial load. Necrotic tissue may be seen as yellow or grey 'slough'

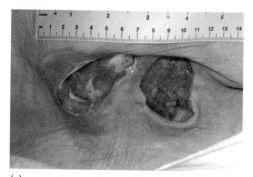

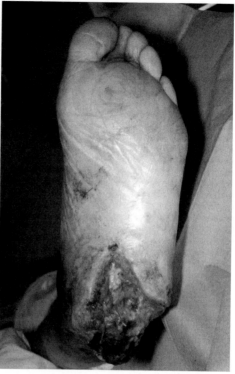

(a)

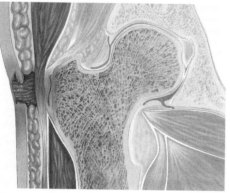

(b)

(a)

Figure 23.14a and b (colour plate 30a and b) *Category/stage III: full thickness skin loss (fat visible).* Full thickness tissue loss. Subcutaneous fat may be visible but bone, tendon or muscle are not exposed. Some slough may be present. May include undermining and tunnelling. Further description: the depth of a Category/Stage III pressure ulcer varies by anatomical location. The bridge of the nose, ear, occiput and malleolus do not have (adipose) subcutaneous tissue and Category/Stage III ulcers can be shallow. In contrast, areas of significant adiposity can develop extremely deep Category/Stage III pressure ulcers. Bone/tendon is not visible or directly palpable.

generally loosely adherent (see Figure 23.16) to the wound surface. Eschar (see Figure 23.17) is also necrotic tissue but is thick, hard, black, and often firmly adherent to the wound. There are several methods of debridement in use though most commonly pressure ulcers are managed through a mixture of sharp debridement and appropriate dressings promoting autolysis:

- Sharp debridement involves removal of necrotic tissue at the bedside or in the treatment room using a scalpel, scissors or curette.
- Surgical debridement in the operating room may be necessary, especially for extensive category 3 or 4 pressure ulcers.
- Autolytic debridement facilitates the body's own mechanism of clearing necrotic tissue and debris by the maintenance of a moist wound environment through the judicious use of appropriate dressings.
- Enzymatic debridement removes necrotic tissue by a variety of enzyme preparations which usually applied topically.

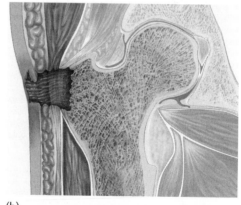

(b)

Figure 23.15a and b (colour plate 31a and b) *Category/stage IV: full thickness tissue loss (muscle/bone visible).* Full thickness tissue loss with exposed bone, tendon or muscle. Slough or eschar may be present. Often include undermining and tunnelling. Further description: the depth of a Category/Stage IV pressure ulcer varies by anatomical location. The bridge of the nose, ear, occiput and malleolus do not have (adipose) subcutaneous tissue and these ulcers can be shallow. Category/Stage IV ulcers can extend into muscle and/or supporting structures (e.g., fascia, tendon or joint capsule) making osteomyelitis or osteitis likely to occur. Exposed bone/muscle is visible or directly palpable.

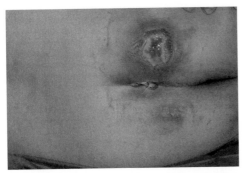

Figure 23.16 (colour plate 32) Slough on buttock pressure ulcer.

- Mechanical debridement is a wet to dry technique, usually using woven cotton gauze. This may lead to damage of healthy tissue when the dressing is removed. It is not widely used in the UK.
- Myiasis involves the use of sterile maggots and may be considered a form of enzymatic therapy associated with a component of mechanical debridement.

A reasonable index of suspicion for infection should be maintained. However, it is important to realize that all pressure ulcers are colonized with bacteria. Only signs of clinical infection, local or systemic, should prompt bacterial culture to confirm the organism and antibiotic sensitivities. During wound infection, the overall number of bacteria within the wound increases due to overgrowth of infecting (virulent) bacteria. Generally, wound infection is associated with the classical clinical signs of infection. In addition, wound infection may be associated with increased wound pain, tenderness, increased wound exudate, a 'beefy' red wound bed, overgranulation, (mal-)odour, and contact bleeding. Depending upon the balance between bacterial virulence and host response, wound infection may progress to cellulitis, bacteraemia, or septicaemia.

Local wound infection (see Figure 23.18) may be treated with topical antimicrobials such as cadexomer, iodine, or silver in appropriate formulations, either as a dressing or an ointment. Systemic treatment of an infected pressure ulcer and/or accompanying cellulitis, bacteraemia, or osteomyelitis should be guided by culture and sensitivity of the organism(s). Broad-spectrum antibiotic therapy should be initiated, reflecting the site and depth of the pressure ulcer while awaiting the results of tissue culture and sensitivity or blood cultures. However, swab results may not accurately reflect deep tissue cultures. Ulcer biopsy, if possible, will yield better tissue cultures.

Organisms commonly responsible for pressure ulcer infection include *Staphylococcus aureus*, enterococci, group B beta haemolytic streptococci, and *Pseudomonas aeruginosa*. Penicillins or macrolides are generally indicated in the first instance, although adherence to local guidelines should be observed. Suspicion of infection with anaerobic bacteria, particularly associated with a deep wound, may require the addition of metronidazole.

A chronic, indolent, non-healing wound may reflect the development of underlying osteomyelitis, often as a result of Gram-negative or anaerobic bacteria. Indeed, bone may be palpable at the base of the wound. Plain radiographs

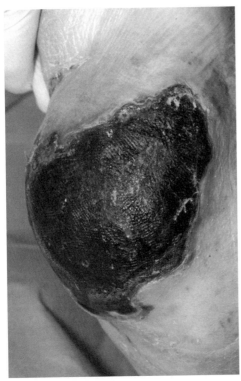

Figure 23.17 (colour plate 33) Eschar on heel pressure ulcer.

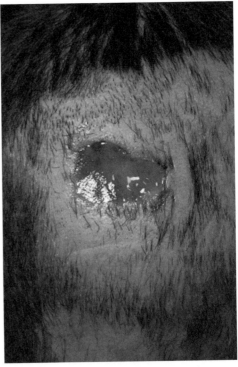

Figure 23.18 (colour plate 34) Locally infected scalp pressure ulcer.

often lack sufficient diagnostic sensitivity and specificity and a bone scan or magnetic resonance imaging may be necessary to aid the diagnosis of osteomyelitis. Treatment is with a prolonged course of antibiotics (an average of 6 weeks, although there is no definitive optimal duration). Surgical debridement of devitalised bone may be necessary.

Topical wound management

Dressings

Although dressings play a major role in the treatment of pressure ulcers, they are unlikely to promote healing in the absence of a holistic approach to management of pressure ulceration. Modern occlusive dressings promote moist wound healing, enhance autolytic debridement, facilitate re-epithelialization, provide a barrier to bacteria and reduce pain associated with pressure ulceration. Pressure ulcer characteristics and classification should be used to choose an appropriate dressing from the multitude available (see Table 23.6). Local and national guidelines should also be considered as should cost, availability, ease of application, and patient preference.

Moisture associated tissue damage (maceration), actual or potential, of skin around the pressure ulcer may be ameliorated by the use of topical barrier preparations (e.g. zinc oxide, titanium dioxide, dimeticone, benzalkonium, or white soft paraffin).

Adjunctive therapies

A variety of other topical treatment modalities are in current use. The negative pressure wound healing device (see Figure 23.19) is increasingly being used to treat deep, cavitating wounds with large amounts of exudate for an average length of 3–4 weeks. After this time, the wound fills considerably with healthy tissue. Conventional dressings are then used to manage the ulcer to complete healing.

Direct contact (capacitative) electrical stimulation has been used in the management of recalcitrant category/stage II, as well as category/stage III and IV pressure ulcers which have not responded to conventional therapy. A variety of other novel modalities, for example hyperbaric oxygen therapy and ultrasound, have been used but evidence of their efficacy is lacking.

Sterile maggots may be used for 2 to 3 days to treat sloughy and infected ulcers. Recombinant growth factors including platelet-derived growth factor (PDGF) and basic fibroblast growth factor (bFGF) have been used to treat category III and IV pressure ulcers. Allogeneic tissue-engineered cultured grafts ('skin substitutes') have similarly been used to treat stage III and IV pressure ulcers in trials. Neither modality is in widespread clinical use.

Table 23.6 Suggested dressing type for different pressure ulcer categories

Pressure ulcer category	Dressing type	Advantages/disadvantages
Minimally exuding I–II	Semi-permeable film	Promote moist environment
		Adheres to healthy skin but not to wound
		Allows visual checks
		May be left in place several days
		No cushioning
		Not for infected or heavily exuding wounds
Low to moderately exuding, non-infected II–III	Foams	Degree of cushioning
		May be left in place 2–3 days
		Needs secondary dressing
Low to moderately exuding II–IV	Hydrogels	Supplies moisture to low exudates wounds
		Useful for cavities and sinuses
		May be left in place several days
		Needs secondary dressing
		May cause maceration
Low to moderately exuding III–IV	Hydrocolloids	Absorbable
		Conformable
		Good in 'difficult areas' – heel, elbow, sacrum
		May be left in place several days
		May cause maceration
Moderate to highly exuding II–IV	Hydrofibres	Useful in cavities, sinuses, undermining wounds
		Highly absorbent
		Non adherent
		May be left in place for several days
		Needs secondary dressing
Moderate to Highly exuding II – IV	Alginates	Useful in cavities, sinuses, undermining wounds
		Highly absorbent
		Needs secondary dressing
		Needs to be changed daily

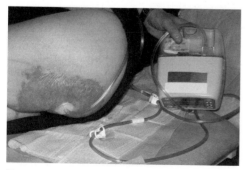

Figure 23.19 (colour plate 35) Negative pressure device *in situ*.

Surgical treatment

Surgical treatment of pressure ulcers is appropriate for those patients whose health outcomes and quality of life would significantly be improved by such intervention. Surgical reconstruction may be suitable for some category III and IV pressure ulcers not responding to conventional conservative management and may improve healing times. A successful outcome is highly dependent on the optimization of the individual's medical and nutritional status. Infected bone must be resected prior to or during surgical closure.

Musculocutaneous and fasciocutaneous flaps are commonly used techniques in the reconstruction of pressure ulcers. The flaps consist of skin, muscle, and a blood supply which fill the defect made by the pressure ulcer. The flaps are able to withstand pressure and shear trauma. They are also particularly useful when treating pressure ulcers

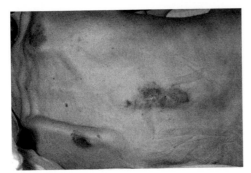

Figure 23.20 (colour plate 36) Pressure ulcers in cachectic patient with terminal illness.

complicated by osteomyelitis by bringing highly vascularized muscle into the area from which the devitalised and infected bone has been excised. Complications include haematoma, seroma, infection, wound infection, flap necrosis, and dehiscence.

Surgical debridement of pressure ulcers (especially extensive categories III and IV ulcers), under general anaesthetic, is sometimes necessary to remove large amounts of necrotic material. This improves the local wound environment and helps promote healing.

Terminal Illness

Individuals with terminal illness are at high risk of pressure ulceration (see Figure 23.20). Prevalence of pressure ulcers in such patients ranges from 37% to 50% and reflect the severity of the underlying disease. Although most pressure ulcers are avoidable, they may reflect the multisystem failure, which often accompanies terminal illness. In these cases, aggressive preventative measures may be inappropriate; patient comfort and dignity should be of prime concern. Symptomatic treatment including comfort, pain relief and odour management should be optimized in liaison with local palliative care services.

Box 23.1 Additional categories for the US

Unstageable/unclassified: full thickness skin or tissue loss – depth unknown

Full thickness tissue loss in which actual depth of the ulcer is completely obscured by slough (yellow, tan, gray, green or brown) and/or eschar (tan, brown or black) in the wound bed. Further description: until enough slough and/or eschar are removed to expose the base of the wound, the true depth cannot be determined; but it will be either a Category/Stage III or IV. Stable (dry, adherent, intact without erythema, or fluctuance) eschar on the heels serves as 'the body's natural (biological) cover' and should not be removed.

Suspected deep tissue injury: depth unknown

Purple or maroon localized area of discoloured intact skin or blood-filled blister due to damage of underlying soft tissue from pressure and/or shear. Further description: the area may be preceded by tissue that is painful, firm, mushy, boggy, warmer, or cooler than adjacent tissue. Deep tissue injury may be difficult to detect in individuals with dark skin tones. Evolution may include a thin blister over a dark wound bed. The wound may further evolve and become covered by thin eschar. Evolution may be rapid exposing additional layers of tissue even with treatment.

Further reading

Allman RM, Goode PS, Patrick MM, et al.AA. (1995). Pressure ulcer risk factors among hospitalized patients with activity limitation. *JAMA* **273**: 865–70.

Ayello EA, Mezey M, Amella EJ (1997). Educational assessment and teaching of older clients with pressure ulcers. *Clin Geriatr Med* **13**: 483–96.

Bar CA, Pathy MSJ (1998). Pressure Ulcers. In (Pathy MSJ ed.) *Principles and Practice of Geriatric Medicine*, 3rd edn. London, Wiley.

Barbenel JC, Ferguson-Pell MW, Kennedy R (1986). Mobility of elderly patients in bed. Measurement and association with patient condition. *J Am Geriatr Soc* **34**: 633–6.

Bauer C, Geriach MA, Doughty D (2000). Care of metastatic skin lesions. *J Wound Ostomy Continence Nurs* **27**: 247–57-51.

Bennett G, Dealey C, Posnett J (2004). the cost of pressure ulcers in the U.K. *Age Ageing* **33**: 230–5.

Bourdel-Marchasson I, Barateau M, Rondeau V, et al. (2000). A multi-center trial of the effects of oral nutritional supplementation in critically ill older inpatients. GAGE Group. Groupe Aquitain Geriatrique d'Evaluation. *Nutrition* **16**: 1–5.

Carter DM, Balin AK (1983). Dermatological aspects of aging. *Med Clin North Am* **67**: 531–43.

Clark M, Watts S (1994). The incidence of pressure sores within a National Health Service Trust hospital during 1991. *J Adv Nurs* **20**: 33–6.

Collier M (1996). Pressure reducing mattresses. *J Wound Care* **5**: 207–11.

Collins F (2004). A guide to the selection of specialist beds and mattresses. *J Wound Care/Therapy weekly*, 14–18.

Exton-Smith AN, Sherwin RW (1961). The prevention of pressure sores. Significance of spontaneous bodily movements. *Lancet* **2**: 1124–6.

Hatcliffe S, Dawe R (1996). Implementing 'A Vision for the Future' targets in a hospice. *Nurs Stand* **10**: 44–6.

Hatcliffe S, Dawe R (1996). How patients see symptoms. *Nurs Times* **92**: 61–3.

Hatcliffe S, Dawe R (1996). Monitoring pressure sores in a palliative care setting. *Int J Pall Nurs* **2**: 182–6.

Lazarus GS, Cooper DM, Knighton DR, et al. (1994). Definitions and guidelines for assessment of wounds and evaluation of healing. *Arch Dermatol* **130**: 489–93.

Mathus-Vliegen EM (2004). Old age, malnutrition, and pressure sores: an ill-fated alliance. *J Gerontol A Biol Sci Med Sci* **59**: 355–60.

Stotts NA, Rodeheaver GT, Thomas DR, et al. (2001). An instrument to measure healing in pressure ulcers: development and validation of the pressure ulcer scale for healing (PUSH). *J Gerontol A Biol Sci Med Sci* **56**: M795–9.

The National Institute for Health and Clinical Excellence (NICE).

Thomas DR, Goode PS, Tarquine PH, et al. (1996). Hospital-acquired pressure ulcers and risk of death. *J Am Geriatr Soc* **44**: 1435–40.

Tissue Viability Society in the UK: the National Pressure Ulcer Advisory Panel (NPUAP) in the USA European Pressure Ulcer Advisory Panel (EPUAP).

Vanderwee K, Clark M, Dealey C, et al. (2007). Pressure ulcer prevalence in Europe: a pilot study. *J Eval Clin Pract* **13**: 227–35.

Vowden KR, Vowden P (2009). The prevalence, management and outcome for acute wounds indentified in a wound care survey within one English health care district. *J Tissue Viability* **18**: 7–12.

Cancer in old age

Association of cancer and ageing

Background

The incidence of malignant tumours increases progressively with age, both in animals and in humans. Cancer is a common cause of disability and death in older people: over 50% of malignant neoplasms occur in persons over 70 years. Two major hypotheses have been proposed to explain the association of cancer and age. The first hypothesis holds that this association is a consequence of the duration of carcinogenesis. The second proposes that age-related progressive changes in the internal milieu of the organism may provide an increasingly favourable environment for the initiation of new neoplasms and for the growth of already existent, but latent, malignant cells. These mechanisms may also include proliferative senescence, as the senescent cells loses the ability to undergo apoptosis, and produce substances favouring cancer growth and metastases.

Susceptibility to carcinogenesis at different age

There are age-related differences in sensitivity to carcinogens in some tissues. Thus, with age, susceptibility to carcinogens in murine mammary gland, bowels, thyroid, ovary, soft tissues, cervix, and vagina increases, whereas in lung and haemopoietic tissues it remains stable. The effective dose of carcinogen requiring metabolic activation may vary significantly in old and young organisms because the activity of the enzymes necessary for carcinogen activation in the liver and/or target tissue(s) may change with age. Critical factors that determine the susceptibility of a tissue to carcinogenesis include DNA synthesis and proliferative activity of that tissue at the time of carcinogen exposure, and the efficacy of repair of damaged DNA. The homeostatic regulation of cell numbers in normal tissues reflects a precise balance between cell proliferation and cell death.

Ageing and multi-stage carcinogenesis

Both carcinogenesis and ageing are associated with genomic alterations, which may act synergistically in causing cancer. In particular, three key age-related changes in DNA metabolism may favour cell transformation and cancer growth. These changes are genetic instability, DNA hypomethylation, and formation of DNA adducts. Genetic instability involves activation of genes that are normally suppressed, such as the cellular protooncogenes, and/or inactivation of some tumour suppression genes (p53, Rb, etc.). DNA hypomethylation is characteristic of ageing and of transformed cells. Hypomethylation, a potential mechanism of oncogene activation, may result in spontaneous deamination of cytosine and consequent base transition. Accumulation of inappropriate base pairs may cause cell transformation by activation of cellular proto-oncogenes. Age-related abnormalities of DNA metabolism may be, to some extent, tissue and gene specific. Within the same cell, different DNA segments express different degrees of age-related hypomethylation. The uneven distribution of hypomethylation may underlie selective overexpression of proto oncogenes by senescent cells.

The damage caused by endogenous reactive oxygen species (ROS) has been proposed as a major contributor to both ageing and cancer. ROS may induce mutations in proto oncogenes. A variety of cell defence systems are involved in protecting macromolecules against the devastating action of ROS. These systems include antioxidant enzymes (superoxide dismutase, catalase, glutathione peroxidase, glutathione reductase, and glucose-6 phosphate dehydrogenase), some vitamins (alpha-tocopherol, ascorbic acid), uric acid, and the pineal indole hormone, melatonin. Accumulation with age of some spontaneous mutations can induce genome instability and, hence, increase the sensitivity to carcinogens and/or tumour promoters.

Carcinogenesis is a multistage process: neoplastic transformation implies the engagement of a cell through sequential stages, and different agents may affect the transition between continuous stages. Multistage carcinogenesis is accompanied by disturbances in tissue homeostasis and perturbations in nervous, hormonal, and metabolic factors which may affect antitumour resistance. The development of these changes depends on the susceptibility of various systems to a carcinogen and on the dose of the carcinogen. Changes in the microenvironment may condition key carcinogenic events and determine the duration of each carcinogenic stage, and sometimes they may even reverse the process of carcinogenesis. These microenvironmental changes influence the proliferation rate of transformed cells together, the total duration of carcinogenesis, and, consequently, the latent period of tumour development. Cross-talk between mesenchyme and epithelium has been described as a known driver of differentiation and development. Changes in stromal behaviour can promote epithelial transformation.

Cellular senescence and carcinogenesis

In contrast to germ cells and certain stem cells, the majority of somatic cell types have a limited proliferative life span. These limit may have evolved as a protective mechanism against cancer, although it may also cause accumulation of cells at the end of their replicative life span that may be responsible for the ageing process and increase the susceptibility to carcinogenesis. It is worth noting that data has been accumulated on a loss of stem cell regenerative capacity within aged niches. It was shown that senescent human fibroblasts stimulate premalignant and malignant, but not normal, epithelial cells to proliferate in culture and form tumours in nude mice.

There is increasing evidence that age-related changes in tumour microenvironment might also play a significant role. It is important to stress that in every tissue, the number of events occurring in the stem cell before its complete transformation is variable and depends on many factors, in particular the rate of ageing of the target tissue and its regulatory system(s). This model is consistent with the analysis of age-related distribution of tumour incidence in different sites in both humans and laboratory animals.

Carcinogens accelerate ageing

Given the similarity of molecular changes of ageing and carcinogenesis, it is reasonable to ask whether and how carcinogens may affect ageing. Chronic inhalation of tobacco smoke caused enhanced production of free radicals and signs of accelerated ageing in rats and humans. Ionizing radiation and chemical carcinogens appear to cause disturbances in the internal tissue milieu, similar to those of normal ageing, but at an earlier age. Circadian disruption (shift work or exposure to light at night) causes accelerated ageing and carcinogenesis.

Genetic modifications of ageing and carcinogenesis

Some syndromes of untimely ageing (progeria) are associated with an increased incidence of cancer. Alongside the classical progeria syndromes, some diseases (e.g. sclerocystic ovaries syndrome) are accompanied by disturbances which might be regarded as signs of the intensified ageing. Genetically modified animal models, which are characterized by shortening or extension of the life span, allow us to evaluate the role of ageing genes in mechanisms of carcinogenesis. Practically all models of accelerated ageing show increased tumour incidence and latency shortening.

Cellular senescence has been proposed to contribute to organism ageing. Senescent cells have been shown to accumulate with age in some human tissues. The tissue microenvironment is disrupted by the accumulation of dysfunctional senescent cells. Thus, mutation accumulation may synergize with the accumulation of senescent cells, leading to increasing risk for developing cancer that is a hallmark of mammalian ageing.

According to the multistage model of carcinogenesis, the proportion of partially transformed cells that have progressed through some stages will increase with age. There are evidences of age-related accumulation of 'premalignant' cells in several tissues (skin, lymph node, thymus, spleen, liver, ovary, mammary gland).

There are two strategies of development of the stem cell which could be realized in an organism. One strategy is the cellular differentiation and ageing and, at least, in its individual death (apoptotic or necrotic). Anti-ageing factors support the tissues and maintain functional homeostasis in life-important organs, although when they reach a certain limit, the death of an organism as a whole takes place. Another strategy of the stem cells exposed to exogenous or endogenous harmful factors is through dedifferentiation, immortalization, and the formation of a clone of neoplastic cells. Both strategies are multistage processes, many steps of which are well characterized in relation to the process of carcinogenesis.

Conclusion

In the burst of industrialization, urbanization, and increasing environmental pollution (including light pollution), one may hope only for a partial alleviation of the unfavourable effects on human health. Changes in lifestyle, i.e. in dietary and sexual habits and in smoking and alcohol consumption, may be the most promising approach to achieving a decrease in cancer incidence and an increase in life span. Any factors which normalize the age-related changes in the hormonal status, metabolism, and immunity and thus slow down the realization of the genetic programme of ageing must be most effective in the protection from both premature ageing and cancer. Among these factors are mimetics of calorie restriction (e.g. metformin), melatonin, and some pineal peptides. The influences which protect from the initiating action of damaging agents (antioxidants and antimutagens) may be important additional means of accelerated ageing prevention especially under conditions of an increased risk of exposure to environmental harmful agents.

Further reading

Anisimov VN (1987). *Carcinogenesis and Aging*, vols 1 and 2. Boca Raton, FL, CRC Press.

Anisimov VN (2007). Biology of aging and cancer. *Cancer Control* **14**: 23–31.

Anisimov VN (2009). Carcinogenesis and aging 20 years after: escaping horizon. *Mech Ageing Dev* **130**: 105–21.

Anisimov VN, Sikora E, Pawelec G (2009). Relationships between cancer and aging: multilevel approach. *Biogerontology* **10**: 323–38.

Anisimov VN, Ukraintseva SV, Yashin AI (2005). Cancer in rodents: Does it tell us about cancer in humans? *Nature Rev Cancer* **5**: 807–19.

Balducci L, Ershler WB (2005). Cancer and ageing: a nexus at several levels. *Nat Rev Cancer* **5**: 655–62.

Campisi J, d'Adda di Fagagna F (2007). Cellular senescence: when bad things happen to good cells. *Nat Rev Mol Cell Biol* **8**: 729–40.

DePinho RA (2000). The age of cancer. *Nature* **408**: 248–54.

Hoeijmakers JH, (2007). Genome maintenance mechanisms are critical for preventing cancer as well as other aging-associated diseases. *Mech Ageing Dev* **128**: 460–2.

Serrano M, Blasco MA (2007). Cancer and ageing: convergent and divergent mechanisms. *Nat Rev Mol Cell Biol* **8**: 715–22.

Presentation of cancer in old age

Background

Over 50% of all cancers are diagnosed in individuals aged 70 years or older. Not only do we have an ageing population, but also greater diagnostic certainty when considering malignant disease. The two main sources of cancer statistics are mortality as derived from death certificates and incidence as collected by cancer registries. Unfortunately, both of these sources have increasing inaccuracy as the individual patient ages. Death certificates may fail to document cancer in very frail older individuals, in whom definitive investigations and treatment have not been performed. Cancer registry data may be affected by individuals in whom investigations are felt to be inappropriate or unjustified as a result of frailty, patient wishes, and potentially ageist attitudes. However, determining which of these accounted for the paucity of investigations is often difficult.

When considering the older person with cancer, with increasing age individuals are less likely to present in the way that a younger patient would present and less likely to be investigated; they are more likely to have more advanced disease at presentation; are less likely to be treated with curative intent; and have reduced survival. Although ageist attitudes from patients, family members and healthcare professionals may account for some of the differences witnessed with increasing age, this is not the entire story. The presence of comorbidity leaves oncologists and surgeons with the challenge of dealing with normal ageing, the giants of geriatric medicine, multiple comorbidities, polypharmacy, and the underlying cancer diagnosis. Many older patients present late with resultant reduction in the likelihood of curative therapy. A cancer 'stage-to-age' study in 1981 found a significant positive relationships between age and stage for cancer of the bladder, breast, cervix, kidney, ovary, stomach, and uterus, i.e. the older the patient was, the more likely that he/she would be diagnosed with advanced stage disease. However, this has not always been the finding and older patients may be diagnosed with cancer at less advanced stages, when considering the stomach, pancreas, rectum, and lung in some studies.

Why are older people at risk for delays in diagnosis?

It is sometimes very difficult to recognize the symptoms of cancer in an 80 year old. Many of the symptoms are generalized and include aches and pains, changes in bowel habit, a variety of cutaneous or 'intracavity' lesions, and fatigue.

Lung cancer

Normal ageing results in a gradual decline in pulmonary function. With the decrease in FEV_1 and FVC, the older patient has a reduced respiratory reserve and a reduced ability to clear bronchial secretions. If this is combined with a past history of cigarette smoking, a physician diagnosis of chronic obstructive disease, and a patient diagnosis of 'chest trouble', a further reduction in respiratory function may not trigger a patient to present for further investigations. Chest pain may be attributed to the musculoskeletal system and haemoptysis is a rare and late symptom of lung cancer. The coincidental presence of cardiac decompensation, particularly in those who smoke, may result in a further reason for the patient to ignore worsening symptoms. Although previous reports have highlighted that older people with suspected lung cancer are much less likely to undergo bronchoscopy and definitive investigations, this has improved during the last 20 years, but the UK still has one of the lowest 5-year survival rates for lung cancer and the majority of early deaths are in older individuals.

Although there are no specific papers looking at the presentation of lung cancer in older individuals, a systematic review of the presentation of pneumonia in this age group, may help to guide clinicians. Presentation of pneumonia as 'delirium or confusion' ranges from 15% to 67%, and the absence of cough was particularly prevalent. A persistent cough in the presence of unexplained weight loss will immediately indicate the need for a chest radiograph. A chest infection in an older person should always be followed up, particularly if tiredness, chest or shoulder discomfort, and breathlessness remain after treatment with antibiotics.

Colorectal cancer

Despite screening opportunities for older people, the diagnosis of colorectal tumours is often made following presentation with vague symptoms. Symptomatic anaemia is more commonly seen in older than younger subjects, as is anorexia. Younger subjects with a rectal carcinoma, with symptoms such as tenesmus, abdominal or rectal pain present change in flatus production, or passage of mucus per rectum.

There is evidence that the passage of dark red rectal bleeding or the presence of abdominal mass are the most likely symptoms that result in the older person with colorectal cancer presenting to a primary care physician.

Although many of the symptoms are non-specific and may indicate functional constipation or diverticular disease, the most likely features associated with colorectal cancer are listed in below.

The 10 features most commonly associated with colorectal cancer before diagnosis

- Rectal bleeding
- Weight loss
- Abdominal pain
- Diarrhoea
- Constipation
- Abnormal rectal examination
- Abdominal tenderness
- Haemoglobin <100 g/L
- Positive faecal occult bloods
- Blood glucose >10 mmol/L

Gastric cancer

Although the mean age at presentation with gastric cancer is lower than colorectal or lung tumours, the duration of symptoms is often longer. In some series, dysphagia is present and often attributed to suspected peptic ulcer disease. The finding of anaemia should initiate upper and lower gastrointestinal investigations, and an electrolyte abnormality is reported to be prevalent in some series. A high index of suspicion must be present in patients on aspirin or non-steroidal anti-inflammatory agents. Such patients often attribute or have their symptoms attributed to their underlying medication and are less likely to undergo endoscopy, even in the light of anaemia. The pathogenetic link of *Helicobacter* pylori and gastric cancer is well documented. The eradication of *H. pylori*, particularly in patients without atrophic gastritis or intestinal metaplasia, is particularly useful.

Approximately one-third of patients with gastric tumours are referred as acute emergencies and two-thirds present to the outpatient department. The commonest presentations as an emergency are abdominal pain, vomiting, gastrointestinal bleeding, dysphagia, and a palpable mass. Those patients presenting via the emergency department are more likely to be older, have more advanced disease, and have a reduced duration of survival. Dysphagia, weight loss, and palpable abdominal mass are major independent prognostic factors in gastric cancer, whereas gastrointestinal bleeding, vomiting, and duration of symptoms do not appear to have a significant affect on survival.

Breast cancer

Some older women with breast cancer will be identified through screening, albeit at the patient's request. However the majority of tumours are detected outside of screening programmes. In some series, the mean tumour size is >4 cm and the majority of individuals have evidence of local or more widespread metastasis at presentation.

The non-specific presentation associated with breast cancer is most commonly hypercalcaemia with well-documented 'bones, stones, and abdominal groans'. Unfortunately a small minority of older women will still present with pathological fractures or with symptoms attributable to their hepatic metastases.

Prostate cancer

Some series suggest that up to half of all men may have metastases at the time of presentation with prostate cancer. The most common metastases occur in the bone and result in non-specific 'bone pain', which is often attributed to arthritis by the patient or even their physician. Localized prostatic enlargement results in non-specific urinary symptoms which may also be attributable to prostatic hyperplasia. A prostate-specific antigen (PSA) estimation is mandatory in all individuals with symptoms attributable to outflow obstruction. It must however be remembered that up to 20% of all men with prostate cancer have a normal PSA and therefore identification of prostate cancer requires both PSA and digital rectal examination to be considered in a combined approach. Early involvement of urologists is essential as 'watchful waiting' may be the mainstay of many patients with early disease in whom multiple comorbidities are present.

Conditions associated with malignant disease in older individuals

Although there is little evidence in the benefit of screening for occult cancers, a high level of suspicion needs to be exercised following presentation of patients with certain features. Venous thromboembolism has an established link with cancer and the presence of cancer is a risk factor for the development for venous thromboembolism (VTE). In a small prospective study, 8% of those who presented with VTE were found to have an underlying cancer when extensively investigated with tumour markers, ultrasound, and computed tomography scanning. Although one patient with malignant disease was detected immediately following the VTE diagnosis, in the remainder it was at a later stage during follow-up. Therefore, all older patients with a primary diagnosis of VTE should be followed up in order to detect occult malignancy, although the evidence for this being cost effective or likely to improve prognosis is yet to be established.

Older people often have an asymptomatic presentation of a primary tumour. Symptoms must be investigated even if attributed to other conditions if therapy for that condition fails to improve the clinical situation. Early involvement of the multidisciplinary cancer team is essential if the geriatrician finds evidence of metastatic disease. This enables targeted investigations to focus on the treatable tumours, rather than a random 'hunt the primary' initiative, which is neither helpful to the patient, nor fulfilling for the medical team.

Further reading

Afuwape OO, Irabor DO, Ladipo JK, Ayandipo B (In press). A review of the current profile of gastric cancer presentation in the University College Hospital Ibadan, a tertiary health care institution in the tropics. *J Gastrointest Cancer*.

Blackshaw GR, Stephens MR, Lewis WG, *et al*. (2004). Prognostic significance of acute presentation with emergency complications of gastric cancer. *Gastric Cancer* **7**: 91–6.

Hamilton W, Lancashire R, Sharp D, *et al*. (2009). The risk of colorectal cancer with symptoms at different ages and between sexes: a case-control study. *BMC Med* **7**: 17.

Maconi G, Manes G, Porro GB (2008). Role of symptoms in diagnosis and outcome of gastric cancer. *World J Gastroenterol* **14**: 1149–55.

Rieu V, Chanier S, Philippe P, Ruivard M (2011). Systematic screening for occult cancer in elderly patients with venous thromboembolism: a prospective study. *Intern Med* **41**: 769–75.

Breast cancer

Epidemiology

With 1.15 million new cases per year, breast cancer is the most prevalent cancer and the leading cause of cancer death among women worldwide. The highest incidence is recorded in women over 70 years and these patients also experience the worst relative mortality.

Advanced age at diagnosis is associated with less aggressive tumour biology (hormone receptor-positive, decreased Human Epidermal growth factor Receptor 2 (HER2) expression, lower proliferative index). However, older women are more likely to present with locally advanced tumours. Furthermore, they are less likely to undergo screening, standard staging, and surgical treatment of the primary tumour and they receive adjuvant treatment less frequently. Women over 80 years have higher mortality from early-stage breast cancer than women 67–79 years, even when correcting for comorbidities. Also, older breast cancer patients are less likely to be entered into clinical trials.

Decisions about breast cancer screening in older women are not as straightforward as in younger patients. The following factors need to be considered in the individual patient:

- estimates of life expectancy
- risk of cancer death
- screening outcomes based on published data
- potential harm from screening
- patient's values and preferences.

Surgery

Surgical removal of the tumour is the standard of care for breast cancer independent of the patient's age, although the treatment plan should be tailored to every individual. A geriatric assessment may be useful in delivering individualised treatment. Mortality for breast cancer surgery is negligible (0–0.3%) and there is no excuse for not offering a surgical approach to a patient who is fit for surgery.

Breast conservation is associated with better quality of life and self-esteem, and is preferred by older women. It may often be considered a valid option, provided that the patient is fit and facilities are in place for adjuvant radiotherapy. The target is to excise the primary tumour with sufficient resection margins. However, in patients with a limited life expectancy, the impact of involved margins on the local recurrence rate may be less important.

Mastectomy is indicated when the primary tumour is too large to allow breast preservation, the patient has no interest in breast preservation, or if the patient cannot comply with the adjuvant radiotherapy plan.

Axillary nodes are removed for therapeutic and staging purposes. As sentinel node biopsy is accepted as the standard of care in most cases, axillary dissection is now regarded as inappropriate. A sentinel node biopsy is less traumatizing to the patient and allows a prompt postoperative recovery. However, for frail women with a high-grade primary tumour, a low or intermediate axillary dissection may be suitable, as there are increased risks related to undertaking a second procedure under general anaesthetic in the case of sentinel nodes being positive.

Radiotherapy

As no significant increase in toxicity has been demonstrated for older women, tolerability is not a limiting factor for radiotherapy. Suboptimal and obsolete treatment fields may be associated with a higher risk of non-breast cancer related morbidity, such as cardiac and pulmonary disease.

Adjuvant radiotherapy has been shown to be advantageous and is reported as standard care, regardless of the patient's age. Despite this, postoperative breast irradiation may be debatable in older patients with a low risk of recurrence (small tumour, clear margins, node negative, absence of perineural/lymphovascular invasion, endocrine positive). In these cases, the absolute reduction in local recurrences may be minute and the mortality associated with non-breast cancer related conditions may be higher than the benefit from the additional treatment.

The evidence supporting post-mastectomy irradiation in older women is limited but it is still recommended for large (T3–T4) tumours, more than four positive nodes and when margins are involved. As the survival advantage appears to emerge only after 5 years, chest irradiation should be offered only to women whose life expectancy exceeds 5 years.

Adjuvant hormonal therapy

The effectiveness of hormonal therapy (tamoxifen and aromatase inhibitors) for hormone receptor-positive tumours does not appear to be age related. Tamoxifen represents an excellent treatment modality for older breast cancer patients. There is a lack of data regarding the use of aromatase inhibitors in older patients. Older patients may be more vulnerable to some of the adverse effects of aromatase inhibitors such as muscle and joint pain, osteoporosis and fractures, and cardiovascular events.

Hormonal treatment should be started after completion of chemotherapy. As aromatase inhibitors may cause osteoporosis, the use of bisphosphonates need to be considered when prescribing this drug to older patients with low bone mineral density.

Adjuvant chemotherapy

Individualized decision-making is necessary when considering the use of adjuvant chemotherapy. The patient's absolute benefit, life expectancy, treatment tolerance, and preference should be taken into consideration. Older women with node-positive and hormonal-negative breast cancers are likely to benefit the most.

Standard chemotherapy with fluorouracil or anthracycline is superior to capecitabine in patients with early-stage breast cancer who are 65 years of age or older. In a trial published in 2009, patients who were randomly assigned to capecitabine were twice as likely to relapse and almost twice as likely to die compared with patients receiving standard chemotherapy. However, the benefit must be balanced against more pronounced toxicity. In the absence of cardiovascular contraindications, four courses of an anthracycline-based regimen are usually preferred to fluorouracil. Taxanes could also be added to the treatment in fit high-risk older breast cancer patients.

Trastuzumab, which belongs to the cancer drug group of monoclonal antibodies, may also be offered in older HER2-positive patients when there is no history of heart disease.

Stage IV breast cancer

The treatment goals for older breast cancer patients with stage IV disease are similar to younger patients. Hormonal treatment is the preferred option for hormone receptor-positive cancers, but the use of chemotherapy may be considered when the tumour is hormone receptor-negative or hormone refractory.

Chemotherapeutic drugs with a safer profile are preferred, such as weekly taxane regimens, anthracycline, capecitabine, gemcitabine, and vinorelbine. The doses of these drugs are often reduced in older people, but evidence regarding these adapted dose schedules is lacking. Increased toxicity and only minor survival advantages has been reported for combination chemotherapy when compared with monotherapy.

Key issues

- Patients' and doctors' awareness of breast cancer in the older population needs to be enhanced
- Breast cancer is likely to be undertreated in older patients
- The operative mortality for breast cancer is low
- Radiotherapy seems to be well tolerated in older people
- Tamoxifen works just as well in older as in younger breast cancer patients
- Current standard treatment protocols are not directed towards frail older patients – an individualized geriatric assessment is therefore necessary for treatment decisions
- Increased evidence is needed and would allow for defining standards of care and thus improve outcome

Further reading

Althuis MD, Dozier JM, Anderson WF, et al. (2005). Global trends in breast cancer incidence and mortality 1973–1997. *Int J Epidemiol* **34**: 405–12.

Audisio RA (2004). The surgical risk of elderly patients with cancer. *Surg Oncol* **13**: 169–73.

Bouchardy C, Rapiti E, Fioretta G, et al. (2003). Undertreatment strongly decreases prognosis of breast cancer in elderly women. *J Clin Oncol* **21**: 3580–7.

Clarke M, Collins R, Darby S, et al. (2005). Effects of radiotherapy and of differences in the extent of surgery for early breast cancer on local recurrence and 15-year survival: an overview of the randomised trials. *Lancet* **366**: 2087–106.

Gennari R, Curigliano G, Rotmensz N, et al. (2004). Breast carcinoma in elderly women—features of disease presentation, choice of local and systemic treatments compared with younger postmenopausal patients. *Cancer* **101**: 1302–10.

Giordano SH, Hortobagyi GN, Kau SWC, et al. (2005). Breast cancer treatment guidelines in older women. *J Clin Oncol* **23**: 783–91.

Hughes KS, Schnaper LA, Berry D, et al. (2004). Lumpectomy plus tamoxifen with or without irradiation in women 70 years of age or older with early breast cancer. *N Engl J Med* **351**: 971–7.

Hurria A, Leung D, Trainor K, et al. (2003). Factors influencing treatment patterns of breast cancer patients aged 75 and older. *Crit Rev Oncol Hematol* **46**: 121–6.

Muss HB, Berry DA, Cirrincione CT, et al. (2009). Adjuvant chemotherapy in older women with early-stage breast cancer. *N Engl J Med* **360**: 2055–65.

Schonberg MA, Marcantonio ER, Li D, et al. (2010). Breast cancer among the oldest old: tumor characteristics, treatment choices, and survival. *J Clin Oncol* **28**: 2038–45.

Walter LC, Covinsky KE, (2001). Cancer screening in elderly patients: a framework for individualized decision making. *JAMA* **285**: 2750–6.

Wildiers H, Kunkler I, Biganzoli L, et al. (2007). Management of breast cancer in elderly individuals: recommendations of the International Society of Geriatric Oncology. *Lancet Oncol* **8**(12): 1101-15.

Yancik R, Wesley MN, Ries LAG, et al. (2001). Effect of age and comorbidity in postmenopausal breast cancer patients aged 55 years and older. *JAMA* **285**: 885–92.

Colorectal cancer

Colorectal cancer is a major public health issue. The lifetime probability that a person will develop colorectal cancer is about 6%, and it contributes to 16 000 UK deaths per year. The chance of developing colorectal cancer increases with age, being rare below 50 years. According to a recent paper the incidence per 100 000 in 55–59 year olds is around 103 for men and 77 for women; in 70–74 year olds is around 321 for men and 227 for women. In people over 85 years the incidence is around 498 per 100 000 men and 392 per 100 000 women. These figures are for people with no personal or family history of colorectal cancer, no adenomatous polyps and no inflammatory bowel disease.

The overall 5-year survival rate with colorectal cancer is about 52%. However, survival is very dependent on time of diagnosis: the 5-year survival rate for people with localized disease is over 80%, whereas for people with distant metastases it is 6%. Currently around one-third of cases are detected while the cancer is still localized (see Figure 24.1).

Risk factors

1. Age. 85% of colorectal cancers occur in people over 60 years. Age is the main risk factor.
2. Pre-existing colorectal pathology. This includes previous colorectal malignancies; polyps; inflammatory bowel disease.
3. Dietary factors. A diet low in fibre and high in fat increases risk. A low-fibre diet causes a longer colonic transit time and therefore greater exposure to any carcinogens.
4. Physical activity. A sedentary lifestyle increases the risk.
5. Genetic factors. There are several genetic syndromes which increase the risk of colorectal cancer; however, all genetic causes together account for less than 1% of colorectal cancer cases.

Pathophysiology

More than 95% of colorectal cancers develop from benign adenomatous polyps, with malignant transformation usually requiring 10–30 years. Factors affecting the risk of malignant change of a polyp include its size (polyps over 1.5 cm carry a greater risk), the type of polyp (flat polyps are higher risk than pedunculated polyps), and its histology (villous polyps are more risky than tubular polyps).

Clinical features

Clinical features can be considered in terms of the local effects of the tumour, the effects of secondary deposits, and the general effects of malignant disease.

Local effects include:

- Change in bowel habit. Rectal tumours cause constipation, whereas colon tumours cause alternating diarrhoea and constipation
- The tumour may bleed, resulting in rectal bleeding
- Intestinal obstruction may occur, and this can be either acute, or acute on chronic, and presents with pain, distension, absolute constipation and vomiting
- Bowel perforation can occur

The effects of secondary deposits include:

- jaundice
- hepatomegaly
- abdominal distension due to ascites.

The general effects of malignancy include

- anaemia
- anorexia and weight loss.

Investigations

- Full blood count to detect anaemia caused by bleeding. Liver function tests to assess liver involvement.
- Colonoscopy is the gold standard for investigation and biopsies should be taken for histological examination.
- Ultrasound, CT and MRI may help evaluate tumour size, and local and secondary spread.

Management and prognosis

Treatment of colorectal cancer is by surgical resection of the tumour and its draining lymph nodes. The type of operation required depends on where the tumour is situated within the colon. About 70% of colon cancers are found in the left colon and these may require a left hemicolectomy if situated high in the colon, a sigmoid colectomy if in the lower part of the descending colon, or a Hartmann's procedure if situated at the base of the colon. Until recently radiotherapy and chemotherapy had a limited role in the management of colorectal cancer but many people with Dukes' C tumours now receive postoperative chemotherapy, which reduces the recurrence rate by 40% and the mortality rate by nearly one-third (see Table 24.1).

Screening

The purpose of screening for colorectal cancer is to identify people who are at sufficiently high risk for development and dying from it to warrant intervention (see Table 24.2).

Evidence for the benefits of screening for colorectal cancer

Several large randomized controlled studies have been carried out in Europe and the USA which have provided evidence that screening with faecal occult blood testing (FOBT) every other year significantly reduces colorectal cancer mortality. Analysis of these studies showed compliance of between 60% and 90% in biennial screening and mortality reduction of between 13% and 33% (follow-up periods ranged from 11 to 18 years). The English Bowel Cancer Screening Pilot was set up to assess the feasibility of introducing a national colorectal cancer screening programme based on FOBT into the NHS. A total of 478 250 men and women aged 50–69 were invited for screening. The uptake of FOBT was 56.8%. The overall rate of positive tests was 1.9% and the rate for detecting cancer was 1.62 per 1000 people screened. Following this the NHS bowel cancer screening programme was introduced in England in July 2006.

Current screening recommendations

The UK NHS Bowel Screening Programme currently offers screening every 2 years to everyone aged 60–69. People over 70 can request a kit, but are not sent one automatically. An explanatory letter and FOBT test is sent by post and people who return samples can expect results within 2 weeks.

This programme expects 98% of participants to get a normal result and continue routine screening. 2% will be offered colonoscopy. Four per cent may initially get an

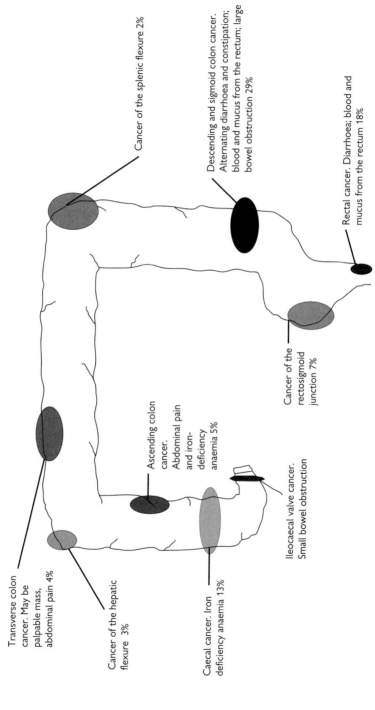

Cancer of the splenic flexure 2%

Descending and sigmoid colon cancer. Alternating diarrhoea and constipation; blood and mucus from the rectum; large bowel obstruction 29%

Rectal cancer. Diarrhoea; blood and mucus from the rectum 18%

Cancer of the rectosigmoid junction 7%

Transverse colon cancer. May be palpable mass, abdominal pain 4%

Cancer of the hepatic flexure 3%

Caecal cancer. Iron deficiency anaemia 13%

Ascending colon cancer. Abdominal pain and iron-deficiency anaemia 5%

Ileocaecal valve cancer. Small bowel obstruction

Figure 24.1 (colour plate 37) Clinical presentation of colorectal cancers by site and the percentages that occur at each site. Data from Cancer Research UK figures for distribution of cases by site within the large bowel. Data relate to diagnoses in England 1997–2000.

Table 24.1 Modified Dukes' classification of colorectal tumours

Stage	Definition	5-year Survival (%)
A	Confined to the mucosa	90
B1	Involves part of the muscle wall	70
B2	Penetrates through muscle wall and reaches the serosa	60
C1	Involves part of the muscle wall; lymph nodes involved	30
C2	Penetrates through the muscle wall and involves serosa; lymph nodes involved	30
D	Distant metastases	6

Table from *Surgery – Crash Course*, Sweetland and Conway, Elsevier, 2004.

unclear result and are advised to repeat the test. The predicted outcomes are that for every 1000 people completing FOBT, about 20 will have a positive FOBT and be offered colonoscopy. Sixteen of these 20 are expected to have the colonoscopy, two of whom are likely to have colorectal cancer.

The procedure for follow-up and removal of polyps depends on their number and size. It is recommended that if the person is low risk (defined as one or two small – i.e. under 1 cm – adenomas) they have another FOBT in 2 years; if they are intermediate risk (three or four small adenomas or an adenoma over 1 cm) they have 3-yearly colonoscopy surveillance until they have had two negative examinations; and if they are high risk (five or more adenomas or three or more adenomas of which at least one is 1 cm or bigger) they have colonoscopy after 12 months, followed by colonoscopy every three years until they have had two negative examinations.

Screening: the pros and cons and future directions in elderly care medicine

As most colorectal cancers develop from benign adenomatous polyps, early detection of these adenomas may be a good basis for screening. However, autopsy studies of people dying from causes other than colorectal cancer have found an incidence of benign colon adenomas ranging from 20% to nearly 50%. These studies also showed that most adenomas do not undergo malignant change, and 75% of people aged 80 have adenomas. By screening for polyps, people who may otherwise have died from unrelated causes may undergo invasive intervention for a condition they would not have developed. It is unclear at present whether screening recommendations should be different for elderly people, both in terms of the actual test used, and whether screening tests are recommended until the end of life or whether there is a point at which the risks begin to outweigh the benefits, either for most people over a certain age or for those in whom tests have so far proved negative.

Table 24.2 Table showing advantages and disadvantages of screening tests for colorectal cancer and considerations in the elderly

Test	Advantages of test	Disadvantages of test	Considerations in screening older people
Faecal occult blood test (FOBT)	Can be carried out at home and is non-invasive. High specificity (98%). Can detect tumours throughout the large bowel. Acceptable to population – in 5 large controlled trials of FOBT in Europe and the USA compliance ranged from 54% to 75%. When evaluated in large-scale, long-term randomized controlled trials, FOBT reduced mortality from colorectal cancer by about 16%. It has been suggested that repeating a positive FOBT will reduce need for follow-up colonoscopies – a study by Kwenter in Gothenburg found the FOBT is positive in 5.9% of people initially but when repeated it reduced to 1.9%.	Low predictive value of positive test (5–10%), as simply detects bleeding and there are many other causes of bleeding. Low sensitivity (50%), as not all cancers bleed. Lowenfels suggests that FOBT misses about half of all malignant large bowel tumours and most polyps. May be less effective for detection of right-sided tumours. Positive FOBT is followed up by colonoscopy which may cause physical health problems. Positive FOBT may cause unnecessary anxiety. Certain foods (e.g. red meat) and medications (e.g. aspirin) may give a false positive result, so must be avoided for three days before the test.	Diverticular disease is the most common cause of gastrointestinal bleeding and is more common in elderly people. It affects two thirds of people over 80 years. Colonic angiodysplasia is a common cause of gastrointestinal bleeding particularly affecting people over 65 years. Anticoagulant therapy increases risks of bleeding, and is more commonly used in elderly people.
Colonoscopy	Entire colon can be visualized. Any lesions seen can be biopsied at the time of colonoscopy. Adenomatous polyps can be removed before they become malignant.	Sedation and full-bowel preparation are necessary. Risk of perforation of 1-2 per 1000 procedures. Colonoscopic screening of the UK population at age 60 would cause over 500 haemorrhages, 150 perforations and 50 deaths per year. Expensive.	Unclear if older people are more at risk of complications. It is believed that risk of perforation may increase with age.

(Continued)

Table 24.2 (Continued)

Test	Advantages of test	Disadvantages of test	Considerations in screening older people
Flexible sigmoidoscopy	Biopsies can be taken. Cheaper than colonoscopy. No full bowel preparation or sedation. Perforation risk lower than colonoscopy.	Only detects cancers in rectosigmoid area. Invasive procedure, with risk of perforation.	Older people at greater risk of perforation than younger people.
Double-contrast barium enema	Entire colon can be visualized by X-rays taken after barium enema given and the colon pumped with air.	Invasive procedure. Lesions detected then require colonoscopy.	Not used in screening.
Virtual colonoscopy	Non-invasive, as involves radiological examination of colon with CT or MRI.	Lesions detected require colonoscopy.	Not enough evidence for use in screening.
DNA stool examination	Sensitivity high (over 90%). Specificity high (over 90%).	Results currently only available from small-scale studies.	Not enough evidence for use in screening.

Review of the evidence for colorectal cancer screening programme in elderly people.

Further reading

Anwar S, Hall C, Elder JB (1998). Screening for colorectal cancer: present, past and future. *Eur J Surg Oncol* **24**: 477–86.

Eddy DM (1990). Screening for colorectal cancer. *Ann Intern Med* **113**: 373–84.

Friedman GD, Selby JV (1990). Colorectal Cancer: have we identified an effective screening strategy? *J Gen Intern Med* **5**: S23–7.

Gatto N, Frucht H, Sundararajan V, et al. (2003). Risk of perforation after colonoscopy and sigmoidoscopy: a population-based study. *J Nat Cancer Inst* **95**: 230–6.

Hart AR, Wicks AC, Mayberry JF (1995). Colorectal cancer screening in asymptomatic populations. *Gut* **36**: 590–8.

Helm JF, Sandler RS (1999). Colorectal cancer screening. *Med Clin North Am* **83**: 1403–20.

Kewenter J, Engaras B, Haglind E, et al. (1990). Value of retesting subjects with a positive Hemoccult in screening for colorectal cancer. *Br J Surg* **77**: 1349–51.

Kronborg O (2003). Screening for colorectal cancer. *Scand J Surg* **92**: 20–4.

Kumar P, Clark M (2002). *Clinical Medicine*. Elsevier.

Lowenfels AB (2002). Fecal occult blood testing as a screening procedure for colorectal cancer. *Ann Oncol* **13**: 40–3.

Macafee DA, Scholefield JH (2003). Population based endoscopic screening for colorectal cancer. *Gut* **52**: 323–26.

NHS Bowel Cancer Screening Programme. www.cancerscreening.nhs.uk/bowel/

Oldenski RJ, Flareau BJ (1992). Colorectal Cancer Screening. *Prim Care* **19**: 621–35.

Sweetland H, Conway K (2004) *Surgery – Crash Course*. Elsevier.

Quarini C, Gosney M (2009). Review of the evidence for colorectal cancer screening programme in elderly people. *Age Ageing* **38**(5): 503–8.

Elder abuse

Elder abuse

Types of abuse

Physical abuse

This includes slapping, punching, kicking, or hitting any individual. These are clear to identify, mainly due to patterns of injury or injuries that appear inconsistent with the story given by the older individual or their carer. Also included within physical abuse is the force feeding of either food, medication, or other substances, as well as inappropriate restraint or sanctions. Inappropriate restraint may at times be difficult to determine, particularly when considering the role of bed rails or straps within a wheelchair. It must be quite clear when any form of restraint is undertaken that it is with the patient's consent or in the patient's best interests, not for the convenience of the carer.

Emotional or psychological abuse

Any intimidation which occurs by either word or deed, constitutes psychological abuse. Harassment or humiliation usually over bodily functions, slowness of action, or in response to cognitive impairment, are all forms of abuse. Cultural discrimination which may be part of enforcing social isolation, also constitutes abuse. The use of blaming, controlling or threats, particularly of abandonment are well documented.

Neglect or deprivation

Deprivation of basic human rights, such as food and clothing, as well as poor provision of medical attention or necessary aids for activities of daily living, are abuse. Any denial of basic right to make informed choices, such as choice of diet, while in either institutional care or hospital care, as well as more complex choices around medical and social care or place of residence, are serious forms of abuse. Inadequate care or neglect of physical and emotional needs at all ages constitutes abuse, as does failing to provide access to social, health or educational services.

Sexual abuse

Any unwanted physical or sexual contact is defined as sexual abuse. This would include everything from a caress or a kiss, through to intercourse with someone who lacks the capacity to consent. The more extreme cases of rape are not only abuse, but also need police intervention. Any indecent exposure or gross indecency, as well as displaying pornographic literature or videos is included within sexual abuse, as is sexual harassment which may be either verbal or physical in nature.

Financial abuse

Any misuse and/or misappropriation of monies, benefits, and/or property.

Discrimination

This includes any situation where a person or group is treated less favourably than another based on their colour, gender, age, sexual orientation, religion, or presence of disability.

Institutional abuse

Abuse that occurs within any institution may fit into any of the above categories. However repeated instances of poor care may be an indication of more serious problems. Neglect and poor professional practice constitutes institutional abuse.

Repeated patient moves from ward to ward and inadequate levels of nursing staff, may also constitute institutional abuse.

Indicators of abuse

Physical abuse

The injuries that occur as a result of physical abuse may only be apparent during detailed physical examination of a vulnerable adult. Injuries may be more severe than one expects from the description of the potential incident which resulted in the injury. This may include broken bones, large numbers of bruises or lacerations of different ages, burns or scalds in areas that are not typically exposed to hot contact. Force feeding may result in injuries to the mouth or a torn frenulum. The withholding of medication may result in worsening of a physical condition, such as heart failure or chronic obstructive pulmonary disease, but may also result in worsening ability to feed oneself or to take drinks or to mobilize in the case of withdrawal of anti-parkinsonian medication.

Emotional or psychological abuse

This may result in extreme nervousness or agitation on the part of the vulnerable adult. It may also result in depression and in extreme cases a victim may attempt suicide.

Neglect or deprivation

This may result in the adult being poorly dressed, usually in clothes inappropriate to the season, and to have poor attention to their personal hygiene. Inadequate food may result in weight loss, pressure sores, fatigue and in extreme cases malnutrition. Social isolation or lack of social service input may result in anxiety and depression.

Sexual abuse

This may result in physical injury or unexplained reactions towards particular individuals.

Financial abuse

This may result in unexplained change in material circumstances e.g. unpaid bills, less food available or consumed, or as a consequence of an individual's attempts to save money, e.g. poor heating and hypothermia.

Institutional abuse

This may result in large numbers of clients being admitted to hospital with similar medical or social care issues. This may include a high prevalence of poor nutrition, pressure sores or anxiety in a number of individuals from one particular care home.

One should remember that frequent or regular visits to the GP, hospital, emergency department, or requiring hospital admission may indicate different forms of abuse. If an individual has frequent or irrational refusal to accept investigation or treatments, such decisions need to be actively explored. If individuals do not wish to return home to a particular individual or setting at the time of discharge, this may be an indication of abuse.

Risk factors

Carer risk factors that increase the risk or likelihood of an abusive situation.

A variety of individuals find themselves in the caring role which may or may not come naturally to them. There are a number of risk factors that must be considered. Any individual with a history of past or present substance misuse, including alcohol, is statistically at an increased risk of abusing. The presence of treated or untreated illness, including carer stress, increases the likelihood of abuse. Recent bereavement, conflicting demands of other family members, chronic ill health, or tiredness all increase risk.

A past history of abuse also increases the likelihood of an individual becoming an abuser.

Factors in a vulnerable adult for increasing the likelihood of them suffering abuse

Although many carers are able to tolerate difficult caring situations, there are some factors that should be borne in mind by healthcare professionals in order to provide support in certain situations. If a vulnerable adult due to physical or mental ill health has a sleep disturbance, which results in them becoming more active during the night, this adds to carer stress and burden. Likewise, the destruction of a physical environment by behavioural issues, as well as wandering and absconding, increase carer stress.

Any physical changes, such as chronic incontinence or extreme physical dependence, increases the risk of abuse by a carer. Unfortunately, factors such as changes in personality or verbal abuse and aggression towards the carer, as well as being non-compliant with the carer's reasonable wishes and desires are trigger behaviours that should be carefully monitored. Underlying psychological issues, such as obsessive behaviour and even self-harm, as well as emotional dependence and changes in an individual's personality, may not only be trigger behaviours, but also may be additional indicators that abuse is already occurring.

Organizational factors that may contribute towards a situation where abuse occurs

The presence of oppressive or even weak management may result in behaviours that border between poor practice and abuse. Not only do inadequate staffing numbers, either in total or in the proportion of those with advanced training, contribute towards abuse, but inadequate staff supervision or support may result in behaviours that are unacceptable becoming common place or even perpetuated. Training should be flexible and supportive aimed at different grades of staff. The presence of rigid routines and closed communication channels, as well as complaints being ignored and not learnt from, are negative organizational factors.

Reporting abuse and how different legislation may help

The Data Protection Act 1998

This covers the recording, storage and sharing of personal information that is either held on paper files or a computer. Such data should only be shared if disclosure is either:

- agreed by the data subject, i.e. the person the information is about
- required by court order or some legal duty
- is necessary to protect the 'vital interests' of the data subject
- necessary to carry out a statutory function such as a duty to assess

In the case of a safeguarding referral, it is clear that information sharing is to protect the 'vital interests' of the subject.

Crime and Disorder Act 1998 (section 115)

This enables anyone, although it does not oblige them, to disclose information to a local authority, NHS body or the police, where disclosure is necessary to prevent or reduce crime. This may be pertinent in the case of systematic financial abuse of an individual in a setting where the perpetrator may repeat this action with more than one vulnerable adult, or when a perpetrator of sexual abuse is identified.

Protection from Harassment Act 1997

Under section 3(3), people can protect themselves from being harassed by applying to the county court for an injunction. If this injunction is broken, the victim can apply for a warrant for the perpetrator to be arrested.

Assault, Occasioning Actual Bodily Harm (ABH section 47) Offences Against the Person Act 1861

This includes any assault which leaves a more serious physical injury which may include extensive or multiple bruising, minor fractures and in the presence of expert evidence, psychiatric injury.

Assault, Occasioning Grievous Bodily Harm (GBH sections 18 and 20 of the Offences Against the Person Act 1861)

This includes any assault which leads to permanent disability, serious disfigurement, compound fracture or blood loss, requiring transfusion.

Medicines Act 1968 (section 58)

It is an offence to administer drugs that have been prescribed for someone else.

Sexual Offences 2003

Under section 3 any sexual assault and under section 1 is rape.

Sections 38–42 prohibit 'sexual activity on the part of the carer with someone who has a mental disorder'

Mental Health Act 1983

Under section 127, any person who is vulnerable due to a mental disorder is protected in two different ways. Firstly, it is an offence for staff at a hospital or mental nursing home to ill-treat or neglect someone who is receiving treatment for a mental disorder, whether as an inpatient or an outpatient. Secondly, it is an offence to ill-treat or neglect mentally disordered person in ones care in any setting. This includes care by relatives, friends, and paid carers. Within this act, 'mental disorders' covers mental illness, learning disability, personality disorder and any other disorder or disability of mind.

Mental Capacity Act 2005

Under section 44, it is an offence to ill-treat or wilfully neglect an incapacitated person one is caring for, either paid or unpaid, for whom one acts under an enduring power of attorney, lasting power of attorney or as deputy. Within this section, the maximum sentence is 5 years in prison.

National Assistance Act 1948

Under section 47, a local council has the power to seek an order from a magistrates' court to authorize the removal from their homes of people at severe risk. This application must be supported by a certificate from a community physician that the person is either:

(a) suffering from grave chronic disease
(b) is elderly or disabled and living in insanitary conditions
(c) is not being properly cared for by him or herself or others and
(d) needs to be removed in his or her interests, or to prevent harm or serious nuisance to others.

Any medical certificate must include a or b and both c and d. The court order may specify removal to a hospital or other place for up to 3 months.

Police and Criminal Evidence Act 1984 (PACE)

PACE together with Codes of Practice, gives suspects who are 'mentally vulnerable' a number of safeguards during any police investigation. This may particularly be the case when abuse has been detected and the perpetrator of a serious incident is also vulnerable.

Safeguarding adults procedures

All concerns about any safeguarding issue must be taken seriously and acted upon in a timely fashion. In the case of urgent medical and/or police involvement outside secondary care, a 999 call may be appropriate. If medical or psychiatric issues are identified, urgent medical attention should be advised. All emergency department staff should act with relevant healthcare professionals to ensure the diagnosis, treatment and investigation of all suspected abuse is performed in a systematic way, recorded for the necessary investigation, with prompt referral to social services. Any individual irrespective of their job title, grade and whether they are acting in a paid or unpaid role, should report concerns as soon as possible and certainly within the same working day to the relevant manager at social services. At no stage should a victim be reassured that concerns remain confidential. They must be informed that although you respect their right to confidentiality, you are unable to keep any matter of abuse a secret. If anyone is unsure as to whether abuse has occurred, it is essential that they seek advice from the safeguarding adult's manager or adult protection coordinator at the local authority social services/community care department.

After ensuring that a potential vulnerable adult has been abused and is safe from further harm, there are certain instances when evidence may be necessary to preserve. As with all areas where police forensic evidence gathering will occur, it is essential to disturb the area as little as possible; if necessary, remove the victims clothing and bag each item separately. In the case of alleged sexual assault, discourage any washing or bathing or use of the toilet, and if necessary put a bed pan or other receptacle within the toilet to collect any material. Do not handle any items which may hold DNA evidence and anything that has been removed should be placed in a dry environment, such as a bin liner, if practical. Do not interview the victim or potential witnesses; this is a police job! Do not do anything that alerts the alleged perpetrator as this may result in them destroying potential evidence. The only time an alleged abuser should be contacted is when it is necessary to safeguard the particular adult or others at risk e.g. by suspending staff during the investigation of an allegation against them.

Recording concerns

It is essential that all recording of information is undertaken as quickly as possible. It is important to record what an individual saw if the abuse was witnessed, or heard if the disclosure was made to them. All recording of a disclosure should be in the exact words and phrases used by the victim and should include any information about where the disclosure occurred and who else was present. Any physical injuries should be recorded on an appropriate body map and the demeanour of the adult making the disclosure should be recorded. At all times, the information should be factual rather than opinion. Any referrals to social services and other agencies should be recorded, along with times and details of contacts.

Remember that as with all reports, notes will later require photocopying and it is essential that your name, together with your role and contact details appear on the report, as well as a signature which is dated and timed.

Origin of Independent Safeguarding Authority (ISA)

The Safeguarding Vulnerable Groups Act 2006, introduced the ISA. In April 2008, this agency began transferring information from the existing PoVA (Protection of Vulnerable Adults) register, to a newer and more wide ranging vetting and barring scheme. From October 2009, the scheme has covered children and vulnerable adults and any person working in these areas is now required to register with the ISA. The scheme is not intended to replace the existing Criminal Records Bureau checks, but to work alongside it and include all staff and volunteers working with vulnerable adults or children.

Vetting and Barring Scheme (VBS)

The VBS was established as a result of the Bichard enquiry. Holly Wells and Jessica Chapman were murdered by Ian Huntley in August 2002. Following this, the Bichard enquiry recommended a new scheme under which everyone who worked with children or vulnerable adults, should be checked and registered. The VBS is a partnership of the ISA and Criminal Records Bureau (CRB). The responsibility of the ISA will be for decision making and maintenance of two barred lists (for each of England, Wales, and Northern Ireland), covering the children's and vulnerable adult sectors. These two new barred lists will replace a number of pre-existing lists. These include the Protection of Children Act (PoCA), List 99 and the Protection of Vulnerable Adults (PoVA) list in England and Wales and in Northern Ireland, the Disqualification from Working with Children (DWC) list, the Unsuitable Person's list (UP) list and the Disqualification from Working with Vulnerable Adults (DWVA) list. In addition, the current system of disqualification orders, which is operated by the Criminal Justice System, will also be replaced.

Practically how have things changed?

From October 2009, there are only two barred lists, both of which will be administered by the ISA, rather than by several government departments. Checking of these new lists can be made as part of the enhanced CRB check. The three lists (PoCA, PoVA, and List 99 have all been replaced).

All employers, including health services, social services and also professional regulators, have a duty to refer any individual to the ISA. The referral of information should be about those who they believe pose a risk to any vulnerable groups. There will be penalties for both barred individuals who seek or undertake work with vulnerable groups and also for any employer who takes them on while knowing that they are barred.

What does this mean for individuals?

From July 2010 all new employees working in roles who have regular contact with vulnerable groups, or those who move jobs to a new provider within such sectors in England, Wales, and Northern Ireland, have been able to register with the ISA and be checked. The new application form is streamed lined to allow ISA registration and a CRB check (including an ISA check). As soon as a person becomes ISA-registered, there will be an ongoing and continuous monitoring to ensure that their status is reassessed against any new information which may come to light. Employers can choose to be continuously informed of changes in an employee's registration status.

What is the ISA?

It is a non-departmental public body that is sponsored by the Home Office. The Home Office also leads on the scheme implementation. It acts as a decision-making element of the vetting and barring scheme and will maintain the two barred lists. The VBS is supported by the legal framework of the Safeguarding Vulnerable Groups Act 2006 and by the Safeguarding Vulnerable Groups (Northern Ireland) Order 2007 in Northern Ireland.

How will this improve safeguarding?

This will become an overarching, large and inclusive system. All barring decisions will be taken by independent experts and will treat equally both paid employees and volunteers. It will ensure that all individuals are first registered with the ISA before beginning any regulated activity and ensure that a barred person will be committing an offence, should they either seek employment or volunteer with potentially vulnerable groups.

Employers have a legal duty to refer appropriate information to the ISA and will be committing an offence if they hire a person in a regulated activity, without first confirming their ISA registration. Employers will be able to check an individual's registration status online and if they have elected to register an interest in an employee, they will be informed if that employee becomes deregistered from the scheme.

'Regulated activity' and 'controlled activity'

A regulated activity is any activity involving contact with children or vulnerable adults of a specified nature (e.g. teaching, training, care, supervision, advice, medical treatment, or in certain circumstances transport) on a frequent, intensive and/or overnight basis. It also includes activity involving contact with children or vulnerable adults in a specified place (e.g. schools, care homes), frequently or intensively.

Controlled activity is defined as covering the work of ancillary support workers in further education, the National Health Service and adult social care (e.g. cleaner, caretaker, catering staff, receptionist) which is done frequently and gives the opportunity for contact with children or vulnerable adults. Also, people working frequently for specified organizations (e.g. local authorities in the exercise of its education or social services function), in roles which gives them the opportunity for access to sensitive records about children or vulnerable adults.

Differences between the ISA and CRB check

A CRB check provides a full picture of a particular individual's criminal history, which for a small group of sensitive roles, is provided to employers. The two types of CRB check are standard and enhanced. From the launch of the new VBS, anyone employed with vulnerable adults in regulated activity will be entitled to an enhanced CRB check. The ISA and CRB processes are intended to run in parallel. The ISA check will only reveal if the person is registered and able to work with children and/or vulnerable adults.

The CRB check will reveal if the person has a criminal record, or if any relevant non-conviction information is available. A person could be registered with the ISA, but still have a criminal record that if known to the employer, would make the person unsuitable to do a particular job.

Further reading

Action on Elder Abuse (2007). *Briefing Paper: The UK Study of Abuse and Neglect of Older People 200*. London: AEA (http://www.elderabuse.org.uk/Prevalence/Briefingpaperprevalence).

Baker AA (1975). Granny battering. *Mod Geriat* **5**: 20–4.

Comijs HC, Pot AM, Smit JH, et al. (1998). Elder abuse in the community: prevalence and consequences. *J Am Geriatr Soc* **46**: 885–8.

Commission for Social Care Inspection (2008). *How Councils Have Assessed their Progress in Delivering Services to Adults Needing Social Care*. London: CSCI (http://www.csci.gov.uk/pdf/1SAS%20Report.pdf).

Cooper C, Selwood A, Livingston G (2008). The prevalence of elder abuse and neglect: a systematic review. *Age Ageing* **37**: 151–60.

Department of Health (2000). *No Secrets: Guidance on Developing and Implementing Multi-agency Policies and Procedures to Protect Vulnerable Adults from Abuse*. London: DoH (http://www.dh.gov.uk/en/Publicationsandstatistics/Publications/PublicationsPolicyAndGuidance/DH_4008486).

Homer AC, Gilleard C (1990). Abuse of elderly people by their carers. *Br Med J* **301**: 1359–62.

O'Keeffe M, Hills A, Doyle M, et al (2007). *UK Study of Abuse and Neglect of Older People. Prevalence Survey Report*. London: National Centre for Social Research (http://www.natcen.ac.uk/natcen/ pages/publications/research_summaries/NC234_RF_OlderPeople_web2.pdf)

Ogg J, Bennett G (1992). Elder abuse in Britain. *Br Med J* **305**: 998–9.

Pillemer K, Finkelhor D (1998). The prevalence of elder abuse: a random sample survey. *Gerontologist* **28**: 51–7.

Podnieks E (1992). National survey on abuse of the elderly in Canada. *J Elder Abuse Negl* **4**: 5–58.

Tomlin S (1988). *Abuse of Elderly People: An Unnecessary and Preventable Problem*. London, British Geriatrics Society.

Wetzels P, Greve W (1996). The elderly as victims of intrafamilial violence—results of a criminologic dark field study. *Z Gerontol Geriatr* **29**: 191–200.

http://www.isa-gov.org.uk

http://www.legislation.gov.uk/ukpga/1998/29/contents

http://www.legislation.gov.uk/ukpga/1998/37/contents

http://www.legislation.gov.uk/ukpga/1997/40/contents

http://www.cps.gov.uk/legal/l_to_o/offences_against_the_person/#P189_14382

http://www.cps.gov.uk/legal/l_to_o/medicines_act_1968/

http://www.legislation.gov.uk/ukpga/2003/42/contents

http://www.dh.gov.uk/en/Publicationsandstatistics/Legislation/Actsandbills/DH_4002034

http://www.legislation.gov.uk/ukpga/2005/9/contents

http://www.dh.gov.uk/en/Publicationsandstatistics/Legislation/Actsandbills/HealthandSocialCareBill/DH_080453

http://www.homeoffice.gov.uk/police/powers/pace-codes/

Gerontechnology

Ambient assisted living at home

Introduction

In Europe, ambient assisted living (AAL, i.e. assistive technology and the related services) has experienced a lot of publicity but is struggling to reach common practice. From a gerontologist's point of view, AAL encompasses both new technologies and related services (in other words, gerontechnologies) that could provide healthy, sick, or disabled older people with a better life in their homes.

Two economic models prevail with regard to telemedicine. Where telemedicine has developed as an added value to a health service, the development of AAL tends to be considered as part of the role of the healthcare bodies. In other nations, such as England, where funding is scarce for the NHS, local authorities, charities, and families tend to have to take charge of the AAL.

AAL technologies are more or less divided in five groups: telealarms; geolocalization; communication technologies; smart games; and robotic devices. Yet these categories often overlap. For example, what is the aim of a telealarm device, such as a pendant alarm? They are mostly recommended for frail people who are alone at times to give them a simple way to send for help in an emergency. They are therefore not only alarm devices but also communication tools - many people sometimes even say that they 'press the button just to have a chat'. Some call these 'false-alarms'. Technical devices can be designed to avoid them, but would it be ethical to stop isolated people who need socializing from getting human contact, when the service sold is actually communication?

Smart domestic devices, such as infrared taps (where water flows automatically on putting ones hands in the bowl) or lights linked to a passive infrared movement sensor, are very simple. Some devices are not perceived as being AAL technology as they are so simple. These include environmentally friendly bulbs that are not at their brightest straight away and are more friendly for people getting up at night to go to the toilet, and cookers that stop if something is burning or spilling over the saucepan.

A good occupational therapist (OT) should know about a wide range of assistive devices and should be able to advise when they are appropriate. This is best achieved in a multidisciplinary approach in order to assist the patient optimise their functioning and participation.

This section will review the different categories outlined above, with some simplified technical aspects and some cases studies. It will then provide some guidelines for when we consider prescribing technology to our patients, and to assist advising their role for people wanting to avoid any loss of autonomy.

Telealarm devices

The UK, through companies like Tunstal, was one of the pioneering countries in the development of telealarms. Local charities which saw the need for their beneficiaries, took part in the distribution and assessments of the technologies.

The first generation of telealarms were simple, telephone-based devices in the shape of a pendant or watch, which would send an alarm to a predefined phone number. Then, back up numbers could be set so that if the first person was not available, it could switch to a second number or an emergency ambulance system. It then became obvious that having a voice contact with the user would help decide on the level of emergency and amount of help required. As previously mentioned, with improvements in the device and its being worn more, combined with them all allowing voice communication, there was a corresponding increase in 'socializing-alarms'. On the other hand, less than 50% of the people wore the device more than 50% of the time, with most leaving it on the bedside table when going to the toilet at night.

Apart from 'false emergencies', a big issue is with not detecting falls and falls due to loss of consciousness, even when the device is worn. For example, it is hard to reach the button on a watch that is trapped under the body after a fall, when you have a broken shoulder and are frightened.

Engineers have been trying to detect falls automatically through various sensors or sensor combinations. Accelerometers, shock detectors and inclinometers are some of the most commonly used. They have been developed around the fundamental issues of a fall involving acceleration with either a tilt or an impact.

However, describing a real human fall is not very easy: a frequent faller will fall as few as three times per year, and combined, this will take only 4 seconds or so. When one compares this to a full year measured in seconds, it is easy to understand how big the challenge is from a biomechanical point of view. A very prominent maker in the field had to withdraw one promising device, as the laboratory tests revealed a huge rate of false alarms. Some improved the devices by detecting movement after the fall, on the basis that a severe fall will cause immobility (even the more if it was a collapse). Others tried to add pulse sensors to have an idea of the associated stress. More recently, work has started to work on a multi-axis accelerometer that is marketed for fall detection, but can also recognise various activities such as standing, seating, and walking, and could be used to detect the increasing falls risk in a frail individual. Unfortunately, those sensors are not yet widely available.

Some work has been done with cameras and virtual image analysis, but the cameras required are still expensive and the results not as good as expected: a home environment is much more changeable than a laboratory, a prison or bank corridor, and dead angles are an issue.

Strategically placed cheap infrared sensors (the same as those used for garage doors) can give information on the patient's activity with little intrusiveness, but data fusion is complex, as they cannot recognise one person from another or a pet.

While it is now possible to differentiate a major fall from a minor fall on a rehabilitation ward, this requires complex analysis and is not suitable outside the research environment at present. Even with the best data fusion, it is not yet possible to detect a fall at the time it occurs, with a 15-minute target being a more feasible goal.

More recently, Steenkeste has developed a network of sensors that can be included in the flooring of a nursing home and tell the staff if a patient just fell and where. Also, where commercial prototypes have been implemented for an acceptable cost, patenting, and royalties issues are delaying the marketing, even if big flooring companies and nursing homes providers have expressed interest. Such 'embedded' systems are transparent to the user and not intrusive, but do not work outdoors.

In summary, available telepresence sensors are press button devices that have to be worn 24 hours per day and 7 days per week by the user. Automatic fall detectors are under investigation, but then they should include a press button for when the user wants help or to make contact for a different reason.

Geolocalization devices

Geolocalization first started with industrial applications, such as the management of a fleet of lorries or taxies and the self-localization of a user (mountain climber, boat skipper, and then smart directions in one car). Five years ago, geolocalization for pets was proposed as a natural evolution of previous applications: from localizing objects or voluntarily localizing yourself to localizing 'escaping' live beings. Then, a Canadian engineer had the experience of losing his father in the cold of winter, and, as a caregiver, considered that 'spying' on his father with a geolocalization device was a negligible intrusion versus the risk of dying in the cold. From this, there came one of the first proper geolocalization devices.

Regarding wandering, there is a lot of reflection on the reasons for this. These can be viewed in three main categories: the patient wants to leave; the patient just wants to go for a walk and the family is 'overcautious'; or the patient wants to go for a walk, gets lost and is unable to come back home. These are three very different issues with different meanings and different ethical implications.

There are two very different types of devices and technologies. The oldest are tags, using active or passive radio waves, with some allowing identification of the wearer (Radio-Frequency IDentification, RFID). They work through relaying information to a central control area when you get close enough to a receiver. If this is the door of the nursing home, the presumption is that you are leaving, and appropriate action can be taken by the nursing home staff.

Industrial or trading makes have to be registered for medical use because of the (now small) risk of interference with pacemakers and other radio-controlled medical devices. This is very important with passive RFID (the simplest and cheaper option), where a metal coil in the label sends back a characteristic radio wave when submitted to a short range magnetic field 'door'.

The other family of geolocalization devices is based on triangulation of an active radio source. It works outdoors (if you are not in a cave or a deep valley) and is based on GPS navigation system or on GSM triangulation (localization of your mobile phone according to the closest relays). Their precision is limited from a few meters, in the best possible test conditions, to over a hundred yards. The big problem is the ratio between the tracking capabilities (i.e. number of dots on a map with the smallest possible time interval) and the weight in batteries and portability (acceptability) of the device.

Currently, the biggest issue is the service: who gets the tracking and what should they do with it when the localization starts. For example, a patient with moderately severe Alzheimer's disease lived 20 miles away from his daughter. He lived in the country and had always been a 'hunter gatherer' type. He went for walks and would get lost more than once a week. Meanwhile, the local police got fed up with searching for him and contacted his daughter. They rented a geolocalization system from a well-respected telephone company, only to send it back within a few weeks. While it was localizing the man effectively, the

daughter was working. Meanwhile, she could not pass on responsibility to her mother, who suffered from intermittent episodes of psychosis.

Some see geolocalization as part of an integrated home service package, with someone able to help the user, even if only through their availability on the phone (most devices include a mobile), such as to guide patients with mild cognitive impairment where they want to go. This approach is typically more acceptable for the patient.

Communication technologies

Unfortunately, unless you have used a mobile phone for some time, the most obvious smart communication device is often useless for many older people. The buttons are much too small when you have arthritis or poor vision, and the touch screens do not work all the time due to skin dryness.

A number of companies are looking into simplified computer interfaces that make it easier for computer-naive users to use web-conferencing or to email their relatives. In France, a company run by a former nursing home manager is proposing an integrated service pack based on a television set as the web-conferencing physical interface. They monitor indoor temperatures, provide home delivery services through an arrangement with local retailers, and can put you in contact with your physician. The service is coordinated by a friendly web-conferencing-based call centre.

The next emerging issue is to ensure that those in their 60s and 70s go on using their computer, and continue to benefit from the wide information and services they get through the Internet. For this population, there are two main issues - physical accessibility (mouse, keypad, screen display) and accessibility to software and websites.

Double clicking is a major issue and should be avoided whenever possible (most of the time this can be set in the parameters). The mouse can be adapted and usually, for people with arthritis, a bigger mouse is better. Having a single button can help, as can trackballs (a kind of reversed mouse were the user is spinning a big ball instead of moving the mouse). Touch screens are difficult to use and experience is showing that older people (even those not so frail) struggle with multipoint technology (where you may move different objects on the same screen at the same time). They tend to have a difficulty maintaining the finger contact required for moving an object, or touch the screen with other parts of the hand at the same time (e.g. palm or the side of another finger).

Shiny screens tend to cause a lot of reflection and so should be avoided. One should bear in mind the visual ergonomic, such that the screen should be at around a 90° angle to the user's line of vision, and not too high or low (position of the neck). Also, there should not be direct light on to the screen, but correct ambient lighting. The keypad or mouse should be on a table, positioned so that the patient's shoulders are relaxed, arms close to vertical, elbow at an angle between 90° and 110° and wrist in slight dorsal flexion. It is important that correct sound is provided; the microphones of laptop computers are often insufficient and proper external baffles are often required for web-conferencing purposes (this also applies to teleconferencing during home telemedicine).

Regarding software interfaces, the most useful are the 3WAC accessibility rules for websites that were developed for the handicapped. One important point is to use a dark background to minimize glare, which should soon become common practice with its being implemented by new energy saving technologies. Size and letter font are important, and Verdana 14 without serif is recommended.

A new method of pointing (click and magnetisation) has been assessed to move an object to a predefined target in patients with either mild cognitive impairment (MCI) or Alzheimer's Disease (AD) and a control group. One trial looked at a simulation of moving sugar from a table to a cup of coffee. Where the usual drag and drop failed even in the MCI group, there was a significant success rate of over 50% in AD patients, including patients scoring down to 12/30 on Mini-Mental State Examination (MMSE).

Further developments include the development of a computer use 'clinic,' through collaboration between a geriatrician with physical medicine training and a human-computer interface specialist with an experience in handicap to help people maintain their communication capabilities. It is based on assessment of the patients' impairments, and then observing them when they try different devices or settings. One simple example is with helping to treat the depression of an 80 year old woman with chloroquine related sight problems and hemiplegia (without cognitive impairment). She was able to resume use of her computer by simply changing the settings of her Microsoft Word to black background and white verdana font.

There is a huge lot of research and development to do in human computer interaction for older people that will benefit users of all ages.

Games

The smartgames market was taken by a storm in 2008 by Nintendo's Wii. It combined convivial games, which are often revived family games, with various haptic interfaces mimicking the tools you would use in the real world (e.g. racquet, rod, boxing gloves). The games are very usable, based on activities that the people already know, and the display on a big screen is easy to arrange.

Geriatricians are mostly interested in two aspects that built the success of the Wii concept and prior to that, the cognitive training aspect with the portable Nintendo DS, namely the 'exergaming.' This combines playing the game with some level of exercising and 'edutainment,' where a cognitive activity is built into the playing environment. The people in charge of entertaining retirement and nursing home residents, as well as physiotherapists, soon saw the potential. Due to the huge sales and wide use, side effects were soon being published, from tendonitis (mostly due to the absence of resistance force in the use of the interfaces) to a former boxer who had to stop using the boxing game, because he was recovering a bit too much of his former pugnacity! From a physical point of view, the risk is that there is no resistance feedback from the interfaces, thus potentially resulting in an excessive range of motion for joints or muscles and the risk of sustaining injury through this.

The Wii Balance Board has been tested with a force platform as standard. A force platform is a device used to assess gait, where one stands on a kind of scales with pressure sensors detecting where the barocentre of the pressures applied by feet is located and how it is moving. The reliability of the measure of the length of the path of the centre of pressure was tested. The tests showed a good reproducibility (both in the Wii and between the Wii and force platform). The physical activity can reach the significant level of brisk walking (3.6 metabolic equivalents) in the older population. This has been shown to have good

acceptability and improvements in balance after 1 month in a small population of community fallers aged over 70. Further research is needed to confirm the consistency of the effects on balance and to see if activity level and the number of falls are improved.

Exergaming appears to be an enjoyable way of maintaining some activity with the related benefits of good humour. Moreover, grandparents (or great-grandparents, even with some handicap) and grandchildren can again play together, with no-one being outdated.

Regarding edutainment, the possible effects are as difficult and speculative as those of cognitive stimulation as a whole. However, participation in social activities would realistically not do any harm and if computers can improve social interaction through a better acceptance, then, clearly, this is something to make the most of, though research is still needed to objectively demonstrate these benefits.

Robotics

Since the name first appeared with Josef Čapek in 1920, 'robot' is highly emotional. From a practical point of view, a robot is a device with a predetermined task and an ability to adapt to some level to the prevailing condition to achieve its task more efficiently.

The robot (see Figure 26.1) has sensors, which are linked to a microprocessor (or even a computer) where the information from them is screened. The collected information is implemented in a command law. The command law (software), dictates the manner in which the data from the sensors will affect the behaviour of the robot. The command law answers mechanical, energetic, security and operational requirements. That law will drive the actuators. Usually, a robot has additional 'mechanical' securities to avoid accidents, which are independent from the command law (e.g. a mechanical switch to prevent the actuator exceeding its nominal load, soft bumpers, range limitations on arms). Most of the robots in this application domain run on low tension electrical energy, usually on batteries or through an alternating current adaptor.

With regard to service robots for personal and private use, they can be classified according to three axes. Their function could be: to address a physical function (e.g. walking aids); inform the user or the caregiver; or fulfil an emotional goal (either fun or loneliness). The categories may overlap (e.g. a robot that both informs and functions as an emotional 'companion'). Then, the robot could be either humanoid (even an android) or lifelike, or resembling a tool. 'Augmented' tools we would call 'smart', such as a smart

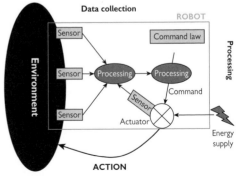

Figure 26.1 Demonstrating the components that make a robot.

walker, may often not be perceived as being robots in the home-environment; they may even be called 'pervasive' – the best-selling personal robots are vacuum-cleaners. Finally, the robot is either mobile or immobile. The avatars that translate spoken language into sign language, such as those giving information in railways stations, are still robots.

Tool robots are readily accepted when they address a specific need and are usable. Usability is optimised by an iterative approach, whereby the prototypes go back and forth from the lab to the user. Lacey developed Guido, his smart walker for those with both a sight and walking problem, after seeing the difficulties of a friend he visited in a nursing-home. However, economical issues prevail when such robots cost much more than an electric wheelchair, thus closing the market.

Companion robots are deemed acceptable *a priori* according to how end-users (patients) or their relatives (caregivers) reacted to a presentation of the possible designs and tasks. Acceptability tends to be confirmed by field experiments, such as with the NurseBot Pearl that could walk residents through their nursing home. At the University of Connecticut, researchers are considering how a robot could behave ethically when reminding a patient to take his pills; this could definitely help with acceptance but this is a task, already difficult for a well-trained nurse, so there is a lot of work involved with developing a functional command law for the robot.

Emotional robots are available on the market. Odetti found reasonable acceptability for the AIBO (Artificial Intelligence roBOt) robot-dog in 28 older people with mild cognitive troubles (MMSE >23). The acceptance rates were higher for people interested in technology. A few studies are considering the potential use of emotional (toy) robots to improve communication in people with cognitive impairment. Tamura studied the effects of either a motor-driven toy dog or an early version of AIBO either plain or dressed in a fluffy cloth on a small group with an average age of 84 years and with severe dementia. Both generated some interaction, with the time spent touching or caring for AIBO being slightly less (but the interaction between the occupational therapist and AIBO was significantly higher than with the toy dog). Wearing cloth or not made little difference. Under certain circumstances and for certain people, AIBO can have some benefits, as reported in three cases, two of elderly handicapped ladies who found it gave them some occupation, and a gentleman suffering from a stroke who felt less lonely and would even occasionally sing a song to the AIBO.

The unanswered questions are, would a robot be able to do better than a doll or automat? Would it be able to do as well as a well trained dog? What would be the related cost? There is still room for a lot of development work.

Conclusion

The old, the frail, the sick, and the disabled deserve new technologies that could help them. For many reasons, from cost to availability to awareness of what is available, our patients are still not benefitting from technologies that already exist. The drug market is organised so that any new drug can be prescribed easily as soon as it is authorised; physicians must insist that health authorities take into account the need of patients for assistive technologies and ambient assisted living. There should be special registration procedures, usable by small and medium sized companies providing these technologies, which would facilitate getting a proper register of what is available. From this, we could then prescribe according to the international classifications of functionalities or diseases.

Further reading

Clark RA, Bryant AL, Pua Y, et al. (2010). Validity and reliability of the Nintendo Wii Balance Board for assessment of standing balance. *Gait Posture* **31**: 307–10.

Graves LE, Ridgers ND, Williams K, et al. (2010). The physiological cost and enjoyment of Wii Fit in adolescents, young adults, and older adults. *J Phys Act Health* **7**: 393–401.

Lacey G, MacNamara S (2000). User involvement in the design and evaluation of a smart mobility aid. *J Rehabil Res Dev* **37**: 709–23.

Montemerlo M, Pineau P, Roy N, et al. (2002). Experiences with a Mobile Robotic Guide for the Elderly. In *AAAI02*. Edmonton: AAAI Press

Odetti L, Anerdi G, Barbieri MP, et al. (2007). Preliminary experiments on the acceptability of animaloid companion robots by older people with early dementia. *Conf Proc IEEE Eng Med Biol Soc* 1816–19.

Tamura T, Yonemitsu S, Itoh A, et al. (2004). Is an entertainment robot useful in the care of elderly people with severe dementia? *J Gerontol A Biol Sci Med Sci* **59**: 83–5.

The Ethical Robot. University of Connecticut, (2010). (http://today.uconn.edu/?p=24249).

Vigouroux V, Rumeau P, Vella F, et al. (2009). Studying Point-Select-Drag interaction techniques for older people with cognitive impairment (regular paper). In: . San Diego, Springer-Verlag, pp. 422–8.

Williams MA, Soiza RL, Jenkinson AM, et al. (2010). EXercising with Computers in Later Life (EXCELL) - pilot and feasibility study of the acceptability of the Nintendo(R) WiiFit in community-dwelling fallers. *BMC Res Notes* **3**: 238.

Telehealth to support health promotion and management of disease

What is telehealth?

If telecare can be described as a service that uses remote monitoring of the environment and an individual's domestic activities to support independence in the home, then telehealth is a service that provides remote monitoring of physiological parameters and their management to support wellbeing and good health in the community. Thus, while telecare services can reduce anxiety and the need for residential care by offering advice and rapid response to emergency situations in the home then telehealth services will help people to exercise self-care and avoid the need for medical intervention. Telehealth will also make people more independent because it reduces the need for NHS resources such as visits to the GP surgery, home visits by nurses and out-of-hours staff, and emergency visits by paramedics. It also prevents many unscheduled hospital admission.

It may be apparent that telecare and telehealth are very closely linked and, for many people, it may be impossible to distinguish between the needs for a service that are medical or social in nature; these include events such as falls, medication mismanagement, support for people with dementia, and issues of incontinence or enuresis. This supports the idea that an integration of telecare/health services will be inevitable as technology matures and as protocols for the sharing of information between local authority social services departments and the NHS improve and become more robust. Currently, telecare services are dominated by alarms based on devices that detect environmental or behavioural problems at an early stage. First generation telehealth would be analogous to this but with sensors attached to the individual and measuring vital signs, or the interaction of the individual with medical devices or systems. Table 26.1 describes a number of potential telehealth alarm sensors, some of which are already available in telecare systems. Others are likely to follow soon, though it is possible that the communication system that links an alarm to a responder will follow alternative paths, especially as medical emergencies can happen at any time and in any place.

Of particular relevance for telehealth alerts is the different levels of response protocol required to ensure that the most appropriate and timely intervention is made. Many medical emergencies that may be flagged up in this way will require the attention of a paramedic, a GP or a specialist nurse (rather than a family member or a support worker). In many such cases, a presentation at the emergency department will be the only safe option. Telehealth is therefore different from telephone advice lines such as NHS Direct as the alert has been raised by the equipment rather than by the patient. Advice and information may not be the priority. It follows that telehealth may not therefore reduce the demands on the health service but may ensure that they are called at an

Table 26.1 Medical and socio-medical emergencies to be managed using alarm telecare/health

Emergency Situations	Role of Sensor	Response
Cardiac arrest/arrhythmia	Detect loss of pulse or irregular rhythm	Paramedic – hospital
Blocked/displaced catheter	Detect that flow of urine has stopped	Paramedic or nurse
Mental health incident	Detect a change in behaviour or activity	Medication – hospital
Instability in walking	Identify increased sway or wobble	Clinic
Asthma attacks	Detect change in breathing rate and depth	Paramedic; GP
Epileptic seizures	Detect convulsions and associated sounds	Support staff
Incontinence/enuresis	Detect moisture or leakage	Support staff
Medication concordance	Remind, and confirm taking of tablets	Pharmacist; GP
Slip, trip or fall	Detect impact and subsequent status	Support staff; paramedic
Wandering	Identify movement out of home at night	Support staff; police
Fever and delirium	Measure elevated temperature	Paramedic - hospital
Hypothermia	Measure very low body temperature	Paramedic - hospital
Heat stress	Identify behavioural change at high temperature	Support staff; paramedic
Nutrition	Measure changes in weight or in dietary intake	Support staff; dietician
Stroke or TIA	Identify absence of body movement	Paramedic - hospital
Fluid retention	Measure weight change overnight	Nurse; GP
Hypoglycaemic incidents	Detect changes in rate of sweating and pulse	Support staff; paramedic – hospital
Pressure area emergency	Measure time spent in particular lying position	Support staff; nurse
Breathing problems	Measure blood oxygen level	Paramedic; GP - hospital

earlier stage, thus improving the prospects for an optimum outcome.

Long-term conditions

Before modern medicine, including the ready availability of antibiotics, people used to die from acute diseases such as pneumonia, tuberculosis, diphtheria, and enteritis and from accidents and other conditions that might be detected at an early stage using appropriate telehealth sensors of the type shown in Table 26.1. Most sudden-onset conditions are curable by allopathic medicine. Other diseases of a chronic nature, such as asthma, congestive heart failure, and diabetes, were not considered to be priorities for many years due, in part, to the fact that they rarely led to immediate death.

Table 26.2 describes the main differences between chronic disease and those that are considered to be acute. The most significant difference is that chronic diseases are long-term conditions which imply many years of suffering, and a high burden to the health and social care system. An ageing population will inevitably result in an increasing burden; chronic disease is likely to overtake acute illness in terms of overall hospital admissions, GP appointments, medication needs, and every other measure of healthcare costs over the next few years. It is vital that more efficient management techniques are developed, and that more emphasis is given to avoiding the development of such diseases, and patients recruited in understanding both the causes and the implications of their lifestyle decisions and their impact on such disease.

Many illnesses that we describe as long-term conditions can now be considered to be either lifestyle diseases or diseases of our environment (i.e. caused in some way by man). Table 26.3 shows the top 12 long-term conditions of the developed world as measured by the number of QALYs (years of quality life) that are lost to them annually. Before the turn of the century, these 12 conditions accounted for nearly half the number of QALYs lost in the developed world. This proportion is likely to increase in the future, and the drain on health services will be considerable without improved prevention and management strategies. Telehealth can play a vital role.

Vital signs monitoring

Vital signs, or signs of life, include a number of objective measures for a person: temperature, respiratory rate, heart beat (pulse), and blood pressure. In the past, these measurements were performed by medical staff using instruments such as a thermometer and a stethoscope and

Table 26.2 A comparison of chronic and acute diseases

Factor	Chronic	Acute
Duration	Long term	Limited (a few days/weeks)
Onset	Slow	Rapid
Causes	Several and changing	Usually one only
Diagnosis	Uncertain	Accurate
Outcome	No complete cure	Complete cure possible
Interventions	Often indecisive	Usually effective
Effect of age on prevalence	Increasing likelihood	Generally none

Table 26.3 Top 12 long-term conditions

	Name	Comments
1	Coronary heart disease (CHD)	A failure to supply adequate circulation to the cardiac muscle and surrounding tissue - already the most common form of disease affecting the heart and an important cause of premature death
2	Stroke	Linked to advanced age, high blood pressure, smoking, embolism, diabetes mellitus, lack of exercise, being overweight, and having high cholesterol
3	Chronic obstructive pulmonary disease (COPD)	Condition may result from chronic bronchitis, emphysema, asthma, or chronic bronchiolitis. Cigarette smoking and air pollution are major risk factors.
4	Depression	Low mood and/or loss of interest in activities, accompanied by emotional, cognitive, physical/behavioural symptoms.
5	Lung cancer	Directly related to active/passive smoking in the majority of cases.
6	Diabetes	There are four types of diabetes mellitus. Type I diabetes is called insulin-dependent diabetes and appears at any age. Type II usually develops in overweight adults.
7	Arthritis	Most common forms are osteoarthritis (degenerative joint disease) and rheumatoid arthritis (immune system attacks the joints).
8	Colorectal cancer	Colon cancer or large bowel cancer includes cancerous growths in the colon, rectum and appendix.
9	Asthma	Associated with excess mucus production causing coughing and difficulty breathing due to inflammation of the airways.
10	Kidney disease	Can be due to loss of function or changes to structure of the kidneys often presenting alongside other chronic disease.
11	Oral diseases	Affect people's teeth, gums and supporting bone and soft tissues (including the tongue, lips and mouth).
12	Osteoporosis	Loss of bone density and strength causing fractures, especially to the hip, wrist and spine.

a sphygmanometer. Hospitals have been using bedside monitors for a number of years enabling measurements to be performed and displayed on a continuous basis. These allow additional devices to be employed that are of significance to the monitoring of particular functions relevant

Table 26.4 Vital signs measurements relevant to telehealth

Vital sign measure	Application
Temperature	Indication of an infection and to check for fever (pyrexia or a febrile condition), detection of hypothermia
ECG	To determine heart rate and detect cardiac arrhythmia or irregular durations or intervals in signatures
Blood pressure	Monitor the effect of medication and lifestyle changes on hypertension, and determine whether blood pressure falls at night compared to the day
Breathing rate	To detect hyperventilation or abnormally low rates
Peak expiratory flow	To monitor breathing and help predict an asthma attack or chest infection; to determine when medication or emergency care is needed
Blood oxygenation	To identify low levels of blood oxygen caused by an exacerbation of COPD or other disease leading to inability to perform domestic tasks
Blood sugar level	To measure how well diabetes is being controlled through lifestyle habits and/or medication.
Cholesterol level	To monitor risk of stroke or heart attack
Blood INR	To determine the clotting tendency of blood, in the measure of warfarin dosage, liver damage, and vitamin K status.
Body weight	To detect sudden changes in weight caused by the collection of fluid risking heart failure

to some types of disease. Table 26.4 describes these measurements and their relevance.

Over the past 20 years, more portable systems have been designed that can be deployed in the home environment by the patient on their own (or with the help of family or other untrained support workers). In this case, the focus is on data collection at a set time of day, and its transmission to a remote server which clinicians can access in order to monitor the patient's condition when appropriate. In the majority of cases, daily analysis of the vital signs data may not be necessary, so a triage is necessary to ensure that the clinicians are made aware of any deterioration in condition. Software is able to perform the 'teletriage' provided that the responsible clinician has established relevant alert thresholds. This is not a trivial task, as normal ranges of measurements of vital signs change with age and medical condition, and incorrect threshold can lead to unnecessary alerts or a failure to detect a problem at an early stage. The results of the teletriage software are often sent to a 24 telecare monitoring centre for non-clinical triage before alerts are sent to medical staff. This is to eliminate spurious results caused by equipment failure or by not performing the measurement procedures correctly.

Second generation telehealth equipment uses a home data hub to which peripheral sensors and measurement devices may be attached. This may be directly or through a wireless arrangement such as Bluetooth. During measurement sessions, usually in the morning, the hub will communicate with the patient using a visual display and/or spoken instructions (usually demanded in the first language of the patient). In addition to the objective measures collected from peripheral devices, newer telehealth systems are capable of asking a number of subjective questions of the patient. These are tailored to their condition and their circumstances. Some systems ask a basic set of three to six questions every day each requiring a simple yes or no answer. If the answer suggests that a problem situation is emerging (e.g. the patient states that they are feeling worse than they did yesterday) then this will be flagged during triage so that an intervention may occur. Others systems employ more complex decision trees where a particular answer may lead to further questions and specific advice being offered. In each case, the telehealth system provides an early indication of emerging problems, enabling the patient and their medical support team to intervene with rescue packages that have a high likelihood of succeeding in avoiding escalation and a need for hospitalization. Examples of success will be described later.

Predictive tools

In order to use telehealth systems as efficiently as possible in dealing with people who have long-term conditions, it is necessary to find cases where the disease management approach involving telehealth may be most relevant. The patient population is usually defined in terms of four levels of complexity (see Figure 26.2) where the lowest level is the entire population and the highest level include those most complex cases.

Popular predictive tools include:

- Hospital Admission Risk programme (HARP) – a system developed in Australia
- High-impact User Manager – developed by Dr Foster Intelligence
- Probability of repeat admissions (Pra) tool – an older US instrument
- Patient At Risk of Re-hospitalization (PARR) – a series of three case-finding algorithms that use a hospital admission as a trigger.

PARR1

The PARR1 algorithm focuses on triggering admissions for specific 'reference' conditions (such as congestive heart disease, chronic obstructive pulmonary disease and diabetes) where improved management in the form of case management and social services interventions may help prevent/avoid future hospitalizations.

PARR2

The PARR2 algorithm uses any emergency admission as a trigger and is not limited to admission for a 'reference' condition. Because it focuses on a larger number of patients, it produces risk scores for more patients than PARR1, but produces a higher rate of 'false positives'.

Combined Predictive Model

This integrates accident and emergency, inpatient, outpatient and GP data sources to predict risk of admission to hospital across an entire patient population including both those that have experienced a recent hospital admission and those who are at very high risk of doing so in the future.

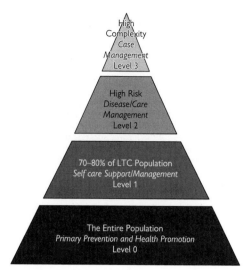

Figure 26.2 The pyramid of care.

There are three main techniques that have been used to identify high-risk patients:
- **Threshold modelling** – identifies patients who meet a specific criterion. Used widely in case-finding. Not accurate in a general population, but better in a specific clinical context, such as those at risk of coronary heart disease.
- **Clinical knowledge** – instinct and training are used to identify individuals to benefit from intervention, but identifies those at high risk rather than in the future.
- **Predictive modelling** – establishes associations between sets of variables to predict future outcomes. The technique appears to be more effective – so tools have been developed to help clinicians select patients for telehealth.

PRISM

This is software employed by the NHS in Wales to provide the Combined Predictive Model with a very usable front-end. This will identify all patients in level 3, for example, where co-ordination of care across the sectors could lead to benefits for patients and services. It further allows potential savings to be modelled by focusing interventions in the most appropriate ways.

The benefits of Predictive Modelling become apparent when telehealth and other Chronic Disease Management interventions are targeted at those patients who are most likely to benefit in terms of reduced numbers of inpatient admissions (emergency and scheduled), and GP appointments.

Health promotion and telecoaching

Telehealth systems provide the information that can lead to early interventions that enable exacerbations of ill-health in people with chronic disease to be managed more effectively. In some cases this means reducing the likelihood of hospitalization or reducing the number of days spent in hospital once admitted. In other cases, spotting a trend can prevent a dangerous situation from developing. However, an analysis of actual data can reveal the type of actions or behaviour that is putting the patient's health at risk. This offers an opportunity to offer advice and information in order to improve an individual's health, and the more advanced telehealth systems can provide such advice in the form of video technology.

One of the more direct approaches that are possible with telehealth is the monitoring of physical activity and calorie use each day. This involves the patient wearing a small accelerometer device which detects movement, its magnitude and duration, converting it into the number of steps and the number of calories consumed as a function of time. By comparing the calorie use with a planned programme, the feedback can provide encouragement to the patient to maintain their current exercise level or to increase it. A number of weight reduction programmes are based on these principles, and are also suitable for people who are at risk of diabetes or who have an obesity

problem. Similar devices can be used to monitor the duration and quality of sleep which is known to play an important role in supporting health improvement.

Although the use of technology to provide motivation and information is known to be useful for many younger patients, other are more susceptible to a human intervention. This is the basis of the motivational interviewing (MI) technique or telecoaching where telephone-based support is provided by life coaches or by trained nurses. They can provide regular but infrequent support to help with smoking cessation plans and with attempts to improve diet and increase activity levels, whilst intervening also at times when the remote monitoring has detected adverse effects such as an increase in weight or a reduction in the number of calories consumed.

In extreme cases, therapy and exercise sessions can be conducted using remote cameras which allow the coach to observe the actions of several patients simultaneously offering encouragement as and when needed. In the future, robotic devices will be available to support rehabilitation classes in the home, offering the physical resistance that a personal trainer might afford if they were present.

Evidence

The benefits of telephone support and help lines have been established over a period of over 20 years for a large number of different illnesses including mental health problems and other long-term conditions. These show that teleconsultations have broadly similar outcomes to support services provided directly by nursing staff. They have been shown to be successful in supporting people who have had surgery, mental health issues, and a wide range of long-term conditions.

Since telemonitoring was first used in the USA in the 1990s, there have been several studies that have looked at the changes in health service utilization compared with normal care. However, most have compared the outcomes with those during a period prior to the introduction of the technology. This can lead to a number of confounders including different frequencies of exacerbations as a function of season (or weather). In the same way, some of the largest trials in the US focused on military veterans who were necessarily different to the general population for a number of reasons including their male to female ratio, and their likely compliance with a new treatment regimen; ex-military staff are more likely to do as they are told than the rest of the population! (especially if their care is provided free of charge).

There have been few examples of Randomised Controlled Trials due to the difficulties in establishing the necessary evaluation protocols and the scale needed for statistical significance. However, the English Whole System Demonstrator project which will report in 2011 aims to provide the strongest possible evidence that telehealth is safe, popular, leads to reduced use of resources and better outcomes. Though not confined to older people, this project offered 1800 people with chronic heart failure (CHF), chronic obstructive pulmonary disease (COPD), or diabetes the latest telehealth monitors in an attempt to provide enhanced case management.

Two examples of impressive reductions in health service utilizations are:

- NHS South East Essex Community Healthcare, At home…. Not alone project:
  - 11.8% reduction in the length of Community Matron face-to-face visits
  - 75% reduction in A&E visits
  - 83% reduction in hospital admissions
  - 72% reduction in 999 calls
  - 56% reduction in GP visits
- Ministry of Health and Long-Term Care and Canada Health Infoway project during which 800) patients were provided with touch screen monitors and peripherals for a 4-month period:
  - Home visits during fell by 66% for CHF patients & 64% for COPD patients
  - Emergency Department visits fell 72% for CHF patients & 74% for COPD patients.
  - Walk-in clinic visits fell by between 95 and 97%.

M-health and the future

Telehealth and telecare services have all been focused on supporting an individual in their own home. This is partly due to the fact that many patients are confined to their homes because of their ill-health but has also been due to the equipment being too large and cumbersome to being carried around. The need for mains electricity and a fixed telephone lines has also influenced the ability to perform vital signs measurements away from the home.

Over the past few years, there has been a trend for equipment to become smaller and more lightweight. Peripherals have linked wirelessly with the control unit so that items can be located in different rooms. Sensors are being integrated into items of clothing or into furniture or bedding so that monitoring can be performed continuously and without any form of intervention from the patient. The potential for sensors to be swallowed so that they can operate from inside the body is being investigated, as is the use of cameras that can detect pulse, breathing rate and blood oxygen level by analysing small movements in the chest wall, and changing facial colours over time. These promote the collection of data on the body using a mobile device which has memory, processing power and the ability to transmit either raw data or processed information (in the form of alerts) to a relevant

Table 26.5 Smart phone applications (SPAs) for supporting people with long-term conditions

Application	Relevance to long-term conditions
Fall/convulsive seizure detection	Enables people with epilepsy to go out knowing that they can be detected and located automatically if they suffer a seizure
Blood sugar and activity measurements	Automatic data entry and measurement of activity level giving trend information and advice for diabetics
Continuous monitoring of cardiac activity	Immediate notification of heart attack and arrhythmia, and changes in periods and timings for people with CHF
Peak flow measurement	Automatic data entry and analysis of lung function showing asthmatics how their measurements compare with the norm
Pulse oximetry	Direct coupling of Blue-tooth enabled device to indicate exacerbation in cases of COPD
Monitoring of well-being and use of smart phone	A non-invasive method of detecting incidences of depression and other mental health problems
Alarm interface for standalone sensor devices	Relaying of alerts for conditions such as hypoglycaemia for people with type 1 diabetes

clinician. A modern smart phone has this potential, and is being considered as the basis for m-care and m-health services.

Basic mobile phones have been used to collect and transmit vital signs information such as blood glucose levels for a number of years. Similarly, SMS and voice messages have been used to provide feedback and reminder messages both in the developed world and in Third World nations where there is little fixed telephone line infrastructure, and even less medical support. The opportunities for using smart phones are far more exciting and ideally suited to the support of patients who suffer from long term conditions. In particular, they are seen as a must have item by many adults, they are portable and carried at all times, and they offer advanced features at low cost.

Table 26.5 lists some examples of downloadable 'applications' that may be relevant to telehealth monitoring. The cost of the applications is small, and smart phones are becoming affordable with contracts of 18 to 24 months costing rather less than the monitoring charges for conventional telehealth systems.

The exact way in which smart phones and their applications will be provided remains a matter of discussions, especially with respect to:

- Data security – can personal information be 'stolen' and used by insurance companies as a reason for increasing premiums
- Reliability – should a physician have confidence in measurements taken by the patient themselves in unknown settings and without confirmation that they were relaxed
- Increasing demand for self-care – the worried well are already using internet facilities to search for diagnoses and remedies.

Irrespective of the way that patients using their mobile phones, this technology will become relevant to physician as an ubiquitous display medium, ideal for sharing scans, x-ray images and photographs but also to initiate mobile teleconferencing with colleagues and peers. The same device will become a source of reference both through downloaded apps and through web searches.

Telecare to support independent living

Telecare is the umbrella term given to all connected systems that are used in the home environment plus an increasing number of electronic aids to daily living which play an important role in supported needs that would otherwise be unmet without bringing in additional human resources in the form of homecare services.

Telecare as an assistive technology

Aids to independence can be classified into four main groups:

- Adaptations to the home environment – these are fixed installations that include grab rails, ramps, level access showers, and large mechanical or electro-mechanical modifications including through-floor lifts and stair lifts. Occupational therapists usually provide the expertise to design changes of this type, though the time taken to implement the changes can lead to some people having to stay longer in hospital than may be otherwise necessary (delayed transfer of care).
- Aids to daily living – these are generally portable devices ranging from walking sticks and frames through to boxes for storing medication, pill crushers and cutters, and a variety of gadgets that help people with any form of disability from performing domestic tasks. Although a deficit may be identified by a health or social care professional, most people recognise that they need some low-level support, but may be unsure what it best to buy from a range of catalogues or from pharmacies.
- Environmental control systems – people who have major physical or communication problems struggle to perform a number of basic tasks such as operating electrical appliances, making a phone call and opening or closing doors or windows. Environmental control systems and speech synthesisers enable them to maintain a level of independence in performing tasks with technological support. Systems are very personalised and are expensive both to purchase and to maintain because of their vital role in supporting independence.
- Connected systems – these are alarms, switches and various other peripherals and sensors that connect to each other and to a separate alarm device in order to provide an alert to the user or his carers, remote of otherwise, in the event of a dangerous situation occurring. The systems generally use low power radio transmissions in a narrow frequency band that has been allocated to such applications. This avoids interference and makes alarm transmissions and reception extremely reliable. However, much higher bandwidths can be used for sharing large amounts of data including video.

The future demand for telecare devices is likely to be so great that they will become consumer items, perhaps sold by DIY stores and similar retail outlets. Certainly, prices should be low and standard solutions available for rapid installation so that people being discharged from hospital following accident or illness may go home with their telecare devices or may have other devices installed in their home before they get there or within a few hours of their return home.

Alarms and telecare services

When health and social care professionals assess an individual's ability to live safely and independently in the community, they are looking fundamentally at their ability to perform the activities of daily living and the risks to their independence and social inclusion when they do so. These depend intimately on the way that they live including whether they live alone, how much informal care support is available, the type of property in which they live, and the type of lifestyle that they choose to follow. Ultimately, they need to think about the level of risk that is likely to exist and the ways that these risks can be either removed or managed. Risk removal is neither necessary nor is it popular with most people as it directly impinges on their freedom to do what they want when they want. Therefore, risk management is the aim of most community care interventions.

Risk is a complex concept which can be measured as the product of the likelihood of an adverse incident occurring (on a scale of zero to one where zero represent no chance while a one represents total certainty) multiplied by the impact of such an event. Impact is also measured from zero to one where zero means that the effect of an incident is trivial, while one means a catastrophe (which may be the death of the client, his or her neighbours or a professional in the worst cases). If both the likelihood of an adverse incident occurring is high, and the potential outcomes is also very serious then the level of risk must be reduced to an acceptable level. In the past, this meant admission to a residential care or nursing home where individual liberties could be restricted to such an extent that the individual would have little opportunity to perform any risky task, however trivial it might sound. This is a form of deskilling which is counter to current principles.

In practice, a telecare sensor provides an early detection of incidents enabling interventions to be performed in a timely manner. For example, Figure 26.3 shows how a fall detector (or an intelligent bed occupancy monitor) may be used to manage a situation where a service user is unable to get up off the ground without help following a slip or a trip. In many cases, the response might include a falls pick-up team rather than paramedics. This team would carry a portable inflatable cushion arrangement which would enable a single responder to lift someone from the ground quickly and gently, thus avoiding the need to go to a hospital emergency department in many cases. The significance of the rapid response is that the faller will not spend hours on the floor which can wreck confidence for independent living and which can result in the need for hospital attention if they had a long lie.

Figure 26.4 shows the processes involved in a Telecare Service that can provide the responses and outcomes described by example in Figure 26.3. There are such services that operate at a national level and operate by third sector or private organisations. They offer economies of scale but may find it difficult to more local needs and preferences, especially with respect to response protocols. Local or regional services tend to be more focused on their own communities and have clearer referral routes for physicians and other specialists to follow in ensuring that a patient receives the best possible service. Most will employ Quality Systems and will be compliant with Codes of Practice that are designed to ensure that processes and protocols are safe and effective.

The choice of which sensors to prescribe may seem obvious but, in practice, may require more knowledge of their

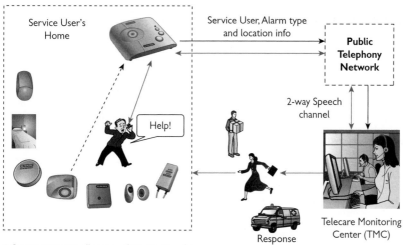

1. Sensor automatically raises alarm to care phone
2. Alarm call raised
3. TMC Operator talks to Service User
4. TMC Operator follows protocol and arranges appropriate response

Figure 26.3 The operational functionality of a basic telecare alarm system.

behaviour and preferences. Indeed, a number of decision-support tools are being offered to help prescribers ensure that they have the best options available, but also to ensure that the elements of telecare selected are inter-operable. This usually means procuring both the sensors and the communication hub (sometime known as the care-phone) from the same vendor – though this issue is likely to resolved in the future when transmissions systems such

as 'Zigbee' replace the existing one way transmission methods.

The most popular telecare sensors include bed occupancy monitors, medication reminder/dispenser instruments, and locator devices that use GPS to detect a vulnerable person (typically with Alzheimer's disease) moving outside an area of safety perhaps in the middle of the night. These devices work with a carephone but can

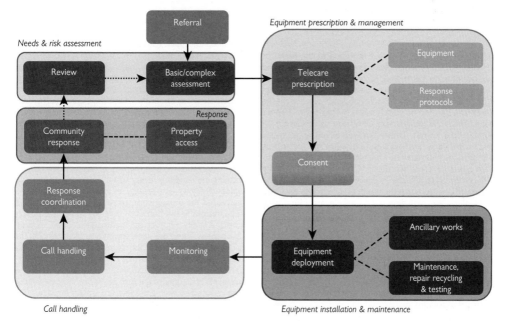

Figure 26.4 Processes involved in providing alarm based telecare service.

Table 26.6 The potential benefits of a telecare alarm service to all stakeholders

Service users	Carers	Social Services	Housing Providers	NHS
Increased choice in managing risk	Improved peace of mind	Reduced care admissions to care homes	Reduced voids in sheltered housing	Reduced hospital admission and readmissions
More responsive approach	Reduced stress	Improved assessment of needs & risks	Increased demand for special housing	Improved medication compliance
Improved Quality of Life	Improved Quality of Life	Fewer delayed transfers of care	Fewer incidents of accidental damage	Fewer ambulance call outs and A&E presentations
Increased independence	Increased independence	Increased capacity of care system	New roles for wardens and support staff	More patients able to perform special care at home
Reduction in overall care costs	Opportunities for respite	Reduced demand for other services	Improved security of properties	Shorter hospital stays and rapid discharge

also link to a local carer who has a pager-type device, or they can use the mobile networks to send alerts by SMS or e-mail to appropriate responders.

Extending the application of telecare
The telecare service shown in Figure 26.3 is an example of a basic alarm arrangement that follows a simple protocol that would be put in place following a referral. The frequency of alarm and the way in which the responses worked would be reviewed regularly and changes made if necessary. This is the form of telecare offered by nearly all service providers and is associated with a wide range of outcomes of the type shown in Table 26.6, with benefits accruing to all the stakeholders.

However, this is an entirely reactionary approach and does little to prevent emergencies from occurring despite the rich environment of data in which the devices sit. Many telecare peripheral devices report information in a simple binary format. They may be door sensors reporting that a door is open or closed, movement sensors reporting activity or inactivity, usage sensors describing whether or not an electrical appliance is switched on or off, and occupancy sensors describing the status of a bed, a chair, a room or a shower cubicle. These data collected over a 24-hour period (or over a number of weeks) can describe an individual's lifestyle in a manner which can confirm the hours of activity, the times when they venture outside, and the number of visitors that they receive. Systems that collect and display this type of information can be used for a period of 4 or 5 weeks to provide a continuous assessment file which can be used to clearly identify long-term support needs and avoid unnecessary admission to residential or nursing care homes. These are web-based applications that, in principle, allow real-time monitoring of status at any time. Such systems can be extended to provide real-time alerts. In some situations, these might be sent by SMS, or e-mail to a family care giver or to the next of kin. However, to ensure that there will be a response on a 24/7 basis, alerts are best directed to a Telecare Monitoring Centre where an appropriate response protocol can be initiated.

Evidence for success
Telecare systems have been introduced widely since 2001 when multi-sensors systems were first tried in West Lothian in Scotland. In those days, the choice of sensors was restricted to environmental detectors such as smoke alarms, flood alarms, gas alarms and temperature extreme alarms, plus some new specialist device such as a worn fall detector, a bed occupancy sensor, an enuresis detector

and a property exit alert. Everyone over the age of 75 was originally offered a standard set of home safety sensors plus a carephone. Also, those who were considered to be particularly frail and people with a cognitive impairment were offered additional devices dependent on an individual assessment. Successive evaluation studies concluded that the systems were extremely popular with the users, but that it had also significantly reduced the level of admissions to residential homes and had also reduced the level of community support that was required.

Elsewhere, telecare services were targeted at different groups using specific items of technology and more focused response protocols. In one study, sensors to detect falls during the day or at night helped to improve the confidence of service users to such an extent that many were able to perform more personal tasks, such as bathing, for themselves. In several studies aimed at supporting people with dementia and their families, there was good evidence to show reduced levels of carer stress and, because the patient was safe despite being allowed to perform most domestic tasks, quality of life was preserved. People who need polypharmacy can be reminded when to take their medication and, when a pill dispensing unit is employed, their compliance improved considerably. The need for check visits disappears and compliance with prescription improves.

In terms of outcomes, many people who might have been offered a place in a residential or nursing care home without telecare can manage well in their own homes, supported by a community care packages that includes technology. Telecare and community equipment are therefore helping to transform social and primary care services.

Future developments in home telecare
The next generation of telecare systems will be based on video interaction. Whilst the idea of having video cameras tracking movement in every room would offend the principles of dignity and privacy of most people, it has not prevented the introduction of so-called 'granny cams' in key locations in the homes of older or vulnerable people, so that a family member can make a 'virtual visit' to check up on them. These are generally private arrangements that fall outside the scope of formal services, which can mean that there may be no formal response mechanism to a perceived emergency situation. This might then mean that the levels of anxiety of the care givers are increased rather than reduced by having the telecare system in place.

A more likely approach, which is already gaining traction, is the use of a telecare hub connected to the television and to the telecommunications network. This set-top box will

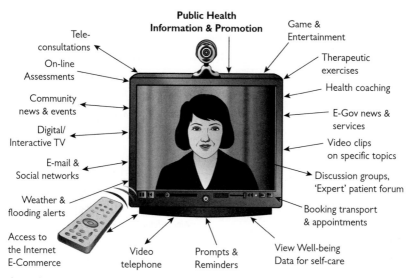

Figure 26.5 Some telecare applications that could be employed through future digital TV systems.

integrate existing digital TV channels and functions with services such as the Internet that would otherwise be delivered through a computer. Whilst an ambition might be to have various telecare radio transmitters and receivers inside the box enabling it to monitor the sensor networks described above and to perform a number of closed loop control functions (such as switching lights and water supplies on and off), such boxes may be a number of years away. In the short term, the boxes are likely to enable digital convergence to occur by providing access to the Web on the TV screen. Alternative approaches may be undertaken in different countries, with some of these boxes integrated into the TV. Figure 26.5 shows a number of applications that could be down-loaded in order to provide the user with a menu of interactive telecare services that may be relevant to their particular need.

The set-top box will either include an integral camera or it will have a socket for an external camera (which could be controlled by the system). This will enable teleconsultations to reduce the need for health and social care professionals and patients to have for meetings. Video telephone calls could also be made to family and friends with opportunities to forge new remote friendships using this medium. Such approaches may play an important role in overcoming social isolation and loneliness that will otherwise be inevitable consequences of an ageing population.

Mobile telecare (mCare)

A telecare system that works only in the home environment might discourage people from going out and enjoying the freedom to enjoy fresh air and exercise that will improve both their health and their mental well-being. It follows that a mobile version of telecare – mCare – will develop that utilises the power of the mobile telephone in providing a communication channel that people can always carry around with them. Hospitals and community physicians, dentists and opticians across the developed world are already using message alerts and SMS reminders to

ensure that patients attend appointments or take their medication. In Africa and other developing countries, where there is little fixed line telephone infrastructure, mobile telephony is already becoming the foundation of

Table 26.7 Smart phones features and applications

Feature	Example applications
Microphone	Electronic stethoscope; cough analysis; alarm relay for remote sensors
Speaker	Hearing aid with replay function; personal hearing test; communication aid for people with speech and language problems; sleep support
Accelerometer	Automatic fall detector; epileptic seizure detector; pedometer and calories used monitor; training for CPR
GPS system	Location of emergency event; location of nearest defibrillator
Magnetometer	Warnings for people with pacemakers and implanted devices
Temperature chip	Hypothermia warnings (coupled with inactivity); heat stress
Camera(s)	Signage for deaf; magnifying glass; colour detector; rash identification
Flash unit (light source)	Non-invasive pulse measurement
Vibration unit	Alarm clock and monitor for deaf; reminder system
Bluetooth and wifi	Vital signs display and relay; fitness monitor; smart home controller
Input connections	Bioharness for vital signs data collection; adaptors for instruments

monitoring and training programmes in health. mHealth applications abound as the benefits of medical advice and action are quickly transferred to otherwise isolated communities.

Most new mobile handsets available today are smart phones. This means that they have operating systems that can run downloadable applications (apps), and a number of built-in features that may be utilised directly for supporting well-being and improving Quality of Life. Table 26.7 list these features together with examples of how they are being utilized in 'apps'.

It is currently unclear how m-care will be offered as a service but it is likely that individuals who already have a smart phone will pay the small sums required to download appropriate applications if they feel that this will satisfy a need. In the same way, a smart phone and some applications could be provided as part of a telecare service alongside home based equipment so that service users are supported by the technology wherever they happen to be. It is likely that physicians will need only to refer their patients to an appropriate service, which can be commissioned to satisfy individual needs including an extended use of telecare and mCare.

The main benefit to the user of mCare technology is that one ubiquitous device can become the means to address any number of current needs, from a hearing aid to a magnifying glass. Experience shows that younger patients are prepared to buy the smart phones and the applications for themselves from 'App stores' run by the phone manufacturers or the network providers. There seems to be no stigma involved in carrying around a smart phone so the challenges of using assistive technology can be relegated to history.

Further reading

Telemedicine and e-Health, Mary Ann Liebert Inc., Publishers. ISSN: 1530-5627 10 Issues Annually Online ISSN: 1556–3669

Journal of Telemedicine and Telecare, Royal Society of Medicine Press Ltd

Journal of Assistive Technologies, Pier Professional, Editor: Chris Abbott. Print ISSN: 1754-9450; Online ISSN: 2042–8723.

Role of the multidisciplinary team

Nursing and the multidisciplinary team

Nurses are specialist professionals present on the wards with the patients for 24 hours every day. They carry out some of the most intimate aspects of care, and are the frontline for anything from medical emergencies to dealing with the emotions of distraught patients and their relatives.

There are core clinical issues that nurses and nursing are developing further expertise in, as research capacity increases and nurses take on specialist and advanced roles in older people's services. The generalist nature of much of nursing practice may be a strength as it enables nursing to 'oil the system' of older people's services. However, although nursing may be considered therapeutically non-specific, significant new insights are allowing us to clarify the nurse's role in both recovery and in rehabilitation.

This chapter will make explicit what the potential contribution of nursing is to medical care within the context of older people's services, and how this may best be incorporated into service delivery. The chapter will include some recommendations about how the nursing contribution can be strengthened within older people's health services.

The nature of nursing care

Although nurses have developed expertise in clinical technical skills, often transferred from doctors, the profession has continued to stress the importance of patient-centred care. Clinical guidelines and patient directives contribute to a governance framework for nurses to expand the technical aspects of their clinical role. However, nursing is an art as well as a science and nurses are concerned with the provision of effective technical care alongside more personal aspects of patient and family support. Nurses facilitate and assist understanding for patients and carers in:

- *Conservation and avoiding Complications* - preserving existing health and function, avoidance/minimization of additional problems, and preparing patients so they are in the best physical health/level of ability to approach the future.
- *Consequences and Challenges* – understanding recovery and considering how to approach future hurdles.
- *Consolation, Combination and Consolidation* – understanding the unpredictability and risks of the future. Also, how to live with a range of complex issues that need to work together.

For the former of these, conservation, nursing practice in older people's services may, as well as providing supportive care in the acute phase of illness, be to help patients perform essential aspects of daily living such as eating, drinking, and personal hygiene until they are able to perform these themselves. However, some may never achieve independence in even basic tasks, and so they or their relatives may need to be supported in understanding the limited goals set (consequences and challenges), and/or in coming to terms with, and planning for these and other needs to be met (consolation, combination and consolidation), for example through social care services. Together these aspects constitute rehabilitation, which is one of the major foci of nursing practice in older people's services both in acute and non-acute settings.

Although rehabilitation is often conceptualized in terms of functional recovery, and to be the specific remit of the allied health professions (AHPs, e.g. physiotherapy, occupational and, speech and language therapy), effective rehabilitation can only truly be achieved through nursing input. The rehabilitation role of nursing is to reinforce the contributions of these AHPs, providing opportunities for practice within other aspects of care, and to maintain an environment and culture that is conducive to rehabilitation.

Nursing continues to debate its role in rehabilitation, particularly in light of the shift away from medical to more social models of rehabilitation by the International Classification of Disability, Health and Function (World Health Organization, 2001). For example, nursing continues to develop understanding about the family and social impact of stroke, and plays a key role in providing education and support to patients and families as they adjust to life with stroke.

Registered and support staff

As a registered profession, nurses undergo a training programme with academic and practical training prescribed by European Union legislation, often within a University degree programme. The proportion of nurses with degrees in the UK has substantially increased in recent years from 17% in 2002 to 31% in 2009.

Clinical services are often supported by staff who will usually have vocational qualifications in aspects of health or social care. The usual model of work distribution involves the delegation of work or tasks for which the Registered Nurse remains professionally accountable.

Although the mix of Registered Nurses to support staff should be driven by the care needs of patients, it is inevitable in a publicly funded service that budgetary constraints and policy such as the EU Directive on Junior Doctor hours will also influence staffing profiles. The challenge for nursing in recent years has been to ensure that these influences, coupled with a transfer of clinical tasks (usually from medicine to nursing), has not meant a dilution of care at the bedside. In 2006, the UK Royal College of Nursing recommended that, in general, the proportion of registered to support staff should be 2:1. Evidence from observational research in the UK and US indicates that higher nurse to patient ratios are associated with lower rates of poor outcomes for patients, including urinary and chest infections and mortality.

Changes in the UK health policy context have provided nursing with the opportunity to develop new roles in both hospital and community settings. The development of specialist and consultant nursing roles has provided opportunities to develop expertise in aspects of clinical care, and service development, education and research. These role developments have not been confined to hospital settings: community matrons have, for example, been appointed to ensure care quality across community settings. Within stroke care, there are increasingly innovative approaches to defining stroke-specific knowledge and understanding, as well as the skills and abilities required. The development of the UK Forum for Stroke Training allows clear definition of roles within a range of settings.

Care provision in older people's services

Within inpatient settings, nurses provide care that is both prescribed by nurses and other professional groups. Care prescribed and delivered by nurses is mostly underpinned by an 'activities of living' approach – doing or supporting patients to undertake those activities of living that they are unable to perform for themselves. This work provides opportunities for nurses to address health risks associated with hospital stays such as tissue viability, falls management, nutritional health, personal safety and infection control.

Nursing also has a role in delivering care prescribed by others, and has the potential to provide useful information, on acceptability and impact, to guide future care planning.

There are some aspects of care provision where nursing is developing considerable practical expertise, such as with managing leg ulcers, although the availability of high-quality evidence of intervention effectiveness may be variable.

Nurses play a key role in the assessment of continence needs, and in developing programmes of care that address both functional and other types of incontinence. Importantly, nurses are the only professional group who have meaningful opportunities to address night time incontinence issues, which can often influence whether patients go home or not. A focus on problems with activities of living such as mobility and eating and drinking means that nurses are well-placed to evaluate and manage tissue viability, falls prevention, nutritional, and hydration needs. These can often be put at risk through hospital admission, and together with infection control, are increasingly public markers of health service quality.

Care management in older people's service

Nurses have a key role in facilitating assessments that pull together the multidisciplinary team (MDT) around an individual patient's care. This may involve making referrals and coordinating the input of the MDT. Meanwhile, nurses are increasingly taking on assessments undertaken by other professional groups: most bedside swallow screening is now undertaken by nurses, rather than speech and language therapists who have been enabled to focus on complex communication problems. Statutory frameworks for continuing healthcare mean that nurses play a role in assessing care needs for both nursing and personal care services.

The services that support older people are complex and often require transitions to be facilitated across care settings, and across phases of patient recovery. Through its generalist role, nursing has a key role in planning for, and supporting patients and families through these transitions which. Maintaining a sense of continuity in care, and being cared for, can be a challenge when a service appears fragmented through changes in staff and care settings, and particularly in complex discharges from hospital and the commencement of palliative care.

Therapeutic nursing in older people

Reflecting the shift in thinking on rehabilitation, nurses play a key role in helping patients and families adjust to the consequences of ill-health. The dearth of clinical psychology services, and the focus on dementia within mental health services for Older People, mean that access to services for depression for example are limited. Nurses have a key role in providing emotional support and more advanced interventions such as motivational interviewing that address this issue.

Central to nursing practice is the development of therapeutic relationships with patients and family members. There are a number of reasons why nurses may be well placed to do this, including the continual presence of nursing within most healthcare settings, and for some patients,

a greater sense of approachability in comparison to other professional groups. These relationships can influence the effectiveness of information giving, education and supportive interventions, and are the basis of maintaining dignity during invasive interventions and often impersonal, complex services.

Nurses have the potential to uncover more hidden issues which may influence the impact and effectiveness of health services. This may include insights into mood and behaviours including diurnal variations (e.g. sundowner syndrome, where patients deteriorate in the evenings, having been models of good behaviour while their doctors are around during the daytime). Nurses are often aware of the best means of calming a patient, from simple things like their awareness of toileting needs through to fears induced by closing curtains reminding them of frightening wartime experiences. Knowledge of overnight care and toileting needs are particularly important when planning a successful discharge to home or ongoing care needs.

Nurses can often be the first to become aware of possible concerns with more serious issues such as abuse, through being able to witness the interactions of patients with, for example, their families, or through their role with managing pressure care.

Teamworking

Teamwork is essential in the delivery of effective and efficient patient care. It requires an appreciation of the actual and potential contributions of all the team members, whose individual contributions should be underpinned by their specialist knowledge and skills. One of the challenges for nursing is that, comparison with many allied health professional groups, they may appear to lack a specific clinical focus. For example, on rehabilitation wards, there tends to be a focus on the specific sessions with the therapists as being the 'rehabilitation', while not the appreciating the vital parts done by the nurses, such as when encouraging the patients to wash and dress themselves independently or helping with difficult transfers and so building strength and confidence with these throughout the week.

There is some evidence in stroke however that suggests that the contribution is not always fully realized. Anecdotally, very different approaches to bringing nurses into decision-making opportunities can be found. In some instances, nurses do not always attend MDT meetings. If nurses do attend, then those with knowledge of the patients under review should contribute, rather than those with ward management responsibility, who for a variety of reasons may not have a full awareness of relevant issues. It is also important that nurses value and articulate their contribution and continue to develop it further through research and development. However, they should also develop and test the effectiveness of new strategies that support multi-disciplinary working.

Conclusion

Although nurses are developing specialist roles in some aspects of patient care, it is essential that these developments and the challenges in maintaining an appropriate skill mix do not dilute the quality of care at the bedside. Rather than diminishing its importance in a multidisciplinary service, the generalist nature of the nursing role can significantly enhance the quality and outcomes of older people's services. Such services should ensure that there are systems in place, such as good team-working, to ensure that these potential benefits are realized.

Further reading

Aiken LH, Clarke SP, Sloane DM, et al. (2002). Hospital nurse staffing and patient mortality, nurse burnout, and job dissatisfaction. *JAMA* **288**: 1987–93

Burton C, Gibbon B (2005). Expanding the role of the stroke nurse: a pragmatic clinical trial. *J Adv Nurs* **52**: 640–50.

Gibbon B, Watkins C, Barer D, et al. (2002). Can staff attitudes to team working in stroke care be improved? *J Adv Nurs* **40**: 105–11

Gibbon B (2003). The contribution of the nurse to stroke units in the United Kingdom. *Journal of Australian Rehabilitation Nurses* **6**: 8–13.

Hindle A, Coates A (2011). *Nursing Care of Older People*. Oxford University Press, Oxford. In press

Kirkevold M (2010). The role of nursing in the rehabilitation of stroke survivors: an extended theoretical account. *Adv Nurs Sci* **33**: e27–e40.

Rafferty AM, Clarke SP, Coles J, et al. (2007). Outcomes of variation in hospital nurse staffing in English hospitals: Cross-sectional analysis of survey data and discharge records. *Int J Nurs Stud* **44**: 175–82.

Redfern SJ, Ross FM (2005). *Nursing Older People*. Churchill Livingstone, Edinburgh.

Royal College of Nursing (2006) *Setting Appropriate Ward Nurse Staffing Levels in NHS Acute Trust*. Royal College of Nursing, London.

Watkins CL, Gibbon B, Cooper H, et al. (2001). Performing interprofessional research: the example of a Team Care Project. *Nurse Researcher* **9**: 29–48.

Watkins CL, Auton MF, Deans CF, et al. (2007). Motivational interviewing early after acute stroke: a randomized, controlled trial. *Stroke* **38**: 1004–9.

Watkins CL, Leathley MJ, Scoular P (2010). Stroke-Specific Education Framework [online], Department of Health, last accessed on 2 November 2010 at URL: http://www.dh.gov.uk/prod_consum_dh/groups/dh_digitalassets/@dh/@en/@ps/@sta/@perf/documents/digitalasset/dh_116343.pdf

Williams J, Perry L, Watkins C, (2010). *Acute Stroke Nursing*. Wiley-Blackwell, Chichester.

World Health Organization (2001). *International Journal of Functioning, Disability and Health*. World Health Organization, Geneva.

Dietetics and the multidisciplinary team

Dietitians are professionals with expert knowledge and skills in the application of nutritional science to the human condition in health and disease. Their skills lie in understanding the complex relationship between nutrients and health and translating this into accessible information and simple strategies that the patient can implement. Their role extends across acute, rehabilitation and community teams and they provide unique skills in the assessment and management of patients and their carers.

Specialist dieticians work with older age groups in both acute and community settings using knowledge and skills acquired through practice and postgraduate training (the British Dietetic Association Nutrition Advisory Group for the Elderly runs an MSc module biannually).

The strategy of promoting food group based nutritional advice provides a useful tool that is cross cultural and highlights the benefits of eating a variety of foods. It is a simple model that can help in the management of common conditions of ageing such as type 2 diabetes, obesity, and hyperlipidaemia.

As the population becomes frailer this strategy of healthy eating needs to be modified to aim for food intake that more closely reflects the individual's requirements for energy, protein, and micronutrients.

Conditions that deteriorate over time (e.g. chronic obstructive pulmonary disease, Parkinson's disease, motor neurone disease, malignancy) or that acutely affect ability to maintain nutritional intake (e.g. stroke, acute delirium) or increase requirements (e.g. fracture, infection) will all impact on nutritional status. These conditions are not mutually exclusive, adding to the complexity of assessing and managing nutrition in these patient groups.

Accurate assessment of nutritional status involves:

- Anthropometric measurement – weight and weight history, height, or a measure appropriate to the patient such as demi-span, ulna length, or knee height. It may also include muscle mass measures such as mid upper arm circumference
- Clinical condition – factors that affect nutrition such as diabetes, coeliac disease, liver or kidney disease, neurological conditions, allergies
- Biochemistry and medication – clinical markers for nutritional status and associated factors (serum folate, iron status, vitamin B12, urea and electrolytes, serum proteins, phosphate, magnesium, calcium, C-reactive protein, and other inflammatory indicators). Current prescribed and non-prescribed medications
- Nutrition – current intake, diet history to include food preference and dislikes, frequency of consumption, portion size, previous experience of dietary change
- Social/cultural/psychological – identify access to foods, others who may influence eating, shopping and cooking ability, storage facilities for food, mental health status, cognitive capacity, and motivation

In developing a picture of the patient and the influences on their diet, it is possible to develop personalized nutrition plans that identify short- and long-term goals for dietary management. Information is often gathered over a period of time prioritising that which will quickly assist with managing the patient's condition.

The holistic picture of the patient is drawn from the experience of health professionals and others working in the multidisciplinary team.

Nursing and medical staff are key to nutritional management in hospitals. The regular contact with patients can alert them to problems that need dietetic input.

Writing nutritional supplements on the drug charts increases the likelihood of the patient being offered them at an appropriate time. Weighing patients and keeping food and fluid charts are essential to help identify concerns about poor intakes or weight loss. Early intervention can help prevent deterioration and speed recovery.

Speech and language therapists (SLTs) assess swallowing ability in neurological conditions. Using this information provision of appropriate textured nutrition can be achieved. SLTs can share communication strategies that will help the patient to be more self determining in their food choices, picture boards and pictorial menus are commonly used to help patients express their preferences and dislikes and can be used to identify when patients prefer to eat if they cannot express this verbally.

Occupational therapists assess skills with activities of daily living including kitchen skills and need for adaptive technologies to improve grip and dexterity. This can be immensely powerful for a patient who has previously been unable to feed themselves and is likely to increase a sense of independence.

Physiotherapists can help with positioning to assist patients at mealtimes. Eating food is much easier sitting at a table at the right height with the correct cutlery and foods a patient has selected for themselves, and gravity helps the food go down if the patient is sitting upright.

As part of the multidisciplinary team the dietitian provides practical solutions to nutritional problems and advises the team on strategies that can positively influence nutritional status. Progress can be monitored through reviewing weight, food records, and biochemistry. Talking with the patient and their carers about how they feel things are going, what is working and what is not helps to ensure that the patient is at the centre of their nutritional care.

For patients who will require artificial nutrition long term (usually via a percutaneous endoscopic gastrostomy (PEG) tube) the dietitian is an essential member of the team. The dietitian liaises with the patient, family, carers, and the wider community team to ensure safe transfer of nutritional care. By talking with the patient, it is possible to identify how and when they prefer feeding, the type of feeding most appropriate (e.g. continuous pump feeding, bolus feeding, supplementing oral intake if appropriate). Identifying the risks associated with feeding, including refeeding syndrome, and responding to the concerns of the wider team, it is possible to address these in a way that manages them appropriately. Training patients and carers prior to discharge enables them to express their concerns about nutrition to the dietitian and for these to be addressed early in their transition, reducing the risk of early readmission as a result of feeding problems.

In clinics, the dietitian may often be part of the wider clinical team in attendance and team discussions on patient management can be more easily resolved without referring on. The addition of nutritional risk assessment to the clinic setting is recommended nationally.

Joint audit programmes that include nutritional standards are regularly undertaken and can help to improve care for patients. BAPEN (www.bapen.org) conducts annual audits of nutritional status in a range of health settings and many dietitians lead on this in their healthcare community.

Developing policy on nutrition, contributing to development of care pathways, strategic programmes for care and research are all within the role of the dietitian.

Dietitians provide training on a range of subjects to healthcare professionals both formally in the classroom and informally in their day to day contact. Multidisciplinary training on nutrition assessment and optimizing nutrition in vulnerable groups helps to give other team members confidence in their skills and provides them with an expert resource when they find themselves in difficulty.

The role of the psychologist in the multidisciplinary team

Acknowledgement of the importance of psychological factors in the mediation of health and illness ensures the inclusion of psychologists as core members of the multidisciplinary team. Broad-based training and endorsement of the biopsychosocial approach to illness are further validations of their appropriate inclusion in the multidisciplinary skills mix.

Recognition of the way in which the ageing process impacts on health and well-being is important to the success of psychological interventions in this age group. An understanding of how this process is related to changes in brain structure and functioning is key to assessment accuracy and treatment efficacy. It is also important to have knowledge of conditions relevant to this group and which include degenerative brain conditions, stroke, chronic pain, arthritis, sleep disturbance, alcohol misuse and depression.

Rehabilitation psychologists typically have training and skills in a number of appropriate areas including developmental and health psychology, psychopathology and neuropsychology. They may be skilled in Cognitive Behaviour Therapy (CBT) and/or other psychological interventions.

Potential roles for psychologists include:

- psychometric assessment
- case formulation and intervention
- advice and support to the multidisciplinary team
- service evaluations, audit and research.

Areas of psychometric assessment include general cognitive functioning as well as psychological adjustment. For the former, the clinician may start with a quick cognitive screen to identify areas which require further detailed assessment (see Table 27.1). A comprehensive evaluation would assess intellectual functioning, information processing (including attention and working memory), memory (including immediate and delayed recall), visuospatial and language abilities, and executive functioning. Executive functions are complex integrated skills which include planning, problem solving, self-monitoring and behavioural modification. They represent the coordinated working of various cognitive processes and neural networks and are therefore highly sensitive to the disruptive effects of brain injuries and conditions affecting cognition. The multi-factorial nature of executive ability means that there is no single psychometric measure that adequately captures the complexity of executive functioning in everyday behaviour. Typically, neuropsychologists sample different components of executive abilities.

Areas to consider in the evaluation of psychological adjustment include mood, coping resources and life satisfaction. Clinicians should also be on the look-out for more significant psychopathology such as paranoia and obsessive-compulsive behaviour.

Psychometric assessment

All psychological formulations and interventions start with an assessment, which may range from a brief bedside consultation to an extensive clinical interview and psychometric evaluation lasting several hours. The more frail patient is often not robust enough for the latter. Psychometric testing provides objective evidence of what deficits are present, which in turn helps target interventions and an objective means of monitoring progress. There is a wide choice of validated assessments, including tests, questionnaires and structured interviews.

Assessment protocols are typically informed by referral questions and service settings. Brief cognitive screening is often carried out by others members of the multidisciplinary team, with the most commonly used tools being the Folstein Mini-Mental State Examination (MMSE), Abbreviated Mental Test Score (AMTS), Addenbrook's Cognitive Examination (Revised) (ACE-R) and Montreal Cognitive Assessment (MOCA). However, these are limited in their scope and application. By definition, they are short and therefore less reliable and can only sample a restricted range of behaviours. Poor sensitivity (i.e. not being able to detect subtle cognitive impairment) is a problem facing measures such as the MMSE. However, an advantage is that they are economical in practice and can be administered by non-psychologist members of the multidisciplinary team.

The use of measures such as the Repeatable Battery for the Assessment of Neuropsychological Status (RBANS) or the Neuropsychological Assessment Battery Screening Module (NAB-Scr) allows for a more robust and comprehensive appraisal of cognitive function with representative sampling of attention, memory, language, visuospatial and executive functions. The referral question and service context will determine if more extensive assessment is required (e.g. Wechsler Memory Scale IV). Intellectual functioning is typically measured with shortened versions of traditional IQ tests or with the Wechsler Abbreviated Scale of Intelligence (WASI-II). Together with functional assessments provided by other members of the multidisciplinary team, these measures can provide an understanding of how an individual's cognitive strengths and weaknesses may impact on their ability to engage in everyday tasks and live independently.

Psychological adjustment may be probed using clinical interview and appropriate questionnaires such as:

- Geriatric Depression Scale (most commonly GDS-15; shorter versions are available)
- Cornell Scale for Depression in Dementia (information from patient and carers)
- Hospital Anxiety and Depression Scale (HADS)
- Patient Health Questionnaire (PHQ-9).
- Stroke Aphasic Depression Questionnaire (SADQ-10) (records observable depressive symptoms such as tearfulness and withdrawal; can be completed by any member of the MDT.)

Some clinical presentations may require a more in-depth assessment using the Clinical Assessment Scales for the

Table 27.1 Psychometric screening tools

Purpose	Cognitive	Mood
Brief screening (5–20 mi)	MMSE	PHQ-9
	MOCA	GDS- Short
	ACE-R	SADQ-10
	Cognistat	HADS
Comprehensive screening (20–45 min)	NAB-Scr	CASE-SF
	RBANS	

Elderly (CASE-SF), a symptom inventory which taps into *DSM-IV* Axis I disorders.

Psychologists may contribute to the assessment of an older adult's ability to resume or maintain independent community living. A number of specific measures have been developed for this purpose and include tools such as the *Community Integration Scale*, *Independent Living Scales* and *Mayo Portland Adjustment Inventory*. Neuropsychological assessment of working memory, executive function, memory and speed of processing may provide predictions of functional independence and success in extended activities of daily living, such as driving.

Case formulation and intervention

Psychologists are trained in a multidimensional approach to understanding health and disability and are able to draw on and integrate diverse bits of information relevant to psychological case formulation. In older adults, this process frequently relies on a clear understanding of the impact of change in health status or life circumstance. Laidlaw *et al.* provide a useful CBT framework for developing an appropriate case formulation. Considerations include personal experiences and beliefs and the way in which these promote adaptive and maladaptive behaviours.

A variety of interventions are appropriate for older adults and include CBT, solution-focused, mindfulness and reminiscence therapies as well as supportive counselling. Modifications to standard therapeutic approaches are often required to accommodate physical and cognitive limitations. Individuals with cognitive impairment represent a particular challenge to CBT therapists as treatment success is often determined by an adequate understanding of cause and effect and sufficient volitional behaviour. This may be lacking in some instances requiring modification to traditional CBT approaches. For example, a CBT protocol could be adapted to incorporate greater structure, expanded explanations and with more immediate follow-up and feedback to maintain focus and compliance. Similarly, greater use of behavioural modelling and alternative communication strategies could be incorporated into the treatment plan of an individual with dysphasia.

Depression, anxiety, pain management and adjustment to physical disability are common treatment targets for individuals in this age group. Working with service users and significant others to maximize psychosocial adjustment is a further important component of rehabilitation and typically complements more specific interventions.

Advice and support to the multidisciplinary team

A lack of progress in rehabilitation can often be attributed to psychological factors affecting service users and/or to limitations in treatment delivery. As team members, psychologists can use their knowledge of individual and group dynamics to help identify barriers to successful outcome and provide colleagues with advice and suggestions on overcoming them. Interventions at a care team level may include the identification and removal of barriers to organizational change and refinement of service delivery. Stress and conflict within multidisciplinary teams may also be identified and resolved with psychological input. With the publication of the *Mental Capacity Act (2005)* and cognisance of the safeguards and rights of individuals receiving health and social care, increasing use is being made of psychological expertise in addressing consent and capacity issues.

Service evaluations, audit and research

Psychologists possess expertise in data analysis and research design, knowledge which allows them to participate in a range of service evaluations, audit and research. Few services offer protected time for this activity but contributions could potentially be made to clinical audits, outcomes research, the evaluation of the cost-effectiveness of commissioned services and issues relevant to the development of new services. Service users are increasingly being placed at the heart of rehabilitation efforts and with skills in interviewing and questionnaire design, psychologists have an important role to play in service evaluation and development.

Further reading

Frank RG, Rosenthal M, Caplan B (eds) (2010). *Handbook of Rehabilitation Psychology*, 2nd edn. APA,

Kennedy P (ed). (2007). *Psychological Management of Physical Disabilities: A Practitioner's Guide*. Routledge.

Laidlaw K, Thompson LW, Dick-Siskin L, Gallagher-Thompson D (2003). *Cognitive Behaviour Therapy with Older People*. Wiley.

Marcotte TD, Grant I (eds) (2010). *Neuropsychology of Everyday Functioning*. Guilford. Chapters 10–12 with further information on how neuropsychological assessments correlate with day to day functioning.

Otto MW, Simon NM, Olantunji BO, Sung SC, Pollack MH (2011). *10-Minute CBT: Integrating Cognitive Behavioural Strategies into Your Practice*. Oxford.

Woods R, Clare L, Eds. (2008). *Handbook of the Clinical Psychology of Ageing* 2nd Ed. Wiley. Chapter 34. Helpful advice and insights into the dynamics of multidisciplinary team working.

Social workers

A social worker is a key member of the multidisciplinary team and is often fundamental in the discharge planning, especially for high-risk and complex discharges. All social workers are qualified to degree level. Social workers in some areas are also called care managers and at times this can cause confusion.

Social workers form relationships with people and assist them to live more successfully within their local communities by helping them find solutions to their problems. Social work involves engaging not only with patients themselves but their families and friends as well as working closely with other organizations including the police, local authority departments, schools, and the probation service.

Social Workers work for a range of organizations, primarily in local authorities, independent organizations, and charities, but some also work for the NHS, such as in hospitals, mental health trusts and community-based settings.

Social workers need a breadth of skills, as they will act as an adviser, advocate, counsellor, and listener. They ascertain personal knowledge about the patient and the family's current circumstances and background details prior to admission. They advise on the timescales for implementing care packages and for discussing alternative forms of care if required. Social Workers set up and manage packages of care in the patient's home providing a wide range of services including personal care, shopping, meal preparation, personal alarm systems, and review these services on a regular basis.

The social worker needs to have a wide knowledge of resources in the community so that they are able to advise the team and the patient about what is available for the patient. The social worker at discharge can:

- Organize respite care – for example, either through sitting services (including overnight support), day care placements, or regular respite care in a nursing or residential home to provide the carer with a break.
- Liaise with voluntary and private agencies to establish the best community support to meet the patient's needs on discharge from hospital, such as arranging carers or community meals.
- Set in place 'safety nets' for high-risk discharges either by directly overseeing the patient's ongoing care or liaising with community colleagues to hand over responsibility of the case if appropriate. Some local authority social services do not have hospital based social work teams, so this process would depend predominantly on how individual local authorities are organized. Many patients are taken home for a 'home visit' prior to discharge. These visits are normally planned by the occupational therapist but the social worker will be involved as part of the discharge planning process. Some patients, particularly those who are confused and are determined to go home, are taken home if the risks are acceptable. If this happens, the social worker will ensure that this is monitored very closely and, if the patient's condition deteriorates, the social worker will arrange a transfer to a care home.
- Overseeing discharge to nursing and residential care homes.

The social worker will become more involved with the patient, especially those who have complex needs. The social worker will complete community care assessments for patients in consultation with the multidisciplinary team, patient and the family. It is important for the social worker to be aware of the patient's own goals and expectations and to be able to assess any risk that the patient may be in. The social worker will then organize the appropriate care, either in the community or in residential or nursing care as required. The social worker will guide and support the family and patient through to placement, including financial advice. They will then go on to work with the patient and family for a period of time to ensure that care plans are meeting their needs in whatever setting and to support patients and families in organizing and reassessing any difficult situations that may arise and will formally review after a set period of time.

Identifying, investigating and monitoring of vulnerable adults

The social worker is responsible for alerting the safeguarding team (every local authority has a safeguarding team) of any possible abuse, including physical and financial abuse. This includes escalation of concerns over care in care homes (such as when a patient is admitted from one with pressure sores) or possible concerns over carers in the community.

Multidisciplinary team (MDT) working

Terminology

Multidisciplinary teams are often discussed in the same context as joint working, interagency work and partnership working. The latter two refer to different agencies working in partnership rather than with the operation of a single team. The term 'joint working', though, is often used to cover teams and agencies.

In all areas of social work and health there are clients who require the help of more than one kind of professional. Older people, people with mental health problems, disabled people, troubled teenagers and families in crisis all require more expertise than one type of professional can offer.

Multidisciplinary teams have evolved at varying speeds in different parts over the past 30 years or so in response to local need, the foresight of individual local authority social work departments and the imperatives of central government. Mental health was among the first professions to adopt them; professionals in this sector work in teams of between eight and 16 people and consist of workers from different professions.

Examples of types of teams (NB councils differ in terminology for team names and team composition)

Hospital teams

Social workers within multidisciplinary teams in hospitals are particularly effective and are integral to the discharge planning process. Many hospitals do not have social work teams and this can result in social work departments in Local Authorities operating an 'in-reach' service to hospitals. This involves community social workers coming into the hospital to assess an individual patient, but not always becoming part of the MDT in the same way as a ward or unit based social worker would. This can cause problems with communication, though does have the advantage of improving continuity of care after discharge.

Community Mental Health Teams (CMHT)

The CMHT is regarded as the model for all multi-disciplinary teams. Approved social workers and community psychiatric nurses are the mainstay of CMHT's. The Mental Health Act 2007 created the role of approved mental health professionals and approved clinicians to take over the role of approved social worker (in the former case). This role will be open to other professionals, not only approved social workers (ASWs).

Standard 7 of the National Standards Framework for Older People states: 'The aim of this standard is to promote good mental health in older people and to treat and support those older people with dementia and depression.'

Older people who have mental health problems have access to integrated mental health services, provided by the NHS and councils to ensure effective diagnosis, treatment and support for them and their carers.

Community Mental Health Teams for Older People work with patients who are over 65 years old and have mental health problems, with the most common diagnosis being dementia. The social worker provides support to the families by introducing them to support groups and other community and voluntary resources. Social workers in these teams have access to mental health day units and are normally based with the hospital team.

Crisis Resolution Team/Home Treatment Teams

These operate for adults with mental health problems so that can remain at home with support. They can consist of occupational therapists, social workers, community psychiatric nurses, and psychologists. The Crisis Resolution Team/Home Treatment Service is a community-based multidisciplinary team, aiming to provide a short-term intensive, safe and effective home based assessment and treatment for adults with severe mental health problems. Where appropriate, the service will be provided as an alternative to inpatient care, working in partnership with other services. The team covers the same boundaries as the Community Mental Health Teams.

The single assessment process

This was introduced in 2003 to reduce the duplication of information gathered by the different teams of healthcare professionals and improve efficiency within the system. Its use clearly implies that older people have their own multidisciplinary teams. In practice this is not always the case and individual professionals still complete their own assessments which can slow down the assessment process and decision making process and may result in delayed discharges of care.

Social work fears

Some social workers have expressed concern that their professional identity could suffer in multidisciplinary teams as other professions may tend to take the lead, notably medical professionals. Research has explored the requirements for the role of social workers in MDTs and found four main themes: models of professional practice; status and power; confidentiality, and information sharing; and relations with external agencies. Frost *et al* argued that social workers were felt to be well situated to meet the challenge, and that social workers in multidisciplinary teams were committed to making them work.

Conclusion

The role of the social worker in the multidisciplinary team brings social expertise, social care law and regulation clarity, community resources information, and access to them. Social workers know the social background of the patient and their family including any difficulties they may be experiencing. The advocacy role carried out by the social worker also ensures that the needs and aspirations of the patient and their family are acknowledged by the multidisciplinary team.

Further reading

Atwal A, Caldwell K (2005). Do all health and social care professionals interact equally: a study of interactions in multidisciplinary teams in the United Kingdom. *Scand J Caring Sci* **19**: 268–73.

Frost N, Robinson M, Anning A. (2005). Social workers in multidisciplinary teams: issues and dilemmas for professional practice. *Child Family Social Work* **10**: 187–96.

Goslyn P, Briggs G. (2009) Social services, community care and benefits. In (Gosney M, Harris T, eds) *Managing Older People in Primary Care. A Practical Guide.* Oxford University Press, pp. 355–68.

The doctor's role within the multidisciplinary team

Older patients' problems do not all fit into the field of expertise of just one health professional. The result is that we work in teams. Each member of the team brings their own perspective, expertise, and experience of working with that patient and with others who have had similar problems. Such a multidisciplinary team (MDT) is the normal way of working for older patients undergoing rehabilitation in a variety of settings.

Use of multidisciplinary teams

- Rehabilitation of older people
- General internal medicine
- Respiratory medicine
- Stroke and neurology
- Rheumatology
- Trauma
- Psychiatry
- Palliative care
- Community services

Constituents of a multidisciplinary team

The make-up of the team may vary, but in general it will consist of a

- doctor
- nurse
- occupational therapist
- physiotherapist
- care manager/social worker.

    Occasionally they contain:

- the patient
- the patient's family or representative
- district nurse
- carers
- dietician
- pharmacist
- psychiatric nurse
- speech and language therapist
- palliative care nurse
- psychologist
- specialist nurse (e.g. Parkinson's disease nurse, heart failure nurse).

The key to an effective MDT is that all of its members are involved in the care of the patients under discussion and know them well, and are not simply representatives.

MDTs in the rehabilitation of older people predate the use of randomized controlled trials, and there is considerable research evidence to support their effectiveness and cost-effectiveness. Because they are deemed so palpably useful and effective by the people who are involved in them, and because the ward can be seen to function less well in the absence of key members, together with the lack of a sensible alternative way of working, they have become the accepted norm.

The role of the doctor in the multidisciplinary team

Leadership and responsibility

Where the team is led by a consultant, it would be usual for that doctor to lead the MDT, both clinically and in terms of service development. This may not always be the case, depending upon the experience and personality of others in the team. Many wards have no regular consultant input, and an MDT may be led by a GP, or perhaps not have a doctor as a regular member, with another clinician leading the team.

The doctor has particular responsibilities to the patient and is legally accountable for his own actions and those of the team in a way that applies far less to others. When things go wrong, and there are complaints or litigation, it is the ward manager and the senior doctor who have to devote most time and energy to this, and may end up in the witness box.

Doctors normally work in a way that involves taking decisions (often with incomplete information) that involve an element of risk. This is a necessary attribute in rehabilitation, as the moment when a patient can make progress with complete safety may never arrive, and decisions have to be taken by the team and the patient about what level of risk is acceptable.

Clinical assessment

An experienced doctor brings particular skills to the MDT. Primarily these are a knowledge and understanding of the patient's condition, and how it is likely to change over time. They need to weigh up the often multiple underlying illnesses and disabilities that the patient has, and determine what the patient's condition and needs are likely to be not just now, but in the near, or sometimes more distant future. For example, a patient not taking an active part in rehabilitation due to vascular dementia may have a different treatment plan from one who appears to be in the same condition, but has dementia due to Lewy body disease, which might respond well to treatment.

Older people find themselves in hospital for a wide variety of reasons. There is a broad spectrum of types of wards that may treat them. Some people may have a fixed disability or slowly progressive illness that requires very little medical input. Others are clinically unstable, possibly approaching the end of their lives, with frequent infections, and cardiac, renal, metabolic, neurological, and respiratory problems. Commonly several of these things coexist making their treatment complex. For the latter group, their medical problems dominate decisions about their future. Between these extremes is a larger group of patients who have multiple medical problems compounded by physical and cognitive frailty, and complex drug regimens. Some of these are also approaching the end of their lives, on a route and on a timescale that is not predictable.

The process of rehabilitation involves the doctor continually reassessing the patient's medical state. Evidence-based treatments may no longer be appropriate for some conditions, may have undesirable effects, or may interact with the patient's other medical problems. Expertise is required in deciding which treatments are important, and which it is right to withhold. These decisions require regular reassessment depending on the patient's progress. During this process the doctor acquires an idea of the patient's direction of travel in terms of their recovery or deterioration. This is critical to the decisions made by the MDT.

Whereas the nurses and therapists are on the ward on a daily basis, the consultant may only see the patients at designated times during a week. This can make it easier to assess progress or lack of it, and where goals are not met, or where there is a decline, to initiate a search for possible causes. These might be medical, such as intercurrent infection or dehydration, or psychological.

Depression is common among patients undergoing rehabilitation, and often overlooked because it is not considered. Some patients are able to mask considerable degrees of cognitive impairment, which always need to be assessed formally.

Limiting treatment and decisions about the end of life
The doctor will have an understanding of how well the patient has responded to treatment, or whether different treatment should be offered, and sometimes why treatment that is available is not appropriate in this case.

Advance care planning involves inviting the patient, where able, to discuss their views about how they would like to be treated in future. The patient should share their views with the family. When the patient is unable to take part, the family may be aware of what their previous views had been, and may hold views of their own, which the team should be aware of, but not be bound by unless there is a relevant, active Lasting Power of Attorney.

Setting the ceiling of medical treatment is a key role for the doctor, who has to declare when a patient should cease active treatment, and move towards palliative care. This needs to be discussed with the patient, when capable of taking part in these discussions, and with the patient's family or representative, as well as other members of the team. The doctor then needs to prescribe appropriate medication at the end of life. Only the doctor is seen as having the authority to make such decisions.

Continuity
In many wards staff rotate from one clinical area to another, and the make-up of the team may change every few weeks. The consultant, together with a senior nurse and the care manager are usually the longest serving members of the team. The consultant is also frequently the most experienced at looking after older people.

Arranging the involvement of others
Involving other medical or surgical specialties in the management of frail older people requires a consideration of the balance between benefits to the patient and the discomfort or inconvenience it might cause them, and this judgement requires an experienced doctor. If the balance is in favour of benefit, the expected outcome needs to be explained to the person coming to see the patient. There may be a reluctance to offer treatments or procedures to frail people, and the seniority of the doctor is often invaluable in this transaction.

Patients may require the services of other agencies – housing, legal services, health or social care services in distant areas etc. Occasionally these agencies are more helpful when dealing with a doctor representing the patient than other staff.

Mental capacity assessment
Many older people have a number of problems when it comes to assessing their capacity. They may have communication difficulties such as dysphasia and deafness, and cognitive problems such as dementia. These assessments are commonly carried out by nursing and therapy staff, but when there are concomitant psychiatric problems such as depression and psychosis, an experienced geriatrician or specialist psychiatric assessment is required.

Education
One important role for the doctor in the MDT is to ensure that all members understand the medical and other aspects of the patient's problems, drawing in the expertise of others in the team. Complex issues of prognosis, multiple physical and mental illnesses, with complex social and legal situations need to be aired at MDT meetings for everyone to have a full understanding of how the patient and their family can be helped. Senior doctors also have an important role in educating junior doctors and students (of medicine, nursing and therapies) on the benefits of working with MDTs.

Management responsibilities
A great deal of time is spent working with management in the organization (and reorganization) of services. Major changes in the working of the ward are commonly led by the doctor, who needs to be in a position to take the team with them in making changes.

Multidisciplinary teams without doctors
There are clinical areas in which there is no doctor in the MDT, for example on nurse-led wards, or wards where there are so many different teams that a multidisciplinary meeting defies organization, or teams working with specialties that show little interest in the patient's discharge plans. Such meetings tend to become more concerned with the process of discharge than with the patient's clinical state, and are less effective. For patients undergoing stroke rehabilitation, there is evidence that adding a doctor to a MDT of a nurse, an occupational therapist, and a physiotherapist leads to a greater consideration of the patient's needs, better goal setting, greater patient involvement, and improved team working

Further reading
Monaghan J, Channell K, McDowell D et al. (2005). Improving patient and carer communication, multidisciplinary team working and goal-setting in stroke rehabilitation. Clin Rehabil 19: 194–9.

Index

Page numbers in *italics* denote figures or tables.